# Best Before Exams

*A Quick Review for Competitive Exams for Nursing Officers*

# Best Before Exams

## *A Quick Review for Competitive Exams for Nursing Officers*

**Useful for Central Govt. and All Other Recruitment Exams**

**Veerabhadrappa G Mendagudli** MSc (N)
Associate Professor
Dr Vithalrao Vikhe Patil Foundations (DVVPF's)
College of Nursing, Ahmednagar, Maharashtra, India

**Viresh S Mahajani** BSc (N)
Staff Nurse
VMMC Medical College and
Shri Chattrapati Shivaji Maharaj Sarvopchar Rugnalay
Solapur, Maharashtra, India

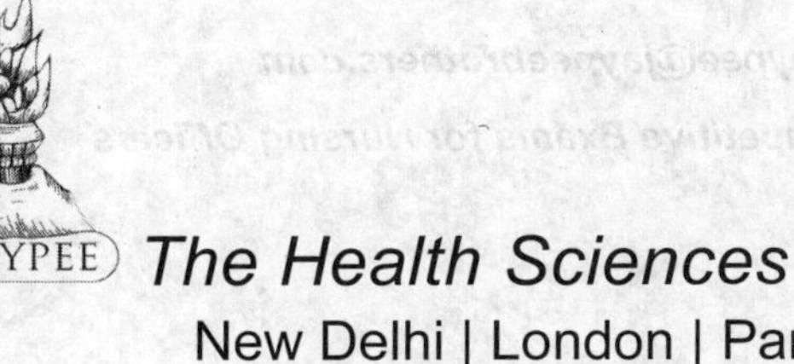

JAYPEE *The Health Sciences Publisher*
New Delhi | London | Panama

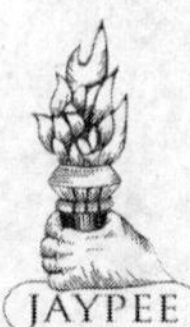

**Jaypee Brothers Medical Publishers (P) Ltd**

## Headquarters

Jaypee Brothers Medical Publishers (P) Ltd
4838/24, Ansari Road, Daryaganj
New Delhi 110 002, India
Phone: +91-11-43574357
Fax: +91-11-43574314
Email: jaypee@jaypeebrothers.com

## Overseas Offices

J.P. Medical Ltd
83 Victoria Street, London
SW1H 0HW (UK)
Phone: +44 20 3170 8910
Fax: +44 (0)20 3008 6180
Email: info@jpmedpub.com

Jaypee-Highlights Medical Publishers Inc
City of Knowledge, Bld. 235, 2nd Floor, Clayton
Panama City, Panama
Phone: +1 507-301-0496
Fax: +1 507-301-0499
Email: cservice@jphmedical.com

Jaypee Brothers Medical Publishers (P) Ltd
17/1-B Babar Road, Block-B, Shaymali
Mohammadpur, Dhaka-1207
Bangladesh
Mobile: +08801912003485
Email: jaypeedhaka@gmail.com

Jaypee Brothers Medical Publishers (P) Ltd
Bhotahity, Kathmandu
Nepal
Phone: +977-9741283608
Email: kathmandu@jaypeebrothers.com

Website: www.jaypeebrothers.com
Website: www.jaypeedigital.com



**Inquiries for bulk sales may be solicited at: *jaypee@jaypeebrothers.com***

***Best Before Exams—A Quick Review for Competitive Exams for Nursing Officers***

*First Edition:* **2018**

***ISBN: 978-93-5270-062-2***

*Printed at* Replika Press Pvt. Ltd.

# Contributors

**Abhijith Diwate**
Deputy Director
Dr Vithalrao Vikhe Patil Foundations
College of Physiotherapy
Ahmednagar, Maharashtra, India

**Anand Heralagi**
Principal
RKM School of Nursing
Vijayapur, Karnataka, India

**Anupama Oak**
Associate Professor
KDA College of Nursing
Mumbai, Maharashtra, India

**Gauri Sunil Mahajani**
Public Health Nurse
Solapur Municipal Corporation
Solapur, Maharashtra, India

**Jeyaseelan Mackam Devadason**
Principal
Annai JKK College of Nursing (TN)
Komarapalayam, Tamil Nadu, India

**Nagarajappa D**
Principal
Kamalnayan Bajaj Nursing College
Aurangabad, Maharashtra, India

**Nayak BB**
Professor and HOD
Department of Pharmacology
DVVPF's Medical College
Ahmednagar, Maharashtra, India

**Sarfraj S Sayyed**
Lecturer
Giriraj Nursing School
Baramati, Maharashtra, India

**Shalmon Chopade**
Principal
BLDEA's Shri BM Patil Institute of Nursing Sciences
Vijayapur, Karnataka, India

**Shivaleela S Sarawad**
Lecturer
Dr Vithalrao Vikhe Patil Foundations
College of Nursing College
Ahmednagar, Maharashtra, India

**Shraddha Gandhi**
Principal
RSC College of Nursing
Gwalior, Madhya Pradesh, India

**Shreenath Kulkarni**
Principal
Dr Vithalrao Vikhe Patil Foundations
College of Physiotherapy
Ahmednagar, Maharashtra, India

**Suchitra A Ratti**
Professor
BLDEA's Shri BM Patil Institute of Nursing Sciences
Vijayapur, Karnataka, India

**Suhas A Shinde**
Associate Professor
Department of Obst/Gyn
Dr Vithalrao Vikhe Patil Foundations Medical College
Ahmednagar, Maharashtra, India

**Urmila G Gavali**
Assistant Professor
Department of Obst/Gyn
Dr Vithalrao Vikhe Patil Foundations Medical College
Ahmednagar, Maharashtra, India

# Preface

*'Do not lose your grip on the dreams of past,*
*You must fight just to bring them alive'*

Presenting with an immense pleasure *Best Before Exams—A Quick Review for Competitive Exams for Nursing Officers,* an ultimate examination preparation kit to fulfil the dreams of students who are preparing for *government jobs.* A single preparatory guide for all different faculties of nursing, covering topics from every corner on different subjects including nursing academics which is a single handed key to success in nursing recruitment exams.

This book contains detail analysis of various thirteen different subjects included in nursing academics and preferred exams alongwith various multiple choice questions for each of them. It also includes diagrammatic representation for certain subjects where it is necessary for better understanding of students. Certain subjects like biochemistry which are untouched in all other recruitment guides due to its complexity is also included with simplicity, has been found important while preparing for exams like AIIMS and NIMHANS. It also contains nine National level recruitment exams solved question paper of recent years including papers from year 2017 and cover about 100 MCQs that have been frequently asked for exams till now and are believed to be repeated in upcoming years too. We promise to bring you the best through this and in all upcoming editions. Henceforth, with genuine wish to help all in fulfilling your wishes that will come true. Thank you all for your support, we are eager to have your feedback and suggestions if any.

**Veerabhadrappa G Mendagudli**
**Viresh S Mahajani**

# Acknowledgments

*'A ship is safe at harbor but that is not the ship is meant for'*

Firstly we would like to thank the Lord Almighty who empowered us to sail our ship in this world of competition and emerged as champions through all tough times. We pray on His feet to show similar favor to all his childrens, and help them to fulfil their dreams.

Then we thank all those who contributed sleepless nights along with us to bring this book in front of you as it is today. It was not an easy task, but was only possible because they stood beside us strongly. This is to all those unsung heroes behind this book who may remain in darkness, henceforth, they are our heroes and will remain the same through our entire life.

Our sincere thanks to Mr Abhijith Diwate, Deputy Director of Dr Vithalrao Vikhe Patil Foundations Medical College and Hospital, Ahmednagar, Maharashtra, India for his constant support and encouragement.

It is our proud privilege to express profound sense of gratitude and heartful thanks to Dr Jeyaseelan Mackam Devadason, Principal at Annai JKK College of Nursing (TN), Prof Shalmon Chopade, Principal and Mrs Suchitra A Ratti, Professor, HOD of CHN Department of BLDEA's Shri BM Patil Institute of Nursing Sciences, Vijayapur, Karnataka, India for their support and encouragement.

Our sincere thanks to sales representatives and staff of Jaypee Brothers Medical Publishers (P) Ltd, New Delhi for giving us an opportunity to publish this book.

# Contents

## Quick Review and MCQs



## Solved Previous Year Question Papers

# QUICK REVIEW

## Human Anatomy Review and Multiple Choice Questions

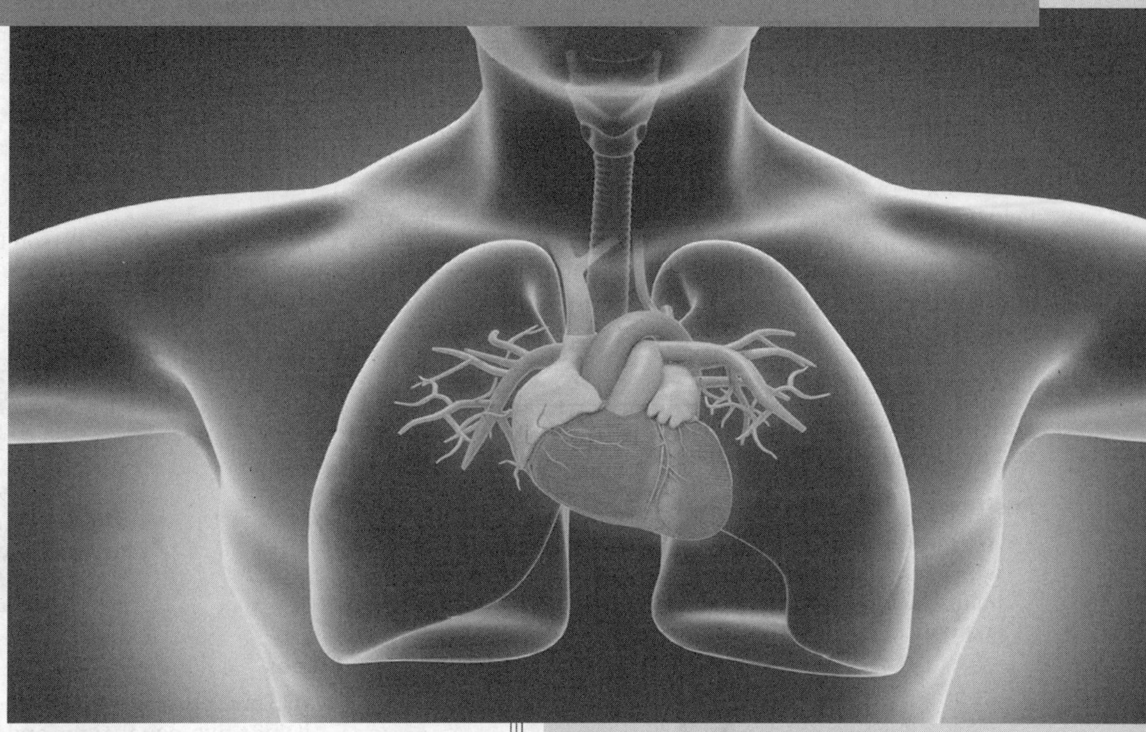

### HIGHLIGHTS

- Introduction
- Language of Anatomy
- Skeleton
- Cardiovascular System
- Nervous System
- Respiratory System
- Gastrointestinal System
- Urinary System
- Multiple Choice Questions

# Anatomy

## INTRODUCTION

Human anatomy is the science which deals with the structure of the human body. The term, 'anatomy', is derived from a Greek word, 'anatome', meaning cutting up. The term 'dissection' is a Latin equivalent of the Greek anatome. However, the two words, anatomy and dissection, are not synonymous. Dissection is a mere technique, whereas anatomy is a wide field of study. Anatomy forms firm foundation of the whole art of medicine and introduces the student to the greater part of medical terminology. 'Anatomy is to physiology as geography is to history, i.e. it describes the theatre in which the action takes place.'

## LANGUAGE OF ANATOMY

Various positions, planes, terms in relation to various regions and movements are described.

### Positions

- *Anatomical position:* When a person is standing straight with eyes looking forwards, both arms by the side of body, palms facing forwards, both feet together, the position is anatomical position.

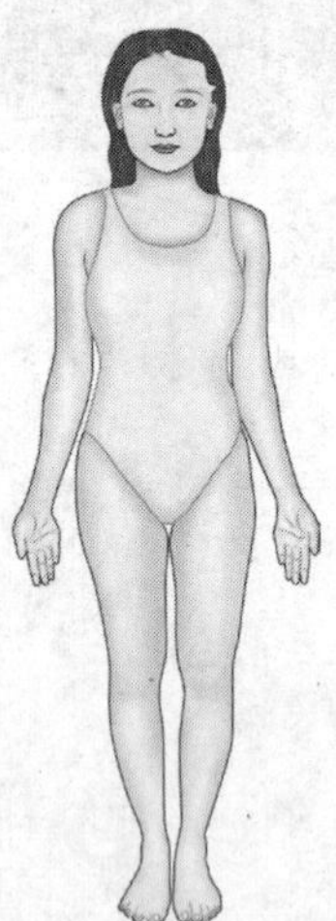

- *Supine position:* When a person is lying on her/his back, arms by the side, palms facing upwards and feet put together, the position is supine position.

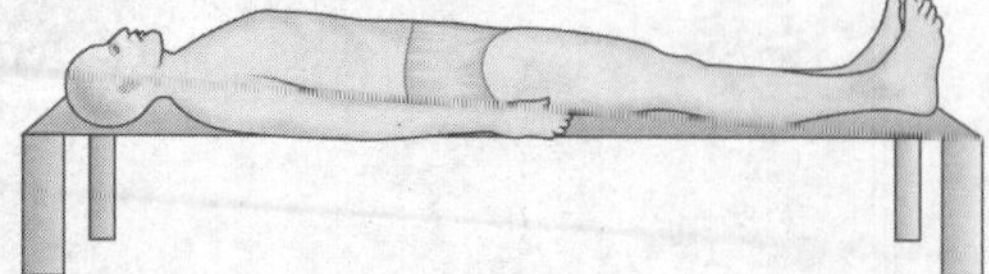

- *Prone position:* Person lying on his/her face, chest and abdomen is said to be in prone position.

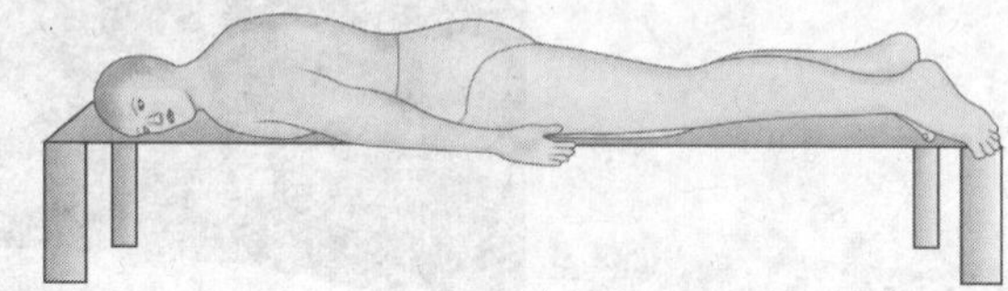

- *Lithotomy position:* Person lying on her back with legs up and feet supported in straps. This position is mostly used during delivery of the baby.

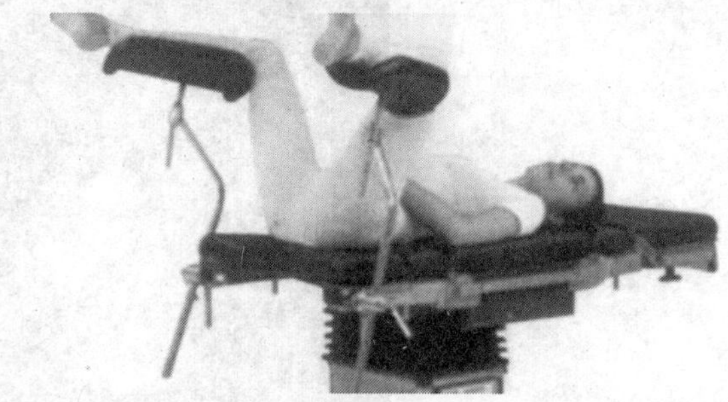

### Planes

- A plane passing through the centre of the body dividing it into two equal right and left halves, is the median or midsagittal plane. Plane parallel to median or midsagittal plane is the ***sagittal plane***.
- A plane at right angles to sagittal or median plane which divides the body into anterior and posterior halves is called a ***coronal plane.***

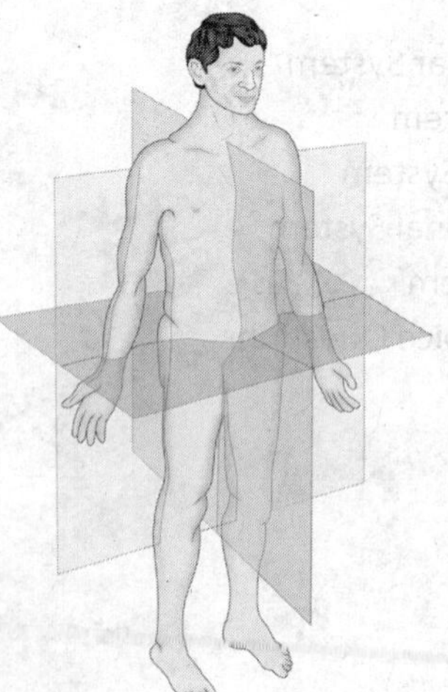

- A plane at right angles to both sagittal and coronal planes which divides the body into upper and lower parts is called a ***transverse plane.***

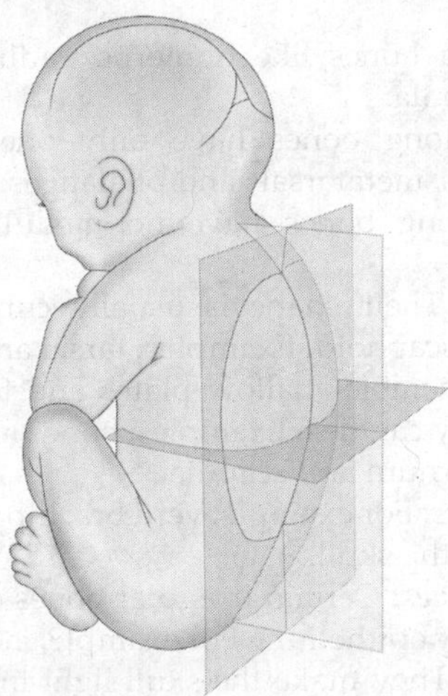

## Terms Used in Relation to Trunk

- ***Ventral*** or ***anterior*** is the front of trunk.
- ***Dorsal*** or ***posterior*** is the back of trunk.
- ***Medial*** is a plane close to the median plane.
- ***Lateral*** is plane away from the median plane.
- ***Proximal/cranial/superior*** is close to the head end of trunk.
- ***Distal/caudal/inferior*** is close to the lower end of the trunk.
- ***Superficial*** is close to skin/towards surface of body.
- ***Deep*** away from skin/away from surface of body.
- ***Ipsilateral*** on the same side of the body as another structure.
- ***Contralateral*** on opposite side of body from another structure.
- ***Invagination*** is projection inside.
- ***Evagination*** is projection outside.

## Terms Used for Describing Vessels

- ***Arteries*** carry oxygenated blood away from the heart, with the exception of the pulmonary and umbilical arteries which carry deoxygenated blood. Arteries resemble trees because they have branches (arterioles).
- ***Veins*** carry deoxygenated blood towards the heart, with the exception of the pulmonary and umbilical veins which carry oxygenated blood. Veins resemble rivers because they have tributaries (venules). Veins have valves to allow unidirectional flow of blood.
- ***Capillaries*** are networks of microscopic vessels connecting arterioles to venules.
- ***Anastomosis*** is a precapillary or postcapillary communication between the neighboring vessels.

## Terms Used in Clinical Anatomy

- The suffix, ***'-itis'***, means inflammation, e.g. appendicitis, tonsillitis, arthritis, neuritis, dermatitis, etc.
- The suffix, ***'-ectomy'***, means removal from the body, e.g. appendectomy, tonsillectomy, gastrectomy, nephrectomy, etc.
- The suffix, ***'-otomy'***, means to open and then close a hollow organ, e.g. laparotomy, hysterotomy, cystotomy, cystolithotomy,etc.
- The suffix, ***'-ostomy'***, means to open hollow organ and leave it open, e.g. cystostomy, colostomy, tracheostomy, etc.
- The suffix, ***'-oma***\means a tumor, e.g. lipoma, osteoma, neurofibroma, hemangioma, carcinoma, etc.
- ***Puberty:*** The age at which the secondary sexual characters develop, being 12–15 years in girls and 13–16 years in boys.
- ***Symptoms*** are subjective complaints of the patient about his disease.
- ***Signs (physical signs)*** are objective findings of the doctor on the patient.
- ***Diagnosis:*** Identification of a disease, or determination of the nature of a disease.
- ***Prognosis:*** Forecasting the probable course and ultimate outcome of a disease.
- ***Pyrexia:*** Fever.
- ***Lesion:*** Injury, or a circumscribed pathologic change in the tissues.
- Inflammation is the local reaction of the tissues to an injury or an abnormal stimulation caused by a physical, chemical, or biologic agent. It is characterized by: (a) Swelling; (b) pain; (c) redness; (d) warmth of heat; and (e) loss of function.
- ***Edema:*** Swelling due to accumulation of fluid in the extracellular space.
- ***Thrombosis:*** Intravascular coagulation (solidification) of blood.
- ***Embolism:*** Occlusion of a vessel by a detached and circulating thrombus (embolus).
- ***Hemorrhage:*** Bleeding which may be external or internal.
- ***Ulcer:*** A localized breach (gap, erosion) in the surface continuity of the skin or mucous membrane.
- ***Sinus:*** A blind track (open at one end) lined by epithelium.
- ***Fistula:*** A track open at both the ends and lined by epithelium.
- ***Necrosis:*** Local death of a tissue or organ due to irreversible damage to the nucleus.
- ***Degeneration:*** A retrogressive change causing deterioration in the structural and functional qualities. It is a reversible process, but may end in necrosis.
- ***Gangrene:*** A form of necrosis (death) combined with putrefaction.
- Infarction: Death (necrosis) of a tissue due to sudden obstruction of its artery of supply (often an end-artery).
- ***Atrophy:*** Diminution in the size of cells, tissue, organ, or a part due to loss of its nutrition.
- ***Dystrophy:*** Diminution in the size due to defective nutrition.
- ***Hypertrophy:*** Increase in the size without any increase in the number of cells.
- ***Hyperplasia:*** Increase in the size due to increase in the number of cells.
- ***Hypoplasia:*** Incomplete development.
- ***Aplasia:*** Failure of development.
- ***Syndrome:*** A group of diverse symptoms and signs constituting together the picture of a disease.

- ***Paralysis:*** Loss of motor power (movement) of a part of body due to denervation or primary disease of the muscles.
- ***Hemiplegia:*** Paralysis of one-half of the body.
- ***Paraplegia:*** Paralysis of both the lower limbs.
- ***Monoplegia:*** Paralysis of any one limb.
- ***Quadriplegia:*** Paralysis of all the four limbs.
- ***Anesthesia:*** Loss of the touch sensibility.
- ***Analgesia:*** Loss of the pain sensibility.
- ***Thermanesthesia:*** Loss of the temperature sensibility.
- ***Hyperesthesia:*** Abnormally increased sensibility.
- ***Paresthesia:*** Perverted feeling of sensations.
- ***Coma:*** Deep unconsciousness.
- ***Tumor (neoplasm):*** A circumscribed, noninflammatory, abnormal growth arising from the body tissues.
- ***Benign:*** Mild illness or growth which does not endanger life.
- ***Malignant:*** Severe form of illness or growth, which is resistant to treatment and ends in death.
- ***Carcinoma:*** Malignant growth arising from the epithelium (ectoderm or endoderm).
- ***Sarcoma:*** Malignant growth arising from connective tissue (mesoderm).
- ***Cancer:*** A general term used to indicate any malignant neoplasm which shows invasiveness and results in death of the patient.
- ***Metastasis:*** Spread of a local disease (like the cancer cells) to distant parts of the body.
- ***Convalescence:*** The recovery period between the end of a disease and restoration to complete health.
- ***Therapy:*** Medical treatment.

## SKELETON

Skeleton includes bones and cartilages. It forms the main supporting framework of the body, and is primarily designed for a more effective production of movements by the attached muscles.

### Functions

- Bones give shape and support to the body, and resist any forms of stress.
- These provide surface for the attachment of muscles, tendons, ligaments, etc.
- These serve as levers for muscular actions.
- The skull, vertebral column and thoracic cage protect brain, spinal cord and thoracic viscera, respectively.
- Bone marrow manufactures blood cells.
- Bones store 97% of the body calcium and phosphorus.
- Bone marrow contains reticuloendothelial cells which are phagocytic in nature and take part in immune responses of the body.
- The larger paranasal air sinuses affect the timber of the voice.

### Classification of Bones

#### According to Shape

- ***Long bones:*** Each long bone has an elongated shaft (diaphysis) and two expanded ends (epiphyses) which are smooth and articular. The shaft typically has 3 surfaces separated by 3 borders, a central medullary cavity, and a nutrient foramen directed away from the growing end. Examples:
  - typical long bones like humerus, radius, ulna, femur, tibia and fibula;
  - miniature long bones have only one epiphysis like metacarpals, metatarsals and phalanges; and
  - modified long bones have no medullary cavity like clavicle.
- ***Short bones:*** Their shape is usually cuboid, cuneiform, trapezoid, or scaphoid. Examples: tarsal and carpal bones.
- ***Flat bones*** resemble shallow plates and form boundaries of certain body cavities. Examples: bones in the vault of the skull, ribs, sternum and scapula.
- ***Irregular bones:*** For example, vertebra, hip bone, and bones in the base of the skull.
- ***Pneumatic bones:*** Certain irregular bones contain large air spaces lined by epithelium. For example, maxilla, sphenoid, ethmoid, etc. They make the skull light in weight, help in resonance of voice, and act as air conditioning chambers for the inspired air.
- ***Sesamoid bones:*** These are bony nodules found embedded in the tendons or joint capsules. They have no periosteum and ossify after birth. They are related to an articular or nonarticular bony surface, and the surfaces of contact are covered with hyaline cartilage and lubricated by a bursa or synovial membrane.
  For example, patella, pisiform, fabella, etc.
  Functions of the sesamoid bones are:
  - to resist pressure;
  - to minimize friction;
  - to alter the direction of pull of the muscle; and
  - to maintain the local circulation.
- ***Accessory (supernumerary) bones*** are not always present. These may occur as ununited epiphyses developed from extra centers of ossification. For example, sutural bones, os trigonum (lateral tubercle of talus), os vesalianum (tuberosity of 5th metatarsal), etc. In medicolegal practice, accessory bones may be mistaken for fractures. However, these are often bilateral, and have smooth surfaces without any callus.
- ***Heterotopic bones:*** Bones sometimes develop in soft tissues. Horse riders develop bones in adductor muscles (rider's bones).

#### Developmental Classification

- ***Membrane (dermal) bones*** ossify in membrane (intramembranous or mesenchymal ossification), and are thus derived from mesenchymal condensations. For example, bones of the vault of skull and facial bones.
  - ***Cartilaginous bones*** ossify in cartilage intracartilaginous or endochondral ossification), and are thus derived from preformed cartilaginous models. For example, bones of limbs, vertebral column and thoracic cage.
  - ***Membrano-cartilaginous bones*** ossify partly in membrane and partly in cartilage. Examples are clavicle, mandible, occipital, temporal, sphenoid.

- *Somatic bones:* Most of the bones are somatic.
  - *Visceral bones:* These develop from pharyngeal arches. Examples are hyoid bones, part of mandible and ear ossicles.

### Regional Classification

- Axial skeleton includes skull, vertebral column, and thoracic cage.
- Appendicular skeleton includes bones of the limbs.

### Structural Classification

- *Macroscopically,* the architecture of bone may be compact or cancellous.
  - Compact bone is dense in texture like ivory, but is extremely porous. It is best developed in the cortex of the long bones. This is an adaptation to bending and twisting forces (a) combination of compression, tension and shear).
  - Cancellous or spongy, or trabecular bone is open in texture, and is made up of a meshwork of trabeculae (rods and plates) between which are marrow containing spaces. The trabecular meshworks are of three primary types, namely—(a) meshwork of rods, (b) meshwork of rods and plates, and (c) meshwork of plates (Singh, 1978).

## Cartilage

### Synonyms

- Chondros (G)
- Gristle

Compare with the terms chondrification, chondrodystrophy, synchondrosis, etc.

### Definition

Cartilage is a connective tissue composed of cells (chondrocytes) and fibers (collagen or yellow elastic) embedded in a firm, gel-like matrix which is rich in a mucopolysaccharide. It is much more elastic than bone.

### General Features

- Cartilage has no blood vessels or lymphatics. The nutrition of cells diffuses through the matrix.
- Cartilage has no nerves. It is, therefore, insensitive.
- Cartilage is surrounded by a fibrous membrane, called perichondrium, which is similar to periosteum in structure and function. The articular cartilage has no perichondrium, so that its regeneration after injury is inadequate.
- When cartilage calcifies, the chondrocytes die and the cartilage is replaced by bone like tissue.

### Types of Cartilage

There are three types of cartilages:

1. Hyaline cartilage
2. Fibrocartilage
3. Elastic cartilage

### Comparison between Bone and Cartilage

| Bone | Cartilage |
|---|---|
| Bone is hard | Cartilage is firm |
| Matrix has inflexible material called ossein | It has chondroitin providing flexibility |
| Matrix possesses calcium salt | Calcium salts not present |
| Bone has rich nerve supply | It does not have nerve supply |
| It is vascular in nature | It is avascular in nature |
| Bone marrow is present | Bone marrow is absent |
| Growth is only by apposition | Growth is appositional and interstitial |

## Joints

### Definition

Joint is a junction between two or more bones or cartilages. It is a device to permit movements. However, immovable joints are primarily meant for growth, and may permit moulding during childbirth.

There are more joints in a child than in an adult because as growth proceeds some of the bones fuse together, e.g. the ilium, ischium and pubis to form the pelvic bone; the two halves of the infant frontal bone, and of the infant mandible; the five sacral vertebrae and the four coccygeal vertebrae.

### Classification of Joints

*Structural Classification*

- Fibrous joints
  - Sutures
  - Syndesmosis
  - Gomphosis
- Cartilaginous joints
  - Primary cartilaginous joints or synchondrosis
  - Secondary cartilaginous joints or symphysis
- Synovial joints
  - Ball-and-socket or spheroidal joints
  - Sellar or saddle joints
  - Condylar or bicondylar joints
  - Ellipsoid joints
  - Hinge joints
  - Pivot or trochoid joints
  - Plane joints

*Functional Classification (According to the Degree of Mobility)*

- Synarthrosis (immovable), like fibrous joints
- Amphiarthrosis (slightly movable), like cartilaginous joints.
- Diarthrosis (freely movable), like synovial joints.

*Synarthroses*

*Synarthroses* are fixed joints at which there is no movement. The articular surfaces are joined by tough fibrous tissue. Often the edges of the bones are dovetailed into one another as in the sutures of the skull.

#### *Amphiarthroses*

***Amphiarthroses*** are joints at which slight movement is possible. A pad of cartilage lies between the bone surfaces, and there are fibrous ligaments to hold the bones and cartilage in place. The cartilages of such joints also act as shock absorbers, e.g. the intervertebral discs between the bodies of the vertebrae, where the cartilage is strengthened by extra collagen fibers.

#### *Diarthroses or Synovial Joints*

***Diarthroses or synovial joints*** are known as freely movable joints, though at some of them the movement is restricted by the shape of the articulating surfaces and by the ligaments which hold the bones together. These ligaments are of elastic connective tissue.

A synovial joint has a fluid-filled cavity between articular surfaces which are covered by articular cartilage. The fluid, known as synovial fluid, produced by the synovial membrane which lines the cavity except for the actual articular surfaces and covers any ligaments or tendons which pass through the joint. Synovial fluid acts as a lubricant. The form of the articulating surfaces controls the type of movement which takes place at any joint.

The movements possible at synovial joints are:

**Angular**

- ***Flexion:*** Decreasing the angle between two bones;
- ***Extension:*** Increasing the angle between two bones.
- ***Abduction:*** moving the part away from the mid-line.
- ***Adduction:*** bringing the part towards the mid-line.

Rotary

- **Rotation:** Turning upon an axis.
- **Circumduction:** Moving the extremity of the part round in a circle so that the whole part inscribes a cone.

Gliding

Gliding one part slides on another.

#### *Regional Classification*

- ***Skull type:*** Immovable.
- ***Vertebral type:*** Slightly movable.
- ***Limb type:*** Freely movable.

#### *According to Number of Articulating Bones*

- ***Simple joint:*** When two bones articulate, e.g. interphalangeal joints.
- ***Compound joint:*** More than two bones articulate within one capsule, e.g. elbow joint, wrist joint.
- ***Complex joint:*** When joint cavity is divided by an intra-articular disc, e.g. temporomandibular joint and sterno-clavicular joint.

## CARDIOVASCULAR SYSTEM

Cardiovascular system is the *transport system* of the body, through which the nutrients are conveyed to places where these are utilized, and the metabolites (waste products) are conveyed to appropriate places from where these are expelled. The conveying medium is a liquid tissue, the blood, which flows in tubular channels called *blood vessels*. The circulation is maintained by the central pumping organ called the *heart*.

### Components

Cardiovascular system is a closed system of tubes made up of the following parts based on their structural and topographical characteristics

- ***Heart:*** It is a four-chambered muscular organ which pumps blood to various parts of the body. Each half of the heart has a receiving chamber called atrium, and a pumping chamber called ventricle.
- ***Arteries:*** These are distributing channels which carry blood away from the heart.
  - They branch like trees on their way to different parts of the body.
  - The large arteries are rich in elastic tissue, but as branching progresses there is an ever-increasing amount of smooth muscle in their walls.
  - The minute branches which are just visible to naked eye are called arterioles.
  - *Angeion* is a Greek word, meaning a vessel (blood vessel or lymph vessel). Its word derivatives are angiology, angiography, hemangioma and thromboangitis obliterans.
- ***Veins:*** These are draining channels which carry blood from different parts of the body back to the heart.
  - Like rivers, the veins are formed by tributaries.
  - The small veins (venules) join together to form larger veins , which in turn unite to form great veins called venae cavae
- ***Capillaries:*** These are networks of microscopic vessels which connect arterioles with the venules.
  - These come in intimate contact with the tissues for a free exchange of nutrients and metabolites across their walls between the blood and the tissue fluid.
  - The metabolites are partly drained by the capillaries and partly by lymphatics.
  - Capillaries are replaced by sinusoids in certain organs, like liver and spleen.

Functionally, the blood vessels can be classified into the following five groups:

1. Distributing vessels, including arteries
2. Resistance vessels, including arterioles and precapillary sphincters
3. Exchange vessels, including capillaries, sinusoids, and postcapillary venules
4. Reservoir (capacitance) vessels, including larger venules and veins
5. Shunts, including various types of anastomoses.

### Types of Circulation of Blood

- ***Systemic (greater) circulation:*** The blood flows from the left ventricle, through various parts of the body, to the right atrium, i.e. from the left to the right side of the heart.
- ***Pulmonary (lesser) circulation:*** The blood flows from the right ventricle, through the lungs, to the left atrium, i.e. from the right to the left side of the heart.
- ***Portal circulation:*** It is a part of systemic circulation, which has the following characteristics:
  - The blood passes through two sets of capillaries before draining into a systemic vein.

- The vein draining the first capillary network is known as portal vein which branches like an artery to form the second set of capillaries or sinusoids. For example, hepatic portal circulation hypothalamo-hypophyseal portal circulation and renal portal circulation.

## Arteries

### Characteristic Features

- Arteries are thick-walled, being uniformly thicker than the accompanying veins, except for the arteries within the cranium and vertebral canal where these are thin.
- Their lumen is smaller than that of the accompanying veins.
- Arteries have no valves.
- An artery is usually accompanied by vein(s) and nerve(s), and the three of them together form the neurovascular bundle which is surrounded and supported by a fibroareolar sheath.

### Types of Arteries and Structure

- *Large arteries of elastic type,* e.g. aorta and its main branches (brachiocephalic, common carotid, subclavian and common iliac) and the pulmonary arteries.
- *Medium and small arteries of muscular type,* e.g. temporal, occipital, radial, popliteal, etc.
- *Smallest arteries of muscular type* are called arterioles. They measure 50–100 micron in diameter. Arterioles divide into terminal arterioles with a diameter of 15–20 micron, and having one or two layers of smooth muscle in their walls. The side branches from terminal arterioles are called metarterioles which measure 10–15 micron at their origin and about 5 micron at their termination. The terminal narrow end of metarteriole is surrounded by a precapillary sphincter which regulates blood flow into the capillary bed. It is important to know that the muscular arterioles are responsible for generating peripheral resistance, and thereby for regulating the diastolic blood pressure.

### Palpable Arteries

Some arteries can be palpated through the skin. These are—common carotid, facial, brachial, radial, abdominal aorta, femoral, posterior tibial and dorsalis pedis.

### Nerve Supply of Arteries

The nerves supplying an artery are called *nervi vascularis*. The nerves are mostly non-myelinated sympathetic fibers which are vasoconstrictor in function. A few fibers are myelinated, and are believed to be sensory to the outer and inner coats of the arteries. Vasodilator innervation is restricted to the following sites:

- The skeletal muscle vessels are dilated by cholinergic sympathetic nerves.
- The exocrine gland vessels are dilated on parasympathetic stimulation.
- The cutaneous vessels are dilated locally to produce the flare (redness) after an injury. The vasodilatation is produced by the afferent impulses in the cutaneous nerves which pass antidromically in their collaterals to the blood vessels (axon reflex).

## Veins

### Characteristic Features

- Veins are thin-walled, being thinner than the arteries.
- Their lumen is larger than that of the accompanying arteries.
- Veins have valves which maintain the unidirectional flow of blood, even against gravity. Since the venous pressure is low (7 mm Hg), the valves are of utmost value in the venous return. However, the valves are absent:
  - In the veins of less than 2 mm diameter.
  - In the venae cavae.
  - In the hepatic, renal, uterine, ovarian (not testicular), cerebral, spinal, pulmonary, and umbilical veins.
- The muscular and elastic tissue content of the venous walls is much less than that of the arteries. This is directly related to the low venous pressure.
- Large veins have dead space around them for their dilatation during increased venous return. The dead space commonly contains the regional lymph nodes.

### Structure of Veins

Veins are made up of usual three coats which are found in the arteries. But the coats are ill-defined, and the muscle and elastic tissue content is poor. In poorly developed tunica media, the amount of collagen fibers is more than the elastic and muscle fibers. The adventitia is thickest and best developed. The smooth muscle is altogether absent:

- in the veins of maternal part of placenta;
- in the cranial venous sinuses and pial veins;
- in the retinal veins;
- in the veins of cancellous bone; and
- in the venous spaces of the corpora cavernosa and corpus spongiosum.

### Blood and Nerve Supply of Veins

The larger veins, like the arteries, are supplied with nutrient vessels called vasa vasorum. But in the veins, the vessels may penetrate up to the intima, probably because of the low venous pressure and the low oxygen tension.

Nerves also are distributed to the veins in the same manner as to the arteries, but are fewer in number.

### Factors Helping in Venous Return

- Overflow from the capillaries, pushed from behind by the arteries (vis-a-tergo).
- Negative intrathoracic pressure sucks the blood into the heart from all over the body.
- Gravity helps venous return in the upper part of the body.
- Arterial pulsations press on the venae comitantes intermittently and drive the venous blood towards the heart.
- Venous valves prevent any regurgitation (back flow) of the luminal blood.

## Capillaries

Capillaries (capillus = hair) are networks of microscopic endothelial tubes interposed between the metarterioles and venules. The true capillaries (without any smooth muscle cell) begin after a transition zone of 50–100 micron beyond the precapillary sphincters. The capillaries are replaced by cavernous (dilated) spaces in the sex organs, splenic pulp and placenta.

### *Size*

The average diameter of a capillary is 6–8 micron, just sufficient to permit the red blood cells to pass through in 'single file'. But the size varies from organ to organ. It is smallest in the brain and intestines, and is largest (20 micron) in the skin and bone marrow.

### Anastomoses

### *Definition*

A precapillary or postcapillary communication between the neighboring vessels is called anastomoses. Circulation through the anastomosis is called collateral circulation.

### Types

- ***Arterial anastomoses*** is the communication between the arteries, or branches of arteries. It may be actual or potential.
  - In ***actual arterial anastomosis*** the arteries meet end to end. For example, palmar arches plantar arch, circle of Willis, intestinal arcades, labial branches of facial arteries.
  - In ***potential arterial anastomoses*** the communication takes place between the terminal arterioles. Such communications can dilate only gradually for collateral circulation. Therefore on sudden occlusion of a main artery, the anastomoses may fail to compensate the loss. The examples are seen in the coronary arteries and the cortical branches of cerebral arteries, etc.
- ***Venous anastomoses*** is the communication between the veins or tributaries of veins. For example, the dorsal venous arches of the hand and foot.
- ***Arteriovenous anastomosis*** (shunt) is the communication between an artery and a vein. It serves the function of phasic activity of the organ. When the organ is active these shunts are closed and the blood circulates through the capillaries. However, when the organ is at rest, the blood bypasses the capillary bed and is shunted back through the arteriovenous anastomosis.The shunt vessel may be straight or coiled, possesses a thick muscular coat, and is under the influence of sympathetic system.

  Shunts of simple structure are found in the skin of nose, lips and external ear; in the mucous membrane of nose and alimentary canal; the coccygeal body; the erectile tissue of sexual organs; the tongue; the thyroid gland and sympathetic ganglia. Specialized arteriovenous anastomoses are found in the skin of digital pads and nail beds. They form a number of small units called *glomera*.

  Preferential 'thoroughfare channels 'are also a kind of shunts. They course through the capillary network. Many true capillaries arise as their side branches.

  One thoroughfare channel with its associated capillaries forms a microcirculatory unit. The size of the unit is variable from 1–2 to 20–30 true capillaries. The number of active units varies from time to time.

### End-Arteries

### *Definition*

Arteries which do not anastomose with their neighbours are called endarteries.

*Examples:*

- Central artery of retina and labyrinthine artery of internal ear are the best examples of an absolute end arteries.
- Central branches of cerebral arteries and vasa recta of mesenteric arteries.
- Arteries of spleen, kidney, lungs and metaphyses of long bones.

### *Importance*

Occlusion of an end-artery causes serious nutritional disturbances resulting in death of the tissue supplied by it. For example, occlusion of central artery of retina results in blindness.

## NERVOUS SYSTEM

Nervous system is the chief controlling and coordinating system of the body. It controls and regulates all activities of the body, whether voluntary or involuntary, and adjusts the individual (organism) to the given surroundings.

### Parts of Nervous System

The nervous system is broadly divided into central and peripheral parts which are continuous with each other. Further subdivisions of each part are given.

- ***Central Nervous System (CNS)*** includes:
  - ***Brain or encephalon,*** which occupies cranial cavity, and contains the higher governing centres.
  - ***Spinal cord or spinal medulla,*** which occupies upper two-thirds of the vertebral canal, and contains many reflex centers.
- ***Peripheral nervous system (PNS)*** is subdivided into the following two components.
  1. ***Cerebrospinal nervous system*** is the somatic component of the peripheral nervous system, which includes 12 pairs of cranial nerves and 31 pairs of spinal nerves. It innervates the somatic structures of the head and neck, limbs and body wall, and mediates somatic sensory and motor functions.
  2. ***Peripheral autonomic nervous system*** is the visceral component of the peripheral nervous system, which includes the visceral or splanchnic nerves that are connected to the CNS through the somatic nerves. It innervates the viscera, glands, blood vessels and nonstriated muscles, and mediates the visceral functions.

  The cerebrospinal and autonomic nervous systems differ from each other in their efferent pathways.

### Cell Types of Nervous System

The nervous tissue is composed of two distinct types of cells:

1. The excitable cells are the nerve cells or neurons
2. The non-excitable cells constitute neuroglia and ependyma in the CNS, and Schwann cells in the PNS.

## Neuron

Hach nerve cell or neuron has a cell body or perikaryon, having a central nucleus and Nissl granules in its cytoplasm.

*Types of Neurons*

Neurons can be classified in several ways.

- According to the number of their processes (neurites) they may be:
  - ***Unipolar***, e.g. mesencephalic nucleus;
  - ***Pseudo-unipolar***, e.g. sensory ganglia or spinal ganglia
  - ***Bipolar***, e.g. spiral and vestibular ganglia and bipolar neurons of retina.
  - ***Multipolar***, neurons in cerebrum and cerebellum.
- According to the length of axon, the neurons are classified as:
  - ***Golgi type I*** neurons, with a long axon; and
  - ***Golgi type II*** neurons (microneurons), with a short or no axon.

## Blood-Brain Barrier

Certain dyes, when injected intravenously, fail to stain the parenchyma of brain and spinal cord, although they pass easily into the non-nervous tissues. However, the same dyes, when injected into the ventricles, enter the brain substances easily. This indicates that a barrier exists at the capillary level between the blood and nerve cells. The possible structures constituting the blood-brain barrier are as follows.

- Capillary endothelium without fenestrations.
- Basement membrane of the endothelium.
- The end feet of astrocytes covering the capillary walls.

The barrier permits a selective passage of blood contents to the nervous tissue, and thus the toxic and harmful substances are ordinarily prevented from reaching the brain.

## Reflex Arc

A reflex arc is the basic functional unit of the nervous system which can perform an integrated neural activity. In its simplest form, i.e. mono-synaptic reflex arc, is made up of:

- A receptor, e.g. skin
- A sensory or afferent neuron
- A motor or efferent neuron
- An effector, e.g. muscle.

The complex forms of reflex arc are polysynaptic due to addition of one or more internuncial neurons (interneurons) in between the afferent and efferent neurons.

An involuntary motor response of the body is called a reflex action. The stretch reflexes (tendon jerks) are the examples of monosynaptic reflexes whereas the withdrawal reflex (response to a painful stimulus) is a polysynaptic reflex.

## Peripheral Nerves

The nerves are solid white cords composed of bundles (fasciculi) of nerve fibers. Each nerve fiber is an axon with its coverings.The nerve fibers are supported and bound together by connective tissue sheaths at different levels of organization of the nerve. The whole nerve trunk is ensheathed by epineurium, each fasciculus by perineurium, and each nerve fiber by a delicate endoneurium. The toughness of a nerve is due to its fibrous sheaths, otherwise the nerve tissue itself is very delicate and friable.

## Spinal Nerves

There are 31 pairs of spinal nerves, including 8 cervical, 12 thoracic, 5 lumbar, 5 sacral, and 1 coccygeal.

## Autonomic Nervous System

Autonomic nervous system controls involuntary activities of the body, like sweating, salivation, peristalsis, etc. It differs fundamentally from the somatic nervous system in having:

- The preganglionic fibers arising from the CNS
- The ganglia for relay of the preganglionic fibers
- The postganglionic fibers arising from the ganglia which supply the effectors (smooth muscles and glands).

In contrast, the somatic nerves after arising from the CNS reach their destination without any interruption.

Autonomic nervous system is divided into two more or less complementary parts, the sympathetic and parasympathetic systems.

The sympathetic activities are widespread and diffuse, and combat the acute emergencies.

The parasympathetic activities are usually discrete and isolated, and provide a comfortable environment.

Both systems function in absolute coordination and adjust the body involuntarily to the given surroundings.

## Sympathetic Nervous System

- It is also known as 'thoracolumbar' outflow because it arises from lateral horn of T1 to L2 segments of the spinal cord.
- The medullated preganglionic fibers (white rami communicantes) arise from the lateral column of the spinal cord, emerge through the ventral rami where the white rami are connected to the ganglia of the sympathetic chain
- Preganglionic fibers relay either in the lateral ganglia (sympathetic chain) or in the collateral ganglia, e.g. the coeliac ganglion. The non-medullated post-ganglionic fibers run for some distance before reaching the organ of supply.
- The adrenal medulla is a unique exception in the body; it is supplied by the preganglionic fibers.
- Sympathetic nerve endings are adrenergic in nature, meaning thereby that noradrenalin is produced for neurotransmission. The only exception to this general rule are the cholinergic sympathetic nerves supplying the sweat glands and skeletal muscle vessels for vasodilatation.
- Functionally, sympathetic nerves are vasomotor (vasoconstrictor), sudomotor (secretomotor to sweat glands), and pilomotor (contract the arrector pili and cause erection of hair) in the skin of limbs and body wall. In addition, sympathetic activity causes dilation of pupil, pale face, dry mouth, tachycardia, rise in blood pressure, inhibition of hollow viscera, and closure of the perineal sphincters. The blood supply to the skeletal muscles, heart and brain is markedly increased. Thus, sympathetic reactions tend to be 'mass reactions', widely diffused in

their effect and that they are directed towards mobilization of the resources of the body for expenditure of energy in dealing with the emergencies or emotional crises (fright, fight, flight).

### Parasympathetic Nervous System

- It is also known as craniosacral outflow because it arises from the brain (mixed with III, VII, IX and X cranial nerves) and sacral.
- The preganglionic fibers are very long, reaching right upto the viscera of supply. The ganglia, called terminal ganglia, are situated mostly on the viscera and, therefore, the postganglionic fibers are very short.
- Parasympathetic nerve endings are cholinergic in nature, similar to the somatic nerves.
- Functionally, parasympathetic activity is seen when the subject is fully relaxed. His pupils are constricted, lenses accommodated, face flushed, mouth moist, pulse slow, blood pressure low, bladder and gut contracting, and the perineal sphincters relaxed.

In general the effects of parasympathetic activity are usually discrete and isolated, and directed towards conservation and restoration of the resources of energy in the body.

## RESPIRATORY SYSTEM

- Respiratory systems allow animals to move oxygen (needed for cellular respiration) into body tissues and remove carbon dioxide (waste product of cellular respiration) from cells.
- 'Respiration' is used several different ways:
  - Cellular respiration is the aerobic breakdown of glucose in the mitochondria to make ATP.
  - Respiratory systems are the organs in animals that exchange gases with the environment.
  - 'Respiration' is an everyday term that is often used to mean 'breathing.'

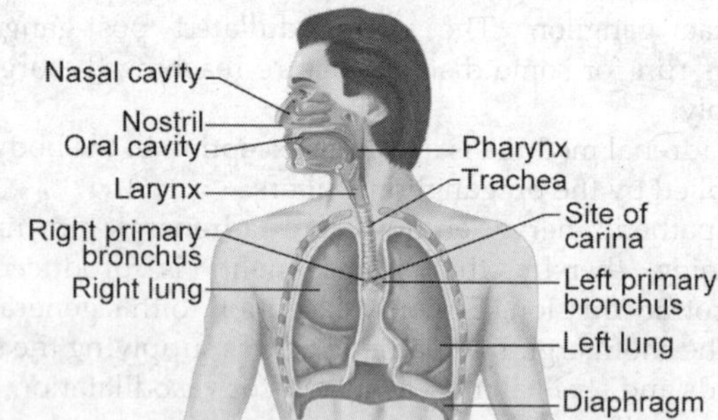


- Consists of the respiratory and conducting zones
- Respiratory zone
  - Site of gas exchange
  - Consists of bronchioles, alveolar ducts, and alveoli
- Conducting zone
  - Provides rigid conduits for air to reach the sites of gas exchange
  - Includes all other respiratory structures (e.g., nose, nasal cavity, pharynx, trachea)
- Respiratory muscles—diaphragm and other muscles that promote ventilation.

### Major Functions of the Respiratory System

- To supply the body with oxygen and dispose of carbon dioxide
- Respiration—four distinct processes must happen
  1. Pulmonary ventilation—moving air into and out of the lungs
  2. External respiration—gas exchange between the lungs and the blood
  3. Transport—transport of oxygen and carbon dioxide between the lungs and tissues
  4. Internal respiration—gas exchange between systemic blood vessels and tissues.

### Respiratory System is Divided into Two Parts

1. Upprer respiratory tract
   - Nose
   - Paranasal sinuses
   - Pharynx
2. Lower respiratory tract
   - Begins with true vocal cords and extends to alveoli
   - Larynx
   - Trachea
   - Main stem bronchi
   - Segmental bronchi
   - Subsegmental bronchi
   - Bronchioles
   - Terminal bronchioles
   - Respiratory bronchioles
   - Alveolar ducts
   - Alveolar sacs
   - Alveoli

### Structure of the Nose

- The nose is divided into two regions:
  1. The external nose, including the root, bridge, dorsum nasi, and apex
  2. The internal nasal cavity
- Philtrum—a shallow vertical groove inferior to the apex
- The external nares (nostrils) are bounded laterally by the alae.

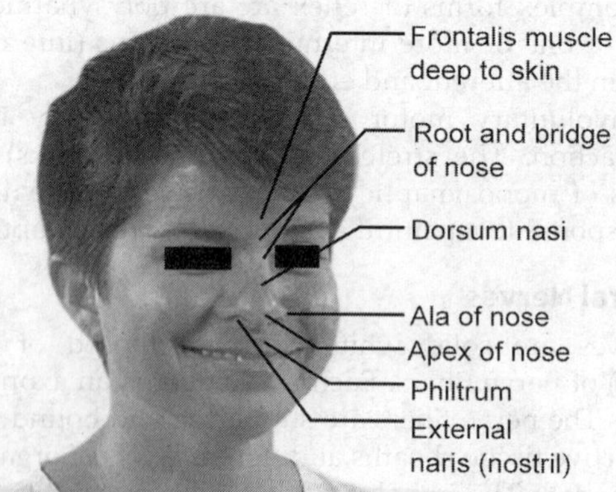

### Nasal Cavity

- Lies in and posterior to the external nose
- Is divided by a midline nasal septum
- Opens posteriorly into the nasal pharynx via internal nares
- The ethmoid and sphenoid bones form the roof
- The floor is formed by the hard and soft palates
- Vestibule—nasal cavity superior to the nares
  - Vibrissae—hairs that filter coarse particles from inspired air
- Olfactory mucosa
  - Lines the superior nasal cavity
  - Contains smell receptors
- Respiratory mucosa
  - Lines the balance of the nasal cavity
  - Glands secrete mucus containing lysozyme and defensins to help destroy bacteria
- Inspired air is:
  - Humidified by the high water content in the nasal cavity
  - Warmed by rich plexuses of capillaries
- Ciliated mucosal cells remove contaminated mucus
- Superior, medial, and inferior conchae:
  - Protrude medially from the lateral walls
  - Increase mucosal area
  - Enhance air turbulence and help filter air
- Sensitive mucosa triggers sneezing when stimulated by irritating particles.

### Functions of the Nasal Mucosa and Conchae

- During inhalation the conchae and nasal mucosa:
  - Filter, heat, and moisten air
- During exhalation these structures:
  - Reclaim heat and moisture
  - Minimize heat and moisture loss

### Paranasal Sinuses

- Sinuses in bones that surround the nasal cavity
- Sinuses lighten the skull and help to warm and moisten the air.

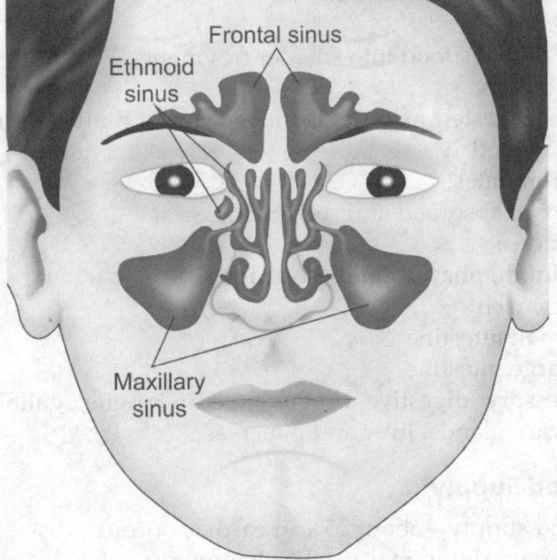


### Pharynx

- Funnel-shaped tube of skeletal muscle that connects to the:
  - Nasal cavity and mouth superiorly
  - Larynx and esophagus inferiorly
- Extends from the base of the skull to the level of the sixth cervical vertebra
- It is divided into three regions
  1. Nasopharynx
  2. Oropharynx
  3. Laryngopharynx.

### Nasopharynx

- Lies posterior to the nasal cavity, inferior to the sphenoid, and superior to the level of the soft palate
- Strictly an air passageway
- Lined with pseudostratified columnar epithelium
- Closes during swallowing to prevent food from entering the nasal cavity
- The pharyngeal tonsil lies high on the posterior wall
- Pharyngotympanic (auditory) tubes open into the lateral walls.

### Oropharynx

- Extends inferiorly from the level of the soft palate to the epiglottis
- Opens to the oral cavity via an archway called the fauces
- Serves as a common passageway for food and air
- The epithelial lining is protective stratified squamous epithelium
- Palatine tonsils lie in the lateral walls of the fauces
- Lingual tonsil covers the base of the tongue.

### Laryngopharynx

- Serves as a common passageway for food and air
- Lies posterior to the upright epiglottis
- Extends to the larynx, where the respiratory and digestive pathways diverge.

### Trachea

- Flexible and mobile tube extending from the larynx into the mediastinum
- Composed of three layers:
  1. Mucosa—made up of goblet cells and ciliated epithelium
  2. Submucosa—connective tissue deep to the mucosa
  3. Adventitia—outermost layer made of C-shaped rings of hyaline cartilage.

### Conducting Zone: Bronchi

- The carina of the last tracheal cartilage marks the end of the trachea and the beginning of the right and left bronchi
- Air reaching the bronchi is:
  - Warm and cleansed of impurities
  - Saturated with water vapor
- Bronchi subdivide into secondary bronchi, each supplying a lobe of the lungs
- Air passages undergo 23 orders of branching in the lungs.

### Bronchial Tree

- Tissue walls of bronchi mimic that of the trachea
- As conducting tubes become smaller, structural changes occur
  - Cartilage support structures change
  - Epithelium types change
  - Amount of smooth muscle increases
- Bronchioles
  - Consist of cuboidal epithelium
  - Have a complete layer of circular smooth muscle
  - Lack cartilage support and mucus-producing cells

### Respiratory Zone

- Defined by the presence of alveoli; begins as terminal bronchioles feed into respiratory bronchioles
- Respiratory bronchioles lead to alveolar ducts, then to terminal clusters of alveolar sacs composed of alveoli
- Approximately 300 million alveoli:
  - Account for most of the lungs' volume
  - Provide tremendous surface area for gas exchange.

### Respiratory Membrane

- This air-blood barrier is composed of:
  - Alveolar and capillary walls
  - Their fused basal laminas
- Alveolar walls:
  - Are a single layer of type I epithelial cells
  - Permit gas exchange by simple diffusion
  - Secrete angiotensin converting enzyme (ACE)
- Type II cells secrete surfactant.

### Alveoli

- Surrounded by fine elastic fibers
- Contain open pores that:
  - Connect adjacent alveoli
  - Allow air pressure throughout the lung to be equalized
- House macrophages that keep alveolar surfaces sterile.

### Gross Anatomy of the Lungs

- Lungs occupy all of the thoracic cavity except the mediastinum
  - Root—site of vascular and bronchial attachments
  - Costal surface—anterior, lateral, and posterior surfaces in contact with the ribs
  - Apex—narrow superior tip
  - Base—inferior surface that rests on the diaphragm
  - Hilus—indentation that contains pulmonary and systemic blood vessels.

### Lungs

- Cardiac notch (impression)—cavity that accommodates the heart
- Left lung—separated into upper and lower lobes by the oblique fissure
- Right lung—separated into three lobes by the oblique and horizontal fissures
- There are 10 bronchopulmonary segments in each lung
- Base, apex (cupula), costal surface, cardiac notch
- Oblique and horizontal fissure in right lung results in 3 lobes
- Oblique fissure only in left lung produces 2 lobes
- Blood vessels and airways enter lungs at hilus
- Forms root of lungs
- Covered with pleura (parietal becomes visceral).

### Blood Supply to Lungs

- Lungs are perfused by two circulations— pulmonary and bronchial
- Pulmonary arteries—supply systemic venous blood to be oxygenated
  - Branch profusely, along with bronchi
  - Ultimately feed into the pulmonary capillary network surrounding the alveoli
- Pulmonary veins—carry oxygenated blood from respiratory zones to the heart
- Bronchial arteries—provide systemic blood to the lung tissue
  - Arise from aorta and enter the lungs at the hilus
  - Supply all lung tissue except the alveoli
- Bronchial veins anastomose with pulmonary veins
- Pulmonary veins carry most venous blood back to the heart.

### Pleurae

- Thin, double-layered serosa
- Parietal pleura
  - Covers the thoracic wall and superior face of the diaphragm
  - Continues around heart and between lungs
- Visceral, or pulmonary, pleura
  - Covers the external lung surface
  - Divides the thoracic cavity into three chambers
    - ➢ The central mediastinum
    - ➢ Two lateral compartments, each containing a lung.

## GASTROINTESTINAL SYSTEM

- Gastrointestinal (GI) tract [alimentary canal] a continuous muscular digestive tube
  - Digests:
    - ➢ Breaks food into smaller fragments
  - Absorbs:
    - ➢ Digested material is moved through mucosa into the blood
  - Eliminates:
    - ➢ Unabsorbed and secreted wastes.
- Includes:
  - Mouth, pharynx and esophagus
  - Stomach
  - Small intestine
  - Large intestine
- Accessory digestive organs—teeth, tongue, gallbladder, salivary glands, liver and pancreas.

### GI Blood Supply

- Blood supply—about 25% of cardiac output
- Arterial: Abdominal aorta (celiac trunk)

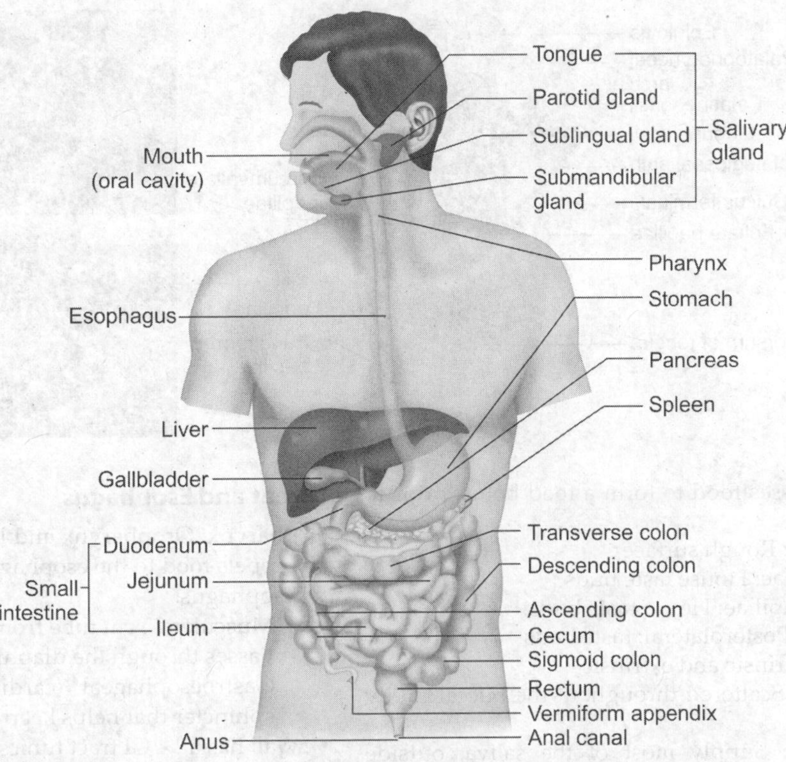


- Celiac trunk (hepatic, splenic and gastric branches which serve the liver, spleen and stomach)
- Celiac trunk (superior and inferior mesenteric branches serve small and large intestine).

## Histology

- GI tract wall has four layers:
  1. Mucosa
  2. Submucosa
  3. Muscularis Externa
  4. Serosa or Adventitia
- Mucosa: The epithelial membrane that lines the GI tract from mouth → anus.
  - Secretes mucous, digestive enzymes and hormones
  - Absorbs nutrients
  - Protects from disease and from the GI contents
- Mucosa; three layers:
  1. Epidermis
  2. Lamina propria (loose connective tissue— contain capillaries and some elements of MALT)
  3. Muscularis mucosa
- Submucosa: Moderately dense CT with blood, nerve, lymph vessels and lymphoid follicles; rich in elastic fibers
- Muscularis externa: Smooth muscle
  - Responsible for peristalsis and segmentation
  - Circular layer
  - Longitudinal layer
  - Sphincters: In some areas the circular layer thickens; act as valves
- Serosa of intraperitoneal organs = visceral peritoneum
- Esophagus has an outer covering of fibrous connective tissue = adventitia
- Retroperitoneal organs: Visceral serosa on the surface facing the peritoneal cavity and adventitia on the surface facing the body wall.

## Nerves

- Intrinsic (local): Short reflex
  - Submucosal nerve plexus: Regulates glands and mucosal muscle
  - Myenteric plexus: Controls GI wall and GI motility
- Extrinsic (CNS): Long reflex
  - Parasympathetic NS: Enhances gut motility and secretion
  - SNS: Inhibits gut motility and secretion

## Functional Anatomy: Mouth

- Mouth: Lips, palate, and tongue
- Mouth cavity = Buccal cavity
- Lips: Extend from inferior margin of the nose to the superior margin of the chin. Red area = red margin, is poorly keratinized and lacks sweat or sebaceous glands.
- Palate:
  - Hard palate: Rigid surface against which food is forced in chewing
  - Soft palate: Muscular structure that rises and blocks off the nasopharynx during swallowing
- Tongue: Muscular tentacle composed of interlaced muscle fibers that grips and repositions food, mixes food with

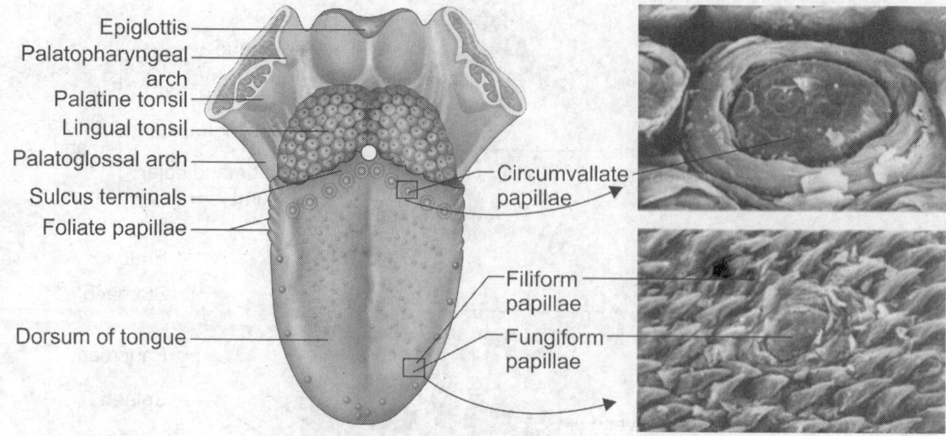


saliva and compresses food to form a food bolus, prior to swallowing.

- Filiform papillae: Rough surface
- Fungiform papillae: House taste buds
- Circumvallate papillae: House taste buds,
- Foliate papillae: Posterolateral; taste buds

- Salivary glands: Intrinsic and extrinsic
  - Intrinsic glands: Scattered throughout the buccal cavity mucosa
  - Extrinsic glands: Supply most of the saliva; outside buccal cavity and supply secretions via ducts:
    - ➢ Parotid
    - ➢ Submandibular
    - ➢ Sublingual
- Composition of saliva:
  - 97–99.5% $H_2O$
  - Electrolytes: pH 6.75–7.0
  - Amylase (digestive enzyme)
  - Proteins: Mucin, lysozyme, and IgA
- Protection from microbes by saliva:
  - IgA: Immunglobulins in secretions
  - Lysozyme: Bacteriostatic (inhibits bacterial growth)
  - Cyanide
  - Defensins: Local antibiotic activity and when activated promote chemotaxis by WBCs
  - Normal flora: Convert salivary components to nitrates then to NO. NO is toxic and bacteriocidal
- Control of salivation:
  - Continuous baseline secretory activity
    - ➢ With food ingestion, salivation increases dramatically
    - ➢ Parasympathetic NS: Chemoreceptors and pressoreceptors stimulate salivatory nuclei to increase salivation
- Teeth:
  - Primary: $\frac{2I\ 1C\ 2M}{2I\ 1C\ 2M} \times 2 = 20$
  - Permanent: $\frac{2I\ 1C\ 2PM\ 3M}{2I\ 1C\ 2PM\ 3M} \times 2 = 32$
  - Structures
    - ➢ Crown: Exposed above gingiva (gum)
    - ➢ Root: Anchored by periodontal ligament to the bone by a fibrous joint (gomphosis).

## Throat and Esophagus

- Pharynx: Oropharynx and laryngopharynx; muscular wall propels food to the esophagus.
- Esophagus:
  - Muscular 25 cm tube from laryngopharynx to stomach
  - Passes through the diaphragm at the esophageal hiatus
  - Gastroesophageal (cardiac) sphincter: A physiologic sphincter that helps keep esophagus closed when empty
- Wall has all 4 GI tract tunics:
  - Epithelial layer changes at the junction with the stomach from stratified squamous epithelium to simple columnar epithelium
    - ➢ Esophageal mucous glands lubricate food bolus
  - Muscularis externa
    - ➢ Superior 1/3 of muscularis externa is skeletal muscle
    - ➢ Middle 1/3 is mixed skeletal and smooth
    - ➢ Lower 1/3 is smooth muscle
  - Adventitia: External covering.

## Stomach

- Cardiac region: Narrow, receives food bolus
- Fundus: Bulge that extends superolaterally to the cardia, reaches the diaphragm
- Body: Mid-portion

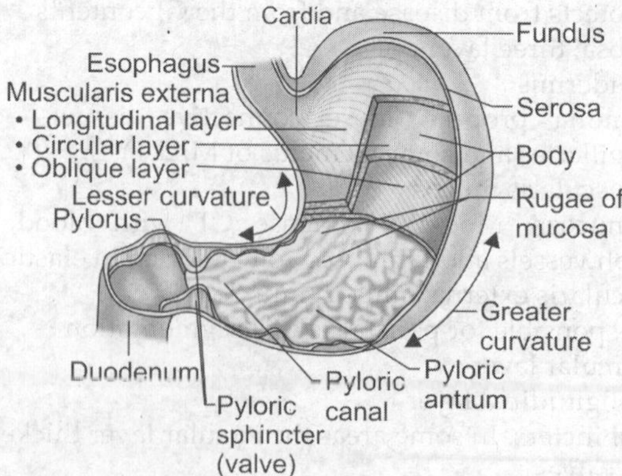

- Pyloric antrum: Funnel shaped portion narrows to form the
  - Pyloric canal > pylorous > pyloric sphincter > small intestine
- Rugae
  - longitudinal mucosal folds
- Volume about 4L
- Gastric glands secrete gastric juices
  - Mucous neck cells: In the duct portion
  - Parietal cells: Mid portion secrete HCl and intrinsic factor for B12 absorption
  - Chief cells: Base of gland; secretes pepsinogen a precursor molecule to pepsin (an enzyme that digests protein)
- Enteroendocrine cells: Secrete multiple hormonal products
  - Gastrin, histamine, endorphins, serotonin, cholecystokinin, and somatostatin, which influence several digestive system organs
- Mucosal barrier: Protects the stomach from its own secretions
  - Viscous mucous overlies a thick coating of $HCO_3$ (rich mucous)
  - Tight junctions between epithelial cell PM of glandular cells are impermeable to HCl
  - Epithelium is replaced every 3–6 days.

### Digestive Processes (Stomach)

- Acts as a holding vessel for ingested food
- Participates in mechanical and chemical digestion
- Propulsion: Delivers its product (chyme) to the small intestine
- Protein digestion: HCl denatures protein
  - HCl activates pepsinogen to pepsin
  - Pepsin breaks peptide bonds of proteins
  - Rennin: An enzyme that breaks down casein (milk protein) secreted in infants
- Intrinsic factor: Required for Vit. B12 absorption (needed to mature RBC);
  - Absence of B12 results in pernicious anemia.

### Small Intestine: Gross Anatomy

- 6–7 m long: From pyloric sphincter to the ileocecal valve
- Three subdivisions:
  1. Duodenum
  2. Jejunum
  3. Ileum
- Duodenum:
  - Curves around the pancreatic head (~25 cm long)
  - Contains the hepatopancreatic ampulla: formed by the merger of the bile duct and the pancreatic duct.
  - Hepatopancreatic sphincter controls admission of bile and pancreatic enzymes to the duodenum
  - Duodenum is retroperitoneal
- Duodenenal regulation of gastric emptying: Feedback mechanisms monitor the contents being delivered from the stomach
  - High fat content
  - Low pH (high acidity)
  - Hypertonicity (high osmolality)
  - All result in decreased stomach emptying.
- Jejunum: Extends from duodenum to ileum (~2.5 m long)
- Ileum: From jejunum to ileocecal valve (~3.6 m long)
- Jejunum and ileum function in absorption;
  - Intraperitoneal
  - Suspended from mesentery whose veins and lymph vessels carry nutrients away from small intestine.

### Small Intestine Wall

- Cell types:
  - Mostly absorptive cells
  - Goblet (mucous) cells increase in number as the small intestine progresses
  - Enteroendocrine cells
  - T-lymphocytes
- Intestinal crypts with cells that secrete intestinal juice and contain Paneth cells that secrete protective lysozyme (antibacterial)
- Peyer's patches: lymphoid follicle in submucosa
- Brunners glands (duodenum) secrete $HCO_3^-$ rich mucous to increase the pH of chyme
- Villus epithelium is replaced every 3–6 days
- Intestinal Juice: Isotonic with blood plasma, slightly alkaline, low enzyme content.

### Liver and Gallbladder

Liver produces bile (fat emulsifier) that is stored in and concentrated by the gallbladder.

- Largest gland
- Four lobes
- Falciform ligament
  - Mesentery supports liver from diaphragm and anterior body wall
  - Separates right (R) and left (L) lobes
- Round ligament fibrous remnant of umbilical vein
- Blood supply
  - Hepatic artery and hepatic portal vein
- Bile
  - drains from biliary ducts to common hepatic duct which fuses with cystic duct from gallbladder to form the bile duct
- Composition of bile: Alkaline solution: Bile salts, bile pigments, cholesterol, fats and phospholipids
  - Bile salts and phospholipids participate in fat absorption
- Bile salts are conserved by enterohepatic circulation
  - Reabsorbed in the ileum
  - Return to liver in hepatic portal blood
  - Re-secreted by the liver
- Bile pigments and bilirubin break down to urobilin then stercobilin
- Gallbladder = a muscular pouch that stores bile and expels bile when needed via the cystic duct and the bile duct.

### Large Intestine: Gross Anatomy

- Ileocecal valve to anus (~1.5 m)
- Teniae coli: 3 ribbons of longitudinal smooth muscle.

- Haustra: Pocket-like segments of large intestine
- Epiploic appendages: Fat filled pouches of visceral peritoneum
- Cecum: Blind pouch (below ileocecal valve)
- Appendix: Attached to cecum (lymphoid)
- Colon: Ascending, transverse, descending, sigmoid
  - Transverse colon and sigmoid colon are intraperitoneal; anchored by mesentery. The rest of the colon is retroperitoneal
- Rectum
- Anal canal.

### Large Intestine: Microscopic Anatomy

- All 4 layers present
- Mucosa: Simple columnar epithelium until anal canal (stratified squamous)
  - No folds or villi. No significant enzyme secretions
  - Crypts: Invaginations of mucosa contain large numbers of goblet cells that secrete mucous for protection and lubrication
- Bacterial flora
  - Ferment indigestible CHO: Produces about 500 mL of gas per day
  - Synthesize B complex vitamins and most vitamin K
- Propulsion:
  - Haustra contractions: Stretch stimulate haustra to contract moving (and mixing) contents to next haustra
  - Mass peristalsis: Long, slow contractile waves moving contents toward rectum (3–4 per day)
  - Gastrocolic reflex: Food intake causes mass peristalsis.

## URINARY SYSTEM

### Urinary System Components

- Kidneys
- Ureters
- Urinary bladder
- Urethra
- Kidneys
- 1% body weight
- Retroperitoneal, posterior abdominal wall
- Adrenal gland anchored superior.

### Three Layers CT Anchor Kidneys

- *Renal capsule*: Collagen fibers covering organ.
- *Adipose capsule*: Adipose cushion around renal capsule.
- *Renal fascia*: Collagen fibers fused to renal capsule and deep fascia of body wall and peritoneum.

Renal ptosis = floating kidney: Starvation or injury, kidney loose from body wall, could twist blood vessels or ureters

- Hilum: Where renal arteries, renal, veins, ureters enter/exit
- Hilum opens to renal sinus
- Renal sinus lined with renal apsule,contiguous with outside.

### Kidney Has Two Layers

1. *Cortex:* Superficial, contact renal capsule, houses filtration structures (nephrons)
2. *Medulla:* 6–18 renal pyramids, parallel bundles of collection tubules, apex, papilla, points toward renal sinus
   - Kidney divided into sections: renal lobes
   - Renal lobe = renal pyramid + surrounding cortex called renal columns, lobe is complete site of urine production.

### Blood Supply and Innervation to Kidney

- Receives 20–25% cardiac output
- Highly vascularized, many capillaries involved in filtration (nephrons)
- Innervation from renal plexus controlled by ANS
- Most is sympathetic to:
  - Adjust rate of urine formation (change BP and flow at nephron)
  - Stimulate release of renin (restricts water and $Na^+$ loss at nephron).

### *Nephron*

- Smallest functional unit of kidney
- More than 1 million per kidney
- Two major parts:
  1. Renal corpuscle = glomerular capsule + glomerulus
  2. Renal tubule = proximal convoluted tubule (PCT) + nephron loop + distal convoluted tubule (DCT).

Two important capillary beds associated with each nephron:

1. Glomerulus: Filtration
2. Peritubular capillaries: Reclaim filtrate, concentrate urine

Both connected to arterioles only (not for $O_2$ exchange) afferent arteriole capillary efferent arteriole.

### *Two Types of Nephrons*

1. Cortical nephrons: Majority, in cortex, short nephron loops
2. Juxtamedullary nephrons: 15%, at cortex/medulla interface, long nephron loops, important for water conservation and concentrated urine.

### *Renal Corpuscle: Site of Filtration*

Two parts:

1. Glomerular capsule: Thin parietal epithelium, forms capsule around glomerulus
2. Glomerulus: Fenestrated capillaries covered by podocytes = visceral epithelium, intertwine to create filtration slits on surface of capillaries, slits smaller than fenestrations in glomerular capillaries to restrict filtration of large molecules.

### *Renal Tubule*

Reabsorption to process raw filtrate into urine—Three parts:

1. PCT: Simple cuboidal epithelium with microvilli, reabsorbs organic nutrients, ions, water, and small plasma proteins from filtrate exiting glomerular capsule.
2. Nephron loop: Simple squamous epithelium, reabsorbs $Na^+$, $Cl^-$, and $H_2O$ from filtrate, important to regulate volume and solute conc. of urine, has descending and ascending limbs.

3. DCT: Simple cuboidal epithelium, flat surface, has four important functions:
   1. Secretion: Removal of wastes from peritubular capillaries into filtrate
   2. Reabsorb $Na^+$ and $Ca^{2+}$ from filtrate
   3. Optional $H_2O$ reabsorption from filtrate under hormonal control
   4. Contribute to formation of juxtaglomerular apparatus.

### *Juxtaglomerular Apparatus (JGA)*

Consists of two cell types:
1. Endocrine cells of DCT = macula densa
2. Granular cells of afferent arteriole = juxtaglomerular cells
   Together cells monitor blood and produce:
   - Renin: Enzyme, restricts $Na^+$ and $H_2O$ at nephron
   - Erythropoietin: Hormone, stimulates RBC production.

### Collecting System

Collecting ducts + papillary ducts nephrons
1 collecting duct (renal pyramid) many collecting ducts 1 papillary duct
- Final osmotic concentration of filtrate adjusted by collecting duct, after this urine is complete and exits kidney:
  - Papillary duct (renal papilla) minor calyx major calyx renal pelvis ureter

Polycystic kidney disease = genetic, cysts form that cause swelling of kidney tubules, compression reduces function.

### *Urine Transport, Storage and Elimination*

- Urine production and modification: Renal tubules and collecting system
- Once in renal pelvis, urine complete, excreted

via ureters, bladder, urethra.
Nephrolithiasis = blockage of urinary passage, e.g. calculi (kidney stone); crystalized deposits of calcium, magnesium, or uric acid, form in renal pelvis, can become lodged in ureters. Large ones may need disruption by a lithotripter.

### Ureters

Connect renal pelvis to urinary bladder wall layers:
- Mucosa with transitional epithelium
- Muscularis with two layers of smooth muscle
- Adventitia, attaches to posterior body wall
  - Contractions occur every 30 sec to force urine toward bladder.

### Urinary Bladder

- Wall folded into rugae when empty (expands)
- Wall layers:
  - Mucosa with transitional epithelium
  - Muscularis with 3 layers of smooth muscle = detrusor muscle (contraction causes expulsion of urine from bladder)
  - Detrusor muscle thickened around urethral opening to create the internal urethral sphincter (provides involuntary control over release of urine)
- Adventitia, fibrous, anchors bladder to pelvic floor.

### Urethra

- Single tube, connects bladder to environment
- Lined with pseudostratified columnar epithelium
- Passes through band of skeletal muscle that forms external urethral sphincter, under voluntary control, relaxation results in micturition.

### Micturition Reflex

- When bladder contains ~200 mL urine, stretch receptors triggered, signal conscious awareness of pressure and stimulates contraction of detrusor muscle
- Voluntary maintenance of contracted external urethral sphincter prevents urination, detrusor will relax (opening will open internal urethral sphincter allowing urination)
- Continued increase in urinary volume will repeatedly trigger reflex
- If volume exceeds ~500 mL, forced relaxation of internal and external urethral sphincters will result in non-voluntary urination/micturition Incontinence = inability to voluntarily control urine excretion, due to: loss of muscle tone, damage to sphincters, damage to nerves or control centers in brain.

### Age-related Changes

- Decline in functional nephrons
- Reduction in GFR (damage or blood flow)
- Reduced sensitivity to ADH = dilute urine
- Problems with micturition
- Incontinence
- Urinary retention (enlarged prostate).

## CRANIAL NERVES AND THEIR FUNCTIONS

The cranial nerves are the 12 pairs of nerves that leave the brain via their own individual apertures in the skull.

### List of the Cranial Nerves

1. CN I: Olfactory (smell)
2. CN II: Optic (sight)
3. CN III: Oculomotor (moves eyelid and eyeball and adjusts the pupil and lens of the eye)
4. CN IV: Trochlear (moves eyeballs)
5. CN V: Trigeminal (facial muscles incl. chewing; facial sensations)
6. CN VI: Abducens (moves eyeballs)
7. CN VII: Facial (taste, tears, saliva, facial expressions)
8. CN VIII: Vestibulocochlear (auditory)
9. CN IX: Glossopharyngeal (swallowing, saliva, taste)
10. CN X: Vagus (Control of PNS e.g. smooth muscles of GI tract)
11. CN XI: Accessory (moving head and shoulders, swallowing)
12. CN XII: Hypoglossal (tongue muscles-speech and swallowing).

More information about the names, numbers and functions of the 12 cranial nerves is summarized in the following table.

| S. No. | Cranial nerve (number and name) | Function(s) of cranial nerve | |
|---|---|---|---|
| 1 | CN I: Olfactory (sensory) | Smell | |
| 2 | CN II: Optic (sensory) | Vision, also called **eyesight**. (Each optic nerve contains approx a million nerve fibers that receive information from the rod and cone cells of the retina.) | |
| 3 | CN III: Oculomotor (mixed, mainly motor) | Moves the eyeball and eyelid, adjusts the **lens of the eye** for near vision and also constricts the **pupil of the eye** via motor fibers distributed to muscles located in and around the **eye**. | |
| | | **Parasympathetic fibers** adjust the size of the pupil and the shape of the lens of the eye. | **Fibers outside the eye** extend to the upper eyelid and the extrinsic muscles that turn the eyeball in different directions, (incl. the superior rectus, medial rectus, inferior rectus and inferior oblique muscles). |
| 4 | CN IV: Trochlear (mixed, mainly motor) | Moves the eyeballs by sending nerve impulses to the superior oblique muscles which are among the group of muscles that rotate the eyeballs in their sockets. (The action of this nerve is coordinated with those of the oculomotor and abducens nerves, i.e. cranial nerves III and VI.) | |
| 5 | CN V: Trigeminal (mixed) | This is largest cranial nerve and splits into the following three divisions, each of which includes both motor and sensory fibers.<br>1. Ophthalmic nerve<br>2. Maxillary nerve<br>3. Mandibular nerve<br>The motor fibers of all 3 divisions control the **facial muscles** involved in chewing. The sensory fibers convey sensations of touch, pain and temperature from the front of the head including the **mouth** and also from the meninges. | |
| 6 | CN VI: Abducens (mixed, mainly motor) | Moves the eyeballs outwards by sending nerve impulses to the lateral rectus muscles. | |
| 7 | CN VII: Facial (mixed) | Sensory fibers are concerned with taste via the taste buds at the front of the tongue. Motor fibers control secretion of tears via the lacrimal glands and saliva via the sublingual salivary glands as well as facial expressions via some of the **muscles of facial expression**. A branch of the facial nerve regulates the tension on the ear ossicles. | |
| 8 | CN VIII: Vestibulocochlear (mixed, mainly sensory) | Two branches: Vestibular nerve (senses equilibrium) and Cochlear nerve (hearing) | |
| | | **Vestibular nerve:** Aids equilibrium by carrying impulses from the semicircular canals—providing info about posture, movement and balance | **Cochlear nerve:** Carries impulses from the cochlea, so is known as the nerve of hearing |
| 9 | CN IX: Glossopharyngeal (mixed) | **Motor fibers**<br>• Modulate swallowing via supply to muscles of the throat (pharynx) area<br>• Parasympathetic control of secretion of saliva (via supply to the parotid salivary glands) | |
| | | **Sensory fibers**<br>• Monitors **blood pressure**<br>• Monitors levels of oxygen and carbon dioxide in **blood**<br>• Coordination of some muscle activity, e.g. in some swallowing muscles<br>• Sensations of taste, touch, pain and temperature from posterior third of the tongue and tissues of the soft palate | |
| 10 | CN X: Vagus (mixed) | **Motor fibers:**<br>• Under conscious control<br>– Stimulates **voluntary muscles** that affect swallowing, coughing and speech.<br>• Under unconscious control<br>– Stimulates the contraction and relaxation of **smooth muscle** in the gastrointestinal tract (GI, also called the **alimentary canal**)<br>– Can trigger reduction (slowing) of heart-rate<br>– Stimulates secretion of digestive fluids | |
| | | **Sensory fibers:**<br>• Monitors **blood pressure**<br>• Monitors levels of oxygen and carbon dioxide in **blood**<br>• Sensations of touch, pain and temperature from throat area<br>• Sensations from visceral organs in thorax and abdomen | |

*Contd...*

*Contd...*

| S. No. | Cranial nerve (number and name) | Function(s) of cranial nerve | |
|---|---|---|---|
| 11 | CN XI: Accessory (mixed, mainly motor) | Arises from two roots, cranial and spinal. | |
| | | **Cranial parts:** Controls swallowing movements because nerve fibers (from the cranial root of cranial nerve XI) join the vagus nerve to form the recurrent laryngeal nerve which supplies the internal laryngeal muscles. | **Spinal Parts:** Governs movement of the head and shoulders by supplying the **sternocleidomastoid** and **trapezius** muscles in the (anterior and posterior) regions of the neck. |
| 12 | CN XII: Hypoglossal (mixed, mainly motor) | Supplies the muscles of the tongue—responsible for the tongue movements involved in speech and swallowing | |

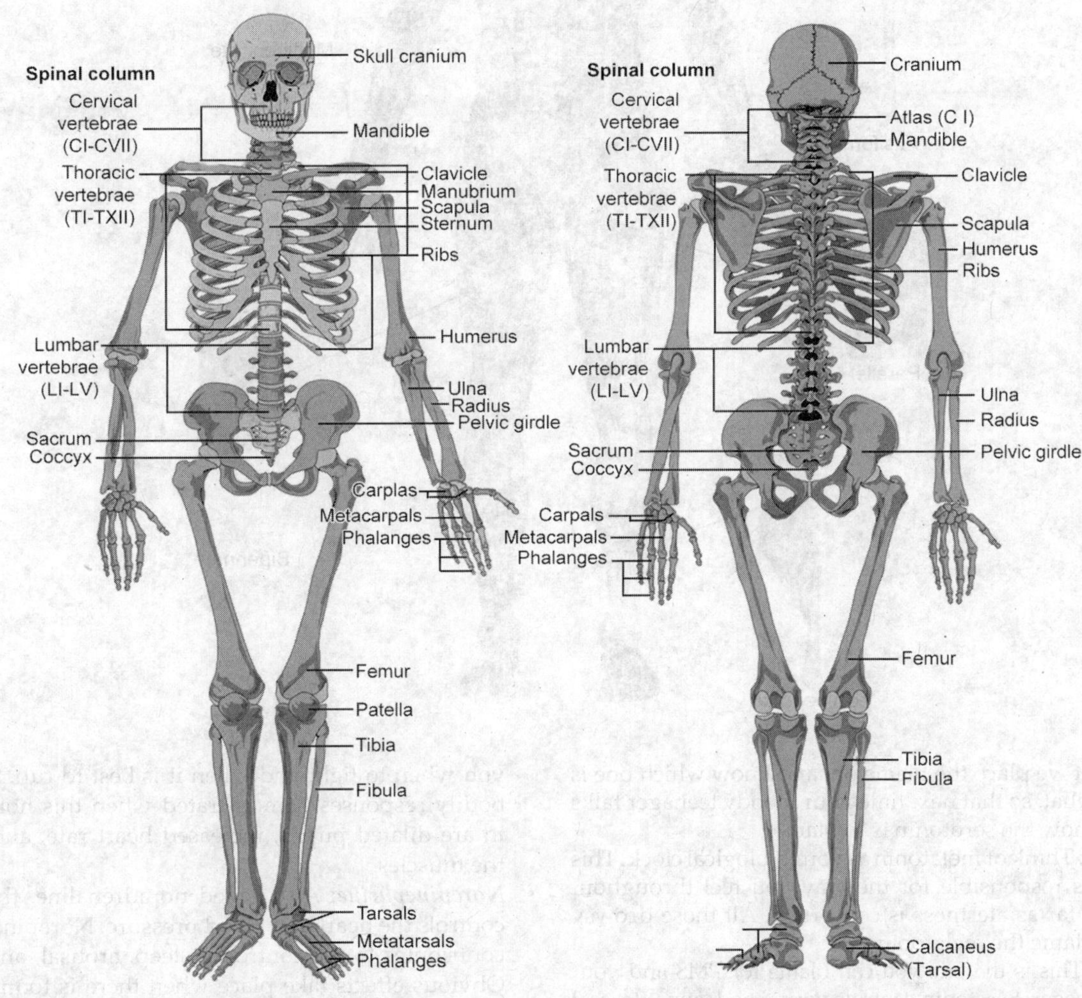


## LIST OF HUMAN HORMONES AND THEIR IMPORTANCE

Hormones; we blame them for an awful lot. When a teenager acts out, 'you know how those hormones are!' When a pregnant woman starts crying at a hot dog commercial, we claim, 'Do not mind her, it is all those hormones.' But how many people actually know what the hormones are that they are referring to? Blaming hormones for all of life's problems has just become a habit instead of something that is really well known.

Some hormones you may have heard of and same may sound like gibberish. The functions of some are relatively easy to understand, while others require a science major. We have assembled a list of some of the more commonly known hormones that are responsible for some of the most major functions of the body. It is about time we got to know the

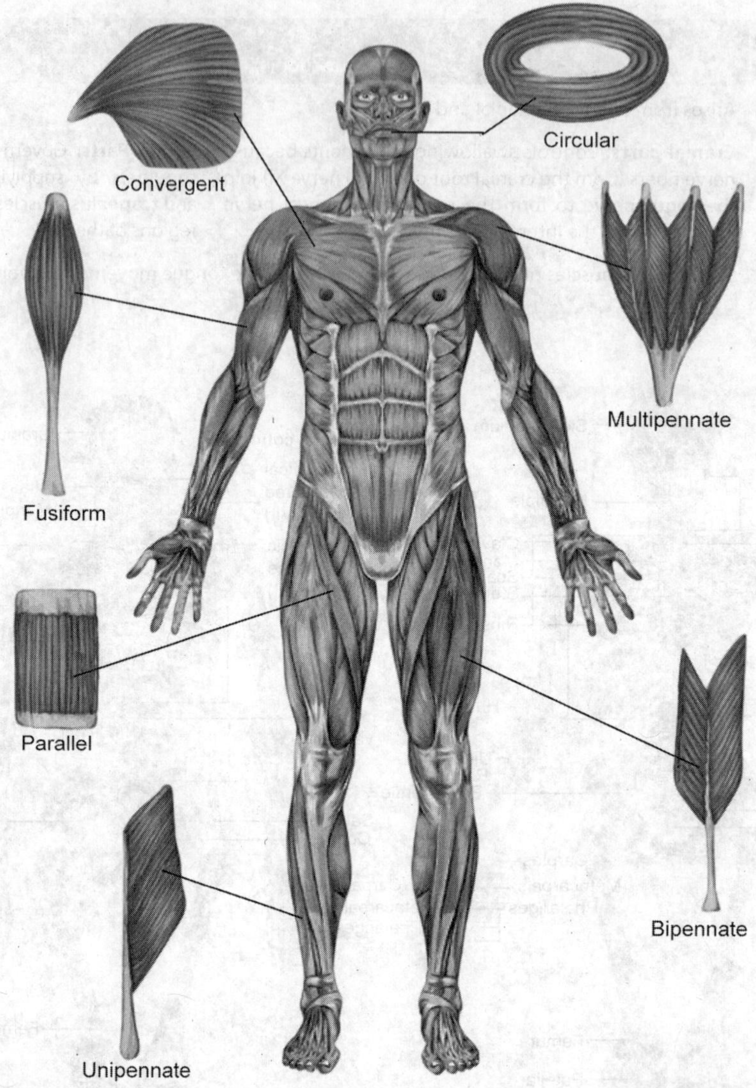


hormones that we place the blame on, and know which one is to blame for what, so that next time your moody teenager talks back, you'll know the serotonin is to blame.

- ***Melatonin***: Think of melatonin as your biological clock. This hormone is responsible for the way you feel throughout the day as far as alertness is concerned. All those drowsy feelings? Blame the melatonin.
- ***Serotonin***: This is the one you can blame for PMS and your moody teenager. Serotonin controls your mood, appetite, and your sleep cycles.
- ***Thyroxin***: A form of thyroid hormone, thyroxin increases the rate of your metabolism and also affects protein synthesis, which is the process that cells go through to build protein.
- ***Epinephrine***: This is one that you have most likely heard of; it is also called adrenaline. Among a whole list of other things, epinephrine is responsible for what is known as the, 'fight or flight' response. This is the hormone that tells you when to fight and when it is best to run. Some of the bodily responses demonstrated when this hormone kicks in are dilated pupils, increased heart rate, and tensing of the muscles.
- ***Norepinephrine***: Also called noradrenaline, this hormone controls the heart and blood pressure. Norepinephrine also contributes to the control of sleep, arousal, and emotions. Obvious effects take place when there is too much or too little of this hormone. Too much gives you an anxious feeling while too little can leave you feeling depressed or sedated.
- ***Dopamine***: This controls the heart rate and also assists in perception; deciphering what is real and what is not.
- ***Antimullerian hormone***: An inhibitor for the release of prolactin, the protein responsible mainly for lactation.
- ***Adiponectin***: This is a protein hormone, it regulates metabolic processes such as the regulation of glucose.

- ***Adrenocorticotropic hormone***: This assists in synthesizing corticosteroids, which are responsible for stress response, blood electrolyte levels, and other physiologic systems.
- ***Angiotensinogen***: Responsible for the narrowing of blood vessels; a process known as vasoconstriction.
- ***Antidiuretic hormone***: This hormone is also known by other names, but it is mainly responsible for retaining water within the kidneys.
- ***Atrial natriuretic peptide***: A peptide hormone secreted by the cells of the heart and other muscles. It is mostly involved with the control of water, sodium, potassium, and fat within the body.
- ***Calcitonin***: Aids in constructing bone and reducing blood calcium.
- ***Cholecystokinin***: Aids in the release of digestive enzymes for the pancreas and acts as an appetite suppressant.
- ***Corticotropin-releasing hormone***: Releases cortisol in response to stress.
- ***Erythropoietin***: Stimulates the production of erythrocytes, which are blood cells responsible for delivering oxygen.
- ***Follicle-stimulating hormone***: Stimulates the follicles within the sex organs of both males and females.
- ***Gastrin***: Secretes gastric acid.
- ***Ghrelin***: Hunger stimulant as well as aiding in the secretion of the growth hormone.
- ***Glucagon***: Helps to increase the blood glucose level.
- ***Growth hormone-releasing hormone***: As its name clearly implies, this hormone releases the growth hormone.
- ***Human chorionic gonadotropin***: Keeps the immune system from attacking a forming embryo during pregnancy.
- ***Growth hormone***: Helps to stimulate growth and the reproduction of cells.
- ***Insulin***: Responsible for several anabolic effects, primarily glucose intake.
- ***Insulin-like growth factor***: Has the same effects as insulin while also regulating the growth and development of cells.
- ***Leptin***: Slows down the appetite while simultaneously speeding up metabolism.
- ***Luteinizing hormone***: Aids ovulation in women and testosterone production in men.
- ***Melanocyte stimulating hormone***: Produce melanocytes, which are responsible for the pigment in skin and hair.
- ***Orexin***: Increases the appetite while also increasing your alertness and energy levels.
- ***Oxytocin***: A hormone that plays a major role in reproduction, it aids in orgasm and is also responsible for the release of breast milk.
- ***Parathyroid hormone***: Among other functions, this hormone is mainly responsible for the activation of Vitamin D.
- ***Prolactin***: A major contributor in sexual satisfaction and the production of breast milk.
- ***Secretin***: Inhibits gastric acid production.
- ***Aldosterone***: Mainly responsible for absorbing sodium in the kidneys to increase the volume of blood within the body.
- ***Testosterone***: The major male hormone, testosterone is responsible for sex drive, development of the sex organs, and the changes that take place during puberty.
- ***Androstenedione***: Essentially estrogen.
- ***Estradiol***: In males, this hormone is responsible for preventing what is basically known as cell death of the germ cells. In females, this hormone is in overdrive. Among other things, estradiol accelerates height and metabolism, maintains the blood vessels and skin, aids in water retention, and even aids in hormone-sensitive cancers.
- ***Progesterone***: A major contributor to the body's support of pregnancy.
- ***Lipotropin***: Stimulates the production of pigment by aiding in melanin production.
- ***Brain natriuretic peptide***: Aids in reducing blood pressure.
- ***Histamine***: A hormone based in the stomach, histamine aids in the secreting of gastric acid.
- ***Endothelin***: Controls muscle contractions within the stomach.
- ***Enkephalin***: Simply a pain regulator.

These are only examples of some of the hormones within the body; there are more complex hormones whose functions are not easily understood. Our bodies (when in proper working order) function like well-oiled machines, and the hormones are a major part of nearly every process. Clearly, hormones are responsible for much more than angry teens, squeaky voices, and weepy pregnant women.

## MULTIPLE CHOICE QUESTIONS

**1. The endocrine part of pancreas consist of:**

(a) Islet of Langerhans
(b) Tubular acne
(c) Columnar cells
(d) Transitional cells

**2. Cirrhosis of liver means:**

(a) Necrosis of liver cells
(b) Inflammation of liver cells
(c) Fibrosis of liver cells
(d) Edema of liver cells

**3. 80% of blood supply to liver is by:**

(a) Hepatic artery
(b) Hepatic vein
(c) Splenic artery
(d) Portal vein

**4. Artery supplying visual area of brain is:**

(a) Posterior cerebral
(b) Middle cerebral
(c) Anterior cerebral
(d) Interior carotid

5. **All the statements are true about coronary arteries EXCEPT:**
(a) Are functionally end arteries
(b) Get filled during systole
(c) Are enlarged Vasa vosa
(d) Are most prone of any arteries to develop atherosclerosis
6. **Paired skull bone are:**
(a) Frontal, parietal (b) Occipital, temporal
(c) Parietal, temporal (d) Sphenoid, ethmoid
7. **Fracture of floor of anterior cranial fossa may cause:**
(a) Discharge of CSF through nose
(b) Black eyes
(c) Bleeding through nose
(d) All of the above
8. **The internal supporting framework of cell is:**
(a) Cytoskeleton (b) Ribosome
(c) Plasma membrane (d) Microfilament
9. **Total number of true ribs in human body are:**
(a) 10 (b) 20
(c) 12 (d) 24
10. **The strongest muscle in human body is:**
(a) Porns major (b) Masseter
(c) Quadratus femoris (d) Biceps brachii
11. **Following are the connective tissue EXCEPT:**
(a) Cartilage (b) Blood
(c) Myocardium (d) White fibrous tissue
12. **The only bone in human body that does not articulate with any other bone:**
(a) Patella (b) Coccyx
(c) Hyoid (d) Stapes
13. **Total pair of spinal nerves are:**
(a) 28 (b) 30
(c) 31 (d) 32
14. **Central nervous system consist of:**
(a) Brain, spinal cord and afferent nerves
(b) Brain and spinal cord
(c) Brain, spinal cord and efferent nerves
(d) Cerebrum, cerebellum and medulla
15. **Bone containing large air spaces lined by epithelium is:**
(a) Long bone (b) Irregular bone
(c) Pneumatic bones (d) Sesamoid bones
16. **Elastic cartilage is present in:**
(a) Trachea (b) Bronchus
(c) Epiglottis (d) Intervertebral disc
17. **Nerve supply of biceps brachial muscle is:**
(a) Musculocutaneous nerve
(b) Radial nerve
(c) Ulnar nerve
(d) Median nerve
18. **Artey used for measuring of blood pressure is:**
(a) Brachial artery
(b) Radial artery
(c) Ulnar nerve
(d) Median nerve
19. **Extension of knee joint is brought about by:**
(a) Quadriceps femoris (b) Hamstring
(c) Gluteus maximus (d) Popliteus
20. **Foot drop is due to injury to:**
(a) Femoral nerve
(b) Obturator nerve
(c) Deep peroneal nerve
(d) Tibial nerve
21. **Right lung contains:**
(a) Eight bronchopulmonary segments
(b) Nine bronchopulmonary segments
(c) Ten bronchopulmonary segments
(d) None of the above
22. **Sternal puncture is done through:**
(a) Upper part of sternal body
(b) Lower half of manubrium
(c) Upper half of manubrium
(d) None of the above
23. **Bile duct opens into the following part of duodenum:**
(a) Superior (b) Descending
(c) Horizontal (d) Ascending
24. **Right testicular vein open into:**
(a) Inferior vena cava (b) Right renal vein
(c) Left renal vein (d) None of the above
25. **Following are the muscle of mastication EXCEPT:**
(a) Massester
(b) Temporalis
(c) Buccinator
(d) Lateral and medial pterygoid
26. **Following air sinuses open into the middle meatus of the nose EXCEPT:**
(a) Frontal (b) Maxillary
(c) Anterior ethmoidal (d) Posterior ethmoidal
27. **Occipital lobe of cerebrum contains:**
(a) Somatomotor area (b) Somatosensory area
(c) Visual area (d) Auditory area
28. **Usually lumbar puncture is done by inserting LP needle between:**
(a) 12th thoracic and 1st lumbar vertebra
(b) 1st and 2nd lumbar vertebra
(c) 3rd and 4th lumbar vertebra
(d) 1st and 2nd sacral vertebra
29. **Superior radio lunar joint is a _____ joint.**
(a) Ball and socket (b) Pivot
(c) Condylar joint (d) Fibrous
30. **Injury to the radial nerve in arm causes:**
(a) Claw hand
(b) Erbs paralysis
(c) Wrist drop
(d) Apr thumb deformity
31. **Anterior part of interventricular septum is supplied by the branch of ____________ artery.**
(a) Right coronary
(b) Left coronary
(c) Circumflex
(d) Right marginal

32. **Inferior vena caval opening in the diaphragm is at the level of ________ vertebra.**
(a) T8 (b) T9
(c) T10 (d) T11

33. **Most dangerous position of appendix is ___.**
(a) Pelvic (b) Splenic
(c) Paracolic (d) Promontoric

34. **Deep inguinal ring is an apparent opening in:**
(a) Fascia transversalis (b) Peritoneum
(c) Internal oblique (d) External oblique

35. **Injury to the common peroneal nerve at the level of neck devils will cause:**
(a) Foot drop
(b) Inability to evert foot
(c) Sensory loss over anterior and lateral aspect of leg and foot
(d) All the above

36. **All are true about sesamoid bone except:**
(a) Developed after birth
(b) Develop in tendons
(c) Periosteum is present
(d) After the pull of muscle

37. **Intramuscular injection in the gluteal regions are given in the________ quadrant.**
(a) Superio medial (b) Superio lateral
(c) Inferio medial (d) Inferio lateral

38. **Hairpin bend are associated with ________ artery.**
(a) Nutrient (b) Periosteal
(c) Epiphyseal (d) Metaphyseal

39. **Blood supply to superio lateral surface of cerebral hemisphere is largely given by ________ artery.**
(a) Anterior cerebral (b) Middle cerebral
(c) Posterior cerebral (d) Anterior choroidal

40. **Age of closure of anterior fontanelle is:**
(a) One month (b) Six months
(c) One year (d) One and half year

41. **Taste of sensation from anterior 2/3 of the tongue is carried by ________ nerve.**
(a) Glossopharyngeal (b) Hypoglossal
(c) Chorda tympani (d) Vagus

42. **Axillary artery is continuation of:**
(a) Brachiocephalic artery
(b) Subclevian artery
(c) Common carotid artery
(d) Aorta

43. **The safe site for giving intranet muscular injection in gluteal region is:**
(a) Upper and inner quadrant
(b) Lower and inner quadrant
(c) Upper and outer quadrant
(d) Lower and outer quadrant

44. **Metacarpal bones are examples of:**
(a) Short bones (b) Irregular bones
(c) Miniature bone (d) Supernumerary bone

45. **The cells lacking nucleus are:**
(a) Mast cells (b) Erythrocytes
(c) Neurons (d) Muscle cells

46. **The member of hematopoietic-lymphoid system is:**
(a) Spleen (b) Adrenal medulla
(c) Kidney (d) Pancreas

47. **The part of male reproductive system, ligated in family planning operation is:**
(a) Testis (b) Prostate
(c) Vas deferens (d) Epididymis

48. **Bile is synthesized in:**
(a) Gallbladder (b) Liver
(c) Bile duct (d) Duodenum

49. **The vein carrying oxygenated blood is:**
(a) Portal vein (b) Renal vein
(c) Great cerebral vein (d) Pulmonary vein

50. **The taste sensation from posterior 1/3rd of tongue are carried by:**
(a) Hypoglossal nerve
(b) Facial nerve
(c) Vagus nerve
(d) Glossopharyngeal nerve

51. **A muscle of leg which is called peripheral heart:**
(a) Poplitial (b) Soleus
(c) Tibialis posterior (d) Gastrocnemius

52. **The safety muscle of the tongue is:**
(a) Genioglossus (b) Hyoglossus
(c) Styloglossus (d) Palatoglossus

53. **The part of lung where exchange of gases takes place is:**
(a) Bronchus (b) Alveoli
(c) Bronchioles (d) Stromal

54. **The insuline is secreted by:**
(a) Pituitary gland (b) Pancreas
(c) Liver (d) Stomach

55. **The fovea on the head of femur gives attachment to:**
(a) Gluteus medius
(b) Iliofemoral ligament
(c) Round ligament
(d) Pubofemoral ligament

56. **An example of compound synovial joint is:**
(a) Shoulder joint (b) Knee joint
(c) Hip joint (d) Interphalangeal joint

57. **All are unpaired cartilages of larynx EXCEPT:**
(a) Thyroid (b) Cricoid
(c) Epiglottis (d) Arytenoid

58. **Cerebrospinal fluid is formed by:**
(a) Arachnoid villi
(b) Arachnoid granulation
(c) Choroid plexus
(d) Cisterna magna

59. **An example of end artery is:**
(a) Femoral artery (b) Coronary artery
(c) Brachial artery (d) Carotid artery

**60. Cervical vertebrae adequate recognised by the presence of:**
(a) Foramen transversarium
(b) Foramen ovals
(c) Foramen magnum
(d) Vertebral foramen

**61. All are the branches of facial artery EXCEPT:**
(a) Submental (b) Superior labial
(c) Transverse facials (d) Lateral nasal

**62. The receptors for hearing are located in:**
(a) Utricle
(b) Saccule
(c) Ampulla of semicircular canals
(d) Spiral organ of Corti

**63. The only long bone lying horizontally is:**
(a) Rib (b) Clavicle
(c) Pelvis (d) Radius

**64. The inner visual layer of serous pericardium is called:**
(a) Endocardium (b) Epicardium
(c) Myocardium (d) Mediastinum

**65. The muscle of the back of the thigh is called:**
(a) Gluteal muscle (b) Popliteal muscle
(c) Hamstring muscle (d) Quadriceps muscle

**66. The total genetic information in a cell is carried by its:**
(a) Mitochondria (b) Ribosome
(c) Chromosome (d) Golgi complex

**67. The arterial supply to retina is by:**
(a) Cilliary artery (b) Central artery
(c) Opthlamic artey (d) Fascial artery

**68. The content of femoral canal is:**
(a) Femoral artery (b) Femoral nerve
(c) Femoral vein (d) Femoral lymph node

**69. All are intracapsular structure of knee joint except:**
(a) Cruciate ligament
(b) Coronary ligament
(c) Meniscofemoral ligament
(d) Tibial collateral ligament

**70. Wrist drop is a result of injury to ______ nerve.**
(a) Median nerve (b) Radial nerve
(c) Ulnar nerve (d) Musculocutaneous nerve

**71. Lymphatic from the testis drain into:**
(a) Internal iliac node
(b) Superficial inguinal node
(c) External iliac node
(d) Para-aortic node

**72. All are site of portacaval anastomosis EXCEPT:**
(a) Lower end of esophagus
(b) Ileocecal junction
(c) Posterior abdominal wall
(d) Base area of liver

**73. Right border of the heart is formed by:**
(a) Right atrium
(b) Right ventricle
(c) Right atrium and right ventricle
(d) Superior vena cava

**74. Sensory supply to face is predominantly by branches of:**
(a) Oculomotor nerve (b) Facial nerve
(c) Trigeminal nerve (d) Accessory nerve

**75. Tongue is supplied by all EXCEPT:**
(a) Lingual (b) Cords tympani
(c) Glossopharyngeal (d) Hypoglossal

**76. Retraction of the protruded mandible is done by:**
(a) Medial pterygoid (b) Lateral pterygoid
(c) Masseter (d) Temporalis

**77. Facial artery is a branch of:**
(a) Common carotid artery
(b) Internal carotid artery
(c) External carotid artery
(d) Subclavian artery

**78. The life span of an RBC is:**
(a) 100 days (b) 120 days
(c) 180 days (d) 80 days

**79. Hypothyroidism in infants leads to:**
(a) Addison's disease (b) Myxedema
(c) Cretinism (d) Thyrotoxicosis

**80. The bond of protein structure that is not broken in denaturation is:**
(a) Hydrogen (b) Peptide
(c) Ionic (d) Disulfide

**81. Sphingomyelins are:**
(a) Essential fatty acids (b) Simple lipids
(c) Compound lipids (d) Derived lipids

**82. Hormone secretion increase:**
(a) Gastric secretion (b) Salivary secretion
(c) Pancreatic secretion (d) Intestinal secretion

**83. Control of motor movement and coordination is due to:**
(a) Vestibular organ (b) Cerebellum
(c) Limbic system (d) Hypothalamus

**84. Correction of hypermetropia is done by prescribing:**
(a) Concave lenses (b) Cylindrical lenses
(c) Convex lenses (d) Planoconcave lenses

**85. Approximate tidal volume is:**
(a) 150 mL (b) 750 mL
(c) 500 mL (d) 1000 mL

**86. Diabetes mellitus is caused by:**
(a) Less secretion of insulin
(b) Excess of glucose intake
(c) Excess of insulin
(d) Excess of protein intake

**87. Functional unit of kidney:**
(a) Sinusoid (b) Pelvis
(c) Glomerulus (d) Calyces

**88. Normal serum bilirubin concentration is:**
(a) 0.2 to 1.0 mg% (b) 2.0 to 3.0 mg%
(c) 1.0 to 2.0 mg % (d) None of the above

**89. Increase in RBC count is known as:**
(a) Anemia (b) Leukemia
(c) Polycythemia (d) Thrombocytopenia

**90. Decrease in platelet count is known as:**
(a) Leucopenia (b) Polycythemia
(c) Anemia (d) Thrombocytopenia

**91. Which vitamin is required for clotting mechanism?**
(a) Vitamin K (b) Vitamin A
(c) Vitamin B (d) Intrinsic factors

**92. Decrease in WBC county is known as:**
(a) Leukemia (b) Leukocytosis
(c) Leucopenia (d) All the above

**93. 4 kcal of energy is liberated after oxidation EXCEPT for:**
(a) Carbohydrates (b) Fats
(c) Protein (d) Glycogen

**94. Following are the pneumatic bones EXCEPT:**
(a) Maxilla (b) Mandible
(c) Frontal (d) Sphenoid

**95. Following vein open into right atrium EXCEPT:**
(a) Superior vena cava (SVC)
(b) Coronary sinus
(c) Inferior vena cava (IVC)
(d) Great cardiac vein

**96. Fertilization of ovum occur in the ___ of fallopian tube.**
(a) Infundibulum (b) Ampulla
(c) Isthmus (d) Intramural part

**97. Hypoglossal nerve supplies all the following muscle EXCEPT:**
(a) Genioglossus (b) Hypoglossus
(b) Palatoglossus (d) Styloglossus

**98. Medial plane divides body into:**
(a) Anterior and posterior plane
(b) Right and left equally
(c) Superior and inferior halves
(d) Also called transverse plane

**99. Mental foramen is an opening in:**
(a) Frontal bone (b) Maxilla
(c) Zygomatic (d) Mandible

**100. Deltoid muscle:**
(a) Insert on deltoid tuberosity of humerus
(b) Initiate abduction
(c) Innervated by musculocutaneous nerve
(d) Forms border of qudrangular space

**101. The femoral canal:**
(a) The medial most compartment of femoral sheet
(b) Contains femoral canal
(c) Is wider in male than female
(d) Has inferior epigastric vessel

**102. Medial longitudinal arch of foot is formed by all EXCEPT:**
(a) Calcaneus (b) Cuboid
(c) Talus (d) Navicular

**103. Head of pancreas is closely related to:**
(a) Second part of duodenum
(b) Left lobe of liver
(c) Spleen
(d) Ascending colon

**104. One of the following is not a carpel bone:**
(a) Capitate (b) Cuboid
(c) Lunate (d) Hamate

**105. Foramen magnum is opening in:**
(a) Parietal bone (b) Sphenoid bone
(c) Occipital bone (d) Temporal bone

**106. Content of carotid sheet are all EXCEPT:**
(a) Internal jugular vein
(b) Common carotid artery
(c) Sympathetic trunk
(d) Vagus nerve

**107. Portal vein is formed by union of:**
(a) Superior mesentric and splenic vein
(b) Splenic vein and inferior vena cava
(c) Superior mesentric and inferior venal cava
(d) Infertvena cava n hepatic vein

**108. Vertebra is ___ type of bone.**
(a) Short (b) Flat
(c) Sesamoid (d) Irregular

**109. The muscle that unlocks the knee joint is:**
(a) Popliteus
(b) Gastrocnemius
(c) Quadriceps femoris
(d) Plantaris

**110. Coronary arteries are the branches of:**
(a) Ascending aorta
(b) Left pulmonary artery
(c) Right pulmonary artery
(d) Brachiocephalic trunk

**111. Transitional epithelium lines the following organ:**
(a) Skin
(b) Jejunum
(c) Second part of duodenum
(d) Urinary bladder

**112. Auditory tube opens into:**
(a) Nasopharynx (b) Nasal cavity
(c) Oral cavity (d) Larynx

**113. Deltoid muscle is supplied by:**
(a) Musculocutaneous nerve
(b) Axillary nerve
(c) Radial nerve
(d) Supracapsular nerve

**114. Covering of the bone is called:**
(a) Perichondrium
(b) Periosteum
(c) Endosteum
(d) Endocardium

**115. Nerve supply of biceps brachii is:**
(a) Radial
(b) Median
(c) Musculocutaneous
(d) Axillary

**116. Winging of scapula is due to paralysis of:**
(a) Serratus anterior (b) Latissimus dorsi
(c) Pectoralis major (d) Deltoid

**117. Nerve supply of gluteus maximus:**
(a) Superior gluteal (b) Inferior gluteal
(c) Femoral (d) Obturator

**118. Floating rib is:**
(a) 7th (b) 8th
(c) 9th (d) 12th

**119. Left lung consist of:**
(a) 2 lobes (b) 3 lobes
(c) 4 lobes (d) 5 lobes

**120. Apex of the heart is formed by:**
(a) Right atrium (b) Left atrium
(c) Right ventricle (d) Left ventricle

**121. Humerus is which type of bone:**
(a) Long (b) Irregular
(c) Short (d) Sesamoid

**122. Nerve related to surgical neck of humerus is:**
(a) Radial (b) Musculocutaneous
(c) Median (d) Axillary

**123. Lining epithelium of the skin is:**
(a) Startified squamous epithelium
(b) Simple squamous epithelium
(c) Transitional epithelium
(d) Simple cuboidal epithelium

**124. Following is an example of elastic cartilage:**
(a) Pinna of the ear
(b) Intervertebral disc
(c) Menisci of knee joint
(d) Articular disc of temporomandibular joint

**125. Following are the features of interior of right atrium EXCEPT:**
(a) Sulcus terminalis
(b) Fossa ovalis
(c) Opening of coronary sinus
(d) Moderator band

**126. Scapula is a ______ type of bone.**
(a) Sesamoid (b) Flat
(c) Irregular (d) Long

**127. One of the following artery is used for measuring BP:**
(a) Ulnar (b) Axillary
(c) Subclavian (d) Brachial

**128. Hip joint is following type of joint:**
(a) Condylar (b) Ball and socket
(c) Plane (d) Saddle

**129. Following opening are present in the right atrium EXCEPT:**
(a) Superior vena cava (SVC)
(b) Inferior vena cava (IVC)
(c) Coronary sinus
(d) Pulmonary trunk

**130. Ulnar nerve is a branch of:**
(a) Medial cord of brachial plexus
(b) Lateral cord of brachial plexus
(c) Posterior cord of brachial plexus
(d) Lower trunk of brachial plexus

**131. How many lumbar vertebrae are present in vertebral column?**
(a) 5 (b) 7
(c) 10 (d) 12

**132. The serious membrane lining the thoracic cavity is called:**
(a) Pericardium (b) Pleura
(c) Synovial membrane (d) Peritoneum

**133. Which of the following is a part of large intestine?**
(a) Jejunum (b) Ileum
(c) Duodenum (d) Cecum

**134. Pulmonary vein open into which chamber of heart:**
(a) Left atrium (b) Left ventricle
(c) Right atrium (d) Right ventricle

**135. Movement towards midline of the body is called as:**
(a) Flexion (b) Abduction
(c) Extension (d) Addiction

**136. Which cavity is present within the cerebral hemispheres?**
(a) Third ventricle (b) Fourth ventricle
(c) Lateral ventricle (d) Cerebral aqueduct

**137. Which of the following is a long bone?**
(a) Vertebrae (b) Metacarpals
(c) Tibia (d) Frontal

**138. The central tendon of respiratory diaphragm is associated with heart:**
(a) Inferiorly (b) Anteriorly
(c) Posteriorly (d) Laterally

**139. Which of the following is not a part of brainstem:**
(a) Midbrain (b) Pond
(c) Medulla oblongata (d) Cerebellum

**140. The length of adult esophagus (in cm) is about:**
(a) 25 (b) 26
(c) 27 (d) 29

**141. Posterior boundary of cranial cavity is formed by which bone?**
(a) Temporal (b) Occipital
(c) Frontal (d) Parietal

**142. Spinal cord extends from foramen magnum to lower border of vertebra:**
(a) T11 (b) T12
(c) L1 (d) L3

**143. All are the layers of scalp EXCEPT:**
(a) Skin and convective tissue
(b) Endosteal layer of dura mater
(c) Aponeurosis
(d) Loose areolar tissue

**144. Superior radio-ulnar joint is ________ variety of joint.**
(a) Ball and socket (b) Condylar
(c) Pivot (d) Fibrous

**145. All the following veins drain into coronary sinus EXCEPT:**
(a) Great cardiac vein (b) Small cardiac vein
(c) Middle cardiac vein (d) Anterior cardiac vein

**146. Left Suprarenal vein drains into:**
(a) Inferior vena cava (b) Left testicular vein.
(c) Left renal vein (d) Splenic vein

**147. All the muscles are abductors of eyeball EXCEPT:**
(a) Medial rectus (b) Superior rectus
(c) Inferior oblique (d) Inferior rectus

**148. Septomarginal band is found in:**
(a) Right atrium (b) Right ventricle
(c) Left atrium (d) Left ventricle

**149. Stomach bed includes all EXCEPT:**
(a) Spleen (b) Pancreas
(c) Splenic artery (d) Right kidney

**150. All of the following are projection fibers EXCEPT:**
(a) Corona radiata (b) Pyramidal tract
(c) External capsule (d) Internal capsule

**151. Following is the fixed part of urinary bladder:**
(a) Base (b) Apex
(c) Neck (d) None of the above

**152. Thyroid gland produces:**
(a) T3 (b) T4
(c) Calcitonin (d) All the above

**153. All of the following are nuclei of cerebellum EXCEPT:**
(a) Dentate (b) Emboliform
(c) Olivary (d) Fastigial

**154. Pisiform is an example of:**
(a) Short bone (b) Irregular bone
(c) Sesamoid bone (d) Flat bone

**155. Apex beat of heart is felt in:**
(a) 3rd Intercostal space
(b) 4th Intercostal space
(c) 5th Intercostal space
(d) 6th Intercostal space

**156. Hilum of the right lung show:**
(a) Two bronchus (b) One bronchial
(c) One vein (d) Two arteries

## ANSWERS

| | | | | | | | | | | | | | | | |
|---|---|---|---|---|---|---|---|---|---|---|---|---|---|---|---|
| **1.** | (a) | **21.** | (c) | **41.** | (c) | **61.** | (c) | **81.** | (c) | **101.** | (a) | **121.** | (a) | **141.** | (b) |
| **2.** | (c) | **22.** | (a) | **42.** | (a) | **62.** | (d) | **82.** | (b) | **102.** | (b) | **122.** | (d) | **142.** | (c) |
| **3.** | (d) | **23.** | (b) | **43.** | (c) | **63.** | (b) | **83.** | (a) | **103.** | (a) | **123.** | (a) | **143.** | (b) |
| **4.** | (d) | **24.** | (a) | **44.** | (a) | **64.** | (b) | **84.** | (c) | **104.** | (b) | **124.** | (a) | **144.** | (c) |
| **5.** | (d) | **25.** | (c) | **45.** | (b) | **65.** | (c) | **85.** | (c) | **105.** | (c) | **125.** | (a) | **145.** | (d) |
| **6.** | (c) | **26.** | (c) | **46.** | (a) | **66.** | (c) | **86.** | (a) | **106.** | (c) | **126.** | (b) | **146.** | (a) |
| **7.** | (a) | **27.** | (c) | **47.** | (c) | **67.** | (c) | **87.** | (c) | **107.** | (c) | **127.** | (d) | **147.** | (a) |
| **8.** | (a) | **28.** | (c) | **48.** | (b) | **68.** | (d) | **88.** | (a) | **108.** | (d) | **128.** | (b) | **148.** | (b) |
| **9.** | (d) | **29.** | (b) | **49.** | (d) | **69.** | (d) | **89.** | (c) | **109.** | (a) | **129.** | (d) | **149.** | (d) |
| **10.** | (b) | **30.** | (c) | **50.** | (d) | **70.** | (b) | **90.** | (d) | **110.** | (a) | **130.** | (a) | **150.** | (c) |
| **11.** | (c) | **31.** | (b) | **51.** | (c) | **71.** | (d) | **91.** | (a) | **111.** | (d) | **131.** | (d) | **151.** | (c) |
| **12.** | (c) | **32.** | (a) | **52.** | (a) | **72.** | (b) | **92.** | (c) | **112.** | (a) | **132.** | (b) | **152.** | (d) |
| **13.** | (c) | **33.** | (b) | **53.** | (b) | **73.** | (c) | **93.** | (b) | **113.** | (b) | **133.** | (d) | **153.** | (c) |
| **14.** | (b) | **34.** | (a) | **54.** | (b) | **74.** | (c) | **94.** | (b) | **114.** | (b) | **134.** | (a) | **154.** | (c) |
| **15.** | (c) | **35.** | (a) | **55.** | (c) | **75.** | (a) | **95.** | (b) | **115.** | (c) | **135.** | (d) | **155.** | (c) |
| **16.** | (c) | **36.** | (c) | **56.** | (b) | **76.** | (c) | **96.** | (b) | **116.** | (a) | **136.** | (b) | **156.** | (c) |
| **17.** | (a) | **37.** | (b) | **57.** | (d) | **77.** | (c) | **97.** | (b) | **117.** | (b) | **137.** | (c) | | |
| **18.** | (a) | **38.** | (b) | **58.** | (c) | **78.** | (b) | **98.** | (b) | **118.** | (d) | **138.** | (a) | | |
| **19.** | (a) | **39.** | (a) | **59.** | (b) | **79.** | (a) | **99.** | (d) | **119.** | (a) | **139.** | (d) | | |
| **20.** | (b) | **40.** | (d) | **60.** | (a) | **80.** | (b) | **100.** | (d) | **120.** | (d) | **140.** | (a) | | |

# QUICK REVIEW

## Human Physiology Review and Multiple Choice Questions

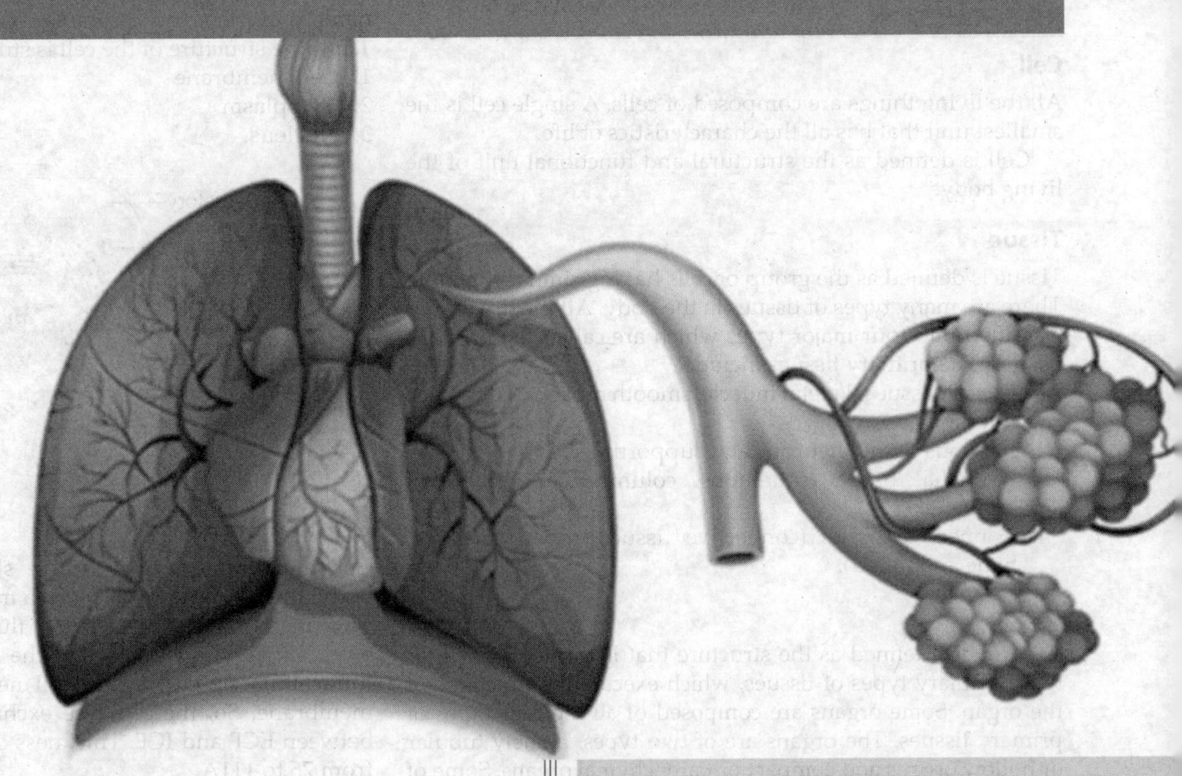

### HIGHLIGHTS

- Introduction
- Structure of the Cell
- Blood
- Digestive System
- Renal Physiology
- Cardiovascular System
- Respiratory System
- Multiple Choice Questions

# Physiology

## INTRODUCTION

### Cell

All the living things are composed of cells. A single cell is the smallest unit that has all the characteristics of life.

Cell is defined as the structural and functional unit of the living body.

### Tissue

Tissue is defined as the group of cells having similar function. There are many types of tissues in the body. All the tissues are classified into four major types which are called the primary tissues. The primary tissues include:

1. Muscle tissue (skeletal muscle, smooth muscle and cardiac muscle)
2. Nervous tissue (neurons and supporting cells)
3. Epithelial tissue (squamous, columnar and cuboidal epithelial cells)
4. Connective tissue (connective tissue proper, cartilage, bone and blood).

### Organ

An organ is defined as the structure that is formed by two or more primary types of tissues, which execute the functions of the organ. Some organs are composed of all the four types of primary tissues. The organs are of two types, namely tubular or hollow organs and compact or parenchymal organs. Some of the organs in the body are brain, heart, lungs, stomach, intestine, liver, gallbladder, pancreas, kidneys, endocrine glands, etc.

### System

The organ system is defined as group of organs that work together to carry out specific functions of the body.

Each system performs a specific function. Digestive system is concerned with digestion of food particles. Excretory system eliminates unwanted substances. Cardiovascular system is responsible for transport of substances between the organs. Respiratory system is concerned with the supply of oxygen and removal of carbon dioxide. Reproductive system is involved in the reproduction of species. Endocrine system is concerned with growth of the body and regulation and maintenance of normal life. Musculoskeletal system is responsible for stability and movements of the body. Nervous system controls the locomotion and other activities including the intellectual functions.

## STRUCTURE OF THE CELL

Each cell is formed by a cell body and a membrane covering the cell body called the cell membrane. Cell body has two parts, namely nucleus and cytoplasm surrounding the nucleus. Thus, the structure of the cell is studied under three headings:

1. Cell membrane
2. Cytoplasm
3. Nucleus.

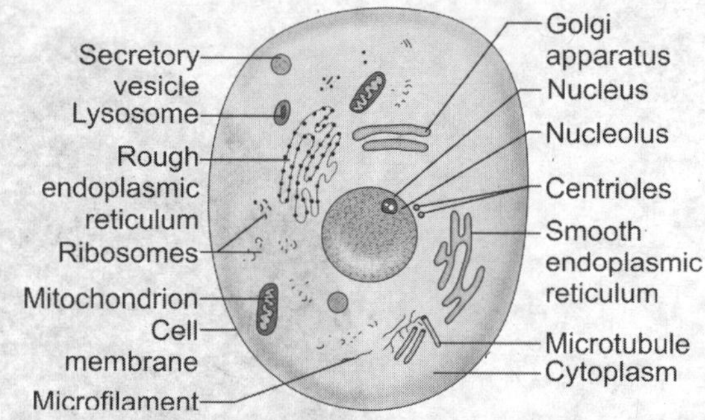


### Cell Membrane

Cell membrane is a protective sheath, enveloping the cell body. It is also known as plasma membrane or plasmalemma. This membrane separates the fluid outside the cell called extracellular fluid (ECF) and the fluid inside the cell called intracellular fluid (ICF). The cell membrane is a semipermeable membrane. So, there is free exchange of certain substances between ECF and ICF. Thickness of the cell membrane varies from 75 to 111Å.

#### *Composition of Cell Membrane*

Cell membrane is composed of three types of substances:

1. Proteins (55%)
2. Lipids (40%)
3. Carbohydrates (5%).

#### *Structural Model of the Cell Membrane*

*Fluid Mosaic Model*

In 1972, SJ Singer and GL Nicholson proposed 'The fluid mosaic model'. According to them, the membrane is a fluid with mosaic of proteins (mosaic means pattern formed by arrangement of different colored pieces of stone, tile, glass or other such materials). This model is accepted by the scientists till now. In this model, the proteins are found to float in the lipid layer instead of forming the layers of the sandwich-type model.

#### *Functions of Cell Membrane*

1. ***Protective function:*** Cell membrane protects the cytoplasm and the organelles present in the cytoplasm.

2. ***Selective permeability:*** Cell membrane acts as a semipermeable membrane, which allows only some substances to pass through it and acts as a barrier for other substances.
3. ***Absorptive function:*** Nutrients are absorbed into the cell through the cell membrane.
4. ***Excretory function:*** Metabolites and other waste products from the cell are excreted out through the cell membrane.
5. ***Exchange of gases:*** Oxygen enters the cell from the blood and carbon dioxide leaves the cell and enters the blood through the cell membrane.
6. ***Maintenance of shape and size of the cell:*** Cell membrane is responsible for the maintenance of shape and size of the cell.

## Cytoplasm

Cytoplasm of the cell is the jellylike material formed by 80% of water. It contains a clear liquid portion called cytosol and various particles of different shape and size. These particles are proteins, carbohydrates, lipids or electrolytes in nature. Cytoplasm also contains many organelles with distinct structure and function.

## *Organelles in Cytoplasm*

Cytoplasmic organelles are the cellular structures embedded in the cytoplasm. Organelles are considered as small organs of the cell. Some organelles are bound by limiting membrane and others do not have limiting membrane. Each organelle is having a definite structure and specific functions.

### *Endoplasmic Reticulum*

Endoplasmic reticulum is a network of tubular and microsomal vesicular structures which are interconnected with one another. The diameter of the lumen is about 400 to 700Å. The endoplasmic reticulum forms the link. The endoplasmic reticulum forms the link.

*Types of Endoplasmic Reticulum*

Endoplasmic reticulum is of two types, namely rough endoplasmic reticulum and smooth endoplasmic reticulum.

Both the types are interconnected and continuous with one another.

Rough Endoplasmic Reticulum

It is the endoplasmic reticulum with rough, bumpy or bead-like appearance. Rough appearance is due to the attachment of granular ribosomes to its outer surface. Hence, it is also called the granular endoplasmic

Smooth Endoplasmic Reticulum

It is the endoplasmic reticulum with smooth appearance. It is also called agranular reticulum. It is formed by many interconnected tubules. So, it is also called tubular endoplasmic reticulum.

Functions of Rough Endoplasmic Reticulum

1. Synthesis of proteins
2. Degradation of worn-out organelles

Functions of Smooth Endoplasmic Reticulum

- Synthesis of non-protein substance
- Role in cellular metabolism
- Storage and metabolism of calcium
- Catabolism and detoxification.

### *Golgi Apparatus*

Golgi apparatus or Golgi body or Golgi complex is a membrane-bound organelle, involved in the processing of proteins. It is present in all the cells except red blood cells.

*Functions of Golgi Apparatus*

Major functions of Golgi apparatus are processing, packing, labeling and delivery of proteins and other molecules like lipids to different parts of the cell.

### *Lysosomes*

Lysosomes are the membrane-bound vesicular organelles found throughout the cytoplasm. The lysosomes are formed by Golgi apparatus. The enzymes synthesized in rough endoplasmic reticulum are processed and packed in the form of small vesicles in the Golgi apparatus. Then, these vesicles are pinched off from Golgi apparatus and become the lysosomes.

*Types of Lysosomes*

Lysosomes are of two types:
1. Primary lysosome, which is pinched off from Golgi apparatus. It is inactive in spite of having hydrolytic enzymes
2. Secondary lysosome, which is the active lysosome. It is formed by the fusion of a primary lysosome with phagosome or endosome.

*Functions of Lysosomes*

Lysosomes are often called 'garbage system' of the cell because of their degradation activity. About 50 different hydrolytic enzymes, known as acid hydroxylases are present in the lysosomes, through which lysosomes execute their functions.

*Important Lysosomal Enzymes*

- Proteases, which hydrolyze the proteins into amino acids
- Lipases, which hydrolyze the lipids into fatty acids and glycerides
- Amylases, which hydrolyze the polysaccharides into glucose
- Nucleases, which hydrolyze the nucleic acids into mononucleotides.

***Specific function of lysosomes:***
- Degradation of macromolecules
- Degradation of worn-out organelles
- Removal of excess of secretory products
- Secretion of perforin, granzymes, melanin and serotonin.

### *Centrosome and Centrioles*

Centrosome is the membrane-bound cellular organelle situated almost in the center of cell, close to nucleus.

It consists of two cylindrical structures called centrioles which are made up of proteins. Centrioles are responsible for the movement of chromosomes during cell division.

### *Secretory Vesicles*

Secretory vesicles are the organelles with limiting membrane and contain the secretory substances. These vesicles are formed in the endoplasmic reticulum and are processed and packed in Golgi apparatus. Secretory vesicles are present throughout the cytoplasm. When necessary, these vesicles are ruptured and secretory substances are released into the cytoplasm.

### *Mitochondrion*

Mitochondrion (plural = mitochondria) is a membrane-bound cytoplasmic organelle concerned with production of energy. It is a rod-shaped or oval-shaped structure with a diameter of 0.5 to 1 μ. It is covered by a bilayered membrane. The outer membrane is smooth and encloses the contents of mitochondrion. This membrane contains various enzymes such as acetyl-CoA synthetase and glycerolphosphate acetyltransferase. The inner membrane is folded in the form of shelf-like inward projections called cristae and it covers the inner matrix space. Cristae contain many enzymes and other protein molecules which are involved in respiration and synthesis of adenosine triphosphate (ATP). Because of these functions, the enzymes and other protein molecules in cristae are collectively known as respiratory chain or electron transport system.

Enzymes and other proteins of respiratory chain

- Succinic dehydrogenase
- Dihydronicotinamide adenine dinucleotide (NADH) dehydrogenase
- Cytochrome oxidase
- Cytochrome C
- ATP synthase.

Inner cavity of mitochondrion is filled with matrix which contains many enzymes. Mitochondrion moves freely in the cytoplasm of the cell. It is capable of reproducing itself. Mitochondrion contains its own deoxyribonucleic acid (DNA), which is responsible for many enzymatic actions. In fact, mitochondrion is the only organelle other than nucleus, which has its own DNA.

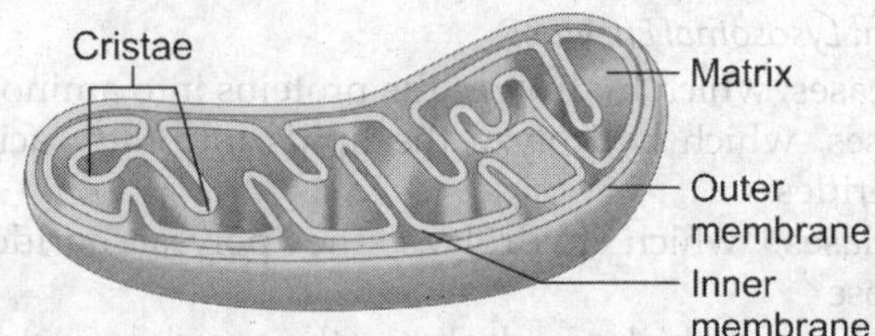


*Functions of Mitochondrion*

- ***Production of energy:*** Mitochondrion is called the 'power house' or 'power plant' of the cell because it produces the energy required for cellular functions.
- ***Synthesis of ATP:*** The components of respiratory chain in mitochondrion are responsible for the synthesis of ATP by utilizing the energy by oxidative phosphorylation.
- ***Other functions:*** Other functions of mitochondria include storage of calcium and detoxification of ammonia in liver.

### *Ribosomes*

Ribosomes are the organelles without limiting membrane. These organelles are granular and small dot-like structures with a diameter of 15 nm. Ribosomes are made up of 35% of proteins and 65% of ribonucleic acid (RNA). RNA present in ribosomes is called ribosomal RNA (rRNA). Ribosomes are concerned with protein synthesis in the cell.

*Functions of Ribosomes*

Ribosomes are called 'protein factories' because of their role in the synthesis of proteins. Messenger RNA (mRNA) carries the genetic code for protein synthesis from nucleus to the ribosomes. The ribosomes, in turn arrange the amino acids into small units of proteins.

## Nucleus

Nucleus is the most prominent and the largest cellular organelle. It has a diameter of 10 μ to 22 μ and occupies about 10% of total volume of the cell.

Nucleus is present in all the cells in the body except the red blood cells. The cells with nucleus are called eukaryotes and those without nucleus are known as prokaryotes. Presence of nucleus is necessary for cell division. Most of the cells have only one nucleus (uninucleated cells). Few types of cells like skeletal muscle cells have many nuclei (multinucleate cells). Generally, the nucleus is located in the center of the cell. It is mostly spherical in shape. However, the shape and situation of nucleus vary in some cells.

### *Structure of Nucleus*

Nucleus is covered by a membrane called nuclear membrane and contains many components. Major components of nucleus are nucleoplasm, chromatin and nucleolus.

*Nuclear Membrane*

Nuclear membrane is double layered and porous in nature. This allows the nucleoplasm to communicate with the cytoplasm.

*Nucleoplasm*

Nucleoplasm is a highly viscous fluid that forms the ground substance of the nucleus. It is similar to cytoplasm present outside the nucleus. Nucleoplasm surrounds chromatin and nucleolus.It contains dense fibrillar network of proteins called the nuclear matrix and many substances such as nucleotides and enzymes. The nuclear matrix forms the structural framework for organizing chromatin. The soluble liquid part of nucleoplasm is known as nuclear hyaloplasm.

*Chromatin*

Chromatin is a thread-like material made up of large molecules of DNA.

*Chromosomes*

Chromosome is the rod-shaped nuclear structure that carries a complete blueprint of all the hereditary characteristics of that species. A chromosome is formed from a single DNA molecule coiled around histone molecules. Each DNA contains many genes.

### *Functions of Nucleus*

Major functions of nucleus are the control of cellular activities and storage of hereditary material. Several processes are involved in the nuclear functions.

Functions of nucleus are:

- Control of all the cell activities that include metabolism, protein synthesis, growth and reproduction (cell division)
- Synthesis of RNA
- Formation of subunits of ribosomes
- Sending genetic instruction to the cytoplasm for protein synthesis through messenger RNA (mRNA)
- Control of the cell division through genes
- Storage of hereditary information (in genes) and transformation of this information from one generation of the species to the next.

## BLOOD

### Introduction

Blood is a connective tissue in fluid form. It is considered as the 'fluid of life' because it carries oxygen from lungs to all parts of the body and carbon dioxide from all parts of the body to the lungs. It is known as 'fluid of growth' because it carries nutritive substances from the digestive system and hormones from endocrine gland to all the tissues. The blood is also called the 'fluid of health' because it protects the body against the diseases and gets rid of the waste products and unwanted substances by transporting them to the excretory organs like kidneys.

### Properties of Blood

- *Color:* Blood is red in color. Arterial blood is scarlet red because it contains more oxygen and venous blood is purple red because of more carbon dioxide.
- *Volume:* Average volume of blood in a normal adult is 5 L. In a newborn baby, the volume is 450 mL. It increases during growth and reaches 5 L at the time of puberty. In females, it is slightly less and is about 4.5 L. It is about 8% of the body weight in a normal young healthy adult, weighing about 70 kg.
- *Reaction and pH:* Blood is slightly alkaline and its pH in normal conditions is 7.4.
- *Specific gravity:* Specific gravity of total blood: 1.052 to 1.061.
  - *Specific gravity blood cells:* 1.092 to 1.101
  - *Specific gravity of plasma:* 1.022 to 1.026
- *Viscosity:* Blood is five times more viscous than water. It is mainly due to red blood cells and plasma proteins.

### Composition of Blood

Blood contains the blood cells which are called formed elements and the liquid portion known as plasma.

#### *Blood Cells*

Three types of cells are present in the blood:

1. Red blood cells or erythrocytes
2. White blood cells or leukocytes
3. Platelets or thrombocytes.

#### *Plasma*

Plasma is a straw-colored clear liquid part of blood. It contains 91 to 92% of water and 8 to 9% of solids. The solids are the organic and the inorganic substances.

#### *Serum*

Serum is the clear straw-colored fluid that oozes from blood clot. When the blood is shed or collected in a container, it clots. In this process, the fibrinogen is converted into fibrin and the blood cells are trapped in this fibrin forming the blood clot. After about 45 minutes, serum oozes out of the blood clot. For clinical investigations, serum is separated from blood cells and clotting elements by centrifuging. Volume of the serum is almost the same as that of plasma (55%). It is different from plasma only by the absence of fibrinogen, i.e. serum contains all the other constituents of plasma except fibrinogen. Fibrinogen is absent in serum because it is converted into fibrin during blood clotting. Thus,

Serum = Plasma – Fibrinogen

### Functions of Blood

- *Nutritive function:* Nutritive substances like glucose, amino acids, lipids and vitamins derived from digested food are absorbed from gastrointestinal tract and carried by blood to different parts of the body for growth and production of energy.
- *Respiratory function:* Transport of respiratory gases is done by the blood. It carries oxygen from alveoli of lungs to different tissues and carbon dioxide from tissues to alveoli.
- *Excretory function:* Waste products formed in the tissues during various metabolic activities are removed by blood and carried to the excretory organs like kidney, skin, liver, etc. for excretion.
- *Transport of hormones and enzymes:* Hormones which are secreted by ductless (endocrine) glands are released directly into the blood. The blood transports these hormones to their target organs/tissues. Blood also transports enzymes.
- *Regulation of water balance:* Water content of the blood is freely interchangeable with interstitial fluid. This helps in the regulation of water content of the body.
- *Regulation of acid-base balance:* Plasma proteins and hemoglobin act as buffers and help in the regulation of acid-base balance.
- *Regulation of body temperature:* Because of the high specific heat of blood, it is responsible for maintaining the thermoregulatory mechanism in the body, i.e. the balance between heat loss and heat gain in the body.
- *Storage function:* Water and some important substances like proteins, glucose, sodium and potassium are constantly required by the tissues. Blood serves as a readymade source for these substances. And, these substances are taken from blood during the conditions like starvation, fluid loss, electrolyte loss, etc.
- *Defensive function:* Blood plays an important role in the defense of the body. The white blood cells are responsible for this function. Neutrophils and monocytes engulf the bacteria by phagocytosis. Lymphocytes are involved in development of immunity.

### Red Blood Cells

Red blood cells (RBCs) are the non-nucleated formed elements in the blood. Red blood cells are also known as erythrocytes (erythros = red). Red color of the red blood cell is due to the presence of the coloring pigment called hemoglobin.

### Normal Value

RBC count ranges between 4 and 5.5 million/cu mm of blood. In adult males, it is 5 million/cu mm and in adult females, it is 4.5 million/cu mm.

### Normal Shape

Normally, the RBCs are disk shaped and biconcave (dumbbell shaped).

### Normal Size

- Diameter: 7.2 μ (6.9 to 7.4 μ).
- Thickness: At the periphery it is thicker with 2.2 μ and at the center it is thinner with 1 μ. This difference in thickness is because of the biconcave shape.
- Surface area: 120 sq μ.
- Volume: 85 to 90 cu μ.

### Normal Structure

Red blood cells are nonnucleated. Only mammal, which has nucleated RBC is camel. Because of the absence of nucleus in human RBC, the DNA is also absent. Other organelles such as mitochondria and Golgi apparatus also are absent in RBC. Because of absence of mitochondria, the energy is produced from glycolytic process. Red cell does not have insulin receptor and so the glucose uptake by this cell is not controlled by insulin.

### Lifespan of Red Blood Cells

Average lifespan of RBC is about 120 days. After the lifetime the senile (old) RBCs are destroyed in reticuloendothelial system.

### Functions of Red Blood Cells

- Transport of oxygen from the lungs to the tissues
- Transport of carbon dioxide from the tissues to the lungs
- Buffering action in blood
- In blood group determination.

### Normal Hemoglobin Content

Average hemoglobin (Hb) content in blood is 14 to 16 g/dL. However, the value varies depending upon the age and sex of the individual.

*Age*

- At birth: 25 g/dL
- After 3rd month: 20 g/dL
- After 1 year: 17 g/dL
- From puberty onwards: 14 to 16 g/dL
- At the time of birth, hemoglobin content is very high because of increased number of RBCs.

*Sex*

- In adult males: 15 g/dL
- In adult females: 14.5 g/dL

### Normal Values of Packed Cell Volume (PCV)

Normal PCV:

- In males = 40 to 45%
- In females = 38 to 42%

## White Blood Cells

### Introduction

White blood cells (WBCs) or leukocytes are the colorless and nucleated formed elements of blood (leuko is derived from Greek word leukos = white). Alternate spelling for leukocytes is leucocytes.

Compared to RBCs, the WBCs are larger in size and lesser in number. Yet functionally, these cells are important like RBCs because of their role in defense mechanism of body and protect the body from invading organisms by acting like soldiers.

### Classification

Some of the WBCs have granules in the cytoplasm. Based on the presence or absence of granules in the cytoplasm, the leukocytes are classified into two groups:

1. Granulocytes which have granules.
2. Agranulocytes which do not have granules

- *Granulocytes:* Depending upon the staining property of granules, the granulocytes are classified into three types:
  - (i) Neutrophils with granules taking both acidic and basic stains.
  - (ii) Eosinophils with granules taking acidic stain.
  - (iii) Basophils with granules taking basic stain.
- *Agranulocytes:* Agranulocytes have plain cytoplasm without granules.
  Agranulocytes are of two types:
  - (i) Monocytes.
  - (ii) Lymphocytes.

### Normal White Blood Cell Count

Total WBC count (TC): 4,000 to 11,000/cu mm of blood.

### Variations in White Blood Cell Count

- *Leukocytosis:* Leukocytosis is the increase in total WBC count. Leukocytosis occurs in both physiological and pathological conditions.
- *Leukopenia:* Leukopenia is the decrease in total WBC count. The term leukopenia is generally used for pathological conditions only.
- *Granulocytosis:* Granulocytosis is the abnormal increase in the number of granulocytes.
- *Granulocytopenia:* Granulocytopenia is the abnormal reduction in the number of granulocytes.
- *Agranulocytosis:* Agranulocytosis is the acute pathological condition characterized by absolute lack of granulocytes.

### Physiological Variations

- *Age:* WBC count is about 20,000 per cu mm in infants and about 10,000 to 15,000 per cu mm of blood in children. In adults, it ranges between 4,000 and 11,000 per cu mm of blood.

- *Sex:* Slightly more in males than in females.
- ***Diurnal variation:*** Minimum in early morning and maximum in the afternoon.
- *Exercise:* Increases slightly.
- *Sleep:* Decreases.
- ***Emotional conditions like anxiety:*** Increases.
- *Pregnancy:* Increases.
- *Menstruation:* Increases.
- *Parturition:* Increases.

## Pathological Variations

All types of leukocytes do not share equally in the increase or decrease of total leukocyte count. In general, the neutrophils and lymphocytes vary in opposite directions.

*Leukocytosis*

Leukocytosis is the increase in total leukocyte (WBC) count. It occurs in conditions such as:
- Infections
- Allergy
- Common cold
- Tuberculosis
- Glandular fever.

*Leukemia*

Leukemia is the condition which is characterized by abnormal and uncontrolled increase in leukocyte count more than 1,000,000/cu mm. It is also called blood cancer.

*Leukopenia*

Leukopenia is the decrease in the total WBC count. It occurs in the following pathological conditions:
- Anaphylactic shock
- Cirrhosis of liver
- Disorders of spleen
- Pernicious anemia
- Typhoid and paratyphoid
- Viral infections.

### Variation in Differential Leukocyte Count

Differential leukocyte count varies in specific diseases.

*Neutrophilia*

Neutrophilia or neutrophilic leukocytosis is the increase in neutrophil count. It occurs in the following conditions:
- Acute infections
- Metabolic disorders
- Injection of foreign proteins
- Injection of vaccines
- Poisoning by chemicals and drugs like lead, mercury, camphor, benzene derivatives, etc.
- Poisoning by insect venom
- After acute hemorrhage.

*Eosinophilia*

Eosinophilia is the increase in eosinophil count and it occurs in:
- Asthma and other allergic conditions
- Blood parasitism (malaria, filariasis)
- Intestinal parasitism
- Scarlet fever.

*Basophilia*

Basophilia is the increase in basophil count and it occurs in:
- Smallpox
- Chickenpox
- Polycythemia vera.

*Monocytosis*

Monocytosis is the increase in monocyte count and it occurs in:
- Tuberculosis
- Syphilis
- Malaria
- Kala-azar
- Glandular fever.

*Lymphocytosis*

Lymphocytosis is the increase in lymphocyte count and it occurs in:
- Diphtheria
- Infectious hepatitis
- Mumps
- Malnutrition
- Rickets
- Syphilis
- Thyrotoxicosis
- Tuberculosis.

*Neutropenia*

Neutropenia is the decrease in neutrophil count. It occurs in:
- Bone marrow disorders
- Tuberculosis
- Typhoid
- Vitamin deficiencies
- Autoimmune diseases.

*Eosinopenia*

Decrease in eosinophil count is called eosinopenia. It occurs in:
- Cushing's syndrome
- Bacterial infections
- Stress
- Prolonged administration of drugs such as steroids, ACTH, epinephrine.

*Basopenia*

Basopenia or basophilic leukopenia is the decrease in basophil count. It occurs in:
- Urticaria (skin disorder)
- Stress
- Prolonged exposure to chemotherapy or radiation therapy.

*Monocytopenia*

Monocytopenia is the decrease in monocyte count. It occurs in:
- Prolonged use of prednisone (immunosuppressant steroid)
- AIDS
- Chronic lymphoid leukemia.

*Lymphocytopenia*

Lymphocytopenia is the decrease in lymphocytes. It occurs in:
- AIDS
- Hodgkin's disease (cancer of the lymphatic system)
- Malnutrition

- Radiation therapy
- Steroid administration.

## Platelets

### Introduction

Platelets or thrombocytes are the formed elements of blood. They are small colorless, non-nucleated and moderately refractive bodies. These formed elements of blood are considered to be the fragments of cytoplasm. Size of platelets:

- Diameter: 2.5 μ (2 to 4 μ)
- Volume: 7.5 cu μ (7 to 8 cu μ)

### Normal Count and Variations

Normal platelet count is 2,50,000/cu mm of blood. It ranges between 2,00,000 and 4,00,000/cu mm of blood.

### Physiological Variations

- Age: Platelets are less in infants (1,50,000 to 2,00,000/cu mm) and reaches normal level at 3rd month after birth.
- Sex: There is no difference in the platelet count between males and females. In females, it is reduced during menstruation.
- High altitude: Platelet count increases.
- After meals: After taking food, the platelet count increases.

### Properties of Platelets

Platelets have three important properties (three 'A's):

1. Adhesiveness
2. Aggregation
3. Agglutination.

### Adhesiveness

Adhesiveness is the property of sticking to a rough surface. During injury of blood vessel, endothelium is damaged and the subendothelial collagen is exposed.

While coming in contact with collagen, platelets are activated and adhere to collagen. Adhesion of platelets involves interaction between von Willebrand factor secreted by damaged endothelium and a receptor protein called glycoprotein Ib situated on the surface of platelet membrane. Other factors which accelerate adhesiveness are collagen, thrombin, ADP, thromboxane A2, calcium ions, P-selectin and vitronectin.

### Aggregation (Grouping of Platelets)

Aggregation is the grouping of platelets. Adhesion is followed by activation of more number of platelets by substances released from dense granules of platelets.

During activation, the platelets change their shape with elongation of long filamentous pseudopodia which are called processes or filopodia. Filopodia help the platelets aggregate together. Activation and aggregation of platelets is accelerated by ADP, thromboxane A2 and platelet-activating factor (PTA: cytokine secreted by neutrophils and monocytes.

### Agglutination

Agglutination is the clumping together of platelets. Aggregated platelets are agglutinated by the actions of some platelet agglutinins and platelet-activating factor.

### Functions of Platelets

Normally, platelets are inactive and execute their actions only when activated. Activated platelets immediately release many substances. This process is known as platelet release reaction. Functions of platelets are carried out by these substances. Functions of platelets are:

- ***Role in blood clotting:*** Platelets are responsible for the formation of intrinsic prothrombin activator. This substance is responsible for the onset of blood clotting.
- ***Role in clot retraction:*** In the blood clot, blood cells including platelets are entrapped in between the fibrin threads. Cytoplasm of platelets contains the contractile proteins, namely actin, myosin and thrombosthenin, which are responsible for clot retraction.
- ***Role in prevention of blood loss (Hemostasis):*** Platelets accelerate the hemostasis by three ways:
  1. Platelets secrete 5-HT, which causes the constriction of blood vessels.
  2. Due to the adhesive property, the platelets seal the damage in blood vessels like capillaries.
  3. By formation of temporary plug, the platelets seal the damage in blood vessels .
- ***Role in repair of ruptured blood vessel:*** Platelet-derived growth factor (PDGF) formed in cytoplasm of platelets is useful for the repair of the endothelium and other structures of the ruptured blood vessels.
- ***Role in defense mechanism:*** By the property of agglutination, platelets encircle the foreign bodies and destroy them.

### Lifespan and Fate of Platelets

Average lifespan of platelets is 10 days. It varies between 8 and 11 days. Platelets are destroyed by tissue macrophage system in spleen. So, splenomegaly (enlargement of spleen) decreases platelet count and splenectomy (removal of spleen) increases platelet count.

### Applied Physiology–Platelet Disorders

Platelet disorders occur because of pathological variation in platelet count and dysfunction of platelets.

Platelet disorders are:

- Thrombocytopenia
- Thrombocytosis
- Thrombocythemia
- Glanzmann's thrombasthenia.
- ***Thrombocytopenia:*** Decrease in platelet count is called thrombocytopenia. It leads to thrombocytopenic purpura. Thrombocytopenia occurs in the following conditions:
  - Acute infections
  - Acute leukemia
  - Aplastic and pernicious anemia
  - Chickenpox
  - Smallpox
  - Splenomegaly
  - Scarlet fever
  - Typhoid
  - Tuberculosis
  - Purpura
  - Gaucher's disease.

- *Thrombocytosis:* Increase in platelet count is called thrombocytosis. Thrombocytosis occurs in the following conditions:
  - Allergic conditions
  - Asphyxia
  - Hemorrhage
  - Bone fractures
  - Surgical operations
  - Splenectomy
  - Rheumatic fever
  - Trauma (wound or injury or damage caused by external force).
- *Thrombocythemia:* Thrombocythemia is the condition with persistent and abnormal increase in platelet count. It occurs in the following conditions:
  - Carcinoma
  - Chronic leukemia
  - Hodgkin's disease.
- *Glanzmann's Thrombasthenia:* Glanzmann's thrombasthenia is an inherited hemorrhagic disorder, caused by structural or functional abnormality of platelets. It leads to thrombasthenic purpura. However, the platelet count is normal. It is characterized by normal clotting time, normal or prolonged bleeding time but defective clot retraction.

## Plasma Proteins

### Introduction

Plasma proteins are:
- Serum albumin
- Serum globulin
- Fibrinogen.

Serum contains only albumin and globulin. Fibrinogen is absent in serum because, it is converted into fibrin during blood clotting. Because of this, the albumin and globulin are usually called serum albumin and serum globulin.

### Normal Values

Normal values of the plasma proteins are:
- Total proteins: 7.3 g/dL (6.4 to 8.3 g/dL)
- Serum albumin: 4.7 g/dL
- Serum globulin: 2.3 g/dL
- Fibrinogen: 0.3 g/dL

### Albumin/Globulin Ratio

Ratio between plasma level of albumin and globulin is called albumin/globulin (A/G) ratio. It is an important indicator of some diseases involving liver or kidney.

Normal A/G ratio is 2 : 1.

### Origin of Plasma Proteins in Embryo

In embryonic stage, the plasma proteins are synthesized by the mesenchyme cells. The albumin is synthesized first and other proteins are synthesized later.

### In Adults

In adults, the plasma proteins are synthesized mainly from reticuloendothelial cells of liver. The plasma proteins are synthesized also from spleen, bone marrow, disintegrating blood cells and general tissue cells.

Gamma globulin is synthesized from B lymphocytes.

### Functions of Plasma Proteins

Plasma proteins are very essential for the body. Following are the functions of plasma proteins:
- *Role in coagulation of blood:* Fibrinogen is essential for the coagulation of blood
- *Role in defense mechanism of body:* Gamma globulins play an important role in the defense mechanism of the body by acting as antibodies (immune substances). These proteins are also called immunoglobulins. Antibodies react with antigens of various microorganisms, which cause diseases like diphtheria, typhoid, streptococcal infections, mumps, influenza, measles, hepatitis, rubella, poliomyelitis, etc.
- *Role in transport mechanism:* Plasma proteins are essential for the transport of various substances in the blood. Albumin, alpha globulin and beta globulin are responsible for the transport of the hormones, enzymes, etc. The alpha and beta globulins play an important role in the transport of metals in the blood.
- *Role in maintenance of osmotic pressure in blood:* At the capillary level, most of the substances are exchanged between the blood and the tissues. However, because of their large size, the plasma proteins cannot pass through the capillary membrane easily and remain in the blood. In the blood, these proteins exert the colloidal osmotic (oncotic) pressure. Osmotic pressure exerted by the plasma proteins is about 25 mm Hg.

  Since the concentration of albumin is more than the other plasma proteins, it exerts maximum pressure. Globulin is the next and fibrinogen exerts least pressure.

  *Importance of osmotic pressure–Starling's hypothesis*

  Osmotic pressure exerted by the plasma proteins plays an important role in the exchange of various substances between blood and the cells through capillary membrane. According to Starling's hypothesis, the net filtration through capillary membrane is proportional to the hydrostatic pressure difference across the membrane minus the oncotic pressure difference.
- *Role in regulation of acid-base balance:* Plasma proteins, particularly the albumin, play an important role in regulating the acid-base balance in the blood. This is because of the virtue of their buffering action. Plasma proteins are responsible for 15% of the buffering capacity of blood.
- *Role in viscosity of blood:* Plasma proteins provide viscosity to the blood, which is important to maintain the blood pressure. Albumin provides maximum viscosity than the other plasma proteins.
- *Role in erythrocyte sedimentation rate (ESR):* Globulin and fibrinogen accelerate the tendency of rouleaux formation by the red blood cells. Rouleaux formation is responsible for ESR, which is an important diagnostic and prognostic tool.
- *Role in suspension stability of red blood cells:* During circulation, the red blood cells remain suspended uniformly

in the blood. This property of the red blood cells is called the suspension stability. Globulin and fibrinogen help in the suspension stability of the red blood cells.

- *Role in production of trephone substances:* Trephone substances are necessary for nourishment of tissue cells in culture. These substances are produced by leukocytes from the plasma proteins.
- *Role as reserve proteins:* During fasting, inadequate food intake or inadequate protein intake, the plasma proteins are utilized by the body tissues as the last source of energy. Plasma proteins are split into amino acids by the tissue macrophages.
  Amino acids are taken back by blood and distributed throughout the body to form cellular protein molecules. Because of this, the plasma proteins are called the reserve proteins.

## Erythropoiesis

### Definition

Erythropoiesis is the process of the origin, development and maturation of erythrocytes. Hemopoiesis or hematopoiesis is the process of origin, development and maturation of all the blood cells.

### Site of Erythropoiesis in Fetal Life

In fetal life, the erythropoiesis occurs in three stages:

1. *Mesoblastic stage:* During the first two months of intrauterine life, the RBCs are produced from mesenchyme of yolk sac.
2. *Hepatic stage:* From third month of intrauterine life, liver is the main organ that produces RBCs. Spleen and lymphoid organs are also involved in erythropoiesis.
3. *Myeloid stage:* During the last three months of intrauterine life, the RBCs are produced from red bone marrow and liver.

### In Newborn Babies, Children and Adults

In newborn babies, growing children and adults, RBCs are produced only from the red bone marrow.

- *Up to the age of 20 years:* RBCs are produced from red bone marrow of all bones (long bones and all the flat bones).
- *After the age of 20 years:* RBCs are produced from membranous bones like vertebra, sternum, ribs, scapula, iliac bones and skull bones and from the ends of long bones. After 20 years of age, the shaft of the long bones becomes yellow bone marrow because of fat deposition and looses the erythropoietic function.
  In adults, liver and spleen may produce the blood cells if the bone marrow is destroyed or fibrosed. Collectively bone marrow is almost equal to liver in size and weight. It is also as active as liver. Though bone marrow is the site of production of all blood cells, comparatively 75% of the bone marrow is involved in the production of leukocytes and only 25% is involved in the production of erythrocytes. But still, the leukocytes are less in number than the erythrocytes, the ratio being 1:500. This is mainly because of the lifespan of these cells. Lifespan of erythrocytes is 120 days whereas the lifespan of leukocytes is very short ranging from 1 to 10 days.

### Stages of Erythropoiesis

Various stages between cotony forming unit-erythrocyte (CFU-E) cells and matured RBCs are:

- Proerythroblast
- Early normoblast
- Intermediate normoblast
- Late normoblast
- Reticulocyte
- Matured erythrocyte.
- *Proerythroblast (megaloblast):* Proerythroblast or megaloblast is the first cell derived from CFU-E. It is very large in size with a diameter of about 20 μ. Its nucleus is large and occupies the cell almost completely. The nucleus has two or more nucleoli and a reticular network. Proerythroblast does not contain hemoglobin. The cytoplasm is basophilic in nature. Proerythroblast multiplies several times and finally forms the cell of next stage called early normoblast. Synthesis of hemoglobin starts in this stage. However, appearance of hemoglobin occurs only in intermediate normoblast.
- *Early normoblast:* The early normoblast is little smaller than proerythroblast with a diameter of about 15 μ. In the nucleus, the nucleoli disappear. Condensation of chromatin network occurs. The condensed network becomes dense. The cytoplasm is basophilic in nature. So, this cell is also called basophilic erythroblast. This cell develops into next stage called intermediate normoblast.
- *Intermediate normoblast:* Cell is smaller than the early normoblast with a diameter of 10 to 12 μ. The nucleus is still present. But, the chromatin network shows further condensation. The hemoglobin starts appearing. Cytoplasm is already basophilic. Now, because of the presence of hemoglobin, it stains with both acidic as well as basic stains. So this cell is called polychromophilic or polychromatic erythroblast. This cell develops into next stage called late normoblast.
- *Late normoblast:* Diameter of the cell decreases further to about 8 to 10 μ. Nucleus becomes very small with very much condensed chromatin network and it is known as ink-spot nucleus. Quantity of hemoglobin increases and the cytoplasm becomes almost acidophilic. So, the cell is now called orthochromatic erythroblast. In the final stage of late normoblast just before it passes to next stage, the nucleus disintegrates and disappears. The process by which nucleus disappears is called pyknosis. The final remnant is extruded from the cell. Late normoblast develops into the next stage called reticulocyte.
- *Reticulocyte:* Reticulocyte is otherwise known as immature RBC. It is slightly larger than matured RBC. The cytoplasm contains the reticular network or reticulum, which is formed by remnants of disintegrated organelles. Due to the reticular network, the cell is called reticulocyte. The reticulum of reticulocyte stains with supravital stain. In newborn babies, the reticulocyte count is 2% to 6% of RBCs,

i.e. 2 to 6 reticulocytes are present for every 100 RBCs. The number of reticulocytes decreases during the first week after birth. Later, the reticulocyte count remains constant at or below 1% of RBCs. The number increases whenever production and release of RBCs increase. Reticulocyte is basophilic due to the presence of remnants of disintegrated Golgi apparatus, mitochondria and other organelles of cytoplasm. During this stage, the cells enter the blood capillaries through capillary membrane from site of production by diapedesis.

- *Matured erythrocyte:* Reticular network disappears and the cell becomes the matured RBC and attains the biconcave shape. The cell decreases in size to 7.2 μ diameter. The matured RBC is with hemoglobin but without nucleus. It requires 7 days for the development and maturation of RBC from proerythroblast. It requires 5 days up to the stage of reticulocyte. Reticulocyte takes 2 more days to become the matured RBC.

### Factors Necessary for Erythropoiesis

Development and maturation of erythrocytes require variety of factors, which are classified into three categories:

1. General factors
2. Maturation factors
3. Factors necessary for hemoglobin formation.

### General Factors

General factors necessary for erythropoiesis are:

- Erythropoietin
- Thyroxine
- Hemopoietic growth factors
- Vitamins.
- *Erythropoietin:* Most important general factor for erythropoiesis is the hormone called erythropoietin. It is also called hemopoietin or erythrocyte stimulating factor.
  - *Chemistry:* Erythropoietin is a glycoprotein with 165 amino acids.
  - *Source of secretion:* Major quantity of erythropoietin is secreted by peritubular capillaries of kidney. A small quantity is also secreted from liver and brain.
  - *Stimulant for secretion:* Hypoxia is the stimulant for the secretion of erythropoietin.
  - *Actions of erythropoietin:* Erythropoietin causes formation and release of new RBCs into circulation.

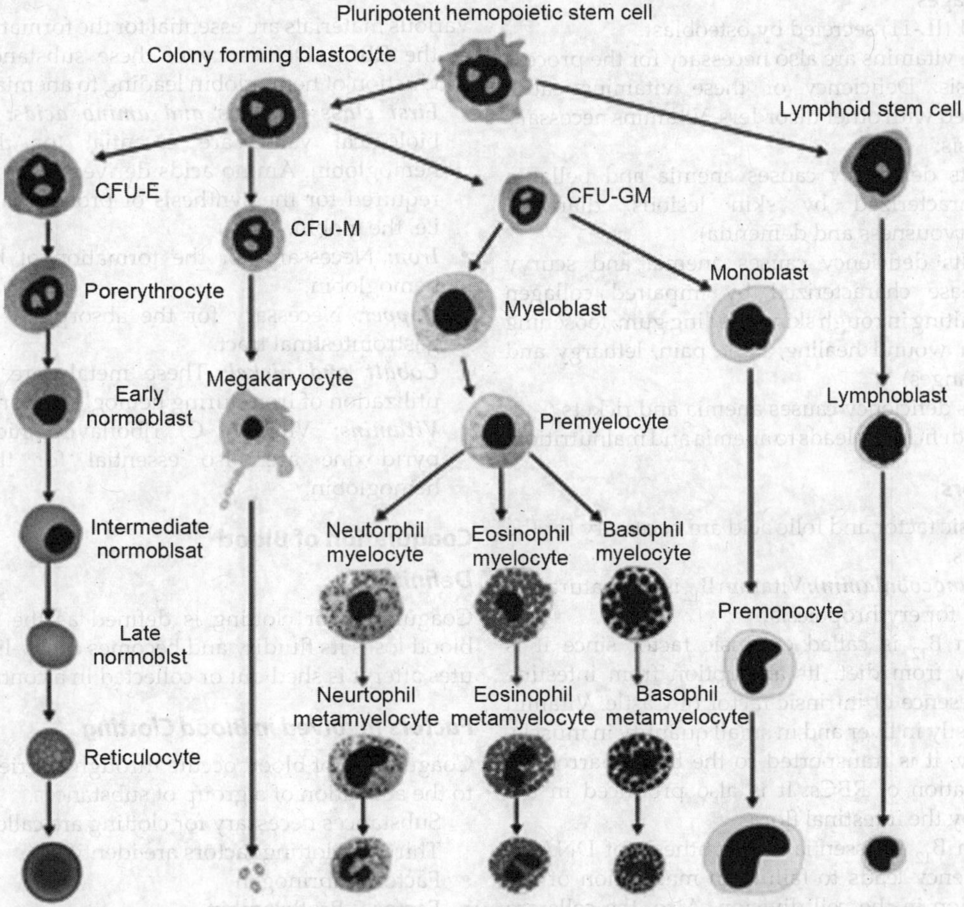

After secretion, it takes 4 to 5 days to show the action. Erythropoietin promotes the following processes:

a. Production of proerythroblasts from CFU-E of the bone marrow
b. Development of proerythroblasts into matured RBCs through the several stages—early normoblast, intermediate normoblast, late normoblast and reticulocyte
c. Release of matured erythrocytes into blood. Even some reticulocytes (immature erythrocytes) are released along with matured RBCs. Blood level of erythropoietin increases in anemia.

- ***Thyroxine:*** Being a general metabolic hormone, thyroxine accelerates the process of erythropoiesis at many levels. So, hyperthyroidism and polycythemia are common.
- ***Hemopoietic growth factors:*** Hemopoietic growth factors or growth inducers are the interleukins and stem cell factor (steel factor). Generally these factors induce the proliferation of PHSCs.

  Interleukins (IL) are glycoproteins, which belong to the cytokines family. Interleukins involved in erythropoiesis:
  - Interleukin-3 (IL-3) secreted by T-cells
  - Interleukin-6 (IL-6) secreted by T-cells, endothelial cells and macrophages
  - Interleukin-11 (IL-11) secreted by osteoblast.
- ***Vitamins:*** Some vitamins are also necessary for the process of erythropoiesis. Deficiency of these vitamins cause anemia associated with other disorders. Vitamins necessary for erythropoiesis:
  - Vitamin B: Its deficiency causes anemia and pellagra (disease characterized by skin lesions, diarrhea, weakness, nervousness and dementia).
  - Vitamin C: Its deficiency causes anemia and scurvy (ancient disease characterized by impaired collagen synthesis resulting in rough skin, bleeding gum, loosening of teeth, poor wound healing, bone pain, lethargy and emotional changes).
  - Vitamin D: Its deficiency causes anemia and rickets.
  - Vitamin E: Its deficiency leads to anemia and malnutrition.

### Maturation Factors

Vitamin $B_{12}$, intrinsic factor and folic acid are necessary for the maturation of RBCs.

- ***Vitamin $B_{12}$ (cyanocobalamin):*** Vitamin $B_{12}$ is the maturation factor necessary for erythropoiesis.

  ***Source:*** Vitamin $B_{12}$ is called extrinsic factor since it is obtained mostly from diet. Its absorption from intestine requires the presence of intrinsic factor of Castle. Vitamin $B_{12}$ is stored mostly in liver and in small quantity in muscle. When necessary, it is transported to the bone marrow to promote maturation of RBCs. It is also produced in the large intestine by the intestinal flora.

  ***Action:*** Vitamin $B_{12}$ is essential for synthesis of DNA in RBCs. Its deficiency leads to failure in maturation of the cell and reduction in the cell division. Also, the cells are larger with fragile and weak cell membrane resulting in macrocytic anemia.

  Deficiency of vitamin $B_{12}$ causes pernicious anemia. So, vitamin $B_{12}$ is called antipernicious factor.
- ***Intrinsic factor of castle:*** Intrinsic factor of castle is produced in gastric mucosa by the parietal cells of the gastric glands. It is essential for the absorption of vitamin $B_{12}$ from intestine. In the absence of intrinsic factor, vitamin $B_{12}$ is not absorbed from intestine. This leads to pernicious anemia. Deficiency of intrinsic factor occurs in:
  - Severe gastritis
  - Ulcer
  - Gastrectomy.

  ***Hematinic principle:*** Hematinic principle is the principle thought to be produced by the action of intrinsic factor on extrinsic factor. It is also called or antianemia principle. It is a maturation factor.
- ***Folic acid:*** Folic acid is also essential for maturation. It is required for the synthesis of DNA. In the absence of folic acid, the synthesis of DNA decreases causing failure of maturation. This leads to anemia in which the cells are larger and appear in megaloblastic (proerythroblastic) stage. And, anemia due to folic acid deficiency is called megaloblastic anemia.

### Factors Necessary for Hemoglobin Formation

Various materials are essential for the formation of hemoglobin in the RBCs. Deficiency of these substances decreases the production of hemoglobin leading to anemia. Such factors are:

- ***First class proteins and amino acids:*** Proteins of high biological value are essential for the formation of hemoglobin. Amino acids derived from these proteins are required for the synthesis of protein part of hemoglobin, i.e. the globin.
- ***Iron:*** Necessary for the formation of heme part of the hemoglobin.
- ***Copper:*** Necessary for the absorption of iron from the gastrointestinal tract.
- ***Cobalt and nickel:*** These metals are essential for the utilization of iron during hemoglobin formation.
- ***Vitamins:*** Vitamin C, riboflavin, nicotinic acid and pyridoxine are also essential for the formation of hemoglobin.

## Coagulation of Blood

### Definition

Coagulation or clotting is defined as the process in which blood loses its fluidity and becomes a jelly-like mass few minutes after it is shed out or collected in a container.

### Factors Involved in Blood Clotting

Coagulation of blood occurs through a series of reactions due to the activation of a group of substances.

Substances necessary for clotting are called clotting factors. Thirteen clotting factors are identified:

- Factor I Fibrinogen
- Factor II Prothrombin
- Factor III Thromboplastin (tissue factor)
- Factor IV Calcium

- Factor V Labile factor (proaccelerin or accelerator globulin)
- Factor VI Presence has not been proved
- Factor VII Stable factor
- Factor VIII Antihemophilic factor (antihemophilic globulin)
- Factor IX Christmas factor
- Factor X Stuart-Prower factor
- Factor XI Plasma thromboplastin antecedent
- Factor XII Hageman factor (Contact factor)
- Factor XIII Fibrin-stabilizing factor (fibrinase)
- Clotting factors were named after the scientists who discovered them or as per the activity, except factor
- Factor IX or Christmas factor was named after the patient in whom it was discovered.

## Sequence of Clotting Mechanism

***Stages of blood clotting:*** In general, blood clotting occurs in three stages:

1. Formation of prothrombin activator
2. Conversion of prothrombin into thrombin
3. Conversion of fibrinogen into fibrin.

*Stage 1: Formation of Prothrombin Activator*

Blood clotting commences with the formation of a substance called prothrombin activator, which converts prothrombin into thrombin. Its formation is initiated by substances produced either within the blood or outside the blood. Thus, formation of prothrombin activator occurs through two pathways:

1. Intrinsic pathway
2. Extrinsic pathway.

1. ***Intrinsic pathway for the formation of prothrombin activator:*** In this pathway, the formation of prothrombin activator is initiated by platelets, which are within the blood itself.

   *Sequence of events in intrinsic pathway*

   - During the injury, the blood vessel is ruptured. Endothelium is damaged and collagen beneath the endothelium is exposed.
   - When factor XII (Hageman factor) comes in contact with collagen, it is converted into activated factor XII in the presence of kallikrein and high molecular weight (HMW) kinogen.
   - The activated factor XII converts factor XI into activated factor XI in the presence of HMW kinogen.
   - The activated factor XI activates factor IX in the presence of factor IV (calcium).
   - Activated factor IX activates factor X in the presence of factor VIII and calcium.
   - When platelet comes in contact with collagen of damaged blood vessel, it gets activated and releases phospholipids.
   - Now the activated factor X reacts with platelet phospholipid and factor V to form prothrombin activator. This needs the presence of calcium ions.
   - Factor V is also activated by positive feedback effect of thrombin (see below).

2. ***Extrinsic pathway for the formation of prothrombin activator:*** In this pathway, the formation of prothrombin activator is initiated by the tissue thromboplastin, which is formed from the injured tissues.

   *Sequence of events in extrinsic pathway*

   - Tissues that are damaged during injury release tissue thromboplastin (factor III). Thromboplastin contains proteins, phospholipid and glycoprotein, which act as proteolytic enzymes.
   - Glycoprotein and phospholipid components of thromboplastin convert factor X into activated factor X, in the presence of factor VII.
   - Activated factor X reacts with factor V and phospholipid component of tissue thromboplastin to form prothrombin activator. This reaction requires the presence of calcium ions.

*Stage 2: Conversion of Prothrombin into Thrombin*

Blood clotting is all about thrombin formation. Once thrombin is formed, it definitely leads to clot formation.

Sequence of events in Stage 2:

- Prothrombin activator that is formed in intrinsic and extrinsic pathways converts prothrombin into thrombin in the presence of calcium (factor IV).
- Once formed thrombin initiates the formation of more thrombin molecules. The initially formed thrombin activates factor V. Factor V in turn accelerates formation of both extrinsic and intrinsic prothrombin activator, which converts prothrombin into thrombin. This effect of thrombin is called positive feedback effect.

*Stage 3: Conversion of Fibrinogen into Fibrin*

The final stage of blood clotting involves the conversion of fibrinogen into fibrin by thrombin.

Sequence of events in stage 3:

- Thrombin converts inactive fibrinogen into activated fibrinogen due to loss of 2 pairs of polypeptides from each fibrinogen molecule. The activated fibrinogen is called fibrin monomer.
- Fibrin monomer polymerizes with other monomer molecules and form loosely arranged strands of fibrin.
- Later these loose strands are modified into dense and tight fibrin threads by fibrin-stabilizing factor (factor XIII) in the presence of calcium ions. All the tight fibrin threads are aggregated to form a meshwork of stable clot.

## Anticlotting Mechanism in the Body

Under physiological conditions, intravascular clotting does not occur. It is because of the presence of some physicochemical factors in the body.

- Physical factors
  - Continuous circulation of blood.
  - Smooth endothelial lining of the blood vessels.
- Chemical factors–natural anticoagulants
  - Presence of natural anticoagulant called heparin that is produced by the liver
  - Production of thrombomodulin by endothelium of the blood vessels (except in brain capillaries). Thrombomodulin is a thrombin-binding protein. It binds with thrombin and forms a thrombomodulin-thrombin complex. This complex activates protein C. Activated protein C along with its cofactor protein S inactivates

Factor V and Factor VIII. Inactivation of these two clotting factors prevents clot formation
- All the clotting factors are in inactive state.

## Anticoagulants

Substances which prevent or postpone coagulation of blood are called anticoagulants. Anticoagulants are of three types:

- Anticoagulants used to prevent blood clotting inside the body, i.e. in vivo.
- Anticoagulants used to prevent clotting of blood that is collected from the body, i.e. in vitro.
- Anticoagulants used to prevent blood clotting both in *vivo* and in *vitro*.

### *Heparin*

Heparin is a naturally produced anticoagulant in the body. It is produced by mast cells which are the wandering cells present immediately outside the capillaries in many tissues or organs that contain more connective tissue. These cells are abundant in liver and lungs. Basophils also secrete heparin.

Heparin is a conjugated polysaccharide. Commercial heparin is prepared from the liver and other organs of animals. Commercial preparation is available in liquid form or dry form as sodium, calcium, ammonium or lithium salts.

*Mechanism of Action of Heparin*

- Heparin:
  - Prevents blood clotting by its antithrombin activity. It directly suppresses the activity of thrombin.
  - Combines with antithrombin III (a protease inhibitor present in circulation) and removes thrombin from circulation
  - Activates antithrombin III
  - Inactivates the active form of other clotting factors like IX, X, XI and XII.

*Uses of Heparin*

Heparin is used as an anticoagulant both in *vivo* and in *vitro*.

*Clinical Use*

Intravenous injection of heparin (0.5 to 1 mg/kg body weight) postpones clotting for 3 to 4 hours (until it is destroyed by the enzyme heparinase). So, it is widely used as an anticoagulant in clinical practice. In clinics, heparin is used for many purposes such as:

- To prevent intravascular blood clotting during surgery.
- While passing the blood through artificial kidney for dialysis.
- During cardiac surgery, which involves heart-lung machine.
- To preserve the blood before transfusion.

*Use in the Laboratory*

Heparin is also used as anticoagulant in vitro while collecting blood for various investigations. About 0.1 to 0.2 mg is sufficient for 1 mL of blood. It is effective for 8 to 12 hours. After that, blood will clot because heparin only delays clotting and does not prevent it. It is the most expensive anticoagulant.

### *Coumarin Derivatives*

Warfarin and dicoumoral are the derivatives of coumarin.

*Mechanism of Action*

Coumarin derivatives prevent blood clotting by inhibiting the action of vitamin K. Vitamin K is essential for the formation of various clotting factors, namely II, VII, IX and X.

*Uses*

Dicoumoral and warfarin are the commonly used oral anticoagulants (in vivo). Warfarin is used to prevent myocardial infarction (heart attack), strokes and thrombosis.

### *Ethylenediaminetetraacetic Acid (EDTA)*

It is a strong anticoagulant. It is available in two forms:

1. Disodium salt ($Na_2$ EDTA).
2. Tripotassium salt ($K_3$ EDTA).

*Mechanism of Action*

These substances prevent blood clotting by removing calcium from blood.

*Uses*

EDTA is used as an anticoagulant both in *vivo* and in *vitro*. It is:

- Commonly administered intravenously, in cases of lead poisoning.
- Used as an anticoagulant in the laboratory (in vitro). About 0.5 to 2.0 mg of EDTA per mL of blood is sufficient to preserve the blood for at least 6 hours. On refrigeration, it can preserve the blood up to 24 hours.

### *Oxalate Compounds*

Oxalate compounds prevent coagulation by forming calcium oxalate, which is precipitated later. Thus, these compounds reduce the blood calcium level.

Earlier sodium and potassium oxalates were used. Nowadays, mixture of ammonium oxalate and potassium oxalate in the ratio of 3 : 2 is used. Each salt is an anticoagulant by itself. But potassium oxalate alone causes shrinkage of RBCs. Ammonium oxalate alone causes swelling of RBCs. But together, these substances do not alter the cellular activity.

*Mechanism of Action*

Oxalate combines with calcium and forms insoluble calcium oxalate. Thus, oxalate removes calcium from blood and lack of calcium prevents coagulation.

*Uses*

Oxalate compounds are used only as in vitro anticoagulants. 2 mg of mixture is necessary for 1 mL of blood. Since oxalate is poisonous, it cannot be used in vivo.

### *Citrates*

Sodium, ammonium and potassium citrates are used as anticoagulants.

*Mechanism of Action*

Citrate combines with calcium in blood to form insoluble calcium citrate. Like oxalate, citrate also removes calcium from blood and lack of calcium prevents coagulation.

*Uses*

Citrate is used as in vitro anticoagulant.

- It is used to store blood in the blood bank as:
  - Acid citrate dextrose (ACD): 1 part of ACD with 4 parts of blood
  - Citrate phosphate dextrose (CPD): 1 part of CPD with 4 parts of blood
- Citrate is also used in laboratory in the form of formol-citrate solution (Dacie's solution) for RBC and platelet counts.

### Other Substances which Prevent Blood Clotting

Peptone, C-type lectin (proteins from venom of viper snake) and hirudin (from the leach *Hirudinaria manillensis*) are the known anticoagulants.

### Procoagulants

Procoagulants or hemostatic agents are the substances which accelerate the process of blood coagulation. Procoagulants are:

#### *Thrombin*

Thrombin is sprayed upon the bleeding surface to arrest bleeding by hastening blood clotting.

#### *Snake Venom*

Venom of some snakes (vipers, cobras and rattle snakes) contains proteolytic enzymes which enhance blood clotting by activating the clotting factors.

#### *Extracts of Lungs and Thymus*

Extract obtained from the lungs and thymus has thromboplastin, which causes rapid blood coagulation.

#### *Sodium or Calcium Alginate*

Sodium or calcium alginate substances enhance blood clotting process by activating the Hageman factor.

#### *Oxidized Cellulose*

Oxidized cellulose causes clotting of blood by activating the Hageman factor.

### Tests for Blood Clotting

Blood clotting tests are used to diagnose blood disorders.

Some tests are also used to monitor the patients treated with anticoagulant drugs such as heparin and warfarin:

- Bleeding time
- Clotting time
- Prothrombin time
- Partial prothrombin time
- International normalized ratio
- Thrombin time.

#### *Bleeding Time*

Bleeding time (BT) is the time interval from oozing of blood after a cut or injury till arrest of bleeding. Usually, it is determined by Duke method using blotting paper or filter paper method. Its normal duration is 3 to 6 minutes. It is prolonged in purpura.

#### *Clotting Time*

Clotting time (CT) is the time interval from oozing of blood after a cut or injury till the formation of clot. It is usually determined by capillary tube method. Its normal duration is 3 to 8 minutes. It is prolonged in hemophilia.

#### *Prothrombin Time*

Prothrombin time (PT) is the time taken by blood to clot after adding tissue thromboplastin to it. Blood is collected and oxalated so that, the calcium is precipitated and prothrombin is not converted into thrombin. Thus, the blood clotting is prevented. Then a large quantity of tissue thromboplastin with calcium is added to this blood. Calcium nullifies the effect of oxalate. The tissue thromboplastin activates prothrombin and blood clotting occurs. During this procedure, the time taken by blood to clot after adding tissue thromboplastin is determined.

It time indicates the total quantity of prothrombin present in the blood.

Normal duration of prothrombin time is 10 to 12 seconds. It is prolonged in deficiency of prothrombin and other factors like factors I, V, VII and X. However, it is normal in hemophilia.

#### *Partial Prothrombin Time or Activated Prothrombin Time*

Partial prothrombin time (PPT) is the time taken for the blood to clot after adding an activator such as phospholipid, along with calcium to it. It is also called activated partial prothrombin time (APTT). This test is useful in monitoring the patients taking anticoagulant drugs.

It is carried out by observing clotting time after adding phospholipid, a surface activator and calcium to a patient's plasma. Phospholipid serves as platelet substitute. Commonly used surface activator is kaolin.

Normal duration of partial prothrombin time is 30 to 45 seconds. It is prolonged in heparin or warfarin therapy (since heparin and warfarin inhibit clotting) and deficiency or inhibition of factors II, V, VIII, IX, X, XI and XII.

#### *International Normalized Ratio*

International normalized ratio (INR) is the rating of a patient's prothrombin time when compared to an average. It measures extrinsic clotting pathway system. INR is useful in monitoring impact of anticoagulant drugs such as warfarin and to adjust the dosage of anticoagulants. Patients with atrial fibrillation are usually treated with warfarin to protect against blood clot, which may cause strokes. These patients should have regular blood tests to know their INR in order to adjust warfarin dosage. Blood takes longer time to clot if INR is higher.

Normal INR is about 1. In patients taking anticoagulant therapy for atrial fibrillation, INR should be between 2 and 3. For patients with heart valve disorders, INR should be between 3 and 4. But, INR greater than 4 indicates that blood is clotting too slowly and there is a risk of uncontrolled blood clotting.

### *Thrombin Time*

Thrombin time (TT) is the time taken for the blood to clot after adding thrombin to it. It is done to investigate the presence of heparin in plasma or to detect fibrinogen abnormalities. This test involves observation of clotting time after adding thrombin to patient's plasma. Normal duration of thrombin time is 12 to 20 seconds. It is prolonged in heparin therapy and during dysfibrinogenemia (abnormal function of fibrinogen with normal fibrinogen level).

## DIGESTIVE SYSTEM

### Introduction

Digestion is defined as the process by which food is broken down into simple chemical substances that can be absorbed and used as nutrients by the body. Most of the substances in the diet cannot be utilized as such. These substances must be broken into smaller particles, so that they can be absorbed into blood and distributed to various parts of the body for utilization. Digestive system is responsible for these functions.

Digestive process is accomplished by mechanical and enzymatic breakdown of food into simpler chemical compounds. A normal young healthy adult consumes about 1 kg of solid diet and about 1 to 2 liter of liquid diet everyday. All these food materials are subjected to digestive process, before being absorbed into blood and distributed to the tissues of the body. Digestive system plays the major role in the digestion and absorption of food substances.

Thus, the functions of digestive system include:
- Ingestion or consumption of food substances
- Breaking them into small particles
- Transport of small particles to different areas of the digestive tract
- Secretion of necessary enzymes and other substances for digestion
- Digestion of the food particles
- Absorption of the digestive products (nutrients)
- Removal of unwanted substances from the body.

### Functional Anatomy of Digestive System

Digestive system is made up of gastrointestinal tract (GI tract) or alimentary canal and accessory organs, which help in the process of digestion and absorption. GI tract is a tubular structure extending from the mouth up to anus, with a length of about 30 feet. It opens to the external environment on both ends. GI tract is formed by two types of organs:

1. ***Primary digestive organs:*** Primary digestive organs are the organs where actual digestion takes place. Primary digestive organs are:
   - Mouth
   - Pharynx
   - Esophagus
   - Stomach
   - Small intestine
   - Large intestine.

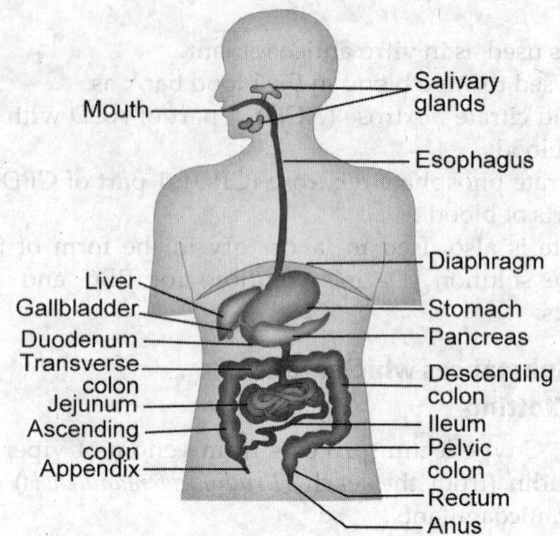


2. ***Accessory digestive organs:*** Accessory digestive organs are those which help primary digestive organs in the process of digestion. Accessory digestive organs are:
   - Teeth
   - Tongue
   - Salivary glands
   - Exocrine part of pancreas
   - Liver
   - Gallbladder.

### Wall of Gastrointestinal Tract

In general, wall of the GI tract is formed by four layers which are from inside out:
1. Mucus layer
2. Submucus layer
3. Muscular layer
4. Serous or fibrous layer.

- ***Mucus layer:*** Mucus layer is the innermost layer of the wall of GI tract. It is also called gastrointestinal mucosa or mucous membrane. It faces the cavity of GI tract. Mucosa has three layer of structures:
  - (i) Epithelial lining
  - (ii) Lamina propria
  - (iii) Muscularis mucosa.
  - ***Epithelial lining:*** Epithelial lining is in contact with the contents of GI tract. The type of cells in this layer varies in different parts of GI tract. The inner surface of mouth, surface of tongue, inner surface of pharynx and esophagus have stratified squamous epithelial cells. However, mucous membrane lining the other parts such as stomach, small intestine and large intestine has columnar epithelial cells.
  - ***Lamina propria:*** Lamina propria is formed by connective tissues, which contain fibroblasts, macrophages, lymphocytes and eosinophils.
  - ***Muscularis mucosa:*** Muscularis mucosa layer consists of a thin layer of smooth muscle fibers. It is absent in mouth and pharynx. It is present from esophagus onwards.
- ***Submucus layer:*** Submucus layer is also present in all parts of GI tract, except the mouth and pharynx. It contains loose

collagen fibers, elastic fibers, reticular fibers and few cells of connective tissue. Blood vessels, lymphatic vessels and nerve plexus are present in this layer.

- *Muscular layer:* Muscular layer in lips, cheeks and wall of pharynx contains skeletal muscle fibers. The esophagus has both skeletal and smooth muscle fibers. Wall of the stomach and intestine is formed by smooth muscle fibers. Smooth muscle fibers in stomach are arranged in three layers:
  (i) Inner oblique layer
  (ii) Middle circular layer
  (iii) Outer longitudinal layer.
  Smooth muscle fibers in the intestine are arranged in two layers:
  (i) Inner circular layer
  (ii) Outer longitudinal layer.
  Auerbach nerve plexus is present in between the circular and longitudinal muscle fibers. The smooth muscle fibers present in inner circular layer of anal canal constitute internal anal sphincter. The external anal sphincter is formed by skeletal muscle fibers.
- *Serous or fibrous layer:* Outermost layer of the wall of GI tract is either serous or fibrous in nature. The serous layer is also called serosa or serous membrane and it is formed by connective tissue and mesoepithelial cells. It covers stomach, small intestine and large intestine.
  The fibrous layer is otherwise called fibrosa and it is formed by connective tissue. It covers pharynx and esophagus.

## Salivary Glands

In humans, the saliva is secreted by three pairs of major (larger) salivary glands and some minor (small) salivary glands.

### Major Salivary Glands

Major glands are:

- Parotid glands
- Submaxillary or submandibular glands
- Sublingual glands.
- *Parotid glands:* Parotid glands are the largest of all salivary glands, situated at the side of the face just below and in front of the ear. Each gland weighs about 20 to 30 g in adults. Secretions from these glands are emptied into the oral cavity by Stensen duct. This duct is about 35 to 40 mm long and opens inside the cheek against the upper second molar tooth.
- *Submaxillary glands:* Submaxillary glands or submandibular glands are located in submaxillary triangle, medial to mandible.
  Each gland weighs about 8 to 10 g. Saliva from these glands is emptied into the oral cavity by Wharton duct, which is about 40 mm long. The duct opens at the side of frenulum of tongue, by means of a small opening on the summit of papilla called caruncula sublingualis.
- *Sublingual glands:* Sublingual glands are the smallest salivary glands situated in the mucosa at the floor of the mouth. Each gland weighs about 2 to 3 g. Saliva from these glands is poured into 5 to 15 small ducts called ducts of Rivinus. These ducts open on small papillae beneath the tongue. One of the ducts is larger and it is called Bartholin duct. It drains the anterior part of the gland and opens on caruncula sublingualis near the opening of submaxillary duct.

### Minor Salivary Glands

- *Lingual mucus glands:* Lingual mucus glands are situated in posterior one third of the tongue, behind circumvallate papillae and at the tip and margins of tongue.
- *Lingual serous glands:* Lingual serous glands are located near circumvallate papillae and filiform papillae.
- *Buccal glands:* Buccal glands or molar glands are present between the mucous membrane and buccinator muscle. Four to five of these are larger and situated outside buccinator, around the terminal part of parotid duct.
- *Labial glands:* Labial glands are situated beneath the mucous membrane around the orifice of mouth.
- *Palatal glands:* Palatal glands are found beneath the mucous membrane of the soft palate.

## Stomach

### Functional Anatomy of Stomach

Stomach is a hollow organ situated just below the diaphragm on the left side in the abdominal cavity.

Volume of empty stomach is 50 mL. Under normal conditions, it can expand to accommodate 1 to 1.5 L of solids and liquids. However, it is capable of expanding still further up to 4 L.

### Parts of Stomach

In humans, stomach has four parts:

1. Cardiac region
2. Fundus
3. Body or corpus
4. Pyloric region.

- *Cardiac region:* Cardiac region is the upper part of the stomach where esophagus opens. The opening is guarded by a sphincter called cardiac sphincter, which opens only towards stomach. This portion is also known as cardiac end.
- *Fundus:* Fundus is a small domeshaped structure. It is elevated above the level of esophageal opening.
- *Body or corpus:* Body is the largest part of stomach forming about 75 to 80% of the whole stomach. It extends from just below the fundus up to the pyloric region.
- *Pyloric region:* Pyloric region has two parts, antrum and pyloric canal. The body of stomach ends in antrum. Junction between body and antrum is marked by an angular notch called incisura angularis. Antrum is continued as the narrow canal, which is called pyloric canal or pyloric end. Pyloric canal opens into first part of small intestine called duodenum. The opening of pyloric canal is guarded by a sphincter called pyloric sphincter. It opens towards duodenum. Stomach has two curvatures. One on the right side is lesser curvature and the other on left side is greater curvature.

### Structure of Stomach Wall

Stomach wall is formed by four layers of structures:

1. ***Outer serous layer:*** Formed by peritoneum.
2. ***Muscular layer:*** Made up of three layers of smooth muscle fibers, namely inner oblique, middle circular and outer longitudinal layers.
3. ***Submucus layer:*** Formed by areolar tissue, blood vessels, lymph vessels and Meissner nerve plexus.
4. ***Inner mucus layer:*** Lined by mucus-secreting columnar epithelial cells. The gastric glands are situated in this layer. Under resting conditions, the mucosa of the stomach is thrown into many folds. These folds are called rugae. The rugae disappear when the stomach is distended after meals. Throughout the inner mucus layer, small depressions called gastric pits are present. Glands of the stomach open into these pits. Inner surface of mucus layer is covered by 2 mm thick mucus.

### Glands of Stomach (Gastric Glands)

Glands of the stomach or gastric glands are tubular structures made up of different types of cells. These glands open into the stomach cavity via gastric pits.

*Classification of Glands of the Stomach*

Gastric glands are classified into three types, on the basis of their location in the stomach:

1. ***Fundic glands or main gastric glands or oxyntic glands:*** Situated in body and fundus of stomach.
2. ***Pyloric glands:*** Present in the pyloric part of the stomach
3. ***Cardiac glands:*** Located in the cardiac region of the stomach.

*Structure of Gastric Glands*

1. ***Fundic glands:*** Fundic glands are considered as the typical gastric glands. These glands are long and tubular. Each gland has three parts, viz. body, neck and isthmus.

Cells of Fundic Glands

- Chief cells or pepsinogen cells
- Parietal cells or oxyntic cells
- Mucus neck cells
- Enterochromaffin (EC) cells or Kulchitsky cells
- Enterochromaffin-like (ECL) cells.

  Parietal cells are different from other cells of the gland because of the presence of canaliculi (singular = canaliculus). Parietal cells empty their secretions into the lumen of the gland through the canaliculi. But, other cells empty their secretions directly into lumen of the gland.

2. ***Pyloric glands:*** Pyloric glands are short and tortuous in nature. These glands are formed by G cells, mucus cells, EC cells and ECL cells.
3. ***Cardiac glands:*** Cardiac glands are also short and tortuous in structure, with many mucus cells. EC cells, ECL cells and chief cells are also present in the cardiac glands.

- ***Enteroendocrine cells:*** Enteroendocrine cells are the hormon-esecreting cells present in the glands or mucosa of gastrointestinal tract, particularly stomach and intestine. The enteroendocrine cells present in gastric glands are G cells, EC cells and ECL cells.

### Functions of Stomach

- Mechanical function
  - ***Storage function:*** Food is stored in the stomach for a long period, i.e. for 3 to 4 hours and emptied into the intestine slowly. The maximum capacity of stomach is up to 1.5 L. Slow emptying of stomach provides enough time for proper digestion and absorption of food substances in the small intestine.
  - ***Formation of chyme:*** Peristaltic movements of stomach mix the bolus with gastric juice and convert it into the semisolid material known as chyme.
- ***Digestive function:*** Refer functions of gastric juice.
- ***Protective function:*** Refer functions of gastric juice.
- ***Hemopoietic function:*** Refer functions of gastric juice.
- ***Excretory function:*** Many substances like toxins, alkaloids and metals are excreted through gastric juice.

### Properties and Composition of Gastric Juice

Gastric juice is a mixture of secretions from different gastric glands.

*Properties of Gastric Juice*

- Volume: 1200 mL/day to 1500 mL/day.
- Reaction: Gastric juice is highly acidic with a pH of 0.9 to 1.2. Acidity of gastric juice is due to the presence of hydrochloric acid.
- Specific gravity: 1.002 to 1.004

*Composition of Gastric Juice*

Gastric juice contains 99.5% of water and 0.5% solids. Solids are organic and inorganic substances.

*Functions of Gastric Juice/Functions of Gastric Glands*

Function of the gastric gland is to secrete gastric juice. Secretory activities of different cells of gastric glands and enteroendocrine cells are listed in:

- ***Digestive function:*** Gastric juice acts mainly on proteins. Proteolytic enzymes of the gastric juice are pepsin and rennin.

  Gastric juice also contains some other enzymes like gastric lipase, gelatinase, urase and gastric amylase.
  - ***Pepsin:*** Pepsin is secreted as inactive pepsinogen. Pepsinogen is converted into pepsin by hydrochloric acid. Optimum pH for activation of pepsinogen is below 6.
  - ***Action of pepsin:*** Pepsin converts proteins into proteoses, peptones and polypeptides. Pepsin also causes curdling and digestion of milk (casein).
  - ***Gastric lipase:*** Gastric lipase is a weak lipolytic enzyme when compared to pancreatic lipase. It is active only when the pH is between 4 and 5 and becomes inactive at a pH below 2.5. Gastric lipase is a tributyrase and it hydrolyzes tributyrin (butter fat) into fatty acids and glycerols.
  - ***Actions of other enzymes of gastric juice:***
    - ***Gelatinase:*** Degrades type I and type V gelatin and type IV and V collagen (which are proteoglycans in meat) into peptides.

- ➢ *Urase:* Acts on urea and produces ammonia.
- ➢ *Gastric amylase:* Degrades starch (but its action is insignificant).
- ➢ *Rennin:* Curdles milk (present in animals only).

- *Hemopoietic function:* Intrinsic factor of Castle, secreted by parietal cells of gastric glands plays an important role in erythropoiesis.
  It is necessary for the absorption of vitamin $B_{12}$ (which is called extrinsic factor) from GI tract into the blood. Vitamin $B_{12}$ is an important maturation factor during erythropoiesis. Absence of intrinsic factor in gastric juice causes deficiency of vitamin B12, leading to pernicious anemia.
- *Protective function–function of mucus:* Mucus is a mucoprotein, secreted by mucus neck cells of the gastric glands and surface mucus cells in fundus, body and other parts of stomach. It protects the gastric wall by the following ways:
  - Protects the stomach wall from irritation or mechanical injury, by virtue of its high viscosity.
  - Prevents the digestive action of pepsin on the wall of the stomach, particularly gastric mucosa.
  - Protects the gastric mucosa from hydrochloric acid of gastric juice because of its alkaline nature and its acid-combining power.
- *Functions of hydrochloric acid:* Hydrochloric acid is present in the gastric juice:
  - Activates pepsinogen into pepsin
  - Kills some of the bacteria entering the stomach along with food substances. This action is called bacteriolytic action
  - Provides acid medium, which is necessary for the action of hormones.

## Functional Anatomy of Liver and Biliary System

Liver is a dual organ having both secretory and excretory functions. It is the largest gland in the body, weighing about 1.5 kg in man. It is located in the upper and right side of the abdominal cavity, immediately beneath diaphragm.

### Liver

- *Hepatic lobes:* Liver is made up of many lobes called hepatic lobes. Each lobe consists of many lobules called hepatic lobules.
- *Hepatic lobules:* Hepatic lobule is the structural and functional unit of liver. There are about 50,000 to 100,000 lobules in the liver. The lobule is a honeycomb-like structure and it is made up of liver cells called hepatocytes.
- *Hepatocytes and hepatic plates:* Hepatocytes are arranged in columns, which form the hepatic plates. Each plate is made up of two columns of cells. In between the two columns of each plate lies a bile canaliculus. In between the neighboring plates, a blood space called sinusoid is present.
  Sinusoid is lined by the endothelial cells. In between the endothelial cells some special macrophages called Kupffer cells are present.
- *Portal triads:* Each lobule is surrounded by many portal triads. Each portal triad consists of three vessels:
  1. A branch of hepatic artery
  2. A branch of portal vein
  3. A tributary of bile duct.

  Branches of hepatic artery and portal vein open into the sinusoid. Sinusoid opens into the central vein. Central vein empties into hepatic vein.

  Bile is secreted by hepatic cells and emptied into bile canaliculus. From canaliculus, the bile enters the tributary of bile duct. Tributaries of bile duct from canaliculi of neighboring lobules unite to form small bile ducts. These small bile ducts join together and finally form left and right hepatic ducts, which emerge out of liver.

### Biliary System

Biliary system or extrahepatic biliary apparatus is formed by gallbladder and extrahepatic bile ducts (bile ducts outside the liver). Right and left hepatic bile ducts which come out of liver join to form common hepatic duct. It unites with the cystic duct from gallbladder to form common bile duct. All these ducts have similar structures.

Common bile duct unites with pancreatic duct to form the common hepatopancreatic duct or ampulla of Vater, which opens into the duodenum.

There is a sphincter called sphincter of Oddi at the lower part of common bile duct, before it joins the pancreatic duct. It is formed by smooth muscle fibers of common bile duct. It is normally kept closed; so the bile secreted from liver enters gallbladder where it is stored.

Upon appropriate stimulation, the sphincter opens and allows flow of bile from gallbladder into the intestine.

### Blood Supply to Liver

Liver receives maximum blood supply of about 1,500 mL/minute. It receives blood from two sources, namely the hepatic artery and portal vein.

#### Hepatic Artery

Hepatic artery arises directly from aorta and supplies oxygenated blood to liver. After entering the liver, the hepatic artery divides into many branches. Each branch enters a portal triad.

#### Portal Vein

Portal vein is formed by superior mesenteric vein and splenic vein. It brings deoxygenated blood from stomach, intestine, spleen and pancreas. Portal blood is rich in monosaccharides and amino acids. It also contains bile salts, bilirubin, urobilinogen and GI hormones. However, the oxygen content is less in portal blood.

Flow of blood from intestine to liver through portal vein is known as enterohepatic circulation. The blood from hepatic artery mixes with blood from portal vein in hepatic sinusoids. Hepatic cells obtain oxygen and nutrients from the sinusoid.

#### Hepatic Vein

Substances synthesized by hepatic cells, waste products and carbon dioxide are discharged into sinusoids. Sinusoids drain them into central vein of the lobule. Central veins from many lobules unite to form bigger veins, which ultimately form hepatic veins (right and left) which open into inferior vena cava.

## Properties and Composition of Bile

*Properties of Bile*

- Volume: 800 to 1,200 mL/day
- Reaction: Alkaline
- pH: 8 to 8.6
- Specific gravity: 1.010 to 1.011
- Color: Golden yellow or green.

*Composition of Bile*

Bile contains 97.6% of water and 2.4% of solids. Solids include organic and inorganic substances.

## Secretion of Bile

Bile is secreted by hepatocytes. The initial bile secreted by hepatocytes contains large quantity of bile acids, bile pigments, cholesterol, lecithin and fatty acids. From hepatocytes, bile is released into canaliculi. From here, it passes through small ducts and hepatic ducts and reaches the common hepatic duct. From common hepatic duct, bile is diverted either directly into the intestine or into the gallbladder. Sodium, bicarbonate and water are added to bile when it passes through the ducts. These substances are secreted by the epithelial cells of the ducts. Addition of sodium, bicarbonate and water increases the total quantity of bile.

## Storage of Bile

Most of the bile from liver enters the gallbladder, where it is stored. It is released from gallbladder into the intestine whenever it is required. When bile is stored in gallbladder, it undergoes many changes both in quality and quantity such as:

- Volume is decreased because of absorption of a large amount of water and electrolytes (except calcium and potassium)
- Concentration of bile salts, bile pigments, cholesterol, fatty acids and lecithin is increased because of absorption of water and electrolytes
- The pH is decreased slightly
- Specific gravity is increased
- Mucin is added to bile

## Bile Salts

Bile salts are the sodium and potassium salts of bile acids, which are conjugated with glycine or taurine.

*Formation of Bile Salts*

Bile salts are formed from bile acids. There are two primary bile acids in human, namely cholic acid and chenodeoxycholic acid, which are formed in liver and enter the intestine through bile. Due to the bacterial action in the intestine, the primary bile acids are converted into secondary bile acids:

- Cholic acid → deoxycholic acid
- Chenodeoxycholic acid → lithocholic acid

Secondary bile acids from intestine are transported back to liver through enterohepatic circulation. In liver, the secondary bile acids are conjugated with glycine (amino acid) or taurin (derivative of an amino acid) and form conjugated bile acids, namely glycocholic acid and taurocholic acids. These bile acids combine with sodium or potassium ions to form the salts, sodium or potassium glycocholate and sodium or potassium taurocholate.

*Enterohepatic Circulation of Bile Salts*

Enterohepatic circulation is the transport of substances from small intestine to liver through portal vein. About 90 to 95% of bile salts from intestine are transported to liver through enterohepatic circulation. Remaining 5 to 10% of the bile salts enter large intestine. Here, the bile salts are converted into deoxycholate and lithocholate, which are excreted in feces.

*Functions of Bile Salts*

Bile salts are required for digestion and absorption of fats in the intestine. The functions of bile salts are:

- ***Emulsification of fats:*** Emulsification is the process by which the fat globules are broken down into minute droplets and made in the form of a milky fluid called emulsion in small intestine, by the action of bile salts.
  Lipolytic enzymes of GI tract cannot digest the fats directly because the fats are insoluble in water due to the surface tension. Bile salts emulsify the fats by reducing the surface tension due to their detergent action. Now the fats can be easily digested by lipolytic enzymes.
  Unemulsified fat usually passes through the intestine and then it is eliminated in feces.
  Emulsification of fats by bile salts needs the presence of lecithin from bile.
- ***Absorption of fats:*** Bile salts help in the absorption of digested fats from intestine into blood. Bile salts combine with fats and make complexes of fats called micelles. The fats in the form of micelles can be absorbed easily.
- ***Choleretic action:*** Bile salts stimulate the secretion of bile from liver. This action is called choleretic action.
- ***Cholagogue action:*** Cholagogue is an agent which causes contraction of gallbladder and release of bile into the intestine. Bile salts act as cholagogues indirectly by stimulating the secretion of hormone cholecystokinin. This hormone causes contraction of gallbladder, resulting in release of bile.
- ***Laxative action:*** Laxative is an agent which induces defecation. Bile salts act as laxatives by stimulating peristaltic movements of the intestine.
- ***Prevention of gallstone formation:*** Bile salts prevent the formation of gallstone by keeping the cholesterol and lecithin in solution. In the absence of bile salts, cholesterol precipitates along with lecithin and forms gallstone.

## Bile Pigments

Bile pigments are the excretory products in bile. Bilirubin and biliverdin are the two bile pigments and bilirubin is the major bile pigment in human beings.

Bile pigments are formed during the breakdown of hemoglobin, which is released from the destroyed RBCs in the reticuloendothelial system.

*Formation and Excretion of Bile Pigments*

Stages of formation and circulation of bile pigments:

- Senile erythrocytes are destroyed in reticuloendothelial system and hemoglobin is released from them.
- Hemoglobin is broken into globin and heme.
- Heme is split into iron and the pigment biliverdin.
- Iron goes to iron pool and is reused.
- First formed pigment biliverdin is reduced to bilirubin.
- Bilirubin is released into blood from the reticuloendothelial cells.
- In blood, the bilirubin is transported by the plasma protein, albumin. Bilirubin circulating in the blood is called free bilirubin or unconjugated bilirubin.
- Within few hours after entering the circulation, the free bilirubin is taken up by the liver cells.
- In the liver, it is conjugated with glucuronic acid to form conjugated bilirubin.
- Conjugated bilirubin is then excreted into intestine through bile.

*Fate of Conjugated Bilirubin*

Stages of excretion of conjugated bilirubin:

- In intestine, 50% of the conjugated bilirubin is converted into urobilinogen by intestinal bacteria.
  First the conjugated bilirubin is deconjugated into free bilirubin, which is later reduced into urobilinogen.
- Remaining 50% of conjugated bilirubin from intestine is absorbed into blood and enters the liver through portal vein (enterohepatic circulation). From liver, it is reexcreted in bile.
- Most of the urobilinogen from intestine enters liver via enterohepatic circulation. Later, it is reexcreted through bile.
- About 5% of urobilinogen is excreted by kidney through urine. In urine, due to exposure to air, the urobilinogen is converted into urobilin by oxidation.
- Some of the urobilinogen is excreted in feces as stercobilinogen. In feces, stercobilinogen is oxidized to stercobilin.

*Normal Plasma Levels of Bilirubin*

Normal bilirubin (total bilirubin) content in plasma is 0.5 to 1.5 mg/dL. When it exceeds 1mg/dL, the condition is called hyperbilirubinemia. When it exceeds 2 mg/dL, jaundice occurs.

## Functions of Bile

Most of the functions of bile are due to the bile salts.

- ***Digestive function:*** Refer functions of bile salts.
- ***Absorptive functions:*** Refer functions of bile salts.
- ***Excretory functions:*** Bile pigments are the major excretory products of the bile. Other substances excreted in bile are:
  - Heavy metals like copper and iron
  - Some bacteria like typhoid bacteria
  - Some toxins
  - Cholesterol
  - Lecithin
  - Alkaline phosphatase.
- ***Laxative action:*** Bile salts act as laxatives.
- ***Antiseptic action:*** Bile inhibits the growth of certain bacteria in the lumen of intestine by its natural detergent action.
- ***Choleretic action:*** Bile salts have the choleretic action.
- ***Maintenance of pH in gastrointestinal tract:*** As bile is highly alkaline, it neutralizes the acid chime which enters the intestine from stomach. Thus, an optimum pH is maintained for the action of digestive enzymes.
- ***Prevention of gallstone formation:*** Refer function of bile salts.
- ***Lubrication function:*** The mucin in bile acts as a lubricant for the chyme in intestine.
- ***Cholagogue action:*** Bile salts act as cholagogues.

## Functions of Liver

Liver is the largest gland and one of the vital organs of the body. It performs many vital metabolic and homeostatic functions, which are summarized below.

- ***Metabolic function:*** Liver is the organ where maximum metabolic reactions such as metabolism of carbohydrates, proteins, fats, vitamins and many hormones are carried out.
- ***Storage function:*** Many substances like glycogen, amino acids, iron, folic acid and vitamins A, $B_{12}$ and D are stored in liver.
- ***Synthetic function:*** Liver produces glucose by gluconeogenesis. It synthesizes all the plasma proteins and other proteins (except immunoglobulins) such as clotting factors, complement factors and hormone-binding proteins. It also synthesizes steroids, somatomedin and heparin.
- ***Secretion of bile:*** Liver secretes bile which contains bile salts, bile pigments, cholesterol, fatty acids and lecithin. The functions of bile are mainly due to bile salts. Bile salts are required for digestion and absorption of fats in the intestine. Bile helps to carry away waste products and breakdown fats, which are excreted through feces or urine.
- ***Excretory function:*** Liver excretes cholesterol, bile pigments, heavy metals (like lead, arsenic and bismuth), toxins, bacteria and virus (like that of yellow fever) through bile.
- ***Heat production:*** Enormous amount of heat is produced in the liver because of metabolic reactions. Liver is the organ where maximum heat is produced.
- ***Hemopoietic function:*** In fetus (hepatic stage), liver produces the blood cells. It stores vitamin $B_{12}$ necessary for erythropoiesis and iron necessary for synthesis of hemoglobin. Liver produces thrombopoietin that promotes production of thrombocytes.
- ***Hemolytic function:*** The senile RBCs after a lifespan of 120 days are destroyed by reticuloendothelial cells (Kupffer cells) of liver.
- ***Inactivation of hormones and drugs:*** Liver catabolizes the hormones such as growth hormone, parathormone, cortisol, insulin, glucagon and estrogen. It also inactivates the drugs, particularly the fat-soluble drugs. The fat-soluble drugs are converted into water-soluble substances, which are excreted through bile or urine.
- ***Defensive and detoxification functions:*** Reticuloendothelial cells (Kupffer cells) of the liver play an important role

in the defense of the body. Liver is also involved in the detoxification of the foreign bodies.
- Foreign bodies such as bacteria or antigens are swallowed and digested by reticuloendothelial cells of liver by means of phagocytosis.
- Reticuloendothelial cells of liver also produce substances like interleukins and tumor necrosis factors, which activate the immune system of the body.
- Liver cells are involved in the removal of toxic property of various harmful substances. Removal of toxic property of the harmful agent is known as detoxification.

  Detoxification in liver occurs in two ways:
- Total destruction of the substances by means of metabolic degradation.
- Conversion of toxic substances into nontoxic materials by means of conjugation with glucuronic acid or sulfates.

## Gallbladder

Bile secreted from liver is stored in gallbladder. The capacity of gallbladder is approximately 50 mL.

Gallbladder is not essential for life and it is removed (cholecystectomy) in patients suffering from gallbladder dysfunction. After cholecystectomy, patients do not suffer from any major disadvantage. In some species, gallbladder is absent.

### *Functions of Gallbladder*

Major functions of gallbladder are the storage and concentration of bile.

- ***Storage of bile:*** Bile is continuously secreted from liver. But it is released into intestine only intermittently and most of the bile is stored in gallbladder till it is required.
- ***Concentration of bile:*** Bile is concentrated while it is stored in gallbladder.

  The mucosa of gallbladder rapidly reabsorbs water and electrolytes, except calcium and potassium. But the bile salts, bile pigments, cholesterol and lecithin are not reabsorbed. So, the concentration of these substances in bile increases 5 to 10 times.
- ***Alteration of pH of bile:*** The pH of bile decreases from 8–8.6 to 7–7.6 and it becomes less alkaline when it is stored in gallbladder.
- ***Secretion of mucin:*** Gallbladder secretes mucin and adds it to bile. When bile is released into the intestine, mucin acts as a lubricant for movement of chyme in the intestine.
- ***Maintenance of pressure in biliary system:*** Due to the concentrating capacity, gallbladder maintains a pressure of about 7 cm $H_2O$ in biliary system. This pressure in the biliary system is essential for the release of bile into the intestine.

## RENAL PHYSIOLOGY

### Kidney

### *Introduction*

Excretion is the process by which the unwanted substances and metabolic wastes are eliminated from the body.

A large amount of waste materials and carbon dioxide are produced in the tissues during metabolic process. In addition, residue of undigested food, heavy metals, drugs, toxic substances and pathogenic organisms like bacteria are also present in the body. All these substances must be removed to keep the body in healthy condition. Various systems/organs in the body are involved in performing the excretory function, viz.

- Digestive system excretes food residues in the form of feces. Some bacteria and toxic substances also are excreted through feces.
- Lungs remove carbon dioxide and water vapor.
- Skin excretes water, salts and some wastes. It also removes heat from the body.
- Liver excretes many substances like bile pigments, heavy metals, drugs, toxins, bacteria, etc. through bile.

Although various organs are involved in removal of wastes from the body, their excretory capacity is limited. But renal system or urinary system has maximum excretory capacity and so it plays a major role in homeostasis. Renal system includes:

- A pair of kidneys
- Ureters
- Urinary bladder
- Urethra.

Kidneys produce the urine. Ureters transport the urine to urinary bladder. Urinary bladder stores the urine until it is voided (emptied). Urine is voided from bladder through urethra.

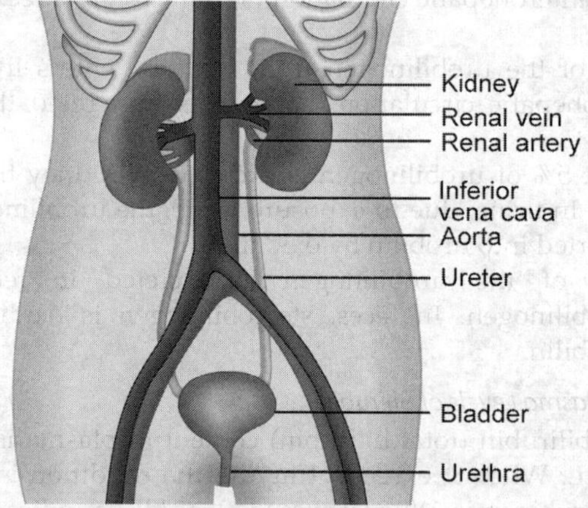


### *Functions of Kidney*

Kidneys perform several vital functions besides formation of urine. By excreting urine, kidneys play the principal role in homeostasis. Thus, the functions of kidney are:

#### *Role in Homeostasis*

Primary function of kidneys is homeostasis. It is accomplished by the formation of urine. During the formation of urine, kidneys regulate various activities in the body, which are concerned with homeostasis such as:

- ***Excretion of waste products:*** Kidneys excrete the unwanted waste products, which are formed during metabolic activities:

- Urea (end product of amino acid metabolism)
- Uric acid (end product of nucleic acid metabolism)
- Creatinine (end product of metabolism in muscles)
- Bilirubin (end product of hemoglobin degradation)
- Products of metabolism of other substances. Kidneys also excrete harmful foreign chemical substances such as toxins, drugs, heavy metals pesticides, etc.

• ***Maintenance of water balance:*** Kidneys maintain the water balance in the body by conserving water when it is decreased and excreting water when it is excess in the body. This is an important process for homeostasis.
• ***Maintenance of electrolyte balance:*** Maintenance of electrolyte balance, especially sodium is in relation to water balance. Kidneys retain sodium if the osmolarity of body water decreases and eliminate sodium when osmolarity increases.
• ***Maintenance of acid–base balance:*** The pH of the blood and body fluids should be maintained within narrow range for healthy living. It is achieved by the function of kidney. Body is under constant threat to develop acidosis, because of production of lot of acids during metabolic activities. However, it is prevented by kidneys, lungs and blood buffers, which eliminate these acids. Among these organs, kidneys play major role in preventing acidosis. In fact, kidneys are the only organs, which are capable of eliminating certain metabolic acids like sulfuric and phosphoric acids.

*Hemopoietic Function*

Kidneys stimulate the production of erythrocytes by secreting erythropoietin. Erythropoietin is the important stimulating factor for erythropoiesis. Kidney also secretes another factor called thrombopoietin, which stimulates the production of thrombocytes.

*Endocrine Function*

Kidneys secrete many hormonal substances in addition to erythropoietin and thrombopoietin. Hormones secreted by kidneys:
• Erythropoietin
• Thrombopoietin
• Renin
• 1, 25-dihydroxycholecalciferol (calcitriol)
• Prostaglandins.

*Regulation of Blood Pressure*

Kidneys play an important role in the long-term regulation of arterial blood pressure by two ways:
• By regulating the volume of extracellular fluid
• Through renin-angiotensin mechanism.

*Regulation of Blood Calcium Level*

Kidneys play a role in the regulation of blood calcium level by activating 1,25-dihydroxycholecalciferol into vitamin D. Vitamin D is necessary for the absorption of calcium from intestine.

## *Functional Anatomy of Kidney*

Kidney is a compound tubular gland covered by a connective tissue capsule. There is a depression on the medial border of kidney called hilum, through which renal artery, renal veins, nerves and ureter pass.

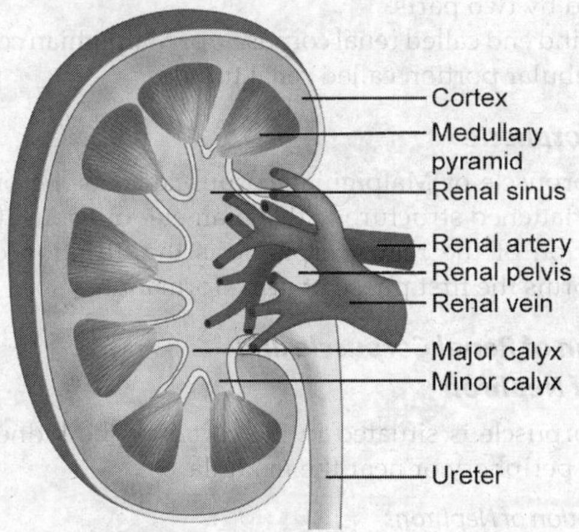


*Different Layers of Kidney*

Components of kidney are arranged in three layers:
1. Outer cortex
2. Inner medulla
3. Renal sinus.

1. ***Outer cortex:*** Cortex is dark and granular in appearance. It contains renal corpuscles and convoluted tubules. At intervals, cortical tissue penetrates medulla in the form of columns, which are called renal columns or columns of Bertini.
2. ***Inner medulla:*** Medulla contains tubular and vascular structures arranged in parallel radial lines. Medullary mass is divided into 8 to 18 medullary or Malpighian pyramids. Broad base of each pyramid is in contact with cortex and the apex projects into minor calyx.
3. ***Renal sinus:*** Renal sinus consists of the following structures:
   - Upper expanded part of ureter called renal pelvis
   - Subdivisions of pelvis: 2 or 3 major calyces and about 8 minor calyces
   - Branches of nerves, arteries and tributaries of veins
   - Loose connective tissues and fat.

*Tubular Structures of Kidney*

Kidney is made up of closely arranged tubular structures called uriniferous tubules. Blood vessels and interstitial connective tissues are interposed between these tubules. Uriniferous tubules include:
• Terminal or secretary tubules called nephrons, which are concerned with formation of urine.
• Collecting ducts or tubules, which are concerned with transport of urine from nephrons to pelvis of ureter.
• Collecting ducts unite to form ducts of Bellini, which open into minor calyces through papilla.

## Nephron

### *Introduction*

Nephron is defined as the structural and functional unit of kidney. Each kidney consists of 1 to 1.3 millions of nephrons.

The number of nephrons starts decreasing after about 45 to 50 years of age at the rate of 0.8 to 1% every year. Each nephron is formed by two parts:

1. A blind end called renal corpuscle or Malpighian corpuscle.
2. A tubular portion called renal tubule.

### Renal Corpuscle

Renal corpuscle or Malpighian corpuscle is a spheroidal and slightly flattened structure with a diameter of about 200 μ.

Function of the renal corpuscle is the filtration of blood which forms the first phase of urine formation.

### Situation of Renal Corpuscle and Types of Nephron

Renal corpuscle is situated in the cortex of the kidney either near the periphery or near the medulla.

#### *Classification of Nephrons*

Based on the situation of renal corpuscle, the nephrons are classified into two types:

1. Cortical nephrons or superficial nephrons: Nephrons having the corpuscles in outer cortex of the kidney near the periphery. In human kidneys, 85% nephrons are cortical nephrons.
2. Juxtamedullary nephrons: Nephrons having the corpuscles in inner cortex near medulla or corticomedullary junction.

### Structure of Renal Corpuscle

Renal corpuscle is formed by two portions:

1. Glomerulus
2. Bowman capsule.

#### *Glomerulus*

Glomerulus is a tuft of capillaries enclosed by Bowman capsule. It consists of glomerular capillaries interposed between afferent arteriole on one end and efferent arteriole on the other end. Thus, the vascular system in the glomerulus is purely arterial.

Glomerular capillaries arise from the afferent arteriole. After entering the Bowman capsule, the afferent arteriole divides into 4 or 5 large capillaries. Each large capillary subdivides into many small capillaries. These small capillaries are arranged in irregular loops and form anastomosis. All the smaller capillaries finally reunite to form the efferent arteriole, which leaves the Bowman capsule.

Diameter of the efferent arteriole is less than that of afferent arteriole. This difference in diameter has got functional significance.

#### Functional Histology

Glomerular capillaries are made up of single layer of endothelial cells, which are attached to a basement membrane. Endothelium has many pores called fenestrae or filtration pores. Diameter of each pore is 0.1 μ. Presence of the fenestra is the evidence of the filtration function of the glomerulus.

#### *Bowman Capsule*

Bowman capsule is a capsular structure, which encloses the glomerulus. It is formed by two layers:

1. Inner visceral layer
2. Outer parietal layer.

Visceral layer covers the glomerular capillaries. It is continued as the parietal layer at the visceral pole. Parietal layer is continued with the wall of the tubular portion of nephron. The cleft-like space between the visceral and parietal layers is continued as the lumen of the tubular portion.

Functional anatomy of Bowman capsule resembles a funnel with filter paper. Diameter of Bowman capsule is 200 μ.

#### Functional Histology

Both the layers of Bowman capsule are composed of a single layer of flattened epithelial cells resting on a basement membrane. Basement membrane of the visceral layer fuses with the basement membrane of glomerular capillaries on which the capillary endothelial cells are arranged. Thus, the basement membranes, which are fused together, form the separation between the glomerular capillary endothelium and the epithelium of visceral layer of Bowman capsule. Epithelial cells of the visceral layer fuse with the basement membrane but the fusion is not complete.

Each cell is connected with basement membrane by cytoplasmic extensions of epithelial cells called pedicles or feet. These pedicles are arranged in an interdigitating manner leaving small cleft-like spaces in between. The cleft-like space is called slit pore. Epithelial cells with pedicles are called podocytes.

### Tubular Portion of Nephron

Tubular portion of nephron is the continuation of Bowman capsule. It is made up of three parts:

1. Proximal convoluted tubule
2. Loop of Henle
3. Distal convoluted tubule.

#### *Proximal Convoluted Tubule*

Proximal convoluted tubule is the coiled portion arising from Bowman capsule. It is situated in the cortex. It is continued as descending limb of loop of Henle. Length of proximal convoluted tubule is 14 mm and the diameter is 55 μ. Proximal convoluted tubule is continued as loop of Henle.

#### Functional Histology

Proximal convoluted tubule is formed by single layer of cuboidal epithelial cells. Characteristic feature of these cells is the presence of hair-like projections directed towards the lumen of the tubule. Because of the presence of these projections, the epithelial cells are called brush-bordered cells.

#### *Loop of Henle*

Loop of Henle consists of:

- Descending limb
- Hairpin bend
- Ascending limb.
- ***Descending limb:*** Descending limb of loop of Henle is made up of two segments:
  1. Thick descending segment
  2. Thin descending segment.
  - ***Thick descending segment:*** Thick descending segment is the direct continuation of the proximal convoluted

tubule. It descends down into medulla. It has a length of 6 mm and a diameter of 55 μ.

It is formed by brushbordered cuboidal epithelial cells.

- *Thin descending segment:* Thick descending segment is continued as thin descending segment. It is formed by flattened epithelial cells without brush border and it is continued as hairpin bend of the loop.

- ***Hairpin bend:*** Hairpin bend formed by flattened epithelial cells without brush border and it is continued as the ascending limb of loop of Henle.
- ***Ascending limb:*** Ascending limb or segment of Henle loop has two parts:
  1. Thin ascending segment
  2. Thick ascending segment.
  - *Thin ascending segment:* Thin ascending segment is the continuation of hairpin bend. It is also lined by flattened epithelial cells without brush border.

Total length of thin descending segment, hairpin bend and thin ascending segment of Henle loop is 10 to 15 mm and the diameter is 15 μ. Thin ascending segment is continued as thick ascending segment.

- *Thick ascending segment:* Thick ascending segment is about 9 mm long with a diameter of 30 μ. Thick ascending segment is lined by cuboidal epithelial cells without brush border.

  The terminal portion of thick ascending segment, which runs between the afferent and efferent arterioles of the same nephrons forms the macula densa. Macula densa is the part of juxtaglomerular apparatus. Thick ascending segment ascends to the cortex and continues as distal convoluted tubule.

- ***Length and extent of loop of Henle:*** Length and the extent of the loop of Henle vary in different nephrons:
  - In cortical nephrons, it is short and the hairpin bend penetrates only up to outer medulla.
  - In juxtamedullary nephrons, this is long and the hairpin bend extends deep into the inner medulla. In some nephrons, it even runs up to the papilla.

*Distal Convoluted Tubule*

Distal convoluted tubule is the continuation of thick ascending segment and occupies the cortex of kidney.

It is continued as collecting duct. The length of the distal convoluted tubule is 14.5 to 15 mm. It has a diameter of 22 to 50 μ.

Functional Histology

Distal convoluted tubule is lined by single layer of cuboidal epithelial cells without brush border. Epithelial cells in distal convoluted tubule are called intercalated cells (I cells).

### Collecting Duct

Distal convoluted tubule continues as the initial or arched collecting duct, which is in cortex. The lower part of the collecting duct lies in medulla. Seven to ten initial collecting ducts unite to form the straight collecting duct, which passes through medulla.

Length of the collecting duct is 20 to 22 mm and its diameter varies between 40 and 200 μ. Collecting duct is formed by cuboidal or columnar epithelial cells.

*Functional Histology*

Collecting duct is formed by two types of epithelial cells:
1. Principal or P cells
2. Intercalated or I cells.

These two types of cells have some functional significance.

### Passage of Urine

At the inner zone of medulla, the straight collecting ducts from each medullary pyramid unite to form papillary ducts or ducts of Bellini, which open into a 'V' shaped area called papilla. Urine from each medullary pyramid is collected in the papilla. From here it is drained into a minor calyx. Three or four minor calyces unite to form one major calyx. Each kidney has got about 8 minor calyces and 2 to 3 major calyces.

From minor calyces urine passes through major calyces, which open into the pelvis of the ureter. Pelvis is the expanded portion of ureter present in the renal sinus. From renal pelvis, urine passes through remaining portion of ureter and reaches urinary bladder.

## Juxtaglomerular Apparatus

### Definition

Juxtaglomerular apparatus is a specialized organ situated near the glomerulus of each nephron (juxta = near).

### Functions of Juxtaglomerular Apparatus

Primary function of juxtaglomerular apparatus is the secretion of hormones. It also regulates the glomerular blood flow and glomerular filtration rate.

*Secretion of Hormones*

Juxtaglomerular apparatus secretes two hormones:
1. Renin
2. Prostaglandin.

Renin

Juxtaglomerular cells secrete renin. Renin is a peptide with 340 amino acids. Along with angiotensins, rennin forms the renin-angiotensin system, which is a hormone system that plays an important role in the maintenance of blood pressure.

- ***Stimulants for renin secretion:*** Secretion of renin is stimulated by four factors:
  (i) Fall in arterial blood pressure
  (ii) Reduction in the ECF volume
  (iii) Increased sympathetic activity
  (iv) Decreased load of sodium and chloride in macula densa.
- ***Renin-angiotensin system:*** When renin is released into the blood, it acts on a specific plasma protein called angiotensinogen or rennin substrate. It is the α2-globulin. By the activity of renin, the angiotensinogen is converted into a decapeptide called angiotensin I. Angiotensin I is converted into angiotensin II, which is an octapeptide by the activity of angiotensin-converting enzyme (ACE) secreted from lungs. Most of the conversion of angiotensin I into angiotensin II takes place in lungs. Angiotensin II has a short half-life of about 1 to 2 minutes. Then it is rapidly degraded into a heptapeptide called angiotensin III by

angiotensinases, which are present in RBCs and vascular beds in many tissues. Angiotensin III is converted into angiotensin IV, which is a hexapeptide.

- *Actions of angiotensins*
  - ***Angiotensin I:*** Angiotensin I is physiologically inactive and serves only as the precursor of angiotensin II.
  - ***Angiotensin II:*** Angiotensin II is the most active form. Its actions are:

    On blood vessels:
    - Angiotensin II increases arterial blood pressure by directly acting on the blood vessels and causing vasoconstriction. It is a potent constrictor of arterioles. Earlier, when its other actions were not found it was called hypertensin.
    - It increases blood pressure indirectly by increasing the release of noradrenaline from postganglionic sympathetic fibers. Noradrenaline is a general vasoconstrictor.

    On adrenal cortex:
    - It stimulates zona glomerulosa of adrenal cortex to secrete aldosterone. Aldosterone acts on renal tubules and increases retention of sodium, which is also responsible for elevation of blood pressure.

    On kidney:
    - Angiotensin II regulates glomerular filtration rate by two ways:
      (i) It constricts the efferent arteriole, which causes decrease in filtration after an initial increase
      (ii) It contracts the glomerular mesangial cells leading to decrease in surface area of glomerular capillaries and filtration
    - It increases sodium reabsorption from renal tubules. This action is more predominant on proximal tubules.

    On brain:
    - Angiotensin II inhibits the baroreceptor reflex and thereby indirectly increases the blood pressure. Baroreceptor reflex is responsible for decreasing the blood pressure.
    - It increases water intake by stimulating the thirst center.
    - It increases the secretion of orticotropin-releasing hormone (CRH) from hypothalamus. CRH in turn increases secretion of adrenocorticotropic hormone (ACTH) from pituitary.
    - It increases secretion of antidiuretic hormone (ADH) from hypothalamus.

    ***Other actions:*** Angiotensin II acts as a growth factor in heart and it is thought to cause muscular hypertrophy and cardiac enlargement.
  - ***Angiotensin III:*** Angiotensin III increases the blood pressure and stimulates aldosterone secretion from adrenal cortex. It has 100% adrenocortical stimulating activity and 40% vasopressor activity of angiotensin II.
  - ***Angiotensin IV:*** It also has adrenocortical stimulating and vasopressor activities.

Prostaglandin

Extraglomerular mesangial cells of juxtaglomerular apparatus secrete prostaglandin. Prostaglandin is also secreted by interstitial cells of medulla called type I medullary interstitial cells.

*Secretion of Other Substances*

- Extraglomerular mesangial cells of juxtaglomerular apparatus secrete cytokines like interleukin-2 and tumor necrosis factor.
- Macula densa secretes thromboxane $A_2$.

*Regulation of Glomerular Blood Flow and Glomerular Filtration Rate*

Macula densa of juxtaglomerular apparatus plays an important role in the feedback mechanism called tubuloglomerular feedback mechanism, which regulates the renal blood flow and glomerular filtration rate.

## Urine Formation

### Introduction

Urine formation is a blood cleansing function. Normally, about 1,300 mL of blood (26% of cardiac output) enters the kidneys. Kidneys excrete the unwanted substances along with water from the blood as urine. Normal urinary output is 1 to 1.5 L/day.

### Processes of Urine Formation

When blood passes through glomerular capillaries, the plasma is filtered into the Bowman capsule. This process is called glomerular filtration. Filtrate from Bowman capsule passes through the tubular portion of the nephron. While passing through the tubule, the filtrate undergoes various changes both in quality and in quantity. Many wanted substances like glucose, amino acids, water and electrolytes are reabsorbed from the tubules. This process is called tubular reabsorption. And, some unwanted substances are secreted into the tubule from peritubular blood vessels. This process is called tubular secretion or excretion. Thus, the urine formation includes three processes:

1. Glomerular filtration
2. Tubular reabsorption
3. Tubular secretion.

Among these three processes filtration is the function of the glomerulus. Reabsorption and secretion are the functions of tubular portion of the nephron.

## Glomerular Filtration

### Introduction

Glomerular filtration is the process by which the blood is filtered while passing through the glomerular capillaries by filtration membrane. It is the first process of urine formation. The structure of filtration membrane is well suited for filtration.

### Filtration Membrane

Filtration membrane is formed by three layers:

1 Glomerular capillary membrane
2. Basement membrane
3. Visceral layer of Bowman capsule.

1. ***Glomerular capillary membrane:*** Glomerular capillary membrane is formed by single layer of endothelial cells,

which are attached to the basement membrane. The capillary membrane has many pores called fenestrae or filtration pores with a diameter of 0.1μ.

2. *Basement membrane:* Basement membrane of glomerular capillaries and the basement membrane of visceral layer of Bowman capsule fuse together. The fused basement membrane separates the endothelium of glomerular capillary and the epithelium of visceral layer of Bowman capsule.
3. *Visceral layer of Bowman capsule:* This layer is formed by a single layer of flattened epithelial cells resting on a basement membrane. Each cell is connected with the basement membrane by cytoplasmic extensions called pedicles or feet. Epithelial cells with pedicles are called podocytes. Pedicles interdigitate leaving small cleft-like spaces in between. The cleftlike space is called slit pore or filtration slit. Filtration takes place through these slit pores.

### Process of Glomerular Filtration

When blood passes through glomerular capillar ies, the plasma is filtered into the Bowman capsule. All the substances of plasma are filtered except the plasma proteins. The filtered fluid is called glomerular filtrate.

### Ultrafiltration

Glomerular filtration is called ultrafiltration because even the minute particles are filtered. But, the plasma proteins are not filtered due to their large molecular size. The protein molecules are larger than the slit pores present in the endothelium of capillaries. Thus, the glomerular filtrate contains all the substances present in plasma except the plasma proteins.

### Glomerular Filtration Rate

Glomerular filtration rate (GFR) is defined as the total quantity of filtrate formed in all the nephrons of both the kidneys in the given unit of time.

Normal GFR is 125 mL/minute or about 180 L/day.

### Pressures Determining Filtration

Pressures, which determine the GFR are:

1. Glomerular capillary pressure
2. Colloidal osmotic pressure in the glomeruli
3. Hydrostatic pressure in the Bowman capsule.

These pressures determine the GFR by either favoring or opposing the filtration.

1. *Glomerular capillary pressure:* Glomerular capillary pressure is the pressure exerted by the blood in glomerular capillaries. It is about 60 mm Hg and, varies between 45 and 70 mm Hg. Glomerular capillary pressure is the highest capillary pressure in the body. This pressure favors glomerular filtration.
2. *Colloidal osmotic pressure:* It is the pressure exerted by plasma proteins in the glomeruli. The plasma proteins are not filtered through the glomerular capillaries and remain in the glomerular capillaries. These proteins develop the colloidal osmotic pressure, which is about 25 mm Hg. It opposes glomerular filtration.
3. *Hydrostatic pressure in bowman capsule:* It is the pressure exerted by the filtrate in Bowman capsule. It is also called capsular pressure. It is about 15 mm Hg. It also opposes glomerular filtration.

### Factors Regulating (Affecting) GFR

1. *Renal blood flow:* It is the most important factor that is necessary for glomerular filtration. GFR is directly proportional to renal blood flow. Normal blood flow to both the kidneys is 1,300 mL/minute. The renal blood flow itself is controlled by autoregulation.
2. *Tubuloglomerular feedback:* Tubuloglomerular feedback is the mechanism that regulates GFR through renal tubule and macula densa. Macula densa of juxtaglomerular apparatus in the terminal portion of thick ascending limb is sensitive to the sodium chloride in the tubular fluid.

When the glomerular filtrate passes through the terminal portion of thick ascending segment, macula densa acts like a sensor. It detects the concentration of sodium chloride in the tubular fluid and accordingly alters the glomerular blood flow and GFR. Macula densa detects the sodium chloride concentration via $Na^{+}K^{+}$ $2Cl^{-}$ cotransporter (NKCC2).

When the concentration of sodium chloride increases in the filtrate. When GFR increases, concentration of sodium chloride increases in the filtrate. Macula densa releases adenosine from ATP. Adenosine causes constriction of afferent arteriole. So the blood flow through glomerulus decreases leading to decrease in GFR. Adenosine acts on afferent arteriole via adenosine A1 receptors.

There are several other factors, which increase or decrease the sensitivity of tubuloglomerular feedback. Factors increasing the sensitivity of tubuloglomerular feedback:

- Adenosine
- Thromboxane
- Prostaglandin $E_2$
- Hydroxyeicosatetraenoic acid.

Factors decreasing the sensitivity of tubuloglomerular feedback:

- Atrial natriuretic peptide
- Prostaglandin $I_2$
- Cyclic AMP (cAMP)
- Nitrous oxide.

*When the concentration of sodium chloride decreases in the filtrate.*

When GFR decreases, concentration of sodium chloride decreases in the filtrate. Macula densa secretes prostaglandin ($PGE_2$), bradykinin and renin. $PGE_2$ and bradykinin cause dilatation of afferent arteriole. Renin induces the formation of angiotensin II, which causes constriction of efferent arteriole. The dilatation of afferent arteriole and constriction of efferent arteriole leads to increase in glomerular blood flow and GFR.

3. *Glomerular capillary pressure:* Glomerular filtration rate is directly proportional to glomerular capillary pressure. Normal glomerular capillary pressure is 60 mm Hg. When glomerular capillary pressure increases, the GFR also increases. Capillary pressure, in turn depends upon the renal blood flow and arterial blood pressure.

4. *Colloidal osmotic pressure:* Glomerular filtration rate is inversely proportional to colloidal osmotic pressure, which is exerted by plasma proteins in the glomerular capillary blood. Normal colloidal osmotic pressure is 25 mm Hg. When colloidal osmotic pressure increases as in the case of dehydration or increased plasma protein level GFR decreases. When colloidal osmotic pressure is low as in hypoproteinemia, GFR increases.
5. *Hydrostatic pressure in Bowman capsule:* GFR is inversely proportional to this. Normally, it is 15 mm Hg. When the hydrostatic pressure increases in the Bowman capsule, it decreases GFR. Hydrostatic pressure in Bowman capsule increases in conditions like obstruction of urethra and edema of kidney beneath renal capsule.
6. *Constriction of afferent arteriole:* Constriction of afferent arteriole reduces the blood flow to the glomerular capillaries, which in turn reduces GFR.
7. *Constriction of efferent arteriole:* If efferent arteriole is constricted, initially the GFR increases because of stagnation of blood in the capillaries. Later when all the substances are filtered from this blood, further filtration does not occur. It is because, the efferent arteriolar constriction prevents outflow of blood from glomerulus and no fresh blood enters the glomerulus for filtration.
8. *Systemic arterial pressure:* Renal blood flow and GFR are not affected as long as the mean arterial blood pressure is in between 60 and 180 mm Hg due to the autoregulatory mechanism. Variation in pressure above 180 mm Hg or below 60 mm Hg affects the renal blood flow and GFR accordingly, because the autoregulatory mechanism fails beyond this range.
9. *Sympathetic stimulation:* Afferent and efferent arterioles are supplied by sympathetic nerves. The mild or moderate stimulation of sympathetic nerves does not cause any significant change either in renal blood flow or GFR.

   Strong sympathetic stimulation causes severe constriction of the blood vessels by releasing the neurotransmitter substance, noradrenaline. The effect is more severe on the efferent arterioles than on the afferent arterioles. So, initially there is increase in filtration but later it decreases. However, if the stimulation is continued for more than 30 minutes, there is recovery of both renal blood flow and GFR. It is because of reduction in sympathetic neurotransmitter.
10. *Surface area of capillary membrane:* GFR is directly proportional to the surface area of the capillary membrane. If the glomerular capillary membrane is affected as in the cases of some renal diseases, the surface area for filtration decreases. So there is reduction in GFR.
11. *Permeability of capillary membrane:* GFR is directly proportional to the permeability of glomerular capillary membrane. In many abnormal conditions like hypoxia, lack of blood supply, presence of toxic agents, etc. the permeability of the capillary membrane increases. In such conditions, even plasma proteins are filtered and excreted in urine.
12. *Contraction of glomerular mesangial cells:* Glomerular mesangial cells are situated in between the glomerular capillaries. Contraction of these cells decreases surface area of capillaries resulting in reduction in GFR.
13. *Hormonal and other factors:* Many hormones and other secretory factors alter GFR by affecting the blood flow through glomerulus.

    Factors increasing GFR by vasodilatation:
    - Atrial natriuretic peptide
    - Brain natriuretic peptide
    - cAMP
    - Dopamine
    - Endothelial-derived nitric oxide
    - Prostaglandin ($PGE_2$).

    Factors decreasing GFR by vasoconstriction:
    - Angiotensin II
    - Endothelins
    - Noradrenaline
    - Platelet-activating factor
    - Platelet-derived growth factor
    - Prostaglandin ($PGF_2$).

## Tubular Reabsorption

### Introduction

Tubular reabsorption is the process by which water and other substances are transported from renal tubules back to the blood. When the glomerular filtrate flows through the tubular portion of nephron, both quantitative and qualitative changes occur. Large quantity of water (more than 99%), electrolytes and other substances are reabsorbed by the tubular epithelial cells. The reabsorbed substances move into the interstitial fluid of renal medulla. And, from here, the substances move into the blood in peritubular capillaries.

Since the substances are taken back into the blood from the glomerular filtrate, the entire process is called tubular reabsorption.

### Selective Reabsorption

Tubular reabsorption is known as selective reabsorption because the tubular cells reabsorb only the substances necessary for the body. Essential substances such as glucose, amino acids and vitamins are completely reabsorbed from renal tubule. Whereas the unwanted substances like metabolic waste products are not reabsorbed and excreted through urine.

### Mechanism of Reabsorption

Basic transport mechanisms involved in tubular reabsorption are of two types:
1. Active reabsorption
2. Passive reabsorption.

1. *Active Reabsorption:* Active reabsorption is the movement of molecules against the electrochemical (uphill) gradient. It needs liberation of energy, which is derived from ATP.

   *Substances reabsorbed actively:* Substances reabsorbed actively from the renal tubule are sodium, calcium, potassium, phosphates, sulfates, bicarbonates, glucose, amino acids, ascorbic acid, uric acid and ketone bodies.
2. *Passive reabsorption:* Passive reabsorption is the movement of molecules along the electrochemical

(downhill) gradient. This process does not need energy.

***Substances reabsorbed passively:*** Substances reabsorbed passively are chloride, urea and water.

### *Routes of Reabsorption*

Reabsorption of substances from tubular lumen into the peritubular capillary occurs by two routes:

1. Trancelluar route
2. Paracellular route.

1. ***Transcellular route:*** In this route the substances move through the cell. It includes transport of substances from:
   - Tubular lumen into tubular cell through apical (luminal) surface of the cell membrane
   - Tubular cell into interstitial fluid
   - Interstitial fluid into capillary.
2. ***Paracelluar Route:*** In this route, the substances move through the intercellular space. It includes transport of substances from:
   - Tubular lumen into interstitial fluid present in lateral intercellular space through the tight junction between the cells
   - Interstitial fluid into capillary.

### *Site of Reabsorption*

Reabsorption of the substances occurs in almost all the segments of tubular portion of nephron.

1. ***Substances reabsorbed from proximal convoluted tubule:*** About 7/8 of the filtrate (about 88%) is reabsorbed in proximal convoluted tubule. The brush border of epithelial cells in proximal convoluted tubule increases the surface area and facilitates the reabsorption. Substances reabsorbed from proximal convoluted tubule are glucose, amino acids, sodium, potassium, calcium, bicarbonates, chlorides, phosphates, urea, uric acid and water.
2. ***Substances reabsorbed from loop of henle:*** Substances reabsorbed from loop of Henle are sodium and chloride.
3. ***Substances reabsorbed from distal convoluted tubule:*** Sodium, calcium, bicarbonate and water are reabsorbed from distal convoluted tubule.

### *Regulation of Tubular Reabsorption*

Tubular reabsorption is regulated by three factors:

1. ***Glomerulotubular balance:*** Glomerulotubular balance is the balance between the filtration and reabsorption of solutes and water in kidney.

   When GFR increases, the tubular load of solutes and water in the proximal convoluted tubule is increased. It is followed by increase in the reabsorption of solutes and water. This process helps in the constant reabsorption of solute particularly sodium and water from renal tubule.

   ***Mechanism of glomerulotubular balance:*** Glomerulotubular balance occurs because of osmotic pressure in the peritubular capillaries. When GFR increases, more amount of plasma proteins accumulate in the glomerulus. Consequently, the osmotic pressure increases in the blood by the time it reaches efferent arteriole and peritubular capillaries. The elevated osmotic pressure in the peritubular capillaries increases reabsorption of sodium and water from the tubule into the capillary blood.
2. ***Hormonal factors:*** Hormones, which regulate GFR are as follows:
   - ***Aldosterone:*** It increases sodium reabsorption in ascending limb, distal convoluted tubule and collectmg duct.
   - ***Angiotensin II:*** It increases sodium reabsorption In proximal tubule, thick ascending limb, distal tubule and collecting duct (mainly in proximal convoluted tubule).
   - ***Antidiuretic hormone:*** It increases water reabsorption in distal convoluted tubule and collecting duct.
   - ***Atrial natriuretic factor:*** It decreases sodium reabsorption.
   - ***Brain natriuretic factor:*** It decreases sodium reabsorption.
   - ***Parathormone:*** It increases reabsorption of calcium, magnesium and hydrogen decreases phosphate reabsorption.
   - ***Calcitonin:*** It decreases calcium reabsorption.
3. ***Nervous Factor:*** Activation of sympathetic nervous system increases the tubular reabsorption (particularly of sodium) from renal tubules. It also increases the tubular reabsorption indirectly by stimulating secretion of renin from juxtaglomerular cells. Renin causes formation of angiotensin II, which increases the sodium reabsorption.

## Tubular Secretion

### *Introduction*

Tubular secretion is the process by which the substances are transported from blood into renal tubules. It is also called tubular excretion. In addition to reabsorption from renal tubules, some substances are also secreted into the lumen from the peritubular capillaries through the tubular epithelial cells.

Dye phenol red was the first substance found to be secreted in renal tubules in experimental conditions.

Later many other substances were found to be secreted. Such substances are:

- Para-aminohippuric acid (PAH)
- Diodrast
- 5-hydroxyindoleacetic acid (5HIAA)
- Amino derivatives
- Penicillin.

### *Substances Secreted in Different Segments of Renal Tubules*

- Potassium is secreted actively by sodium-potassium pump in proximal and distal convoluted tubules and collecting ducts.
- Ammonia is secreted in the proximal convoluted tubule.
- Hydrogen ions are secreted in the proximal and distal convoluted tubules. Maximum hydrogen ion secretion occurs in proximal tubule.
- Urea is secreted in loop of Henle. Thus, urine is formed in nephron by the processes of glomerular filtration, selective reabsorption and tubular secretion.

## Properties and Composition of Normal Urine

### *Properties of Urine*

- Volume: 1,000 to 1,500 mL/day
- Reaction: Slightly acidic with pH of 4.5 to 6
- Specific gravity: 1.010 to 1.025
- Osmolarity: 1,200 mOsm/L
- Color: Normally, straw colored
- Odor: Fresh urine has light aromatic odor.

If stored for some time, the odor becomes stronger due to bacterial decomposition.

### *Composition of Urine*

Urine consists of water and solids. Solids include organic and inorganic substances.

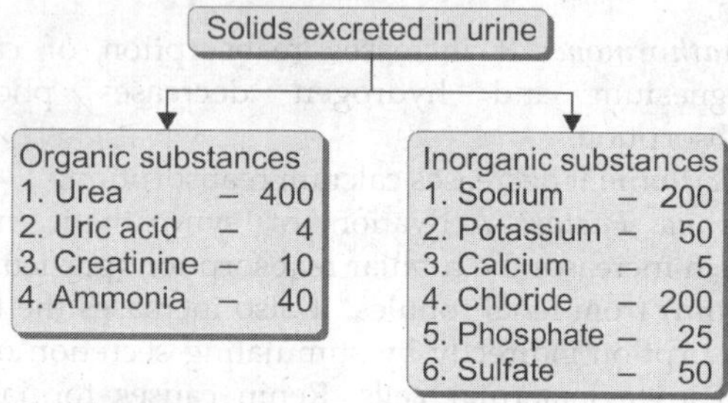


## CARDIOVASCULAR SYSTEM

### Introduction

Cardiovascular system includes heart and blood vessels. Heart pumps blood into the blood vessels.

Blood vessels circulate the blood throughout the body. Blood transports nutrients and oxygen to the tissues and removes carbon dioxide and waste products from the tissues.

### Heart

Heart is a muscular organ that pumps blood throughout the circulatory system. It is situated in between two lungs in the mediastinum. It is made up of four chambers, two atria and two ventricles. The musculature of ventricles is thicker than that of atria. Force of contraction of heart depends upon the muscles.

### *Right Side of the Heart*

Right side of the heart has two chambers, right atrium and right ventricle. Right atrium is a thin walled and low pressure chamber. It has got the pacemaker known as sinoatrial node that produces cardiac impulses and atrioventricular node that conducts the impulses to the ventricles. Right atrium receives venous (deoxygenated) blood via two large veins:

1. Superior vena cava that returns venous blood from the head, neck and upper limbs.
2. Inferior vena cava that returns venous blood from lower parts of the body. Right atrium communicates with right ventricle through tricuspid valve. Wall of right ventricle is thick. Venous blood from the right atrium enters the right ventricle through this valve. From the right ventricle, pulmonary artery arises. It carries the venous blood from right ventricle to lungs. In the lungs, the deoxygenated blood is oxygenated.

### *Left Side of the Heart*

Left side of the heart has two chambers, left atrium and left ventricle. Left atrium is a thin walled and low pressure chamber. It receives oxygenated blood from the lungs through pulmonary veins. This is the only exception in the body, where an artery carries venous blood and vein carries the arterial blood. Blood from left atrium enters the left ventricle through mitral valve (bicuspid valve). Wall of the left ventricle is very thick. Left ventricle pumps the arterial blood to different parts of the body through systemic aorta.

### *Septa of the Heart*

Right and left atria are separated from one another by a fibrous septum called interatrial septum. Right and left ventricles are separated from one another by interventricular septum. The upper part of this septum is a membranous structure, whereas the lower part of it is muscular in nature.

### *Layers of Wall of the Heart*

Heart is made up of three layers of tissues:

1. Outer pericardium
2. Middle myocardium
3. Inner endocardium.

### *Pericardium*

Pericardium is the outer covering of the heart. It is made up of two layers:

- Outer parietal pericardium
- Inner visceral pericardium.

The space between the two layers is called pericardial cavity or pericardial space and it contains a thin film of fluid.

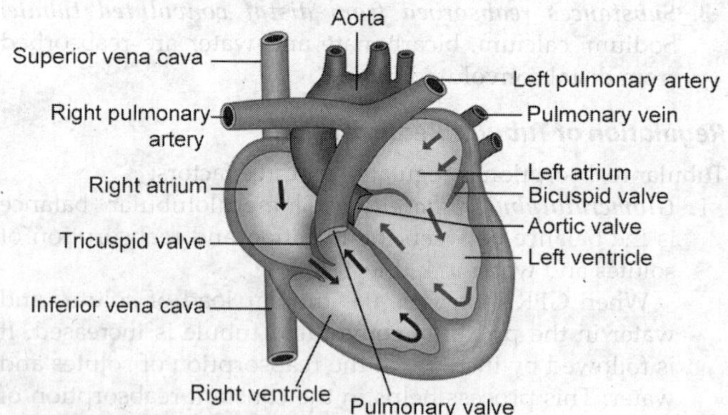


### *Myocardium*

Myocardium is the middle layer of wall of the heart and it is formed by cardiac muscle fibers or cardiac myocytes. Myocardium forms the bulk of the heart and it is responsible for pumping action of the heart. Unlike skeletal muscle fibers, the cardiac muscle fibers are involuntary in nature.

Myocardium has three types of muscle fibers:
1. Muscle fibers which form contractile unit of heart
2. Muscle fibers which form pacemaker
3. Muscle fibers which form conductive system.

### *Endocardium*

Endocardium is the innermost layer of heart wall. It is a thin, smooth and glistening membrane. It is formed by a single layer of endothelial cells, lining the inner surface of the heart. Endocardium continues as endothelium of the blood vessels.

### *Valves of the Heart*

There are four valves in human heart. Two valves are in between atria and the ventricles called atrioventricular valves. Other two are the semilunar valves, placed at the opening of blood vessels arising from ventricles, namely systemic aorta and pulmonary artery. Valves of the heart permit the flow of blood through heart in only one direction.

*Atrioventricular Valves*

Left atrioventricular valve is otherwise known as mitral valve or bicuspid valve. It is formed by two valvular cusps or flaps. Right atrioventricular valve is known as tricuspid valve and it is formed by three cusps.

Brim of the atrioventricular valves is attached to atrioventricular ring, which is the fibrous connection between the atria and ventricles. Cusps of the valves are attached to papillary muscles by means of chordate tendineae. Papillary muscles arise from inner surface of the ventricles. Papillary muscles play an important role in closure of the cusps and in preventing the backflow of blood from ventricle to atria during ventricular contraction. Atrioventricular valves open only towards ventricles and prevent the backflow of blood into atria.

*Semilunar Valves*

Semilunar valves are present at the openings of systemic aorta and pulmonary artery and are known as aortic valve and pulmonary valve respectively. Because of the half moon shape, these two valves are called semilunar valves. Semilunar valves are made up of three flaps. Semilular valves open only towards the aorta and pulmonary artery and prevent the backflow of blood into the ventricles.

## Blood Vessels

Vessels of circulatory system are the aorta, arteries, arterioles, capillaries, venules, veins and venae cavae.

### *Arterial System*

Arterial system comprises the aorta, arteries and arterioles. Walls of the aorta and arteries are formed by three layers:
1. Outer tunica adventitia, which is made up of connective tissue layer. It is the continuation of fibrous layer of parietal pericardium.
2. Middle tunica media, which is formed by smooth muscles.
3. Inner tunica intima, which is made up of endothelium. It is the continuation of endocardium. Aorta, arteries and arterioles have two laminae of elastic tissues:

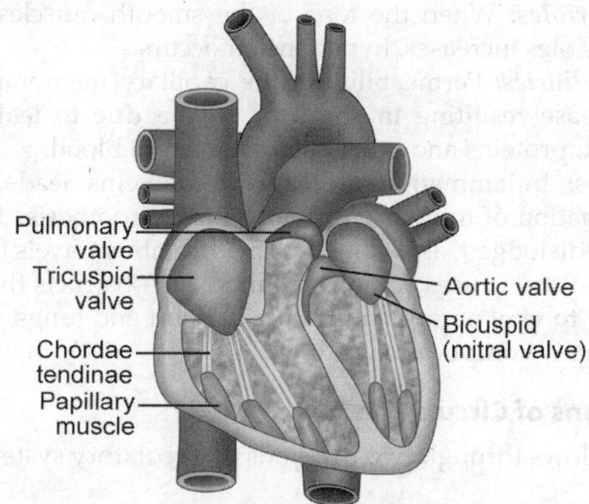


- External elastic lamina between tunica adventitia and tunica media
- Internal elastic lamina between tunica media and tunica intima. Aorta and arteries have more elastic tissues and the arterioles have more smooth muscles. Arterial branches become narrower and their walls become thinner while reaching the periphery. Aorta has got the maximum diameter of about 25 mm. Diameter of the arteries is gradually decreased and at the end arteries, it is about 4 mm. It further decreases to 30 μ in the arterioles and ends up with 10 μ in the terminal arterioles. Resistance (peripheral resistance) is offered to blood flow in the arterioles and so these vessels are called resistant vessels.

Arterioles are continued as capillaries, which are small, thin walled vessels having a diameter of about 5 to 8 μ. Capillaries are functionally very important because, the exchange of materials between the blood and the tissues occurs through these vessels.

### *Venous System*

From the capillaries, venous system starts and it includes venules, veins and venae cavae. Capillaries end in venules, which are the smaller vessels with thin muscular wall than the arterioles. Diameter of the venules is about 20 μ. At a time, a large quantity of blood is held in venules and hence the venules are called capacitance vessels. Venules are continued as veins, which have the diameter of 5 mm. Veins form superior and inferior venae cavae, which have a diameter of about 30 mm.

Walls of the veins and venae cavae are made up of inner endothelium, elastic tissues, smooth muscles and outer connective tissue layer. In the veins and venae cavae, the elastic tissue is less but the smooth muscle fibers are more.

### *Complications in Blood Vessels*

- *Aorta and arteries:* Arterial blood vessels are highly susceptible for arteriosclerosis and atherosclerosis. Arteriosclerosis is the disease of the arteries, associated with hardening, thickening and loss of elasticity in the wall of the vessels. Atherosclerosis is the disease marked by the narrowing of lumen of arterial vessel due to deposition of cholesterol.

- *Arterioles:* When the tone of the smooth muscles in the arterioles increases, hypertension occurs.
- *Capillaries:* Permeability of the capillary membrane may increase resulting in shock or edema due to leakage of fluid, proteins and other substances from blood.
- *Veins:* Inflammation of the wall of veins leads to the formation of intravascular clot called thrombosis. The clot gets dislodged, as thrombus. The thrombus travels through blood and causes embolism. Embolism obstructs the blood flow to vital organs such as brain, heart and lungs, leading to many complications.

## Divisions of Circulation

Blood flows through two divisions of circulatory system:

### Systemic Circulation

Systemic circulation is otherwise known as greater circulation. Blood pumped from left ventricle passes through a series of blood vessels, arterial system and reaches the tissues. Exchange of various substances between blood and the tissues occurs at the capillaries.

After exchange of materials, blood enters the venous system and returns to right atrium of the heart. From right atrium, blood enters the right ventricle.

Thus, through systemic circulation, oxygenated blood is supplied from heart to the tissues and venous blood returns to the heart from tissues.

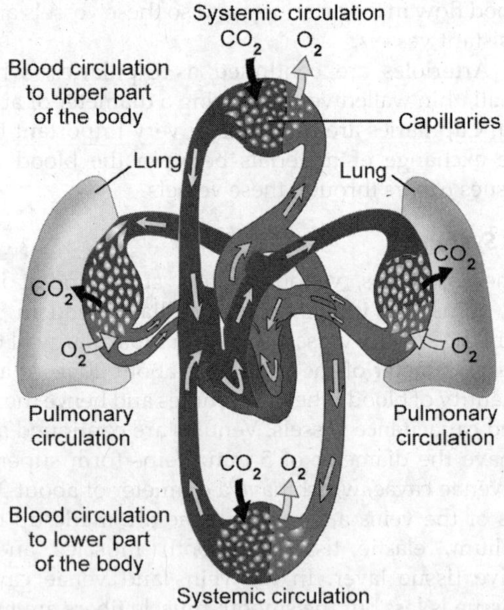


### Pulmonary Circulation

Pulmonary circulation is otherwise called lesser circulation. Blood is pumped from right ventricle to lungs through pulmonary artery. Exchange of gases occurs between blood and alveoli of the lungs at pulmonary capillaries. Oxygenated blood returns to left atrium through the pulmonary veins. Thus, left side of the heart contains oxygenated or arterial blood and the right side of the heart contains deoxygenated or venous blood.

## Cardiac Cycle

### Definition

Cardiac cycle is defined as the succession of (sequence of) coordinated events taking place in the heart during each beat. Each heartbeat consists of two major periods called systole and diastole. During systole, heart contracts and pumps the blood through arteries.

During diastole, heart relaxes and blood is filled in the heart. All these changes are repeated during every heartbeat, in a cyclic manner.

### Events of Cardiac Cycle

Events of cardiac cycle are classified into two:
1. Atrial events
2. Ventricular events.

### Divisions and Duration of Cardiac Cycle

When the heart beats at a normal rate of 72/minute, duration of each cardiac cycle is about 0.8 second.

### Atrial Events

Atrial events are divided into two divisions:
1. Atrial systole = 0.11 (0.1) sec
2. Atrial diastole = 0.69 (0.7) sec.

### Ventricular Events

Ventricular events are divided into two divisions:
1. Ventricular systole = 0.27 (0.3) sec
2. Ventricular diastole = 0.53 (0.5) sec.

In clinical practice, the term 'systole' refers to ventricular systole and 'diastole' refers to ventricular diastole. Ventricular systole is divided into two subdivisions and ventricular diastole is divided into five subdivisions.

#### *Ventricular Systole*

Time (second)
1. Isometric contraction = 0.05 sec
2. Ejection period = 0.22 sec

= 0.27 sec

#### *Ventricular Diastole*

1. Protodiastole = 0.04 sec
2. Isometric relaxation = 0.08 sec
3. Rapid filling = 0.11 sec
4. Slow filling = 0.19 sec
5. Last rapid filling = 0.11 sec

= 0.53 sec

Among the atrial events, atrial systole occurs during the last phase of ventricular diastole. Atrial diastole is not considered as a separate phase, since it coincides with the whole of ventricular systole and earlier part of ventricular diastole.

### Description of Atrial Events

#### *Atrial Systole*

Atrial systole is also known as last rapid filling phase or presystole. It is usually considered as the last phase of ventricular diastole. Its duration is 0.11 second.

During this period, only a small amount, i.e. 10% of blood is forced from atria into ventricles. Atrial systole is not essential for the maintenance of circulation. Many persons with atrial fibrillation survive for years, without suffering from circulatory insufficiency. However, such persons feel difficult to cope up with physical stress like exercise.

- ***Pressure and volume changes:*** During atrial systole, the intraatrial pressure increases.
  Intraventricular pressure and ventricular volume also increase but slightly.
- ***Fourth heart sound:*** Contraction of atrial musculature causes the production of fourth heart sound.

### *Atrial Diastole*

After atrial systole, the atrial diastole starts. Simultaneously, ventricular systole also starts. Atrial diastole lasts for about 0.7 sec (accurate duration is 0.69 sec).

This long atrial diastole is necessary because, this is the period during which atrial filling takes place. Right atrium receives deoxygenated blood from all over the body through superior and inferior venae cavae. Left atrium receives oxygenated blood from lungs through pulmonary veins.

- ***Atrial events vs ventricular events:*** Out of 0.7 sec of atrial diastole, first 0.3 sec (0.27 sec accurately) coincides with ventricular systole. Then, ventricular diastole starts and it lasts for about 0.5 sec (0.53 sec accurately). Later part of atrial diastole coincides with ventricular diastole for about 0.4 sec. So, the heart relaxes as a whole for 0.4 sec. shows the correlation between atrial and ventricular events of cardiac cycle.

## Description of Ventricular Events

### *Isometric Contraction Period*

Isometric contraction period in cardiac cycle is the first phase of ventricular systole. It lasts for 0.05 second. Isometric contraction is the type of muscular ontraction characterized by increase in tension, without any change in the length of muscle fibers. Isometric contraction of ventricular muscle is also called isovolumetric contraction. Immediately after atrial systole, the atrioventricular valves are closed due to increase in ventricular pressure. Semilunar valves are already closed. Now, ventricles contract as closed cavities, in such a way that there is no change in the volume of ventricular chambers or in the length of muscle fibers. Only the tension increases in ventricular musculature.Because of increased tension in ventricular musculature during isometric contraction, the pressure increases sharply inside the ventricles.

#### First Heart Sound

Closure of atrioventricular valves at the beginning of this phase produces first heart sound.

#### Significance of Isometric Contraction

During isometric contraction period, the ventricular pressure increases greatly. When this pressure increases above the pressure in the aorta and pulmonary artery, the semilunar valves open. Thus, the pressure rise in ventricle, caused by isometric contraction is responsible for the opening of semilunar valves, leading to ejection of blood from the ventricles into aorta and pulmonary artery.

### *Ejection Period*

Due to the opening of semilunar valves and isotonic contraction of ventricles, blood is ejected out of both the ventricles. Hence, this period is called ejection period.

Duration of this period is 0.22 second. Ejection period is of two stages:

#### First Stage or Rapid Ejection Period

First stage starts immediately after the opening of semilunar valves. During this stage, a large amount of blood is rapidly ejected from both the ventricles. It lasts for 0.13 second.

#### Second Stage or Slow Ejection Period

During this stage, the blood is ejected slowly with much less force. Duration of this period is 0.09 second.

- ***End-systolic volume:*** Ventricles are not emptied at the end of ejection period and some amount of blood remains in each ventricle. Amount of blood remaining in ventricles at the end of ejection period (i.e. at the end of systole) is called endsystolic volume. It is 60 to 80 mL per ventricle.
  - ***Measurement of end-systolic volume:*** Endsystolic volume is measured by radionuclide angiocardiography (multigated acquisition–MUGA scan) and echocardiography. It is also measured by cardiac catheterization, computed tomography (CT) scan and magnetic resonance imaging (MRI).
- ***Ejection Fraction:*** Ejection fraction refers to the fraction (or portion) of end-diastolic volume (see below) that is ejected out by each ventricle per beat. From 130 to 150 mL of end-diastolic volume, 70 mL is ejected out by each ventricle (stroke volume). Normal ejection fraction is 60 to 65%.
  - ***Determination of ejection fraction:*** Ejection fraction ($E_f$) is the stroke volume divided by end-diastolic volume expressed in percentage. Stroke volume (SV) is, end-diastolic volume (EDV) minus endsystolic volume (ESV).

  Ejection fraction is calculated as:

$$SV = EDV - ESV$$

$$E_f = \frac{SV}{EDV}$$

Where, $E_f$ = Ejection fraction
SV = Stroke volume
EDV = End-diastolic volume
ESV = End-systolic volume.

- ***Significance of determining ejection fraction:*** Ejection fraction is the measure of left ventricular function. Clinically, it is considered as an important index for assessing the ventricular contractility. Ejection fraction decreases in myocardial infarction and cardiomyopathy.

### *Protodiastole*

Protodiastole is the first stage of ventricular diastole, hence the name protodiastole. Duration of this period is 0.04 second. Due to the ejection of blood, the pressure in aorta and pulmonary artery increases and pressure in ventricles drops. When intraventricular pressure becomes less than the pressure in aorta and pulmonary artery, the semilunar valves close. Atrioventricular valves are already closed. No other change occurs in the heart during this period. Thus, protodiastole indicates only the end of systole and beginning of diastole.

Second Heart Sound

Closure of semilunar valves during this phase produces second heart sound

*Isometric Relaxation Period*

Isometric relaxation is the type of muscular relaxation, characterized by decrease in tension without any change in the length of muscle fibers. Isometric relaxation of ventricular muscle is also called isovolumetric relaxation. During isometric relaxation period, once again all the valves of the heart are closed. Now, both the ventricles relax as closed cavities without any change in volume or length of the muscle fiber. Intraventricular pressure decreases during this period. Duration of isometric relaxation period is 0.08 second.

Significance of Isometric Relaxation

During isometric relaxation period, the ventricular pressure decreases greatly. When the ventricular pressure becomes less than the pressure in the atria, the atrioventricular valves open. Thus, the fall in pressure in the ventricles, caused by isometric relaxation is responsible for the opening of atrioventricular valves, resulting in filling of ventricles.

*Rapid Filling Phase*

When atrionventricular valves are opened, there is a sudden rush of blood (which is accumulated in atria during atrial diastole) from atria into ventricles. So, this period is called the first rapid filling period. Ventricles also relax isotonically. About 70% of filling takes place during this phase, which lasts for 0.11 second.

Third Heart Sound

Rushing of blood into ventricles during this phase causes production of third heart sound.

*Slow Filling Phase*

After the sudden rush of blood, the ventricular filling becomes slow. Now, it is called the slow filling. It is also called diastasis. About 20% of filling occurs in this phase. Duration of slow filling phase is 0.19 second.

*Last Rapid Filling Phase*

Last rapid filling phase occurs because of atrial systole. After slow filling period, the atria contract and push a small amount of blood into ventricles. About 10% of ventricular filling takes place during this period. Flow of additional amount of blood into ventricle due to atrial systole is called atrial kick.

Enddiastolic Volume

Enddiastolic volume is the amount of blood remaining in each ventricle at the end of diastole. It is about 130 to 150 mL per ventricle.

- ***Measurement of enddiastolic volume:*** It is measured by the same methods, which are used to measure end-systolic volume.

## Electrocardiogram (ECG)

### *Definitions*

- ***Electrocardiography:*** Electrocardiography is the technique by which electrical activities of the heart are studied. The spread of excitation through myocardium produces local electrical potential. This low-intensity current flows through the body, which acts as a volume conductor. This current can be picked up from surface of the body by using suitable electrodes and recorded in the form of electrocardiogram. This technique was discovered by Dutch physiologist, Einthoven Willem, who is considered the father of electrocardiogram (ECG).
- ***Electrocardiograph:*** It is the instrument (machine) by which electrical activities of the heart are recorded.
- ***Electrocardiogram:*** Electrocardiogram (ECG or EKG from electrocardiogram in Dutch) is the record or graphical registration of electrical activities of the heart, which occur prior to the onset of mechanical activities. It is the summed electrical activity of all cardiac muscle fibers recorded from surface of the body.

### *Uses of ECG*

Electrocardiogram is useful in determining and diagnosing the following:

- Heart rate
- Heart rhythm
- Abnormal electrical conduction
- Poor blood flow to heart muscle (ischemia)
- Heart attack
- Coronary artery disease
- Hypertrophy of heart chambers.

### *Electrocardiographic Grid*

The paper that is used for recording ECG is called ECG paper. ECG machine amplifies the electrical signals produced from the heart and records these signals on a moving ECG paper.

Electrocardiographic grid refers to the markings (lines) on ECG paper. ECG paper has horizontal and vertical lines at regular intervals of 1 mm. Every 5th line (5 mm) is thickened.

*Duration*

Time duration of different ECG waves is plotted horizontally on X-axis.

On X-axis

- 1 mm = 0.04 second
- 5 mm = 0.20 second

*Amplitude*

Amplitude of ECG waves is plotted vertically on Y-axis.

On Y-axis

- 1 mm = 0.1 mV
- 5 mm = 0.5 mV

*Speed of The Paper*

Movement of paper through the machine can be adjusted by two speeds, 25 mm/second and 50 mm/second. Usually, speed of the paper during recording is fixed at 25 mm/second. If heart rate is very high, speed of the paper is changed to 50 mm/second.

### *ECG Leads*

ECG is recorded by placing series of electrodes on the surface of the body. These electrodes are called ECG leads and are connected to the ECG machine.

Electrodes are fixed on the limbs. Usually, right arm, left arm and left leg are chosen. Heart is said to be in the center of an imaginary equilateral triangle drawn by connecting the roots of these three limbs. This triangle is called Einthoven triangle.

*Einthoven Triangle and Einthoven*

***Law:*** Einthoven triangle is defined as an equilateral triangle that is used as a model of standard limb leads used to record electrocardiogram. Heart is presumed to lie in the center of Einthoven triangle. Electrical potential generated from the heart appears simultaneously on the roots of the three limbs, namely the left arm, right arm and the left leg. ECG is recorded in 12 leads, which are generally classified into two categories.

1. Bipolar leads
2. Unipolar leads.

Bipolar Limb Leads

Bipolar limb leads are otherwise known as standard limb leads. Two limbs are connected to obtain these leads and both the electrodes are active recording electrodes, i.e. one electrode is positive and the other one is negative. Standard limb leads are of three types:

(i) Limb lead I
(ii) Limb lead II
(iii) Limb lead III.

- ***Lead I:*** Lead I is obtained by connecting right arm and left arm. Right arm is connected to the negative terminal of the instrument and the left arm is connected to the positive terminal.
- ***Lead II:*** Lead II is obtained by connecting right arm and left leg. Right arm is connected to the negative terminal of the instrument and the left leg is connected to the positive terminal.
- ***Lead III:*** Lead III is obtained by connecting left arm and left leg. Left arm is connected to the negative terminal of the instrument and the left leg is connected to the positive terminal.

Unipolar Leads

Here, one electrode is active electrode and the other one is an indifferent electrode. Active electrode is positive and the indifferent electrode is serving as a composite negative electrode.

Unipolar leads are of two types:

1. Unipolar limb leads
2. Unipolar chest leads.

1. ***Unipolar limb leads:*** Unipolar limb leads are also called augmented limb leads or augmented voltage leads. Active electrode is connected to one of the limbs. Indifferent electrode is obtained by connecting the other two limbs through a resistance. Unipolar limb leads are of three types:
   (i) aVR lead
   (ii) aVL lead
   (iii) aVF lead.
   - ***aVR lead:*** Active electrode is from right arm. Indifferent electrode is obtained by connecting left arm and left leg.
   - ***aVL lead:*** Active electrode is from left arm. Indifferent electrode is obtained by connecting right arm and left leg.
   - ***aVF lead:*** Active electrode is from left leg (foot). Indifferent electrode is obtained by connecting the two upper limbs.
2. ***Unipolar chest leads:*** Chest leads are also called 'V' leads or precardial chest leads. Indifferent electrode is obtained by connecting the three limbs, viz. left arm, left leg and right arm, through a resistance of 5000 ohms. Active electrode is placed on six points over the chest. This electrode is known as the chest electrode and the six points over the chest are called $V_1$, $V_2$, $V_3$, $V_4$, $V_5$ and $V_6$. V indicates vector, which shows the direction of current flow.

   Position of chest leads:

- $V_1$: Over 4th intercostal space near right sternal margin
- $V_2$: Over 4th intercostal space near left sternal margin
- $V_3$: In between $V_2$ and $V_4$
- $V_4$: Over left 5th intercostal space on the mid clavicular line
- $V_5$: Over left 5th intercostal space on the anterior axillary line
- $V_6$: Over left 5th intercostal space on the mid axillary line.

## Waves of Normal ECG

Normal ECG consists of waves, complexes, intervals and segments. Waves of ECG recorded by limb lead II are considered as the typical waves. Normal electrocardiogram has the following waves, namely P, Q, R, S and T. Einthoven had named the waves of ECG starting from the middle of the English alphabets (P) instead of starting from the beginning (A).

Major Complexes in ECG

- 'P' wave, the atrial complex
- 'QRS' complex, the initial ventricular complex
- 'T' wave, the final ventricular complex
- 'QRST', the ventricular complex.

'P' Wave

'P' wave is a positive wave and the first wave in ECG. It is also called atrial complex.

- Cause: 'P' wave is produced due to the depolarization of atrial musculature. Depolarization spreads from SA node to all parts of atrial musculature. Atrial repolarization is not recorded as a separate wave in ECG because it merges with ventricular repolarization (QRS complex).
- ***Duration:*** Normal duration of 'P' wave is 0.1 second.
- ***Amplitude:*** Normal amplitude of 'P' wave is 0.1 to 0.12 mV.
- ***Morphology:*** 'P' wave is normally positive (upright) in leads I, II, aVF, V4, V5 and V6. It is normally negative (inverted) in aVR. It is variable in the remaining leads, i.e. it may be positive, negative, biphasic or flat.
- ***Clinical significance:*** Variation in the duration, amplitude and morphology of 'P' wave helps in the diagnosis of several cardiac problems such as:

1. Right atrial hypertrophy: 'P' wave is tall (more than 2.5 mm) in lead II. It is usually pointed.
2. Left atrial dilatation or hypertrophy: It is tall and broad based or M shaped.
3. Atrial extrasystole: Small and shapeless 'P' wave, followed by a small compensatory pause.

4. Hyperkalemia: 'P' wave is absent or small.
5. Atrial fibrillation: 'P' wave is absent.
6. Middle AV nodal rhythm: 'P' wave is absent.
7. Sinoatrial block: 'P' wave is inverted or absent.
8. Atrial paroxysmal tachycardia: 'P' wave is inverted.
9. Lower AV nodal rhythm: 'P' wave appears after QRS complex.

### 'QRS' Complex

'QRS' complex is also called the initial ventricular complex. 'Q' wave is a small negative wave. It is continued as the tall 'R' wave, which is a positive wave. 'R' wave is followed by a small negative wave, the 'S' wave.

- ***Cause:*** 'QRS' complex is due to depolarization of ventricular musculature. 'Q' wave is due to the depolarization of basal portion of interventricular septum. 'R' wave is due to the depolarization of apical portion of interventricular septum and apical portion of ventricular muscle. 'S' wave is due to the depolarization of basal portion of ventricular muscle near the atrioventricular ring.
- ***Duration:*** Normal duration of 'QRS' complex is between 0.08 and 0.10 second.
- ***Amplitude:***
  - Amplitude of 'Q' wave = 0.1 to 0.2 mV.
  - Amplitude of 'R' wave = 1 mV.
  - Amplitude of 'S' wave = 0.4 mV.
- ***Morphology:*** 'Q' wave is normally small with amplitude of 4 mm or less. It is less than 25% of amplitude of 'R' wave in leads I, II, aVL, V5 and V6. In the remaining leads, its amplitude is < 0.2 mm.

  From chest leads V1 to V6, 'R' wave becomes gradually larger. It is smaller in V6 than V5. 'S' wave is large in V1 and larger in V2. It gradually becomes smaller from V3 to V6.
- ***Clinical significance:*** Variation in the duration, amplitude and morphology of 'QRS' complex helps in the diagnosis of several cardiac problems such as:
  1. Bundle branch block: QRS is prolonged or deformed
  2. Hyperkalemia: QRS is prolonged.

### 'T' Wave

'T' wave is the final ventricular complex and is a positive wave.

- Cause: 'T' wave is due to the repolarization of ventricular musculature.
- Duration: Normal duration of 'T' wave is 0.2 second.
- Amplitude: Normal amplitude of 'T' wave is 0.3 mV.
- Morphology: 'T' wave is normally positive in leads I, II and $V_5$ and $V_6$. It is normally inverted in lead aVR. It is variable in the other leads, i.e. it is positive, negative or flat.
- ***Clinical significance:*** Variation in duration, amplitude and morphology of 'T' wave helps in the diagnosis of several cardiac problems such as:
  - Acute myocardial ischemia: Hyperacute 'T' wave develops. Hyperacute 'T' wave refers to a tall and broad-based 'T' wave, with slight asymmetry.
  - Old age, hyperventilation, anxiety, myocardial infarction, left ventricular hypertrophy and pericarditis: 'T' wave is small, flat or inverted
  - Hypokalemia: 'T' wave is small, flat or inverted
  - Hyperkalemia: 'T' wave is tall and tented.

### 'U' Wave

'U' wave is not always seen. It is also an insignificant wave in ECG. It is supposed to be due to repolarization of papillary muscle.

- ***Clinical significance:*** Appearance of 'U' wave in ECG indicates some clinical conditions such as:
  - *Hypercalcemia, thyrotoxicosis and hypokalemia:* 'U' wave appears. It is very prominent in hypokalemia.
  - *Myocardial ischemia:* Inverted 'U' wave appears.

## Intervals and Segments of ECG

### 'P-R' Interval

- 'P-R' interval is the interval between the onset of 'P' wave and onset of 'Q' wave.
- 'P-R' interval signifies the atrial depolarization and conduction of impulses through AV node. It shows the duration of conduction of the impulses from the SA node to ventricles through atrial muscle and AV node.
- 'P' wave represents the atrial depolarization. Short isoelectric (zero voltage) period after the end of 'P' wave represents the time taken for the passage of depolarization within AV node.

#### Duration

Normal duration of 'P-R interval' is 0.18 second and varies between 0.12 and 0.2 second. If it is more than 0.2 second, it signifies the delay in the conduction of impulse from SA node to the ventricles. Usually, the delay occurs in the AV node. So it is called the AV nodal delay.

#### Clinical Significance

Variation in the duration of 'P-R' intervals helps in the diagnosis of several cardiac problems such as:

1. It is prolonged in bradycardia and first degree heart block
2. It is shortened in tachycardia, Wolf-Parkinson-White syndrome, Lown-Ganong-Levine syndrome, Duchenne muscular dystrophy and type II glycogen storage disease.

### *'Q-T' Interval*

- 'Q-T' interval is the interval between the onset of 'Q' wave and the end of 'T' wave.
- 'Q-T' interval indicates the ventricular depolarization and ventricular repolarization, i.e. it signifies the electrical activity in ventricles.

#### Duration

Normal duration of Q-T interval is between 0.4 and 0.42 second.

#### Clinical Significance

1. 'Q-T' interval is prolonged in long 'Q-T' syndrome, myocardial infarction, myocarditis, hypocalcemia and hypothyroidism
2. 'Q-T' interval is shortened in short 'Q-T' syndrome and hypercalcemia.

### *'S-T' Segment*

'S-T' segment is the time interval between the end of 'S' wave and the onset of 'T' wave. It is an isoelectric period.

J Point

The point where 'S-T' segment starts is called 'J' point. It is the junction between the QRS complex and 'S-T' segment.

Duration of 'S-T' Segment

Normal duration of 'S-T' segment is 0.08 second.

Clinical Significance

Variation in the duration of 'S-T' segment and its deviation from isoelectric base indicates the pathological conditions such as:

1. Elevation of 'S-T' segment occurs in anterior or inferior myocardial infarction, left bundle branch block and acute pericarditis. In athletes, 'S-T' segment is usually elevated.
2. Depression of 'S-T' segment occurs in acute myocardial ischemia, posterior myocardial infarction, ventricular hypertrophy and hypokalemia.
3. 'S-T' segment is prolonged in hypocalcemia.
4. 'S-T' segment is shortened in hypercalcemia.

*'R-R' Interval*

'R-R' interval is the time interval between two consecutive 'R' waves.

Significance

'R-R' interval signifies the duration of one cardiac cycle.

Duration

Normal duration of 'R-R' interval is 0.8 second.

Significance of Measuring 'R-R' Interval

Measurement of 'R-R' interval helps to calculate:

- Heart rate
- Heart rate variability.
- ***Heart rate:*** Heart rate is calculated by measuring the number of 'R' waves per unit time.
  - ***Calculation of heart rate:*** Time is plotted horizontally (X-axis). On X-axis, interval between two thick lines is 0.2 sec (see above). Time duration for 30 thick lines is 6 seconds. Number of 'R' waves (QRS complexes) in 6 seconds (30 thick lines) is counted and multiplied by 10 to obtain heart rate. For the sake of convenience, the ECG paper has special time marking at every 3 seconds. So it is easy to find the time duration of 6 seconds.
- ***Heart rate variability:*** Heart rate variability (HRV) refers to the beat-to-beat variations. Under resting conditions, the ECG of healthy individuals exhibits some periodic variation in 'R-R' intervals. This rhythmic phenomenon is known as respiratory sinus arrhythmia (RSA), since it fluctuates with the phases of respiration. 'R-R' interval decreases during inspiration and increases during expiration.
  - ***Significance of heart rate variability:*** HRV decreases in many clinical conditions like:
    - Cardiovascular dysfunctions such as hypertension
    - Diabetes mellitus
    - Psychiatric problems such as panic and anxiety.

## Cardiac Output

### *Introduction*

Cardiac output is the amount of blood pumped from each ventricle. Usually, it refers to left ventricular output through aorta. Cardiac output is the most important factor in cardiovascular system, because rate of blood flow through different parts of the body depends upon cardiac output.

### *Definitions and Normal Values*

Usually, cardiac output is expressed in three ways:

1. Stroke volume
2. Minute volume
3. Cardiac index.

However, in routine clinical practice, cardiac output refers to minute volume.

*Stroke Volume*

Stroke volume is the amount of blood pumped out by each ventricle during each beat.

Normal value: 70 mL (60 to 80 mL) when the heart rate is normal (72/minute).

*Minute Volume*

Minute volume is the amount of blood pumped out by each ventricle in 1 minute. It is the product of stroke volume and heart rate:

Minute volume = Stroke volume × Heart rate

Normal value: 5 L/ventricle/minute.

*Cardiac Index*

Cardiac index is the minute volume expressed in relation to square meter of body surface area. It is defined as the amount of blood pumped out per ventricle/minute/square meter of the body surface area.

Normal value: 2.8 ± 0.3 L/square meter of body surface area/minute (in an adult with average body surface area of 1.734 square meter and normal minute volume of 5 L/minute).

### *Ejection Fraction*

Ejection fraction is the fraction of end-diastolic volume that is ejected out by each ventricle. Normal ejection fraction is 60 to 65%.

### *Cardiac Reserve*

Cardiac reserve is the maximum amount of blood that can be pumped out by heart above the normal value. Cardiac reserve plays an important role in increasing the cardiac output during the conditions like exercise.

It is essential to withstand the stress of exercise. Cardiac reserve is usually expressed in percentage.

In a normal young healthy adult, the cardiac reserve is 300 to 400%. In old age, it is about 200 to 250%.

It increases to 500 to 600% in athletes. In cardiac diseases, the cardiac reserve is minimum or nil.

### *Distribution of Cardiac Output*

The whole amount of blood pumped out by the right ventricle goes to lungs. But, the blood pumped by the left ventricle is distributed to different parts of the body.

Fraction of cardiac output distributed to a particular region or organ depends upon the metabolic activities of that region or organ.

Distribution of blood pumped out of left ventricle heart, which pumps the blood to all other organs, receives the least amount of blood. Liver receives maximum amount of blood.

## *Factors Maintaining Cardiac Output*

Cardiac output is maintained (determined) by four factors:
1. Venous return
2. Force of contraction
3. Heart rate
4. Peripheral resistance.

### *Venous Return*

Venous return is the amount of blood which is returned to heart from different parts of the body. When it increases, the ventricular filling and cardiac output are increased. Thus, cardiac output is directly proportional to venous return, provided the other factors (force of contraction, heart rate and peripheral resistance) remain constant.

Venous return in turn, depends upon five factors:
(i) Respiratory pump
(ii) Muscle pump
(iii) Gravity
(iv) Venous pressure
(v) Sympathetic tone.

#### Respiratory Pump

Respiratory pump is the respiratory activity that helps the return of blood, to heart during inspiration. It is also called abdominothoracic pump. During inspiration, thoracic cavity expands and makes the intrathoracic pressure more negative. It increases the diameter of inferior vena cava, resulting in increased venous return.

At the same time, descent of diaphragm increases the intra-abdominal pressure, which compresses abdominal veins and pushes the blood upward towards the heart and thereby the venous return is increased.

Respiratory pump is much stronger in forced respiration and in severe muscular exercise.

#### Muscle Pump

Muscle pump is the muscular activity that helps in return of the blood to heart. During muscular activities, the veins are compressed or squeezed. Due to the presence of valves in veins, during compression the blood is moved towards the heart. When muscular activity increases, the venous return is more.

When the skeletal muscles contract, the vein located in between the muscles is compressed. Valve of the vein proximal to the contracting muscles is opened and the blood is propelled towards the heart.

Valve of the vein distal to the muscles is closed by the back flow of blood.

During relaxation of the muscles, the valve proximal to muscles closes and prevents the back flow of blood. The valve distal to the muscles opens and allows the blood to flow upwards.

#### Gravity

Gravitational force reduces the venous return. When a person stands for a long period, gravity causes pooling of blood in the legs, which is called venous pooling. Because of venous pooling, the amount of blood returning to heart decreases.

#### Venous Pressure

Venous pressure also affects the venous return. Pressure in the venules is 12 to 18 mm Hg. In the smaller and larger veins, the pressure gradually decreases. In the great veins, i.e. inferior vena cava and superior vena cava, the pressure falls to about 5.5 mm Hg. At the junction of venae cavae and right atrium, it is about 4.6 mm Hg. Pressure in the right atrium is still low and it alters during cardiac action. It falls to zero during atrial diastole. This pressure gradient at every part of venous tree helps as a driving force for venous return.

#### Sympathetic Tone

Venous return is aided by sympathetic or vasomotor tone, which causes constriction of venules. Venoconstriction pushes the blood towards heart.

### *Force of Contraction*

Cardiac output is directly proportional to the force of contraction, provided the other three factors remain constant. According to Frank-Starling law, force of contraction of heart is directly proportional to the initial length of muscle fibers, before the onset of contraction.

Force of contraction depends upon preload and afterload.

#### Preload

Preload is the stretching of the cardiac muscle fibers at the end of diastole, just before contraction. It is due to increase in ventricular pressure caused by filling of blood during diastole. Stretching of muscle fibers increases their length, which increases the force of contraction and cardiac output.

Thus, force of contraction of heart and cardiac output are directly proportional to preload.

#### Afterload

Afterload is the force against which ventricles must contract and eject the blood. Force is determined by the arterial pressure. At the end of isometric contraction period, semilunar valves are opened and blood is ejected into the aorta and pulmonary artery. So, the pressure increases in these two vessels. Now, the ventricles have to work against this pressure for further ejection. Thus, the afterload for left ventricle is determined by aortic pressure and afterload for right ventricular pressure is determined by pressure in pulmonary artery.

Force of contraction of heart and cardiac output are inversely proportional to afterload.

### *Heart Rate*

Cardiac output is directly proportional to heart rate provided, the other three factors remain constant.

Moderate change in heart rate does not alter the cardiac output. If there is a marked increase in heart rate, cardiac output is increased. If there is marked decrease in heart rate, cardiac output is decreased.

### *Peripheral Resistance*

Peripheral resistance is the resistance offered to blood flow at the peripheral blood vessels. Peripheral resistance is the resistance or load against which the heart has to pump the blood. So, the cardiac output is inversely proportional to peripheral resistance.

Resistance is offered at arterioles so, the arterioles are called resistant vessels. In the body, maximum peripheral resistance is offered at the splanchnic region.

## Arterial Blood Pressure

### *Definitions and Normal Values*

Arterial blood pressure is defined as the lateral pressure exerted by the column of blood on wall of arteries.

The pressure is exerted when blood flows through the arteries. Generally, the term 'blood pressure' refers to arterial blood pressure.

Arterial blood pressure is expressed in four different terms:

*Systolic Blood Pressure*

Systolic blood pressure (systolic pressure) is defined as the maximum pressure exerted in the arteries during systole of heart.

Normal systolic pressure: 120 mm Hg (110 to 140 mm Hg).

*Diastolic Blood Pressure*

Diastolic blood pressure (diastolic pressure) is defined as the minimum pressure exerted in the arteries during diastole of heart.

Normal diastolic pressure: 80 mm Hg (60 to 80 mm Hg).

*Pulse Pressure*

Pulse pressure is the difference between the systolic pressure and diastolic pressure. Normal pulse pressure: 40 mm Hg (120 – 80 = 40).

*Mean Arterial Blood Pressure*

Mean arterial blood pressure is the average pressure existing in the arteries. It is not the arithmetic mean of systolic and diastolic pressures. It is the diastolic pressure plus one third of pulse pressure. To determine the mean pressure, diastolic pressure is considered than the systolic pressure. It is because, the diastolic period of cardiac cycle is longer (0.53 second) than the systolic period (0.27 second).

Normal mean arterial pressure: 93 mm Hg (80 + 13 = 93).

Formula to calculate mean arterial blood pressure:

Mean arterial blood pressure

= Diastolic pressure + 1/3 of pulse pressure

$$= 80 + \frac{40}{3} = 93.3 \text{ mm Hg}$$

### *Variations*

Blood pressure is altered in physiological and pathological conditions. Systolic pressure is subjected for variations easily and quickly and its variation occurs in a wider range. Diastolic pressure is not subjected for easy and quick variations and its variation occurs in a narrow range.

*Physiological Variations*

1. *Age:* Arterial blood pressure increases as age advances.
   Systolic pressure in different age
   - Newborn: 70 mm Hg
   - After 1 month: 85 mm Hg
   - After 6 month: 90 mm Hg
   - After 1 year: 95 mm Hg
   - At puberty: 120 mm Hg
   - At 50 years: 140 mm Hg
   - At 70 years: 160 mm Hg
   - At 80 years: 180 mm Hg

   Diastolic pressure in different age
   - Newborn: 40 mm Hg
   - After 1 month: 45 mm Hg
   - After 6 month: 50 mm Hg
   - After 1 year: 55 mm Hg
   - At puberty: 80 mm Hg
   - At 50 years: 85 mm Hg
   - At 70 years: 90 mm Hg
   - At 80 years: 95 mm Hg
2. ***Sex:*** In females, up to the period of menopause, arterial pressure is 5 mm Hg, less than in males of same age. After menopause, the pressure in females becomes equal to that in males of same age.
3. ***Body built:*** Pressure is more in obese persons than in lean persons.
4. ***Diurnal variation:*** In early morning, the pressure is slightly low. It gradually increases and reaches the maximum at noon. It becomes low in evening.
5. ***After meals:*** Arterial blood pressure is increased for few hours after meals due to increase in cardiac output.
6. ***During sleep:*** Usually, the pressure is reduced up to 15 to 20 mm Hg during deep sleep. However, it increases slightly during sleep associated with dreams.
7. ***Emotional conditions:*** During excitement or anxiety, the blood pressure is increased due to release of adrenaline.
8. ***After exercise:*** After moderate exercise, systolic pressure increases by 20 to 30 mm Hg above the basal level due to increase in rate and force of contraction and stroke volume. Normally, diastolic pressure is not affected by moderate exercise. It is because, the diastolic pressure depends upon peripheral resistance, which is not altered by moderate exercise.
   After severe muscular exercise, systolic pressure rises by 40 to 50 mm Hg above the basal level. But, the diastolic pressure reduces because the peripheral resistance decreases in severe muscular exercise.

*Pathological Variations*

Pathological variations of arterial blood pressure are hypertension and hypotension.

### *Determinants of Arterial Blood Pressure–Factors Maintaining Arterial Blood Pressure*

Some factors are necessary to maintain normal blood pressure. These factors are called local factors, mechanical factors or determinants of blood pressure.

*Types of Local Factors*

Local factors are divided into two types:

1. Central factors, which are pertaining to the heart:
   - Cardiac output
   - Heart rate

2. Peripheral factors, which are pertaining to blood and blood vessels:
   - Peripheral resistance
   - Blood volume
   - Venous return
   - Elasticity of blood vessels
   - Velocity of blood flow
   - Diameter of blood vessels
   - Viscosity of blood.

*Central Factors*

***Cardiac output:*** Systolic pressure is directly proportional to cardiac output. Whenever the cardiac output increases, the systolic pressure is increased and when cardiac output is less, the systolic pressure is reduced. Cardiac output increases in muscular exercise, emotional conditions, etc. So in these conditions, the systolic pressure is increased. In conditions like myocardial infarction, the cardiac output decreases, resulting in fall in systolic pressure.

***Heart rate:*** Moderate changes in heart rate do not affect arterial blood pressure much. However, marked alteration in the heart rate affects the blood pressure by altering cardiac output.

*Peripheral Factors*

Peripheral Resistance

Peripheral resistance is the important factor, which maintains diastolic pressure. Diastolic pressure is directly proportional to peripheral resistance. Peripheral resistance is the resistance offered to the blood flow at the periphery. Resistance is offered at arterioles, which are called the resistant vessels. When peripheral resistance increases, diastolic pressure is increased and when peripheral resistance decreases, the diastolic pressure is decreased. Arterial blood pressure is directly proportional to:

- Cardiac output
- Heart rate
- Peripheral resistance
- Blood volume
- Venous return
- Velocity of blood flow
- Viscosity of blood

Arterial blood pressure is inversely proportional to:

- Elasticity of blood vessel
- Diameter of blood vessel

Blood Volume

Blood pressure is directly proportional to blood volume.

Blood volume maintains the blood pressure through the venous return and cardiac output. If the blood volume increases, there is an increase in venous return and cardiac output, resulting in elevation of blood pressure.

Venous Return

Blood pressure is directly proportional to venous return. When venous return increases, there is an increase in ventricular filling and cardiac output, resulting in elevation of arterial blood pressure.

Elasticity of Blood Vessels

Blood pressure is inversely proportional to the elasticity of blood vessels. Due to elastic property, the blood vessels are distensible and are able to maintain the pressure. When the elastic property is lost, the blood vessels become rigid (arteriosclerosis) and pressure increases as in old age. Deposition of cholesterol, fatty acids and calcium ions produce rigidity of blood vessels and atherosclerosis, leading to increased blood pressure.

Velocity of Blood Flow

Pressure in a blood vessel is directly proportional to the velocity of blood flow. If the velocity of blood flow increases, the resistance is increased. So, the pressure is increased.

Diameter of Blood Vessels

Arterial blood pressure is inversely proportional to the diameter of blood vessel. If the diameter decreases, the peripheral resistance increases, leading to increase in the pressure.

Viscosity of Blood

Arterial blood pressure is directly proportional to the viscosity of blood. When viscosity of blood increases, the frictional resistance is increased and this increases the pressure.

## Coronary Circulation

### *Distribution of Coronary Blood Vessels*

*Coronary Arteries*

Heart muscle is supplied by two coronary arteries, namely right and left coronary arteries, which are the first branches of aorta. Arteries encircle the heart in the manner of a crown, hence the name coronary arteries (Latin word corona = crown).

*Right and Left Coronary Arteries*

Right coronary artery supplies whole of the right ventricle and posterior portion of left ventricle. Left coronary artery supplies mainly the anterior and lateral parts of left ventricle. There are many variations in diameter of coronary arteries.

*Variations in Coronary Arteries*

- In 50 to 60% of human beings, the right coronary artery is larger (right dominant) and supplies more blood to heart than left coronary artery.
- In 15 to 20% of human beings, the left coronary artery is larger (left dominant).
- In 20 to 30% of human beings, both arteries supply almost equal amount of blood.

*Branches of Coronary Arteries*

Coronary arteries divide and subdivide into smaller branches, which run all along the surface of the heart.

Smaller branches are called epicardiac arteries and give rise to further smaller branches known as final arteries or intramural vessels. Final arteries run at right angles through the heart muscle, near the inner aspect of wall of the heart.

### *Venous Drainage*

Venous drainage from heart muscle is by three types of vessels.

1. ***Coronary sinus:*** Coronary sinus is the larger vein draining 75% of total coronary flow. It drains blood from left side of the heart and opens into right atrium near tricuspid valve.

2. *Anterior coronary veins:* Anterior coronary veins drain blood from right side of the heart and open directly into right atrium.
3. *Thebesian veins:* Thebesian veins drain deoxygenated blood from myocardium, directly into the concerned chamber of the heart.

### Physiological Shunt

Physiological shunt is the diverted route (diversion), through which the venous (deoxygenated) blood is mixed with arterial blood. Deoxygenated blood flowing from thebesian veins into cardiac chambers makes up the part of normal physiological shunt. Other component of physiological shunt is the drainage of deoxygenated blood from bronchial circulation into pulmonary vein, without being oxygenated.

### Normal Coronary Blood Flow

Normal blood flow through coronary circulation is about 200 mL/minute. It forms 4% of cardiac output. It is about 65 to 70 mL/minute/100 g of cardiac muscle.

### Factors Regulating Coronary Blood Flow

*Autoregulation*

Like any other organ, heart also has the capacity to regulate its own blood flow by autoregulation. Coronary blood flow is not affected when mean arterial pressure varies between 60 and 150 mm Hg. Several factors are involved in the autoregulation mechanism. Coronary blood flow is regulated mainly by local vascular response to the needs of cardiac muscle. Factors regulating coronary blood flow:

1. Need for oxygen
2. Metabolic factors
3. Coronary perfusion pressure
4. Nervous factors.

1. *Need for Oxygen:* Oxygen is the most important factor maintaining blood flow through the coronary blood vessels. Amount of blood passing through coronary circulation is directly proportional to the consumption of oxygen by cardiac muscle.
   Even in resting condition, a large amount of oxygen, i.e. 70 to 80% is consumed from the blood by heart muscle than by any other tissues. In conditions associated with increased cardiac activity, the need for oxygen increases enormously.
   Thus, the need for oxygen, i.e. hypoxia immediately causes coronary vasodilatation and increases the blood flow to heart.
2. *Metabolic Factors:* Coronary vasodilatation during hypoxic conditions occurs because of some metabolic products, which increase the coronary blood flow by vasodilatation.
   *Reactive hyperemia:* Reactive hyperemia is the increase in blood flow due to the vasodilator effects of metabolites.
   *Metabolic Products which Increase the Coronary Blood Flow*
   *Adenosine:* Adenosine is a potent vasodilator and it increases the blood flow to cardiac muscle. During hypoxia, ATP in the muscle is degraded in large amount, forming ADP. Some ADP molecules are further degraded into adenosine, which is released into tissue fluids of heart muscle.
   *Other substances:* Other substances which increase the coronary blood flow by vasodilatation are:
   - Potassium
   - Hydrogen
   - Carbon dioxide
   - Adenosine phosphate compounds.
3. *Coronary Perfusion Pressure:* Perfusion pressure is the balance between mean arterial pressure and venous pressure. Thus, coronary perfusion pressure is the balance between mean arterial pressure in aorta and the right atrial pressure. Since right aterial pressure is low, the mean arterial pressure becomes the major factor that maintains the coronary blood flow. Range of mean arterial pressure at which the coronary blood flow can be maintained is given above.
4. *Nervous Factors:* Coronary blood vessels are innervated both by parasympathetic and sympathetic divisions of autonomic nervous system. It is not known whether the autonomic nerves have direct effect on blood flow in various conditions. However, these nerves influence the coronary blood flow indirectly by acting on the musculature of heart.
   For example, stimulation of sympathetic nerves increases the rate and force of contraction of heart. This in turn, causes liberation of more metabolites which dilate the blood vessels and increase the coronary blood flow. Similarly, when parasympathetic nerves are stimulated, the cardiac functions are inhibited and the production of metabolites is less. Coronary blood flow decreases.

## Fetal Circulation and Respiration

### Introduction

Fetal circulation is different from that of adults because of the presence of placenta. Since fetal lungs are nonfunctioning, placenta is responsible for exchange of gases between fetal blood and mother's blood. So, the blood from right ventricle is diverted to placenta.

Development of heart is completed at 4th week of intrauterine life and it starts beating at the rate of 65 per minute. Along with heart, the blood vessels also develop. Heart rate gradually increases and reaches the maximum rate of about 140 beats per minute just before birth. Fetus is connected with the mother through placenta. Fetal blood passes to placenta through umbilical vessels and the maternal blood runs through uterine vessels. These two sets of blood vessels lie in close proximity in the placenta through which exchange of substances takes place between mother's blood and fetal blood. However, there is no direct admixture of maternal and fetal blood.

### Blood Vessels in Fetus

As fetal lungs are non-functioning, there is no necessity of large amount of blood to be pumped into lungs.

Instead, the fetal heart pumps large quantity of blood into the placenta for exchange of substances. From placenta, the umbilical veins collect the blood, which has more oxygen and nutrients. Umbilical vein passes through liver. Some amount of blood is supplied to liver from umbilical vein. However, a large quantity of blood is diverted from umbilical vein into the inferior vena cava through ductus venosus. Liver receives blood from portal vein also.

In liver, the oxygenated blood mixes slightly with deoxygenated blood and enters the right atrium via inferior vena cava. From right atrium, major portion of blood is diverted into left atrium via foramen ovale.

Foramen ovale is an opening in intra-atrial septum. Blood from upper part of the body enters the right atrium through superior vena cava. From right atrium, blood enters right ventricle. From here, blood is pumped into pulmonary artery. From pulmonary artery, blood enters the systemic aorta through ductus arteriosus.

Only a small quantity of blood is supplied to fetal lungs. Blood from left ventricle is pumped into aorta.

Fifty percent of blood from aorta reaches the placenta through umbilical arteries.

### *Fetal Lungs*

Pulmonary vascular resistance is the resistance offered to blood flow through pulmonary vascular bed. This resistance is very high in fetus because of the non-functioning of fetal lungs. The high resistance in fetal lungs increases the pressure in the blood vessels of lungs. Because of the high pressure, the blood is diverted from pulmonary artery into aorta via ductus arteriosus.

### *Changes in Circulation and Respiration after Birth: Neonatal Circulation and Respiration*

1. *First Breath of the Child:* When fetus is delivered and umbilical cord is cut and tied, the lungs start functioning. When placental blood flow is cut off, there is sudden hypoxia and hypercapnia. Now, left atrium. It causes increase in the left atrial pressure. Simultaneously, due to stoppage of blood from placenta, pressure in inferior vena cava is decreased. It leads to fall in right atrial pressure. Thus, the pressure in right atrium is less and the pressure in left atrium is already high. This causes the closure of foramen ovale. Within few days after birth, the foramen ovale closes completely and fuses with the atrial wall.
2. *Reversal of Blood Flow in Ductus Arteriosus:* In fetus, since pulmonary arterial pressure is very high, the blood passes from pulmonary artery into aorta via ductus arteriosus. However, in neonatal life, since the systemic arterial pressure is more than pulmonary arterial pressure, the blood passes in opposite direction in ductus arteriosus, i.e. from systemic aorta into pulmonary aorta. The reversed flow in ductus arteriosus is heard as continuous murmur in infants.
3. *Closure of Ductus Venosus:* Due to the contraction of smooth muscle near junction between umbilical vein and ductus venosus, the constriction and closure of ductus venosus occurs. Later, the ductus venosus becomes fibrous band.
4. *Closure of Ductus Arteriosus:* Ductus arteriosus starts closing due to narrowing. It closes completely after 2 days and the adult type of circulation starts. In some rare cases, the ductus arteriosus does not close. It remains intact producing a continuous murmur. This condition with intact ductus arteriosus is known as patent ductus arteriosus.

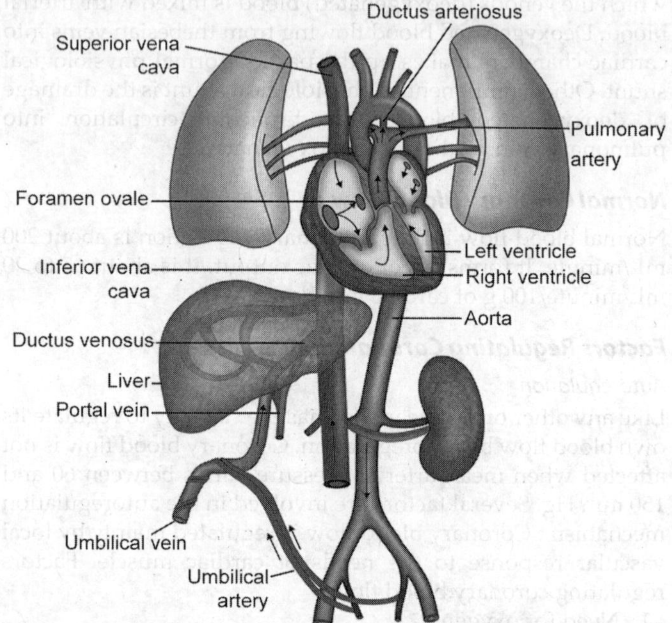


## RESPIRATORY SYSTEM

### Introduction

Respiration is the process by which oxygen is taken in and carbon dioxide is given out. The first breath takes place only after birth. Fetal lungs are non-functional.

So, during intrauterine life the exchange of gases between fetal blood and mother's blood occurs through placenta.

After the first breath, the respiratory process continues throughout the life. Permanent stoppage of respiration occurs only at death.

### *Normal Respiratory Rate at Different Age*

- Newborn: 30 to 60/minute
- Early childhood: 20 to 40/minute
- Late childhood: 15 to 25/minute
- Adult: 12 to 16/minute.

### Types of Respiration

Respiration is classified into two types:

1. External respiration that involves exchange of respiratory gases, i.e. oxygen and carbon dioxide between lungs and blood.
2. Internal respiration which involves exchange of gases between blood and tissues.

## Phases of Respiration

Respiration occurs in two phases:

1. Inspiration during which air enters the lungs from atmosphere.
2. Expiration during which air leaves the lungs. During normal breathing, inspiration is an active process and expiration is a passive process.

## Functional Anatomy of Respiratory Tract

Respiratory tract is the anatomical structure through which air moves in and out. It includes nose, pharynx, larynx, trachea, bronchi and lungs.

### *Pleura*

Each lung is enclosed by a bilayered serous membrane called pleura or pleural sac. Pleura has two layers namely inner visceral and outer parietal layers. Visceral layer is attached firmly to the surface of the lungs.

At hilum, it is continuous with parietal layer, which is attached to the wall of thoracic cavity.

*Intrapleural Space or Pleural Cavity*

Intrapleural space or pleural cavity is the narrow space in between the two layers of pleura.

*Intrapleural Fluid*

Intrapleural space contains a thin film of serous fluid called intrapleural fluid, which is secreted by the visceral layer of the pleura.

Functions of intrapleural fluid:

1. It functions as the lubricant to prevent friction between two layers of pleura.
2. It is involved in creating the negative pressure called intrapleural pressure within intrapleural space.

*Pleural Cavity in Abnormal Conditions*

In some pathological conditions, the pleural cavity expands with accumulation of air (pneumothorax), water (hydrothorax), blood (hemothorax) or pus (pyothorax).

### *Tracheobronchial Tree*

Trachea and bronchi are together called tracheobronchial tree. It forms a part of air passage.

*Components of Tracheobronchial Tree*

1. Trachea bifurcates into two main or primary bronchi called right and left bronchi.
2. Each primary bronchus enters the lungs and divides into secondary bronchi.
3. Secondary bronchi divide into tertiary bronchi. In right lung, there are 10 tertiary bronchi and in left lung, there are eight tertiary bronchi.
4. Tertiary bronchi divide several times with reduction in length and diameter into many generations of bronchioles.
5. When the diameter of bronchiole becomes 1 mm or less, it is called terminal bronchiole.
6. Terminal bronchiole continues or divides into respiratory bronchioles, which have a diameter of 0.5 mm.

### *Upper and Lower Respiratory Tracts*

Generally, respiratory tract is divided into two parts:

1. Upper respiratory tract that includes all the structures from nose up to vocal cords; vocal cords are the folds of mucous membrane within larynx that vibrates to produce the voice.
2. Lower respiratory tract, which includes trachea.

## Respiratory Unit

Parenchyma of lungs is formed by respiratory unit that forms the terminal portion of respiratory tract. Respiratory unit is defined as the structural and functional unit of lung. Exchange of gases occurs only in this part of the respiratory tract.

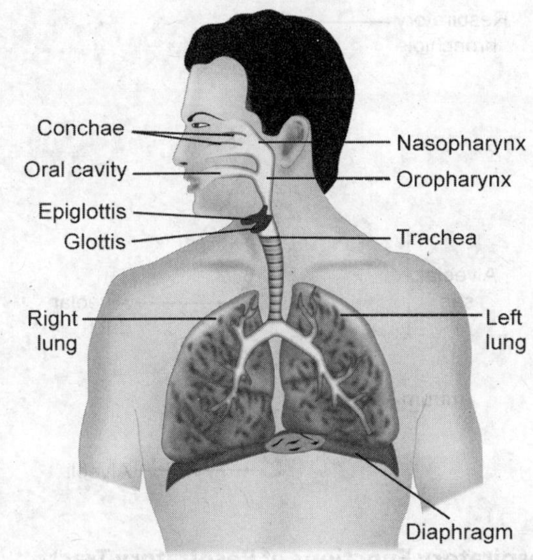


## Structure of Respiratory Unit

Respiratory unit starts from the respiratory bronchioles Each respiratory bronchiole divides into alveolar ducts. Each alveolar duct enters an enlarged structure called the alveolar sac. Space inside the alveolar sac is called antrum. Alveolar sac consists of a cluster of alveoli. Few alveoli are present in the wall of alveolar duct also. Thus, respiratory unit includes:

1. Respiratory bronchioles
2. Alveolar ducts
3. Alveolar sacs
4. Antrum
5. Alveoli.

Each alveolus is like a pouch with the diameter of about 0.2 to 0.5 mm. It is lined by epithelial cells.

*Alveolar Cells or Pneumocytes*

Alveolar epithelium consists of alveolar cells or pneumocytes, which are of two types namely type I alveolar cells and type II alveolar cells.

Type I Alveolar Cells

Type I alveolar cells are the squamous epithelial cells forming about 95% of the total number of cells. These cells form the site of gaseous exchange between the alveolus and blood.

Type II Alveolar Cells

Type II alveolar cells are cuboidal in nature and form about 5% of alveolar cells. These cells are also called granular pneumocytes. Type II alveolar cells secrete alveolar fluid and surfactant.

### *Respiratory Membrane*

Respiratory membrane is the membranous structure through which the exchange of gases occurs.

Respiratory membrane separates air in the alveoli from the blood in capillary. It is formed by the alveolar membrane and capillary membrane. Respiratory membrane has a surface area of 70 square meter and thickness of 0.5 micron.

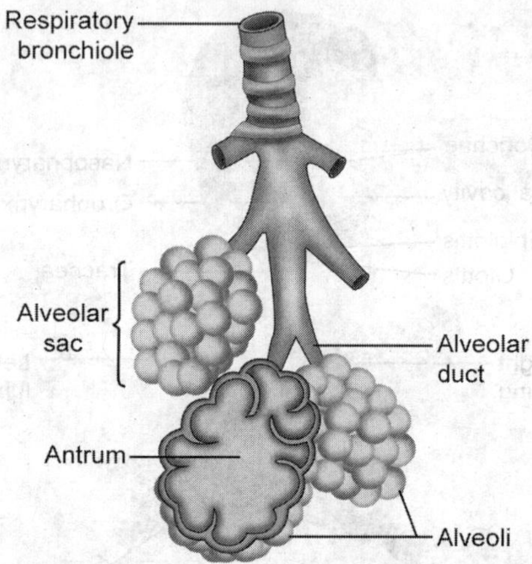


### Non-respiratory Functions of Respiratory Tract

Besides primary function of gaseous exchange, the respiratory tract is involved in several non-respiratory functions of the body. Particularly, the lungs function as a defense barrier and metabolic organs, which synthesize some important compounds. Non-respiratory functions of the respiratory tract are:

1. ***Olfaction:*** Olfactory receptors present in the mucous membrane of nostril are responsible for olfactory sensation.
2. ***Vocalization:*** Along with other structures, larynx forms the speech apparatus. However, larynx alone plays major role in the process of vocalization. Therefore, it is called sound box.
3. ***Prevention of Dust Particles:*** Dust particles, which enter the nostrils from air, are prevented from reaching the lungs by filtration action of the hairs in nasal mucous membrane. Small particles, which escape the hairs, are held by the mucus secreted by nasal mucous membrane. Those dust particles, which escape nasal hairs and nasal mucous membrane, are removed by the phagocytic action of macrophages in the alveoli.

   Particles, which escape the protective mechanisms in nose and alveoli are thrown out by cough reflex and sneezing reflex.
4. ***Defense Mechanism:*** Lungs play important role in the immunological defense system of the body. Defense functions of the lungs are performed by their own defenses and by the presence of various types of cells in mucous membrane lining the alveoli of lungs. These cells are leukocytes, macrophages, mast cells, natural killer cells and dendritic cells.
   - ***Lung's own defenses:*** Epithelial cells lining the air passage secrete some innate immune factors called defensins and cathelicidins. These substances are the antimicrobial peptides, which play an important role in lung's natural defenses.
   - ***Defense through leukocytes:*** Leukocytes, particularly the neutrophils and lymphocytes present in the alveoli of lungs provide defense mechanism against bacteria and virus. Neutrophils kill the bacteria by phagocytosis. Lymphocytes develop immunity against bacteria.
   - ***Defense through macrophages:*** Macrophages engulf the dust particles and the pathogens, which enter the alveoli and thereby act as scavengers in lungs. Macrophages are also involved in the development of immunity by functioning as antigen presenting cells. When foreign organisms invade the body, the macrophages and other antigen presenting cells kill them. Later, the antigen from the organisms is digested into polypeptides. Polypeptide products are presented to T lymphocytes and B lymphocytes by the macrophages.

     Macrophages secrete interleukins, tumor necrosis factors (TNF) and chemokines. Interleukins and TNF activate the general immune system of the body. Chemokines attract the white blood cells towards the site of any inflammation.
   - ***Defense through mast cell:*** Mast cell is a large cell resembling the basophil. Mast cell produces the hypersensitivity reactions like allergy and anaphylaxis. It secretes heparin, histamine, serotonin and hydrolytic enzymes.
   - ***Defense through natural killer (NK) cell:*** NK cell is a large granular cell, considered as the third type of lymphocyte. Usually NK cell is present in lungs and other lymphoid organs. Its granules contain hydrolytic enzymes, which destroy the microorganisms.

     NK cell is said to be the first line of defense in specific immunity particularly against viruses. It destroys the viruses and viral infected or damaged cells, which may form the tumors. It also destroys the malignant cells and prevents development of cancerous tumors. NK cells secrete interferons and the tumor necrosis factors.
   - ***Defense through dendritic cells:*** Dendritic cells in the lungs play important role in immunity. Along with macrophages, these cells function as antigen presenting cells.
5. ***Maintenance of Water Balance:*** Respiratory tract plays a role in water loss mechanism. During expiration, water evaporates through the expired air and some amount of body water is lost by this process.
6. ***Regulation of Body Temperature:*** During expiration, along with water, heat is also lost from the body. Thus, respiratory tract plays a role in heat loss mechanism.

7. ***Regulation of Acid-Base Balance:*** Lungs play a role in maintenance of acid-base balance of the body by regulating the carbon dioxide content in blood. Carbon dioxide is produced during various metabolic reactions in the tissues of the body. When it enters the blood, carbon dioxide combines with water to form carbonic acid. Since carbonic acid is unstable, it splits into hydrogen and bicarbonate ions.

   $CO_2 + H_2O \rightarrow H_2CO_3 \rightarrow H^+ + HCO_3^-$

   Entire reaction is reversed in lungs when carbon dioxide is removed from blood into the alveoli of lungs.

   $H^+ + HCO_3^- \rightarrow H_2CO_3 \rightarrow CO_2 + H_2O$

   As carbon dioxide is a volatile gas, it is practically blown out by ventilation. When metabolic activities are accelerated, more amount of carbon dioxide is produced in the tissues.

   Concentration of hydrogen ion is also increased. This leads to reduction in pH. Increased hydrogen ion concentration causes increased pulmonary ventilation (hyperventilation) by acting through various mechanisms like chemoreceptors in aortic and carotid bodies and in medulla of the brain. Due to hyperventilation, excess of carbon dioxide is removed from body fluids and the pH is brought back to normal.
8. ***Anticoagulant Function:*** Mast cells in lungs secrete heparin. Heparin is an anticoagulant and it prevents the intravascular clotting.
9. ***Secretion of Angiotensin-converting Enzyme:*** Endothelial cells of the pulmonary capillaries secrete the angiotensin-converting enzyme (ACE). It converts the angiotensin I into active angiotensin II, which plays an important role in the regulation of ECF volume and blood pressure.
10. ***Synthesis of Hormonal Substances:*** Lung tissues are also known to synthesize the hormonal substances, prostaglandins, acetylcholine and serotonin which have many physiological actions in the body including regulation of blood pressure.

## Respiratory Protective Reflexes

Respiratory protective reflexes are the reflexes that protect lungs and air passage from foreign particles.Respiratory process is modified by these reflexes in order to eliminate the foreign particles or to prevent the entry of these particles into the respiratory tract.

Following are the respiratory protective reflexes:

### *Cough Reflex*

Cough is a modified respiratory process characterized by forced expiration. It is a protective reflex and it is caused by irritation of respiratory tract and some other areas such as external auditory canal.

*Causes*

Cough is produced mainly by irritant agents. It is also produced by several disorders such as cardiac disorders (congestive heart failure), pulmonary disorders (chronic obstructive pulmonary disease–COPD) and tumor in thorax, which may exert pressure on larynx, trachea, bronchi or lungs.

*Mechanism*

Cough begins with deep inspiration followed by forced expiration with closed glottis. This increases the intrapleural pressure above 100 mm Hg. Then, glottis opens suddenly with explosive outflow of air at a high velocity. Velocity of the airflow may reach 960 km/hour.

It causes expulsion of irritant substances out of the respiratory tract.

*Reflex Pathway*

Receptors that initiate the cough are situated in several locations such as nose, paranasal sinuses, larynx, pharynx, trachea, bronchi, pleura, diaphragm, pericardium, stomach, external auditory canal and tympanic membrane.

Afferent nerve fibers pass via vagus, trigeminal, glossopharyngeal and phrenic nerves. The center for cough reflex is in the medulla oblongata.

Efferent nerve fibers arising from the medullary center pass through the vagus, phrenic and spinal motor nerves. These nerve fibers activate the primary and accessory respiratory muscles.

### *Sneezing Reflex*

Sneezing is also a modified respiratory process characterized by forced expiration. It is a protective reflex caused by irritation of nasal mucous membrane.

*Causes*

Irritation of the nasal mucous membrane occurs because of dust particles, debris, mechanical obstruction of the airway and excess fluid accumulation in the nasal passages.

*Mechanism*

Sneezing starts with deep inspiration, followed by forceful expiratory effort with opened glottis resulting in expulsion of irritant agents out of respiratory tract.

*Reflex Pathway*

Sneezing is initiated by the irritation of nasal mucous membrane, the olfactory receptors and trigeminal nerve endings present in the nasal mucosa.

Afferent nerve fibers pass through the trigeminal and olfactory nerves. Sneezing center is in medulla oblongata. It is located diffusely in spinal nucleus of trigeminal nerve, nucleus solitarius and the reticular formation of medulla.

Efferent nerve fibers from the medullary center pass via trigeminal, facial, glossopharyngeal, vagus and intercostal nerves. These nerve fibers activate the pharyngeal, tracheal and respiratory muscles.

### *Swallowing (Deglutition) Reflex*

Swallowing reflex is a respiratory protective reflex that prevents entrance of food particles into the air passage during swallowing.

While swallowing of the food, the respiration is arrested for a while. Temporary arrest of respiration is called apnea. Arrest of breathing during swallowing is called swallowing apnea or deglutition apnea. It takes place during pharyngeal stage, i.e. second stage of deglutition and prevents entry of food particles into the respiratory tract.

## Mechanics of Respiration

### Respiratory Movements

*Introduction*

Respiration occurs in two phases namely inspiration and expiration.

During inspiration, thoracic cage enlarges and lungs expand so that air enters the lungs easily. During expiration, the thoracic cage and lungs decrease in size and attain the preinspiratory position so that air leaves the lungs easily.

During normal quiet breathing, inspiration is the active process and expiration is the passive process.

*Muscles of Respiration*

Respiratory muscles are of two types:

1. Inspiratory muscles
2. Expiratory muscles.

However, respiratory muscles are generally classified into two types:

1. Primary or major respiratory muscles, which are responsible for change in size of thoracic cage during normal quiet breathing
2. Accessory respiratory muscles that help primary respiratory muscles during forced respiration.

*Inspiratory Muscles*

Muscles involved in inspiratory movements are known as inspiratory muscles.

Primary Inspiratory Muscles

Primary inspiratory muscles are the diaphragm, which is supplied by phrenic nerve (C3 to C5) and external intercostal muscles, supplied by intercostal nerves (T1 to T11).

Accessory Inspiratory Muscles

Sternocleidomastoid, scalene, anterior serrati, elevators of scapulae and pectorals are the accessory inspiratory muscles.

*Expiratory Muscles*

Primary Expiratory Muscles

Primary expiratory muscles are the internal intercostals muscles, which are innervated by intercostal nerves. Accessory expiratory muscles

Accessory expiratory muscles are the abdominal muscles.

### Movements of Thoracic Cage

Inspiration causes enlargement of thoracic cage. Thoracic cage enlarges because of increase in all diameters, viz. anteroposterior, transverse and vertical diameters.

Anteroposterior and transverse diameters of thoracic cage are increased by the elevation of ribs. Vertical diameter is increased by the descent of diaphragm.

In general, change in the size of thoracic cavity occurs because of the movements of four units of structures:

1. ***Thoracic Lid:*** Thoracic lid is formed by manubrium sterni and the first pair of ribs. It is also called thoracic operculum. Movement of thoracic lid increases the anteroposterior diameter of thoracic cage. Due to the contraction of scalene muscles, the first ribs move upwards to a more horizontal position. This increases the anteroposterior diameter of upper thoracic cage.
2. ***Upper Costal Series:*** Upper costal series is constituted by second to sixth pair of ribs. Movement of upper costal series increases the anteroposterior and transverse diameter of the thoracic cage. Movement of upper costal series is of two types:
   (i) ***Pump handle movement:*** Contraction of external intercostal muscles causes elevation of these ribs and upward and forward movement of sternum. This movement is called pump handle movement. It increases anteroposterior diameter of the thoracic cage.
   (ii) ***Bucket handle movement:*** Simultaneously, the central portions of these ribs (arches of ribs) move upwards and outwards to a more horizontal position. This movement is called bucket handle movement and it increases the transverse diameter of thoracic cage.
3. ***Lower Costal Series:*** Lower costal series includes seventh to tenth pair of ribs. Movement of lower costal series increases the transverse diameter of thoracic cage by bucket handle movement.
   ***Bucket handle movement:*** Lower costal series of ribs also show bucket handle movement by swinging outward and upward. This movement increases the transverse diameter of the thoracic cage.
   Eleventh and twelfth pairs of ribs are the floating ribs. These ribs are not involved in changing the size of thoracic cage.
4. ***Diaphragm:*** Movement of diaphragm increases the vertical diameter of thoracic cage. Normally, before inspiration the diaphragm is dome shaped with convexity facing upwards. During inspiration, due to the contraction, muscle fibers are shortened. But the central tendinous portion is drawn downwards so the diaphragm is flattened.

Flattening of diaphragm increases the vertical diameter of the thoracic cage.

### Movements of Lungs

During inspiration, due to the enlargement of thoracic cage, the negative pressure is increased in the thoracic cavity. It causes expansion of the lungs. During expiration, the thoracic cavity decreases in size to the preinspiratory position. Pressure in the thoracic cage also comes back to the preinspiratory level. It compresses the lung tissues so that, the air is expelled out of lungs.

*Collapsing Tendency of Lungs*

Lungs are under constant threat to collapse even in resting conditions because of certain factors.

Factors Causing Collapsing Tendency of Lungs

Two factors are responsible for the collapsing tendency of lungs:

1. ***Elastic property of lung tissues:*** Elastic tissues of lungs show constant recoiling tendency and try to collapse the lungs.
2. ***Surface tension:*** It is the tension exerted by the fluid secreted from alveolar epithelium on the surface of alveolar membrane.

   Fortunately, there are some factors, which save the lungs from collapsing.

*Factors Preventing Collapsing Tendency of Lungs*

In spite of elastic property of lungs and surface tension in the alveoli of lungs, the collapsing tendency of lungs is prevented by two factors:

1. ***Intrapleural pressure:*** It is the pressure in the pleural cavity, which is always negative (see below). Because of negativity, it keeps the lungs expanded and prevents the collapsing tendency of lungs produced by the elastic tissues.
2. ***Surfactant:*** It is a substance secreted in alveolar epithelium. It reduces surface tension and prevents the collapsing tendency produced by surface tension.

*Surfactant*

Surfactant is a surface acting material or agent that is responsible for lowering the surface tension of a fluid.

Surfactant that lines the epithelium of the alveoli in lungs is known as pulmonary surfactant and it decreases the surface tension on the alveolar membrane.

Source of Secretion of Pulmonary Surfactant

Pulmonary surfactant is secreted by two types of cells:

1. Type II alveolar epithelial cells in the lungs, which are called surfactant secreting alveolar cells or pneumocytes. Characteristic feature of these cells is the presence of microvilli on their alveolar surface.
2. Clara cells, which are situated in the bronchioles. These cells are also called bronchiolar exocrine cells.

Chemistry of Surfactant

Surfactant is a lipoprotein complex formed by lipids especially phospholipids, proteins and ions.

1. ***Phospholipids:*** Phospholipids form about 75% of the surfactant. Major phospholipid present in the surfactant is dipalmitoylphosphatidylcholine (DPPC).
2. ***Other lipids:*** Other lipid substances of surfactant are triglycerides and phosphatidylglycerol (PG).
3. ***Proteins:*** Proteins of the surfactant are called specific surfactant proteins (SP). There are four main surfactant proteins, called SPA, SPB, SPC and SPD. SPA and SPD are hydrophilic, while SPB and SPC are hydrophobic. Surfactant proteins are vital components of surfactant and the surfactant becomes inactive in the absence of proteins.
4. ***Ions:*** Ions present in the surfactant are mostly calcium ions.

Formation of Surfactant

Type II alveolar epithelial cells and Clara cells have a special type of membrane bound organelles called lamellar bodies, which form the intracellular source of surfactant. Laminar bodies contain surfactant phospholipids and surfactant proteins. These materials are synthesized in endoplasmic reticulum and stored in laminar bodies.

By means of exocytosis, lipids and proteins of lamellar bodies are released into surface fluid lining the alveoli. Here, in the presence of surfactant proteins and calcium, the phospholipids are arranged into a lattice (meshwork) structure called tubular myelin. Tubular myelin is in turn converted into surfactant in the form of a film that spreads over the entire surface of alveoli.

Most of the surfactant is absorbed into the type II alveolar cells, catabolized and the products are loaded into lamellar bodies for recycling.

Factors Necessary for The Formation and Spreading of Surfactant

Formation of surfactant requires many substances. Forma tion of tubular myelin requires DPPC, PG and the hydrophobic proteins, SPB and SPC.

Formation of surfactant film requires SPB, SPC and PG. Type II alveolar epithelial cells occupy only about 5% of alveolar surface. However, the surfactant must spread over the entire alveolar surface. It is facilitated by PG and calcium ions.

Glucocorticoids play important role in the formation of surfactant.

Functions of Surfactant

- Surfactant reduces the surface tension in the alveoli of lungs and prevents collapsing tendency of lungs.

  ***Surfactant acts by the following mechanism:*** Phospholipid molecule in the surfactant has two portions. One portion of the molecule is hydrophilic.

  This portion dissolves in water and lines the alveoli. Other portion is hydrophobic and it is directed towards the alveolar air. This surface of the phospholipid along with other portion spreads over the alveoli and reduces the surface tension. SPB and SPC play active role in this process.
- Surfactant is responsible for stabilization of the alveoli, which is necessary to withstand the collapsing tendency.
- It plays an important role in the inflation of lungs after birth. In fetus, the secretion of surfactant begins after the 3rd month. Until birth, the lungs are solid and not expanded. Soon after birth, the first breath starts because of the stimulation of respiratory centers by hypoxia and hypercapnea. Although the respiratory movements are attempted by the infant, the lungs tend to collapse repeatedly. And, the presence of surfactant in the alveoli prevents the lungs from collapsing.
- Another important function of surfactant is its role in defense within the lungs against infection and inflammation. Hydrophilic proteins SPA and SPD destroy the bacteria and viruses by means of opsonization. These two proteins also control the formation of inflammatory mediators.

Effect of Deficiency of Surfactant–respiratory Distress Syndrome

Absence of surfactant in infants, causes collapse of lungs and the condition is called respiratory distress syndrome or hyaline membrane disease. Deficiency of surfactant occurs in adults also and it is called adult respiratory distress syndrome (ARDS).

In addition, the deficiency of surfactant increases the susceptibility for bacterial and viral infections.

## Respiratory Pressures

Two types of pressures are exerted in the thoracic cavity and lungs during process of respiration:

1. Intrapleural pressure or intrathoracic pressure
2. Intra-alveolar pressure or intrapulmonary pressure.

### *Intrapleural Pressure*

*Definition*

Intrapleural pressure is the pressure existing in pleural cavity, that is, in between the visceral and parietal layers of pleura. It is exerted by the suction of the fluid that lines the pleural cavity. It is also called intrathoracic pressure since it is exerted in the whole of thoracic cavity.

*Normal Values*

Respiratory pressures are always expressed in relation to atmospheric pressure, which is 760 mm Hg. Under physiological conditions, the intrapleural pressure is always negative.

Normal values are:

1. At the end of normal inspiration: –6 mm Hg (760 – 6 = 754 mm Hg)
2. At the end of normal expiration: –2 mm Hg (760 – 2 = 758 mm Hg)
3. At the end of forced inspiration: –30 mm Hg
4. At the end of forced inspiration with closed glottis (Müller maneuver): –70 mm Hg
5. At the end of forced expiration with closed glottis (Valsalva maneuver): +50 mm Hg.

*Cause for Negativity of Intrapleural Pressure*

Pleural cavity is always lined by a thin layer of fluid that is secreted by the visceral layer of pleura. This fluid is constantly pumped from the pleural cavity into the lymphatic vessels. Pumping of fluid creates the negative pressure in the pleural cavity. Intrapleural pressure becomes positive in Valsalva maneuver and in some pathological conditions such as pneumothorax, hydrothorax, hemothorax and pyothorax.

*Measurement*

Intrapleural pressure is measured by direct method and indirect method. In the direct method, the intrapleural pressure is determined by introducing a needle into the pleural cavity and connecting the needle to a mercury manometer. In indirect method, intrapleural pressure is measured by introducing the esophageal balloon, which is connected to a manometer. Intrapleural pressure is considered as equivalent to the pressure existing in the esophagus.

*Significance of Intrapleural Pressure*

Throughout the respiratory cycle intrapleural pressure remains lower than intra-alveolar pressure. This keeps the lungs always inflated.

Intrapleural pressure has two important functions:

1. It prevents the collapsing tendency of lungs
2. Because of the negative pressure in thoracic region, larger veins and vena cava are enlarged, i.e. dilated. Also, the negative pressure acts like suction pump and pulls the venous blood from lower part of body towards the heart against gravity. Thus, the intrapleural pressure is responsible for venous return. So, it is called the respiratory pump for venous return.

### *Intra-alveolar Pressure*

*Definition*

Intra-alveolar pressure is the pressure existing in the alveoli of the lungs. It is also known as intrapulmonary pressure.

*Normal Values*

Normally, intra-alveolar pressure is equal to the atmospheric pressure, which is 760 mm Hg. It becomes negative during inspiration and positive during expiration.

Normal values are:

1. During normal inspiration: –1 mm Hg (760 – 1 = 759 mm Hg)
2. During normal expiration: +1 mm Hg (760 + 1 = 761 mm Hg)
3. At the end of inspiration and expiration: Equal to atmospheric pressure (760 mm Hg)
4. During forced inspiration with closed glottis (Müller maneuver): –80 mm Hg
5. During forced expiration with closed glottis (Valsalva maneuver): +100 mm Hg.

*Measurement*

Intra-alveolar pressure is measured by using plethysmograph.

*Significance of Intra-alveolar Pressure*

1. Intra-alveolar pressure causes flow of air in and out of alveoli. During inspiration, the intra-alveolar pressure becomes negative, so the atmospheric air enters the alveoli. During expiration, intra-alveolar pressure becomes positive. So, air is expelled out of alveoli.
2. Intra-alveolar pressure also helps in exchange of gases between the alveolar air and the blood.

*Transpulmonary Pressure*

Transpulmonary pressure is the pressure difference between intra-alveolar pressure and intrapleural pressure. It is the measure of elastic forces in lungs, which is responsible for collapsing tendency of lungs.

## Pulmonary Function Tests

### *Introduction*

Pulmonary function tests or lung function tests are useful in assessing the functional status of the respiratory system both in physiological and pathological conditions.

Lung function tests are based on the measurement of volume of air breathed in and out in quiet breathing and forced breathing. These tests are carried out mostly by using spirometer.

### *Types of Lung Function Tests*

Lung function tests are of two types: 1. Static lung function tests and 2. dynamic lung function tests

*Static Lung Function Tests*

Static lung function tests are based on volume of air that flows into or out of lungs. These tests do not depend upon the rate at which air flows. Static lung function tests include static lung volumes and static lung capacities.

*Dynamic Lung Function Tests*

Dynamic lung function tests are based on time, i.e. the rate at which air flows into or out of lungs. These tests include forced vital capacity, forced expiratory volume, maximum ventilation volume and peak expiratory flow. Dynamic lung function tests are useful in determining the severity of obstructive and restrictive lung diseases.

## Lung Volumes

Static lung volumes are the volumes of air breathed by an individual. Each of these volumes represents the volume of air present in the lung under a specified static condition (specific position of thorax). Static lung volumes are of four types:

### *Tidal Volume*

Tidal volume (TV) is the volume of air breathed in and out of lungs in a single normal quiet respiration. Tidal volume signifies the normal depth of breathing.

*Normal Value*

500 mL (0.5 L).

### *Inspiratory Reserve Volume*

Inspiratory reserve volume (IRV) is an additional volume of air that can be inspired forcefully after the end of normal inspiration.

*Normal Value*

3,300 mL (3.3 L).

### *Expiratory Reserve Volume*

Expiratory reserve volume (EVR) is the additional volume of air that can be expired out forcefully, after normal expiration.

*Normal Value*

1,000 mL (1 L).

### *Residual Volume*

Residual volume (RV) is the volume of air remaining in lungs even after forced expiration. Normally, lungs cannot be emptied completely even by forceful expiration. Some quantity of air always remains in the lungs even after the forced expiration. Residual volume is significant because of two reasons:

1. It helps to aerate the blood in between breathing and during expiration
2. It maintains the contour of the lungs.

*Normal Value*

1,200 mL (1.2 L)

## Lung Capacities

Static lung capacities are the combination of two or more lung volumes. Static lung capacities are of four types:

### *Inspiratory Capacity*

Inspiratory capacity (IC) is the maximum volume of air that is inspired after normal expiration (end expiratory position). It includes tidal volume (TV) and inspiratory reserve volume (IRV).

$$IC = TV + IRV$$
$$= 500 + 3{,}300 = 3{,}800 \text{ mL}$$

### *Vital Capacity (VC)*

Vital capacity (VC) is the maximum volume of air that can be expelled out forcefully after a deep (maximal) inspiration. VC includes inspiratory reserve volume, tidal volume (ERV) and expiratory reserve volume (RV).

$$VC = IRV + TV + ERV$$
$$= 3{,}300 + 500 + 1{,}000 = 4{,}800 \text{ mL}$$

Vital capacity is significant physiologically and its determination is useful in clinical diagnosis as explained later in this chapter.

### *Functional Residual Capacity*

Functional residual capacity (FRC) is the volume of air remaining in lungs after normal expiration (after normal tidal expiration). Functional residual capacity includes expiratory reserve volume (ERV) and residual volume (RV).

$$FRC = ERV + RV$$
$$= 1{,}000 + 1{,}200 = 2{,}200 \text{ mL}$$

### *Total Lung Capacity*

Total lung capacity (TLC) is the volume of air present in lungs after a deep (maximal) inspiration. It includes all the volumes.

$$TLC = IRV + TV + ERV + RV$$
$$= 3{,}300 + 500 + 1{,}000 + 1{,}200$$
$$= 6{,}000 \text{ mL}$$

## Measurement of Lung Volumes and Capacities

Spirometry is the method to measure lung volumes and capacities. Simple instrument used for this purpose is called spirometer. Modified spirometer is known as respirometer. Nowadays plethysmograph is also used to measure lung volumes and capacities.

## Spirometer

Spirometer is made up of metal and it contains two chambers namely outer chamber and inner chamber. Outer chamber is called the water chamber because it is filled with water. A floating drum is immersed in the water in an inverted position. Drum is counterbalanced by a weight. Weight is attached to the top of the inverted drum by means of string or chain. A pen with ink is attached to the counterweight. Pen is made to write on a calibrated paper, which is fixed to a recording device.

Inner chamber is inverted and has a small hole at the top. A long metal tube passes through the inner chamber from the bottom towards the top. Upper end of this tube reaches the top portion of the inner chamber.

Then the tube passes through a hole at the top of inner chamber and penetrates into outer water chamber above the level of water. A rubber tube is connected to the outer end of the metal tube. At the other end of this rubber tube, a mouthpiece is attached. Subject respires through this mouthpiece by closing the nose with a nose clip.

When the subject breathes with spirometer, during expiration, drum moves up and the counterweight comes down. Reverse of this occurs when the subject breathes the air from the spirometer, i.e. during inspiration. Upward and downward movements of the counterweight are recorded in the form of a graph. Upward deflection of the curve in the graph shows inspiration and the downward deflection denotes expiration.

Spirometer is used only for a single breath. Repeated cycles of respiration cannot be recorded by using this instrument because carbon dioxide accumulates in the spirometer and oxygen or fresh air cannot be provided to the subject.

### *Respirometer*

Respirometer is the modified spirometer. It has provision for removal of carbon dioxide and supply of oxygen.

Carbon dioxide is removed by placing soda lime inside the instrument. Oxygen is supplied to the instrument from the oxygen cylinder, by a suitable valve system. Oxygen is filled in the inverted drum above water level and the subject can breathe in and out with instrument for about 6 minutes and recording can be done continuously.

### *Spirogram*

Spirogram is the graphical record of lung volumes and capacities using spirometer. Upward deflection of the spirogram denotes inspiration and the downward curve indicates expiration. In order to determine the lung volumes and capacities, following four levels are to be noted in spirogram:

1. Normal end expiratory level
2. Normal end inspiratory level
3. Maximum expiratory level
4. Maximum inspiratory level.

### *Computerized Spirometer*

Computerized spirometer is the solid state electronic equipment. It does not contain a drum or water chamber. Subject has to respire into a sophisticated transducer, which is connected to the instrument by means of a cable.

### *Disadvantages of Spirometry*

By using simple spirometer, respirometer or computerized spirometer, not all the lung volumes and lung capacities can be measured.

Volume, which cannot be measured by spirometry, is the residual volume. Capacities, which include residual volume also cannot be measured. Capacities that include residual volume are functional residual capacity and total lung capacity.

Volume and capacities, which cannot be measured by spirometry, are measured by nitrogen washout technique or helium dilution technique or by body plethysmograph.

## Vital Capacity

### *Definition*

Vital capacity is the maximum volume of air that can be expelled out of lungs forcefully after a maximal or deep inspiration.

### *Lung Volumes Included in Vital Capacity*

Vital capacity includes inspiratory reserve volume, tidal volume and expiratory reserve volume.

### *Normal Value*

$$VC = IRV + TV + ERV$$
$$= 3{,}300 + 500 + 1{,}000 = 4{,}800 \text{ mL}.$$

### *Variations of Vital Capacity*

*Physiological Variations*

1. Sex: In females, vital capacity is less than in males.
2. Body built: Vital capacity is slightly more in heavily built persons.
3. Posture: Vital capacity is more in standing position and less in lying position.
4. Athletes: Vital capacity is more in athletes.
5. Occupation: Vital capacity is decreased in people with sedentary jobs. It is increased in persons who play musical wind instruments such as bugle and flute.

*Pathological Variations*

Vital capacity is decreased in the following respiratory diseases:

1. Asthma
2. Emphysema
3. Weakness or paralysis of respiratory muscle
4. Pulmonary congestion
5. Pneumonia
6. Pneumothorax
7. Hemothorax
8. Pyothorax
9. Hydrothorax
10. Pulmonary edema
11. Pulmonary tuberculosis.

*Measurement*

Vital capacity is measured by spirometry. The subject is asked to take a deep inspiration and expire forcefully.

## Forced Vital Capacity

Forced vital capacity (FVC) is the volume of air that can be exhaled forcefully and rapidly after a maximal or deep inspiration. It is a dynamic lung capacity.

Normally FVC is equal to VC. However in some pulmonary diseases, FVC is decreased.

## Forced Expiratory Volume or Timed Vital Capacity

### *Definition*

Forced expiratory volume (FEV) is the volume of air, which can be expired forcefully in a given unit of time (after a deep inspiration). It is also called timed vital capacity or forced expiratory vital capacity (FEVC). It is a dynamic lung volume.

- FEV1 = Volume of air expired forcefully in 1 second
- FEV2 = Volume of air expired forcefully in 2 seconds
- FEV3 = Volume of air expired forcefully in 3 seconds.

### *Normal Values*

Forced expiratory volume in persons with normal respiratory functions is as follows:

- $FEV_1$ = 83% of total vital capacity
- $FEV_2$ = 94% of total vital capacity
- $FEV_3$ = 97% of total vital capacity
- After 3rd second = 100% of total vital capacity.

### *Significance of Determining Forced Expiratory Volume*

Vital capacity may be almost normal in some of the respiratory diseases. However, the FEV has great diagnostic value, as it is decreased significantly in some respiratory diseases.

It is very much decreased in obstructive diseases like asthma and emphysema. It is slightly reduced in some restrictive respiratory diseases like fibrosis of lungs.

## Respiratory Minute Volume

### *Definition*

Respiratory minute volume (RMV) is the volume of air breathed in and out of lungs every minute. It is the product of tidal volume (TV) and respiratory rate (RR).

$$RMV = TV \times RR$$
$$= 500 \times 12 = 6{,}000 \text{ mL}$$

### *Normal Value*

Normal respiratory minute volume is 6 L.

### *Variations*

Respiratory minute volume increases in physiological conditions such as voluntary hyperventilation, exercise and emotional conditions. It is reduced in respiratory diseases.

## Maximum Breathing Capacity or Maximum Ventilation Volume

### *Definition*

Maximum breathing capacity (MBC) is the maximum volume of air, which can be breathed in and out of lungs by forceful respiration (hyperventilation: increase in rate and force of respiration) per minute. It is also called maximum ventilation volume (MVV).

MBC is a dynamic lung capacity and it is reduced in respiratory diseases.

### *Normal Value*

In healthy adult male, it is 150 to 170 L/minute and in females, it is 80 to 100 L/minute.

### *Measurement*

Subject is asked to breathe forcefully and rapidly with a respirometer for 15 seconds. Volume of air inspired and expired is measured from the spirogram. From this value, the MBC is calculated for 1 minute.

For example,

- MBC in 12 seconds = 32 L
- MBC per minute = $\frac{32}{12} \times 60$ L = 160 L

## Peak Expiratory Flow Rate

### *Definition*

Peak expiratory flow rate (PEFR) is the maximum rate at which the air can be expired after a deep inspiration.

### *Normal Value*

In normal persons, it is 400 L/minute.

### *Measurement*

Peak expiratory flow rate is measured by using Wright peak flow meter or a mini peak flow meter.

### *Significance of Determining PEFR*

Determination of PEFR rate is useful for assessing the respiratory diseases especially to differentiate the obstructive and restrictive diseases. Generally, PEFR is reduced in all type of respiratory disease. However, reduction is more significant in the obstructive diseases than in the restrictive diseases.

Thus, in restrictive diseases, the PEFR is 200 L/minute and in obstructive diseases, it is only 100 L/minute.

## Restrictive and Obstructive Respiratory Diseases

Diseases of respiratory tract are classified into two types:

These two types of respiratory diseases are determined by lung functions tests, particularly FEV.

### *Restrictive Respiratory Disease*

Restrictive respiratory disease is the abnormal respiratory condition characterized by difficulty in inspiration.

Expiration is not affected. Restrictive respiratory disease may be because of abnormality of lungs, thoracic cavity or/ and nervous system.

### *Obstructive Respiratory Disease*

Obstructive respiratory disease is the abnormal respiratory condition characterized by difficulty in expiration.

- Restrictive respiratory diseases
  - Poliomyelitis
  - Myasthenia gravis
  - Flail chest (broken ribs)
  - Paralysis of diaphragm
  - Spinal cord diseases
  - Pleural effusion.
- Obstructive respiratory diseases
  - Asthma
  - Chronic bronchitis
  - Emphysema
  - Cystic fibrosis
  - Laryngotracheobronchitis
  - Epiglottis

- Tumors
- Severe cough and cold with phlegm.

## Ventilation

In general, the word 'ventilation' refers to circulation of replacement of air or gas in a space. In respiratory physiology, ventilation is the rate at which air enters or leaves the lungs. Ventilation in respiratory physiology is of two types:

### Pulmonary Ventilation

*Definition*

Pulmonary ventilation is defined as the volume of air moving in and out of respiratory tract in a given unit of time during quiet breathing. It is also called minute ventilation or respiratory minute volume (RMV).

Pulmonary ventilation is a cyclic process, by which fresh air enters the lungs and an equal volume of air leaves the lungs.

*Normal Value and Calculation*

Normal value of pulmonary ventilation is 6,000 mL (6 L)/minute. It is the product of tidal volume (TV) and the rate of respiration (RR).

It is calculated by the formula:

- Pulmonary ventilation = Tidal volume × Respiratory rate = 500 mL × 12/minute = 6,000 mL/minute.

### Alveolar Ventilation

***Definition:*** Alveolar ventilation is the amount of air utilized for gaseous exchange every minute.

Alveolar ventilation is different from pulmonary ventilation. In pulmonary ventilation, 6 L of air moves in and out of respiratory tract every minute. But the whole volume of air is not utilized for exchange of gases. Volume of air subjected for exchange of gases is the alveolar ventilation. Air trapped in the respiratory passage (dead space) does not take part in gaseous exchange.

*Normal Value and Calculation*

Normal value of alveolar ventilation is 4,200 mL (4.2 L)/minute.

It is calculated by the formula: Alveolar ventilation = (Tidal volume – Dead space) × Respiratory rate = (500 – 150) mL × 12/minute = 4,200 mL (4.2 L)/minute.

## Dead Space

***Definition:*** Dead space is defined as the part of the respiratory tract, where gaseous exchange does not take place. Air present in the dead space is called dead space air.

### Types of Dead Space

Dead space is of two types:

*Anatomical Dead Space*

Anatomical dead space extends from nose up to terminal bronchiole. It includes nose, pharynx, trachea, bronchi and branches of bronchi up to terminal bronchioles. These structures serve only as the passage for air movement. Gaseous exchange does not take place in these structures.

*Physiological Dead Space*

Physiological dead space includes anatomical dead space plus two additional volumes.

Additional volumes included in physiological dead space are:

1. Air in the alveoli, which are non-functioning. In some respiratory diseases, alveoli do not function because of dysfunction or destruction of alveolar membrane.
2. Air in the alveoli, which do not receive dequate blood flow. Gaseous exchange does not take place during inadequate blood supply.

These two additional volumes are generally considered as wasted ventilation.

Wasted Ventilation and Wasted Air

Wasted ventilation is the volume of air that ventilates physiological dead space. Wasted air refers to air that is not utilized for gaseous exchange. Dead space air is generally considered as wasted air.

### Normal Value of Dead Space

Volume of normal dead space is 150 mL. Under normal conditions, physiological dead space is equal to anatomical dead space. It is because, all the alveoli are functioning and all the alveoli receive adequate blood flow in normal conditions.

Physiological dead space increases during respiratory diseases, which affect the pulmonary blood flow or the alveoli.

## MULTIPLE CHOICE QUESTIONS

**1. Cardiac output for man under normal basal conditions would be close to:**
(a) 2.5 L (b) 5 L
(c) 7.5 L (d) 9 L

**2. Alzheimer's disease is related to loss of:**
(a) Memory (b) Motor function
(c) Pain sensation (d) Posture regulations

**3. Immunoglobulin involved in body allergic reaction:**
(a) Ig A (b) Ig E
(c) Ig M (d) Ig D

**4. Following substance are ketogenic:**
(a) Fatty acids (b) Leucine
(c) Lysine (d) All of the above

**5. Cerebrospinal fluid is secreted by:**
(a) Choroid plexus (b) Arachnoid villa
(c) Neurons (d) Neuroglia

**6. Absence of 'P' wave in an ECG would indicate blockage of impulse from:**
(a) SA node (b) AV node
(c) Bundle of His (d) Purkinje fibers

**7. Pain sensation is carried by:**
(a) Dorsal column (b) Anterolateral pathways
(c) Pyramidal tract (d) Spinocerebellar tract

**8. In 28 days menstrual cycle ovulation will occur on:**
(a) 5th day (b) 10th day
(c) 14th day (d) 20th day

**9. Severe stimulation of sympathetic system will:**
(a) Increase GFR (b) Decrease GFR
(c) No effect on GFR (d) Lead to shut down

**10. Plasma pH is:**
(a) 7.4 (b) 7.0
(c) 6.8 (d) 6.4

**11. Starch and glycogen are polymers of:**
(a) Fructose (b) Maltose
(c) Glucose (d) Galactose

**12. Antidiuretic hormone act on:**
(a) Proximal convoluted tubule
(b) Distal convoluted tubule
(c) Loop of Henle
(d) Collecting duct

**13. Active transport across a cell membrane occur:**
(a) Along the concentration gradient
(b) Along electrical gradient
(c) Against concentration gradient
(d) None of the above

**14. pH of fasting whole gastric juice is:**
(a) 7 (b) 7.4
(c) 0.9 to 1.3 (d) 14

**15. The duration of cardiac cycle is seconds, with heart of 72 b/m is**
(a) 0.4 (b) 0.8
(c) 1.2 (d) 1.6

**16. Hyperthyroidism cause all EXCEPT:**
(a) Increase in BMR
(b) Increase in body weight
(c) Increased body temperature
(d) Increase heart rate

**17. Glomerular filtration rate (GFR) in human is normally (in mL/min):**
(a) 50 (b) 75
(c) 125 (d) 250

**18. RBC of blood group 'O' contain following antigen:**
(a) Antigen A (b) Both (a) and (b).
(c) Antigen B (d) None of the above

**19. Neurotransmitters at neuromuscular junction is:**
(a) Adrenaline (b) Dopamine
(c) Noradrenaline (d) Acetylcholine

**20. Proliferative phase (First half) of menstrual cycle is maintained by:**
(a) Estrogen (b) Progesterone
(c) Androgen (d) Prolactin

**21. Ovulation occurs approximately between the following days of menstrual cycle:**
(a) 10 to 12 (b) 14 to 16
(c) 20 to 22 (d) 6 to 10

**22. Daylight vision (photopic vision) is the function of:**
(a) Rods
(b) Cones
(c) Ganglionic cells in retina
(d) Pigment cells of retina

**23. Corpus callosum is an example of ______ variety of white fibers:**
(a) Projection (b) Commissural
(c) Association (d) All of the above

**24. Reticulocytes:**
(a) Are nucleated RBC's
(b) Normally are 10% of circulating RBC's
(c) Are devoid of hemoglobin
(d) Count is an indicator of bone marrow activity

**25. Sense of proprioception is carried by:**
(a) Dorsal column
(b) Spinothalamic tract
(c) Posterior spinocerebellar tract
(d) Anterior spinocerebellar tract

**26. Fovea of the eye:**
(a) Has the lowest light threshold
(b) Has the highest light threshold
(c) Contains only rods
(d) Contains only red and green cones

**27. Amount of air left in the lung after forceful expiration is:**
(a) Dead space
(b) Residual volume
(c) Functional residual capacity
(d) Vital capacity

**28. Hematocrit of 41% means that in the sample of blood analysed:**
(a) 41% of hemoglobin is in plasma
(b) Blood has 41% hemoglobin
(c) 59% of the hemoglobin in plasma
(d) 41% of blood in plasma

**29. The most biologically active iodothyronine secreted by the thyroid follicle is:**
(a) T4 (b) T3
(c) MIT (d) DIT

**30. The first step in stoppage of bleeding from small cut is:**
(a) Platelet plug formation
(b) Local vascular spasm
(c) Clot retraction
(d) Fibrin formation

**31. The total air that can be expelled out of lung after maximal aspiration is known as:**
(a) Vital capacity (b) Tidal volume
(c) Total lung capacity (d) Inspiratory capacity

**32. Progesterone is secreted by:**
(a) Vaginal epithelium (b) Corpus luteum
(c) Adrenal medulla (d) Endometrium

**33. Erythropoiesis requires all the following EXCEPT:**
(a) Vitamin B (b) Folic acid
(c) Iron (d) Retinol

**34. Which of the following transport system does not require carriers?**
(a) Simple diffusion
(b) Facilitated diffusion
(c) Primary active transport
(d) Secondary active transport

**35. Troponin-C:**
(a) Is the contractile protein in skeletal muscle
(b) Is calcium binding protein
(c) Contains globular head
(d) Is the active site on actine filament

**36. The biconcave shape of RBC is due to:**
(a) Elastin (b) Spectrin
(c) Myosin (d) Tropomyosin

**37. Which is not a muscle of inspiration?**
(a) Diaphragm
(b) Internal intercostal muscle
(c) Sternomastoid
(d) External intercostal muscle

**38. Physiological respiratory dead space in adult is:**
(a) 105 mL (b) 150 mL
(c) 125 mL (d) 200 mL

**39. Hydrochloric acid in stomach is produced by:**
(a) Goblet cells (b) Cardiac cells
(c) Parietal cells (d) None of the above

**40. Glomerular filtration rate in adult is approximately:**
(a) 50 mL/min (b) 125 mL/min
(c) 75 mL/min (d) 250 mL/min

**41. Maximum amount of water is absorbed in the following part of renal tubule:**
(a) Proximal convoluted tubule
(b) Ascending limb of loop of Henle
(c) Distal convoluted tubule
(d) Descending limb of loop of Henle

**42. Center for regulation of body temperature lies in:**
(a) Cerebellum (b) Thalamus
(c) Spinal cord (d) Hypothalamus

**43. In muscular exercise following changes occurs EXCEPT:**
(a) Increased heart rate
(b) Decreased cardiac output
(c) Increased systolic pressure
(d) Increased blood flow to skeletal muscle

**44. Vasomotor center is situated in:**
(a) Pons (b) Medulla
(c) Spinal cord (d) Midbrain

**45. HIV-Virus in human blood affects following cells:**
(a) RBC's (b) T lymphocytes
(c) B lymphocyte (d) Eosinophils

**46. Normal calcium level is (in mg%):**
(a) 5–6 (b) 7–8
(c) 9–11 (d) 15

**47. Parkinsonism is disease due to defect in:**
(a) Basal ganglia (b) Cerebral cortex
(c) Cerebellum (d) Hypothalamus

**48. Site for protein synthesis in cell is:**
(a) Mitochondria (b) Lysosomes
(c) Golgi complex (d) Ribosome

**49. Following features are found in hyperthyroidism EXCEPT:**
(a) Enlarged thyroid gland
(b) Increase in heart rate
(c) Decreased BMR
(d) Exopthalmos

**50. Average duration of menstrual cycle is (in day's):**
(a) 28 (b) 25
(c) 20 (d) 14

**51. Pancreatic juice rich in bicarbonate ions is secreted in response to:**
(a) CCK-PZ (b) Secretin
(c) HCl (d) Gastrine

**52. Renin is secreted by:**
(a) Lungs (b) Thyroid gland
(c) Kidney (d) Liver

**53. Following are the functions of cerebellum EXCEPT:**
(a) Regulation of food intake
(b) Co-ordination
(c) Regulation of voluntary activities
(d) Maintenance of equilibrium

**54. Mechanism of production of first heart sound is:**
(a) Closure of A-V valve
(b) Opening of A-V valve
(c) Closure of semilunar valve
(d) Opening of semilunar valve

**55. Delay in conduction of cardiac impulse occurs at:**
(a) SA node (b) AV node
(c) Bundle of His (d) Purkinje fibers

**56. Permanent method of contraception in females is:**
(a) Oral contraceptive pills
(b) Copper T
(c) Vasectomy
(d) Tubectomy

**57. Following is true for surfactant EXCEPT:**
(a) It is surface reducing agent
(b) Secreted by alveolar cells
(c) Dipalmitoyl lecithin
(d) Required for diffusion of gases

**58. Hormone required for milk ejection**
(a) Oxytocin (b) Prolactin
(c) Estrogen (d) Progesterone

**59. The kidney normally secrets:**
(a) Erythropoietin (b) Renin
(c) Both (d) None

**60. The refractive error, hypermetropia may be corrected by following lens:**
(a) Convex (b) Concave
(c) Cylindrical (d) Plain glasses

**61. The following is the sensory function of organ of Corti:**
(a) Smell (b) Taste
(c) Vision (d) Hearing

62. **The following endocrine gland regulates the basal metabolic rate:**
(a) Adrenal cortex (b) Thyroid
(c) Anterior pituitary (d) Thymus

63. **The following is known as exchange vessel:**
(a) Arteries (b) Arterioles
(c) Capillaries (d) Venules

64. **The normal partial pressure of oxygen ($PO_2$) in arterial blood is:**
(a) 45 mm Hg (b) 65 mm Hg
(c) 95 mm Hg (d) 105 mm Hg

65. **The following is the site for RBC formation in adult:**
(a) Liver (b) Spleen
(c) Kidney (d) Bone marrow

66. **Power house of cell is:**
(a) Nucleus
(b) Sarcoplasmic reticulum
(c) Golgi complex
(d) Mitochondria

67. **The hormone aldosterone is secreted by:**
(a) Thyroid gland (b) Adrenal cortex
(c) Anterior pituitary (d) Thymus

68. **Normal range of pH of extracellular fluid is:**
(a) 7.36–7.45 (b) 6.1–6.5
(c) 8.2–8.5 (d) 6.1–7.2

69. **Intracellular fluid is rich in:**
(a) Sodium (b) Potassium
(c) Calcium (d) Bicarbonate

70. **Vitamin $B_{12}$ is absorbed:**
(a) In combination with intrinsic factors
(b) In stomach
(c) Along with fat
(d) In large intestine

71. **Erythropoiesis:**
(a) Occurs in human blood vessels
(b) Is stimulated by hypoxia
(c) Is unaffected by age and sex
(d) Takes place in liver and spleen in adult

72. **Jaundice is yellowish discoloration seen in:**
(a) Hemolytic disease of newborn
(b) Mismatch blood transfusion
(c) Liver disease
(d) All of the above

73. **Difference in hemoglobin in fetal and adult is:**
(a) Color (b) Structure of heme
(c) Affinity to oxygen (d) Formation of iron

74. **Duration of cardiac cycle is equal to:**
(a) Circulation
(b) RR interval
(c) Interval between first and second heart sound
(d) PR interval

75. **Plasma protein playing a major role in process of coagulation:**
(a) Prealbumin (b) Albumin
(c) Globulin (d) Fibrinogen

76. **Intrinsic factors is secreted by:**
(a) Stomach (b) Pancreas
(c) Liver (d) Small intestine

77. **Process of facilitated diffusion:**
(a) Requires energy
(b) Requires carrier
(c) Occurs against concentration gradient
(d) All of the above

78. **The number of nephron in each kidney, in millions:**
(a) One (b) Two
(c) Three (d) Four

79. **Movement of oxygen from alveoli to pulmonary capillaries is brought about by:**
(a) Primary active transport
(b) Secondary active transport
(c) Filtration
(d) Simple diffusion

80. **The AV nodal delay is:**
(a) 0.09 sec (b) 0.05 sec
(c) 0.02 sec (d) 0.01 sec

81. **Macrophages are the mature form of:**
(a) Neutrophils (b) Eosinophils
(c) Basophils (d) Monocytes

82. **Hemoglobin first appears in RBC in _______ stage:**
(a) Early normoblast
(b) Intermediate normoblast
(c) Late normoblast
(d) Pronormoblast

83. **During skeletal muscle contraction there is decrease in length of:**
(a) A band (b) H band
(c) Actin filament (d) Myosin filament

84. **Heart rate is maximum in:**
(a) Adult (b) Newborn
(c) Fetus (d) Old aged

85. **RBC does not contain:**
(a) Nucleus
(b) Mitochondria
(c) Endoplasmic reticulum
(d) All of the above

86. **Glucose is co- transported into cell with:**
(a) Na (b) Ka
(c) Ca (d) $H^+$

87. **Plasma protein with highest molecular weight is:**
(a) Albumin (b) Globulin
(c) Fibrinogen (d) Prothrombin

88. **Spontaneous respiration cease after:**
(a) Transaction of brain above pons
(b) Transaction of brainstem at lower end of medulla
(c) Transaction of vagus nerve
(d) Transaction of vagus nerve and brainstem above the pons

89. **In human body heparin is secreted by:**
(a) Lymphocytes (b) Neutrophils
(c) Basophils (d) RBC

**90. Cell mediation immunity is provided by:**
(a) T- lymphocytes
(b) B- lymphocytes
(c) Plasma cells
(d) Monocytes

**91. Enlargement of thyroid gland is called:**
(a) Tetany
(b) Tumor
(c) Goiter
(d) Callus

**92. Organ that act as reservoir of bile:**
(a) Liver
(b) Gallbladder
(c) Pancreas
(d) Stomach

**93. Testosterone is secreted by:**
(a) Kidney
(b) Testis
(c) Ovaries
(d) Pancreas

**94. Pepsin is responsible for digestion of:**
(a) Fats
(b) Protein
(c) Carbohydrates
(d) Cholesterol

**95. An example of active transport is:**
(a) Simple diffusion
(b) Facilitated diffusion
(c) Osmosis
(d) Na-K pump

**96. Number of spinal nerve in human beings:**
(a) 11 pairs
(b) 31 pairs
(c) 21 pairs
(d) 41 pairs

**97. The membrane covering the heart is:**
(a) Peritoneum
(b) Pleura
(c) Periosteum
(d) Pericardium

**98. Center for swallowing reflex is located in:**
(a) Pons
(b) Medulla
(c) Cerebellum
(d) Basal ganglia

**99. Which of the following is called voluntary striated muscle?**
(a) Cardiac muscle
(b) Smooth muscle
(c) Skeletal muscle
(d) Plain muscle

**100. Which hormone is secreted by pancreas?**
(a) Insulin
(b) Adrenaline
(c) Vasopressin
(d) Gastrin

**101. Hemophilia A is caused due to deficiency of:**
(a) Factor III
(b) Factor IV
(c) Factor VIII
(d) Factor XI

**102. Thick filament of skeletal muscle is made up of:**
(a) Actin
(b) Myosin
(c) Troponin
(d) Tropomyosin

**103. Spermatogenesis takes on an average:**
(a) 60 days
(b) 88 days
(c) 74 days
(d) 102 days

**104. All of the following about sympathetic nerve supply to heart is true:**
(a) By sympathetic nerve cells
(b) Its stimulation decrease heart rate
(c) Its stimulation increase force of contraction
(d) Controlled by vasomotor center

**105. Bulk of reabsorption of GFR occurs in:**
(a) Proximal convoluted tubule
(b) Loop of Henle
(c) Collecting tubule
(d) Distal convoluted tubule

**106. Sounds intensity is measured in:**
(a) Diopters
(b) Pounds
(c) Dalton
(d) Decibels

**107. Renin is secreted by:**
(a) Cells in macula densa
(b) Cells in distal tubule
(c) Cells in proximal tubule
(d) Juxtaglomerular cells

**108. Most of the $CO_2$ transported in blood is:**
(a) Dissolved in plasma
(b) Bound to $Cl^-$
(c) In $HCO3^-$ form
(d) In carbamino compound formed from Hb

## ANSWERS

| | | | | | | | | | | | |
|---|---|---|---|---|---|---|---|---|---|---|---|
| **1.** | (b) | **21.** | (b) | **41.** | (a) | **61.** | (d) | **81.** | (d) | **101.** | (c) |
| **2.** | (a) | **22.** | (b) | **42.** | (d) | **62.** | (b) | **82.** | (b) | **102.** | (b) |
| **3.** | (b) | **23.** | (b) | **43.** | (b) | **63.** | (c) | **83.** | (b) | **103.** | (c) |
| **4.** | (a) | **24.** | (d) | **44.** | (b) | **64.** | (c) | **84.** | (c) | **104.** | (b) |
| **5.** | (a) | **25.** | (a) | **45.** | (b) | **65.** | (d) | **85.** | (d) | **105.** | (a) |
| **6.** | (a) | **26.** | (d) | **46.** | (c) | **66.** | (d) | **86.** | (a) | **106.** | (d) |
| **7.** | (a) | **27.** | (c) | **47.** | (a) | **67.** | (b) | **87.** | (a) | **107.** | (d) |
| **8.** | (b) | **28.** | (a) | **48.** | (d) | **68.** | (a) | **88.** | (b) | **108.** | (d) |
| **9.** | (a) | **29.** | (a) | **49.** | (b) | **69.** | (b) | **89.** | (a) | | |
| **10.** | (a) | **30.** | (b) | **50.** | (a) | **70.** | (a) | **90.** | (a) | | |
| **11.** | (c) | **31.** | (a) | **51.** | (c) | **71.** | (b) | **91.** | (c) | | |
| **12.** | (b) | **32.** | (b) | **52.** | (c) | **72.** | (d) | **92.** | (b) | | |
| **13.** | (c) | **33.** | (d) | **53.** | (a) | **73.** | (b) | **93.** | (b) | | |
| **14.** | (c) | **34.** | (a) | **54.** | (c) | **74.** | (b) | **94.** | (c) | | |
| **15.** | (b) | **35.** | (b) | **55.** | (b) | **75.** | (d) | **95.** | (d) | | |
| **16.** | (d) | **36.** | (b) | **56.** | (d) | **76.** | (a) | **96.** | (b) | | |
| **17.** | (c) | **37.** | (c) | **57.** | (d) | **77.** | (c) | **97.** | (d) | | |
| **18.** | (d) | **38.** | (b) | **58.** | (a) | **78.** | (a) | **98.** | (b) | | |
| **19.** | (d) | **39.** | (c) | **59.** | (c) | **79.** | (d) | **99.** | (c) | | |
| **20.** | (a) | **40.** | (b) | **60.** | (a) | **80.** | (c) | **100.** | (a) | | |

# QUICK REVIEW

## Foundation of Nursing Review and Multiple Choice Questions

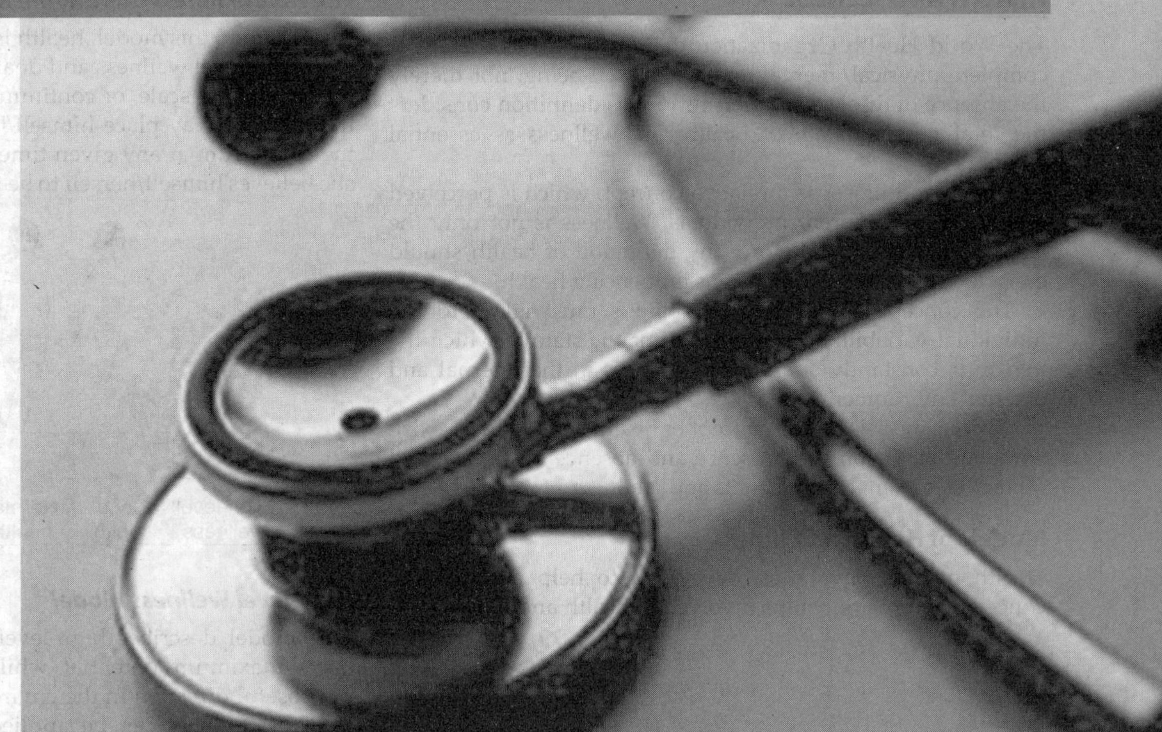

### HIGHLIGHTS

- Health and Illness
- Communication and Interpersonal Relationships in Nursing
- Principles and Practices of Nursing
- Nursing Process
- Admission of the Patient
- Health Assessment and Physical Examination
- Sterilizations and Disinfection
- Biomedical Waste Management
- First Aid and Emergency Kit
- Multiple Choice Questions

# Foundation of Nursing

## HEALTH AND ILLNESS

The World Health Organization defines health as a state of complete physical, mental and social well-being, not merely the absence of disease and infirmity. This definition considers the total persons state of health and wellness as essential component.

Health and illness is a relative concept, which is perceived differently by different individuals. Wellness is not only the absence of disease; therefore, any definition of health should consider the different dimensions influencing health.

The concept of health and wellness must allow for an individual variability. Health is a dynamic state in which the person is constantly adapting to changes in the internal and external environment.

Various models on the concept of health and wellness exist. Some are based on the presence and absence of disease and others on holism, health beliefs and wellness.

### Models of Health and Illness

Health models have been developed to help describe the concepts and relationships involved in health and illness.

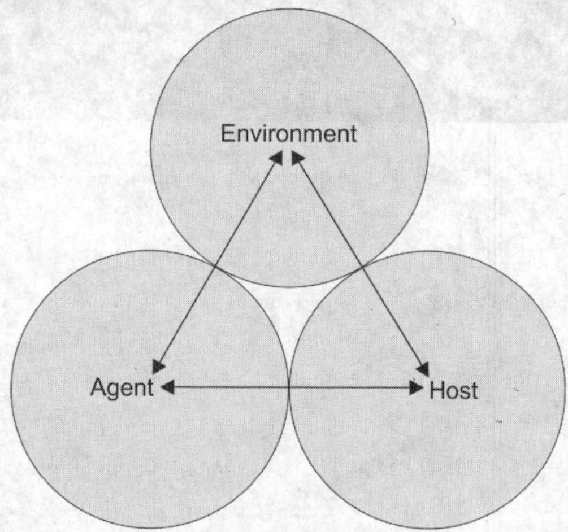


#### *Host–agent-environment Model*

According to this model health is an ever-changing state and health and illness depends on interaction of host, agent and environmental factors. These factors are constantly in interaction and a combination of factors increases the possibility of illness. When the agent, host and environment variables are in equilibrium health is maintained. On the other hand when the balance is disrupted disease occurs.

#### *The Health Illness Continuum Model*

According to this model, health is a constantly changing state, with high level wellness and death being in the opposite ends of a graduated scale, or continuum. The nurse must be aware that a client may place himself/herself at different points on the continuum at any given time depending on how well he/she believes himself/herself to be functioning for his/her illness

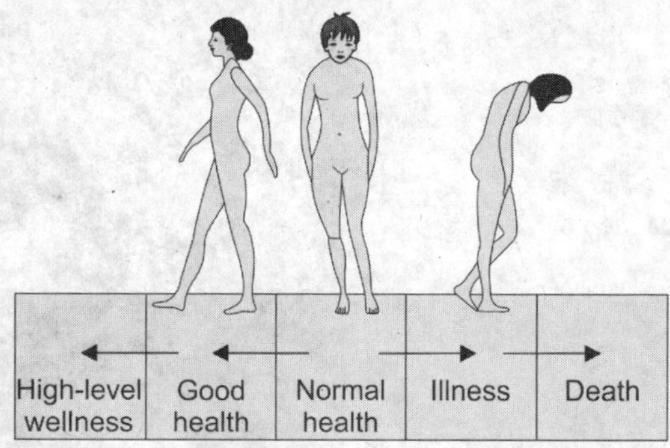


#### *High-level Wellness Model*

This model describes high-level wellness as functioning to one's maximum potential while maintaining balance and purposeful direction in the environment. The concept of high level of wellness can be applied to the individual, family, community, environment, and society.

In high-level wellness model human beings are viewed as having five aspects:

1. Each individual is functioning as a total personality
2. Each person possess dynamic energy
3. Each person is at peace with inner and outer worlds
4. Each person has a relationship between energy use and self integration
5. Each person has an inner world and an outer world. These five processes help the person know who and what he/she is. This model is holistic, allowing the nurse to care for the total person with regard for all dimensional factors affecting the person's state of being as he/she strives to reach maximum potential.

#### *Health Belief Model*

The health belief model is based on what people perceive, or believe, to be true about them in relation to health. This model is based on three components:

1. Perceived susceptibility to a disease
2. Perceived seriousness of a disease
3. Perceived value of action.

This model states that whether or not a person practices a particular health behavior can be understood by knowing two factors:

1. The degree to which the person perceives a personal health threat
2. The perception that a particular health practice will be effective in reducing that threat.

The perception of a personal health threat is itself influenced by at least three factors:

1. General health values, which include interest, and concern about health
2. Specific beliefs about vulnerability to a particular health problem
3. Beliefs about the consequence of the health problem.

Whether or not the perception of a threat leads to changing health behavior also depends on whether a person thinks a particular health practice will be effective against the health problem in question and whether or not the cost of undertaking that measure exceeds the benefits of the measure. The health belief model enable nurses to understand why people practice health behavior and also to predict some of the circumstances under which people's health behavior will change.

### Factors Affecting Health and Illness

- *Physical dimension:* Genetic make up, age, developmental level, race and sex.
- *Emotional dimension:* How the mind and body interact to affect to body function and to respond to body conditions also influences health. For example, long term stress affects the body systems, anxiety affects health habits and conversely calm acceptance and relaxation can actually change body responses to illness.
- *Intellectual dimension:* Encompasses cognitive abilities, educational background and past experiences.
- *Environmental dimension:* The environment has many influences on health and illness. Housing sanitation, climate, pollution of air, food and water are aspects of the environmental dimension.
- *Sociocultural dimension:* Health practices are strongly influenced by a person's economic level, lifestyle, family and culture.
- *Spiritual dimension:* Spiritual and religious beliefs and values are important components of how a person behaves in health and illness.

## COMMUNICATION AND INTERPERSONAL RELATIONSHIPS IN NURSING

### Communication

- Communication is a complex process of sending and receiving verbal and nonverbal messages.
- Allows for exchange of information, feelings, needs and preferences
- The process of creating common understanding
- The process of sharing information
- The process of generating and transmitting meanings.

### Purposes of Communication

- Information
- Education
- Persuasion
- Entertainment.

### Goals of Communication: Shared Meaning

- Mutual understanding of the meaning of the message.
- Feedback/response indicates if the meaning of the message was communicated as intended.

### Types of Communication

People communicate in a variety of ways.

1. *Verbal communication:* It is an exchange of information using words and includes both the spoken and the written word. Verbal communication depends on language. Language is a prescribed way of using words so that people can share information effectively. Both spoken and written communication reveal a great deal about a person. Conscious use of spoken or written word. Choice of words can reflect age, education, developmental level, and culture.

   Feelings can be expressed through tone, pace, etc. The verbal form of communication is used extensively by nurses when speaking with clients, giving oral reports to other nurses, writing care plans and recording in nursing progress reports.

   *Characteristics: simple, brief, clear, well timed, relevant, adaptable, credible.*
2. *Nonverbal communication:* It is the exchange of information without the use of words. It is communication through gestures, facial expressions, posture, body movement, voice tone, rate of speech, eye contact. It is generally accepted that non-verbal communication expresses more of true meaning of a message than verbal communication. Therefore, nurses must be aware of both the nonverbal messages they send and receive from clients.

   Nonverbal is less conscious than verbal, requires systematic observation and valid interpretation.
3. *Metacommunication:* It is a message about a message. It includes anything that is taken into account when interpreting what is happening, such as the role of the communicator, the nonverbal messages sent and the context of the communication taking place.

### Relationship between Verbal and Nonverbal Communications

*Congruency:* Are verbal and nonverbal messages consistent? Nurse states observations and validates the communication.

### *Levels of Communication*

- Intrapersonal
- Interpersonal
- Public.

### Communication Model

A conceptual model makes the abstraction of communication more concrete. A model provides form and utility through which nursing knowledge can be iterated.

### A Communication Model

We have said that models add concreteness to a concept in addition to having a form and utility of their own. The communication model comprises six elements:

1. The referent
2. The source encoder
3. The message
4. The channel
5. The receiver decoder
6. Feedback

Every encounter we have with another person, whether spontaneous or deliberate, begins with an idea—a reason for engaging in a verbal exchange. Our model must begin with what idea, referent. A referent may be one of "a wide range of objects, situations ideas, or experiences" Any one of these items or a combination of them prompts the source encoder to initiate action in order to convey the message engendered by the referent.

The *source encoder* is a term that describes a person who communicates with another. Our ability to form, use and understand the messages we transmit is continually influenced by numerous factors, it includes our communication skills, our attitudes, our levels of knowledge, and our sociocultural system. These factors are never static; indeed they are always changing, always being modified as we change and are modified by the events that surround us. Whenever we act in the role of the source-encoder we must consider these influences in order to understand not only our own communication, but also the communicative behavior of others.

Our ability to transmit the experiences we encounter is limited, if we do not poses the ability to encode them in a form recognizable by others. The vocal mechanisms used in speech, the motor skills used in writing, and the language peculiar to a specific culture are encoding skills possessed to some degree by every human being.

Similarly, the use of gestures and other nonverbal behaviors is an encoding ability that often bridges the verbal gaps encountered by people who speak different languages.

The ideas and experiences we have, as the source encoder is, at this stage, still intangible. To make them come alive we must change that intangible invention into an actual physical product, which in the communication model is labeled the *message*. Regardless of the physical product be it a sketch, a letter, or a conversation of our ideas and our experiences.

All of us are aware that a message does not just appear.

Every day we deliver messages of varying kinds and lengths as if we actually knew what operations were involved. In order to convey a message, we must arrange it so that it has some resemblance of recognizable order. In the English language, this requirement is filled by the sentence because it is a series of words in connected speech or writing forming the grammatically complete expression of a single thought. The order established through sentences is the *message code*. Whatever the code is – a sentence, picture or music – its expression becomes the *message content*. Finally, a message can be sent unless consideration is given to the manner in which we convey the desired message *treatment*. *Message treatment* is the decision made in selecting and arranging both codes and content.

Once decisions have been made on the codes and contents of message, we must route the message across a *channel*. Because the cannel in the model involves the senses of hearing, seeing, touching, smelling and tasting, the sensory channel selected must be appropriate to the message we wish to convey.

The receiver decoder is one of the last links in our communication model. Behind this label is the person to whom the message is directed, that other individual who has been influenced by the same factors of communication, knowledge, attitudes, and sociocultural systems as we have been. Since no two people perceive an event or share their perceptions of that event in the same way, it is crucial to any verbal interaction that the receiver decoder understands what we mean to convey. Our intent is not enough. We must aim for precision in our communication. The success with which we convey our thoughts determines how they will be absorbed and translated by the receiver decoder. Then the receiver provides some form of *feedback*, which allows us to determine the success or failure of our communication efforts.

### Importance of Language and Experience in the Communication Process

Language distinguishes humans from other animals. It is used not only to communicate but also to develop the person's view of life and the world. Thus, language and experiences are closely related. A person's view of the world is developed through several kinds of filters. Such filters consist of the sight, hearing, touch, taste and smell. Stimuli processed through these receptor systems enable the person to experience the outside world and through language such experiences can be compared with others' experiences. Another filter through which a person experiences the world is the particular language system into which the person is socialized. Words and sentences give meaning to things and events. Language allows us to conceptualize the world.

A third filter through which a person experiences the world is his or her unique personal history. Every human has a set of experiences that are unique. Cultural background, personal history, family relationships, the person's place in the sibling ranking, the type of parenting received, the genetic makeup of the person, and other factors.

Both nurse and clients bring language and personal experiences into the communication that occurs between them. The interaction between a nurse and clients is productive when a method of communication is at work that identifies and uses common meanings.

Developing a common understanding is the underlying aim of communication.

Two over riding principles that guide communication are:

1. ***Clarity in words*** and sentences used to clarify events when they occur within the frame of reference and common experience of both nurse and clients.

2. *Clarity in communication* occurs when language is used as a tool for the promotion of coherence or connections of ideas expressed.

## Basic Characteristics of Communication

- Communication is a continuous and reciprocal process in which both the sender and the receiver of messages participate simultaneously.
- Communicating person receives and sends messages through verbal and nonverbal means.
- Verbal and nonverbal communication occurs simultaneously.
- Nonverbal communication is more likely to be involuntary. It intends to be less under control of the person sending the message than verbal communication. Nonverbal communication is considered as being a more accurate expression of true feelings. Nonverbal communication often helps a person understand subtle and hidden meanings in what is being said verbally. There is a proverb that says 'Action speaks more than thousand words'.
- Communicating persons respond to messages they receive. This form of feedback is especially important to validate information in order to learn whether the message was received accurately.
- The message cannot always be assumed to mean what the receiver believes it to mean or what the sender intended to mean. Validation is necessary to determine the accuracy of not only the message but also the meaning of the message.
- Exchanging message requires knowledge.
- Past experiences influence messages, sent and interpretation.
- Communication is influenced by the way people feel at the moment or about the subject.

## Communication Techniques in Nursing

**Conversation Skills:**

- Control the tone of your voice so that you are conveying exactly what you mean to say.
- Be knowledgably about the topic of conversation and have accurate information
- Be flexible
- Be clear and concise
- Avoid words that may be interpreted differently
- Be truthful
- Keep an open mind
- Take advantage of available opportunities.

*Listening Skills:* It is a skill that involves both hearing and interpreting what is said. It requires attention and concentration to sort out, evaluate, and validate clues so that one understands the true meanings of what is being said. Listening requires concentrating on the client and what is being said.

### *Techniques to Improve Listening Skills*

- Whenever possible sit when communicating with a client
- Be alert but relaxed and take sufficient time so that the client feels at ease during the conversation
- If culturally appropriate maintain eye contact with the client
- Indicate that you are paying attention to what the client is saying
- Think before responding to the client
- Listen for themes in the client's comments.

*Use of silence:* The nurse can use silence appropriately by taking the time to wait for the client to initiate or continue speaking.

During period of silence, the nurse has the opportunity to observe the clients verbal and nonverbal messages simultaneously.

Periods of silence during communication demonstrating comfort and contentment in the nurse-client relationship.

## Factors that Influence Communication

- Perceptions
- Values
- Background
- Knowledge
- Roles and relationships
- Environmental setting

## Interviewing Techniques

Interview is a major tool in nursing for the collection of data during the assessment step of the nursing process.

*Purpose:* To obtain accurate and throughout information.

### *Techniques*

- Open-ended question
- Closed question
- Validation question
- Clarifying question
- Reflective question
- Sequencing question
- Directing question.

### *Interpersonal Skills in Nursing*

Interpersonal skills are communication skills required for positive relationships between persons. These skills are essential for a nurse to establish and promote good nurse client relationship.

Some of the interpersonal skills are:

- Warmth and friendliness
- Openness
- Empathy
- Competence
- Consideration of client variable

### *Factors Facilitating Positive Interaction*

- Have a purpose for interaction
- Choose a comfortable environment
- Provide privacy
- Confidentiality
- Client focus.

## Communication and the Nursing Process

Communication is one of the instruments of data collection and implementation in the nursing process.

The steps of the nursing process can also be applied in the process of communication.

### Helping Relationship

The helping relationship is sometimes called therapeutic or client nurse relationship.

The goals of a helping relationship between a nurse and a client are determined cooperatively and are defined in terms of the client's needs. Broadly speaking common goals might include:
- Increased independence
- Greater feelings of worth
- Improved physical well-being.

#### *Basic Characteristics of a Helping Relationship*

- Dynamic
- Purposeful and time limited
- The person providing the assistance in a helping relationship assumes the dominant role.

#### *Phases of a Helping Relationship*

- *Orientation phase:* The assessment phase of the nursing process, during this phase:
  - The roles of both persons in the relationship are clarified
  - An agreement about the relationship is established. The agreement is usually a simple verbal exchange or, occasionally, a written document
  - An orientation to health agency, its facilities and administration routines.
- *Working phase:*
  - Client and nurse work together the needs of the client identified during the orientation phase
  - Interaction is the essence of the working phase
  - The nurse as caregiver, teacher and counselor provides what ever the assistance needed to achieve the mutually agreed goal.
- *Termination phase:*
  - Happen at change of shift time
  - When the client is discharged
  - When the nurse leaves for vacation.

## PRINCIPLES AND PRACTICES OF NURSING

Nursing is a major component of the health care delivery system and nurses make up the largest employment group within the system.

Nursing services are necessary for every patient seeking care of various types including primary, secondary, tertiary and restorative. As nursing is an important part of health care delivery system, the nurses need to understand the system to effectively deliver quality care within it.

*Nursing:* Nursing is the process of recognizing, understanding and meeting the health needs of any person or society and is based on a constantly changing body of scientific knowledge.

### Definition of Nursing

Different people have defined nursing differently. However, in this unit we will see some of the common definitions of nursing:

- Nursing is provision of optimal conditions to enhance the person's reparative processes and prevent the reparative process from being interrupted.
- The practice of nursing is defined as diagnosing and treating human response to actual or potential health problems through such services as case finding, health teaching, health counseling and provision of support to or restoration of life and well-being and executing medical regimes prescribed by licensed or otherwise legally authorized physician or dentist.
- Nursing is directed to ward meeting both the health and illness need and man who is viewed holistically as having physical, emotional, psychological intellectual, social and spiritual.
- Nursing is a humanistic science dedicated to compassionate concern with maintaining and promoting health, preventing illness and caring for and rehabilitating the sick and disabled.
- Nursing is a deliberate action, a function of the practical intelligence of nurses and action to bring about humanely desirable conditions in persons and their environments.
- As a practice discipline nursing scientific body of knowledge is used to provide an essential service to people, that is to promote ability to affect health positively.

### History and Development of Nursing

It is difficult to trace the exact origin of the nursing profession. However, moral action is the historical basis for the creation, evolution and practice of nursing.

### Nursing in Ancient Civilization

The early record of ancient civilization offers little information about those who care for the sick. During this time beliefs, about the cause of disease were embedded in superstition and magic and thus treatment often involved magical cures.

- Ancient Egyptians developed community planning and strict hygienic rules to control communicable diseases. The first recorded Nurses were seen.
- In the Babylonian civilization, there were references to tasks and practices traditionally provided by nurses. Nurses are mentioned occasionally in old testament as women who provide care for infant, for the sick and dying and as midwives who assisted during pregnancy and delivery.
- In ancient Rome, care of the sick and injuries was advanced in Mythology and reality. Although medicine as a science was developed. There was little evidence of establishing a foundation for nursing.
- The ancient Greeks gods were believed to have special healing power. In 460 BC Hippocrates born and credited with being the Father of medicine. He proved that illness had natural cause and not to be of a religious or magical cause. Hippocrates first proposed such concepts as physical assessment, medical ethics, patient–centered care and observation and reporting. He emphasized the importance of patient care that contributed a lot for the groundwork of nursing.
- In ancient India, male nurses staffed early hospitals and women served as midwives and nursed ill family members.

### Nursing in the Middle Ages

During this time, monasticism and other religious groups offered the only opportunities for men and women to pursue careers in nursing. It was the Christian value of 'love the neighbor as the self' that had a significant impact on the development of western nursing. The principle of caring was established with Christ's parable of Good Samaritan providing care for a tired and injured stranger.

In the third and fourth centuries several wealthy matrons of Roman empire, including Marcella, Fabiola and Paula, converted to Christianity and used their wealth to provide house of care and healing (the fore runner of hospital) for the poor, the sick and homeless.

Women were not the sole providers of nursing service in the third century in Rome. There was an organization of men called the 'Parabalani' Brotherhood. This group of men provided care to the sick and dying from the great plague in Alexandria.

### Dark Age of Nursing

In this period Monasteries were closed and the work of women in religious order was nearly ended. The few women who cared for the sick during this time were prisoners or prostitutes who had little or no training in nursing. Because of this, nursing was considered as the most minimal of all tasks, and had little acceptance and prestige.

### The Development of Modern Nursing

Three images influenced the development of modern nursing. Ursuline Sisters of Quebec organized the first training for nurses. Theodore Flender revived the deaconess movement and opened a School in Kaiserwerth, Germany, which was training nurses. Elizabeth Fry established the institute of Nursing Sisters. But in the latter half of eighteenth century Florence Nightingale the founder of modern nursing changed the form and direction of nursing and succeeded in establishing it as a respected profession. She was born to wealthy and intellectual family in 1820. In spite of opposition from her family and restrictive societal code for affluent young English woman to be a nurse Nightingale believed she was called by God to help others and to improve the well-being of mankind. In 1847, she received three month's training at Kaiserwerth.

In 1853 she studied in Paris with sister of charity, after which she returned to England to assume the position of super intendment of a charity hospital. Nightingale worked to free nursing from the bonds of the church. She saw nursing as a separate profession from the church, yet she began her career as the result of the mystic experience.

During the Crimean war, Florence Nightingale was asked to recruit a contingent of female nurses. The Jamaica nurse Mary Grant was the first nurse recruited to provide care to the sick and injured in the Crimean war. The achievements of Florence Nightingale in the war were so outstanding that she was recognized by the queen of England who awarded her the Order of Merit.

When she returned to England she established the Nightingale School of Nursing, which was opened in 1860. The school served as a model for other training schools. Its graduates traveled to other counties to manage hospitals and nursing training programs.

## NURSING PROCESS

### Definition of Nursing Process

The definition of the nursing process is a professional nurses approach to identify diagnose, and treat human responses to health and illness (American Nurses Association 2003).

It is a deliberate intellectual activity whereby the practice of nursing is approached in an orderly, systematic manner of patient care, in a dynamic, continuous method to assist the patient to achieve and maintain health.

The nursing process is an orderly systematic manner of determining the patient's problems, making plans to solve them, initiating the plan or assigning others to implement it and evaluating the extent to which the plan was effective in resolving the problems identified.

The nursing process is a systematic method for assessing health status, diagnosing health care needs, formulating a plan of care, initiating plan and evaluating the effectiveness of plan.

### Steps in Nursing Process

- Assessment
- Diagnosis
- Planning
- Implementation
- Evaluation

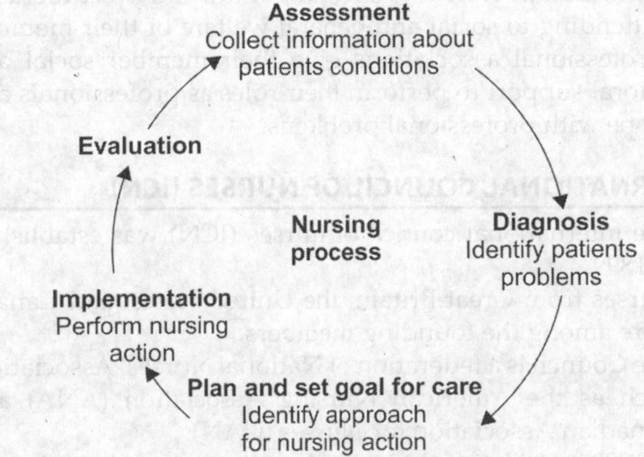


***Assessment:*** This refers to a systematic collection of data, to assist in identifying needs and problems.

Data are collected in a systematic fashion, utilizing the interview or nursing history, physical examinations, laboratory results and other resources.

***Diagnosis:*** Nursing diagnosis is a clinical judgment about individual family or community responses to actual and potential health problems and life processes. During this phase, the data collected during assessment are critically analyzed and interpreted. Conclusions are drawn regarding the patient's needs, problems, concerns and human responses.

***Planning:*** Planning is a systematic approach in developing a plan of action based on a careful assessment.

Strategies are developed to prevent, minimize or connect the problems identified in the nursing diagnosis.

It consists of several steps including establishing priorities, setting objectives, writing interventions, recording outcomes of nursing interventions in an organized fashion to complete the nursing care plan.

***Implementation:*** It refers to carry out a plan that is based on careful assessment of need. It is the initiation and completion of action necessary to achieve the outcomes or objectives.

***Evaluation:*** It is an ongoing process that determines the extent to which the goal has been achieved.

The nurses assess the progress of the patient, institute corrective measures if required, and revise the nursing care plan.

### Nursing Association

The nursing association must perform the following five functions for the preservation and development of its profession:

1. Defining and regulating the profession through setting and enforcing standard of education and practice for generalist and specialist.
2. Developing the knowledge base for practice in its broadest and narrowest components.
3. Transmitting values norms, knowledge, and skill to nursing students, new graduates and members of the profession for application in practice.
4. Communicating and advocating the value and contribution of field to several publics and constituencies.
5. Attending to social and general welfare of their member. Professional associations give their member social and moral support to perform their roles as professionals and cope with professional problems.

## INTERNATIONAL COUNCIL OF NURSES (ICN)

- The international council of nurses (ICN) was established in 1899.
- Nurses from Great Britain, the United States, and Canada were among the founding members.
- The Council is a federation of National Nurses' Association, Such as the American Nursing Association (ANA) and Canadian Association for Nurses (CAN).
- In 1993, 111 National Nurses Associations representing 1.4 million Nurses worldwide were affiliated with the ICN.
- The ICN provides an organization through which member of National Nursing Association can work together to promote the health of people and the care of the sick.

***The Objectives of ICN are:***

- To improve the standers and states of Nursing
- To promote the development of strong National Nurses' Association
- To serve as the authoritative voice for Nurses and the nursing profession worldwide.

***The Ethiopian Nurses Association (ENA)*** was established on 6th May, 1952, in Addis Ababa by the Ethiopian government. Her Royal excellence princess Tenagnework Haile Seilassie was the patron of the association.

- There were 15 (fifteen) member when 1st constituted.
- Then the members increased to 80, including some international nurses at 1965.

***The aim of the Ethiopian Nurses Association was:***

- Discuss and solve problems affecting nurses.
- Setting higher standards in nursing.

The Ethiopian Nurses Association becomes a member of ICN in May 1957. In 1958, the first ENA publication was started, in the form of pamphlet. Signed an agreement with CAN in March 11, 1990 EC. The association has 18 (eighteen) branches in different region and schools. Publish 'voice of nursing' magazine every 6 months.

### Ethiopian Nursing Council

The Ethiopian nursing council was established in 1954. It was responsible for setting examination for nurses, licensing nurses and midwives, registering nurses, and monitoring standard of care. It acted as the official liaison between the ministry of public health and the ENA.

The functions of Ethiopian nursing council were:

- To study nursing needs
- Participating in health planning
- To develop nursing policies
- Making accreditations regarding nursing, midwifery and auxiliary nursing.
- Responsible for recommending disciplinary action against nursing personnel
- To advise on ethical issue concerning nurses and nursing practice.
- Responsible for licensing nurses for revoking (removable) such as licenses as result of malpractices.
- Promoted the training of nursing personnel.

## ADMISSION OF THE PATIENT

The entrance of a patient into a health care agency such as a hospital or a private clinic is termed as admission. A patient enters the hospital by himself or he may be brought to the hospital by his relatives, friends, and neighbors or others.

Mentally ill patients, persons, who have tried to commit suicide and accident patients, are admitted through a legal process.

- Evaluation
- Planning
- Diagnosis
- Assessment
- Implementation
- Knowledge
- Attitude.

### Experience Nursing Process Standards

All ill person enters the hospital to get his disorder cured when a healthy individual gets admitted into a hospital for a day or for investigations and observations and in order to find whether he is suffering from any illness which has not been manifested by any external signs and symptoms.

Patients who have become seriously ill suddenly, come the hospital without having had any time to settle their family work affairs.

Hence, they are not only worried and anxious about the illness, but also are upset about various other problems affect their family. Nurses must understand their physical and mental problems and be very kind and understanding.

***Need for good reception of the patient:*** A nurse has an important role to play in the reception the patient to the hospital. The following are the purposes of this procedure: (1) Prepare the patient both physically and mentally for his stay in the hospital. (2) To help the patient to be comfortable and to provide him with a clean and safe environment. (3) To give a good impression of the hospital and its service so that the patient will fully cooperate with the treatment and nursing care.

A patient may be coming to hospital for the first time. He leaves his familiar home surrounding and his loved ones and comes to an unknown place and to unknown people. Any change in human life is anxiety producing and is viewed with fear.

Added to this, his physical condition gives him fear and anxiety. Hence, it is the nurse's duty to receive the patient, kindly sympathetically and with an understanding of his illness. If he is admitted, he is given a diet sheet and sent to the ward. If he is too ill and needs immediate attention he is given emergency treatment and then transported to the ward.

As soon as the patient comes to the ward, receive him, his relatives and his friends as if you are receiving your guests into your home. Ask them to be seated while you prepare the bed ready for the patient.

If the patient is in a serious condition, the ward nurse is informed in advance about the arrival of the patient, so that the patient does not have to wait till the bed is made ready.

***Need for orientation to place and people:*** Inform the patient and his relatives about the hospital routine, the hospital rules, the general set up of the ward and the personnel working in the ward.

Inform the patient's relatives about the time of visiting hours and supply them with visiting passes.

If the patient is seriously ill give the relative a special pass so that he will be able to stay with the patient in the hospital.

***Need for admission assessment:*** Do a good assessment of his physical condition in order to plan his care. If his physical state needs immediate treatment report to physician and prepare your patient for physical examination and carry out the treatment, which the physician prescribes after the physical examination.

### Orientation to the Ward

The patient who is not very ill, are allowed to move about can be taken round the ward. Introduce the other patients to him and vice versa, and also with the nursing personnel working in the ward. Orient the patient to the whole ward, duty room, toilet rooms, and the unit prepared for him. After making the patient to be seated comfortably explained the hospital policies, procedures, and routines to the patients and his relatives. Tell him what is expected from him. Explain to him the time for meals serving, the doctors visit, visiting time the prayer service, if any and other hospitals routines.

### Care of Belongings

It is always good policy to discourage patients to keep/valuable things and money with them. Send the valuables to home through relatives. If he does not have anyone with him, enter the description of items in the register and send the valuables to the office for safe custody. Get the patient's signature or thumb impression in the register. However, inform the patient that he will get back his valuables on discharge.

It is important that you take care of the patient's clothing, should see that the clothing are cleaned and stored away with proper label or send them home for a fresh set of clean clothes.

However, encourage, patients to use hospital clothing. If a patient is suffering from infectious disease, see that the clothing are disinfected and cleaned before they are sent home or stored away.

## DISCHARGING OF THE PATIENT

Discharge is a preparation of a patient and discharge records to leave the hospital.

***Purpose:*** (1) To ensure continuity of care to the patient after discharge. (2) To assist the patient in discharge process.

***Guidelines:*** The patients are discharged from the hospital in one of the following ways.

***Discharge to home:*** The discharge to home or another hospital or another unit with in the hospital is initiated by the doctor who advises the patient that he is well enough to leave the hospital or requires treatment in another unit within the hospital or in an another hospital.

***Discharge to another hospital or another unit within the hospital*** (referral). When a patient or family is not satisfied with the treatment or care given and wants to leave the hospital against the medical advice in such cases the patient or the relative is asked to sign a statement that he is going or taking the patient on his own will and responsibility.

***Discharge against medical advice (AMA):*** Patient leaves the hospital against the medical officer's advice, when a patient escapes from the hospital without the knowledge of the hospital staff and without signing the said statement he is treated as absconded in the records.

***Nurses Responsibility:*** Inform the patient and the relatives a day or two days before the discharge. Get the discharge slip prepared after checking the vital signs and examining the patient. The nurse should see that the patients personnel hygiene is maintained, he is dressed in home clothes and has taken meals.

Hand over the patient's belonging and any valuable, which have been kept safety, to the patient or the relative under proper receipt. Complete the unit admission and discharge registered case sheet and other records. Hand over the case sheet and other records medical record department under proper receipt. Inform the hospital authorities about the discharge if the patient is medicolegal.

Hand over the discharge slip to the patient or relative and explain about the treatment and the diet to be taken at home, follow up visit and inform to bring the discharge slip on every visits, any special advices pertaining to condition. See that the patient receives all the medicines as per discharge slip. Check the hospital things before the patient leaves the ward. Place the patient in the wheel chair or stretcher according to the patient's condition until he leaves the hospital. Immediately after the patient leaves, reorganize the patient unit.

## BED AND BED MAKING

Bed making is an art. Skillful bed making contributes materially to the patient's comfort. Clean and comfortable bed includes the patient's unit in the hospital.

*Purpose:* (1) To provide clean and comfortable bed to the patient. (2) To observe and prevent patient's complications. (3) To save time, effort and material. (4) To provide a neat appearance of the ward/unit. (5) To adapt the needs of the patient.

*Types of bed:* The beds are of two types, ordinary and special beds.

*Open (simple) bed:* This is prepared for an ambulatory patient.

*Indication:* (1) Provide a clean smooth comfortable bed to the patient.

*Closed (unoccupied) bed:* This is an empty bed in which the top covers are arranged in such a way that all linen beneath the counterpane or bedspread is full protected from dust and dirt until the admission of new patient. On arrival of the patient, this bed is converted into open bed.

*Indication:* Keep the bed ready for receiving the new patient.

*Occupied bed:* This bed is prepared for bedridden patient, lying in the bed.

*Indication:* Provide a clean and comfortable bed with the least disturbance of the patient in it.

### Special Beds

*Admission bed:* This is prepared for the newly admitted patient.

*Indications:* (1) Provide minimum disturbance to the patient during admission, bath and physical examination. (2) Protect bed linen during admission, bath and leave a fresh bed immediately ready for the use.

*Postoperative bed:* This is prepared for the patient who has undergone surgery.

*Indications:* (1) Protect bed linen from vomiting, bleeding, drainage and discharges. (2) Provide warmth and comfort to the patient to prevent shock.

*Fracture bed:* This is a hard firm bed designed for the patient with fracture particularly of spine, pelvis or femur.

*Indications:* (1) Aid in immobilizing the fracture, (2) Prevent unnecessary pain, (3) Provide warmth and comfort to the patient, (4) Prevent undue sagging of the mattress.

*Plaster beds:* This is a hard bed designed for the patient with plaster.

*Indications:* (1) Aid in immobilizing the part until the plaster dries, (2) Aid in drying the plaster in correct position and shape, (3) Provide warmth to dry the plaster and keep the patient comfortable.

*Amputation or stump bed:* In this type of bed the top bed-clothes are divided or split. This is known as amputation or stump bed when it is used for the patient with amputation of legs.

*Indications:* (1) Avoid disturbance to the patient during constant observation, repeated applications or treatments are necessary for abdomen or lower limbs, (2) Take the weight of the clothes off the side of the amputated limb or stump, (3) Keep the stump in good position, (4) Watch stump for hemorrhage constantly and apply a tourniquet instantly if necessary.

*Cardiac bed:* This is prepared for a patient with heart disease.

*Indications:* (1) Relieve dyspnea, (2) Assist in recovery of the patient, (3) Provide comfort to the patient, (4) Prevent complications.

*Rheumatism or renal bed:* This is prepared to provide extra warmth to the patient.

*Indications:* (1) Provide extra warmth to the body incase of general debility and shock, (2) Provide comfort to the aching joints in patients with acute rheumatism. (3) Improve perspiration for excretion of waste products in case of nephritis.

*Burns bed:* This is prepared for a patient with burns.

*Indications:* (1) Prevent infection to the burnt area, (2) Help in healing of the burnt area, (3) Provide comfort to the patient, (4) Prevent the patient from sticking to the sheet as a result of exudates oozing from the burnt area.

The beds must be versatile and adaptable to different needs of the patients with following arrangements.

*Side rails:* These are used to prevent the patient from falling out of bed, protect the restless patient, provide the patient support to grasp and hold when moving about.

*Hand cranks:* These are located at the foot of bed and used to adjust the height of bed, raise or lower the head, foot or knee sections in order to maintain various bed positions for treatment or comfort.

*Special attachments:* The attachments of various poles, frames and equipment for traction are used to modify the beds to meet various needs of the patient for treatment and comfort.

### Therapeutic Environment

- Maintaining and creating trustful supporting relationship in care of patients.
- It is clearly and genuinely communicating and performing care activity.
- Allowing the supportive group in care of patients.
- Acceptance of patients feelings and values and worthy as whole.
- Assist the patient and family in identifying supportive groups. Maintaining a safe and secured environment.
- Reinforce progress in behavior or self care activities or terminating the relationship.
- Encourage evaluation of progress between nurse and the patient.

### Psychosocial Environment

Mental comfort is provided for the patient by eliminating his fear, anxiety and worry. He should receive sympathy and consideration from the nursing and medical staff. His relatives should avoid unpleasant news to him while he is in the hospital. Meeting his spiritual needs may help to give him mental peace and comfort again.

## Body Mechanics and Positioning

**Definition:** Body mechanics means the cooriented use of the body parts to produce motion and maintain equilibrium in relation to both internal and external forces. Posture is the relationship of the various parts of the body in activity or at rest. Position in patient in corrected body alignment means to give proper support to the body in order to maintain muscle tone and eliminate strain.

***Purpose of good body mechanics and posture:*** (1) To provide maximum comfort and relaxation, (2) To aid in normal body function, (3) To prevent contractures and neuromuscular deformities and complications, (4) To conserve maximum possible energy by preventing unnecessary strain.

***Standing position:*** In correct standing position the head is held erect, back is kept straight as much as possible, chest is put forward, shoulders are kept back, elbows are slightly flexed, wrists are extended, fingers are slightly flexed, abdomen is drawn inward and kept flat, knees are slightly flexed, and are pointing ahead and parallel to each other about 3 inches apart.

Knowledge of correct standing position is necessary because all other positions are modifications of standing position. When a nurse helps the patient to sit or lie down in bed, she follows the principles of correct standing position and keeps patient's body in good alignment.

***Sitting position:*** In sitting position, the weight of the body is balanced by ischial tuberosities the buttocks and the thighs. Elbows are flexed and supported, hips are flexed at right angles to the trunk, knees are flexed at right angles to the thighs, and angles are flexed to right angles to the legs and are flat on floor. Back is held erect and the back and buttocks are supported by the back of the chair.

## POSITIONS USED FOR PATIENTS

***Dorsal position:*** Patient is flat on the bed with legs extended and arms at the sides of the body. This is not a comfortable position, as the curves of the body are not supported.

***Dorsal recumbent position:*** This is called back lying position. This is a modification of standing position. The only difference being, the patient is in horizontal position instead of vertical. Patient lies flat on his back with a pillow under his head. A small pad is placed in the hollow of the back, and the knees are slightly flexed. A soft pillow is arranged under the knees. A footboard is provided to prevent foot drop. Arms are kept at the sides of the body. Most of the patients are nursed in this position.

***Lateral position:*** Patient lies on his side with spine straight. The knees are flexed; the upper knees are more flexed than the lower one. Pillows may be provided for the head, in between the legs, and to support back and abdomen. The lower arm is kept above the head and the upper arm is placed on a pillow in front. The arms and legs do not bear the weight of the body. This position is used for general comfort, rest and relaxation. During back care, patient is placed in lateral position.

***Left lateral position:*** It is used for vaginal, perineal and rectal examinations, and the post operative patients are kept in lateral position in order to maintain a clear airway.

***Jackknife position:*** Patients lies on his back with his shoulders slightly elevated. The hips and knees are flexed and brought up to the abdomen and chest. The position is useful to perform a lumbar puncture.

***Knee-chest position:*** The patient knees on the bed and then lowers his head, shoulders and chest and rests them on the bed. Head is turned to one side, and kept on a pillow. The thighs are kept vertical. Arms are crossed above the head. This position is useful for performing vaginal and rectal examinations and for correcting displaced uterus or other organs.

***Lithotomy position:*** The patient is kept on his back. Head and shoulders rest on a small soft pillow. Knees are flexed well and buttocks are brought over to the edge of the bed. If it is used for a long period, the legs are supported by stirrups, attached to the table. The position is used for examination or operations on rectum and genital organs.

***Prone position:*** Patient lies flat on his abdomen with head kept on a pillow and turned to one side. Pillows are kept under the waist and under the lower legs. The arms are flexed at the elbow and kept above the head. This position is used when there is bedsore or burns or an injury at the back and as a change of position for patients which fractured spine.

***Sims' position or semi prone position:*** This is a modified left lateral position. The patient lies on the left side. Head, shoulders and chest are turned forward so that her chest rests on the pillow. The right knee is well flexed and rests on the bed in front. The left knee is slightly flexed and is positioned behind the right knee. This position is useful for performing vaginal examinations and for rests and relaxation.

***Fowler's position:*** Patient is in a partially sitting position. The back of the bed is elevated to 45 degrees with the aid of a backrest and pillow or by adjustment of the cot. Patient's back shoulder and head are supported well. The knees are flexed and supported with a pillow or by cot adjustment. A footrest is provided to prevent foot drop. Patients are not kept in this position for long time, since there is always the danger of thrombus formation. This position is used for patients with dyspnea (difficulty in breathing), distended abdomen, abdominal surgery, cardiothoracic disorders and ascites. The position is also useful while passing Ryle's tube and while performing tapping of ascites fluid.

***Trendelenburg position:*** The patient lies on this back with the foot at the bed elevated on wooden blocks. Patient's head and trunk are lower than the legs.

***Reverse Trendelenburg Position:*** The head and shoulders are at a higher level than the hips, legs and feet. This position is used for reducing intracranial pressure and for other treatment measure.

***Basic Nursing Care:*** Patient and his environment including the bed comprises of patients unit, which needs to be maintained facilitating hygiene environment helping the cure process.

## HYGIENIC NEEDS – PERSONAL HYGIENE

***Definition:*** The word hygiene refers to 'the science of health and its maintenance, the prevention of disease, and sanitary practices'. Personal hygiene is the activity of self-care, including bathing and grooming. Care of the skin, hair, nails, mouth, teeth, eyes, ears, nasal cavities, and perineal and genital areas.

Factors influencing personal hygiene practices:

- *Development level:* Children learn most of their hygiene practices at home and in their personal environment. They modify their behaviour with other family members. Many of these behaviours stick with them throughout life. The advancing age, hormonal levels and changes in the integumentary system often require hygienic practices.
- *Cultural background:* Norms related to hygiene practices differ from culture to culture. For example, North American culture places a high value on personal cleanliness and people have a habit of bathing daily whereas people from other culture may or may not consider bathing as a daily practice.
- *Socio economic status:* Financial status often affects a person's ability to purchase hygiene products.
- *Religion:* Some religions observe specific rules related to personal hygiene.
- *Health status:* Persons who are ill are often unable to attend to personal hygiene activities, either because they have a low energy supply or a specific physical deficit.

## SAFETY AND COMFORT NEEDS

The environment in which the patient is placed should be comfortable and safe, and it should contribute to his well-beings and should not retard his recovery.

Safety means protection from possible injury. Many factors contribute toward the safety of patients in the hospital. The hospital buildings should be structurally sound for ensuring safety for patients with physical limitations such as, blind, aged or handicapped.

The nursing personnel must be safety conscious, and they should take all efforts to prevent accidents in the hospital. She should report all accidents promptly and take measures to prevent them from happening.

*Comfort:* Comfort is a sense of mental and physical well-being. Physical comfort gets affected due to a dirty and wet bed and lack of body alignment. High temperature and humidity, poor ventilation, too much noise, unpleasant odors and glaring lighting make the patient uncomfortable. To promote comfort for the patients, certain mechanical devices can be used. Pillows can be used for giving support for the various part of the body. Sometimes – patient feels comfortable in a propped up position. In a hospital, a backrest is provided for the patient to keep him in a sitting position.

For relaxation of abdominal muscles, when patients are in pain or after an abdominal operation, knees can be kept flexed by means of a knee rest.

A pillow or a blanket or sheet rolled as a pillow can be improvised as a knee rest. Patients should not be kept with flexed knees for a long period. His circulation may get affected. Hence his position is changed frequently.

For supporting feet and for preventing foot drop, foot rests are used. This device keeps the feet at right angles to the leg and prevents deformities. Footrest can be improvised with sandbags.

Other devices used as comfort measures are air rings or cotton rings and air cushions, air mattress, water mattress are to prevent pressure ulcer.

Mental comfort is provided for the patient by eliminating his fear, anxiety and worry. He should receive sympathy and consideration from the nursing and medical staff. His relatives should avoid unpleasant news to him while he is in the hospital. Meeting his spiritual needs may help to give him mental peace and comfort again.

*Mechanical devices for comfort measures:* To hospitals use many mechanical devices for ensuring safety/patients.

*Bed bars (side rails):* These are used to prevent patients from falling out of bed. Patients who require this safety measure are postoperative patients, unconscious, semiconscious mentally disturbed, sedated, blind or children or very old patients.

*Back rest:* These are usually made of metals. These are used to support the back of the patient in upright position.

*Over bed table:* The table such as the cardiac table is placed in front of the patient and the top of the table is adjusted to the desired height. As pillow is arranged on the top of the table so that the patient can lean forward on it for support. When he wants to take food, read or write.

### Footboards

*Foot rests:* These are made of wood and are L shaped, so that one end can be slipped under the mattress to hold the other end in a firm upright position. The patient is placed in supine position to rest the bottoms of the feet flat against the surface of the footboard (covered with sheet).

These are used to prevent foot drop by maintaining good alignment.

*Sandbags:* These are canvas, rubber or plastic bags filled with sand and are 1, 5 and 10 lbs in weight.

These are used to immobilize the body part, placing them snugly next to the part. For example, on either side of the feet to maintain the position of the feet on the footboard, immobilize the fractured limb.

*Blocks (shock blocks):* These are made of wood, may be high or low. These are placed under the foot of the bed for various reasons, e.g. surgical shock, traction and postural drainage. This may be placed under the head of bed to promote drainage and improve cerebral circulation.

*Hand rolls:* These are made of cloth that is rolled into a cylinder about 45 inches long and 23 inches in diameter and stuffed firmly. These are used to keep the fingers form being held in a tight fist leading to flexion contracture in patients who are unable to move the hands due to paralysis, injury or disease.

*Thigh rolls:* These are made by folding a sheet to a desired length of 23 feet and then rolled into a tight cylinder. These are used to support the hips and thighs, preventing them outward rotation and keeping the feet in good alignment, in case of paralysis, fracture of the femur or hip surgery. To use the roll, place the lose end (flap) under the patients hips and thighs with the role under the flap end and then tucking snugly along the hip and thigh.

*Cradle:* These are mostly semicircular in shape, made of wood or metal. These are used to prevent the weight of top bedclothes on patient's feet and toes. To use the cradle, place it over the bottom bedclothes and the top bedclothes are then brought over the cradle. These are used for patients affected by burns.

*Restraints* are devices used to prevent agitated patients, persons who get out of bed at night in their sleep and small children, from falling out of bed.

*Wire mesh* for windows and doors are fixed to prevent insects.

*Safety measures:* Patients should be safeguarded from fire accidents and from careless application of heat. Fire accidents occur mainly due to allowing patients to smoke in bed. Use of faulty electric appliances and careless use of oxygen cylinders. Patient may get injured from careless application of hot water bags, electric pads and application of medications on the skin. Poisonous drugs should be kept under lock and key with specific red label.

Patients may come to harm through bacteriological sources, insects and rodents. Food and water should be made safe for consumption. Insects and rodents should be eliminated.

## ACTIVITIES AND EXERCISES

Activities and exercises are necessary for healthy living. Activities usually performed in a day like eating, dressing, grooming, bathing, brushing, etc. are called activities of daily living.

*Activities of daily living:* It is essential for meeting the day to day needs. When a person does not meet these activities, it is the caregiver's responsibilities to meet their needs. According to their health status the degree of assistance required will vary those who are recording sick needs, total assistance in order to meet their daily needs. Exercise is the performance of physical exertion for improvement of health or the correction of physical deformity.

*Benefits of exercise:* (1) Exercise strengthens muscles, (2) helps to prevent constipation, (3) increases appetite, (4) improves sleep, (5) stimulates blood circulation, (6) improves lung ventilation, (7) prevents obesity, (8) promotes physical and mental well-being, (9) promotes urinary function, (10) it regulates body temperature.

*Types of exercise:* There are two types of exercises. They are:

1. *Active exercise:* Active exercise is a type of physical activity accomplished by the patient without assistance. These exercises help the patient to attain the normal physiological function of the body.
   - Deep breathing and coughing exercise for complete lung expansion usually done by postoperative patient.
   - Exercise of the limbs through full range of motion which includes flexion, extension, adduction, abduction and rotation
   - Moving in bed to change the position
   - Foot exercise to prevent foot drop and toe deformities.
   - Abdominal and gluteal contraction exercise.
2. *Passive exercise:* In passive exercise, the movements or activity is carried out by another person and the patient makes no voluntary effort to assist or resist the action. The passive exercises are usually carried out by the physiotherapist or the nurse. The performance of certain nursing procedures such as bathing the patient, giving back care and changing the position, etc. provides some passive exercise for the patient. Passive exercise is useful for patient with restricted movements, deformities and unconsciousness.

### Moving, Shifting and Lifting Patient

As nurses you may be required to move and lift patients. An important point you have to bear in mind while moving patients is that you must observe correct body mechanic for your patients as well as for yourself.

While lifting heavy objects, it is wise to stand with your feet while apart and firmly on the floor.

The weight should be lifted close to the body. Flex your knees so that your strong muscles of the legs bear the weight of the object.

*Purposes:* (1) To perform the task efficiently.
(2) To avoid the patient from unnecessary effort.
(3) To prevent from strain and back injuries.
(4) To promote circulation and muscular tone.

*Moving upward or downward:* Two nurses are required to do this activity. One nurse places her one hand under the patient's shoulder and the other hand under the lumbar region.

The other nurse stands on the other side of the bed and does the same as the first nurse. The patient, if he is able, is asked to flex the knee and push against the matters with heels. Both nurses together bring the patient up.

*Moving from one side of bed to another:* Move pillows towards the side of the bed. Place your one arm under the shoulders and the other under the lumbar region.

Move upper part of the body to the side of the bed. Then keep one arm under the lumbar region and the other under the thighs and move the middle part of the body of the side of the bed. Lastly place one arm under the thighs and the other under the ankles and move the lower part of the body to the side of the bed. See whether the whole body is straight and in good alignment.

*Turning on side:* Before turning move the patient a little away from the center. If he is to be turned on the left side, you stand at his left. Keep his right arm crossed on the chest and right leg crossed over the left leg. Flex the right knee slightly keep one hand on the patient's right shoulder and the other on his right hip and gently roll him to left lateral position.

*Moving patients from stretcher to bed:* Keep the head of the stretcher at right angles to the foot of the bed. Three nurses are needed.

All stand on the same side of the stretcher one nurse places her arms under the patient's head and shoulders, another keeps her anus under the hips, the third has her arms under the thighs and legs.

All together lift the patient, turn and place him on the bed. The lifters observe body mechanics for themselves. They keep their backs straight, flex their knees and place their one foot forward while transferring the patient.

## OXYGEN NEEDS

Oxygen is administered whenever there is deficiency in the blood is shown by cyanosis. Patients with respiratory dysfunction are treated with oxygen therapy to relieve anoxemia or hypoxemia. The normal amount of oxygen in the blood must be in the range of 80 to 100 mm Hg. If it falls below 60 mm of Hg irreversible physiological effect may take place. The brain cells receive 20 percent of the body's oxygen supply and can live only for 3 to 5 minutes if their oxygen supply cut off.

***Purpose:*** To supply oxygen in conditions when there is interference with the normal oxygenation of the blood.

***Indications for oxygen inhalation:*** (1) Breathlessness due to asthma, pulmonary embolism, emphysema, cardiac insufficiencies, etc. (2) Obstructed airway due to growth, enlarged thyroid, (3) Cyanosis, (4) Shock and circulatory failure, (5) After severe hemorrhage, (6) Anemia, (7) Patients under anesthesia, (8) Asphyxia due to any reason, e.g. drowning, inhalation of poisonous gases, hanging etc., (9) Poisoning with chemicals that alter the tissues ability to utilize oxygen, e.g. cyanide poisoning, (10) Carbon monoxide poisoning, (11) Postoperative chest surgery and thyroidectomies, (12) Insufficient oxygen in atmosphere, (13) Air hunger.

***Methods of oxygen administration:*** Administration of oxygen depends upon the condition of the patient, the concentration desired, the facility available and the preference of the doctor. It can be given by following ways:

***Oxygen by nasal catheter:*** This is the usual method of administering oxygen to the patients in the ward. The nasal catheter is inserted into the nostril reaching upto the uvula. The catheter is taped on the forehead to keep it in place. The nasal catheter permits free movement for the patient and nursing care may be given with much more ease.

***Oxygen by BLB mask:*** When oxygen concentration of over 25% is needed or when oxygen is given under pressure the mask is used. If the mask does not fit snugly over the face, oxygen will be lost from the mask. It is useful for the patients who are unable to breathe through the nose. Flow of 8 to 12 litres oxygen will be sufficient to maintain the concentration of oxygen to 25 to 60%.

BLB (Boothby, Lovelace and Bulbalian) is a rubber mask. It is made to fit over the nose or nose and mouth. The reservoir bag is attached to it.

***Oxygen by Tent:*** It consists of a canopy over the patient's which may cover the patient partially or totally. It is connected to a supply of oxygen. The canopies are transparent, so that the nurse can observe the patient. The lower portion of the canopy is tucked under the bed to prevent the escape of oxygen.

***Oxygen cylinders and accessories:*** Oxygen is supplied in cylinders or tanks. It is stored under a pressure of 2200 lbs 1000 kg per sq. inch. Piped in oxygen is stored under oxygen cylinder are low pressure about 50 to 60 lbs per sq. inch. The oxygen cylinders are painted black with white neck.

The Wolf's bottle has two holed rubber cork in which two glass tubes are inserted—one short and one long. The long tube is attached by rubber tubing to oxygen cylinder. The short tube is attached by rubber tubing and glass connection to a nasal catheter. The large valve of the cylinder is opened with keys. There is a regulator to regulate the flow.

***Care of oxygen cylinders:***

- Handle the cylinder with care.
- Oxygen stand should be used to prevent falling and causing injury to someone or to the equipment.
- It should be always placed at the head of the bed.
- Oxygen does not cause fire but it supports combustion. So avoid any source of fire from the cylinder for fear of fire.
- Visitors and other patients may need to be reminded. Hang 'No smoking' board to the oxygen cylinder.
- Oxygen cylinders should be stored in a cool temperature, because high temperature can cause expansion of the gas with consequent loss of gas through the safety valve.
- Do not use electric appliances close to oxygen.
- Oil or grease should not be used on the regulator, because in the presence of high oxygen concentration, oil is likely to catch the fire and the cylinder may explore.
- Mark empty cylinder, replace protection cap, and set aside from full cylinders.
- Inspect the apparatus at frequent intervals and make sure that it is in working condition. The nurse should learn the working of cylinders, its regulators, etc. before handling the apparatus.

***Precautions:***

- Giving oxygen is an emergency procedure, so it should be ready for 24 hours.
- The nurse should see that the cylinders are full and all the apparatus is in working condition, the key is attached with the cylinder in a bag.
- There should not be any leakage in rubber tubing.
- There should be written order for $O_2$ inhalation and specific must be prescribed to avoid oxygen toxicity.
- Use regulator to reduce the pressure of the oxygen in the cylinder to a safer level.
- Measure the flow in liters per minute. Adjust the flow of oxygen 2 to 4 liters per minute for adults when the nasal catheter is used.
- Use sterile or disposable nasal catheters to avoid infection.
- The catheter should be changed at least every 8 hourly to avoid blockage of catheter.
- The catheter may be taped to the forehead for the comfort of the patient and to keep it in place.
- Patient's nostrils should be lubricated with petroleum jelly, if there is any sign of irritation.
- Oxygen administration must never be stopped until the cause of hypoxia is reversed.
- If nurse is leaving the patient for short period, leave a call bell near the patient.
- The premature babies should be given oxygen inhalation only for a short time and at a very low concentration to avoid retrolental fibroplasia.
- Observe the patient, receiving oxygen inhalation continuously to detect early signs of oxygen toxicity.
- Since oxygen helps in combustion, fire precautions are to be taken when the oxygen is on flow.

## Elimination Needs

***Definition:*** *Elimination* is the process by which waste products are removed from the bowel and bladder by means of feces and urine.

***Factors affecting bowel and bladder elimination:*** Age, dietary intake, fluid intake, physical activity, psychological factors, position during defecation, pain, pregnancy, surgery, anesthesia and diagnostic test.

*Common bowel elimination problems:* Constipation, impaction, diarrhea, incontinence, flatulence, hemorrhoids and bowel diversion.

*Common bladder elimination problems:* Incontinence, urinary retention.

## Summary

- Nursing is the process of recognizing, understanding and meeting the health needs of any person or society and is based on a constantly changing body of scientific knowledge.
- There are five steps in nursing process. They are assessment, diagnosis, planning, implementation, evaluation.
- Application of nursing process
- The entrance of a patient into a health care agency is termed as admission.
- Nurses responsibilities are to inform the patient and the relatives a day or two before the discharge (a) Get the discharge slip prepared after checking the vital signs and examining the patient, (b) The nurse should see that the patients' personnel hygiene is maintained, he is dressed in home clothes and has taken meals. (c) Hand over the patient's belonging and any valuable, which have been kept safety, to the patient or the relative under proper receipt.
- Skilful bed making contributes materially to the patient's comfort
- Beds are of two types ordinary, and special beds
- Body mechanics means the cooriented use of the body parts to produce motion and maintain equilibrium in relation to both internal and external forces.
- The hygiene refers to the science of health and its maintenance the prevention of disease, and sanitary practices.
- Comfort is a sense of mental and physical well-being
- Restraints are used to prevent agitated patient's who get out of bed at night in their sleep and small children, when falling out of bed.
- While lifting heavy objects flex your knees so that your strong muscles of the legs bear the weight of the object.
- Patients with respiratory dysfunction are treated with oxygen therapy to relieve 'anoxemia or hypoxemia'. The normal amount of oxygen in the blood must be in the range of 80 to 100 mm.
- Oxygen can be administered by the ways of nasal catheter, BLB mask, and an oxygen tent.
- Elimination is the process by which waste products are removed from the bowel and bladder by means of feces and urine.
- Exercise is the performance of physical exertion for improvement of health or the correction of physical deformity.

# HEALTH ASSESSMENT AND PHYSICAL EXAMINATION

## Definition of Physical Examination

It is defined as a complete assessment of a patient's physical and mental status.

## Purposes of Physical Examination

(1) To gather baseline data about the clients health. (2) To supplement confirm or repute data obtained in the nursing history. (3) To confirm and identify nursing diagnoses. (4) To make clinical judgment about a clients. (5) Changing health status and management. (6) To evaluate and physiological outcomes of care. (7) It offers an opportunity for health teaching (breast and testicular self examination).

*Indications of Physical Examination:* It is done in hospitals and during home visits, on admission, before and after diagnostic and therapeutic procedure, on discharge, on follow up, health campus.

## Methods of Physical Examination

*Observation of the patient:* Webster's dictionary defines observation as 'the act or power of noticing'.

Nurses are with the patients throughout day and night. Your report of observation is very valuable in helping the physician to arrive at proper diagnosis and treatment. The essence of good nursing depends largely on intelligent observation. It is through observation you notice your patients' deviations from normal condition.

Your observation and prompt actions may help patients from getting into serious complications such as hemorrhage and other similar problems. Your plan of nursing care also depends upon good observation.

Good observation depends on your intelligence and knowledge. Skill in observation is acquired through careful training in using your senses namely, seeing, hearing, touching and smelling.

It is through the sense of seeing you observe whether the patient is walking with difficulty, whether he is in pain and whether he has any other visible problems.

From hearing the sound of his breathing you will able to understand whether the patient is having difficulty in breathing. Touching the patient reveals whether his body temperature is raised above normal or whether the skin is of normal texture or not. Your sense of smell tells you the nature of discharge from wounds and body cavities.

Observation is a continuous process as a patient's condition is never static. It changes continuously. These changes are noticed through careful observation. A nurse's observation includes not only the physical condition of the patient, but also his psychological aspects. Your observation becomes meaningful when it is accompanied by questioning. To come to clear interpretations of your observations, you have to question your patient so that you will be able to find out the problems experienced by the patient.

Through observation you identify the objective symptoms of your patient. Changes in color of the skin, pulse, respiration, discharges from body cavities and changes in speech are some of the examples of objective symptoms.

Pain nausea, fear, anxiety, dizziness and itching are identified by questioning the patient. These are examples of subjective symptoms.

Certain symptoms cannot be identified by observation or questioning. For example, some special techniques are needed to note changes in temperature, pulse, respiration and blood pressure; X-rays and laboratory tests are used for finding out changes in structure and functions of various systems of the human body.

Physicians use methods such as inspection, palpation, percussion and auscultation for observation of patient's condition.

*Inspection* is observing with eye.

*Palpation* is the art of feeling with the hand.

*Percussion and auscultation* depend on the production of sound.

*Percussion* is tapping an area to produce sounds.

*Auscultation* is listening to sounds within the body with a stethoscope. It is the art of hearing the heart sound, bowel movement etc.

*Olfaction:* Sense of smell, (odor).

## Principles of Physical Examination

*Head to foot examination:* When a patient comes to the hospital or clinic, do an overall observation of the patient, note down his problems, report to the senior nurse and write your observations in the nurse's record sheet.

Use the following as a guide for your observation and for estimation of your patient's condition.

- *The general structure of the body:* Whether he is obese, malnourished, acutely ill or chronically ill. Whether he is weak and unable to walk or walks with aid whether he is in pain. Note the color of the skin—pale, jaundiced.
- *Mental status and level of consciousness:* Whether the patient is cheerful or depressed, anxious and worried, irritate, afraid or sad. Whether oriented to place, person and time. Whether fully conscious, drowsy or comatose.
- *Hair and scalp:* Whether the hair is clean, thick, thin, matted, dirty or coarse. Whether there is any lesion, dandruff, pediculi or nits on the scalp.
- *Eyes:* Whether the eyes are protruding, sunken or crossed. Whether the color is abnormal reddish or yellow. Whether there is swelling, discharge, abnormal watering, pain, burning, itching, photophobia or headache. Whether the vision is normal or poor. Whether the patient uses glasses.
- *Face:* Whether the face is pale, flushed or jaundiced. Whether there is swelling, ulcers, rashes or injuries. Whether his eyes are swollen or sunken.
- *Mouth:* Whether his breath smells of drugs or alcohol or has a bad smell. Whether the gum is inflamed, swollen, bleeding or ulcerated. Whether the lips are cyanotic, dry swollen, cracked or ulcerated. Whether the teeth are loose, broken, artificial or irregularly arranged. Whether he has any toothache. Whether the taste is impaired, or disturbed. Whether the tongue is dry, cracked, coated, inflamed, ulcerated, blistered, fissured or swollen.
- *Throat:* Whether the patient has any ulcer, inflammation or pain. Whether he has any difficulty in swallowing.
- *Speech:* Whether the speech is absent. Whether he has any difficulty in speech stammering or incoherent. Whether the voice is hoarse or weak.
- *Nose:* Whether there is any deformity, swelling or discharge of mucous, blood or pus. Whether the sense of smell is present or absent.
- *Ears:* Whether he is able to hear or not. Whether there is collection of wax in the ear. Whether the patient experiences any ringing or buzzing sounds, dizziness, itching or pricking.
- *Neck:* Whether the patient has pain and difficulty in moving the neck. Whether there is any swelling or distended vein.
- *Chest:* Whether the patient suffers from cough. Whether the sputum is of abnormal color or quantity. Whether the breathing is labored or normal.
- *Breast:* Whether there are any abnormalities in the shape and size. Whether there are any lumps or discharge from the nipples.
- *Abdomen:* Whether it is soft, tender, distended, hard, swollen, flabby or protruding. Whether he has any nausea, vomiting or pain. Whether his appetite is normal or not.
- *Back:* Any swelling lump or any sore/ulcer at the back.
- *Upper extremities:* Whether the nails are broken or brittle. Whether there is clubbing of fingertips, tremors of hands, swelling of extremities, pain in the joints or any other abnormality, all range of motions present.
- *Lower extremities:* Normal in shape and size,any deformity, all range of motions present.
- *Skin:* Whether there are any sores, wounds, rashes or scales. Whether the skin is dry, moist, hot, cold or clammy.
- *Excretions and discharges:* Whether the color, consistency, amount, odor, and characteristics of stools, urine, sputum, perspiration, vomitus and vaginal discharge are normal or abnormal. Whether patient gets any pain or any other discomfort during excretion.

*Charting:* The nurses are required to report and record their observations. Show reports her findings to the professional nurse and to the physician.

Recording of the observations is called charting. The nurses should chart their observations correctly. All chartings should be brief, concise, account and complete.

Charting helps physicians, nurses and others to understand the condition and progress of the patient. The chart is also used for legal procedures and research.

A patient's chart includes records maintained by physicians and nurses. A nurse should be able to maintain records related to nursing and she should be able to understand the notes made by physicians and others.

## Physiological Assessment

*Vital signs:* Temperature, pulse respiratory rate and oxygen saturation, blood pressure, pain are called vital signs as indicators of health status. These measures indicate effectiveness of circulation, respiratory, neural and endocrine function because of their importance they are referred to as vital signs.

*Temperature:* Degree of heat maintained by the body. It is the balance between the heats produced and heat lost.

*Oral temperature:* 98.6°F (37°C)

*Rectal temperature/tympanic:* 99.6°F (37.5°C)

*Axillary temperature:* 97.6°F (36.4°C)

*Fever:* It occurs because of heat loss. Mechanisms are unable to keep pace with excess heat production, resulting in an abnormal raise in body temperature.

***Thermometer (clinical thermometer):*** It is used for measuring body temperature

***Thermometer is of two types:*** (1) Basing on the materials. (2) Basing on the route.

***Basing on materials*** (a) Electronic thermometer (b) Disposable thermometer (c) Glass thermometer (d) Temperature sensitive strip

***Basing on the route:*** (a) Oral temperature (b) Rectal temperature (c) Tympanic thermometer

***The common sites for taking body temperature:*** To get accurate measurement of the body temperature, the bulb of the thermometer must be placed where it can be completely surrounded by body tissue and where there are blood vessels situated near the surface. The temperature may vary if the bulb of the thermometer comes in contact with clothing, air, moisture etc. The common sites for ranking body temperature are mouth, groin, rectum, axilla.

Each device measures temperature using the Celsius or Fahrenheit scale. Following formulas are used in converting values

To convert Fahrenheit into Celsius

C = (F–32) × 5/9

E.g. convert 104°F into Celsius

C = (104 – 32) × 5/9

C = 72 × 5/9 = 40°C

To convert Celsius into Fahrenheit

F = C × 9/5 + 32

E.g. convert 37°C to Fahrenheit

= (37 × 9/5) + 32

= 66.6 + 32 = 98.6°F

***Contraindication for rectal method:***

- The patients who had rectal surgery or inflammation of the rectum
- The patients who are having diarrhea
- When the rectum is packed with fecal matter
- Patient who are having some kind of treatments, e.g. bowel wash enemia, etc.

***Contraindications for the oral method:*** Patients who are:

- Extremely nervous
- Delirious
- Unconscious
- Hysterical and mentally confused
- Patient having convulsion mouth breathe
- Patients who have injuries
- Inflammation of operation in the mouth
- Children under the age of 6 years
- Extremely weak patient.

## Types of Fever

Terms used to describe the types and phases of fever.

***Onset:*** Onset or invasion of fever is the period when the body temperature is rising and it may be a sudden or gradual process.

***Fastigium or stadium:*** Fastigium or stadium of fever is the period when the body temperature has reached its returning to normal. The fever may subside suddenly (decline by crisis or gradually (decline by lysis).

***Crisis:*** Crisis is sudden return to normal temperature from a very high temperature within a few hours of days.

***True crisis:*** The temperature falls suddenly within few hours and touches normal, accompanied by a marked improvement in the patient's condition.

***Subnormal temperature:*** When the body temperature falls below normal it is called subnormal temperature. The temperature may vary between 95° to 98°F or 35 to 36.7°C.

***Hyperthermia:*** When the body temperature is raised to 105°F or above it is called hyperthermia.

***Hypothermia:*** If the temperature falls below 95 or 35°C, the condition is called hypothermia.

***False crisis:*** A sudden fall in temperature not accompanied by an improvement in the general condition is called false crisis. It may be dangerous signal and not a sign of improvement.

***Lysis:*** The temperature falls in a zigzag manner for two or three days of a week before reaching normal during which time the other symptoms also gradually disappear.

***Constant fever or continuous fever:*** Constant fever or continuous fever is one in which the temperature varies not more than two degrees between morning and evening and it does not reach normal for a period of days of weeks.

***Remittent fever:*** Remittent fever is a fever characterized by variations of more than two degrees between morning and evening but does not reach normal level.

***Intermittent or quotidian fever:*** The temperature raises from normal or subnormal to high fever and back at regular intervals. The interval may vary from few hours to three days. Usually the temperature is higher in the evening than the morning.

***Inverse fever:*** In this type, the highest range of temperature is recorded in the morning hours and the lowest in the evening which is contrary to that found in the normal course of fever.

***Hectic fever:*** When the difference between the high and low point is very great, the fever is called hectic or swinging fever.

***Relapsing fever:*** Relapsing fever is one in which there are brief febrile period followed by one or more days of normal temperature.

***Irregular fever:*** When the fever is entirely irregular in its course, it cannot be classified under any one of the fevers described above and it is called irregular fever.

***Rigor:*** Rigor is sudden severe attack of shivering in which the body temperature rises rapidly to a stage of hyperpyrexia as seen in malaria.

***Low pyrexia:*** In low pyrexia the fever does not rise above 99 to 100°F or 37.2 to 37.8°C.

***Moderate pyrexia:*** The body temperature remains between 100 to 103°F or 37.8 to 39.4°C.

***High pyrexia:*** The temperature remains between 103 and 105°F or 39.4 and 40.6°C.

***Hyperpyrexia:*** The temperature goes above 105°F.

***Frequency of taking temperature in the hospital:*** Frequency of taking temperature is determined by the condition of the patient. For patients who are not seriously ill, it needs to be taken in the morning and evening. The temperature is to be checked every 4 hours of even more frequently for those who are actually ill, who are having high fever, and postoperative patients. If the temperature is taken by rectum or axilla, it should be specified in the chart.

*Fever (Pyrexa):* Fever or pyrexia is defined as the rise in body temperature above 99°F (37.2°C). The cause of fever are infections, diseases of the nervous system, certain malignant neoplasms, blood diseases such as leukemia, embolism and thrombosis, heat stroke from exposure to hot environment, dehydration, surgical trauma and crushing injuries, skin abnormalities that interfere with heat loss, allergic reactions to foreign proteins and pyrogens, etc.

In fever, all the systems of the body are affected. It may vary with the nature of the diseases.

*Respiratory system:* Shallow and rapid breathing.

*Circulatory system:* Increased pulse rate and palpitation.

*Alimentary system:* Dry mouth, coated tongue, loss of appetite, nausea, vomiting, constipation, or diarrhea.

*Urinary system:* Diminished urinary output, burning micturition, high colored urine.

*Nervous system:* Headache, restlessness, irritability, insomnia, convulsions, delirium

*Musculoskeletal system:* Heavy sweating, hot flushes, goose flush, shivering or rigors.

*Integumentry system:* Heavy sweating, hot flushes, goose flush, shivering or rigors.

Fever is not a disease but it is a sign. Fever is a protective function of the body, 'because the rise in temperature prevents the growth of organisms causing the disease. Fever, if not too high hastens the destruction of bacteria by increasing phagocytes, and by producing immune bodies. A temperature of 104 to 105°F for several hours will destroy the organisms of syphilis and gonorrhea. The range in the body temperature within which the cells can function efficiently is between 34 and 41°C (94 to 106°F) the central nervous system is extremely sensitive to the temperature variations. Irreversible changes may occur in the nervous system if the body temperature goes above 41°C or below 34°C.

## Care in Fevers

- *Regulation of the body temperature:* Care of the patients in fevers focuses on reducing the elevated body temperature. When the patients temperature is moderately elevated, various methods of reducing the temperature be started. The room temperature should be maintained at a comfortable temperature. The room should be well ventilated. The blankets and excess clothing should be removed but prevent the patient from getting drafts. The various method used for cooling the body are:
  - Exposure to cool air by an electric fan
  - Administration of cool drinks
  - Application of cold compress and ice bags
  - Cold sponging and cold packs
  - Cold bath
  - Ice cold lavages and enemas
  - Use of hypothermic blankets of mattresses.

  When surface cooling is used, treatment is directed at not only cooling the body but also preventing shivering. Shivering must be prevented because it increases metabolic activity, produces heat, increases the oxygen usage markedly, increases circulation, may cause hyperventilation and respiratory alkalosis. It takes longer time to reduce body temperature in a shivering patient.
- *Meeting the nutritional need:* The cellular metabolism is greatly increased during fever. The oxygen consumption in the body tissues approximately 13 percent for each centigrade degree of rise in temperature of 7 percent for each Fahrenheit degree, therefore, a high caloric diet is indicated in fevers.

Since the digestive process is slowed down, the diet should be easily digestible and palatable. Most of the patients prefer fluid diet.

Unless it is contraindicated, the fluid intake is increased to 3000 mL in 24 hours to prevent dehydration and to eliminate the waste products.

*Care in rigor:* Rigor is characterized by three stages:

1. ***The first stage or cold stages:*** The patient shivers uncontrollably. The skin is cold, face is pinched and pale, the pulse is feeble and rapid. The temperature rises rapidly to 103°F (39.4°C) or above. In this stage, cover the patient with blankets and apply warmth with hot water bags. Give warm drinks. Protect the patient from falling.
2. ***The second stage or hot stage:*** The skin feels hot and dry, and patient feels very thirsty. The shivering stops. The patient may be restless. The temperature may continue to rise during the second stage, remove all the blankets and hot appliances. Cover him only with a thin blanket. Give him cool drinks. Cold compresses are applied to the head to relieve congestion and headache. The temperature is carefully recorded every 10 to 15 minutes. Watch pulse and respirations carefully. If the temperature goes very high 105°F (40.5°C) cold sponging may be started. Watch for the early signs of sweating.
3. ***The third stage or stage sweating:*** The patient sweats profusely. The temperature falls. The pulse improves. Acute discomforts are diminished. The patient may go into state of shock and collapse if not cared properly.

## Pulse

*Definition of pulse:* The pulse is the palpable bounding of blood flow noted at various parts on the body. Pulse is rhythmic fluctuation of fluid pressure against the arterial wall created by the pumping action of the heart muscle by placing fingers over an artery particularly at the location where it crosses the bond.

### Sites for Checking Pulse

- Temporal artery
- Carotid artery
- Brachial artery
- Radial artery
- Femoral artery
- Popliteal artery
- Dorsalis pedis
- Posterior tibial artery

***Apical pulse auscultated in adult:*** Apical pulse is palpated to count pulse rate in infants.

### Characteristics of Pulse

- ***Rate:*** It is number of pulse beats in a minute. Normal rate in adult is 80 to 100 per minute.
- ***Rhythm:*** It refers to regularity of the beats, beats are spaced at regular intervals they are said to be regular. Interval varies between the beats it is called irregular.
- ***Strength:*** The strength/amplitude of a pulse reflects the volume of blood ejected against the arterial wall.
- ***Volume:*** It refers to the fullness of the artery. It is the force of the blood felt at each beat.
- ***Tension:*** It is the degree of compressibility.
- ***Equality:*** It refers to assess both radial pulses and compare the characteristics of both.
- ***Principles:*** Exercise, emotion and anxiety will cause increased pulse rate, finger tips sensitive to touch will fell the pulsation. Moderate pressure allow one to feel superficial radical artery characteristics of the pulse vary with individuals.

### Factors Involved in Pulse

- ***Age:*** The heart rhythm in infants and children often varies markedly with respiration.
- ***Autonomic nervous system:*** Stimulation of the pare sympathetic nervous system results in decreasing in the pulse rate. Stimulation of sympathetic nervous system results in an increased pulse rate.
- ***Medications:*** Certain cardiac medication such as digoxin decreases heart rate.

## Respiration

***Meaning of respiration:*** Respiration is the mechanism of body uses to exchange gases between the atmosphere and blood and the cells.

***Rate:*** Rate is the number of full respiration in a minute, normal rate is 16–20 breaths/minute.

***Depth of respiration:*** Normal average man at rest inspires and exhales about 500 cc of air with each respiration. If more than this quantity of air passes out in and out of the lungs the respiration is said to be deep.

***Rhythm:*** In normal respiration rhythm is normal.

### Various Sites of Respiration

- Chest
- Abdomen

### Factors Involved in Respiration

- ***Age:*** Normal growth from infancy to adulthood results in a larger lung capacity as lung capacity increases the respiratory rate decreases. Medications narcotic decreases respiratory rate and depth.
- ***Stress:*** Stress increases the rate and depth of respiration.
- ***Exercise:*** It increases rate and depth of the air decreases to meet the body's need for additional oxygen.
- ***Altitude:*** The oxygen content of the air decreases as the altitude increases.
- ***Gender:*** Men normally have larger lung capacity than women.
- ***Body position:*** A straight erect position promotes full chest expansion. A slopped as slumped position impairs ventilator movement.
- ***Fever:*** During fever the respiratory rate may be increased because heat can be lost from lungs.

## Blood Pressure

***Definition:*** Blood pressure is the pressure exerted by blood on the wall of a blood vessel. The normal range of blood pressure is 120/80 mm of Hg in adult.

When the ventricles are contraction, the pressure is at its highest this is known as the 'Systolic Pressure'. 'Diastolic Pressure' is when the ventricles are relaxing and the blood pressure is at its lowest.

***Hypertension:*** When the systolic pressure is above the normal level.

***Hypotension:*** When the systolic pressure is below the normal range.

***Purposes:*** (1) To acquire a baseline. (2) Monitor for fluctuation. (3) To diagnose disease. (4) To assess the cardiovascular system. (5) To monitor the effects of medication.

***Types of equipment required:***

***Mercury Sphygmomanometer:*** This is the simplest and most accurate and economical device for measuring blood pressure as long as it is used correctly.

***Aneroid sphygmomanometer:*** There register pressure through a bellows and lever system, which is more indicate than the mercury reservoir and column.

***Automatic digital sphygmomanometer:*** There remove some of the human error from BP measurement, but observer training is still necessary.

## Pain

***Definition:*** Whatever the person says it is existing whenever the existing person says it does. (MC Caffery 1999)

Pain is the fifth vital sign.

***Characteristics of pain:***

- ***Severity:*** Ranges from no pain to excruciating pain.
- ***Timing:*** Duration and onset of pain.
- ***Location:*** Body area involved.
- ***Quality:*** What the patient feels the pain is.
- ***Personal meaning:*** How affects the persons daily life.

***Factors increasing and decreasing pain:*** Age, gender, activity, rest, sleep, diet, culture, home remedies, drugs, alcohol, diversional activities like listening to music, watching TV, yoga, meditation, etc.

***Pain assessment:*** Pain intensity scale.

***Faces pain scale revised:*** This instrument has 6 faces depicting expressions that range from contented to obvious distress. The patient is asked to point to the face that most closely resembles the intensity of his or her pain.

- Simple Descriptive Pain Intensity Scale
- Numeric Pain Intensity Scale
- Visual Analog Scale
- No pain as bad as it could be possible or unbarrable pain.

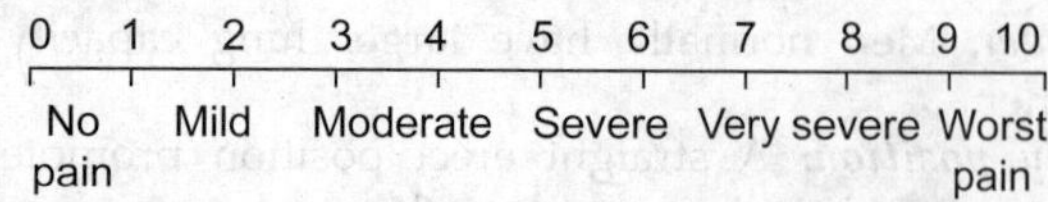


## Testing and Examination

### Urine

*Characteristics of urine:*

- ***Color:*** Normal urine ranges from pale, straw colors amber, depending on its concentration.

  Bleeding from the kidneys or ureters causes urine to become dark red, bleeding from the bladder or urethra causes bright red urine.

  Dark amber urine may be a result of high concentrations of bilirubin caused by liver dysfunction.
- ***Clarity:*** the normal urine appears transparent at voiding. Urine that stands several minutes in a container becomes cloudy renal disease. Many appear cloudy or foamy because of high protein concentrations.
- ***Odor:*** Urine has a characteristics odor. The more concentrated the urine the stronger the odor.

*Characteristics of normal urine:*

- ***Volume:*** One to two liters in 24 hours but varies.
- ***Color:*** Yellow or amber but varies.
- ***Turbidity:*** Transparent when freshly voided but becomes turbid (cloudy) upon standing.
- ***Odor:*** Urine has a characteristic odor. The more concentration the urine the stronger the odor.
- ***pH:*** 4.6 and 8.0 average 6.0 but varies.
- ***Specific gravity:*** 1.001 to 1.035.

*Common Urine Tests*

***Urine testing:*** The nurse often collects urine specimens for laboratory testing. The type of test determines the method of collection.

***Specimen collection:*** The nurse collects random clean voided or mid stream, sterile, and timed specimens.

***Urinalysis:*** The laboratory performs a urinalysis on a specimen obtained by any of the previously described methods. The specimen should be examined as soon as possible, preferably within 2 hrs.

***Specific gravity:*** The specific gravity is the weight or degree of concentration of a substance compared with an equal volume of water.

***Urine culture:*** A urine culture requires a sterile or clean voided sample of urine. It takes approximately 24 to 48 hours before the laboratory can report findings of bacterial growth.

*Urine Test*

***Purposes of sugar test:*** Testing the urine for the persons and the amount of sugar provides the doctors with information about the amount of insulin needed by the patient.

***Purpose of acetone test:*** Acetone is an abnormal finding that indicates that the body has begun to break down stored fats to use for energy, since it is not able to use the sugar.

***Purpose of albumin test:*** High albumin excretion is a prognostic of renal failure and complications such as myocardial infarction.

*Indications for Sugar, Acetone and Albumin*

Sugar in the urine indicates diabetes mellitus. In pregnancy when the renal threshold is lowered, the sugar is found in the urine.

Acetone is found in the urine of people loosing weight or in starvation.

Albuminuria is presently the most reliable early indicator of adverse renal and cardiovascular events in diabetic patients. The consensus is that screening and intervention for albuminuria are worthwhile in patients with insulin dependent diabetes, more often in type I diabetes mellitus than type II. Increased albumin excretion suggests the onset of diabetic nephropathy.

Testing the urine for glucose and acetone is generally done four times a day. The most accurate method is to obtain a double voided urine specimen in which the first voided is set aside and the patient is asked to void a short time later. This second voiding consists of the most recently produced urine from the kidney and is the best indicator of the amount of sugar being excreted at that moment not of urine that may have been in the bladder for hours. If the patient has a Foley's catheter the urine specimen should be taken from the tubing, which contains the latest formed urine not from the drainage bag.

An albumin testing usually requires a 24-hour specimen without preservatives. Some laboratories will accept a random specimen.

*Preparation of the Patient*

- On the previous day explain the procedure to the patient.
- Explain the patient when the urine to collect how to collect and the amount to be collected.
- Provide an appropriate container and demonstrate to him how to use it.
- Instruct him not to contaminate the outside of the bottle.
- Ask the patient to wash the internal genitalia with soap and water and rinse it with water.
- If the patient is unable to do himself the nurse assists him.

*Preparation of Articles*

Correct collection and preparation of urinary specimens for diagnostic testing contributes to accurate test results. Bedside tests for urine glucose and acetone must be done precisely according to the direction to obtain accurate results. Timing of the reading is crucial and the result may be incorrect if the reading is taken too early or too late.

*Patient Family Teaching*

- Encourage reporting for routine urinalysis and follow up examination
- Advise avoidance of any medicine unless specifically prescribed
- Teach the patient and family the importance of fluid intake
- Teach the patient and family how to perform the test.

*Patient Condition*

Presence of sugar in the urine about 140–180 mg/100 mL of blood is glycosuria. Presence of ketone in the urine is ketonuria.

| Characteristics | Normal findings | Special classification |
|---|---|---|
| Volume | Variable | The diet high is roughage produces more feces than a soft, bland diet. Consistently large diarrheal stools suggest a disorder in the small bowel, small and frequent stools with urgency to pass them suggest a disorder of the left colon or rectum. |
| Color | Infant: Yellow<br>Adult: Brown | The brown color of the stool is due to stercobilin, a bile pigment derivative. The rapid rate of peristalsis in the infant causes the stool to be yellow. The color of the stool is influenced by diet. For example, the stool will be almost black if the person eats red meat and dark green vegetables, such as spinach. The stool will be light brown if the diet is high in milk and milk products and low in meat. The absence of bile may cause the stool to appear whiter or clay-colored. Certain drugs influence the color of the stool. For example, iron salts cause the stool to be black. Antacids cause it to be whitish. Bleeding high in the intestinal tract causes a stool to be black owing to the digestion of the blood. Bleeding in lower intestinal tract will result in fresh blood in the stool. |
| Odor | Aromatic, may be affected by foods ingested | Excessive putrefaction causes a strong odor. The presence of blood in the stool causes a unique odor. |
| Consistency | Soft, semi-solid, and formed | The consistency of the stool is influenced by fluid and food. |

## Stool

*Sample of the Label*

Name of the Patient: ____________

Ward/Bed No. ____________

Age: ____________ Sex: ____________

OP/IP: ____________

Name of Specimen: ____________

____________

Nature of Test to be Done: ____________

____________

Date of Collection: ____________

____________

*Abnormality of Stool*

Blood in stool different forms are:

- ***Hematochezia:*** Passage of bright red blood per rectum mixed with or without stool, for example, hemorrhoids, anal fissure and fistula, trauma, ischemic colitis, diverticulitis, polyps, malignancy, etc.
- ***Melena:*** Characteristics are black tarry (sticky) stool (use to production of acid hematin). Offensive (acid hematin is altered by bacteria). Semisolid in consistency. Usually associated with vertigo, dizziness or syncopal attack during defecation. Causes are: (1) Duodenal ulcer and (2) carcinoma of the stomach.
- ***Occult blood causes are:*** Intake of NSAID, hookworm infestation and colorectal cancer, etc.

## Sputum

Sputum is the mucous secretion from the lungs, bronchi, and trachea. It is important to differentiate it from saliva, the clear liquid secreted by the salivary glands in the mouth, sometimes referred to 'spit'. 30 ounces of mucus produced/day. Healthy individuals do not produce sputum. Clients need to cough to bring sputum up from the lungs, bronchi, and trachea into the mouth in order to expectorate into a collecting container.

Document amount of sputum collected, color, odor, consistency (thick, tenacious, watery) and presence of hemoptysis'.

***Sputum production:*** Sputum production with coughing is not normal. Question the client about sputum color (clear, yellow, green, rusty, bloody) and odor.

***Quality:*** Watery, stingy, frothy, thick.

***Quantity:*** Teaspoon, tablespoon, cup. Document in client's medical record any changes in color, odor, quality, or quantity. Assertion whether sputum is produced only often the lying in a certain position.

The amount of sputum produced is increased several disorder, for instance. Clients with bronchitis may expectorate several cups of sputum daily.

## Summary


- Physical examination is defined as complete assessment of a patient's physical and mental status.
- The methods of physical examination are inspection, palpation, percussion, auscultation, and olfaction.
- The recording of the observations is called charting.
- Temperature is degree of heat maintained by the body. It is the balance between the heat produced and heat lost.
- The common sites for taking body temperature are mouth, groin, rectum, axilla.
- Fever or pyrexia is defined as the rise in body temperature above 99°F (37.2°C).
- Crisis is sudden return to normal temperature from a very high temperature within a few hours of days.
- Rigor is sudden severe attack of shivering in which the body temperature rises rapidly to a stage of hyperpyrexia as seen in malaria.
- Pulse is rhythmic fluctuation of fluid pressure against the arterial wall created by the pumping action of the heart muscle by placing fingers over an artery particularly at the location where it cross the bond.
- Respiration is the mechanism of body uses to exchange gases between the atmosphere and blood and the cells.
- Blood pressure is the pressure exerted by blood on the wall of a blood vessel.

- ***Hypertension:*** when the systolic pressure is above the normal level.
- ***Hypotension:*** when the systolic pressure is below the normal range.
- Bleeding from the kidneys or ureters causes urine to become dark red, bleeding from the bladder or urethra causes a bright red urine.
- Absence of bile may cause the stool to appear whiter or clay color.
- The amount of sputum produced is increased several disorder, for instance. Clients with bronchitis may expectorate several cups of sputum daily.

## Medical and Surgical Asepsis

The concept of asepsis (freedom from organisms) is important for all health care workers who have direct or indirect patient contact. Nurses are the persons who have frequent contact with the patients to provide care for 24 hours. It is the responsibility of the nurse to be aware of the patients at risk of developing infectious and also a duty to protect them with aseptic techniques.

## Definition of Asepsis

Asepsis is the practice to reduce or eliminate contaminants (such as bacteria, viruses, fungi and parasites) from entering the operative field is surgery or medicine to prevent infection.
**Definition of aseptic techniques:** Aseptic technique is the effort to keep a client as free from hospital microorganisms as possible.

## Principles of Asepsis

Three things that are extremely important in achieving asepsis are the reduction of time, trauma and trash.

1. ***Time:*** The time taken for any medical or surgical procedure is an important factor. Longer the time taken, have the possibility of greater exposure to contamination.
2. ***Trauma:*** Trauma occurred due to rough handling, excessive dead space, foreign bodies will contribute to infection.
3. ***Trash:*** It refers to contamination by bacteria or foreign matter.

Essential components of maintaining asepsis in a hospital include:
(1) Handwashing, (2) Utilizing gloves, gown and mask as indicated, (3) Cleaning equipment. (4) Handling linens are ways that prevent germs from spreading.

## Types of Asepsis

The two types of aseptic techniques the nurse practices are medical and surgical asepsis.
***Medical asepsis:*** It is a clean technique which includes procedure used to reduce the micro- organisms and prevent their spread. For example, changing patient's bed linen daily, handwashing.
***Surgical asepsis:*** It is a sterile technique which includes procedures used to eliminate the microorganisms. Sterile technique is used where sterile instruments are used, e.g. in operation theater.

***Medical asepsis:*** Medical asepsis is commonly referred as clean technique. The goal is to reduce the number of pathogens or prevent the transmission of pathogens from one person to another.

Techniques used should be appropriate to interrupt the spread of the known pathogen.
***Guidelines for maintaining medical asepsis:*** (1) Thorough hand washing is basic technique for infectious control. (2) Know about patient's susceptibility to infection, e.g. age, nutritional status, stress, etc. (3) Never use aseptic technique haphazardly. (4) Protect health workers from exposure to infectious agents. (5) Aware of the body sites where nosocomial infectious can occur. Proper usage of protective devices like gowns, gloves, masks and protective eye wear. Procedures should follow the principles of techniques, so as to interrupt the transmission of microorganisms.
***Surgical asepsis:*** Surgical asepsis is a sterile technique to eliminate all microorganisms including spores and pathogens, from an object and to protect an area from microorganisms. Surgical asepsis is used in operating room, delivery room, certain diagnostic testing areas, certain procedures like insertion of urinary catheter, sterile dressing changes, preparing an injectable medication, etc. When following surgical asepsis, areas are considered contaminated if they are touched by any object that is not also sterile. While doing the procedure, it is necessary to explain the procedure to the patients to facilitate their cooperation. Inform the patient which objects and areas may not be touched and direct the patient to avoid sudden movements that might contaminate the equipment. This helps the patient assist in maintaining the sterility of procedure.

## Basic Principles of Surgical Asepsis

- Sterile object remains sterile when touched only by another sterile object.
- Only sterile objects may be placed on a sterile field.
- An object held below a person's waist is contaminated. Nurses never turn their backs on a sterile tray.
- A sterile object becomes contaminated by prolonged exposure to air.
- Avoid talking, coughing, sneezing over sterile field or object.
- When a sterile surface comes in contact with a wet contaminated surface, the sterile object becomes contaminated by capillary action.
- The edges of sterile field or container are considered to be contaminated.
- Use dry, sterile forceps when necessary. Forceps soaked in disinfectant are not considered sterile.

***Use of gloves:*** Gloves, not substitute for good hand hygiene. It should worn only once and discarded appropriately. It is more important to perform good hand hygiene before and after using gloves. Gloves provide a barrier but are not impenetrable.
***Gloves are used for the following situations:***

- High risk setting like operating room, labor room.
- Handling the sterile surgical instruments.

- While doing the aseptic procedures like catheterization, suctioning, bowel irrigation, dressing the wound, etc.
- While doing some of the diagnostic procedures like thoracentesis, liver biopsy, renal biopsy, lumbar puncture, etc.
- While caring the patients with infectious diseases.
- While handling the blood and blood products.

*Use of aprons:* Aprons are usually worn to prevent soiling of the nurse's clothing by the patient's blood and body fluids. They provide barrier protection and are worn before entering the patient's room.

Gown is worn only once and is then discarded appropriately. Gown is prepared by cloth or water proof materials. If a gown becomes heavily soiled or moistened with blood or body fluids when caring for a patient, remove it, perform through hand hygiene and put on a clean gown.

*Use of masks:* Masks help prevent the wearer from inhaling large particle aerosols, which usually travel short distances and small particle droplet nuclei, which can remain suspended in the air and travel longer distances. Masks prevent the nurses to touch eyes, nose and mouth, thus limiting the contact of organisms with mucous membranes. Masks practices are used in various situations like sometimes the patient's visitors also have to be used when they are with patients who have respiratory infections. Sometime, the patients with immunosuppressive drug need to wear mask for specific precautions when transported outside the room.

A mask is worn only once and never lowered around the neck and then brought back over the mouth and nose for reuse. It should certainly be changed before it becomes damp from the wearer's exhalations.

## STERILIZATIONS AND DISINFECTION

Disinfection is the destruction usually by chemicals of pathogenic organisms not including bacterial spores.

### Guidelines to be Considered

- Some organisms are carries to destroy than others.
- The greater the number of organisms, the longer it takes to destroy them.
- The type of equipment to be disinfected or sterilizes makes a difference.
- Items used for certain procedures must be sterile.

### Methods of Sterilization

- *Heat:* It is rapid and reliable method to destroy the small and heat resistant objects.
- *Chemicals:* It is slow, corrosive and used for heat sensitive objects for large surfaces.
- *Filtration:* It requires membrane filtration apparatus and only used for liquids.
- *Irradiation:* Ionizing irradiation is reliable but expensive and it is used to sterilize the rooms.

A. *Tyndallization:* Repeated steaming at 100 degree centigrade of culture media on each of three successive days, allowing spores to germinate and to be subsequently killed.

B. *Boiling:* This method is suitable for enamel, metal, glass and rubber wares. Bowl sterilizers are used for large articles, instrument sterilizers for smaller articles.

***Points to remember:***

- See that articles are quite clean, and completely immersed in the water, which also must be clean.
- Only after the water comes to the boil start timing. If more articles are added, the sterilizing time must begin again.
- Boil vigorously for 5 minutes. Boiling will not kill spores.
- Remove articles with sterile cheatle or other lifting forceps. On to a sterile surface.

C. *Autoclaving:* This is a reliable method and may be used for most articles. The autoclave is a metal chamber with an outer jacket and a lid or door, which can be firmly clamped. Steam is generated by heating water in a boiler or in the outer jacket. Air is evacuated from the chamber either by displacement with steam, or by a vacuum attachment. Then the steam is allowed to build up pressure, usually 15 or 20 lbs per square inch, and is kept at that pressure, usually for 15 to 30 minutes. Then the heat is turned off, the steam evacuated, and the contents the autoclave.

***Points to remember:***

- All articles should be clean and dry before packing. Any organic matter such as blood or pus prevents penetration of steam.
- The holes in drums must be open when placing into the autoclave, and closed immediately on taking them out.
- Bundles should be not too large and not tightly packed. Steam should be able to penetrate to the center.
- Rubber gloves cannot stand high temperature and long sterilizing. Autoclave them separately at 15 lbs pressure for 15 minutes.
- To autoclave bottles of fluid, loosen the screw caps. Evacuate the steam slowly.

***General instructions:***

- The articles being sterilized should withstand high temperature.
- The wrapper and the container should allow penetration of the steam into the article.
- The inner chamber must not be too full nor the contents arranged too compactly. Bundles and drums must be packed loose. Cans or jars must be opened and turned on their sides so that steam can easily penetrate the contents.
- The temperature and pressure of the steam should be high enough to kill all the microorganisms including spores. The usual temperature is 121°C and the pressure is 1.05 kg/cm$^2$.
- The destruction of a bacteria depends upon the length of time the articles are exposed to steam under pressure. The minimum time is 30 minutes. If the pressure is increased the exposure time can be reduced.
- In operating an autoclave, it is important to remember that all the air in the inner chamber must be driven out and entirely replaced by steam. Otherwise although the gauge may show a pressure of 15 lbs, this pressure would be caused by a mixture of steam and air and the temperature would be lower than that of the steam alone.
- The articles should be left in the autoclave for a short time after the procedure is over to dry the materials.

***Working of the autoclave:*** Autoclave is the name given to a sterilizer that utilizes saturated steam under pressure (saturated means the steam exerts maximum pressure for water at the given time).

The steam is used in the autoclave for two reasons:

1. When steam is held in a closed container, it is compressed and the temperature rises far above that of the boiling point of water.
2. Steam is able to penetrate porous materials very rapidly, provided that, it is not impeded by unsuitable wrappers or by air trapped within fabrics or hollow instruments.

An autoclave consists of an outer chamber and an inner chamber, which can be tightly closed by a safety lock. The steam is introduced first into the outer chamber until the desired temperature is reached. At this point, the steam is turned into the inner chamber which is packed with articles that are to be sterilized.

As the steam enters the inner chamber, the air is forced out through the valves. The steam is kept flowing into the inner chamber until the desired temperature is reached. It is very important to note the temperature as well as the pressure of the inner chamber. When the desired levels are reached, it should be maintained to the desired length of time (Temp: 121°C, pressure: 1.05 kg/cm$^2$ and the exposure time is 30 minutes).

The removal of air from an autoclave, during the sterilization process is important for two reasons:

1. Air left in the center of a pack or in the cannula of a catheter will prevent the steam from coming into direct contact with the center of the pack or to the lumen of the catheter. Failure to contact means failure to sterilize.
2. Air mixed with steam reduces the temperature of the steam.

At the end of the period, the steam supply is shut off, but the door is not opened until the pressure gauge is at zero and the temperature has fallen to 100°C. This allows the liquids to cool to a point when they will not escape from their containers with the reduction of pressure and it also helps to dry the packaged goods.

**D.** ***Dry heat:*** Sterilizing of glassware including syringes is often done in a hot air oven, at 160 degree centigrade for one hour. Spores as well as organisms are killed. Rubber will not stand up to this heat.

This method is efficient if heat penetrates through dressings, towels and gown.

Two methods are used:

1. ***Incineration:*** Used for disposal of dressings, laboratory media and human tissues and used oil.
   Hospital incinerator may cause unacceptable environmental pollution.
2. ***Hot air oven:*** It is used for objects which cannot tolerate moisture. Mostly used for glassware, oils, powders.

***Methods of disinfection:*** Destruction of organisms by chemical is used in the following circumstances:

- ***Environmental:*** Disinfection of excreta, floors, furniture, linen and fabrics.
- ***Instruments/equipment:*** Sterilization of heat sensitive objects in contact with patient.
- ***Skin and wounds:*** Removal of pathogens.
- ***Food medication:*** Preservation in prevention of spoilage.
- ***Water:*** Removal of pathogens.
- ***Vaccines:*** Destruction of organisms or denaturation of toxins.

***Chemical sterilization:*** It is the method used for eye instruments and other delicate instruments.

### Points to Remember

- The articles must be clean and free from pus, blood or oil.
- They must be completely immersed in the disinfectant.
- The disinfectant should be of a certain strength and the articles must be in contact with it for a certain length of time.
- After sterilization, articles must be well rinsed in sterile water before use.

### Fumigation or Gas Sterilization

Total surface exposure to formaldehyde gas under conditions of controlled humidity, temperature and time exposure will destroy all vegetative forms of bacteria, viruses and most of the spores. The best results can be obtained with high concentrations of gas, humidity above 60% and temperature of not less than 18°C. The exposure time varies one to sixteen hours. The agents that are commonly used for the fumigation are formalin tablets, ethylene oxide liquids, etc.

The disadvantages of the gas sterilization are that it has a pungent smell, it is irritant to the eyes, skin and mucus membrane.

### Ultraviolet Light Sterilization

Ultraviolet sterilization is effective for disinfecting working surfaces and air inside the rooms.

*Disadvantages*

- Light travels in straight lines and does not penetrate. Only the surface of an object in direct line with ultraviolet source is irradiated. Any bacteria in shadows are unaffected. All surfaces should be exposed to the rays. Ultraviolet rays do not penetrate the liquids.
- Prolonged exposure to the ultraviolet rays causes conjunctival damage. To prevent this, dark glasses should be worn.
- It is also injurious to the skin and tissues.
- It is expensive. The cheapest form of ultraviolet radiation is obtained free from the sun. Gama rays have the greatest power of penetration and is used for the sterilization of plastic items such as disposable syringes and catheters which will not withstand heat sterilization and sharp instruments such as hypodermic needles, and scalpel blades. The greatest advantage of this method is that the articles can be packed before sterilization in individual sealed plastic packs or aluminum foils which avoids any handling and possible recontamination after sterilization.

### Principles of Disinfection

- Only objects which cannot be heat treated.
- It is important to remove grease and proteins before use.

- Dilution of concentration should be accurately measured.
- Dilutions should be made aseptically.
- Disinfectants should be appropriately chosen for their purpose, cost antimicrobial range, toxicity and corrosiveness.
- Disinfectants for general cleaning are a waste of money.

### Types of Chemicals

A. *Alkylating agents:* They are capable of killing bacteria, spores and viruses. They are the acceptable chemical alternative to usual heat treatment.

They include:

- *Formaldehyde:* used for instruments and machines sterilization.
- *Glutaraldehyde:* used for instrument sterilization.
- *Ethylene oxide:* used for rubber and plastics articles sterilization.
- *Propiolactone:* Used for gaseous sterilization.

B. *Phenols:* It includes acids and semisynthetic compounds in soap solution. It is some what toxic with a unpleasant smell. It is used for general purpose disinfectants for contaminated surfaces. It has no activity on spores.

*Advantages of disinfection:* This is the method used to sterilize the articles that are destroyed by head and the metallic objects prone to corrosion. This is the most easy method of disinfecting articles.

*Disadvantages:* This method does not ensure sterilization, because the disinfectants does not destroy the spores. Some disinfectants are injurious to the skin and articles.

### Important Points to Remember

- The disinfectant chosen should be efficient to destroy pathogens.
- They should be used in correct strength.
- The articles should be fully submerged in it.
- They are placed for a sufficient length of time.
- They should not be injurious to the skin and articles.
- The article should be thoroughly cleansed to remove the organic material which will protect the bacteria against the action of disinfectants.
- The disinfectant should be inexpensive.
- Instruments soaked in germicides must be adequately rinsed with sterile water before being used.

### Handling of Sterile Articles

- Always wear a mask when handling sterile articles.
- Sterilized articles must be kept in containers or on sterile towels, and kept covered till used.
  Never allow contact of unsterile with sterile articles.
- Make sure there is no dampness. As this could make the things unsterile.
- Never allow any unsterile article including the arms and hands, to pass over a sterile field.
- Never touch the inside of a package or container with your fingers. Use the cheatle forceps.
- To pull a cork from a bottle of sterile field, take care not to contaminate the inside part of the cork nor inside the rim of the inner side up, and then replace it without delay.
- When lifting a cover from a sterile container, lay it down with the inner side up, then replace it without delay.
- To carry a sterile bowl or other container, hold it with your hands underneath, and do not touch the rim.

### Rules for use of Cheatle Forceps

- The sterile jar holding the forceps must be cleaned, resterilized and filled with fresh antiseptic lotion daily. The cheatle forceps should be cleaned and autoclaved or boiled.
- When in use, keep the forceps at elbow level and pointed downwards, because if you lift it upwards the solution may run on to your hand and then back to the forceps, making it unsterile.
- Put the forceps back into the jar immediately after use. Replace carefully without touching the rim of the jar. If the forceps becomes contaminated in any way, it must be resterilized before being put back into the jar.

### Preparing Articles for Sterilization

A convenient method often used to be prepared with sets of the instruments, swabs, sponges, dressings, towels and sutures needed form each type of operation or sterile procedure. These sets are packed into drums, bundles, or on trays, labeled and kept ready for sterilization. The articles should be carefully arranged so that those needed first are on top. They must be loosely packed for steam to penetrate. Drums must have the perforations opened. Bundles should have a double wrapper or close woven cloth or of paper.

Dressings, swabs and sponges are usually made of several thicknesses of surgical gauze. Raw edges must be folded in, swabs and dressings are again folded to the desired size. Sponges used for abdominal surgery need to be large, stitched around the edges and a piece of tape sewed to one corner. When an artery forceps is clipped to the end of the tape, there is no risk of the sponge being left inside the abdomen.

Packing gauze is made in various sizes. Use gauze four times the width of the desired packing.

Fold the edges so that they meet in the middle, and again fold down the center, and roll.

Cotton wool is prepared in various ways. Cotton balls of various sizes are prepared by rolling between the palms. Some may be needed for internal surgery, and for this the cotton ball must be covered with gauze and tied. This type of swab is grasped with a long handled forceps. Cotton squares of various sizes are to be cut for use in dressing wounds. Some may require to be covered with gauze.

*Instruments:* Surgical instruments should be washed first in cold water, then in warm water with a detergent after use. Use a brush to clean well especially between the teeth of artery forceps and clamps. To be properly sterilized, there should be no trace of dried blood or discharge. Rinse in clean water, then boil for 5 minutes and dry well.

Sharp instruments, knives and needles should be dealt with separately, taking care to avoid cuts and puncture wounds.

*Syringes and needles:* As soon as possible after use, draw up some water into the syringe and push enough through each needle to make sure they are not blocked. Infected syringes (used for withdrawing blood or pus) should be washed immediately in a cold disinfectant solution. Next wash the syringes and needles in warm soapy water, using a bottle brush for the barrel. Rinse in clean water. Take care not to get barrels and plungers mixed. But keep them always paired together.

Needles should be examined carefully for sharpness. The tips may be rubbed carefully on a sharpening stone. Take care not to prick your finger as infection may be transmitted in this way.

Rubber tubing after use should be cleaned with cold water, then with hot soapy water. Then rinsed. The inside must be thoroughly clean. Then it is boiled, and hung over a rail to drain. Put away loosely coiled, to avoid kinking. Rubber catheters should be cleaned by running cold water, boil for 5 minutes, then dry, with a towel or by hanging up.

## BIOMEDICAL WASTE MANAGEMENT

Biomedical waste is the waste, which is generated by hospital, nursing homes, clinic, dispensaries, veterinary institution, animal house, pathological laboratory and blood bank and is not degradable.

### Classification of Waste

#### *General Waste*

- General sweeping
- Kitchen waste
- Packing material
- Paper pieces
- Waste from laundry, kitchen, wards and laboratory.

#### *Infectious Waste*

- Human anatomical waste (human tissue, organ and body parts).
- Microbiology and microtechnology waste (waste from laboratory cultures, stocks or specimens of microorganisms lie or attenuated vaccines, human and animal cell culture used in research and industrial laboratories, waste from production of biological, toxins, dishes, and devices used for transfer of cultures).
- Solid waste (items contaminated with blood and body fluids including cotton, ressing, soiled plaster casts, linen, beddings, other materials contaminated).

#### *Sharps*

- Hypodermic needles, stitching needles, needles attached with tubing.
- Scalpel blades, razors, nails, etc.
- Broken glass materials, syringes, blood vials, edges of slides and cover slips in contact with infectious agents.

### Segregation, Packing, Transporting

- Biomedical waste shall not be mixed with other wastes.
- Biomedical waste shall be segregate into containers/bags at the point of generation prior to its storage, transportation, treatment and disposal. The containers shall be labeled.
- Notwithstanding anything contained in the Motor Vehicles Act, 1988, or rules there under, untreated biomedical waste shall be transported only in such vehicle as may be authorized for the purpose by the competent authority as specified by the government.
- No untreated biomedical waste shall be kept stored beyond a period of 48 hours: provides that if for any reason it becomes necessary to store the waste beyond such period, the authorized person must take permission of the prescribing authority and take measures to ensure that the waste does not adversely affect human health and the environment.

### Measures to Minimize Health Risk due to Medial Waste

- Use appropriate protecting clothing like apron, thick layer gloves, long boot with thick sole, face masks, eye glasses when required, with arrangement of disinfection and disposal arrangement for staff handling hospital waste.
- Popularize use of color and emblem code on container bags.
- Introduce monitoring and surveillance for problem areas or high risk areas.
- Constitute a hospital acquired infection control committee.
- Incinerator.
- Conforms to pollution control board norms.
- Built in safety.
- Easy to operate and maintain.
- Minimum site work.
- Shredder for plastic materials (plastic, bottles, syringes, IV sets, etc.) cuts plastic waste into small pieces of 1 cm size chips thus ensuring that syringes, and other plastic material are rendered nonrecyclable.
- Segregation of waste from hospital, kitchen, canteen and houses inside the hospital premises is collected from house to house and transported to vermicomposting site.

### Categories of Biomedical Waste

#### *Category I Human Anatomical Waste*

Waste human tissue

- Human organs
- Human body parts,
  Treatment and disposal incineration/deep burial
- Color coding yellow
- Container plastic bag.

#### *Category II Animal Waste*

Waste animal tissues, organs, body parts carcasses bleeding parts, fluid blood, experimental used in research, waste generated by veterinary, hospitals, colleges, discharge from hospitals, animal house.

Treatment and disposal incineration/deep burial.

- Color coding yellow
- Container plastic bag.

#### *Category III Microbiology and Biotechnology*

Waste from laboratory culture, stocks or specimens of microorganisms, live or attenuated vaccines human and animal cell culture used in research and infectious agents from research and industrial laboratories, waste from production of biological, toxins, dishes and devices used for transfer of cultures.

Treatment and disposal local autoclaving/microwaving/ incineration.

- Colour coding yellow/red
- Container plastic bag/disinfected container.

### *Category IV Waste Sharps*

Waste, needles, syringes, scalpels, blades, glass, etc. that may cause puncture and cuts. This include both used and unused sharps.

Treatment and disposal disinfection chemical treatment with 1% hypochlorite solution/local autoclaving/shredding.

- Color coding blue/white translucent
- Container plastic bag/puncture proof container.

### *Category V Discarded Medicines and Cytotoxic Drugs*

Waste comprising of outdated contaminated and discarded medicines.

Treatment and disposal incineration/destruction and drugs disposal in secured landfills.

- Color coding black
- Container plastic bag.

### *Category VI Solid Waste*

Waste items contaminated with blood and body fluids including cotton, dressings, soiled plaster casts, linen, beddings, other material contaminated with blood.

Treatment and disposal incineration autoclaving/micro-waving.

- Color coding yellow/red
- Container plastic bag/disinfected container.

### *Category VII Solid Waste*

Waste generated from disposable items other than the waste sharps such as tubings, catheters, intravenous sets, etc.

Treatment and disposal disinfection by chemical treatment with 1% hypochlorite solution autoclaving/microwaving and multilation/shredding.

- Color coding red
- Container plastic bag/disinfected container.

### *Category VIII Liquid Waste*

Waste generated from laboratory and washing cleaning, housekeeping and disinfecting activities.

Treatment and disposal disinfection by chemical treatment with 1% hypochlorite solution and discharge into drains.

### *Category IX Incineration Ash*

Waste ash from incineration of any biomedical waste, treatment and disposal, disposal in municipal landfill.

- Color coding black
- Container plastic bag.

### *Category X Chemical Waste*

Chemical used in production in biologicals, chemicals used in disinfection, as insecticides, etc.

Treatment and disposal chemical treatment with 1% hypochlorite solution and discharge into drains for liquids and secured landfill for solids.

- Color coding black for solids
- Container plastic bag.

### Summary

Nurses are the persons who have frequent contact with the patients to provide care for 24 hours.

It is the responsibility of the nurse to be aware of the patients at risk of developing infectious and also a duty to protect them with aseptic techniques.

- Asepsis is the practice to reduce or eliminate contaminants (such as bacteria, viruses, fungi and parasites) from entering the operative field is surgery or medicine to prevent infection.
- Three things that are extremely important in achieving asepsis are the reduction of time, trauma and trash.
- The two types of aseptic techniques the nurse practises are medical and surgical asepsis.
- Medical asepsis is a clean technique which includes procedure used to reduce the microorganisms and prevent their spread. Examples are changing patient's bed linen daily, hand washing.
- It is a sterile technique which procedures used to eliminate the microorganisms. Sterile technique is used where sterile instruments are used, e.g. in operation theater.
- Disinfection is the destruction usually by chemicals of pathogenic organisms not including bacterial spores.
- The three main methods of sterilization are heat, chemicals, irradiation and filtration.
- The methods of disinfection are environmental, equipment, skin and wound, food medication, water and vaccine.
- The types of chemicals used for disinfection are alkylating agents and phenol.

## FIRST AID

**Definition:** First Aid is the initial assistance or treatment given to someone who is injured or suddenly taken ill.

**Aims:** First aid treatment is given to a casualty: (1) To preserve life. (2) To prevent worsening of the condition (3) To promote recovery.

### Rules and Principles of First Aid

(1) Get to the scene quickly, to help in saving life. (2) If the cause of the accident is still there, remove it or the casualty from danger. (3) Be calm, methodical and quick but gentle in handling the casualty. (4) As far as possible keep the casualty where he is until everything is ready for transporting him, (5) Look for the following and treat this first (a) Failure of Breathing. (b) Bleeding. (c) Unconsciousness. (6) Reassure the casualty and others present to reduce shock, (7) See that the casualty is in best position to aid recovery, (8) Clear the cloud tactfully. The casualty needs fresh air. Any other first aider present may help you. Get help also to call the police, direct traffic, etc. as needed. (9) Diagnose injuries and give first aid that is essential. Make use of available first aid equipment. If there is none, improvise the material at hand. (10) Arrange for medical aid as soon as possible, for careful transport, and for informing relatives. (11) Stay with the casualty, continuing to observe and give care until handing over

to the doctor. (12) Do not attempt too much: do the minimum first aid so that the conditions does not become worse and life can be saved. (13) Do not remove clothing unnecessarily, as this may add to shock. (14) Do not give anything by mouth to a casualty who is unconscious, who may have an internal injury or who may soon be given an anesthesia.

## First Aid in Emergency Situations

### Fire

Rapid and clear thinking at a fire is vital. Fire spreads very quickly so your first priority is to warn any people at risk. If in a building, activate the nearest fire alarm. You should also alert the emergency services at once. Panic spreads fast among people trapped in fire. Encourage the people to evacuate the area. Do not delay or reenter a burning building to collect personal possessions. Ignition an electric spark or naked flame) a source of fuel/petrol, wood or fabric and oxygen (air).
***Clothing on Fire:*** Always follow this procedure: (1) Stop, drop and roll. (2) Stop the casualty panicking, running around or going outside. (3) If possible, wrap the casualty tightly in a coat, curtain, blanket or heavy fabric. (4) Roll the casualty along the ground until the flames have been smothered. (5) If water is available cool the burn with the liquid.

### Burns

Skin plays key roles in protecting the body from injury, infection and in maintaining body temperature.

The skin consists of two layers. The outer layer (epidermis) and the inner layer (dermis) and fatty tissue (subcutaneous fat) the epidermis is protected by an oily substance called sebum secreted from sebaceous glands which keeps the skin supple and water proof.

The dermis contains the blood vessels, nerves, muscles sebaceous glands, sweat glands, hair follicles ends of the sensory nerves (sensations like heat, cold, touch, pain) blood vessels supply nutrients and regulates the body temperature.
***Depth of burns:*** Burns are classified according to the depth of the skin damage. There are 3 depths.
***Superficial:*** Only epidermis, e.g. sunburn.
***Partial thickness:*** Destroys epidermis, pain, blister formation.
***Full thickness:*** No pain sensation, skin scared. Need urgent medical attention.

*Assessing a Burn*

***Assess for:*** Pain, difficulty in breathing, signs of shock.
***Aims:*** (1) To stop the burning and relieve pain. (2) To maintain an open airway. (3) To minimize the risk of infection. (4) To arrange urgent removal to hospital. (5) Principles to be followed stop, drop and roll. (6) Help the casualty to lie down. (7) Continue cooling the affected area (8) Cover the injured area with sterile/clean cloth to protect from infection. (9) Monitor the vital signs level of response. (10) Do not break the blisters. (11) Do not apply ointments leads to infection. (12) While waiting for help to arrive, reassure the casualty and see for shock.
***Electrical burn:*** Burns may occur when electricity passes through the body. Burns may be caused by a lightning strike by high-low voltage electric current. An electric shock can also cause cardiac arrest. If the casualty is unconscious, make sure that the casualty is in safe area, open the casualty's airway and check for breathing and do CPR. Do not approach the casualty of high voltage electricity until the current has been switched off and isolated.
***Chemical burns:*** Most corrosive, strong chemicals are in industry. Chemical burns are always serious and casualty needs urgent hospital treatment. Never attempt to neutralize acid or alkali burns unless trained to do. Chemical burn to the eye, first aider is to wash out the eye so that the chemical is diluted and dispersed. Do not allow the casualty to touch the injured eye or forcibly remove the contact lens.
***Sunburn:*** Caused by over exposure to sun. Reddened skin, pain and blistering. If there is extensive blistering seek medical advice.
***Heat exhaustion:*** Caused by Joss of salt and water from the body through excessive sweating.

Complaints of headache, dizziness, confusion loss of appetite and nausea, sweating with pale and clammy skin, cramps in the arm, legs and abdomen, rapid pulse and breathing. Help the casualty to a cool place. Give him plenty of water, weak salt solution. Monitor the vital signs. Be prepared to give CPR if necessary. Transfer the casualty if necessary.
***Heat stroke:*** This condition is caused by failure of body temperature regulation in the brain. Usually due to high fever or prolonged exposure to heat. Headache, dizziness, discomfort, restlessness, hot and flushed, dry skin, bounding pulse, high temperature above 104°F (40°C).

*Types of Burn Causes of the Burn*

***Dry burn:*** Flames, contact with hot objects, scald steam, hot liquids
***Electrical Burn:*** High voltage currents over head cables lighting strikes
***Cold injury:*** Frost bite
***Chemical burn:*** Industrial chemicals, inhaled fumes and corrosive gases, chemical agents
***Radiation burns:*** Sunburn, over exposure to ultraviolet rays, expose to radioactive sources.
***Management:*** (1) Quickly remove the casualty to a cool place warp the casualty in a cold, wet sheet until the temperature comes down to 100°F or give cold sponge. (2) Monitor and record the vital signs. (3) If the casualty becomes unconscious prepared to give CPR. If the casualty is breathing normally place him in a recovery position.

### Fractures

A fracture is a break in continuity of a bone, this may vary from a crack to a complete break.

*Causes of Fractures*

***Direct force:*** A bone can be fractured at the point where the force of a blow is applied.
***Indirect force:*** The bone breaks away from the spot of application of force, e.g. fracture of the clavicle without a stretched hand while falling open and closed fractures.

In an open fracture, one of the broken bone ends may pierce the skin surface or there may be a wound at the fracture site. An open fracture carries a high risk of infection. In closed fracture, the skin above the fracture in intact. However bones may be displaced causes damage to the internal organs.

May cause bleeding (internal) and suffer shock.

*Types of Fractures*

***Green stick fractures:*** Closed fracture mostly it occurs in children.

***Complicated fractures:*** They occur when the jagged ends of the bone fragments damage blood vessels, nerves or a joint, broken bones in the chest may penetrate the lung, heart or liver. In fractures of the skull the brain is usually damaged.

***Depressed fractures:*** These occur in the skull when the broken ends of the bones are pressed inwards.

***Comminuted fractures:*** In these cases, the bone is broken into several fragments. This is serious because there will be muscle damage with more bleeding at the fracture site.

***Impacted fractures:*** After a heavy fall, the fracture may be impacted by the force, e.g. spinal injury falling from tree.

***Pathological fractures:*** These occur when the bone is weakened by loss of calcium, infection or cancer. Minimal cause a break in such cases. In old age the bones are more brittle, and may break spontaneously due to calcium loss which is part of the ageing process.

***Stress fractures:*** Stress caused by repeated minor trauma as in athletic training involved in strenuous training, such as jogging or marathon running.

***Management:*** (1) Advise the casualty to keep ready to received patient. (2) Support the injured part for immobilization. Splints can be used for the support of the area. (3) Dressing to be done and do bandaging to the injured part. (4) Arrange to transport the casualty to hospital as necessary. Treat for shock. (5) Monitor the vital signs.

## Drowning

Drowning is a condition of suffocation which may lead to death, due to airway spasm or water entering into the airway during swimming or when in water.

Drowning is a silent killer. People who are drowned may not be able to call for help because they expend all their energy to breathe or to keep the head over water. Be alert for signs that someone may be in trouble. A swimmer flailing his or her arms. Displaying uneven swimming motions. Lying face down in water. Only the head, showing above water with mouth open.

***The drowning sequence:*** Begins with panic or struggle followed by submersion with breath holding, then water swallowing before passing out, within 3 minutes of being under water, loss of consciousness, within 5 minutes, brain suffers damage, then the heart goes into irregular rhythm before it stops breathing.

***Signs:*** Abdominal distension and vomiting. Bluish or pale skin of the face and lips. Cough with clear or frothy pink sputum. Decreased consciousness or unconsciousness. Labored or no breathing. Weak or no heart beat.

***First Aid:*** (1) Reaching the victim. (2) Reach from ashore. (3) If you cannot reach a person, wade closer. (4) Throw an object that floats with a line to the victim (throw and tow). (5) Use a boat if one is available. (6) If not use must swim to the person, use a towel/board for him to hold. (7) Stabilize the victim in water. (8) Keep the victims head and body aligned, place one hand in the middle of his back. (9) Your arm directly over the victims head. (10) Place your other hand under the victim's upper arm, near the shoulder. (11) Slowly and carefully rotate the victim over in the water, by lifting the shoulder and rotating it over. (12) Support the victim in neutral position in water and start mouth to mouth ventilation. (13) If in deep water, give the occasional breathe of air while towing the casualty ashore.

***Additional care measures:*** (1) When you can place him on a firm surface, check breathing and pulse and continue resuscitation if necessary. (2) As soon as the casualty begins breathing, place in recovery position. (3) Keep the casualty warm. (4) If possible, remove wet clothing and dry him off. (5) Cover with spare clothes and/or towels. (6) If needed treat for hypothermia. (7) Arrange removal to the hospital. (8) Transport in a stretcher case, maintaining the treatment position.

## Hemorrhage

Hemorrhage or bleeding is a flow of blood from an artery, vein or capillary.

*Types of Hemorrhage*

***Arterial bleeding:*** Blood is bright red in color. It spurts at each contraction.

***Venous bleeding:*** Blood is dark red in color. It does not spurt. Steady flow.

***Capillary bleeding:*** Blood is red in color. It does not spurt. Slow in flow.

***Effects of hemorrhage:*** The loss of red blood cells causes a lack of oxygen to the tissues of the body. A decrease in blood volume causes decrease in blood pressure. The heart's pumping rate increases to compensate for reduced blood pressure. The force of the heart beat is reduced since there is less blood to pump.

***How to recognize external bleeding:*** Evidence of major external blood loss. Symptoms and signs of shock. Casualty complains of thirst, blurring vision, fainting, giddiness. Face and lips become pale, skin feels cold and clammy, pulse faster and weaker, restlessness, breathing shallow (air hunger). Unconsciousness may occur.

***Internal bleeding:*** Wounds that have penetrated skull. Wound that have penetrated the chest on abdomen. Signs and symptoms of shock. Blood may appear from one of the body orifices like nose, ear, mouth, rectum, urethra, vagina.

***Management:*** Control bleeding as soon as possible. Keep the wound clean and dress it to minimize blood loss and prevent infection. Quickly transfer the casualty to hospital.

*How to Control Bleeding*

***Direct pressure:*** Place your hand directly over the wound and apply pressure, firm and steady until the bleeding stops. Tie a bandage firmly enough to control bleeding but not so tight to cut off the circulation. Immobilize the injured part. Never replace any dressing once it is applied. If the dressing is soaked, place another dressing and hold both in place with firm pressure.

***Elevation:*** Elevate the bleeding part of the body above the level of the heart so that the flow of blood will slow down in that part and blood clothing take place.

***Pressure points:*** Applying pressure over the pressure points pressing over the underlying bone pressure points on the arms (brachial pressure point) on the groin (femoral pressure point).

***Applying a tourniquet:*** A standard tourniquet is a piece of web belting about 36" long with a buckle device to hold it tightly in place when applied. This is used to stop bleeding. Care to be taken not to cut off the circulation.

***Management:*** Apply direct pressure over the wound with your fingers and palms, with clean pad/cloth you can ask the casualty to apply direct pressure herself. Elevate and support the injured part above the level of the casualty's heart to reduce blood loss. If you suspect the casualty is going into shock, raise and support her legs so that they are above the level of her heart. Secure the dressing with bandage. Tie it with pressure not too tightly to cut off the circulation. Further bleeding still occurs, put on the another bandage over the previous one. Monitor the vital signs. Watch for the signs for shock. Dial for an ambulance and transport the casualty to hospital till then the first aider should not leave the casualty until taken over by doctor or nurse.

***Bleeding from the nose (epistaxis):*** Bleeding occurs from the blood vessels inside the nostrils.

Bleeding coming from nose is also a sign of fractured skull. Make the casualty to sit with the head bent forward, loosen the tight clothing around the neck. Allow the blood to drain from the nostrils. Ask the casualty to breathe through her mouth and to pinch the soft part of the nostril for 10 minutes. If the bleeding restarts tell the casualty to reapply pressure. If bleeding follows a head injury, the blood may appear thin and watery. It is a serious sign because it indicates skull fracture. Tell the casualty to pinch her nose.

Advise her not to speak, swallow, cough spit because she may disturb the blood clots that have formed in the nose. Give her clean cloth to wipe off the dribbling. Advise the casualty to rest quietly for few hours. Avoid exertion, blowing of nose at least four hours so as to not to disturb the clot. If after 30 minutes also bleeding persists or recurs, seek medical aid.

## Shock

Shock occurs with every accident or sudden illness. The nervous system is affected and later if the condition of shock continues, the circulation of blood gradually fails and the patient dies. Prompt first aid treatment is needed to prevent shock increasing, and to help the patient to recover from the primary shock.

***Signs, symptoms and treatment of shock:*** A shocked person may only feel a little faint, weak and cold. And look pale, or he may collapse with signs and symptoms as follows: (1) He feels faint, weak and giddy. (2) The skin feels cold and damp there is sweating even in cold weather. (3) Color is paled and cyanosed (4) He will usually vomit. (5) The pulse is weak and become rapid. (6) He may be restless, mentally confused, and become unconscious in later stages.

*Treatment*

- Reassure the casualty if he is conscious
- Lay him on his back with the head low. If shock is severe, raise the lower part of the body unless is injury to the head nor chest.
- Loosens tight clothing, but do not remove clothing
- If he feels cold, cover him with the blanket, but do not try to warm him by any means
- Offer him a warm sweet drink, e.g. tea or coffee, unless there is internal injury or he is not fully conscious.
- Keep him quiet, and undisturbed, giving only essential first aid treatment for injuries. Avoid causing pain.
- If there are severe injuries, or shock increases, get the casualty to the health center or hospital without delay. He urgently needs IV fluids.

***Electrical shock:*** If an electrical current or lighting flash passes through a person's body. The effects may be mild or so severe as to cause immediate death. There may be failure of respiration while the heart continues to beat. There may be burns where the body was in contact with a live wire.

### Aims of First Aid Treatment

- Have the source of electricity switched off.
- Check breathing, and give artificial respiration immediately if he is not breathing.
- Treat any burns.

## Bandaging and Splinting

***Purposes:*** (1) To secure dressing in position, (2) To form slings for support. (3) To secure pads.

***Roller bandages:*** These bandages are made of cotton, gauze crepe, elastic fabric or linen are wrapped around the injured in spiral turns, figure of eight. To improvise, material may be torn into strips of the required length and width.

***Width required:*** For finger 2.5 cm  
For head and arm 6 cm  
For the leg, about 9 cm  
For the body 15 cm  
The bandages should be tightly and evenly rolled.

***Rules for applying roller bandages:*** Face the casualty, except for bandages the head or back of the neck. When bandaging the left limb, hold the roll of bandage in the right hand and vice versa. Apply the outer side of the bandage to the part, and unroll no more than 5 cm at a time. To bandage a limb, work from below upwards, and from inside towards the outside over the front of the limb. See that the bandage is neither too tight nor too loose. Each layer should cover two thirds of the previous layer of bandage. Finish in front, not over the wound, and fix the end with a safety pin, sticking plaster, stitching, or by tearing the end into two tails and tying. The completed bandage should be comfortable, look neat and fulfill its purpose with no restriction of circulation.

*Patterns Used in Bandaging*

***Circular turns***, as used for head and trunk.

***Simple spiral,*** for parts of uniform thickness, e.g. fingers, wrist.

***Reverse spiral***, used on limbs where the thickness of the part various, e.g. forearm, leg.

***Figure-of-Eight:*** This may be used on limbs instead of the reverse spiral, also for the hand and foot.
***Spica,*** used for the shoulder, hip and thumb.
***Divergent spica,*** for a flexed joint, e.g. elbow, knee, heel.
***Recurrent,*** to cover tips of fingers or a stump special bandages such **as capeline** for the head, eye bandage, ear and breast bandages.
***Choosing the correct size:*** Before applying a roller bandage, check suitable width for the injured area.
***Applying a roller bandage:*** Keep the roller part of the bandage (head) upper most as your work (the unrolled part) is called the 'tail'.Stand in front of the casualty except in cape line (head bandaging and eye bandage are applied standing behind the client). Support the part while bandaging. Learn to use both hands equally, changing the bandage hand to hand. Work from below to upwards.

Finish off securely with either reef knot, safety pin, bandage clip, adhesive tap. Tucking in the end.
***Splinting:*** Splints can be made out of wood, cardboard, iron rods used to support the fractured part and for immoblization.
***Triangular bandages:*** They have various use in first aid. To make two bandages, take a 1 meter square piece of strong cotton cloth, cut in across from corner, and hem the edges. The long side is called the 'base', and the corner opposite to it the 'point', The bandages may be applied opened out or it can be folded into a 'broad' or 'narrow' bandages. A reef knot is used to tie the ends of the bandage, because it is flat and will not slip. The rule for tying a reef knot is 'right over left, then left over right'. If you keep this rule you cannot go wrong.

**Slings** are used to support or limit movement of the upper limb, in cases of injury or inflammation.

Three types of slings are used:

- ***Large arm sling:*** This is used in cases of simple rib fracture and for fracture of the forearm. When applied, only the finger tips should show, the whole arm being well supported.
- ***Collar and cuff sling:*** This supports the wrist only. With the casualty's forearm flexed and fingers touching the opposite shoulder, a clove hitch, made from a narrow bandage, is placed round his wrist. The ends of the bandages are taken around the neck and tied in the hollow just above the collar bone, on the injured side.
- ***Triangular sling:*** This supports the arm with the hand well raised. It gives relief from pain when used in fracture of the collar bone. First place the open bandage across the chest with the point beyond the elbow and one end over the hand. Tuck the base comfortably under the forearm. Take the end behind the elbow across the back and tie to the first end with the knot just in front of the shoulder, on the uninjured side. Fold in the point and fix the bandage with the safety pin.

***Improvised slings:*** The lower edge of the casualty's coat or shirt may be turned up and pinned to support the arm, or the hand may be passed inside a buttoned up coat. A muffler, tie or other suitable cloth may be used to support the arm.
***Bandage for the scalp:*** Place the open bandage on the head with the point at the back. Fold a narrow hem at the base, place it just above the eyebrows, then take the two ends backwards, cross them below the occiput with the point underneath, then back to the forehead where they are tied. Draw the point down and then upwards, and fix it with a safety pin.

## Effects of Extreme Heat

People can be identified as high risk in relation to heat and heat related illness. There are 3 types of heat related illness:

1. Heat stroke
2. Heat exhaustion
3. Heat cramps

### Heat Stroke or Sun Stroke

This condition is caused by failure of body temperature regulation in the brain. Usually due to high fever or prolonged exposure to heat. Heat stroke may be caused by high temperature in factories or furnaces.
***Signs and symptoms:*** Headache, dizziness, discomfort, restlessness, hot and flushed, dry skin, bounding pulse, high temperature above 104°F (40°C ), rapid unconsciousness.
***First aid:***

- Remove the patient to dry and shady place, loosening his collar, and other tight clothing.
- Rise the head and upper part of the body.
- Sprinkle cool water on his body or wrap him in a wet sheet and fan him.
- Keep on taking body temperature every 10 minutes.
- After the body temperature fallen to 102°F wrap him in a dry sheet and keep fan him.
- If the patient is conscious, cool water mixed with salt and glucose for drinking.
- Remove to the hospital.

### Heat Exhaustion

It is caused by too high temperature in the atmosphere directly by the sun, or due to hard work and confinement in a close, hot atmosphere like factories, etc.
***Signs and symptoms:***

- Headache, dizziness, nausea, vomiting, and sometimes abdominal cramps, or cramps in the limbs.
- Face in pale with cold sweat
- Pulse is weak
- Shallow breathing
- Temperature is normal or slightly raised
- Sometimes there is unconsciousness
- There may be a shock
- Loss of appetite.

***First aid:***

- Remove the patient to a cool place
- Place him flat on his back
- Loosen his clothing
- Give him plenty of salted water (¼ liter every ½ hourly)
- Observe the patient.

### Heat Cramps

These are intermittent, painful contractions of skeleton muscles. These cramps occurs the fluid lost in sweat by drinking water but do not replace sodium. Sodium depletion is responsible for the cramps.

Heat cramps usually occur in muscles that have been involved in a strenuous activity. Body temperature is normal and the serum sodium may be normal or low.

*First aid:*

- Replace the sodium with salt tablets or an electrolyte solution.
- Adding salt in the diet will prevent heat cramps.

### Points to Prevent Heat Injury

- Limiting the strenuous activities in the hot weather
- Stay indoor and wear a minimum of clothing's during heat waves.
- When temperatures are unusually high, outdoor activities should be canceled.
- Wear clothes that are loose fitting, light in color and cover the body as much as possible when outdoor
- Loose weight if you are obese
- Avoid heavy exercise
- Use measures to improve ventilation and reduce heat by shades
- Cooking should be done in early morning or late evening to avoid heating up the house during the hot part of the day
- Fans and vents over stoves and ovens should be used to help remove heat from the house.
- Eating more salts, but must be accompanied by an increased amount of fluids.
- Drink lot of water, even the person with cardiovascular disease who might otherwise be limiting fluids.

*Effects of extreme cold:* Effects of extreme cold are common in person who live or work in a climate where temperature falls below 32°F or are in high altitudes.

### Frost Bite

Frost bite occurs when the body is exposed to extreme cold temperature, i.e. ice crystals forming inside the cell can result in permanent circulatory and tissue damage. Body areas susceptible to frost bite are the ear lobes, tip of the nose, fingers and toes.

*Signs and symptoms:*

- The exposed part becomes cold, painful and ultimately numb
- Color first is red, then become white which may later lead to gangrene
- Injured area is white, waxy and firm to tough. Patient uses sensation in the affected area.

*Nursing action:* Gradual warming measures, analgesia, and protection of the injured area.

*First aid:*

- Remove all wet or tight clothing from the frost bitten area
- Carry the patient to a closed room without a fire and undress him carefully
- Remove tight gloves, boots, shocks, rings, etc. from the body
- Do not rub the frozen part with snow or anything else
- Put him to bed and cover him snugly with a dry cloth
- Give him warm drinks
- If face or ear is affected, cover the frozen patch with a gloved hand until normal color and sensation return
- Send for a physician immediately.

### Important Points to Prevent Cold Injury

- Plan activities carefully to minimize exposure
- Dress for the weather
- Avoid vigorous washing of the face
- Saving the beard until after the day's outing
- Apply protective cream to the face prior to exposure
- Wear several layers of loose warm clothing
- Use hand protection. Mittens are generally more effective than gloves
- Avoid alcohol and cigarette
- Avoid becoming unduly fatigue
- Do not use snow, ice, cold water
- If freezing occurs, avoid thawing the part until refreezing is eliminated as a threat.

### Bites and Stings

Bites from sharp, pointed teeth cause deep puncture, wounds that carry germs into the tissues.

*Snake bite:* Commonly two types of snakes are found in our country.

1. Colubrine
2. Viper

All snakes are not poisonous. Identification of the snake is important to enable to give appropriate treatment to be given. If the snake has been killed, it should be taken with the casualty to the hospital most of the people die from fear.

*Signs and symptoms:*

- A pair of puncture marks
- Severe pain, redness, swelling at the site of the bite
- Drowsiness
- Dimness of vision
- Breathing difficulty
- Unable to speak
- Increased salivation
- Convulsions
- Shock
- Weakness of hands and legs, loss of sensation, watering of mouth, slow respiration and weak pulse.

*First aid:*

- Help the casualty to lie down. Reassure her
- Wash the wound
- Slash the wound with knife
- Immobilize the affected part
- Treat for shock
- Resuscitation, if difficulty in breathing
- Shift the casualty to hospital immediately
- Take the killed snake, if available, for proper management.

*Scorpion bites:* Generally scorpion can be seen in the moist dark places and in rainy season. Though the scorpions are not seriously poisonous but sometimes persons can become unconscious.

*Signs and symptoms:*

- Severe burning
- Intolerable increasing pain in the bitten area
- Giddiness
- Vomiting
- Unconsciousness.

*First aid:*
- Patient should make to lie comfortably and soothing cream applied.
- If the patient is unconsciousness, send him to doctor or hospital.
- If a big blister is seen after 6–12 hours and it burst by itself, do the dressing with antibiotic cream.

***Dog bite:*** A rabid animal is aggressive, drooling saliva, must be approached with care. The most serious infection risk is rabies, a potentially fatal viral infection of the nervous system. The virus is carried in the saliva of the infected animal. Tetanus is also a potential risk following any animal bite. The dog should be watched for 10 days. If the dog is healthy after this period then there is no danger of rabies.

*Symptoms:*
- Headache, nausea, vomiting, fever
- Restlessness, confusion
- Difficulty in swallowing
- Foul smelling of the mouth
- Hydrophobia
- Difficulty in drinking water
- Aerophobia
- Respiratory paralysis.

*First aid:*
- Thorough washing of the bitten area and wash the wound with soap and water (detergent solution) for 5–10 minutes.
- Dress the wound with clean sterile gauze or cloth. Apply antibiotic cream.
- Shift the casualty immediately to the hospital.
- The dog should be kept under observation for 10 days.

***Cat bite:*** Cats keep roaming around the houses but if they are disturbed and touched they become violent and can attack. It causes two types of wounds
1. On biting with teeth
2. Scratches by the nails

***First aid:*** Wash the wound and apply the dressing properly.

***Rat bite:*** Rats are harm to the human-being in different ways.
- The flea found on their body spread a dangerous disease called plague.
- Sometimes they scrap the palm of the hand or foot of sleeping person.

***Signs and symptoms:*** Fever

*First aid:*
- Wound should be washed and dressed properly.
- Patient should be sent to the hospital.

***Bees and wasp bite:*** Insect such as bee and Wasp the bite is painful rather than dangerous. Starting pain will be there later mild swelling and redness appears.

*Signs and symptoms:*
- Local pain, itching and severe swelling
- Low blood pressure
- Unconsciousness.

*First aid:*
- To relieve the pain try to remove the sting with tweezer.
- Treatment of the local area.
- Bee venom is acid neutralize with ammonia, soda wasp venom is alkaline neutralize with vinegar.
- To relieve pain and swelling apply cold compress.
- Send the patient to the hospital.

***Ticks and mites bites:*** Tick is a small insect like bed bug. It is about half or one centimeter long. It has a terrible capacity to stick to the body and keep sucking the blood during this period it spreads germs of certain diseases in the body by which tularemie, rocky mountain spotted fever.

***Signs and symptoms:*** Typhus fever

*First aid:*
- The tick or mite has bitten and it is sticked should be immediately removed
- Should be pulled forcefully
- Apply burning cigaret on the dorsal surface
- Apply oil turpentine or kerosene to remove the tick or mite
- The wound should be washed with soap and water
- Apply antibiotic cream
- Apply bandage.

***Spider bite:*** There are 2 types of spider. 1. Black spider, 2. Tarantula. Black spider is more poisonous. Tarantula is big, hairy and less poisonous.

*Signs and symptoms:*
- Redness
- Severe pain
- Local swelling
- Stomach cramps
- Muscle hardness
- The face, legs and hands looks swollen
- Breathlessness and shock.

*First aid:*
- Patient should make to lie in a comfortable position
- Should be covered with blanket or bed sheet
- A cloth or rope should be tight at a distance from the bitten area. So, the blood is not absorbed in other parts of the body
- If the patient is conscious, give coffee or tea to drink
- Bitten area should be cleaned and bandaged
- Send him to the hospital.

***Leech bite:*** Leech is generally found in tanks, rivers, moist and muddy places. It sucks quite a large amount of blood.

*First aid:*
- Apply a burning stick or cigaret on the dorsal surface
- Wash the wound and apply bandage.

***Fish stings:*** Two breeds of thorny fish viz. sting ray fish and jelly fish and generally harm to the humans by stinging.

***Signs and symptoms:*** Severe pain

*First aid:*
- The sting should take it out by scratching the skin
- Wash the wound and do the dressing
- Apply cold bandages of ammonia and water to get relieve from the burning sensation
- If the pain is severe, get the medical aid.

## Poisoning

Poison is a substance which is taken into the body in sufficient quantity may cause temporary or permanent damage. They may be consumed, accidentally (by mistake, by ignorance), for suicidal purpose, intentionally for killing enemies.

***Routes of taking poisons:*** (1) Eating or drinking poisonous substance by mouth. (2) By inhaling gases, fumes, chemical vapors. (3) By injection into the skin as result of bites, e.g. snake bites, hypodermic injection. (4) Absorption through skin, e.g. poisonous sprays. Another common type of self poisoning is termed para suicide. A young person who is emotionally distributed may take such as pain killer or sleeping tablets. The object is to obtain attention and to try and solve the emotional problem, rather than to take their life.

*Recognition:* (1) Depends on the poison. (2) Vomiting, sometimes blood stained. (3) Impaired consciousness. (4) Pain or burning sensation. (5) Empty containers in the area. (6) History of ingestion/exposure.

### Household Poisoning

- Almost every household contains poisonous substances, such as bleach, paint stripper, glue, paraffin, insecticides, pesticides, alcohol, petroleum products, acids, alkalis, sedatives, etc.
- Dilute or weaken the poisonous substances.
- Excess water should be given to weakened their concentrated state except acid poisoning.
- The poisonous substances can be taken out of the body by inducing vomiting. Mixing two tablespoons of salt in one glass of water or two teaspoons of soda bicarb in a glass of water or by mixing one teaspoon of mustard water powder in lukewarm water. If the above substances are not available then lukewarm water alone is also useful.
- In all cases of poisoning seek the medical help, call the doctor immediately.

### Hypnotics

- Heroines and barbiturates can lead to sleep, deep coma by which the respiration is slowed down.
- Take out the poisonous medicines by inducing vomiting or weaken those substances by giving more water to drink.
- Keep the person awakened who is sleeping with the effect of sleeping pills.

### Gas Poisoning

It arises with inhalation of poisonous gases such carbon monoxide, carbon dioxide, inflammable gases, steam of ammonia, etc.

*The effects of these poisonous gases:*
- Reduce the amount of oxygen inhaled air
- Affects the oxygen caring capacity of blood
- Damage the mucous membrane of the respiratory tract, not allowing the oxygen absorbed in the blood from the lungs.

*Signs and symptoms:*
- Dizziness
- Tightening of chest
- Loss of consciousness
- Meiosis
- Respiratory failure
- Falling in blood pressure and pulse
- Twitching and convulsion
- Asphyxia
- Cyanosis
- Circulatory collapse.

*First aid:*
- Bring the patient in the open air
- Keep the patient warm under blanket or bedsheet
- If the respiratory process stopped, start giving artificial respiration
- There is no quick improvement, make an arrangement to send him to hospital.

### Food Poisoning

Food poisoning occurs due to contaminated water, food substances, unboiled and uncleaned vegetables, contaminated kulfi, milk and cream products contains bacteria, it produces toxins.

*Signs and symptoms:*
- Nausea and vomiting
- Cramping abdominal pains
- Diarrhea
- Headache
- Fever
- Features of shock
- Collapse.

*First aid:* The main aim of first aid is to eliminate the poison, give bland fluids such as water, diluted fruit juice or weak tea. The poisonous effect can be weakened by inducing vomiting. But with constant vomiting and diarrhea, the water and electrolyte balance of the body gets disturbed which results in to the weakness and condition of shock arises, the patient should be sent to the doctor and hospital immediately.

### Alcohol Poisoning

Alcohol (ethanol) is a drug that depresses the activity of the central nervous system.

Small quantities generally produce only a slight change of mood.

*Dangers of alcohol poisoning:*
- An unconscious casualty is in danger of inhaling and choking on vomit.
- Hypothermia can occur when exposed to cold.
- Misdiagnosed.

*Signs and symptoms:*
- A strong smell of alcohol
- Unconsciousness
- A flushed and moist face
- Deep, noisy breathing
- A full, bounding pulse.

*First aid:* If a person is intoxication of liquor, he should be made to sit and vomit. After this, give him strong tea or coffee. If the patient is unconscious and the symptoms of head injury are seen, arrange to send him to the hospital immediately.

### Datura Poisoning

This poisoning is due to consumption of seeds of tree 'datura' which may be eaten unknowingly or accidentally or may be due to consumption of belladonna alkaloids containing medicine.

*First aid:*
- Keep the patient in cool, dark and silent room and control the severe movements patiently.

- Vomiting should not be induced in conditions of unconsciousness and cramps.
- Cold bandages should be applied.
- Artificial respiration can be given if necessary.

***Protective measures:***

- Medicine bottles and packets should be clearly labeled and unlabeled bottles should not be used and destroyed.
- Toxic medicines should be labeled poison and keep it in locked almirah.
- The label on the bottle should be read before taking the medicine, during measuring the dose and while keeping the bottle back to the place.
- Cleaning agents should be labeled.
- To avoid food poisoning food should be prepared with cleanliness and kept covered. Adequate cooking and boiling to be done.

### Lead Poisoning

More industrial workers are exposed to lead, as it is most commonly used metal in industries. Most cases of industrial lead poisoning is due to inhalation of fumes and dust of lead or its compounds.

***Symptoms:*** Insomnia, headache, mental confusion, metallic taste, stomach burning, constipation followed by diarrhea, convulsions, muscular weakness, skin, cold and cyanotic.

***First aid:***

- Keep the person quiet.
- Gastric lavage with magnesium or sodium sulfate and analgesics for pain. Maintain fluid and electrolyte balance.
- Diazepam for convulsions.
- Calcium ethylene diaminotetraacetic acid is the specific antidote.
- Adequate urine flow.
- Reduce or eliminate exposure to lead.

### Mercury Poisoning

It occurs in the occupations related to crushing, roasting and condensation of mercury from ore, manufacture of paints, chlorine, caustic soda, paper and pulp.

***Symptoms:*** Tremor, gingivitis, disturbed sleep, burning sensation in mouth, throat, abdominal pain, nausea and vomiting, diarrhea and bloody stools. Weak rapid pulse, slow shallow respiration, cold and clammy skin.

***First aid:***

- Egg white, milk or flour by mouth.
- Lavage with activated charcoal.
- Dimercaprol IM penicillamine.
- Demulcents and analgesics.
- Treat for shock/acute renal failure.

### Cyanide Poisoning

Cyanides are among the most common and most deadly poisons known.

***Symptoms:*** Utter a cry, unconscious, rapid respiration, later slow and gasping. Death usually within 5 minutes.

Smaller doses acrid taste, choking, anxiety, dizziness, headache and convulsions with frothiness.

***First aid:***

- Immediate emesis and gastric lavage no delay. Inhale amyl nitrate immediately 1530 seconds every 23 minutes
- IV sodium nitrite 300 mg in 10 mL of water at rate of 2.5–5 mL this is being done simultaneously
- 12.5 g (50 mL of 25% solution) of sodium thiosulfate to be administered slowly IV for 10 min.
- Artificial respiration
- Recumbent position.

### Turpentine Poisoning

It is derived from various coniferous, pine trees, which yields a volatile oil, as oil turpentine which is used in the preparation of paints, varnishes and in medicine. Turpentine poisoning usually occurs by inhalation.

***Symptoms:*** Warm or burning sensation in the gullet and stomach, followed by cramping, vomiting and diarrhea, weak respiration and pulse. Irritation of urinary tract and CNS.

***First aid:***

- Gastric lavage.
- Soothing drinks and stimulants.
- Increase fluid intake.

***Radiation hazards:*** Many industries use radium and other radioactive substances and these exposures will lead to various hazards.

***Effects of radiation:*** Acute burns, dermatitis, blood dyscrasias, malignancies, genetic effects, lung cancer, affects the eyes, intense conjunctivitis, keratitis.

***Prevention:***

- Avoid direct contact.
- Wear X-ray thick shield during exposure.
- Monitor film badge or pocket electrometer frequently for every 6 months.
- Adequate ventilation in working area.
- Replacement and periodic examination of workers for every 2 months.
- Pregnant woman should avoid exposure.

***Noise induced hearing loss:*** Everyone in industry is concerned about industrial noise and its effect on the hearing in workers. But noise problem is generally a neglected subject.

***Hearing conservation program:*** The principles involved in HCP are outlined below:

- Noise survey
- Audiometry
- Hazard evaluation
- Noise reduction
- Hearing protective devices.

***First aid in establishment:*** Employers should develop appropriate first aid arrangement in their undertakings. Regulation and their associated code of practices be evolved which should apply to virtually all people at work and cover first aid regulation.

Employers should prepare a written statement of policy on first aid, covering employees and bring it to the notice of all concerned.

***First aid room:*** Guidance on the requirement of first aid rooms is contained in the Factories Act, 1948. This is to provide treatment for minor injuries, ambulance should be there and well equipped first aid box to be there.

***Control measures to avoid risk of occupational diseases:***
- Pre employment medical examination
- Periodical medical examination
- Change of job assignment
- Education
- Use of personal protective appliances where required
- Substitution
- Enclosure
- Employment
- Monitoring of work environment
- Adopting engineering control measures
- Good housekeeping and good ventilation.

## Foreign Bodies

***Foreign bodies in the skin:*** Small foreign bodies (wood splinters, shards of glass) usually cause minor puncture wounds with little or no bleeding. If foreign bodies deeply embedded in a wound is not be removed by a first aided, it may cause further injury.

***Splinters:*** Small splinters of wood, metal or glass in the skin particularly of the hands, feet and knees are common injuries. It should be drawn out by using tweezers.

***First aid:***
- Clean area around the splinter with soap and water
- Sterilize a pair or tweezers by passing them through a flame
- Grasp the splinter as close to the skin as possible
- Squeeze the wound to encourage a little bleeding
- Apply an adhesive dressing 'plaster'.

***Foreign bodies in the eye:*** Sand particles, dust, small pieces of glass, coal, emery stone, metal, usually enter the eye as foreign bodies. These particles get situated under the eye lids or eye balls.

***Signs and Symptoms:***
- Pain and irritation
- Watery eyes
- Photophobia

***First aid:***
- Try to take out only those foreign bodies which are lying only on the surface area of the eyes.
- In an emergency condition, it becomes necessary to take out foreign bodies then the hand should be washed properly and cotton piece or soft handkerchief should be made wet with a corner made pointed and then the foreign body should be taken out with a help of pointer end.
- If the foreign body in the middle portion do not try to take it out because this can lead to great harm. The eyes should be closed, padded and then patient should be sent to the hospital.
- The foreign body sometimes comes out when the hairs of the lower eye lid get rubbed with the upper under part of the eye.
- Do not rub the eyes vigorously.
- Examine the eyes carefully with soft hands.

***Foreign bodies in the ear:*** The cases of foreign bodies in the ear occur generally in children like peas, buttons, seeds, flies, mosquitoes or bedbugs.

***First aid:***
- Never use pin or piece of wire to take out foreign bodies from the ear.
- Mosquitoes, bedbugs or flies die by putting olive oil or soda bicarb in lukewarm water in to the ears.
- Send the person to hospital.

***Foreign bodies in the nose:*** Certain foreign bodies like pieces of betel nuts, grains or peas and other seeds enter the nose.

***First aid:***
- Putting olive oil or weather oil in the nose either the foreign body comes out or irritation of the nose subsides.
- Do not sneeze forcefully.
- Send the person to hospital.

***Foreign bodies in the throat:*** Generally in the throat or upper part of the respiratory tract, some pieces of food, small bones of fish, coins or artificial teeth or other things can enter.

***First aid:***
- Generally the foreign body not seen in the throat and even if it is seen then do not try to take it out by finger or other measures.
- Bend the person down and by patting on the shoulder the things comes out
- Artificial respiration
- Send the patient to the hospital.

***Foreign bodies in the stomach:*** The introduction of foreign bodies into the stomach are generally found in the children like buttons, seeds of fruits, coins, safety pins.

***First aid:***
- No immediate risk
- Get eliminated during evacuation
- No need to give laxatives.

## Car Accident

The situations look of victims inspect the victims for bleeding, asphyxia or burning car prevent further accident. Put out fire with a rug, soil or sand turn off car lights and switch off the igniter. Apply the brakes or blocks the wheels with a bulky object set warnings – a red reflector triangle and a white scarf or newspaper along the road up to 200 yards either side of the accident at night wear boldly white.

***The patient:*** Patient should be protected by supporting neck and jaw with a collar made from a newspaper thickly folded to form a rigid but pliable support about 3 by 12 inches and inserted into a stocking.

Extracting the patient from a buckled car especially if the doors are jammed and if the injuries include fractured spine and limbs. Leave it to the expects of police, ambulance, fire brigade, rescue doctors.

***The car first aid kit***
- Kit should be kept in a well closed but easily opened, clearly labeled, metal or plastic box
- Triangular bandages
- Women discarded stockings
- White gauze

- Gamgee tissue (in large pieces 12 inches by 18 inches)
- Cotton elastic or crepe bandages
- Adhesive tape
- Scissors and a rescue blanket.

*When breaks do not work – what to do:* Pump the break pedal park means the parking break use it but do not jam it. It can cause a spin shift into a lower gear side swipe something a guard rail or curb, some bushes, even parked car.

*Six things to do before help arrives:* Avoid a second collision. Do not pack behind the wreck, or on the opposite side of the road.

Reduce the chance of fire by turning off the ignition. Assist the injured. Get the victims out of danger. Get help. Call the police or ambulance. Search the area for victims who might have been thrown from the cars involved.

## CARDIOPULMONARY RESUSCITATION (CPR)

Resuscitation includes all measures that are applied to revive patients who have stopped breathing suddenly and unexpectedly due to either respiratory or cardiac failure. Cardiac arrest is one of the common causes for cardio-respiratory failure.

When a person stops breathing spontaneously, his heart also stops beating. Clinical dearth occurs within 4 to 6 minutes, the cells of the brain. Which are sensitivity to the paucity of oxygen begin to deteriorate. If the oxygen supply is not restored, the patient suffer irreversible brain damage and biological death occurs.

*Cardiorespiratory failure:* The respiratory and cardiovascular systems are interdependent. The heart consumed more oxygen per minute than any other organ in the body, because it is constantly beating. Consequently, when the lungs stops working, the heart fail occurs. Conversely, the ventilation of the lungs fail soon after the heart stops. This is because the respiratory center in the medulla oblongata cannot function without the continuous supply that is normally transported to it by the cardiovascular system.

### Sequence of Cardiopulmonary Resuscitation

A – Airway, B – Breathing, C – Circulation.

#### *General Instruction*

- CPR techniques are used in persons whose respirations and circulation of blood have suddenly and unexpectedly stopped.
- The immediate responsibilities of the resuscitator are:
  - To recognize the signs of cardiac arrest.
  - To protect the patients brain from anoxia.
  - To call for help.
- The CPR must be initiated within 3 to 4 minutes in order to prevent permanent brain damage.
- The CPR techniques should not be discontinued for more than 5 seconds before normal circulation and ventilation of lungs are established.
- Before CPR is attempted in a patient, make sure that the airway is clear.
- Cardiac compressions help to stimulate the circulation.
- The artificial breathing and the cardiac massage should correspond to the normal respiration and pulse rate. The ratio of cardiac compression to ventilation rate is 5:1, i.e. 5 cardiac compression to one ventilation. Cardiac compression given at the rate of 60 per minute. Ventilations are given at the rate of 12 per minute.
- When there are two rescuers, both position themselves on either sides of the victims, i.e. one rescuer does artificial ventilation while the other does external cardiac compressions. The ratio of cardiac compression to ventilation rate is 15:2.
- The circulation of blood is initiated with the external cardiac massage because, the pressure exerted on the pliable sternum squeezes the heart against the spine forcing blood out of the heart into aorta.
- Watch for complications that may occur during the cardiopulmonary resuscitation.
- Discontinue the procedure only when you are sure that the respirations and circulation as re-established.
- Patient's viral signs are watched constantly over a period of 24 to 48 hours after the cardiac arrest, because of the danger of recurring another cardiac arrest at any time.
- A nasogastric incubation and aspiration of gastric contents are necessary for a patient with full stomach to prevent vomiting and aspiration of vomitus into the lungs.

#### *Complications*

- Damage to the cervical spine due to hyperextension of the neck.
- Fracture of the rib and xiphoid process.
- Hemopericardium.
- Pneumothorax.
- Intra-abdominal hemorrhage.
- Gastric distention of air.
- Aspiration of the vomitus into the lungs.

## EMERGENCY KIT

An emergency bag or kit will help you to provide emergency care and treatment in an efficient way. The contents of an emergency bag will vary considerably according to place of practice, proximity of a primary health center, medical clinic or hospital, your individual preference for practice in a specialty area only; and standing orders for administration of medicines, injections, or any other treatment in an emergency. Some nurses may wish to add or delete items from the list of suggested items given in the following section.

The emergency bag should be a portable one, with compartments and pockets with flaps. Replacement of each item as soon as possible after use is imperative to avoid wasting time looking for items in an emergency. Check the bag regularly replenish when necessary and keep items in the same place.

### Emergency Bag Contents

#### *Items and Description Quantity*

For Flashlight, (Medical use) 1

Assessment Tongue spatula 1

Thermometer 1

Aneroid sphygmomanometer 1
Stethoscope 1
Gloves, rubber 1 pair
Small writing pad 1
Pen 1

### *Items and Description Quantity*

For Emergency Bandages, assorted sizes 6
Care Treatment Bandage triangular 2
Gauze pads, individually packed, sterile 6
Adhesive dressing strips (bandaid)
1 packet
Cotton tipped applicators 6
Cotton wool, small packet 1
Adhesive tape 1 roll
Safety pins, assorted sizes 1 dozen
Eyepads 2
Splints, light wood, plywood 2
Bottles, screw topped, wide mouthed (for specimen) 2
Catheters, plastic or rubber, urethral 2
Gastric lavage tube, rubber, medium size 1
Tourniquet or rubber tubing strip 1
Intravenous drip set, disposable type with needle 1 set
Hypodermic syringe 2 mL 1
Hypodermic syringe 5 mL 1
Hypodermic needles no. 26, 24, 22 sizes 4
File for cutting ampoules 1
Pocket knife 1
Scalpel 1
Scissors blunt tipped 1
Scissors sharp pointed 1
Forceps, artery clamps 2
Forceps, dissecting 1
Dextran or dextrose solution (as intravenous drip starter in non-breakable flask or bag) 500 mL.
Oral rehydration power 2 packets
Tetanus Toxoid 5 mL. vial 1 vial
Injection Adrenalin 1:1000 1 mL. 2 ampoules
Injection Pethidine 100 mg in 2 mL. 1 ampoule
Injection Morphine Sulfate 30 mg in 2 mL. 1 ampoule
Injection Atropine Sulfate 1 mg in 1 mL. 1 ampoule
Combined Injection Morphine Sulfate andAtropine Sulfate 1 ampoules.

### Oral Medications

Antihistamines tablet, e.g. Avil, Phenergan, Benadryl
Antispasmodics tablet, e.g. Spasmindon, Belladonna
Antiemetics Tablet, e.g. Siquil, Stemetil
Analgesics Tablet, e.g. Aspirin, Dispirin, Crocin, Paracetamol, Novalgin
Antiasthmatics Tablet, e.g. Aminophylline, Ephedrine
Antacid Tablet, e.g. Aludrox, Gelusil.

### Topical Medications for External Application

Rectified Spirit 30 mL 1 bottle
Tincture benzoin 30 mL 1 bottle
Tincture Iodine, weak 1 bottle
Lotion Calamine 30 mL 1 bottle
Lignocaine/Xylocaine ointment 9% 1 tube.

### Eye Ointment

Tetracycline Eye Ointment 1% 1 tube.

### Summary

- First aid is the initial assistance or treatment given to someone who is injured or suddenly taken ill.
- Do not delay or reenter a burning building to personal possessions.
- Burns according to the depths are superficial, partial thickness, full thickness.
- Chemical burn to the eye, first aider is to wash out the eye so that the chemical is diluted and dispersed.
- A fracture is a break in continuity of a bone, this may vary from a crack to a complete break.
- Poison is a substance which is taken into the body in sufficient quantity may cause temporary or permanent damage.
- Drowning is a condition of suffocation which may lead to death, due to airway spasm or water entering into the airway during swimming or when in water.
- Hemorrhage or bleeding is a flow of blood from an artery,vein or capillary.
- Bandages are made of cotton, gauze crepe, elastic fabric or linen are wrapped around the injured in spiral turns, figure of eight.
- Frost bites occur when the body is exposed to extreme cold temperature.
- Sunburn is caused by over exposure to sun.
- Heat stroke is caused by failure of body temperature in the brain.

## HOSPITAL HOUSEKEEPING

A well-managed housekeeping department can reduce the cost of hospital operation considerably.

If the hospital housekeeping is of poor quality, nursing care suffers, nursing education is adversely affected, efficiency is lowered and the morale is impaired.

### Principles of Good Housekeeping

- The dusting can be done best by a damp duster or by an oiled cloth. A dry duster scatters the dust.
- Dusting is done after sweeping and not before.
- Soap and water are used for cleaning.
- Friction aids in mechanical cleaning. Use brush when cleaning a grooved surface.
- Abrasives are harmful to the painted and polished surface.
- Albuminous materials (e.g. body discharges) are coagulated by the heat. So, it should be removed with cold water.
- Bacteria grow in dark, moist and unclean places
- Exposure to sunlight destroys some bacteria
- Disinfection by chemicals depends upon the cleanliness of the article, the strength of the disinfectant and the length of exposure.
- Effective sterilization depends upon the cleanliness of the articles, the degree of heat and the length of exposure

- Heat, chemicals, abrasives and solvents are harmful to some materials.
- Choosing the correct and the simplest method of cleaning, saves time, material and energy
- Equipment suitable for the purpose for which it is used and in good condition, conveniently located and arranged, saves time material and energy.
- The cleaning articles are stored in a neat and tidy always.

### Cleanliness and Orderliness

Cleanliness and orderliness go hand in hand. Nurses are held responsible for the cleanliness of the wards.

#### Purpose of Cleaning

- To leave a clean polished surface where possible, so that dirt may not be accumulated.
- To remove all dust, dirt and breeding places of microorganisms with the least disturbance to the patient.
- To prolong the life of the articles.
- To keep the articles in such a condition that they are ready for use at any time.
- To maintain the aesthetic factors.

#### Care of Rubber Goods

The rubber goods in common use are mackintosh, hot water bottles, ice caps, ice collars, rubber tubes, catheters, gloves and rubber beds.

Natural and synthetic rubber deteriorate with age, exposure to heat, light, moistures and by chemicals.

Rubber goods should never be dried by artificial heat, nor by contact with the radiator or stove. It should be free from greece and acids.

If autoclaving is used, short periods of exposure are recommended (10–15 minutes).

*Cleaning of rubber mackintosh:*

- Spread the mackintosh on the table or a flat surface and wet with cold water
- Rub the upper surface with soap and water
- Turn the other side rub with soap and water
- If strains are present to be removed
- For disinfection use Lysol or Dettol 1:40
- Hang them on a horizontal cylindrical pole
- Both surfaces absolutely dry powder them
- Store them flat or rolled, never folded
- Store them in a dark cool place.

#### Care of Rubber Gloves

- It is desired that the wearer of the gloves should wash on their hands just before they are removed.
- After removing from the hands, they are washed with soap and cold water, first on the outside then invert and repeat on the inside.
- Rinse well with water both inside and outside
- Holes and tears are discovered by submerging the gloves filled with air in the water. If there are holes, separate the gloves.
- Hang them to dry.
- Turn inside out and dry.
- When both sides are dry, powdered inside and outside and packed in pairs of the same size.
- Steam under pressure is the best method of sterilizing gloves.

#### Care of Rubber Tubes

Catheters vary in size and quality according to the special needs.

*Cleaning of rubber tubes:*

- After use, wash them under running water
- A small quantity of organic matter may be lodged at the eye end. Remove them using a swap stick
- Clean them with the soap and water
- Wash them again under running water
- Boiled tubes for 5 minutes by putting them in the boiled water.
- Dry it by hanging
- When dried, powdered and store them in air tight container
- Reboil or autoclave them before use.

#### Care of Enamel Ware

The articles commonly used are bed pans, urinals, kidney trays, sputum cups, feeding cups and trays.

#### Care of the Bed Pans

- Before emptying the bed pans, inspect the contents. If there are cotton sponges or sanitary pads should be removed by using a forceps.
- Empty the bed pan to a lavatory pan
- Rinse the bed pan with cold water under force
- Wash with soap and warm water using a brush
- To disinfectant the bed pans, soak them in Lysol 1:40
- Bed pans may be placed in direct sun light for few hours
- Keep them dry for the next use on the bed pan track.

#### Care of the Urinals

The urinal should not be left standing for a long-time with urine. It should be cleansed and disinfected by using Lysol solution 1:40.

#### Care of the Kidney Trays

- Before emptying the kidney tray, inspect the contents. If there are cotton sponges or sanitary pads should be removed by using a forceps
- Empty the kidney tray to a lavatory pan
- Rinse the kidney tray with cold water under force
- Wash with soap and warm water using a brush
- To disinfectant the kidney tray, soak them in Lysol 1:40
- Kidney tray may be placed in direct sun light for few hours
- Keep them dry for the next use on the kidney tray track.

#### Care of the Sputum Cups

Non infectious sputum may be emptied lavatory pan.

Infectious sputum should be rendered by boiling or disinfection by chemicals or disposed by burning.

## Care of Instruments

**Care of sharp instruments:** The knifes and scissors are the most commonly used sharp instruments.

Sharp instruments are sterilized by hot air sterilizer exposing into a temperature of 160°C for an hour.

Chemical disinfections can be done by submerging them fully under pure Dettol or other disinfectants.

***Care of other instruments:*** Operation theater instruments should drop into a basin or bucket. Rinse the instruments thoroughly with cold water to remove the blood or other organic matter.

Clean the instruments with sodium carbonate (2%) and hot water.

***Care of glassware:*** Cleaning of the glassware should have a hard smooth surface ground glass susceptible to erosion by water or steam. It should be sterilized with dry heat. Glasswares used for the parenteral therapy should be rinsed with freshly distilled water. When the glass goods are sent for autoclaving or boiling, should be adequately padded to prevent braking by rubbing with hard surfaces.

***Care of syringes and needles:*** Syringes are expensive and common item of the glassware used in the hospital. Rinsing immediately after use to prevent the pistons sticking to the barrels, thus prolonging the life of syringes.

Stuck syringes placed in 25% of aqueous solutions of glycerine and boiled for 10 minutes.

When cleaning and sterilizing the syringes of the same number should be kept together. Sterilization by hot air is the best method of sterilization of glass syringes.

***The important points to remember:***

- After use cold water is forced through the needle with the syringes
- Again wash it with warm water
- If the needles are blocked wire stillest are used to remove
- Needles are sterilized by 10–20 minutes.

***Care of the stainless goods:*** Stainless steel utensils are suitable for almost every other purpose because they are easily cleaned, heat resistant and unbreakable.

## Care of Linen

Care of linen is important and expensive item in the hospital.

### *Rules*

- The linen cup board should be kept in perfect order.
- The cup boards should be locked when not in use.
- Care should be taken to avoid linen being taken home by the patients.
- Stock should be checked at regular intervals.
- All items should be used for the purposes for which they were made.
- Torn linen should not be used on the bed but sent for mending.
- Soiled linen should not be placed on the floor.
- Damp linen should be dried immediately.
- If soiled with urine or motion, these should be rinsed with cold water.
- Remove the strain where straining is unavoidable, old linen should be used.
- The infected linens should be disinfected first.
- Use mackintosh wherever it is necessary to economize the use of linen.

### *General Instructions for Removal of Strains from the Linens*

- Try whether the strains can be removed with cold water.
- The strains which contains proteins such as blood, excreta, milk, pus from the wound are coagulated by the application of heat.
- If the strains contained fatty material, hot water and soak should be used.
- When the strains do not response to the simple methods, bleaching agents may be used such as lemon juice, hydrogen peroxide and bleaching powder.
- Use equal parts of hydrogen peroxide and dilute ammonia and moisture the strain until disappears.

***Blood stains:*** Soak immediately in cold water. When the stains disappear, wash them in warm soapy water. If it is old stain, soak them in a mixture of hydrogen peroxide and ammonia.

For the thick blood stains on the mattress, apply a thick paste of starch and water and allow to stand in the sun. When the paste is dry and discolored, brush off the stain.

***Tea, coffee, coco:*** Linen when it is stained with tea, coffee, and coco, remove it by pouring milk over it.

Washing them in cold water or hot water. Sodium carbonate will remove the stains.

***Rust marks:*** Apply salt and lime juice and exposed to sun light

***Ink strain:*** Sprinkle salt and lime juice and lay in the sun to bleach the strain

***Care of blankets:*** These are expensive articles and do not stand washing or steam disinfections without shrinkage. Blankets should be protected by sheets by under and over it.

Blankets are cleaned by dry cleaning to disinfect them by exposing them to sun light. When storing blankets should be carefully protected from moth using naphthalene balls.

### Care of Mattress and Pillows

Mattress should be brushed at regular and frequent intervals to prevent collection of dust and along the seams. To prevent rusting of the mattress from the wires or springs, use canvass between the mattress and bed sheet. When the patient discharged, mattress should be thoroughly brushed and examine for strains and tears. It should be treated at once. Disinfected by exposing them to sun light.

Pillows should be protected from wet with blood and bodily discharges. They should be protected with mackintoshes when they are used for the patients with bleeding, vomiting, etc.

## Care of Patients Unit

***Care of the flooring:*** Floors are mopped with mops of good quality. Vacuum cleaners may be used.

Most of the floors washed with soap and water.

Wooden floors are kept well polished. They are mopped daily. Water should be wiped of immediately.

Cement floors can be cleaned with hot water and weak solution of sodium carbonate.

Mosaic floors cleaned with mild alkaline solution such as soda, soda bicarb, etc.

*Care of the walls:* Cement and marble walls can be cleaned in the same way as the floors.

*Painted walls:* Never use cleaning solutions that contains a strong alkaline. Painted surface should always be carefully rinsed and dried.

*Daily cleaning:* The patients unit is swept and mopped twice or thrice a day to keep it clean. The furniture should be moved to collect the dust present under them. After sweeping, all the articles are dusted with damp duster, dampened with disinfectant.

*Weekly cleaning:* The roof and walls of the wall should be swept each week to remove the cob webs.

The ceiling fans are dusted with the damp duster. All the furniture should be scrubbed, washed and carbolized.

*Care of the sanitary annex:* Sanitary annex attached to the wards consist of bathing rooms, lavatories, hand washing places, place for washing and storing of bed pans, urinals, etc.

*Bathing room:* The floor should be scrubbed, washed daily to prevent slipping. No water should stagnate in the bathing room.

*Lavatories:* Lavatories pans should be cleaned with vim or sane fresh, using a brush if strains are present, smear a small amount of acid and wash it off. The patients and the relatives should be taught regarding proper use of latrine.

*Hand washing place:* The drains may become blocked by the refuse thrown into the sinks by the patients. They should be told not to throw in to the sink.

## Summary

- Well managed housekeeping department can reduce the cost of hospital operation.
- Effective sterilization depends upon the cleanliness of the articles, the degree of heat and the length of exposure.
- Rubber goods should never be dried by artificial heat or by contact with the radiator or stove.
- For disinfection of rubber mackintosh use Lysol or Dettol 1:40 dilution.
- Holes and tears are discovered by submerging the gloves filled with air or water.
- Steam under pressure is the best method of sterilizing gloves.
- Cleaning of rubber tubes are boiled for 5 minutes by putting them in the boiled water.
- Sterilization by hot air is the best method of sterilization of glass syringes.
- Needles are sterilized by 10–20 minutes.
- Removal of strains from the linens by using equal parts of hydrogen peroxide and dilute ammonia and moisture the strain until disappears.
- Mosaic floors cleaned with mild alkaline solution such as soda, soda bicarb, etc.

## MULTIPLE CHOICE QUESTIONS

**1. Health promotion activities can include:**
(a) Exercise and good nutrition
(b) Smoking and drinking
(c) Unsafe sex
(d) Exposure to air pollution

**2. The first Korotkoff sound indicates:**
(a) Diastolic pressure
(b) Pulse pressure
(c) Systolic pressure
(d) Mean pressure

**3. Positive nitrogen balance would occur in:**
(a) Infection (b) Starvation
(c) Burn injury (d) Pregnancy

**4. Client with apnea experience:**
(a) Difficult respiration requiring more effort
(b) Slowness of breathing followed by rapid respiration
(c) Cessation of breathing which is temporary
(d) Lack of oxygen to body tissue and organ

**5. When feeding tube is first placed in position, verification is done by:**
(a) Auscultation
(b) X-Ray confirmation
(c) pH testing of gastric content
(d) confirmation of distal mark on feeding tube

**6. Circadian rhythm occurs at an interval of:**
(a) 24 hours (b) 48 hours
(c) 36 hours (d) 72 hours

**7. Diminished urinary output is:**
(a) Anuria (b) Oliguria
(c) Dysuria (d) Pyuria

**8. One gram of protein gives:**
(a) 9 kcal (b) 6 kcal
(c) 4 kcal (d) 7 kcal

**9. Causes of cardiac arrest are all except:**
(a) Myocardial infraction
(b) Infection
(c) Drowning
(d) Airway obstruction

**10. The common most site for recording pulse rate is:**
(a) Radial (b) Apical
(c) Brachial (d) Femoral

**11. First school of nursing was started by Florence Nightingale at St Thomas Hospital London, in the year:**
(a) 1820 (b) 1870
(c) 1860 (d) 1850

**12. Steam inhalation is indicated when patient has:**
(a) Chest pain (b) Vomiting
(c) Fever (d) Cough

**13. Nursing registration in India is done by:**
(a) TNAI
(b) State Nursing Council
(c) Indian Nursing Council
(d) International Council of Nursing

**14. In Fowler's position:**
(a) Head end is raised to 30 degree
(b) Head end is raised to 45 degree
(c) Head end is raised to 90 degree
(d) Head end is raised to 15 degree

**15. Body position used for gynecological examination is:**
(a) Prone (b) Supine
(c) Genupectoral (d) Lithotomy

**16. Color of normal urine is:**
(a) Amber (b) Grey
(c) Red (d) Brownish yellow

**17. The process of sanitizing and preserving human remains is:**
(a) Embalming
(b) Autopsy
(c) Harvesting of organ
(d) Euthanasia

**18. Intracellular fluids constitute ________ percentage of body weight:**
(a) 40 (b) 50
(c) 55 (d) 60

**19. A nurse who demonstrate caring by helping family members:**
(a) Make health care decisions for the client
(b) Provides activities of daily living
(c) Become active participants in care
(d) Communicates with the visitor

**20. The purpose of using dilutes hydrogen peroxide for mouth care is:**
(a) To loosen crust (b) As astringent
(c) Antiseptic agent (d) To prevent gingivitis

**21. The client right to refuse treatment is an example of:**
(a) Statuary law (b) Common law
(c) Civil law (d) Nurse practice law

**22. A simple and cost effective method for reducing the risk of stasis of pulmonary secretion and decreased chest wall expansion is:**
(a) Oxygen humidification
(b) Chest physiotherapy
(c) Anti invectives
(d) Frequent change of position

**23. One of the most common electrolytic imbalance is:**
(a) Hyponatremia (b) Hypokalemia
(c) Hyperkalemia (d) Hypernatremia

**24. Poor oxygenation of blood ordinarily will affect the pulse rate and cause it to become:**
(a) Bounding
(b) Irregular
(c) Faster than normal
(d) Slower than normal

**25. The client who is at greater risk of fluid volume deficit is:**
(a) Elderly adult (b) Children
(c) Infants (d) Adults

**26. In which stage of sleep do dream most often occur:**
(a) REM sleep
(b) Stage 2 NREM sleep
(c) Stage 3 NREM sleep
(d) Stage 4 NREM sleep

**27. All of the following are the characteristics of good documentation and reporting EXCEPT:**
(a) Factual (b) Incomplete
(c) Accurate (d) Complete

**28. Recreation is an important aspect of health because:**
(a) It provides good muscle tone
(b) It keeps us happy
(c) A change of activity helps individual to relax
(d) Very few individual enjoy working for living

**29. Physical examination method include the following EXCEPT:**
(a) Palpation (b) Percussion
(c) Auscultation (d) Observation

**30. Formulation of nursing diagnosis is based on:**
(a) Assessment (b) Identification
(c) Clinical nursing skill (d) Medical diagnosis

**31. A medication order should never be implemented if the nurse:**
(a) Does not know the physician
(b) Does not know the patient in detail
(c) Question any part of the medication order
(d) Did not witness the writing of medication order

**32. Professional relationship are:**
(a) Family centered
(b) Personal
(c) Therapeutic
(d) Social process

**33. Application of warm compression is indicated:**
(a) To relieve edema
(b) For the client who is shivering
(c) To promote healing
(d) To prevent pressure sore

**34. Nursing process can be defined as:**
(a) Implementation of nursing care by nurses
(b) Steps, the nurse employs to provide care
(c) A process, the nurse uses to determine the problem
(d) Activities a nurse employee to identify nursing problem

**35. The most accurate assessment of pulse rate would be:**
(a) Carotid pulse (b) Apical pulse
(c) Radial pulse (d) Brachial pulse

**36. The founder of modern nursing is:**
(a) Florence Nightingale
(b) Orem
(c) Callista Roy
(d) Hippocrates

**37. Nursing care plan is:**
(a) Written by the matron in charge
(b) The action plan of care to the individual patient
(c) Same for all patient
(d) The nursing order

**38. The respiratory center is situated in:**
(a) Cerebrum
(b) Cerebellum
(c) Hypothalamus
(d) Medulla oblongata

**39. Best position for using bed pan is:**
(a) Fowler's position (b) Supine position
(c) Prone position (d) Side lying position

**40. Which route gives the most accurate measurement of body temperature:**
(a) Axilla (b) Oral
(c) Rectal (d) Groin

**41. Hyper apnea is:**
(a) An increased rate of respiration
(b) Difficulty in breathing
(c) An increased in depth of respiration
(d) Noisy breathing

**42. Sphygmomanometer is used for measuring the:**
(a) Pulse (b) Temperature
(c) Reparation (d) Blood pressure

**43. The nurse should wear the gloves:**
(a) While having direct contact with blood and body fluid
(b) While taking history from patient
(c) While observing the patient's condition
(d) When infection is spread through air

**44. Breach of legal duty involving injury is known as:**
(a) Negligence (b) Tort
(c) Crime (d) Malpractice

**45. A gown should be worn when:**
(a) Client's hygiene is poor
(b) Client has AIDS or hepatitis
(c) While administering syrup
(d) Blood or body fluid may get into the nurse's cloth performing nursing procedure

**46. Talcum powder is used after bath to:**
(a) Promote comfort
(b) Prevent friction and absorb moisture
(c) Prevent odor
(d) Prevent irritation

**47. Flexion involves:**
(a) Bending the body part
(b) Strengthening the body part
(c) Moving the body part toward the body
(d) Moving the body part away from the body

**48. While giving sponge bath:**
(a) Clean the dirty area first
(b) Move from cleaner part to less cleaner part
(c) Adoptary method
(d) Always be on the right side of the patient

**49. Hierarchy of human needs was identifying by:**
(a) Florence Nightingale
(b) Callista Roy
(c) Abraham Maslow
(d) Virginia Henderson

**50. The formula to convert Fahrenheit to Centigrade scale is:**
(a) C = [32 – F] × 9/5 (b) C = [F – 32] × 5/9
(c) C = [F + 32] × 5/9 (d) C = [F + 32] × 9/5

**51. A Snellen chart is used to assess:**
(a) Hearing (b) Papillary response
(c) Color (d) Vision

**52. Sound caused by air moving through a narrow passage is:**
(a) Wheeze (b) Crackle
(c) Rhonchi (d) Rales

**53. Simple and most effective way to prevent infection:**
(a) Fumigation
(b) Autoclaving
(c) Daily carbolization
(d) Hand washing

**54.The ethical principle that refer to the agreement to keep promises is:**
(a) Beneficence (b) Veracity
(c) Fidelity (d) Nonmaleficence

**55. While giving mouth care to comatose patient, the nurse should assess:**
(a) Gag reflex (b) Range of motion
(c) Neck rigidity (d) Halitosis

**56. Breathing that is normal in rate and depth is:**
(a) Apnea (b) Bradypnea
(c) Orthopnea (d) Eupnea

**57. Normal pH of blood is:**
(a) 7.10 to 7.25 (b) 7.35 to 7.45
(c) 7.45 to 7.60 (d) 7.20 to 7.40

**58. In non-rapid eye movement sleep, stage last for:**
(a) 10 to 20 minutes (b) 20 to 30 minutes
(c) 25 to 35 minutes (d) 40 to 55 minutes

**59. Putting a drop of medicine in the eye is called:**
(a) Inhalation (b) Inunction
(c) Instillation (d) Insertion

**60. Inflammation of vein is called:**
(a) Otitis media (b) Phlebitis
(c) Sinusitis (d) Appendicitis

**61. Nursing Paradigm include:**
(a) Health, person, environment and history
(b) Concept, theory, health and environment
(c) Model, nurse, client and family
(d) Person, health, environment and nursing

**62. During assessment phase of nursing process, the nurse should:**
(a) Propose/formulate hypothesis
(b) Document care
(c) Generate desired outcome
(d) Validate data

**63. Primary prevention of disease includes:**
(a) Health promotion and disease prevention
(b) Early detection of illness
(c) Maintaining health
(d) Prevention and cure of illness

**64. Contributing factor to pressure sore formation are all of the following EXCEPT:**
(a) Pressure (b) Friction
(c) Moisture (d) Fever

**65. History taking is used to collect:**
(a) Objective data (b) Subjective data
(c) Primary data (d) Secondary data

**66. To assess the effectiveness of CPR the nurse look for:**
(a) Radial pulse (b) Temporal pulse
(c) Carotid pulse (d) Brachial pulse

**67. Nurse's day is celebrated on:**
(a) 12 May (b) 12 April
(c) 07 April (d) 07 May

**68. The patient should be given 2 table spoon of milk of magnesia. The nurse would give:**
(a) 5 ml (b) 15 ml
(c) 30 ml (d) 40 ml

**69. The stage in which the individual accepts the loss and beings to look toward the future:**
(a) Denial (b) Anger
(c) Bargaining (d) Acceptance

**70. Health education to the younger adult must be related to the activities of:**
(a) Primary care
(b) Health promotion
(c) Secondary prevention
(d) Rehabilitation

**71. The prescription of medicine Lasix 40 mg OD the nurse administers medication:**
(a) Once a day (b) Twice a day
(c) Thrice a day (d) When required

**72. Blood in urine __________:**
(a) Polyuria (b) Anuria
(c) Hematuria (d) Pyuria

**73. Benedict solution is used for testing urine for the presence of:**
(a) Albumin (b) Sugar
(c) Pus cell (d) Specific gravity

**74. Dyspnea means difficulty in:**
(a) Swallowing (b) Breathing
(c) Urination (d) Digestion

**75. The term 'ENCODER' refers to:**
(a) Sender (b) Receiver
(c) Messenger (d) Message

**76. Instrument used to measure blood pressure:**
(a) Spirometer (b) Manometer
(c) Sphygmomanometer (d) Infusion pump

**77. Total cessation of breathing is called:**
(a) Apnea (b) Cyanosis
(c) Orthopnea (d) Hypercapnea

**78. The temperature of water in hot water bag for a normal adult should be:**
(a) 46–52°C (b) 40.5–45°C
(c) 49–65°C (d) 59–65°C

**79. The exercise in which there is change in muscle tension but no change in muscle length:**
(a) Isotonic exercise (b) Isometric exercise
(c) Dynamic exercise (d) Aerobic exercise

**80. The size of the bandage used for finger is:**
(a) 1 inch (b) 2 inch
(c) 1 cm (d) 2 cm

**81. Lice found on the scalp is known as:**
(a) Pediculus capitis (b) Pediculus pubis
(c) Pediculus corporis (d) Scabies

**82. Which of the following term indicate blood in stool:**
(a) Hemorrhage (b) Hematuria
(c) Melena (d) Hematemesis

**83. Hyperpyrexia indicates a temperature above:**
(a) 102°F (b) 103°F
(c) 104°F (d) 105°F

**84. Skin turgor can be assessed by:**
(a) Indenting with finger tip
(b) Pinching the skin tightly
(c) Touching to detecting moisture
(d) Using special light

**85. Oliguria in adult is urine output less than:**
(a) 500 mL/day (b) 600 mL/day
(c) 1400 mL/day (d) 800 mL/day

**86. Normal body temperature in adult is:**
(a) 98.6°C (b) 100°C
(c) 212°F (d) 98.6°F

**87. Rigor mortis is:**
(a) Reduction in body temperature with loss of skin elasticity after death
(b) Stiffening of body developing 2–4 hours after death
(c) Bluish discoloration of the body after death
(d) Liquifying the body tissue after death

**88. The term ethics refer to:**
(a) Scientific principle (b) Standard of conduct
(c) Nurses pledge (d) Critical thinking

**89. Adaptation theory was developed by:**
(a) Orem (b) Betty Newman
(c) Callista Roy (d) Florence Nightingale

**90. Movement of limb away from the midline of the body is termed as:**
(a) Abduction (b) Adduction
(c) Flexion (d) Extension

**91. Which of the following equipment is used to assess apical pulse?**
(a) Stethoscope (b) Otoscope
(c) Ophthalmoscope (d) Bronchoscope

**92. The focus of hospice care is:**
(a) Promotive (b) Curative
(c) Rehabilitation (d) Palliative

**93. Florence Nightingale was born on:**
(a) 12th May 1820 (b) 12th May 1830
(c) 12th April 1820 (d) 12th April 1830

**94. All of the following are elements of communication EXCEPT:**
(a) Encoder (b) Motivator
(c) Message (d) Decoder

**95. Cheilosis is:**
(a) Drying and cracking of lips
(b) Cracking of nails
(c) Fissure of tongue
(d) Cracking of lips

**96. The best effective way of breaking the chain of infection in the hospital is:**
(a) Hand washing
(b) Wearing gloves
(c) Isolated patient
(d) Providing private room for the patient

**97. Position used to examine the rectum is:**
(a) Knee-chest position (b) Supine
(c) Lithotomy (d) Prone

**98. Anorexia denotes:**
(a) Loss of sleep (b) Loss of appetite
(c) Excessive hunger (d) Excessive thirst

**99. Bluish discoloration of skin due to inadequate oxygenation is:**
(a) Hypoxia (b) Anoxia
(c) Cyanosis (d) Pallor

**100. Which of the following taxonomy is used worldwide for formulating diagnosis?**
(a) NANDA (b) TNAI
(c) ICN (d) INC

**101. Glossitis means:**
(a) Inflammation of oral mucosa
(b) Inflammation of tongue
(c) Inflammation of gums
(d) Inflammation of parotid gland

**102. The nurse is answerable for her own action. This is:**
(a) Responsibility
(b) Accountability
(c) Competence
(d) Negligence

**103. For a blood pressure reading of 140/70 mm of Hg, the pulse pressure is:**
(a) 40 (b) 68
(c) 140 (d) 72

**104. To insert a nasogastric tube, measure the distance from:**
(a) Center of forehead to end of sternum
(b) Tip of nose to end of sternum
(c) Lip to umbilicus
(d) Tip of nose to earlobe and then to the end of sternum

**105. In communication, word should express an idea in a few, simple and clear way. This is called:**
(a) Humor (b) Message
(c) Brevity (d) Pacing

**106. Orientation is checked in terms of the following EXCEPT:**
(a) Time (b) Place
(c) Person (d) Consciousness

**107. In the semi-Fowler's position the head and the trunk is raised to an angle of:**
(a) 15–45° (b) 45–90°
(c) 10–30° (d) 45–60°

**108. The length of standard hospital bed is:**
(a) 6 feet (b) 6.5 feet
(c) 7 feet (d) 7.5 feet

**109. The action of soap is:**
(a) Lubricant
(b) Emollient
(c) Lowers the surface tension
(d) Increase the surface tension of water

**110. One gram of carbohydrate gives:**
(a) 9 kcal (b) 5 kcal
(c) 4 kcal (d) 2 kcal

**111. During surgical hand scrub the hand are scrubbed from:**
(a) Above the elbow (b) Fingertip to elbow
(c) Wrist to fingertip (d) Below the wrist

**112. WHO day is celebrated on:**
(a) 7th April (b) 10th May
(c) 9th April (d) 5th April

**113. The legal definition of death that facilitate organ donation is cessation of:**
(a) Pulse
(b) Respiration
(c) Function of brain
(d) Circulation and respiratory function

**114. Which of the following is not a barrier to effective communication:**
(a) Empathy (b) False reassurance
(c) Defensive behavior (d) Noise

**115. Entire coated tablets are supposed to dissolve in the:**
(a) Small intestine
(b) Stomach
(c) Sublingual mucus membrane
(d) Esophagus

**116. While taking nursing history the nurse promotes communication by:**
(a) Asking 'Why' and 'How' question
(b) Reassuring the patient that there is no cause for alarm
(c) Using broad open ended question
(d) Ask question that can be answered by Yes/No.

**117. Normal intestinal for a contain:**
(a) *E. coli* (b) *S. aureus*
(c) *Clostridium* (d) *Corynebacterium*

**118. Cyanosis is:**
(a) A non-life-threatening event
(b) A late sign of hypoxia
(c) A reliable measure of oxygenation status
(d) An early sign of hypoxia

**119. The priority while providing oral care to an unconscious patient is:**
(a) Prevent aspiration
(b) Prevent mouth odor
(c) Prevent dental caries
(d) Prevent mouth ulceration

**120. The best position given to a breathless patient is:**
(a) Supine (b) Fowler's
(c) Lateral (d) Prone

**121. The heat regulating factor is situated in:**
(a) Cerebrum (b) Cerebellum
(c) Hypothalamus (d) Medulla oblongata

**122. Risk factors are classified into:**
(a) Preventable and non-preventable
(b) Natural and man-made
(c) Treatable and non-treatable
(d) Modifiable and non-modifiable

**123. Maslow's hierarchy of basic needs is useful for planning and implementing nursing care; as it provides a structure for:**
(a) Making accurate nursing diagnosis
(b) Communicating concept
(c) Integrating critical thinking
(d) Establishing priorities of care

**124. Lasix is an example of:**
(a) Anticoagulant (b) Antihypertensive
(c) Diuretic (d) Analgesic

**125. The term nursing process was first published by Id Gyan Orlando in year:**
(a) 1987 (b) 1967
(c) 1950 (d) 1946

**126. A standing order is a:**
(a) Document written and signed by senior nurse
(b) Pre-printed document directing conduct of care in given setting
(c) Protocol to be observed while caring patient in selected clinical area
(d) Physician order documented on patients case chart

**127. To maintain its internal environment at a constant state through:**
(a) Internalization (b) Adaptation
(c) Cellular integrity (d) Homeostasis

**128. Which of the following therapeutic intervention uses moist heat?**
(a) Sitz bath
(b) Infrared light
(c) A commercial hot pack
(d) An aquathermia pad

**129. The internal structure of ear can be visualized using following instrument:**
(a) An otoscope (b) A stethoscope
(c) An ophthalmoscope (d) A tuning fork

**130. A patient's temperature is 38.8° Celsius. The Fahrenheit equivalent:**
(a) 99.8°F (b) 100°F
(c) 101.8°F (d) 103.2°F

**131. The term used to indicate rapid pulse rate:**
(a) Palpitation (b) Bradycardia
(c) Arrhythmia (d) Tachycardia

**132. Which of the following term is used to describe when a person is aware of her own heart beats without feeling pulse:**
(a) Arrhythmia (b) Pulse rhythm
(c) Dysrhythmia (d) Palpitation

**133. Due to which of the following action $KMNO_4$ is used for mouth care:**
(a) Cleansing agent (b) Astringent agent
(c) Oxidizing agent (d) Antiseptic agent

**134. An example of nonverbal communication is:**
(a) Speaking (b) Moaning
(c) Reading (d) Writing

**135. Which of the following system include skin as its main component?**
(a) Immune system (b) Muscular system
(c) Endocrine system (d) Integumentary system

**136. The trade name of the drug refers to:**
(a) Chemical name of the drug
(b) The name given by the manufacturer to the drug
(c) The drug generic name
(d) The action of drug

**137. Which of the following statement is used to describe systolic pressure?**
(a) The phase during which heart is working
(b) The phase during which heart is resting
(c) The pressure in arteries when heart is resting
(d) The pressure in arteries when heart is contracting

**138. The abbreviation 'SOS' used regarding the time of medication administration means:**
(a) Save our soul
(b) If necessary in emergency
(c) At once
(d) Repeat after hours

**139. The scalds are caused due to:**
(a) Electric current
(b) Hot metals
(c) Steam
(d) Friction

**140. The minimum number of times the nurse should check the label when prescribed drug is given to the patient:**
(a) 2 (b) 3
(c) 4 (d) 5

**141. The primary goal of infection control is:**
(a) To control infectious microorganism from reproducing
(b) To control infectious microorganism on one place
(c) To prevent spread of infectious microorganism
(d) Limit microorganism to hospital premises

**142. Narcolepsy is a condition characterized by:**
(a) Excessive anxiety
(b) Excessive sleeping
(c) Excessive fatigue
(d) Excessive sleeplessness

**143. The technique of inspection is best described as:**
(a) Tapping on particular part of the body to produce sound
(b) The sense of feel, touch or press on body
(c) Many senses of examiner to scan (exam) the patient
(d) The sense of hearing to listen only body sound

**144. Which of the following technique is used for breast self-examination?**
(a) Auscultation and percussion
(b) Palpitation and percussion
(c) Inspection and palpitation
(d) Palpitation and auscultation

**145. A persons state of health, wellness and illness depends upon:**
(a) Self-concept (b) Lifestyle
(c) Known risk factor (d) Values and personality

**146. The health status of an individual community is:**
(a) One dimensional
(b) Multifactorial
(c) Determined by agency
(d) Psychosocial status

**147. Presence of certain risk factor:**
(a) Has no role in health practice
(b) Suggest that disease will definitely develop
(c) Increases the chance of developing disease
(d) Increases the chance of progressing disease

**148. Who is the founder of scientific medicine:**
(a) Hippocrates (b) Askipos
(c) Charaka (d) Sushruta

**149. Adult blood pressure is 120/80 mm of Hg normally, the 120 represent:**
(a) Pulse pressure (b) Capillary pressure
(c) Diastolic pressure (d) Systolic pressure

**150. According to primitive people illness was caused by:**
(a) Anger of offended god, evil spirit
(b) Lack of hygiene
(c) Lack of hospital
(d) Invasion organism

**151. Hyperpnea is:**
(a) Increased rate of respiration
(b) Difficulty in breathing
(c) Increase in depth of breathing
(d) Noisy breathing

**152. Early ambulation is ordered in postoperative patient to protect the patient form following postoperative complication:**
(a) Pain (b) Nausea
(c) Wound dehiscence (d) Deep wound thrombosis

**153. Chyluria means:**
(a) Milky white urine (b) Smoky white urine
(c) Pinkish brown urine (d) Bright red color urine

**154. Which of the following nursing skill a nurse needs to obtain accurate information?**
(a) Cognitive skill (b) Teaching skill
(c) Psychomotor skill (d) Interpersonal skill

**155. Grief is the emotional and behavioral response to loss a factor that influence an older adult's grief response is:**
(a) Cultural background
(b) Socio-economic background
(c) Sense of achievement in life
(d) Support available from family member

**156. Failure in professional duty, skill and practice that leads to injury or harm to the client is termed as:**
(a) Malpractice (b) Will
(c) Omission (d) Slander

**157. Infection that results from health care services is referred to as:**
(a) Endogenic infection
(b) Exogeous infection
(c) Nosocomial infection
(d) None of the above

**158. Pathogenicity refers to:**
(a) Capacity of pathogen to cause disease
(b) Accessibility of pathogen to host
(c) Capacity of pathogen to produce toxins
(d) Amount of pathogen present

**159. Subjective data is information obtained from:**
(a) Patient (b) Significant other
(c) Physician (d) Record

**160. Effect of neglected mouth care in illness result in:**
(a) Hemoptysis (b) Parotitis
(c) Oral cancer (d) Stomatitis

**161. Which of the following is part of physical examination:**
(a) Data collection (b) Blood investigation
(c) Auscultation (d) Observation

**162. Acute illness is characterized by:**
(a) Long duration of illness of more than 6 months
(b) Slow progressing illness
(c) Short duration illness with severe illness
(d) Short duration illness with mild symptoms

**163. Foot drop commonly occurs due to:**
(a) Improper position of immobilized patient
(b) Unconsciousness
(c) Generalized weakness
(d) Paraplegia

**164. Patient with heat exhaustion should:**
(a) Avoid drinking fluids
(b) Be covered to prevent shivering
(c) Be cooled as soon as possible
(d) Be given water with salt

**165. The steps in nursing process are all:**
(a) Assessment
(b) Diagnosis
(c) Guidance
(d) Evaluation

**166. The purpose of discharge planning is to:**
(a) Make sure patient takes medications prescribed
(b) Provide medical treatment
(c) Provide health teaching
(d) Ensure continuity of care

**167. An attitude for critical thinking is all EXCEPT:**
(a) Confidence (b) Fearlessness
(c) Risk taking (d) Humility

**168. The purpose of tepid sponge is to:**
(a) Clean the patient's body thoroughly
(b) Induces sleep to the patient
(c) Reduces temperature in febrile patient

**169. Pulse rate less than 60 per minute is known as:**
(a) Tachycardia (b) Water hummer pulse
(c) Dicrotic pulse (d) Bradycardia

**170. The difference between apical pulse and radial pulse is termed as:**
(a) Pulse pressure (b) Asystole
(c) Arrhythmia (d) Pulse deficit

**171. Secondary prevention focuses on all EXCEPT:**
(a) Health risk assessment
(b) Early protection of disease
(c) Health maintenance
(d) Promote interventions

**172. The blood pressure focuses the measurement of:**
(a) Forces of blood against venous wall
(b) Force of blood against arterial wall
(c) Force of blood through the circulation
(d) Flow of blood through heart

**173. The important purpose of change of shift report:**
(a) To maintain standard of care
(b) To adhere to the hospital policy
(c) To ensure continuity of care
(d) To maintain higher quality of care

**174. The nurse detected dull sound while percussing thorax and lungs which indicate:**
(a) A bony structure (b) Air filled cavity
(c) Fluid or solid mass (d) Emphysematous tissue

**175. Potassium deficit in the extracellular fluid is termed as:**
(a) Hyponatremia (b) Hypovolemia
(c) Hypocalcemia (d) Hypokalemia

**176. Which of the technique allows discussion during nurse–patient interview:**
(a) Close ended question
(b) Open ended question
(c) Heading type of question
(d) Problem seeking

**177. Postural drainage includes all EXCEPT:**
(a) Palpation (b) Percussion
(c) Vibration (d) Positioning

**178. Normal heart sound heard on auscultation are:**
(a) $S_0 S_1$ (b) $S_1 S_2$
(c) $S_2 S_3$ (d) $S_3 S_4$

**179. Pulse oximetry measures oxygen level in:**
(a) Muscle (b) Tissue
(c) Venous blood (d) Arterial blood

**180. The normal tidal volume is:**
(a) 3 to 5 mL/kg body weight
(b) 10 to 15 mL/kg body weight
(c) 18 to 20 mL/kg body weight
(d) 2 to 4 mL/kg body weight

**181. Which of the following enema is used to expel the flatus from bowel through rectum and relive ones gaseous distention:**
(a) Retention enema (b) An anthelmintic enema
(c) A carminative enema (d) Medicated enema

**182. In health and illness continuum model the health is believed to be:**
(a) Stable (b) Developing
(c) Dynamic (d) Stagnant

**183. The internal structure of the eye can be visualized by using a/an:**
(a) Otoscope (b) Ophthalmoscope
(c) Stethoscope (d) Tuning fork

**184. The agent, host and environment model of the health and illness is based on the concept of:**
(a) Risk factor
(b) Infectious disease
(c) Health promotion behavior
(d) Stage of illness

**185. For which of the following patient oral temperature can be taken?**
(a) 6 months old infant
(b) Patient receiving oxygen
(c) A 56-year-old health woman
(d) An unconscious patient

**186. A patient having dyspnea, to facilitate respiration the nurse would**
(a) Remove pillow from under the head
(b) Elevate the head end of the bed upto 30–45°
(c) Elevate the foot of bed upto 30–40°
(d) Take blood pressure immediately and hourly

**187. When assessing the abdomen which technique should be conducted after inspection for best evaluation**
(a) Percussion
(b) Palpation
(c) Auscultation
(d) Sequence does not matters

**188. The recommended sequence of removing soiled personal protective equipment when nurse prepare to leave patients room is to remove:**
(a) Gown, goggles, mask, gloves, and exit the room
(b) Gloves, wash hand, remove gown, mask and goggle
(c) Gloves, mask, gown and wash hand
(d) Goggles, mask, gloves and hand wash

**189. During the bath nurse observe that a patient has a dry skin. Which of the following action should be best for the patient?**
(a) Bath the patient and apply spirit
(b) Use an emollient on dry skin
(c) Massage the skin with alcohol
(d) Discourage the fluid intake

**190. Which of the following is the most common site for pressure ulcer when patient is constantly lying in supine position:**
(a) Shoulder (b) Sacrum
(c) Sternum (d) Humerus

**191. Which of the following would the nurse expect to assess as a physiological response to moderate pain:**
(a) Increased pain
(b) Restlessness
(c) Decreased pulse rate
(d) Protection of a painful area

**192. Which term denotes patient's inability to void even though the kidneys are producing urine that enter bladder?**
(a) Urgency (b) Retention
(c) Oliguria (d) Dysuria

**193. The nurse completing anthropometric measurement for a patient collects which of the following information:**
(a) Height and weight
(b) Serum hemoglobin and hematocrit
(c) Diet history
(d) Intake output

**194. The movement of solvent water from an area of lesser concentration to an area of grater solute concentration until equilibrium is established is known as:**
(a) Osmosis (b) Diffusion
(c) Active transport (d) Filtration

**195. Which of the following would the nurse use as the most reliable indicator for patient's fluid balance status?**
(a) Intake and output
(b) Skin turgor
(c) Complete blood count
(d) Daily weight

**196. A nurse caring for an obese 62 years old patient with arthritis, who developed an open reddened area over his sacrum. A priority nursing diagnosis is:**
(a) Imbalance nutrition more than body requirement related to immobilization
(b) Impaired physical mobility related to pain and discomfort
(c) Chronic pain related to immobility
(d) Risk for infection related to alter skin integrity

**197. When using an otoscope to assess the tympanic membrane of an adult the ear canal is straightened by gently pulling the pinna:**
(a) Up and back
(b) Down and forward
(c) Away from examiner
(d) In any direction

**198. With ageing blood pressure is often higher due to:**
(a) Loss of muscle mass
(b) Change in exercise and diet
(c) Decrease peripheral resistance
(d) Decreased elasticity of arterial wall

**199. Which of the following is the most important factor in hand washing:**
(a) Time (b) Friction
(c) Soap (d) Lotion and sprit

**200. Presence of sugar in urine is called:**
(a) Renal threshold (b) Glycosuria
(c) Oliguria (d) Hematuria

**201. One liter is equal to:**
(a) 500 mL (b) 750 mL
(c) 1000 mL (d) 1500 mL

**202. Who is known as Father of Surgery in India:**
(a) Narsimha (b) Sushruta
(c) Bhima (d) Charaka

**203. Implementation of nursing process involve:**
(a) Collection of data
(b) Giving actual nursing care
(c) Measuring effectiveness of nursing care
(d) Systematically developing nursing care plan

**204. Oxygen is stored under pressure of:**
(a) 2200 lbs per sq inch (b) 1500 lbs per sq inch
(c) 2000 lbs per sq inch (d) 1000 lbs per sq inch

**205. On application of ice bag to client with fever, heat is transmitted through:**
(a) Conduction (b) Convection
(c) Evaporation (d) Radiation

**206. The word ethic is derived from Greek word 'ethos' meaning:**
(a) Manners (b) Practice
(c) Guiding line (d) Ethnicity

**207. Premature babies are given oxygen in low concentration to avoid:**
(a) Cardiac failure
(b) Atelectasis
(c) Retrolental fibroplasias
(d) Asphyxia

**208. Increase in depth of respiration:**
(a) Apnea (b) Orthopnea
(c) Hyperpnea (d) Tachypnea

**209. For simple evacuant enema the _____ of solution is used:**
(a) 250 mL (b) 500–1000 mL
(c) 1200 mL (d) 250–500 mL

**210. Stupes are commonly used:**
(a) Relaxing the muscle spasm
(b) Relive pain
(c) Avoid thrombosis
(d) To maintain body flexion

**211. Hydrogen peroxide acts as:**
(a) Cleansing agent (b) Oxidizing agent
(c) Antiseptic agent (d) Bacteriostatic agent

**212. It is complication of local cold application:**
(a) Pain (b) Cyanosis
(c) Burn and blister (d) Infection

**213. The feeding given through opening made on the abdominal wall:**
(a) Gastric gavage (b) Esophageal feeding
(c) Oral feeding (d) RT feeding

## ANSWERS

| **1.** | (a) | **21.** | (c) | **41.** | (c) | **61.** | (a) | **81.** | (a) | **101.** | (b) |
|---|---|---|---|---|---|---|---|---|---|---|---|
| **2.** | (c) | **22.** | (b) | **42.** | (d) | **62.** | (d) | **82.** | (c) | **102.** | (b) |
| **3.** | (d) | **23.** | (b) | **43.** | (a) | **63.** | (a) | **83.** | (d) | **103.** | (c) |
| **4.** | (c) | **24.** | (c) | **44.** | (a) | **64.** | (d) | **84.** | (a) | **104.** | (d) |
| **5.** | (a) | **25.** | (a) | **45.** | (d) | **65.** | (a) | **85.** | (a) | **105.** | (b) |
| **6.** | (a) | **26.** | (a) | **46.** | (b) | **66.** | (c) | **86.** | (d) | **106.** | (d) |
| **7.** | (b) | **27.** | (b) | **47.** | (a) | **67.** | (a) | **87.** | (b) | **107.** | (a) |
| **8.** | (c) | **28.** | (c) | **48.** | (b) | **68.** | (b) | **88.** | (b) | **108.** | (b) |
| **9.** | (d) | **29.** | (d) | **49.** | (c) | **69.** | (d) | **89.** | (c) | **109.** | (c) |
| **10.** | (a) | **30.** | (a) | **50.** | (b) | **70.** | (b) | **90.** | (a) | **110.** | (c) |
| **11.** | (c) | **31.** | (d) | **51.** | (d) | **71.** | (a) | **91.** | (a) | **111.** | (b) |
| **12.** | (d) | **32.** | (c) | **52.** | (a) | **72.** | (c) | **92.** | (d) | **112.** | (a) |
| **13.** | (c) | **33.** | (a) | **53.** | (d) | **73.** | (b) | **93.** | (a) | **113.** | (c) |
| **14.** | (b) | **34.** | (c) | **54.** | (c) | **74.** | (b) | **94.** | (b) | **114.** | (a) |
| **15.** | (a) | **35.** | (b) | **55.** | (a) | **75.** | (a) | **95.** | (d) | **115.** | (a) |
| **16.** | (d) | **36.** | (a) | **56.** | (d) | **76.** | (c) | **96.** | (a) | **116.** | (a) |
| **17.** | (a) | **37.** | (b) | **57.** | (b) | **77.** | (a) | **97.** | (d) | **117.** | (a) |
| **18.** | (c) | **38.** | (d) | **58.** | (a) | **78.** | (b) | **98.** | (b) | **118.** | (b) |
| **19.** | (c) | **39.** | (a) | **59.** | (c) | **79.** | (b) | **99.** | (c) | **119.** | (d) |
| **20.** | (a) | **40.** | (c) | **60.** | (b) | **80.** | (d) | **100.** | (a) | **120.** | (b) |

| **121.** | (c) | **141.** | (c) | **161.** | (c) | **181.** | (c) | **201.** | (c) | | |
|---|---|---|---|---|---|---|---|---|---|---|---|
| **122.** | (d) | **142.** | (d) | **162.** | (c) | **182.** | (c) | **202.** | (b) | | |
| **123.** | (d) | **143.** | (c) | **163.** | (d) | **183.** | (b) | **203.** | (b) | | |
| **124.** | (c) | **144.** | (c) | **164.** | (d) | **184.** | (b) | **204.** | (b) | | |
| **125.** | (c) | **145.** | (b) | **165.** | (c) | **185.** | (c) | **205.** | (a) | | |
| **126.** | (b) | **146.** | (b) | **166.** | (b) | **186.** | (b) | **206.** | (c) | | |
| **127.** | (d) | **147.** | (c) | **167.** | (b) | **187.** | (b) | **207.** | (c) | | |
| **128.** | (a) | **148.** | (a) | **168.** | (c) | **188.** | (c) | **208.** | (b) | | |
| **129.** | (a) | **149.** | (d) | **169.** | (d) | **189.** | (b) | **209.** | (b) | | |
| **130.** | (c) | **150.** | (a) | **170.** | (d) | **190.** | (b) | **210.** | (a) | | |
| **131.** | (d) | **151.** | (c) | **171.** | (b) | **191.** | (b) | **211.** | (b) | | |
| **132.** | (d) | **152.** | (d) | **172.** | (b) | **192.** | (b) | **212.** | (b) | | |
| **133.** | (d) | **153.** | (a) | **173.** | (c) | **193.** | (a) | **213.** | (a) | | |
| **134.** | (b) | **154.** | (d) | **174.** | (d) | **194.** | (a) | | | | |
| **135.** | (d) | **155.** | (d) | **175.** | (d) | **195.** | (a) | | | | |
| **136.** | (b) | **156.** | (a) | **176.** | (b) | **196.** | (d) | | | | |
| **137.** | (d) | **157.** | (c) | **177.** | (c) | **197.** | (a) | | | | |
| **138.** | (b) | **158.** | (a) | **178.** | (b) | **198.** | (d) | | | | |
| **139.** | (c) | **159.** | (a) | **179.** | (d) | **199.** | (b) | | | | |
| **140.** | (b) | **160.** | (d) | **180.** | (a) | **200.** | (b) | | | | |

# QUICK REVIEW

## Microbiology Review and Multiple Choice Questions

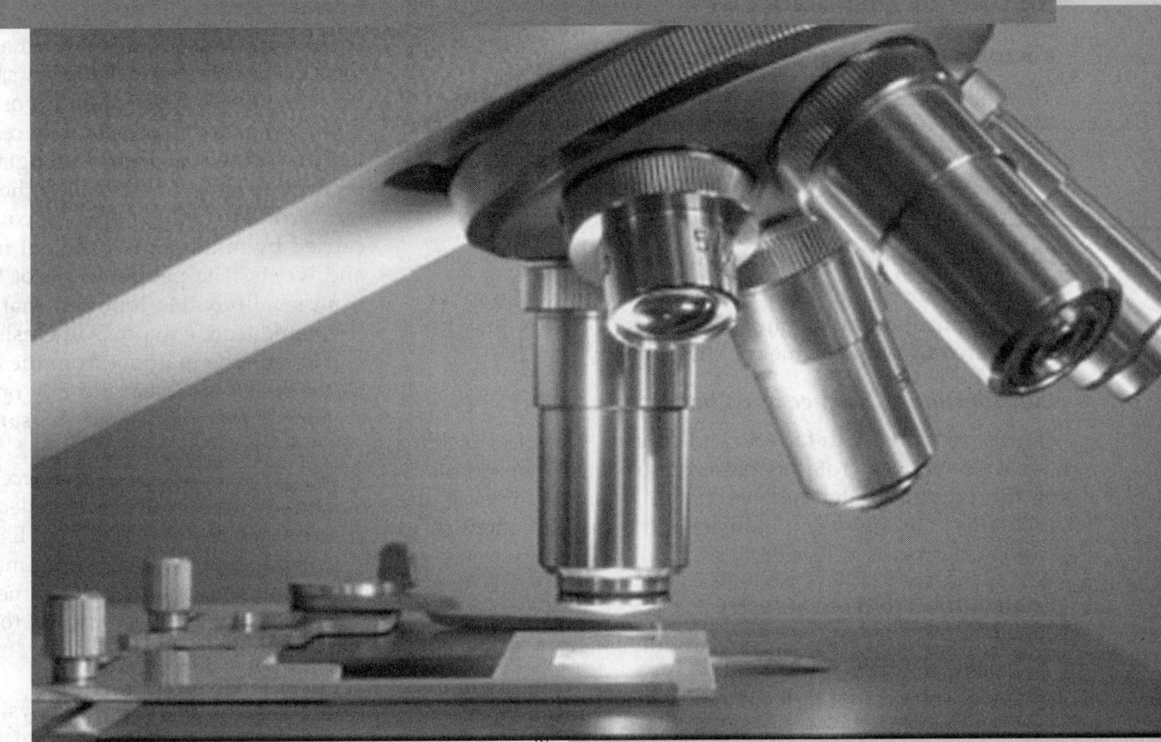

### HIGHLIGHTS

- History of Microbiology
- Stains and Staining Reactions
- Sterilization
- Pure Culture Methods
- Medical Microbiology Microbial Diseases
- Respiratory Tract Infections
- Urinary Tract Infections
- Sexually Transmitted Diseases
- Bacterial Infections of Gastrointestinal Tract
- Types of Clinical Manifestations
- Structure and Development of Immune System
- Multiple Choice Questions

# Microbiology

## HISTORY OF MICROBIOLOGY

### Microbiology

Microbiology is a science that deals with the study of living organisms that cannot be seen by the naked eye. These can be seen with the aid of microscopes, which magnify objects. Many scientists contributed to the science of microbiology.

### Louis Pasteur (1822–1895)

**Louis Pasteur** was a French chemist and a crystallographer.

His contribution to microbiology is so great that he is considered to be the 'Father of Microbiology'.

#### *Contribution to Science as a Chemist*

He was working with tartaric acid crystals. He could pick up the dextro and levo rotatory crystals by seeing the morphology of the crystals. Later he was called to solve some of the problems in fermentation industry and turned his attention to biological process of fermentation.

#### *Contribution to Wine Industry*

- He discovered that alcohol production from grape juice was due to yeast.
- He found out that large amounts of lactic acid production was due to the presence or contamination of rod shaped bacteria.
- He observed that the process of alcohol production, i.e. fermentation took place in the absence of air.
- He coined the terms **aerobic** to describe those organisms requiring air and **anaerobic** to describe those organisms which do not require air for their growth.

#### *Contribution to Modern Microbiology*

Pasteur disproved the theory of spontaneous generation. The theory proposed that living organisms originated spontaneously, particularly from decaying organic matter. He disproved it.

#### *Pasteur's Swan Neck Flask*

Pasteur poured meat infusions into flasks and then drew the top of each flask into a long curved neck that would admit air but not dust. He found that if the infusions were heated, they remained sterile (free from any growth) until they were exposed to dust. He opened them on a dusty road and resealed them and demonstrated the growth of microorganisms in all the flasks. The unopened flasks were sterile.

Thus, he disproved the theory of spontaneous generation.

### Edward Jenner, 1796

It was an ancient observation that persons who had suffered from a specific disease such as smallpox or mumps, resisted the infection on subsequent exposures. They rarely contracted it second time. Such acquired resistance is specific. Edward Jenner—a country doctor in England noted a pustular disease on the hooves of horses called the grease. This was carried by farm workers to the nipples of cows (cowpox). This was again carried by milkmaids. They got inflamed spots on the hands and wrists. The people who got this cowpox were protected from smallpox. He reported that 16 farm workers who had recovered from cowpox were resistant to smallpox infection.

- He took the material from the cowpox and inoculated into the cut of an 8 year old boy on 14 May 1796. Two months later Jenner inoculated the same boy with material taken from smallpox patients.
- This was a dangerous but accepted procedure of that time and the procedure was called variolation. The boy was protected against smallpox. His exposure to the mild disease cowpox had made him immune to the disease smallpox.
- In this manner Jenner began the science of immunology, the study of the body's response to foreign substances.

### Robert Koch (1843–1910)

**Robert Koch** was a German physician.

- For the first time he showed the evidence that a specific germ (Anthrax bacillus) was the cause of a specific disease (splenic fever in sheep).
- He established that a specific germ can cause a specific disease and introduced scientific approach in microbiology.
- He discovered *Bacillus anthracis* (Anthrax bacillus), *Mycobacterium tuberculosis*, and *Vibrio cholerae*.
- He modified Ziehl-Neelsen acid fast staining procedure which was introduced by Ehrlich.
- He devised the solid medium to grow the microorganism to get single colonies.
- He introduced Koch's thread method to find out the efficacy of disinfectants.
- He established certain rules that must be followed to establish a cause and effect relationship between a microorganism and a disease. They are known as **Koch's postulates.**
- He also described the **Koch's phenomenon.**

#### *Koch's Postulates*

Robert Koch developed powerful method to isolate the organisms in pure culture from diseased tissue. He also perfected the techniques of identification of the isolated bacteria.

### *The Need for Koch's Postulates*

In those days, there were no perfect techniques to identify the organisms. Solid media and staining techniques were not available.

So the etiological role of organisms was not known.

To prove the etiology there were not strict criteria. So there was a need to establish criteria.

- The organism should be regularly seen in the lesions of the disease.
- It should be isolated in pure culture on artificial media.
- Inoculation of this culture should produce a similar disease in experimental animals.
- The organism must be recovered from the lesions in these animals.

### *Postulate 1*

- The organism should be found in lesions of the disease.
- All the causative agents of the disease are seen in the particular diseases. If we take *Pneumococci* as example, they are seen in all the pneumonia cases.

### *Postulate 2*

- It should be isolated and grown in solid media.
- *Pneumococci* are grown in solid media and are isolated from the diseases. Some organisms do not grow on solid media or the solid media are not developed yet.
  *Examples, Mycobacterium leprae* and *Treponema pallidum.*

### *Postulate 3*

- The organisms should produce the exact disease in experimental animals.
- Almost all the pathogenic organisms produce the same disease in experimental animals.
- Usually rats, mice, rabbits or guinea pigs are used as experimental animals.
- *Pneumococci* produce pneumonia in animals. *Salmonella* species do not produce typhoid fever in rat, mice or rabbit. So chimpanzee is taken as experimental animal and it produces fever in chimpanzee.

### *Postulate 4*

- It should be isolated from the diseased animal also.
- *Pneumococci* are isolated from the experimental animals also.

### *Modern Addition to Koch's Postulates*

- Today we recognize additional criteria of causal relation between a microorganism and a disease.
- The important one is the demonstration of abnormally high concentration of specific circulating antibodies to the organism in the infected host.
- Or the presence of abnormally high degree of specific immunity or hypersensitivity to the infecting agent in a recently recovered host.

### *Limitations*

Some organisms have not yet been grown in artificial culture media. *Examples, Mycobacterium leprae* and *Treponema pallidum.*

### *Usefulness of Koch's Postulates*

- It is useful in determining pathogenic organisms.
- To differentiate the pathogenic and nonpathogenic micro-organism.
- For the classification of organisms.
- To detect the susceptibility, resistance of the laboratory animals.

### *Conclusion*

Koch has done a valuable work in the field of Microbiology and has made postulates, which have merits, demerits and limitations with modern omission and addition.

## THE COMPOUND LIGHT MICROSCOPE

Anton van Leeuwenhoek of Delft, Holland, constructed simple microscopes composed of double convex glass lenses held between two silver plates. His microscopes could magnify around 50 to 300 times. Microbiologists currently use a variety of light microscopes.

Modern microscopes are all compound microscopes. The light microscopy refers to the use of any kind of microscope that uses visible light to make the specimens observable. The most commonly used light microscopes are:

- Bright-field microscopes
- Dark-field microscopes
- Phase contrast microscopes
- Fluorescence microscopes

Each type of microscope is adapted for certain type of observations.

The standard ordinary light microscope is called a bright-field microscope, because it forms a dark image against a brighter background. A compound microscope with a single eye piece (ocular) is called monocular and with two eye pieces is called binocular.

- A mirror or an electric illuminator is a light source which is located in the base of the microscope.
- There are two focusing knobs, the fine and the coarse adjustment knobs which are located on the arm. These are used to move either the stage or the nosepiece to focus the image.
- The mechanical stage is positioned about halfway up the arm, which allows precise contact of moving the slide.
- The sub stage condenser is mounted within or beneath the stage and focuses a cone of light on the slide. In simpler microscopes, its position is fixed whereas in advanced microscopes it can be adjusted vertically.

The upper part of the microscope arm holds the body assembly.

The nose piece and one or more eyepieces or oculars are attached to it. The body assembly contains a series of mirrors and prisms so that the barrel holding the eyepiece may be tilted for viewing. Three or five objectives with different magnification power are fixed to the nose piece and can be rotated to the position beneath the body assembly. A microscope should always be par focal, i.e. the image should remain in focus when objectives are changed. Light enters the microscope from the base and passes through a blue filter which filters out the long wavelengths of light, leaving the shorter wavelengths and improving the resolution. The light then goes through the condenser which converges the light beams so that they pass through the specimen.

The iris diaphragm controls the amount of light that passes through the specimen and into the objective lens. For higher magnification, greater the amount of light needed to view the specimen clearly. The objective lens magnifies the image before it passes through body tube to the ocular lens in the eyepiece. The ocular of light needed to view the specimen clearly. The objective lens magnifies the image before it passes through body tube to the ocular lens in the eyepiece. The ocular lens further magnifies the image. The total magnification of the light microscope is calculated by multiplying the magnifying power of the objective lens by the magnifying power of the ocular lens.

Representative magnification values for a 10 X ocular are:
Scanning (4X) × (10X) = 40X magnification
Low power (10X) × (10x) = 100X magnification
High dry (40X) × (10X) = 400X magnification
Oil immersion (100X) × (10X) = 1000X magnification

### Microscope Resolution

Objective is the important part in the microscope which is responsible to produce a clear image. The resolution of the objective is most important. Resolution is the capacity of a lens to separate or distinguish between small objects that are close together.

The major factor in the resolution is the wave length of light used. The greatest resolution obtained with light of the shortest wavelength, that is the light at the blue end of the visible spectrum in the range of 450 to 500 nm. The highest resolution possible in a compound light microscope is about 0.2 ìm. That means, the two objects closer together than 0.2 ìm are not resolvable as distinct and separate. The light microscope is equipped with three or four objectives. The working distance of an objective is the distance between the front surface of the lens and the surface of the cover glass or the specimen. Objectives with large numerical apertures and great resolving power have short working distances.

### Numerical Aperture

The resolving power of a light microscope depends on the wavelength of light used and the numerical aperture (NA) of the objective lenses.

The NA of a lens can be increased by:

- Increasing the size of the lens opening and/or
- Increasing the refractive index of the material between the lens and the specimen.

The larger the numerical aperture the better the resolving power. It is important to illuminate the specimens properly to have higher resolution.

The concave mirror in the microscope creates a narrow cone of light and has a small numerical aperture. However, the resolution can be improved with a sub stage condenser.

A wide cone of light through the slide and into the objective lens increases the numerical aperture there by improves the resolution of the microscope.

### Oil Immersion

Oil immersion lens is designed to be in direct contact with the oil placed on the cover slip. An oil immersion lens has a short focal length and hence there is a short working distance between the objective lens and the specimen. Immersion oil has a refractive index closer to that of glass than the refractive index of air, so the use of oil increases the cone of light that enters the objective lens.

Because of refractive index the light passing from the glass into air makes the light to bend.

The light passing from glass through oil does not bend much because the oil has similar refractive index to that of a glass.

The immersion oil with a refractive index of about 1.5 increases the numerical aperture and increases the resolving power of the microscope.

## STAINS AND STAINING REACTIONS

Bacteria are semi-transparent and consist of a clear protoplasmic matter that differs slightly in refractive index from the medium in which they are growing. It is difficult to observe the bacteria in unstained state, except when special methods of illumination are used, to see them in the unstained state.

Stains are useful for the following reasons:

- It makes the microscopic semi-transparent objects visible
- To study the shape and size
- To reveal the presence of various internal and external structures
- To produce specific chemical and physical reaction.

The term stain and dye are not the same. A coloring agent that is used for general purposes is called a dye. The one that is used for biological purposes is called a stain. Based on their chemical behavior, the dyes are classified as acidic, basic and neutral.

An acid (or anionic) dye has a negative charge, e.g. Eosin, Rose Bengal and acid fuchsin. The negatively charged groups are carboxyls (-COOH) and phenolic hydroxyls (-OH). Since they are negatively charged, bind to positively charged cell structures. pH plays an important role in the effectiveness of staining, because the nature and the degree of the charge on cell components change with pH. The anionic dyes stain better under acidic conditions, where the proteins and many other molecules carry a positive charge.

A basic dye (or cationic) carries a positive charge, e.g. methylene blue, basic fuchsin, crystal violet, malachite green, safranin. Basic dyes bind to negatively charged molecules like nucleic acid and many proteins. Since the bacterial cells surfaces are negatively charged, basic dyes are most often used in bacteriology. Basic dyes are normally available as chloride salts.

A neutral dye is a complex salt of a dye acid with a dye base.

The dyes used in bacteriology have two features in common.

1. They have chromophore groups, groups with double bonds, that give the dye its color.
2. They can bind with cells by ionic, covalent or hydrophobic bonding.

Relationship between the type of the dye and its charge when dissociated is summarized.

In positive staining procedure, a stain that has a positively charged chromophore (colored portion of the stain molecule) is attracted to the negatively charged outer surface of the microbial cell. A stain such as methylene blue has a positively charged blue portion of the molecule that stains the microorganism.

In negative staining procedures, a negatively charged chromophore is repelled by the negatively charged microorganisms, resulting in negative or indirect staining of the microbial cell. Nigrosin and Indian ink are frequently used for negative staining of microbial cells, and this type of staining is particularly useful for viewing some structures such as capsules that surround some bacterial cells.

Stains are generally prepared largely as aqueous solutions.

However in some cases, stock solutions are prepared in alcohol, and are diluted with water as needed. Since alcohol removes the stains, pure alcoholic solutions should not be used. Staining solutions are prepared to contain low concentrations of stains rarely exceeding 1%. A very dilute staining solution activity for a long period of time will produce much better results than a more concentrated solution acting for a shorter interval. This procedure has to be followed to reveal internal structure in bacteria.

## Staining Reactions: Interpretation Notes

When the pH of the surroundings of the microbial cells is either neutral or alkaline, all microbial cells have a negative charge on their surface, called the surface charge. Many bacterial cultures produce acids, thereby adding hydrogen ions to a culture medium and decreasing its pH. These hydrogen ions ($H^+$) interact with the surface of the negative charges on the surface. When this happens, the cell surface no longer strongly attracts positively charged dye ions (basic dyes). Thus the microbes from acidic environments stain poorly with basic dyes. For this reason, the basic dyes are made up as alkaline solutions. For example, potassium hydroxide (KOH) is added to solutions of methylene blue to form the stain called Loeffler's Methylene blue.

Some bacteria excrete alkaline materials during growth and this decreases the number of available hydrogen ions in the culture medium. Under such conditions, the cell surface has a greater negative charge, which is more attractive to basic dyes and therefore, allows greater binding, penetration and internal staining of the microbe. Basic dyes stain microorganisms better under neutral or alkaline conditions.

If the dye base molecule has a negative charge, it is repelled by the cell's negatively charged surface. Thus negatively charged dyes neither bind to the cell's surface nor are they able to penetrate into the cell. These are called acid dyes.

The methodology for using acid dyes are different from basic dyes. An acid dye is mixed with a drop of culture smeared on a microscope slide and allowed to air dry. The negatively charged cells are not stained by the negatively charged dye, and they appear as clear area surrounded by a colored background.

Negatively charged dyes used in this way are called negative stains.

Under neutral or alkaline conditions, the negative stains (acidic dyes) work better, because these conditions allow the surface charge to be more negative. Negative stains are of limited usefulness for those using light microscopes, but they can be used to avoid some of the disadvantages of staining with basic dyes.

## Simple Staining

A simple staining solution, contains only one stain, which is dissolved in a solvent. It is applied to the microorganism in one application. The microorganisms give the color characteristic of the staining solution. The purpose of simple staining is to reveal the size and shape of the microorganism. The simple stains that are commonly used by the microbiologists for routine purposes are dilute solution of carbol fuchsin, crystal violet and methylene blue.

Methylene blue is more frequently used than any other stain in bacteriology. It is because of its strong nature and it stains nuclei and nucleic acid granules very intensively. Methylene blue is used for the rapid survey of bacterial population of milk. It is also used for the diagnosis of diphtheria. This stain is incorporated with Eosin in Lactose agar to distinguish typical *E. coli* in contaminated water.

## Differential Staining

In this procedure, more than one dye is employed. Differential staining procedure helps to divide the bacteria into separate groups based on staining characteristics. The two most important differential stains used by bacteriologists are Gram stain and Acidfast stain.

## Gram Staining

The simple staining procedure makes to visualize bacteria clearly, but it does not distinguish between organisms of similar morphology. In 1884, a Danish Physician named, Christian Gram discovered a new technique to differentiate the bacteria of similar morphology. He used two dyes in sequence, each of a different color. The organisms that retain the color of the first dye are called Gram-positive and those that cannot retain the first dye when washed with a decolorizing solution, but then take on the color of the second dye are called Gram-negative. In this method, the fixed bacterial smear is subjected to the following staining regents in the order of sequence listed below:

- Crystal violet
- Iodine solution
- Alcohol (decolorizing agent)
- Safranin.

### Principle

The Gram-positive bacteria will retain the crystal violet and appear deep violet in color. The Gram-negative bacteria lose the crystal violet on decolorization and are counter stained by the safranine and appear red in color. Iodine solution is used as a mordant that fixes the primary stain in or on a substrate by combining with the dye to form an insoluble compound-mordant, for the first stain.

The exact mechanism of action of this staining technique is not clearly understood. However, the most plausible explanations for the reactions are associated with the structure and composition of the cell wall.

The cell walls of Gram-negative bacteria are thinner than that of Gram-positive bacteria and contain a higher percentage of lipid content. During the staining of Gram-negative bacteria, the alcohol treatment extracts the lipid. This results in increased porosity or permeability of the cell wall. The crystal violet-iodine (CV-I) complex, thus can be extracted and the Gram-negative bacteria is decolorized. The cells subsequently take up the color of the counter stain safranin.

The cell walls of Gram-positive bacteria with lower lipid content become dehydrated during alcohol treatment. The pore size decreased, permeability is reduced and the CV-I complex cannot be extracted. Therefore, the Gram-positive cells remain purple-violet.

### Endospore Staining

Endospore formation is a distinguishing feature of the family Bacillaceae, which includes members of the aerobic genus *Bacillus* and the anaerobic genus *Clostridium.* Endospore resists adverse environmental conditions such as dryness, heat and poor nutrient supply. The endospore is a highly retractile body formed within the vegetative bacterial cell at a certain stage of growth.

The size, shape, and position of the spore are relatively constant characteristics of a given species and are therefore, of some value in distinguishing the kind of *Bacillus* from another. The position of the spore in the cell may be central, subterminal or terminal. It may be the same diameter as the cell, smaller or larger causing a swelling of the cell.

Endospores strongly resist application of simple dyes, but once stained are quiet resistant to decolorization. This character suggests one way to make the structure visible. If simple stains are used, the body of the *Bacillus* is deeply colored, whereas the spore is unstained and appears as a clear area in the organism. By vigorous staining procedures the dye can be introduced into the substance of the spore. When thus stained, the spore tends to retain the dye after treatment with decolorizing agents.

To make the distinction clear between the spore and the vegetative portion of the cell, a contrasting counter stain is usually applied in the ordinary fashion and the resulting picture shows the initial stain taken up by the spore and the second stain appear in the cytoplasm. Thus, it makes for a very simple method of distinguishing the endospore from the vegetative cell.

## STERILIZATION

Sterilization is the freeing of an article from all living organisms, including bacteria and their spores.

Sterilization of culture media, containers and instruments is essential in microbiological work for isolation and maintenance of microbes.

In surgery and medicine, the sterilization of instruments, drugs and other supplies is important for the prevention of infection.

Sterilization can be affected in a variety of ways, which can be conveniently categorized as follows:

**Physical methods**

- Heat
  - Dry heat
  - Moist heat
- Radiations
  - Ultraviolet radiations
  - Ionizing radiations
- Filtration

**Chemical methods**

### Sterilization by Heat

Heat can be applied in two forms:

1. The dry heat
2. Moist heat.

### Mechanism of Killing by Dry Heat

- Dry heat kills the organisms by destructive oxidation of essential cell constituents.
- Killing of the most resistant spores by dry heat requires a temperature of about 160°C for 60 minutes.
- Dry heat is employed for glassware; syringes, metal instruments and paper wrapped goods, which are not spoiled by high temperatures.
- It is also used for anhydrous fats, oils and powders that are impermeable to moisture.

### Mechanism of Killing by Moist Heat

- Moist heat kills the organisms by coagulating and denaturing their enzymes and structural protein.
- Sterilization by moist heat of the most resistant spores generally requires 121°C for 15–30 minutes.
- Moist heat is used for the sterilization of culture media, and all other materials through which steam can penetrate.
- Moist heat is more effective than dry heat.
- Sterilization can be done at lower temperatures in a given time at a shorter duration at the same temperature.

### Factors Influencing Sterilization by Heat

- **The temperature and time:** They are inversely related, shorter time is sufficient at high temperatures.
- **Number of microorganisms and spores:** The number of survivors diminished exponentially with the duration of heating.
- Depends on the species, strains and spore forming ability of the microbes.
- Thermal death point is the lowest temperature to give complete killing in aqueous suspension within 10 minutes.
- **Depends on the nature of material:** A high content of organic substances generally tends to protect spores and vegetative organisms against heat.
- Presence of organic or inorganic disinfectants facilitates killing by heat.

- pH also plays an important role in the killing of microorganisms.

## Methods of Sterilization by Dry Heat

### *Red Heat*

Inoculating wires, points of forceps and searing spatulas are sterilized by holding them in the flame of Bunsen burner until they are seen to be red-hot.

### *Flaming*

- This method is used for sterilizing scalpel, mouth of culture tubes, glass slides, etc.
- It involves passing of an article through Bunsen flame without allowing it to become red-hot.

### *Hot Air Oven*

- This is the main means of sterilization by dry heat.
- Exposure at a temperature of 160°C for 1 hour is generally employed.

### *Infrared Radiations*

Source employed is an electrically heated element, the infra red rays are directed on to the object to be sterilized and temperature of 180°C can be obtained.

## Methods of Sterilization by Moist Heat

Moist heat can be employed at:

- Temperature below 100°C
- Temperature of 100°C
- Temperature above 100°C.

### *Moist Heat Below 100°C*

*Examples,* ***Pasteurization of milk:*** In pasteurization of milk the temperature employed is either 63°C for 30 minutes or 72°C for 20 seconds. All nonsporeforming pathogens in milk like *Salmonellae, M tuberculosis* are killed.

### *Moist Heat Above 100°C*

*Sterilization in an Autoclave*

- Autoclaving is the most reliable method.
- It is the method most widely used for sterilization of culture media and surgical supplies.
- When water is boiled within a closed vessel at an increased pressure, the temperature at which it boils and the steam it forms will rise above 100°C
- This principle is used in the autoclave.
- Normally autoclaving is done at 15 lbs. (pounds per sq inch pressure) and 115°C for 15 minutes.

## Sterilization by Filtration

When fluids are passed through bacteria stopping filters, they are made free from bacteria:

- It is useful for making preparations of soluble products of bacterial growth such as toxins.
- Liquids that would be damaged by heat such as serum and antibiotic solutions can be sterilized by filtration.
- Efficient filters should be able to retain Serratia marcescens.

### *Types of Filters*

There are different kinds of filters:

- Earthenware candles—called Berkfeld and Chamberland filters
- Asbestos and asbestos-paper discs filters— called Seitz filters
- Sintered glass filters
- Cellulose membrane filters
- Fiber glass filters.

### *Berkefeld Filters*

- Made from Kieselguhr, a fossil diatomaceous earth
- Three grades of porosity are available:
  1. Veil—coarsest one
  2. N—normal one
  3. W—wenig the finest one.

### *Chamberland Filters*

- Made from unglazed porcelain
- Four grades are available:
  1. L1—clarifying filters
  2. L1a—Big
  3. L2—normal
  4. L3—Finest.

### *Seitz Filter*

- Made up of asbestos pads
- Three grades are available:
  1. K—clarifying filters
  2. Normal
  3. Special EK bacteria stopping filters.

### *Sintered Glass Filters*

- Made from sintered glass
- Different grades available:
  - Grades 1–5
  - Grades 1–2 are for clarifying purpose
  - Grades 3–5 are for sterilization purpose.

### *Membrane Filters*

- Made up of nitrocellulose membranes
- Made with different grades of porosity by adjusting the concentration of constituents.

## Merits and Demerits of Heat Sterilization

### *Merits*

- Sterilization is very effective
- Instruments are standardized to deliver the required effective heat
- Heat deliver system can be monitored effectively with various controls like pressure gauge, temperature meters, etc.
- Established quality control methods available.

### *Demerits*

- Steam impermeable materials like fats, oils and powders cannot be sterilized by autoclaving.

- Heat sensitive materials cannot be sterilized by heat.
  *Examples:*
  - Serum cannot be sterilized
  - Antibiotics
  - Plastic materials
  - Vaccines
  - Rubbers.
- Presence of organic matters interfere with effective sterilization.
- Dangers of explosion when high pressure is used.

## PURE CULTURE METHODS

In the natural environments microorganisms exist in mixed cultures. To establish the role of microbial agent to a disease process, it is essential to demonstrate the organisms or its components in the diseased tissues. To accomplish this, the organism must be cultivated from the tissues. Similarly to know the kinds of organism present in the environment it is necessary to grow them in artificial media. Cultivation of the organism is also essential to obtain pure culture of clone of cells derived from a single cell to perform biochemical differentiation tests and *susceptibility tests* since mixed cultures give misleading results.

### Artificial Culture Media

A medium is an environment which supplies the ingredients necessary for the growth of the organism. Various kinds of media have been prepared in the laboratory to isolate, grow and identify an organism. Depending on the need to isolate and identify an organism from a particular sample or environment, different kinds of media are formulated.

### Kinds of Media

#### *Basal or Supportive Media*

Basal medium is one that contains nutrients that allow the growth of most nonfastidious organism without affording growth advantage to any particular organism over others. Examples: *Nutrient agar* and *Trypticase Soy agar.*

#### *Enrichment Medium*

Enrichment medium is a liquid medium which enhances the growth of certain bacterial species, while inhibiting the growth or prolonging the lag phase of unwanted organisms thus altering the ratio between the two in favor of the required bacterial species.

Example is Selenite F broth for the isolation of *Salmonella* from stool.

To get a pure culture of the organism, any one of the solid media mentioned above is used. In order to get discrete separate colonies, the surface of the medium must be dry. The material is inoculated on the surface by spreading with a sterile loop in such a way that bacteria are ultimately deposited singly. When the bacteria are at a sufficient distance from each other, the whole progeny of each accumulates locally during growth to form a discrete mass or colony which is readily visible to the naked eye. Each colony is presumed to be a pure culture, consisting exclusively of the descendants of a single cell. It may be picked up with a sterile wire to prepare a pure subculture in a fresh medium.

#### *Growth and Colony Characteristics of Bacteria*

The appearances of growths of bacteria in liquid media are generally not distinctive. There is a uniform turbidity in the liquid and little deposit at the bottom. Colony morphology of the isolated bacteria on the solid media has much more value. Attention is paid to the *size* of the colony (diameter in mm), their *outline,* whether circular and entire or indented, or wavy or rhizoid, their elevation low convex, high convex or flat plateau-like, umbonate or nodular, their *translucency,* whether transparent, translucent, or opaque, their *pigmentation,* colorless, white or otherwise pigmented, and whether they produce any *change in the medium* (hemolysis in a blood-containing medium).

*Example:* Colony characteristics of *Staphylococcus aureus* on Nutrient agar.

After aerobic incubation at 37°C for 24 hours, colonies are 1–3 mm in diameter and have a smooth glistening surface, an entire edge, a soft butyrous consistency and an opaque, pigmented appearance.

#### *Growth Characteristics of Yeasts*

- Yeasts are grown on Sabouraud Dextrose agar aerobically.
- Yeasts grow as typical pasty colonies and give out yeasty odor.
- The colony morphology varies with different yeasts.

#### *Growth Characteristics of Filamentous Fungi*

The most common medium used for the isolation of fungi is Sabouraud Dextrose agar. While observing colony morphology, one must note the colors of the surface and the reverse of the colony, the texture of the surface (powdery, granular, woolly, cottony, velvety or glabrous), the topography (elevation, folding, margins, etc.) and the rate of growth.

## MEDICAL MICROBIOLOGY MICROBIAL DISEASES

Thousands of different kinds of microbes are present in all ecological niches. Some are beneficial ones, others are opportunists and some are harmful ones.

Infection is the establishment of the organisms in the tissues resulting in injury or harmful effect to the host. Infections may be endogenous or exogenous. Endogenous infections are contracted from the host himself from the normal flora. Many areas of the body have normal commensal flora. They have many functions. They provide barrier to the infection by competing for nutrition with pathogens. Some produce vitamins which are useful for the host. Some produce colicins to act against pathogens. Generally they do not cause any infection. But there are exceptions. *Streptococcus mitis* is the normal flora of the mouth. It produces infection in the previously damaged heart valves through blood stream after tooth extraction.

*Streptococcus faecalis* causes infective endocarditis and the source is the urinary tract and intestine of the host. Exogenous infections are derived from man, animals and soil. Man gets the infections from patients suffering from diseases.

Some persons may be carriers for the pathogens and they may transmit the diseases to others without getting affected.

Animals are important sources of infection. Such infections are known as zoonotic diseases. Spread of these diseases is usually from animal to animal. Man may be infected as an end host as in rabies. In some cases the infection may spread from man to man as in pneumonic plague.

Soil has also a role in the transmission of infection. Soil is the reservoir for the spores of *Clostridium* species and *Bacillus anthracis*.

### Routes of Spread of Infection

There are five main routes by which a host may become infected.

1. The respiratory route
2. The alimentary tract
3. Genital tract
4. The skin and mucous membrane
5. Placenta.

Organisms causing respiratory infections are as follows:

- *Streptococcus pneumoniae, Haemophilus influenzae, Mycobacterium tuberculosis, Bordetella pertussis* are some of the bacterial pathogens.
- Common cold virus, influenza virus, adenovirus are some of the viruses producing respiratory infections.
- The intestinal diseases like cholera, bacillary dysentery, the enteric fever and bovine tuberculosis are contracted when the organisms are ingested. But in the case of enterovirus infections (poliomyelitis) and Hepatitis though the organisms enter through gastrointestinal system, the effects are seen elsewhere in the body.
- Organisms may be acquired from the skin as in the case of herpes virus infection or through wounds as in tetanus. Wounds may be formed from trauma or thorn pricks or needle stick injury. Organisms may also be introduced through animal bite as in the case of rabies or by insect bites as in dengue, malaria, filariasis, and yellow fever.
- Syphilis, gonorrhea, hepatitis B and AIDS are some of the sexually transmitted diseases. *Treponema pallidum, Neisseria gonorrhoeae*, hepatitis B virus and human immunodeficiency virus (HIV) are the etiologic agents respectively.
- Bacteria like *T. pallidum*, viruses like rubella, cytomegalovirus, parasite like *Toxoplasma gondii* are some of the organisms that enter through placenta and cause disease in the newborn.

### Interaction between Host and Microbe

- Pathogenicity refers to the ability of the organism to cause disease.
- Virulence is the quantitative measure of this property. Virulence is not generally attributable to a single property but depends on several parameters related to the organism, the host and their interaction.
- Microbes first enter the body, survive then multiply, elaborate many factors and produce the disease.

### Virulence Factors

- ***Pili:*** Pili are useful for the attachment of the organisms on the epithelial cells.
- ***Capsule:*** Capsules down regulate the secretion of cytokine. They inhibit leukocyte accumulation. They also induce the suppressor T cells and inhibit lymphoproliferation.
- ***Intracellular residence:*** The following microorganisms reside intracellularly and try to avoid host defense mechanisms. They are *M. tuberculosis, M. leprae, S. typhi, T. gondii, L. donovani, H. capsulatum*.
- ***Production of enzymes:*** Some enzymes like proteases, DNAses, and phospholipases are produced and they help in disruption of cell structures and to hydrolyse host tissues. In *Aspergillus* species proteases help in invasion.
- ***Toxins:*** Bacteria produce both exotoxins and endotoxins which play an important role in the pathogenesis of disease. Exotoxins are produced by some organisms like *C. diphtheriae, C. tetani, C. botulinum*. The exotoxin produced by *V. cholerae* acts on the intestine and is called enterotoxin. The toxin produced by one type of *Escherichia coli* causes acute gastroenteritis. Endotoxins are lipopolysaccharide cell wall of Gram negative bacteria. They induce production of cytokines by different cells of immune system. Coagulation system and complement system are activated. They also affect various organs like kidney, heart and lungs leading to organ failure.
- ***Antigenic variation:*** Microorganisms evade the host immune responses by changing their surface antigens. *N. gonorrhoeae* very often changes its outer membrane protein. Antigenic drift and shift are common in influenza viruses. *Trypanosoma brucei* are covered with thick protein coats which undergo antigenic change during infection. Some organisms produce surface proteins that are similar to host proteins or coat themselves with host proteins that they are mistaken for part of the host itself. The distinction between the commensal and the organisms associated with disease is subtle. The definition of normal flora or pathogen is derived from the resultant complex interaction between the organism and its host.

## RESPIRATORY TRACT INFECTIONS

The lower respiratory tract is sterile. However the upper respiratory tract, the nose and throat are colonized by many organisms.

### Normal Flora of Respiratory Tract

These organisms are: *Staphylococci, Streptococci, Pneumococci, Hemophilus* and *Neisseria*.

#### *Normal Defenses against Infections*

- ***Arrangement of nose:*** There is no direct entry of air
- ***Bronchoconstriction:*** Helps the organisms to be trapped
- ***Cough reflex:*** Expels the microbes outside
- ***Mucociliary blanket:*** Traps the organisms
- ***Mucosal factors:*** Kill the organisms
  - Nonspecific
    - ***Lysozyme:*** Cell wall of gram-positive organism are lysed
    - ***Influenza virus inhibitors:***
    - ***Resident macrophages:*** Kill the organism
  - Specific
    - *Secretory IgA antibody:* Gives first line of defense.

### *Predisposing Factors for Respiratory Tract Infections*

- Ciliated epithelial cell damage due to:
  - Viruses
  - Chemicals
  - Smoking
- Fluid accumulation
- Decreased activity of macrophages

All these factors help in the establishment of the microbes in the respiratory tract.

### *Alveoli*

*Streptococcus pneumoniae M tuberculosis Mycoplasma pneumoniae, Chlamydia pneumoiae.*

### Types of Respiratory Infections

Respiratory infections can be conveniently classified into upper respiratory and lower respiratory infections.

### Upper Respiratory Tract Infections (URTI)

- ***Infections of the paranasal sinuses:*** URTI may cause inflammation of the maxillary sinuses. Bacterial infection also occurs in association with obstruction. The bacteria involved are *Streptococcus pneumoniae, Haemophilus influenzae, Staphylococcus aureus, Streptococcus pyogenes.*
- ***Otitis media:*** This is the result of direct spread of pathogens from the throat via the Eustachian tube. In young, it may be due to *Streptococcus pneumoniae, Haemophilus influenzae, Streptococcus pyogenes*. In old people, it may be due to *Streptococcus pneumoniae, Staphylococcus aureus.*
- ***Sore throat:*** It occurs in the following conditions:
  - Prodromal stages of infectious diseases
  - Diphtheria
  - Vincent infections
  - Sore throat syndrome.

### *Prodromal Stages of Infectious Diseases*

Many viral diseases are acquired via the respiratory tract. Signs and symptoms appear in the mouth and throat. But the target organs may be different.

*Example,* in measles and chickenpox, the mucosae of the upper respiratory tract and mouth are infected before the target organs show full clinical picture. In measles, Koplik's spots appear in buccal mucosa.

### *Diphtheria*

Diphtheria is an acute inflammatory condition of the upper respiratory tract usually the throat. It is caused by *Corynebacterium diphtheriae*. The organisms multiply in the throat and produce a powerful toxin. The toxin acts on myocardium, adrenal glands and nerve endings.

*Laboratory Diagnosis*

**Throat swab is collected:**

- Smear is stained by Gram and Albert stains
  - In positive cases Gram-positive bacilli seen
  - Albert stain shows bacilli with metachromatic granules
- Material is inoculated into blood agar, Loeffler's serum medium and potassium tellurite agars
- Suspected colonies are identified by biochemical test using serum sugars
- Toxigenicity test is done by agar gel precipitation test (Elek's test) and by guinea pig inoculation test.

*Prophylaxis*

- Active immunization is done.
- DPT (Diphtheria, Pertussis and Tetanus) immunization should be given in three doses:
  - 1st dose at third month
  - 2nd dose at 6–8 weeks after the first dose
  - 3rd dose 4–5 months after the 2 dose.
- A booster is given omitting the pertussis at school entry.

*Treatment*

Large dose of antitoxin must be given to confirmed cases. Antibiotics are given to eradicate the organisms.

### *Vincent's Infection*

- Vincent's spirochetes are *Borreliae.*
- They are present as normal flora of the mouth.
- In association with fusiform bacteria they can cause infection.
- Generally infection occurs during malnutrition.
- The infection is called **Vincent's angina.**

### *Sore Throat Syndrome*

Sore throat syndrome is caused by *Streptococcus pyogenes*.

Based on the cell wall polysaccharide of beta hemolytic *Streptococci* they are put in different groups. *Streptococcus pyogenes* belongs to group A. It causes wide range of pyogenic infections in the respiratory tract and skin and life threatening soft tissue infections. Post streptococcal infections may result in adverse immunological reactions leading to rheumatic heart disease or acute glomerulonephritis.

*Laboratory Diagnosis*

For the laboratory diagnosis specimens like throat swab and pus are collected and inoculated in blood agar. The organism is identified by hemolytic property, and serological tests.

Penicillin is the drug of choice for the treatment of streptococcal infections.

*Lower Respiratory Tract Infections*

Many organisms cause lower respiratory tract infections which you will be studying in later classes.

## URINARY TRACT INFECTIONS

Infections of the kidney, ureter and bladder constitute urinary tract infections (UTI). When infections occur in the kidney and ureter it is called upper urinary tract infections and bladder downwards it is called lower urinary tract infections.

### Structure of UTI

Urinary tract infection is common in females than in males. The urethra in females are shorter and wider and is less effective in preventing the bacteria entering the bladder. Sexual intercourse is a predisposing factor. High incidence is seen in pregnant women because of hormonal changes and impairment of urine flow due to pressure on the urinary tract. Other causes of urinary stagnation predispose UTI, such as urethral obstruction, urinary stones, congenital malformation and neurological disorders. Most UTI are caused by organisms originating from the patient's own fecal flora.

### Organisms Causing UTI

For convenience the organisms causing urinary tract infections can be classified into the following:

- ***Organisms most commonly involved are:*** *Escherichia coli, Klebsiella pneumoniae, Proteus mirabilis* and other *Proteus spp, Enterococcus faecalis, Pseudomonas aeruginosa, Staphylococcus saprophyticus* and *S. aureus*.
- ***Uncommon organisms are:*** *Enterobacter species, Serratia spp, Providencia spp*, other nonfermenters.
- ***Rare organisms are:*** Streptococci other than group A, *Candida albicans, Candida glabrata*, etc.

### Laboratory Diagnosis of UTI

Mid-stream urine is collected and transported to the laboratory immediately. If there is any delay expected it should be refrigerated. A quantitative culture should be performed to know the number of gram negative organisms present. A count of more than 100,000 (105/mL) organisms per mL of urine in pure culture is indicative of UTI. For the isolated organisms antibiotic susceptibility testing must be done and appropriate treatment should be given.

## INFECTIONS OF THE CENTRAL NERVOUS SYSTEM

Infecting agents reach the central nervous system (CNS) from the blood or by direct invasion or by ascending through the nerves. The infection of the CNS can be classified as encephalitis and meningitis.

### Meningitis: Etiological Agents

Meningitis is the inflammation of the membranes covering the brain (meninges). This can be caused by a wide range of microorganisms. This can be classified as follows.

### Acute Pyogenic Meningitis

This condition is related to the age of the patients. Coliform bacilli and group B streptococci are common cause in neonates.

*Hemophilus* and *Neisseria meningitidis* are frequently seen in children.

*H. influenzae* and *Str. pneumoniae* are commonly found in adults.

*N. meningitidis* can cause infections in all age groups. Other organisms involved are *Str.pyogenes, S. aureus, Salmonella* species, *Listeria*.

### Pathogenesis and Epidemiology

- ***Neonatal meningitis:*** In early days, it was caused by *Str. pyogenes* and *S. aureus*. But in later years coliform bacilli are most commonly found. Coliform meningitis results in congenital deformities and the source of the organisms can be genitourinary tract, lungs and umbilicus.
- ***Hemophilus meningitis:*** This occurs mainly in young children between the ages of 3 months to 5 years. Protection before 3 months is given by maternal antibody and after 5 months by acquired immunity. Infection spreads through bloodstream.
- ***Meningococcal meningitis (N. meningitidis):*** The organism enters the body via the naso-pharynx, where they may produce localized inflammatory reaction or remain silent. By two ways they may reach the meninges:
  1. They spread directly along the spaces between the sheath and the branches of the olfactory nerve that pierce the cribriform plate.
  2. The organisms invade the bloodstream, either produce transient bacteremia or multiply in the blood. They cause lesions in the skin, adrenal glands, joints and meninges. There are nine groups of meningococci. Infections spread to one another by close contact.
- ***Pneumococcal meningitis:*** Subsequent to some conditions like lobar pneumonia, otitis media, or infection of the para nasal sinus, or injury to skull, *Streptococcus pneumoniae* multiplies in the blood and spread to the meninges.
- ***Meningitis due to other bacteria:*** *Staphylococcus* and *Streptococcus pyogenes* reach the meninges via blood or directly from the exterior after a trauma.
- ***Tuberculous meningitis:*** This occurs in a severe form in young children and is secondary to a tuberculous focus elsewhere in the body. The bacilli reach the meninges via the blood.

### Laboratory Diagnosis

Laboratory diagnosis is made by isolation and identification of specific organism from blood and cerebrospinal fluid (CSF). Antigen can be detected by counter immunoelectrophoresis or latex agglutination test. Blood cultures are useful in 50% cases. Gram stain and acid fast stains are useful in demonstrating the bacteria in the CSF. Fluorescence microscopy is useful for *tuberculous meningitis*. Fontana's staining is useful for spirochetes like *Leptospira, Borrelia* and *Treponema*.

Once organisms are grown, they are identified by standard biochemical tests. Treatment will depend on the nature of the organisms and the antibiotic susceptibility pattern.

### Viral Meningitis

Viruses are the most frequent cause of meningitis. Most cases are due to enteroviruses, ECHO and Coxsackie viruses. Mumps virus can cause meningitis in children.

- ***Pathogenesis:*** Viruses enter by oral or respiratory routes. They establish a silent initial focus somewhere in the nasopharynx or in small bowel. The spread occurs through lymph to the blood. They mainly multiply in lymphoreticular system. The infection is detectable after 5 days. The virus is free in the plasma. They affect the meninges and they may spread to other parts also. This time fever and neck stiffness occur. At this time the virus appears in the throat and gut also. Serum antibody appears about this time.

- *Diagnosis:* Specimens of throat secretions, feces, CSF, are collected during acute phase. During convalescent period feces may be obtained. Enteroviruses can be isolated in tissue cultures. No specific therapy is available.

## SEXUALLY TRANSMITTED DISEASES

Sexually transmitted diseases are the most common communicable diseases after common cold. They are transmitted through sexual contact. They can be classified into the following:

- Bacterial
- Viral
- Parasitic
- Fungal diseases

### Bacterial Diseases

The following are some of the sexually transmitted bacterial diseases.

- Syphilis
- Gonorrhea
- Chancroid
- Chlamydial diseases

The sexually transmitted viral diseases are:

- AIDS
- Hepatitis B
- Warts.

Trichomoniasis and genital candidiasis are the parasitic and fungal diseases respectively.

### Syphilis

*Treponema pallidum* is the organism that causes syphilis. Treponemes are slender spirochetes with fine spirals and pointed or round ends. The pathogenic treponemes have not yet been cultivated in artificial media.

#### *Pathogenesis*

*T. pallidum* is transmitted from one partner to another through intact or damaged mucosa. The organisms establish at the point of entrance and multiply within the next 3 months and a chancre appears.

This is the primary lesion and may disappear. This stage is called *primary syphilis. Secondary syphilis* occurs in two to 6 months after the primary syphilis. Because of the multiplication of the organisms secondary lesions appear on the skin. Spirochetes are abundant in these lesions. Usually the lesions heal spontaneously. In few cases *tertiary syphilis* appears later. This causes chronic granulomata known as gummata in the brain, bone, skin and internal organs. Late manifestations are degeneration of brain cells and destruction of nerve fibers. Tertiary lesions contain few spirochetes.

Infection during pregnancy can be transmitted to the fetus. This causes congenital syphilis.

#### *Laboratory Diagnosis*

Exudates from primary and secondary lesions are collected for examination. They are examined by dark field microscopy for spirochetes and stained by silver staining method to show the spirochetes.

Blood is collected for serological tests to demonstrate antibodies.

Serological tests are divided into two groups viz. nonspecific and specific tests.

In the nonspecific test antibodies to cardiolipin which develop during the infection are demonstrated. The test is called VDRL test.

In the specific test, antibodies developed against *T. pallidum* are demonstrated. *Treponema pallidum* immobilization test (TPI), fluorescent treponemal antibody absorption test (FTA-AB), and *Treponema pallidum* hemagglutination test (TPHA) are some of the specific tests used for the diagnosis of syphilis.

Penicillin is the drug of choice for treatment. For control, all discovered cases must be promptly treated and contacts also must be treated. Sex hygiene, and prophylaxis at the time of exposure are some other control measures. Sexually transmitted diseases can be transmitted simultaneously. Therefore, it is necessary to consider the possibility of syphilis when any other sexually transmitted disease is found.

### Gonorrhea

Gonorrhea is a sexually transmitted infection of columnar and transitional epithelium caused by *Neisseria gonorrhoeae*. The urethra, endocervix, anal canal, pharynx and conjunctivae may be infected directly.

Systemic infection may lead to arthritis, tenosynovitis, dermatitis, endocarditis and meningitis.

#### *Organism*

*Neisseria gonorrhoeae* are gram negative diplococci, kidney shaped, the concave side face each other, nonmotile. Grows on enriched medium in presence of 5–10% $CO_2$.

#### *Pathogenesis*

Anterior urethra is mainly affected in men. Anterior urethra and cervix are affected in women. In advanced infection it affects the prostate, seminal vesicles and epididymis in men and uterus and fallopian tubes are affected in women. Rectal infection and throat carriage occur in both. Gonococcal ophthalmia neonatorum is an infection of the eye of the newborn, is acquired during the passage through infected birth canal. The conjunctivitis progresses and if untreated results in blindness.

To prevent this instillation of tetracycline, erythromycin or silver nitrate solution into the conjunctival sac of the newborn is compulsory.

Gonococcal bacteremia leads to skin lesions on the hands, fore arms, feet, and tenosynovitis and suppurative arthritis.

#### *Laboratory Diagnosis*

Pus and secretions are taken from urethra, cervix, rectum, conjunctiva, throat or synovial fluid for smear and culture. Cultures are to be done immediately after the collection of specimens.

- *Treatment:* Penicillin is given. If the organisms are resistant, after performing antimicrobial susceptibility testing, appropriate drug is given.

- *Chancroid: Haemophilus ducreyi* causes irregular ulcers in the genitalia. It produces chancroid or soft chancre. This is a venereal disease or sexually transmitted disease. *H. ducreyi* is a gram negative bacilli. Chancroid is treated with sulphonamides. If resistant, erythromycin and cotrimoxazole are used.
- *Chlamydial disease:* There are many serotypes in Chlamydia. Some of them cause genital infections. Lymphogranuloma venereum is one of chlamydial sexually transmitted diseases. First a vesicle develops and the lesion ulcerates in the genitals. The inguinal lymph nodes enlarge, suppurate and release pus through multiple sinus tracts. If not treated it will lead to other complications. Sulfonamides and tetracycline are used for the treatment.

### Trichomoniasis

This is caused by *Trichomonas vaginalis*. Trichomonads are flagellate protozoa with 3–5 anterior flagella, other organelles are an undulating membrane.

In female the infection is limited to vulva, vagina and cervix. It usually does not extend to uterus. The mucosal surface may be painful, inflamed, eroded and covered with a frothy yellow or cream colored discharge. In males the prostate, seminal vesicle and the urethra may be infected.

Trichomoniasis is treated with topical and systemic metronidazole.

The patients sexual partner should be examined and treated simultaneously.

Trichomoniasis is treated with topical and systemic metronidazole.

The patients sexual partner should be examined and treated simultaneously.

### Genital Candidiasis

The most common cause of genital candidiasis is due to *Candida albicans*. Generally, it is a commensal in the vagina. When infection occurs white membranous patches are produced in the vagina and vulva.

Thick or watery vaginal discharge is seen. Gram's stain can identify the yeast like cells. Nystatin or miconazole or ketoconazole are used.

### Viral Agents

#### *AIDS (Acquired Immunodeficiency Syndrome)*

Human immunodeficiency virus (HIV) is the etiologic agent of AIDS. It belongs to the lenti virus subgroup which includes slow viruses.

The virus has central nucleoprotein core that contains single stranded RNA genome. The enzyme reverse transcriptase is associated with the viral RNA. This RNA is transcribed into single stranded DNA and then to double stranded DNA.

The virus core is surrounded by a protein shell this is again covered by a lipid bilayer which contains envelope proteins.

#### *Pathogenesis*

Transmission is by sexual contact, through blood and blood products-transfusion and injection. After entry it comes in contact with T4 lymphocytes. T4 cells are damaged and are decreased in mumber and T4 : T8 ratio is reversed. Because helper cells are affected, humoral immunity is also affected. AIDS patients are unable to respond to new antigen. Macrophage monocyte functions are affected because of lack of secretion of activation factors.

Within few weeks of infection, low grade fever, malaise, headache, lymphadenopathy are seen. All persons pass through a period of symptomless infection for several months or years. They show positive antibody tests and are infectious. Lymph nodes are enlarged in some people. Then it leads to other opportunistic infections like oral candidiasis, salmonellosis, tuberculosis. Persons suffer from fatigue, unexplained fever, persistent diarrhea, and weight loss. Finally they reach the stage called AIDS.

#### *Laboratory Diagnosis: Immunological Tests*

Total white blood cell count: Usually below 200/mm$^3$. T4 cell count is less. Lowered cell mediated immunity is seen.

#### *Specific Tests*

Viral antibody detection is performed by ELISA test and confirmed by Western blot test. Virus can be isolated from infected lymphocytes.

#### *Prevention*

- Multipartner sex should be avoided.
- Safer sex should be practiced.
- Blood should be screened before transfusion.
- Sharing of needles should be avoided.

#### *Parasitic Agent*

*Trichomonas vaginalis* is the organism that is transmitted through sexual contact.

## BACTERIAL SKIN AND WOUND INFECTIONS

- Wound can be defied as any interruption of continuity of external or internal surfaces caused by violence.
- Wounds may occur following: Surgery, trauma or injections.
- Wound infections may occur mainly after surgical procedures.
- Wound sepsis is the result of cross infection from human sources and from other outside sources.

### Bacteria Associated with Wound Infections

Many bacteria are associated with wound infection.

The normal flora may also cause infection.

The most common bacteria of the skin are: Staphylococci and various streptococci, *Sarcina spp*, anaerobic diphtheroids, gram negative rods and others. The nutrition is derived from:

- Sweat
- Amino acids peptides from the skin
- Fatty acids from the sebaceous glands of the skin.

### Factors Determining the Ecology of the Skin Bacteria

Four main factors determine the ecology of skin bacteria:

1. The climate: The temperature and humidity
2. The effect of free fatty acids

3. Other bacterial inhibitors
4. Maintenance of the flora by products of skin secretions.

### Defense against Infection

- *Intact skin:* Normal uninterrupted skin provides protection against invasion by bacteria.
- *Lysozyme in sweat:* The enzyme lysozyme provides protection against gram positive bacteria by lysing the cell wall.
- IgA antibodies in the sweat and secretions provide first line of defense against infection.
- Inhibitors like unsaturated fatty acids provide protection against bacteria.
- Bacteriocins produced by the normal flora prevent the establishment of other bacteria.

### Factors Responsible for Wound Infections

- *Host factors:* The following factors help the organisms to survive and produce the infections:
  - Extremes of age
  - Diabetes mellitus
  - Steroid therapy
  - Obesity
  - Malnutrition
  - Immunocompromised individual
  - Presence of remote infection at the time of surgery.
- *Exogenous factors:*
  - Use of unsterile instruments
  - Surgeons hands/from health workers
  - Air/hospital environments.
- *Endogenous factors:*
  - Wound contamination from the patient source: from the normal flora
  - Wound penetrating through structures containing normal flora
  - Surgical procedures involving mucous membranes harboring normal flora
  - Patients carrying pathogens in their nose, throat, axilla, etc.

### Etiological Agents

- *P. aeruginosa*
- *Staph. aureus*
- *Proteus spp*
- Member of enterobacteriaceae
- Anaerobic organisms
- Anaerobic cocci
- Bacteroides.

### Postoperative Infections

- Gas gangrene organisms
- *S. aureus*
- *Cl. tetani.*

### Route of Entry

Wounds may occur following:

- Surgery
- Trauma
- Injections.

Wound infections may occur mainly after surgical procedures. Wound sepsis is the result of cross infection from human sources and from other outside sources.

### Mechanisms of Damage

- Organisms enter through the skin, multiply there and produce the disease in the skin. For example, impetigo, abscess and cellulitis are caused by *Staphylococcus aureus* and *Streptococcus pyogenes*. As soon as the organisms enter the skin they multiply and produce various toxins that kill the cells and produce cellulites. Further damage leads to necrosis and ulcer formation.
- Organisms multiply in the skin and produce disease in internal organs. For example, some group A streptococci multiply in the skin and produce disease known as acute glomerulo-nephritis causing damage to the kidneys. Sometimes *C. diphtheriae* may multiply in the skin and affect the heart due to the toxin.
- Sometimes organism may multiply in the skin and produce the toxin which affect the CNS and the effects are seen. In the case of *Clostridium tetani,* convulsions and paralysis occur due to the production of a powerful toxin.

### Laboratory Diagnosis

Pus and wound swabs are cultured for the aerobic and anaerobic organisms and are identified using appropriate biochemical tests.

## BACTERIAL INFECTIONS OF GASTROINTESTINAL TRACT

Many organisms cause gastrointestinal infections. The most important ones are organisms belonging to the genera *Salmonella, Shigella* and *Vibrio* and certain types of *Escherichia coli.* These are acquired by oral route.

### Acute Gastroenteritis Due to Shigella

Organisms belonging to the genus *Shigella* produce bacillary dysentery. They are gram negative bacilli, nonmotile organisms. There are four species, *Shigella dysenteriae, Sh. flexneri, Sh. boydii,* and *Sh. sonnei.*

#### *Pathogenesis*

The infection is limited to the gastrointestinal tract. Bloodstream invasion is rare. Infection is communicable. Invasion of the mucosal epithelium leads to the formation of micro-abscesses in the wall of the large intestine and ileum which finally results in necrosis of the mucous membrane, ulceration, bleeding and formation of pseudomembrane on the ulcer area. This consists of fibrin, leukocytes, cell debris, necrotic mucous membrane and bacteria.

#### *Toxins of Shigella*

- *Endotoxin:* Upon autolysis, the organisms release LPS which causes the irritation of the bowel wall.
- *Shigella dysenteriae* produces exotoxin which is a heat labile toxin that affects the gut and CNS. It acts as enterotoxin and increases the local concentration of cyclic adenosine monophosphate (AMP) and results in intense and prolonged hypersecretion of water and chlorides and inhibits the re-absorption of sodium.

The gut lumen is distended with fluid, hypermotility and causes diarrhea. As a neurotoxin, it acts on CNS and causes meningismus and coma mainly in children.

*Shigella* produce an early non bloody, voluminous diarrhea and later dysentery with blood, mucous and pus in stools.

### *Laboratory Diagnosis*

Fresh stool, mucus flek and rectal swabs are collected for culture.

Large number of leucocytes, RBC may be seen microscopically.

Selective media like Salmonella shigella agar, deoxycholate citrate agar are used. The organisms are non lactose fermenters and are identified by biochemical test and with specific antisera. Ciprofloxacin is used for the treatment nowadays.

### Acute Gastroenteritis due to Escherichia Coli

Generally *E. coli* is a normal flora of the gut of man. But it may sometimes cause gastrointestinal disease. It may range from mild, selflimiting diarrhea to hemorrhagic colitis. Such stains fall into five groups with specific serotypes and with different **pathogenic mechanisms:**

1. ***Enteropathogenic E. coli (EPEC):*** These cause infantile enteritis in children.
2. ***Enterotoxigenic E. coli (ETEC):*** These cause community acquired diarrheal disease in areas of poor hygiene. It is responsible for traveller's diarrhea.
3. ***Enteroinvasive E. coli (EIEC):*** It causes an illness similar to *Shigella* dysentery in all age groups.
4. ***Verotoxin producing E. coli (VTEC):*** It causes hemorrhagic colitis and hemolytic uremic syndrome.
5. ***Enteroaggregative E. coli (EggEC):*** It causes chronic diarrheal disease.

Contaminated food and water supplies are the most important vehicles of these organisms. Infantile enteritis in hospitals are transmitted through patient to patients, through the hands of attendants and contaminated feeds. VTEC infections are acquired through meat, unpasteurized milk and direct contact with animals.

### *Laboratory Diagnosis*

*E. coli* organisms are grown and their pathogenic characteristics are identified by appropriate tests.

### *Prevention*

Avoid exposure to infectious agents. Fluid and electrolyte imbalance must be corrected early. Strict hygiene is essential in hospitals.

Food borne infections should be avoided by processing and handling cooked meat products separately from raw materials.

## SUPERFICIAL MYCOSIS AND DERMATOMYCOSIS

Thousands of fungi both yeasts and filamentous fungi are present in the environment. About 100 of them cause disease in man and animals.

Only very few species like dermatophytes and *Candida* are transmitted from man to man. Generally the fungal infections are classified into superficial, cutaneous, subcutaneous, and systemic mycoses. Infections of skin, hair and nails may be chronic and resistant to treatment but do not affect the general health of the patients.

### Superficial Mycosis

- ***Tinea versicolor:*** Tinea versicolor is a mild infection of skin. The fungus *Malassezia furfur* grows in the **stratum corneum** of the skin as spherical thick skinned budding cells and short, bent hyphe. It does not cause any pathological signs.

  Fine browny scales appear on the chest, back, abdomen, neck and upper arm. In brown skinned people it produces white patches and in whites brown patches which are of cosmetic importance only.
- ***Tinea nigra:*** Tinea nigra is a condition in which blackish macular area appears on the palmar or plantar surface of the skin. This condition is caused by *Exophiala werneckii*. The infected skin can be removed mechanically or chemically.
- ***Piedra:*** Black piedra is a condition in which black nodules are formed around the scalp hair by *Piedraia hortae*.

  In white piedra, *Trichosporon cutaneum* causes the formation of soft, white nodules around axillary, pubic, beard and scalp hair.

### Dermatomycosis

Dermatomycosis is also known as cutaneous mycosis. It is caused by dermatophytes. They infect superficial keratinized tissues such as skin, hair, and nails. They do not invade deeper tissues.

Dermatophytes are closely related fungi and are classified into three genera:

1. *Trichophyton*
2. *Microsporon*
3. *Epidermophyton.*

These genera are identified by their characteristic morphology of micro and macro conidia produced on Sabouraud's dextrose agar. The infection produced by dermatophytes is called Tinea. In *Tinea corporis* the infection is present in non-hairy, smooth skin.

In *tinea pedis* infection is present in the inter digital spaces on feet. When the infection is present in the groin it is called *tinea cruris* where as when seen on the head it is called *tinea capitis*. *Tinea barbae* is the infection of the beard hair, and Tinea unguium is infection of the nail.

### *Laboratory Diagnosis*

Specimens consists of both skin and nail scrapings and hair plucked from the involved areas. Specimens are examined in a drop of 10% KOH. In skin or nails, branching filaments or chains of arthrospores are seen. Specimens are also inoculated on SDA medium and the fungi identified.

Fungal skin infections are treated with miconazole cream or with griseofulvin.

## AMEBIASIS

- Amebiasis is an infection due to *E. histolytica*
- It occurs only among human and selected primates
- Commonly *E. histolytica* produce intestinal and extra intestinal infections

- Amebiasis is transmitted by oral ingestion of materials containing cyst of *E. histolytica*.

## Morphology of the Organism

### *Trophozoites*

*Entamoeba histolytica* and *Entamoeba coli* have both trophozoites and cyst stages. The cytoplasms of *E. histolytica* is glossy, contains red cells and spherical vacuoles. The nucleus has small central karyosome and fine regular chromatin granules lining the periphery of nuclear membrane. *Entamoeba coli* has granular cytoplasm which contains bacteria and other inclusions and ellipsoid vacuoles. Nucleus has eccentric nucleolus and coarse beaded chromatin at the periphery.

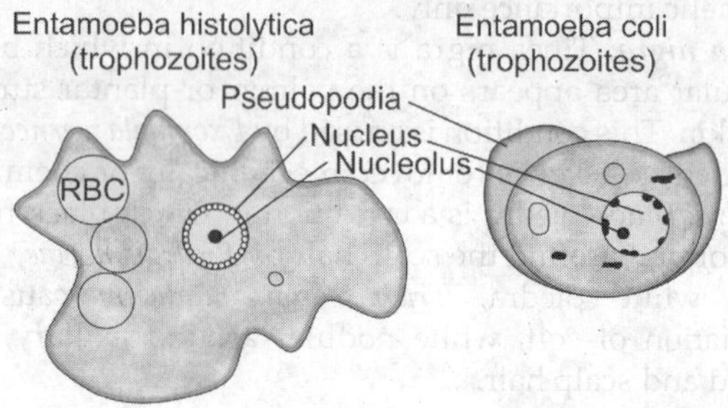


### *Cysts*

Cysts are round, nuclear morphology is similar to trophozoites.

One to four nuclei are seen in *E. histolytica* and eight nuclei are present in *Entamoeba coli* cysts.

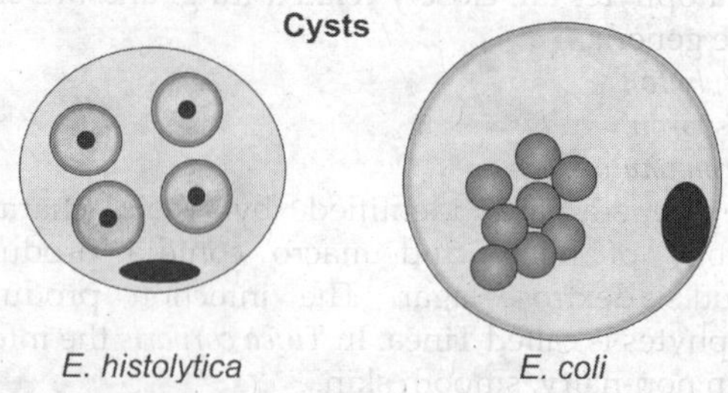


### *Clinical Manifestations of the Disease*

Both intestinal and extra intestinal amebiasis have an incubation period of more than one week (several weeks).

## TYPES OF CLINICAL MANIFESTATIONS

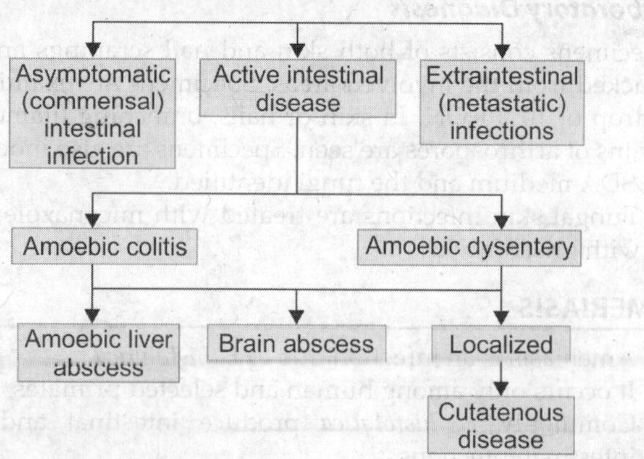


## Asymptomatic Intestinal Infections

- Persons show no symptoms
- They pass cysts in stool.

## Active Intestinal Disease

- Minority of persons with intestinal infection develop diarrheal disease
- They pass red cells and pus in stool
- The symptoms and signs are:
  - Less severe form
    - Fever
    - Abdominal pain
    - Tenesmus
  - More sever form
    - Symptoms similar to ulcerative colitis
    - Peritonitis
    - Secondary intestinal perforations
    - Toxic mega colon.

## Pathology

Parasites produce flask-shaped ulcers in which the base is wider than neck at the epithelial surface.

Organisms are present on the edge of the ulcer.

## Laboratory Diagnosis

- *Direct method:* Demonstration of organism or components of the organisms
- *Indirect method:* Demonstration of response to organisms.

### *Direct Method*

*Wet mount:*
- Saline—Trophozoites, cysts
- Iodine—Cysts
- LCB—Cysts.

- *Stains:* Iodine staining
  - Iron hematoxylin stain
  - Trichrome stain
  - Immunofluorescence staining.
- *Culture:* Non-axenic and axenic culture methods are used.

### *Indirect Methods*

Demonstration of response to organism.

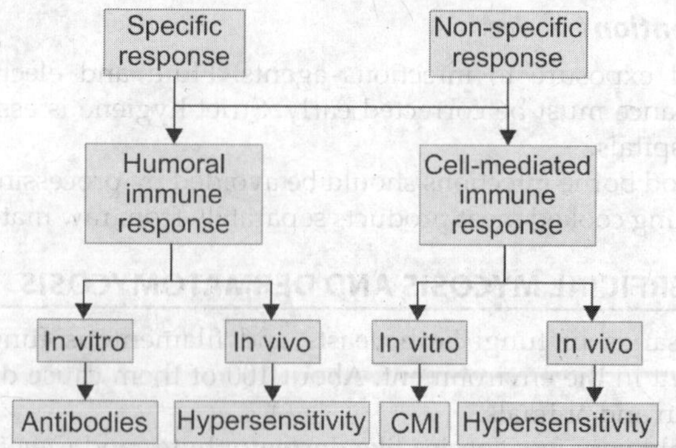

### *Epidemiology, Prevention and Control*

- Cysts are ingested through contaminated food and water
- Flies transfer the cysts from infected stools to food
- Control measures consist of improving environmental and food sanitation
- Carriers must be barred from food handling
- Metronidazole is the drug used for symptomatic amebiasis.

## MALARIA

Malaria is a mosquito borne parasitic disease characterized by episodes of fever, chills, and rigors which occur typically and periodically every third day.

### Etiological Agents

Four species of *Plasmodium* cause Malaria in man. They are:

1. *P vivax*
2. *P falciparum*
3. *P malariae*
4. *P ovale.*

### Life Cycle of Malarial Parasite

- Following the bite of an infected mosquito the sporozoites are introduced into the body.
- The parasites first invade the cells of the liver.
- They multiply by the process of schizogony.
- After 6–12 days merozoites are released into the blood.
- The parasites invade the RBC.
- Inside the RBC they continue to multiply and release merozoites.
- Some parasites transform into macro and micro gametocytes which are taken by the mosquitoes.
- Inside the mosquitoes further multiplication leads to the production of sporozoites.

### Clinical Features

The clinical features of malaria are due to the blood stage parasites.

There is fever with rigor, headache, myalgia, arthralgia, nausea and abdominal pain seen in malaria. Due to rupture of RBC there is anemia. Mild enlargement of spleen is seen.

### Laboratory Diagnosis of Malaria

Presence of malarial parasites in the blood confirms the diagnosis of malaria. A thickly spread blood film is useful for spotting the parasites. Thinly spread films help in the accurate identification of the species. Blood films are stained by either Giemsa or Leishman stains.

Concentration technique like QBC are also available for the diagnosis.

### *Treatment*

Antimalarial drugs are used primarily to eliminate the asexual and blood parasites. Treatment also must be given to eliminate liver stage parasites (Hypnozoites) that could give rise to relapse infection.

The drug of choice is chloroquine. To prevent relapse primaquine is used.

## POLIOMYELITIS

Poliomyelitis is an acute illness with pain and flaccid paralysis affecting mainly lower limbs and is caused by three polioviruses (poliovirus 1, 2 and 3).

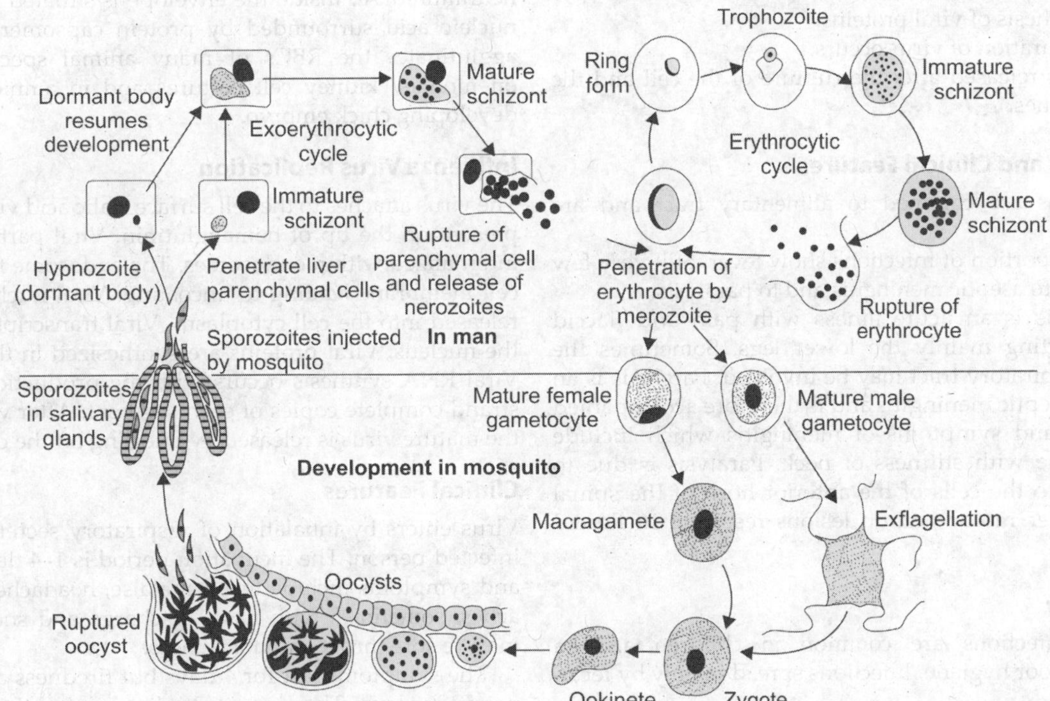

Polioviruses belong to the family of enteroviruses which multiply in the gut and rarely cause intestinal symptoms.

### Characteristics of Enteroviruses—Poliovirus

These viruses enter the body via ingestion by mouth. They multiply in the lymphoid tissues of the alimentary tract including the pharynx.

From the gut they enter the blood (viremia) or shed into the lumen of the intestine.

### Virology

Poliovirus belongs to picornavirus (pico = small + RNA).

They are RNA viruses, having single stranded positive sense RNA.

Viruses are small roughly spherical particles, 25–30 nm in size, stable at acid pH.

They grow rapidly in tissue cultures and produce cytopathic effects.

### Replication of Poliovirus

- Poliovirus attaches to the specific receptors on the cell surface. If the cell is not possessing the receptor it is not susceptible to infection.
- The virus enters the cell by micropinocytosis.
- Then uncoating of capsid proteins occurs. The viral RNA is released into the cytoplasm.
- Viral RNA is a plus strand and it can act as a messenger RNA. So early translation (protein synthesis) occurs.
- At the same time viral RNA synthesis also occurs.
- During this time a vesicle is formed inside the cells.
- Inside the vesicle assembly of viral components occur.
- Afterwards late viral RNA translation occurs leading to further synthesis of viral proteins.
- Finally maturation of virus occurs.
- The virus is released after the rupture of the cell and the cycle continues.

### Pathogenesis and Clinical Features

Most infections are confined to alimentary tract and are symptomless.

A small proportion of infections show fever. Still very few cases progress to aseptic meningitis and to paralysis.

Poliomyelitis is an acute illness with pain and flaccid paralysis affecting mainly the lower legs. Sometimes the muscles of respiratory tract may be involved. Paralysis is an extension of aseptic meningitis and is therefore accompanied by the signs and symptoms of meningitis which include fever, headache with stiffness of neck. Paralysis is due to viral damage to the cells of the anterior horn of the spinal cord with lower motor neuron lesions resulting in flaccid paralysis.

### Epidemiology

Enterovirus infections are common in children and in conditions of poor hygiene. Infections spread mainly by fecal-oral route.

### Laboratory Diagnosis and Control

Feces, throat swab and blood are collected for viral isolation.

These specimens are inoculated into monkey kidney cell cultures and observed for cytopathic effects. The virus can be identified by neutralization using specific antiserum.

### Control

Two types of vaccines are available for three polioviruses.

1. ***Sabin live attenuated virus vaccines:*** It is administered in three oral doses.
2. ***Salk inactivated virus vaccine:*** It contains three polioviruses inactivated by formalin and is given in three injections.

## INFLUENZA

Influenza is one of the great epidemic diseases. From time to time it becomes pandemic and spreads throughout the world.

Influenza virus belongs to the family Orthomyxoviridae. Three immunological types are known. They are influenza type A, B and C viruses. Influenza type A is highly variable antigenically and is responsible for most cases of epidemic influenza, B shows less variation and causes less frequent epidemics, C is antigenically stable and causes only mild infection.

### Structure of the Virus

Influenza virus is a RNA virus. There are eight separate single stranded negative sense fragments. Each segment is a gene and codes for a different protein viz. hemagglutinin and neuraminidase, etc. Viruses are roughly spherical particles, medium size, 80–100 nm, with an envelope. The envelope contains radially projecting spikes of virus hemagglutinin and neuraminidase. Inside the envelope is situated nucleocapsid, nucleic acid surrounded by protein capsomeres. The virus agglutinates the RBCs of many animal species. It grows on monkey kidney cell cultures and in amniotic cavity of developing chick embryo.

### Influenza Virus Replication

The virus attaches to the cell surface sialic acid via the receptor present on the tip of hemagglutinin. Viral particles are then internalized within endosomes. The endosome fuses with the cell membrane leading to uncoating. Viral nucleocapsids are released into the cell cytoplasm. Viral transcription occurs in the nucleus. Viral proteins are synthesized in the cytoplasm. Viral RNA synthesis occurs with the production of positive strand complete copies of each segment. After viral assembly the mature virus is released by budding off the cell.

### Clinical Features

Virus enters by inhalation of respiratory secretions from an infected person. The incubation period is 1–4 days. The signs and symptoms include fever, malaise, headache, generalized aches, sometimes with nasal discharge and sneezing. There may be sore throat and hoarseness.

The symptoms last for 4 days but tiredness and weakness persist for long. The virus multiplies in superficial epithelium of the upper and lower respiratory tract. Influenza causes damage to cilia and desquamation of the epithelium. Few patients may develop pneumonia.

Secondary bacterial infections may also be seen.

### Control

Influenza virus undergoes antigenic variations from time to time.

Epidemics are due to the emergence of new virus strains containing new hemagglutinin and neuraminidase. When major change occurs it is called antigenic shift. If minor change occurs it is called antigenic drift. At the time of pandemic, the speed with which new strain spreads makes it difficult to prepare sufficient quantity of vaccine. Current vaccine contains inactivated virus grown in eggs and either purified or disrupted and purified. It is given subcutaneously and the protection is short lived.

## RABIES

- Rabies is a zoonotic disease. Animals act as reservoir of infection.
- Man gets the infection from the animals.
- Rabies is a lethal form of encephalitis caused by rabies virus, transmitted through the bite of an infected animal usually a dog.

### Properties of the Virus

- The virus is bullet shaped
- It is covered by a membranous envelope
- Has protruding spikes 10 nm long
- Spike is composed of a single glycoprotein
- The genome is single stranded RNA—is a minus strand RNA
- Genome contains RNA dependent RNA polymerase
- When freshly isolated from a case, the virus is called 'street' virus
  - It can multiply in neural and non-neural tissues.
- Serial brain to brain passage in rabbits yields a fixed virus
  - It cannot multiply in non-neural tissue.

### Pathogenesis and Pathology

- Virus is introduced into the tissue by the bite of a rabid animal
  - Canines
  - Bats, etc.
- Virus multiplies in the muscle or connective tissue.
- Infection ascends through the tissue spaces of the sensory nerves to the CNS.
- It multiplies in the CNS
- Spreads though peripheral nerves to salivary glands and tissues.
- Rabies virus has not been isolated from the blood of an infected person.
- The incubation period depends on:
  - Amount of viral inoculum
  - Severity of the bite
  - The distance the virus has to travel from its point of entry to the brain
  - If bitten on the face, higher attack rate and shorter incubation period seen
- There is nerve cell destruction in the cortex, mid brain, basal ganglion, pons and medulla
- It produces cytoplasmic inclusion bodies in nerve cells called Negri bodies.

### Clinical Features

The incubation period is from 4 to 12 weeks, sometimes it may be much longer. If the bite wound is in the neck or head the incubation period is shorter.

The virus spreads from the wound to the central nervous system through nerves.

### Symptoms

The symptoms may be either furious or dumb. In the furious type, the patient shows the symptoms of excitement, with tremor, muscular contractions and convulsions. When there is spasm of muscle of swallowing, patients show fear of water and hence the name hydrophobia is also given to rabies.

In the dumb type of rabies, ascending paralysis is seen involving the muscles of swallowing speech and respiration.

Virus is present in saliva, skin and eyes and brain.

The disease is always fatal following convulsions.

### Epidemiology

Rabies is a natural infection seen in dogs, cats, bats and carnivorous animals such as foxes and wolves. Man acquires the infection generally from infected dogs. Virus is present in the saliva of the infected dog. Infected dog dies within ten days. If the dog remain healthy for ten days after biting, it can be regarded as being free of the virus at the time of biting. Aerosol infection has been recorded as a result of laboratory accident. Human patients do not seem to be a source of infection.

### Diagnosis

#### *Direct Demonstration of Virus*

Specimens such as hair bearing skin from the back of neck, corneal impression smears and brain tissue are examined for virus by immunofluorescence.

Intracytoplasmic inclusion body called Negri body can be demonstrated by conventional microscopy.

#### *Virus Isolation*

Attempt to isolate the virus from brain tissue, saliva, CSF and urine from patients can be made by inoculating into mice and the animal is observed for convulsions, paralysis and postmortem examinations for Negri bodies in the brain tissue.

#### *Vaccination*

Rabies vaccine was first developed by Pasteur in 1885. It consisted of virus attenuated by drying the spinal cord of infected rabbits for varying length of time over KOH. Wild rabies virus is called street virus and attenuated virus is called fixed virus. All vaccines prepared for human use contain inactivated virus.

Now human diploid cell vaccine (HDCV) is used for vaccination.

It contains inactivated virus grown on WI38 or MRC-5 diploid human embryo lung cells.

## STRUCTURE AND DEVELOPMENT OF IMMUNE SYSTEM

### Immunity

Immune system consists of lymphoid cells (both T and B cells) and lymphoid organs. Cells that make up the immune system are distributed throughout the body. They occur predominantly in lymphoreticular organs. These include: Bone marrow, thymus, lymph nodes, spleen, mucosa associated lymphoid tissues. The cells occupy the intricacies of networks formed by reticular cells and fibers supporting framework. The cells involved in the immune function are: Lymphocytes, monocytes, macrophages of tissues, endothelial cells, mast cells, basophils, eosinophils, neutrophils, etc. All cells are derived from pluripotent, self-renewing stem cells of the bone marrow.

### *Organs of Immune System*

Based on the different roles they perform, lymphoid organs can be classified into:

- Primary or central lymphoid organs
- Secondary or peripheral lymphoid organs. Primary lymphoid organs include:
  - Thymus
  - Bone marrow
  - Bursa of Fabricius in birds.

In the primary lymphoid organs, the T and B cells mature into antigen recognizing lymphocytes. Secondary lymphoid organs include lymph nodes, spleen and mucosa associated lymphoid tissue.

### *Thymus Gland*

The thymus gland is a bilobed structure. During fetal development the size of the thymus gland increases and reaches its maximum at birth. After birth the thymus begins to decrease in size and undergoes atrophy with aging.

*Cortex*

The cortex contains epithelial cells. It is densely populated with lymphocytes of various sizes. Most of the lymphocytes in thymus are immature.

*Medulla*

T lymphocytes mature in the cortex and migrate into the medulla.

They leave the medulla and enter the peripheral blood circulation.. Then they are transported to the secondary lymphoid organs.

*Function of the Thymus Gland*

- The primary function of the thymus is the production of Thymic lymphocytes
- Thymus is the major site for lymphocyte proliferation in the body
- One percent of the lymphocytes produced in the thymus leave the thymus, others are destroyed.
- Lymphocytes produced in the thymus are called T lymphocytes or T cells
- In the thymus the lymphocytes are educated so that they can produce cell mediated immune (CMI) response against foreign antigens
- Immature lymphocytes mature in the thymus and acquire different cell differentiation (CD) molecules on their surface.

*Effects of Thymectomy (Removal of Thymus)*

Removal of thymus is called thymectomy. Thymus can be removed either in the neonates or in adults.

Neonatal thymectomy results in an immediate severe reduction in the quality and quantity of T lymphocytes.

Adult thymectomy could result in deficiency of T cell, after the eventual death of T cells that originally populated the secondary lymphoid organs.

Thymectomy affects CMI primarily. It also diminishes antibody response to certain antigens.

### *Bone Marrow*

*Bursa of Fabricius*

It is a primary lymphoid organ of birds which is situated near the cloaca. It consists of lymphoid centers that contain epithelial cells and lymphocytes. These lymphocytes are antibody producing cells. The B cells undergo maturation in this organ. Like thymus the bursa is largest at hatching and undergoes atrophy with maturation.

- Mammals do not have bursa of Fabricius.
- A structure in mammals that functions equivalent to that of birds is the bone marrow.

*Functions of Bursa of Fabricius*

- It produces B lymphocytes. These are responsible for antibody production and humoral immunity.
- These B cells mature and go to the peripheral lymphoid organs and are seeded there.
- Following appropriate antigenic stimulation, B lymphocytes transform into plasma cells and produce antibodies.

### *Secondary Lymphoid Organs*

*Lymph Node*

Lymph nodes are small ovoid structures found in various regions throughout the body. They form channels called as lymphatic channels through which lymph flows.

A Lymph node is surrounded by a fibrous capsule. It has an outer cortex and inner medulla.

*Cortex*

In the cortex the lymphocytes accumulate into primary and secondary follicles. These follicles contain lymphocytes and macrophages.

*Medulla*

In the medulla the lymphocytes are arranged as elongated branching bands or medullary cords. The cortical follicles and medullary cords contain B lymphocytes and constitute bursa/bone marrow dependent areas. Between the cortical follicles and medullary cords, there is a broad, ill-defined intermediate zone called para cortical area. The para cortical area contains T lymphocytes and constitutes the thymus dependent area.

*Functions of Lymph Node*

- Lymph nodes act as filter for lymph
- Phagocytosis of foreign particles takes place in lymph node
- They help the proliferation and circulation of T and B cells
- They enlarge following local antigenic stimulus
- The plasma cells secrete antibodies
- Lymph node is highly efficient in trapping antigen.

*Spleen*

Spleen is the largest of the lymphoid organs. It has a capsule from which descent trabeculae dividing the organ into several interconnected compartments. Spleen is made up of white pulp and red pulp.

*White Pulp*

The splenic artery travels along the trabeculae. On entering the spleen the artery divides into arterioles which are surrounded by lymphoid tissues. This part is called white pulp. White pulp is rich in lymphoid cells.

*Red Pulp*

It is called red pulp because of the red blood cells. Macrophages also are present in this area.

*Functions of Spleen*

- The spleen serves as the graveyard for red blood cells
- The white pulp is rich in T cells and B cells
- The T cells are seen peripherally and the B cells are seen centrally
- After an antigenic stimulus the germinal center containing large number of B cells and plasma cells appear in the periarteriolar areas and almost replace T cells.

*Mucosa Associated Lymphoid Tissue*

The mucosa lining the alimentary, respiratory, genitourinary and other surfaces is exposed to antigens. So these areas have rich collection of lymphoid cells.

These lymphoid cells are called Peyer's patches or scattered isolated lymphoid follicles. These are called as mucosa associated lymphoid tissue (MALT).

Lymphoid tissues in the gut, i.e. from the adenoids and tonsils up to the follicles of colon are called gut associated lymphoid tissues (GALT).

*Functions of MALT and GALT*

- They contain lymphoid and phagocytic cells and a special cell called M cells.
- Both B and T cells are present.
- Predominant antibody produced is IgA in the mucosal lining. Others such as IgG, IgM, and IgE are also produced.
- IgA antibodies provide first line of defense against infectious agents.

## CELLS OF THE IMMUNE SYSTEM

Immune system consists of many organs and different cell types.

The cells of the immune system develop from pluripotent stem cells from bone marrow. The hematopoietic stem cells give rise to red blood cells. White blood cells develop through two different pathways. The lymphoid lineage produces both T and B lymphocytes, and Natural killer (NK) cells. The myeloid lineage produces monocytes, macrophages, granulocytes, basophils, eosinophils, neutrophils, platelets and also mast cells.

### Lymphocytes

#### T Cells

*Origin*

All cells of lymphoid system arise from the pluripotent stem cells from the bone marrow.

*Maturation*

Maturation of T cells takes place in different stages. Thymus secretes a humoral factor that attracts the T cells to the thymus.

*Stage I*

- Pro T cells or early thymocytes.
- They are present in thymic cortex.
- These are the earliest recognizable thymocytes. They contain cell differentiation molecules CD2 and CD7. CD3 proteins are present in the cytoplasm. Transferrin molecule is also present.

*Stage II*

***Intermediate or common thymocytes:*** These are present in thymic cortex. They constitute 85% of lymphocytes at this stage. Additional markers like CD1, CD4 and CD8 are also present. They are called double positive cells because they contain both CD4 and CD8 markers. Genes coding for the $\alpha$ chain of TCR2 molecules are rearranged in these thymocytes.

*Stage III*

***Mature thymocytes:*** This development takes place in thymic medulla. There is loss of CD1, CD38 and transferrin molecules.

CD3 molecule is present on the cell membrane in association with TCR2 molecules. There is distinction of two cell markers CD4 and CD8. The T cells that possess CD4 are called CD4 T cells and the ones possessing CD8 are called CD8 T cells.

*Functional Subsets of T Cells*

Based on their functions the T cells are subdivided into the following:

- T helper cell
- T suppressor cells
- T cytotoxic cells
- T cells involved in delayed-type hypersensitivity (DTH) reaction.

### B Cell Development

*Pre B Cells to Mature B Cells*

B cells like other blood cells arise from pluripotent hematopoietic stem cells. In embryogenesis, the first B cell lineage makes heavy chain but not light chain. More differentiated cells called pre B cells are detected in the fetal liver about half way through gestation. They appear as large and small lymphocytes with cytoplasmic IgM without surface immunoglobulin (Ig) molecules. Similar cells are seen in small numbers in adult bone marrow indicating that B cells continue to arise from stem cells throughout the life.

*Immature B Cells*

Pre B cells give rise to immature B cells which have surface IgM (sIgM). They lack several other surface molecules.

*Mature B Cells*

These arise from immature B cells. They contain two or more surface Ig isotypes along with sIgM. They also have Fc receptors and complement receptors.

They are not easily made tolerant. In the terminal differentiation the mature B cells are stimulated by T dependent antigen to develop into plasma cells which secrete antibody molecules.

## INNATE AND ADAPTIVE IMMUNITY

Immunity is a state of protection from infectious diseases. It has two components namely nonspecific and specific immunities. The nonspecific component is called ***innate immunity***. Innate immunity is defined as disease resistance mechanisms that are not specific to a particular pathogen. The specific component is called ***acquired immunity or adaptive immunity***.

***Adaptive immunity*** shows a high degree of specificity and memory and requires more time to develop. Innate immunity provides the ***first line of defense*** during the critical period just after the host's exposure to a pathogen. A healthy individual when exposed to a variety of microorganisms the innate immunity clears most of them within a few days. During this time the adaptive immune response is not triggered.

However if the innate immunity fails and the microorganisms try to invade the tissues the specific immune response of adaptive immunity is triggered.

Innate and adaptive immunity do not operate independently. They function as a highly interactive and cooperative systems.

Innate immunity consists of four types of defensive barriers namely anatomic, physiologic, phagocytic and inflammatory barriers.

## FACTORS CONTRIBUTING TO INNATE IMMUNITY: STRUCTURE AND ROLE PLAYED

### Anatomic Barriers

In the first line of defense against infection, physical and anatomic barriers try to prevent the entry of pathogens. The skin and the surface of mucous membranes effectively prevent the entry.

Many pathogens enter the body by binding to and penetrating mucous membranes, overcoming the protective effects.

### Skin

The skin consists of two distinct layers. A thinner outer layer is called the ***epidermis*** and a thicker inner layer is called the ***dermis***.

The epidermis contains many layers of tightly packed epithelial cells.

The outermost epidermal layer consists of dead cells and is filled with a hydrophobic protein called keratin. The dermis, which is composed of connective tissue contains blood vessels, hair follicles, sebaceous glands, and sweat glands. The sebaceous glands are associated with the hair follicles and produce an oily secretion called ***sebum***. Sebum consists of lactic acid and fatty acids. These acids maintain the pH of the skin between 3 and 5. This low pH inhibits the growth of most microorganisms.

Intact skin prevents the entry of pathogens and also its low pH inhibits most bacterial growth. Breaks in the skin, even small ones, result in the entry of pathogens to cause infections. The skin is also penetrated by biting insects (mosquitoes, mites, ticks, fleas, flies); if these insects harbor pathogenic organisms, they can introduce the pathogens into the body as they feed.

### Mucous Membranes

The conjunctiva and the alimentary, respiratory, urogenital tracts are lined by mucous membranes. These membranes consist of an outer epithelial layer and an underlying layer of connective tissue. A number of nonspecific defense mechanisms exist to prevent the entry of pathogens.

For example, saliva, tears, and mucous secretions act to wash away potential invaders. They contain antibacterial and antiviral substances.

The viscous fluid called mucus, which is secreted by epithelial cells entraps foreign microorganisms. In the respiratory and gastrointestinal tract, the mucus membrane is covered by cilia. The synchronous movement of cilia propels mucus-entrapped microorganisms towards the exterior from these tissues. In addition, nonpathogenic organisms tend to colonize epithelial cells of mucosal surfaces. These normal flora generally compete with pathogens for attachment sites on the epithelial cell surface and for necessary nutrients. Mucus also contains the enzyme lysozyme which lyses the bacterial cell. Mucoproteins present in the mucus also inhibit the hemagglutinins of influenza virus.

Many pathogens enter the body by binding to and penetrating mucous membranes, overcoming the protective effects.

### Physiologic Barriers

The following act as physiologic barriers of innate immune response:

- Antibodies against blood group antigens
- Alternate pathway of complement system
- Macrophages
- Interferons
- $\gamma\delta$ cells
- CD5-B cells

Also, the physiologic barriers that contribute to innate immunity include temperature, pH and various soluble factors. Many animal species are not susceptible to certain diseases simply because their normal body temperature inhibits the growth of the pathogens. Chicken for example have innate immunity to anthrax because their high body temperature inhibits the growth of the bacteria. Gastric acidity acts as physiologic barrier to infection because very few ingested microorganisms can survive the low pH of the stomach contents. In the mouth, streptococci produce peroxides that compete with bacteria for iron and enhance respiratory activity in neutrophils. Many soluble factors contribute to nonspecific immunity such as the enzyme lysozyme, interferon, and complement.

The flushing action of urine combined with the low pH of the urinogenital tract prevents the pathogens from establishing in the urogenital tract. Desquamation of epithelial cells from the vaginal wall in adult women provides a substrate for lactobacilli growth. These bacteria produce lactic acid, and also compete with pathogenic bacteria for nutrients and space.

The flushing action of milk in the mammary gland that contains lactenins, bacterial inhibitors, iron binding protein lactoferrin lactoperoxidase, and IgA enhancers also contributes to innate immunity. Phagocytic cells released into the mammary gland caused in response to irritation due to sucking contributes to phagocytic action, lactoferrins and hydrogen peroxide.

- ***Antimicrobial peptides:*** Cells of many animals produce antimicrobial substances that act as endogenous natural antibiotics or disinfectants.
  These micropeptides take many forms.
- ***α-Defensins:*** There are six known human alpha defensins. Four belong to neutrophils and the other two are present in vagina and cervix.
- ***β-Defensins:*** Large amounts of β-Defensins appear in Henley's loop, distal and collecting tubules of kidney and also in the vagina, cervix, uterus and fallopian tubes. These peptides have broad spectrum, salt-sensitive antibacterial activity and show synergy with lysozyme and lactoferrin.
- ***Cathelicidins:*** Humans express only one cathelicidin, a prepropeptide that is released after neutrophil elastase action.
- ***Protegrins:*** They are broad-spectrum antimicrobial peptides found in porcine neutrophils, where they are stored as cathelin containing precursors.
- ***Granulysin:*** They are found in granules of human cytolytic T lymphocytes and natural killer cells. They act in combination with perforins, gain access to intracellular compartment of microbes and kill them.
- ***Histatins:*** These are small histidine-rich human salivary proteins that display moderate activity against *Candida albicans* at acidic pH and also have antifungal actions.
- ***Lysozyme:*** It is a hydrolytic enzyme found in mucus secretions and tears, and is able to cleave the peptidoglycan layer of the bacterial cell wall.
- ***Interferon:*** Comprises a group of proteins produced by virus-infected cells. One of the many functions of the interferons is the ability to bind to nearby cells. It also induces a generalized antiviral state.

There are three different types of interferons:

1. IFN-α
2. IFN-β
3. IFN-γ.

They are synthesized by leucocytes on exposure to viruses, fibroblasts and effector T cells on induction respectively. The second effect of interferons in host defense is to increase expression of the MHC class I complex and TAP transporter proteins, enhancing the ability of virus-infected cells to present viral peptides to CD-8 cells. The third property is the activation of natural killer cells.

**Complement** is a group of serum proteins that circulate in an inactive state. A variety of specific and nonspecific immunologic mechanisms can convert the inactive forms of complement proteins into active form. When activated complement can cause damage to the membranes of pathogenic organisms, so that they are either destroyed or phagocytosed and cleared.

## Phagocytic Barriers

Another important innate defense mechanism is the ingestion of extracellular particulate material by phagocytosis. Phagocytosis is a phenomenon in which there is uptake of material by a cell from its environment. In phagocytosis, a cell's plasma membrane expands around the particulate material to form large vesicles called phagosomes.

Most phagocytosis is conducted by specialized cells, such as blood monocytes, neutrophils, and tissue macrophages. Phagocytosis may be enhanced by a variety of factors collectively termed as ***opsonins*** which consist of antibodies and various serum components of complement.

***Polymorphonuclear (PMN) leucocytes*** also referred to as granulocytes include basophils, mast cells, eosinophils and neutrophils.

These short-lived phagocytic cells contain lysosomes filled with hydrolytic enzymes. They play a major role in protection against infection.

*Macrophages:* These cells enter the blood as monocytes and migrate to different tissues. In these tissues they undergo different changes.

The monocyte is a small, spherical cell with few projections, abundant cytoplasm, little endoplasmic reticulum, and many granules. Macrophages of different tissues have different names. In liver they are called Kupffer cells, in lungs—alveolar macrophages, in spleen–splenic macrophages, in brain—microglial cells, etc.

Macrophages have the following functions:

- They phagocytose particles from the environment.
- Process antigens and present to T cells, thus function as ***antigen-presenting cells.***

Certain cytotoxic or killer cells destroy the target cell not by phagocytosis but by releasing biologically potent molecules. Such killer cells include the cytotoxic T lymphocytes and *Natural killer cells* (NK Cells).

## Inflammatory Barriers

Tissue damage caused by a wound or by an invading pathogenic microorganism induces a complex sequence of events collectively called as the ***inflammatory response.*** As early as the first century AD, the Roman physician Celsus described the 'five cardinal signs of infection' as *rubor* (redness), *tumor* (swelling), *calor* (heat), *dolor* (pain) and *function laesa* (loss of function).

The cardinal signs of inflammation reflect the major events of an inflammatory response.

- *Vasodilation:* An increase in the diameter of blood vessels of nearby capillaries occurs. The vessels that carry blood away from the affected area constrict. This results in engorgement of the capillary network. The engorged capillaries are responsible for tissue redness (erythema) and in increase in tissue temperature.
- An increase in capillary permeability facilitates an influx of fluid and cells from the engorged capillaries into the tissue. The fluid that accumulates (exudates) has a much higher protein content. Accumulation of fluid contributes to tissue swelling (edema).
- Influx of phagocytes from the capillaries into the tissue is facilitated by the increased capillary permeability. As phagocytic cells accumulate at the site and begin to phagocytose bacteria, they release lytic enzymes, which can damage nearby healthy cells. The accumulation of dead cells, digested material, and fluid forms a substance called pus.

The events in the inflammatory response are initiated by a complex series of events. During the inflammatory response, many chemical mediators are released, in response to tissue damage. They are called **acute-phase proteins.** The concentrations of these proteins increase dramatically in tissue-damaging infections. C-reactive protein is a major acute-phase protein produced by the liver. Another mediator of the inflammatory response is **histamine,** a chemical released by a variety of cells in response to tissue damage. Histamine causes vasodilation and increased permeability. Another important group of inflammatory mediators are called **kinins.** They are normally present in blood plasma in an inactive form. Tissue injury activates these peptides, which then cause vasodilation and increased permeability. A particular kinin, called bradykinin, also stimulates pain receptors in the skin. Vasodilation and the increase in capillary permeability in an injured tissue also enable enzymes of the blood-clotting system to enter the tissue. These enzymes activate an enzyme cascade that results in the deposition of insoluble strands of **fibrin.** The fibrin strands wall off the injured area from the rest of the body and serve to prevent the spread of infection.

Once the inflammatory response has subsided and most of the debris has been cleared away by phagocytic cells, tissue repair and regeneration of new tissue begins. Capillaries grow into the fibrin of a blood clot. New connective tissue cells, called fibroblasts and capillaries accumulate, and scar tissue forms.

### *Collaboration between Innate and Adaptive Immunity*

Innate and Adaptive immunity do not operate in total independence of each other. They cooperate in important ways to produce more effective immunity. For example, the encounter between macrophages and microbes can generate antigen presenting cells that stimulate and direct adaptive immune responses. This facilitates the participation of the adaptive immune system in the elimination of the pathogen.

Macrophages also secrete immunoregulatory hormone-like molecules, called cytokines. The cytokines and other signals generated by innate immunity play important roles in triggering lymphocyte responses.

The adaptive immune system produces signals and components that stimulate and increase the effectiveness of innate responses. There is increase in the ability of macrophages to kill the microbes they have ingested. The production of antibodies against an invading pathogen also has important effects on the recruitment of the complement system to the defense of the host. By binding to the pathogen, antibodies mark it as a target for attack by complement, and the complex of antibody and pathogen is also a potent activator of this attack.

Thus, these two systems, nonspecific and specific immunity, form an interactive and mutually supportive network that erects an effective and formidable barrier to infection.

## ADAPTIVE IMMUNITY

Immunity is the resistance shown by the host towards injury caused by microorganisms and their products. Immunity can be classified into two types. They are innate or natural immunity and acquired or adaptive immunity.

Innate immunity is the resistance to infections which individuals possess due to their genetic makeup. Innate immunity is again divided into two types. They are specific and non-specific.

Acquired or adaptive immunity which occurs after exposure to an infectious agent is specific and is mediated by either antibodies or lymphoid cells. It can be passive or active.

### Passive Immunity

Passive immunity is transmitted by antibodies preformed in another host. It is of two types. They are natural passive and artificial passive immunity. In natural passive immunity the antibodies which are formed in mother are transferred to fetus. They give protection to the newborn babies for three months. In artificial passive immunity the preformed antibodies are administered to the persons. For example, anti- tetanus serum is used as passive immunization against tetanus. It provides immediate and temporary protection.

### Active Immunity

It is produced directly by the immune system of the host. Also it is induced by contact with antigen and give long lasting protection.

The immune response is of two types. They are humoral immunity and cell mediated immunity.

It is produced directly by the immune system of the host. Also it is induced by contact with antigen and give long lasting protection. The immune response is of two types. They are humoral immunity and cell mediated immunity.

Adaptive or acquired immunity forms the hosts second line of defense.

When microorganisms overcome or circumvent the innate, nonspecific defense mechanism or deliberately administered as vaccines, they encounter the adaptive immunity.

### Definition

Adaptive (acquired) immunity, refers to antigen-specific defense mechanisms that take several days to become protective and are designed to remove a specific antigen.

This is the immunity one develops throughout life. Six major characteristics of acquired immunity are:

1. ***Specificity:*** It shows exquisite specificity for distinct molecules against which it is induced and does not recognize other molecules.
2. ***Self-nonself discrimination or tolerance:*** It can discriminate self-antigens belonging to the individuals own body and are made tolerant to these self-antigens. Under very rare circumstances they react to the self- antigens body and are made tolerant to these self-antigens.
3. ***Inducible:*** Adaptive immune response can be induced artificially.
4. ***Diversity:*** Different types of microbes induce responses in different ways so that diverse responses are generated.
5. ***Memory:*** Adaptive immune response has the ability to remember and respond more vigorously to repeated exposure to the same microbe.
6. ***Self-limiting:*** Adaptive immunity usually improves upon repeated exposure to a given infection.

Adaptive immunity involves the following:

- Antigen-presenting cells (APCs) such as macrophages and dendritic cells
- The activation and proliferation of antigen-specific B-lymphocytes
- The activation and proliferation of antigen-specific T-lymphocytes
- And the production of antibody molecules, cytotoxic T-lymphocytes (CTLs), activated macrophages and NK cells, and cytokines. There are two major branches of the adaptive immune responses: Humoral immunity and cell-mediated immunity.
  - ***Humoral immunity:*** Humoral immunity involves the production of antibody molecules in response to an antigen and is mediated by B-lymphocytes.
  - ***Cell-mediated immunity:*** Cell-mediated immunity involves the production of cytotoxic T-lymphocytes, activated macrophages, activated NK cells, and cytokines in response to an antigen.

## Humoral Immune System

B cells develop in bone marrow. These B cells have membrane bound antibody as a receptor for antigen. Each B cell makes one kind of antibody. B cells differentiate into plasma cells, which produce large amounts of soluble antibody.

## Cellular Immune System

Helper T cells mature in the thymus and contain a single T cell receptor for antigen. Helper T cell activation requires recognition of antigen and a co-stimulatory signal from the innate immune system.

Helper T cells contain a surface protein called CD4 and must be activated by the antigen presenting dendritic cells of the innate immune system.

## Fate of Antigens

Antigens are of two types namely complete antigens and incomplete antigens. Complete antigens are substances when introduced into the body induce an immune response. Incomplete antigens do not induce immune response but they react with preformed antibodies and are called **haptens.**

The mechanisms by which the complete antigens are destroyed depend on factors such as:

- Physical nature of antigens
- Chemical nature of antigen
- Dose of antigen
- Route of entry
- Antigen presentation.

### *Physical Nature of Antigen*

Particulate antigens are removed from the circulation by two phases, one by a non-immune phase and another by immune phase. In the non-immune phase antigen is removed by phagocytic cells and in the immune phase antigen-antibody complexes are formed.

With soluble antigens three phases are seen. In the phase of equilibrium, the antigen is diffused into extravascular spaces. In the metabolic phase the antigen level falls down due to catabolic decay and during immune elimination the antigen is eliminated by antigen antibody reactions.

### *Chemical Nature of Antigen*

Protein antigens are eliminated within weeks. Polysaccharide antigens are eliminated slowly. It takes several months to destroy them.

### *Dose of Antigen*

Macrophages modulate the dose of antigens so that they are not too low or too high.

### *Route of Entry*

Antigens introduced intravenously are localized in spleen, liver bone marrow, kidneys and lungs and are killed by reticuloendothelial cells mainly tissue macrophages.

Antigens introduced subcutaneously are localized in lymph nodes.

### *Presentation of Antigen*

Presentation of antigens to the immunocompetent cells is carried out by macrophages and dendritic cells.

*Adjuvants*

Adjuvants are substances which enhance the immune responses. Immunocompetent B lymphocytes recognize antigens and produce antibodies. For this recognition it requires T cell help. Once B cell contacts its specific antigen, it undergoes clonal proliferation and is converted into plasma cells and secretes antibody.

## ANTIBODIES

Antibodies are glycoprotein molecules which are produced in response to an antigen, and reacts specifically with it in an observable manner.

- Tiselius in 1937 analyzed serum by free zone electrophoresis and characterized proteins at pH 8.6. All proteins have negative charge and move towards anode.

- Tiselius and Kabat analyzed rabbit's hyperimmune sera before and after absorption with immunizing agent.
  - After absorption there was pronounced decrease in γ globulin.
  - Hence antibody activity was traced down to γ globulin.

## Immunoglobulin

- γ globulin is not a homogeneous protein
- In 1964 WHO international agreement selected the generic name Ig for all antibody containing proteins
- They subdivided Ig into different classes.

### *Immunoglobulin Classes*

In man 5 major classes of Ig are described:

1. *IgG:* The major serum component
2. *IgM:* Macroglobulin
3. *IgA:* Present predominantly in secretions
4. *IgD:* Important cell membrane receptor form
5. *SgE:* Antibody involved in hypersensitivity reaction.

## Characterization of Antibodies

- Early physical chemical studies were done with IgG from horse, rabbit and human
- Important structural features were predicted even before sophisticated studies were available
- Molecular weight was calculated from sedimentation and diffusion studies
- Asymmetrical and or non-globular form by viscosity studies
- Globular domain structure from unique susceptibility to proteolytic enzymes
- Two antigen binding sites by hapten antibody reactions
- Thus early studies predicted three functional domains and have been confirmed.

## Structure of Antibodies

- Before going into the structure of antibody, one must know the structure of proteins
- Proteins are made from amino acids
- Amino acids form poly peptide chains
- Polypeptides form proteins
- Proteins have 3 dimensional structure:
  - If any change in the primary sequence of amino acid in polypeptide
  - Or in three dimensional structure there is change in the property.

## Digestion with Enzymes

- Rodney and Porter digested rabbit Ig with the enzyme papain
- It cleaved the molecule and produced two major fractions and a small amount of short peptides.

## Before/After Absorption

- One fraction (MW 45,000) still possessed antigen binding site and was named as fragment antibody binding (Fab)
- The other fragment could be crystallized, and was called Fragment crystallized (Fc)
- Fab possessed antigen binding site but was monovalent
- Possessed one reactive site
- Could not cross link antigen molecule
- When one added up the molecular weights of Fab and Fc fragments, plus the observation that the Fab was monovalent, it appeared that the original antibody contained.
- Two Fab fragments and one Fc fragment.

## General Formula for Antibody

- The general formula for antibody is (H2 L2)
- The Igs are made of 2 heavy chains and 2 light chains
- These are held together by covalent bonds
- These bonds are interchain disulphide bridges
- Each chain is made of a number of loops
- These loops are known as domains
- Each domain is formed by intrachain disulphide bonds
- There are 2 loop sections per L chain and 4 loop sections per H chain
- There are two terminals in each chain:
  - One is called C terminus
  - Other is called N terminus.

## Digestion with Papain and Pepsin

- When antibody molecule was treated with enzyme pepsin, it was cleaved in different fashion
- A large fragment with two antigen binding sites and smaller fragments
- The larger fragment was called (Fab) 2 fragment.

### *Light Chain*

- C terminus contains the constant region
- N terminus contains the variable region
- L chain is named as Kappa (κ) and lambda (λ)
  - Contains two domains
  - Domain at N terminus is variable domain of light chain called VL
  - Domain at C terminus is constant domain called CL.

### *Types of Heavy Chain*

- There are 5 different types of H chains
- Based on the type of H chain the classes of antibody is determined
- They are:
  - γ Gamma—IgG
  - α Alpha—IgA
  - μ Mu—IgM
  - ξ Epsilon—IgE
  - δ Delta—IgD.

#### *Properties and Functions of IgM*

- IgM is the main immunoglobulin produced early in primary immune response
- It is present on the surface of all uncommitted B lymphocytes
- IgM is a pentamer and the valence is 10
- IgM is the most efficient immunoglobulin in agglutination, complement fixation and other antigen antibody reactions
- It plays an important role in the defense against bacterial and viral diseases
- It does not cross placenta.

*IgG*

- It has two identical antigen binding sites and is bivalent
- There are four subclasses namely IgG1, IgG2, IgG3 and IgG4
- IgG is the predominant antibody in secondary immune response
- It plays an important role in defense against bacteria, viruses
- It also neutralizes toxins
- It crosses placenta and is found in large quantities in newborns.

*IgA*

- IgA is found mainly in secretions like milk, tears, saliva and secretions of respiratory, intestinal and genital tracts.
- It protects the mucus membranes against microbial attack.
- As many microbes enter the body through these mucus membranes, IgA offers the first line of defense.
- Each IgA molecule consists of two H2L2 units and a J chain and a secretory component.
- The secretory component is a polypeptide synthesized by epithelial cells and it helps IgA to pass the mucosal surface.

*IgE*

- IgE antibody is present in increased quantities in allergic individuals.
- The Fc portions of the molecule binds to mast cells and eosinophils.
- When this antibody combines with its antigen on the mast cell surface, it leads to allergic response.

*IgD*

- IgD has no antibody function
- It may act as antigen receptor on cells
- In serum it is present in only trace amounts.

## EXERCISE

### Antigen-Antibody Reactions

### *Antigen*

Antigen is defined as foreign substance capable of inducing a specific immune response, which is also called immunogen.

### *Antibody*

It is a protein produced from plasma cell consisting of two identical heavy chains and light chains that recognizes a particular epitope on an antigen and reacts with it in an observable manner.

Antigens and antibodies combine with each other specifically in an observable manner. The reactions between antigens and antibodies are useful in many ways.

- They form the basis of antibody mediated immunity against infectious diseases.
- They cause tissue injury in some type of hypersensitivity reactions and autoimmune diseases.
- In the laboratory, they help:
  - In the diagnosis of infections
  - In epidemiological surveys
  - In the identification of infectious agents and noninfectious agents such as enzymes. In general these reactions can be used for the identification of either antigens or antibodies. Antigen-antibody reactions in vitro are known as serological reactions.

### *Stages Involved in Antigen-antibody Reactions*

The reaction between antigen and antibody occurs in three stages.

1. *Primary stage:* The primary stage is the initial reaction between the two, without any visible effects. This reaction is rapid, occurs even at low temperatures and obeys the general law of physical chemistry and thermodynamics. The reaction is reversible, the combination between antigen and antibody molecules being effected by the weaker intramolecular forces such as van der Waals forces, ionic bonds and hydrogen bonding rather than by the firmer covalent bonding. The primary reaction can be detected by estimating free and bound antigen or antibody separately in the reaction mixture.
2. *Secondary stage:* The secondary stage leads to demonstrable events such as precipitation, agglutination, lysis of cells, killing of live antigens, neutralization reactions, complement fixation and enhancement of phagocytosis. Thus the antigen causing agglutination was called agglutinin that causing precipitation precipitin. Thus the antibody causing agglutination was called agglutinogen, that causing precipitin precipitinogen.
3. *Tertiary stage:* Some antigen-antibody reactions occurring in vivo initiate chain reactions that lead to neutralization or destruction of injurious antigens, or to tissue damage. These are the tertiary reactions and include humoral immunity against infectious disease as well as clinical allergy and other immunological diseases.

### *General Features of Antigen-antibody Reactions*

Antigen-antibody reactions have the following general characteristics:

- The reaction is specific. An antigen combines only with its homologous antibody and vice versa. The specificity, however is not absolute and cross reaction may occur due to antigenic similarity and relatedness.
- Entire molecules react and not fragments.
- There is no denaturation of the antigen or the antibody during the reaction.
- The combination occurs at the surface.
- The combination is firm but reversible. The firmness of the union is influenced by the affinity and the avidity of the reaction. Affinity refers to the intensity if interaction between the Antigen and Antibody. Avidity is the strength of the bond after the formation of the complexes.
- Both antigens and antibodies participate in the formation of agglutinates or precipitates.
- Antigens and antibodies can combine in varying proportion.

### *Measurement of Antignen and Antibody*

Many methods are available for the measurement of antigen and antibody participating in the reactions.

Measurement may be in terms of mass or more commonly as units or titer.

The antibody titer of a serum is the highest dilution of the serum which gives an observable reaction with antigen in the particular reaction.

The titer of a serum is influenced by the nature and the type and conditions of the test.

There are two important parameters of serological tests. They are sensitivity and specificity. Sensitivity refers to the ability of the test to detect even very minute quantity of the antigen or antibody.

Specificity refers to the ability of the test to detect reactions between homologous antigens and antibodies only.

### *Types of Antigen-antibody Reactions*

- Precipitation
- Agglutination
- Neutralization

### *Agglutination Reaction*

When a particulate antigen is mixed with its antibody in the presence of electrolytes at a suitable temperature and pH, the particles are clumped together or agglutinated.

Agglutination is more sensitive than precipitation for the detection of antibodies. The same principles govern agglutination and precipitation.

Agglutination occurs optimally when antigens and antibodies react in equivalent proportions. The zone phenomenon may be seen when either an antibody or antigen is in excess.

Incomplete or monovalent antibodies do not cause agglutination, though they combine with the antigen. They may act as blocking antibodies, inhibiting agglutination by the complete antibody added subsequently.

### *Types of Agglutination Reactions*

- Slide agglutination
- Tube agglutination
- Passive agglutination
- Hemagglutination

*Slide Agglutination*

When a drop of the appropriate antiserum is added to a smooth, uniform suspension of a particulate antigen in the drop of a saline on a slide or tile, agglutination takes place. A positive result is indicated by the clumping together of the particles and the clearing of the drop. Mixing the antigen and the antiserum with a loop or gently rocking the slide facilitates the reaction. Depending on the titer of the serum, agglutination may occur instantly or within seconds. Clumping occurring after a minute may be due to drying of the fluid and should be disregarded.

It is essential to have on the same slide a control consisting of the antigen suspension in saline, without the antiserum, to ensure that the antigen is not agglutinable. Agglutination is usually visible to the naked eye but may sometimes require confirmation under the microscope.

Slide agglutination is a routine procedure for the identification of many bacterial isolates from clinical specimens. It is also the method used for blood grouping and cross matching.

*Tube Agglutination*

This is a standard quantitative method for the measurement of antibodies. When a fixed volume of a particulate antigen suspension is added to an equal volume of serial dilution of an antiserum in test tubes, the agglutination titer of the serum can be estimated. Tube agglutination is routinely employed for the serological diagnosis of typhoid, brucellosis and rickettsial fever. Widal agglutination test is done for typhoid, Brucella agglutination test is done for Brucellosis and Weil-Felix test is done for rickettsial infections.

## PRECIPITATION REACTIONS

When a soluble antigen combines with its antibody in the presence of electrolytes (NaCl) at a suitable temperature and pH the precipitation of antigen and antibody complex occurs.

Precipitation occurs most rapidly and abundantly in which antigen and antibody are present in equivalent proportion. In the preceding tubes in which the antigen is excess and in the latter tube antibody is in excess the precipitation will be weak or even absent.

### Quantitative Precipitation Test

Marrack (1934) proposed the lattice hypothesis to explain the mechanism of precipitation. According to this concept, multivalent antigen combines with bivalent antibody in varying proportions. Precipitation results when a layer of lattice is formed consisting of alternating antigen and antibody molecules. This is possible only at zone of equivalence.

In the zones of antigen and antibody, excess, the lattice does not exist.

### Application of Precipitation Reaction

The precipitation test may be carried out either as qualitative or as a quantitative test. It is used for detecting antigen and antibody. It is therefore, used in application in the identification of blood and seminal stains and also in testing of food adulteration. The following types of precipitation tests are in common use:

- ***Ring test***
  - *Ascoli test:* This is used for the detection of bacterial antigen anthrax in tissues /organs of dead animals or man.
  - It can be used for Lancefield grouping of Streptococci.
- ***Slide test:*** In a clean slide a drop of antigen is taken and a drop of antibody is mixed. Floccules appear. VDRL slide test for syphilis is done in this way.
- ***Tube test:*** Antigen and antibody are allowed to react in the tubes to form precipitates. Khan test for syphilis is done in this way.
- ***Precipitation test in gels:*** Immunodiffusion is usually performed in a soft 1% agar gel.

  Antigen and antibody react in thin gel to form a line of precipitate.

### Types of Immunodiffusion

Single diffusion in one dimension (oudin procedure): Antibody is incorporated in agar gel in a test tube. The antigen solution is layered over it. The antigen diffuses downward through the agar gel forming a line of precipitation.

### *Double Diffusion in One Dimension (Oakley-Fulthorpe Procedue)*

Antibody is incorporated in a gel in the tube. Above the antibody a column of plain agar is placed. Antigen is placed on top of this.

The antigen and antibody move towards each other in the column of plain agar and form the precipitation line.

### *Single Diffusion in Two Dimensions (Radial Immunodiffusion)*

In this test the antibody is incorporated in the agar gel. Wells are cut in the gel. Antigen is added to the wells. The antigen diffuses radially from the well and forms ring shaped bands of precipitation concentrically around the well. The diameter of the halo gives the estimate of the concentration of the antigen.

It is used to estimate the concentration of the classes of immunoglobulin in the serum.

### *Double Diffusion in Two Dimensions*

Agar gel is poured on a slide and wells are cut. Antiserum is placed in the central well different antigens are placed in the surrounding wells.

Antigens and antibodies move towards each other and form precipitin lines. Different types of precipitin lines are formed. If the two adjacent antigens are identical, the lines of precipitate will fuse together.

If they are not identical the lines will cross each other. If there is partial identity there will be a spur formation.

This test can be used for comparing different antigen and antibody systems.

Other types of immunoprecipitation tests in gel are immunoelectrophoresis, electroimmunodiffusion and crossed immunoelectrophoresis, etc.

## MULTIPLE CHOICE QUESTIONS

**1. Antiseptic techniques in surgery were introduced by:**
(a) John Tyndall (b) Ivanovosky
(c) Loeffler (d) Joseph Lister

**2. Which decolorizer is used in Gram's Staining?**
(a) Sulfuric acid (b) Hydrochloric acid
(c) Alcohol (d) Picric acid

**3. Which of the following is organ of locomotion in bacteria?**
(a) Pili (b) Flagella
(c) Cilia (d) Pseudopodia

**4. The chemical agent used for fumigation of operation theaters:**
(a) Alcohol (b) Iodine
(c) Formaldehyde (d) Phenol

**5. Rice water stool are characteristic of diarrhea due to:**
(a) Shigella (b) Pseudomonas
(c) Vibrio cholerae (d) Proteus vulgaris

**6. Common cause of pyogenic meningitis in younger children are all EXCEPT:**
(a) Streptococcus pneumoniae
(b) H influenzae
(c) N meningitidis
(d) Streptococcus viridians

**7. Hydrophobia is characteristic of which viral disease?**
(a) Hepatitis (b) Polio
(c) Rabies (d) Herpes

**8. Infective form of *E. histolytica* is:**
(a) Uninucleated cyst (b) Binucleated
(c) Trophozoite (d) Quadrinucleated cyst

**9. Which of the following antibody denotes recent infection?**
(a) IgG (b) IgA
(c) IgD (d) IgM

**10. Which fungus causes oral thrush in bottle fed infants?**
(a) Cryptococcus (b) Penicillium
(c) Candida (d) Histoplasma

**11. Which serological test is done for diagnosis of typhus fever?**
(a) Weil-Felix (b) ASO
(c) Widal (d) VDRL

**12. Man act as definitive host in the following parasite EXCEPT:**
(a) Leishmania (b) Plasmodium
(c) W. Bancrofti (d) Taenia

**13. Which of the following is affected by dermatophytes?**
(a) Hair (b) Skin
(c) Nail (d) All the above

**14. Bacteria static agents means:**
(a) Which kills bacteria
(b) Inhibits the growth of bacteria
(c) Stimulates the growth of bacteria
(d) None of the above

**15. Which of the following is anaerobic culture medium?**
(a) Alkaline peptone medium
(b) Bile medium
(c) Robertson's cooked meat medium
(d) Nutrient medium

**16. Infection with which of the following parasite causes Iron deficiency anemia?**
(a) Ascaris lumbricoides
(b) Taenia solium
(c) Enterobius vermicularis
(d) Ancylostoma duodenale

**17. Which of the following organism causes sexually transmitted diseases?**
(a) N. gonorrhoeae (b) Chlamydia
(c) Treponema pallidum (d) Nocardia

**18. Which parasite causes filariasis in man?**
(a) Giardia
(b) Ancylostoma duodenale
(c) Wuchereria bancrofti
(d) Leishmania

**19. Universal safety precautions should be followed for:**
(a) All patients
(b) Hospitalized patient
(c) HIV infected patients
(d) HIV and HBV infected patients

**20. Media most commonly used for the isolation of fungi is:**
(a) Sabourauds dextrose agar
(b) MacConkey agar
(c) Loeffiler serum slope
(d) Lowenstein-Jensen medium

**21. Virus contain:**
(a) DNA (b) RNA
(c) Both A and B (d) Either A or B

**22. The commonly used transport media for anaerobes:**
(a) Hartleys broth (b) Alkaline peptone water
(c) RCM (d) All the above

**23. Cigar bundle appearance on microscopy is a feature of:**
(a) C. Diphtheriae (b) M. Leprae
(c) Cl. Perfringens (d) N. Gonorrhoeae

**24. Number of bacteria present in per mL of urine to consider it as significant bacteriuria is greater than or equal to:**
(a) 100 (b) 1000
(c) 10000 (d) 100000

**25. Blood agar is an example of:**
(a) Transport medium
(b) Differential medium
(c) Enrichment medium
(d) Enriched medium

**26. Disposal of soiled dressing is done in:**
(a) Red bag (b) Yellow bag
(c) Black bag (d) Brown bag

**27. Which hepatitis is transmitted through feco-oral route?**
(a) A (b) B
(c) C (d) D

**28. Which bacteria show Chinese letter appearance?**
(a) Bordetella
(b) Corynebacterium
(c) Mycobacterium leprea
(d) Clostridium

**29. Commonest source of staphylococcal infection is:**
(a) Fomites (b) Vectors
(c) Human carriers (d) Infected animals

**30. Poliovirus enter human body through:**
(a) Inhalation (b) Ingestion
(c) Skin cut (d) Sexual route

**31. Following are suitable disinfectants for skin EXCEPT:**
(a) Ethanol (b) Dettol
(c) Formalin (d) Savlon

**32. Following are live vaccine EXCEPT:**
(a) OPV (b) BCG
(c) MMR (d) TAB

**33. Enterobius vermicularis is commonly known as:**
(a) Round worm (b) Hook worm
(c) Tape worm (d) Pin worm

**34. Which of the following is known as acid fast bacilli?**
(a) Corynebacterium (b) Mycobacterium
(c) Mycoplasma (d) Bacillus anthracis

**35. Which organism can grow in disinfectants and antiseptic lotions kept in hospital used?**
(a) Proteus (b) Salmonella
(c) Pseudomonas (d) Klebsiella

**36. Arrangement of streptococci is in:**
(a) Clusters (b) Chains
(c) Pairs (d) Cigar bundle appearance

**37. Dengue is caused by bite of:**
(a) Tick (b) Mite
(c) Louse (d) Mosquito

**38. When flagella are distributed all around the bacterial cell, the arrangement is known as:**
(a) Monotrichous (b) Lophotrichous
(c) Amphitrichous (d) Peritrichous

**39. Non-infectious waste is disposed in _____ color coded bags.**
(a) Red (b) Yellow
(c) Black (d) Blue transparent

**40. Samples for microbiological (bacteriological) investigations should be sent in:**
(a) Cork screw container (b) Sterile container
(c) Washed container (d) Plugged container

**41. Microscopic examination of peripheral blood smear is used to demonstrate:**
(a) Microfilaria (b) Malaria parasite
(c) Trypanosomes (d) All the above

**42. Common opportunistic infections seen in HIV/AIDS patient include:**
(a) Toxoplasmosis (b) Herpes
(c) Candidiasis (d) All the above

**43. The enzyme coagulase is produced by:**
(a) Staphylococcus aureus
(b) Staphylococcus epidermidis
(c) Micrococcus
(d) Streptococcus pyogenes

**44. The discovery of compound microscope is attributed to:**
(a) Antou van Leeuwenhoek
(b) Robert Koch
(c) Louis Pasteur
(d) Joseph Lister

**45. Cultivation of virus can be done using following method EXCEPT:**
(a) Embryonated egg inoculation
(b) Culture media
(c) Animal inoculation
(d) Cell culture

**46. The reaction of soluble antigen with homologous antibody is known as:**
(a) Agglutination (b) Precipitation
(c) Neutralization (d) Complement fixation

**47. The commonest cause of non-suppurative lesion like acute rheumatic fever is:**
(a) Streptococcus viridians
(b) Streptococcus pneumonia
(c) Streptococcus pyogenes
(d) Staphylococcus aureus

**48. Drumstick appearance is a characteristic morphology of:**
(a) Clostridium perfringens
(b) Clostridium tetani
(c) Clostridium bifermentans
(d) Clostridium tertium

**49. The selective media for isolation of salmonella is:**
(a) Mannitol sugar agar
(b) Wilson-blair medium
(c) TCBS
(d) Chocolate agar

**50. The counter stain used for Ziehl-Neelsen stain is:**
(a) Methylene blue (b) Carbol fuchsin
(c) Neutral blue (d) Gentian violet

**51. In bacteria growth curve exponential growth of bacteria occurs in:**
(a) Lag phase (b) Log phase
(c) Stationary phase (d) Phase of decline

**52. The antibody which can pass through placenta is:**
(a) IgA (b) IgE
(c) IgM (d) IgG

**53. Bacteria that grows at 55°C are known as:**
(a) Psychrophiles (b) Thermophiles
(c) Halophiles (d) Mesophiles

**54. The term 'steatorrhea' is used to describe stool containing:**
(a) Blood (b) Fat
(c) Mucus (d) Parasite

**55. The size of RBC's increases after they are infected with:**
(a) Plasmodium ovale
(b) Plasmodium vivax
(c) Plasmodium falciparum
(d) Plasmodium malariae

**56. Indian ink preparation is used for demonstration of:**
(a) Candida albicans
(b) Penicillium
(c) Cryptococcus neoformans
(d) Mucor

**57. Bacteria was first observed and described by:**
(a) Antonu van Leeuwenhoek
(b) Louis Pasteur
(c) Joseph lister
(d) Robert Koch

**58. Sporulation of bacteria occurs in:**
(a) Lag phase (b) Log phase
(c) Stationary phase (d) Phase of decline

**59. Commonly used holding time and temperature of autoclave is:**
(a) 145°C for 20 mins (b) 121°C for 26 mins
(c) 121°C for 15 mins (d) 170°C for 10 mins

**60. Cold sterilization is achieved by:**
(a) Gamma rays (b) Pasteurization
(c) UV rays (d) Tyandallization

**61. The technique of sterilization and development of steam sterilizer, hot air oven and autoclave was introduced by:**
(a) Joseph Lister (b) Louis Pasteur
(c) Robert Hook (d) Robert Koch

**62. Period between inoculation of bacteria in a culture medium and beginning of multiplication is known as:**
(a) Lag phase (b) Log phase
(c) Stationary phase (d) Phase of decline

**63. The center of protein synthesis in bacteria are:**
(a) Episomes (b) Mesosomes
(c) Ribosomes (d) Volutin granules

**64. Teichoic acid is typically present in cell wall of:**
(a) Gram positive bacteria
(b) Gram negative bacteria
(c) Fungi
(d) Viruses

**65. Potassium tellurite (KT) medium is an example of:**
(a) Enrich medium (b) Enrichment medium
(c) Selective medium (d) Complex medium

**66. McIntosh–Filde's jar is used for culturing:**
(a) Anaerobes (b) Fungi
(c) Parasite (d) Viruses

**67. In a health care setting measures which will best prevent nosocomial infection is:**
(a) Use of apron (b) Use of gloves
(c) Use of mask (d) Handwashing

**68. Best disinfectant for general use in ward and critical area is:**
(a) Glutaraldehyde (b) Phenol
(c) Savlon (d) Sodium hypochlorite

**69. Temperature of hot air oven:**
(a) 100°C (b) 121°C
(c) 160°C (d) 200°C

**70. Following are waterborne infections EXCEPT:**
(a) Cholera (b) Hepatitis C
(c) Hepatitis E (d) Typhoid fever

**71. Following are example of agglutination reaction:**
(a) Paul-Bunnell test (b) Weil-Felix test
(c) Widal test (d) VDRL test

**72. Following are examples of live vaccines EXCEPT:**
(a) Chickenpox vaccine (b) Measles vaccine
(c) Mumps vaccines (d) Salk polio vaccine

**73. Examples of bacillus is:**
(a) Streptococcus viridans
(b) Neisseria pneumonia
(c) Proteus vulgaris
(d) None of the above

**74. Example of Gram positive, spore bearing anaerobes is:**
(a) Lactobacilli
(b) Klebsiella pneumoniae
(c) Bacillus anthracis
(d) Clostridium perfringens

**75. Typhus fever is caused by:**
(a) Chlamydiae (b) Mycoplasma
(c) Rickettsiae (d) Spirochaetes

**76. Type of hypersensitivity reaction which is mediated by IgE is:**
(a) Type I (b) Type II
(c) Type III (d) Type IV

**77. Superficial fungal infection is caused by:**
(a) Cryptococcus neoformans
(b) Histoplasma capsulatum
(c) Pityriasis versicolor
(d) Rhinosporidium seeberi

**78. Causative agent of syphilis is:**
(a) Borrelia vincentü
(b) Leptospira Spp
(c) Mycoplasma hominis
(d) Treponema pallidum

**79. Alexander Fleming is credited with the accidental discovery of:**
(a) Antituberculine drugs
(b) Penicillin
(c) Qunine
(d) Sulfonamides

**80. Disposable plastic syringes can be sterilized by:**
(a) Ethylene oxide (b) Formaldehyde gas
(c) Halogen (d) Phenolic compounds

**81. Albert stain is used to detect:**
(a) Chlamydiae
(b) Clostridium welchii
(c) Cornybacterium diphtheria
(d) Rickettsiae

**82. Measures which may NOT contribute significantly to control hospital acquired infection is:**
(a) Biomedical waste management
(b) Handwashing
(c) Insertion of IV line under aseptic precautions
(d) Regular disinfection of utensils

**83. Fungi are usually cultured on:**
(a) Blood agar
(b) L-J media
(c) MacConkey's medium
(d) Sabouraud's medium

**84. Bacteria that needs carbon dioxide for growth are:**
(a) Capnophilic (b) Mesophilic
(c) Psychrophilic (d) Thermophilic

**85. All of the following contribute to bacterial pathogenicity EXCEPT:**
(a) Adhesion
(b) Presence of plasmids
(c) Toxigenicity
(d) Presence of volutin granules

**86. Common name of Necator americanus is:**
(a) Roundworm (b) Hookworm
(c) Tapeworm (d) Guinea worm

**87. Which species of plasmodium causes malignant tertian malaria?**
(a) P vivax (b) P falciparum
(c) P ovale (d) P maleriae

**88. Which of the following causes diarrhea?**
(a) Trypanosome (b) Leishmania
(c) Giardia (d) Toxoplasma

**89. BCG vaccine is prepared from:**
(a) Mycobacterium bovis
(b) Mycobacterium tuberculosis
(c) Mycobacterium avium
(d) Mycobacterium xenopi

**90. Sexual mode of reproduction occurs in:**
(a) Accidental host
(b) Definitive host
(c) Intermediate host
(d) None of the above

**91. Example of pigment producing bacteria is:**
(a) Staphylococcus
(b) Pseudomonas
(c) Atypical mycobacterium
(d) All the above

**92. An active motile form of protozoa is termed as:**
(a) Cyst (b) Merozoite
(c) Schizont (d) Trophozoit

**93. Detection of HIV during window period can be done by:**
(a) PCR (b) P 24 antigen
(c) Viral culture (d) All the above

**94. Efficiency of autoclave is checked by:**
(a) Bacillus subtilis
(b) Bacillus stearothermophilus
(c) Clostridium perfringens
(d) Clostridium tetani

**95. NIH swab is used in laboratory diagnosis of infection caused by:**
(a) Ascaris lumbricoides
(b) Enterobius vermicularis
(c) Strongyloides stercoralis
(d) Trichuris trichiura

**96. Usual dose of purified protein derivative (PPD) in Mantoux test is:**
(a) 0.5 IU (b) 5 IU
(c) 50 IU (d) 500 IU

**97. Example of true yeast:**
(a) Candida albicans
(b) Cryptococcus neoformans
(c) Histoplasma capsulatum
(d) None of the above

**98. Best specimen for isolation of salmonella in first week of illness is:**
(a) Blood (b) CSF
(c) Feces (d) Urine

99. **Typhus fever is diagnosed by:**
(a) Dick test (b) Shick test
(c) Weil-Felix staining (d) Widal test

100. **Plague is transmitted by:**
(a) Mites (b) Rat fleas
(c) Sand fleas (d) Ticks

101. **The generation time of bacteria is generally:**
(a) 20 sec (b) 20 min
(c) 20 hrs (d) 21 days

102. **The commonest site of extraintestinal amebiasis is:**
(a) Spleen (b) Liver
(c) Kidney (d) All the above

103. **Operation theaters are sterilized by:**
(a) Ethylene oxide gas
(b) Washing with soap and water
(c) Carbolic acid spraying
(d) Formaldehyde fumigation

104. **AIDS is caused by virus that damages:**
(a) Lymphocytes stem cells
(b) B lymphocytes
(c) $CD_4$ lymphocytes
(d) $CD_8$ lymphocytes

105. **The following are physical methods of sterilization 'EXCEPT':**
(a) Flaming
(b) Sunlight
(c) Gamma radiation
(d) Phenol

106. **The best method of disposing infective hospital material is:**
(a) Radiation
(b) Boiling
(c) Flaming
(d) Incineration

107. **Cerebral malaria is caused by:**
(a) P vivax
(b) P falciparum
(c) P ovale
(d) P malariae

108. **The largest virus is:**
(a) Pox
(b) Foot and mouth disease
(c) HIV
(d) Rabies

109. **The optimum pH of most pathogenic bacteria is:**
(a) 5.4
(b) 7.4
(c) 6.0
(d) 9.0

110. **Resistance acquired by an individual during life is:**
(a) Innate immunity
(b) Acquired immunity
(c) Non-specific immunity
(d) Natural immunity

111. **An association in which parasite derives benefits from host and also produces injury is called:**
(a) Symbiosis
(b) Commensalism
(c) Parasitism
(d) Adaptation

112. **Plague is caused by:**
(a) Yersinia
(b) Pasteurella
(c) Francisella
(d) Edwardsiella

113. **Louis Pasteur's contribution includes:**
(a) Introduced solid media
(b) Discovered rabies vaccine
(c) Discovered tubercle bacillus
(d) Cultured diphtheria bacillus

114. **Bacteria whose optimal temperature growth is 37°C are known as:**
(a) Capnophilic
(b) Psychrophiles
(c) Thermophils
(d) None of the above

115. **Bacterial spore formation is meant for:**
(a) Reproduction
(b) Multiplication
(c) Survival
(d) Toxin production

116. **Bacteria multiply by:**
(a) Sporulation
(b) Binary fission
(c) Budding
(d) None of the above

117. **Food poisoning is caused by:**
(a) S typhi
(b) S paratyphi A
(c) S paratyphi B
(d) S typhimurium

118. **Which of the following mosquitoes act as vector of Chikungunya virus?**
(a) Aedes
(b) Anopheles
(c) Culex
(d) None of the above

119. **Which of the commonest mode of transmission of HIV?**
(a) Sexual
(b) Parenteral
(c) Perinatal
(d) Oral

120. **Shape of rabies virus:**
(a) Polygonal
(b) Bullet shape
(c) Spherical
(d) Tubular

## ANSWERS

| 1. | (d) | 21. | (d) | 41. | (d) | 61. | (b) | 81. | (c) | 101. | (b) |
|---|---|---|---|---|---|---|---|---|---|---|---|
| 2. | (c) | 22. | (c) | 42. | (d) | 62. | (a) | 82. | (d) | 102. | (b) |
| 3. | (b) | 23. | (b) | 43. | (a) | 63. | (c) | 83. | (d) | 103. | (d) |
| 4. | (c) | 24. | (d) | 44. | (a) | 64. | (a) | 84. | (a) | 104. | (c) |
| 5. | (c) | 25. | (d) | 45. | (b) | 65. | (c) | 85. | (a) | 105. | (d) |
| 6. | (b) | 26. | (a) | 46. | (b) | 66. | (a) | 86. | (b) | 106. | (d) |
| 7. | (c) | 27. | (a) | 47. | (c) | 67. | (d) | 87. | (b) | 107. | (b) |
| 8. | (c) | 28. | (b) | 48. | (d) | 68. | (a) | 88. | (c) | 108. | (c) |
| 9. | (d) | 29. | (c) | 49. | (b) | 69. | (c) | 89. | (a) | 109. | (a) |
| 10. | (c) | 30. | (b) | 50. | (b) | 70. | (b) | 90. | (c) | 110. | (b) |
| 11. | (a) | 31. | (c) | 51. | (b) | 71. | (c) | 91. | (a) | 111. | (c) |
| 12. | (b) | 32. | (d) | 52. | (d) | 72. | (a) | 92. | (d) | 112. | (a) |
| 13. | (b) | 33. | (d) | 53. | (b) | 73. | (c) | 93. | (a) | 113. | (b) |
| 14. | (b) | 34. | (b) | 54. | (b) | 74. | (d) | 94. | (b) | 114. | (d) |
| 15. | (c) | 35. | (a) | 55. | (c) | 75. | (c) | 95. | (a) | 115. | (c) |
| 16. | (a) | 36. | (b) | 56. | (c) | 76. | (a) | 96. | (b) | 116. | (b) |
| 17. | (b) | 37. | (d) | 57. | (a) | 77. | (c) | 97. | (b) | 117. | (a) |
| 18. | (c) | 38. | (d) | 58. | (d) | 78. | (d) | 98. | (c) | 118. | (a) |
| 19. | (d) | 39. | (d) | 59. | (c) | 79. | (b) | 99. | (c) | 119. | (a) |
| 20. | (a) | 40. | (b) | 60. | (a) | 80. | (a) | 100. | (b) | 120. | (b) |

# QUICK REVIEW

## Nutrition Review and Multiple Choice Questions

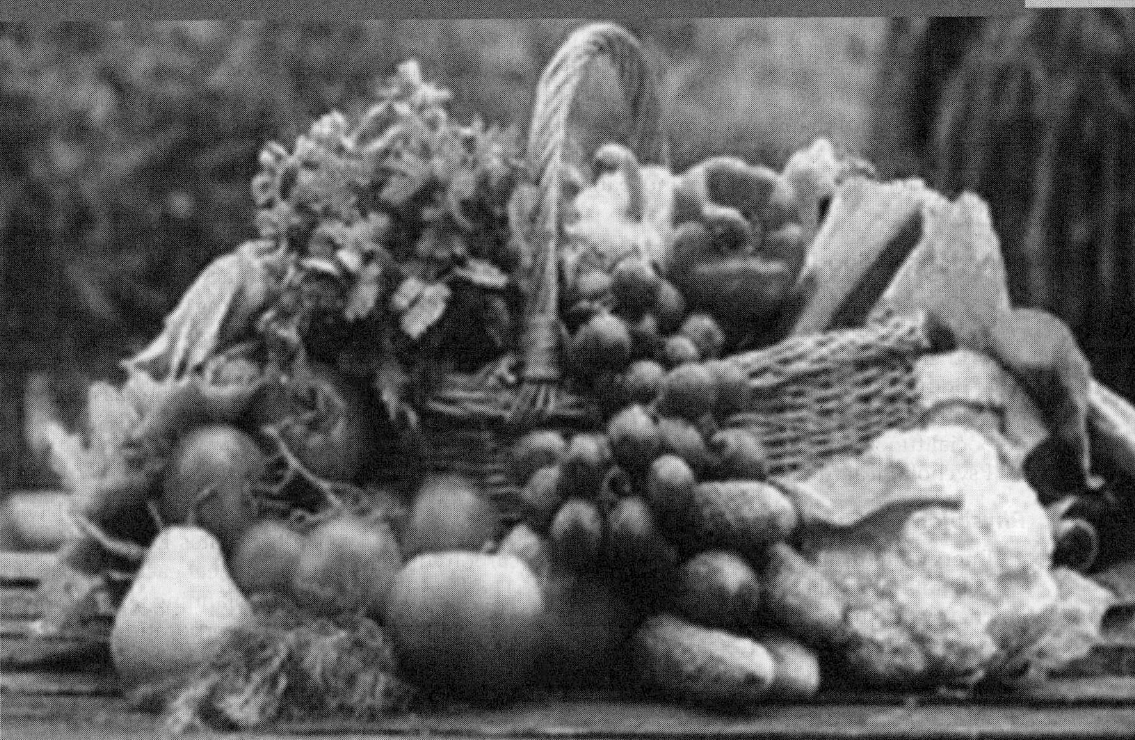

### HIGHLIGHTS

- Food Groups: A Guide in Menu Planning
- Cooking Methods: Merits and Demerits
- Carbohydrates
- Protein
- Lipid
- Energy
- Minerals and Vitamins
- Water
- Multiple Choice Questions

# Nutrition and Dietetics

## FOOD GROUPS: A GUIDE IN MENU PLANNING

Food is the basic necessity of man. It is a mixture of different nutrients such as carbohydrate, protein, fat, vitamins and minerals. These nutrients are essential for growth, development and maintenance of good health throughout life.

They also play a vital role in meeting the special needs of pregnant and lactating women and patients recovering from illness.

### Functions of Food

Food may be classified according to their functions in the body.
- Physiological functions
  - Energy-yielding foods (carbohydrate, protein, fat)
  - Body building foods (protein)
  - Protective foods (vitamins and minerals)
- Social functions
- Psychological functions.

### *Physiological Functions of Food*

- **Energy-yielding foods:** Foods rich in carbohydrates and fats are called energy yielding foods. They provide energy to sustain the involuntary processes essential for continuance of life, to carry out various professional, household and recreational activities and to convert food ingested into usable nutrients in the body.
  The energy needed is supplied by the oxidation of foods consumed. Cereals, roots and tubers, dried fruits, oils, butter and ghee are all good sources of energy.
- **Body building foods:** Foods rich in protein are called body building foods. Milk, meat, eggs and fish are rich in proteins of high quality. Pulses and nuts are good sources of protein but the protein is not of high quality. These foods help to maintain life and promote growth. They also supply energy.
- **Protective and regulatory foods:** Foods rich in protein, minerals and vitamins are known as protective and regulatory foods. They are essential for health and regulate activities such as maintenance of body temperature, muscle contraction, control of water balance, clotting of blood, removal of waste products from the body and maintaining heartbeat. Milk, egg, liver, fruits and vegetables are protective foods.

### *Social Functions of Food*

Food has always been the central part of our community, social, cultural and religious life. It has been an expression of love, friendship and happiness at religious, social and family get-togethers.

### *Psychological Functions of Food*

In addition to satisfying physical and social needs, foods also satisfy certain emotional needs of human beings. These include a sense of security, love and acceptance. For example, preparation of delicious foods for family members is a token of love and affection.

### *Significance of the Five-food Group System*

The five food group system can be used for the following purposes:
- Planning wholesome balanced menus to achieve nutritional adequacy.
- Assessing nutritional status—a brief diet history of an individual can disclose inadequacies of food and nutrients from any of the five groups.

  Based on the assessment, nutrition education can be imparted to the individual.

### Food Pyramid

The food guide pyramid was introduced in 1992 by USDA (United States Department of Agriculture) as a general plan of what to eat each day. The food guide pyramid is a valuable tool for planning a health promoting diet.

By incorporating the principle of balance, variety and moderation, an individual can still eat their favorite foods while following the food guide pyramid.

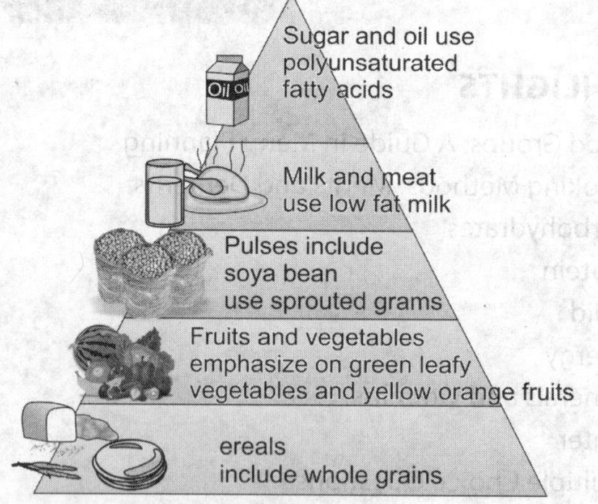


***Balance:*** It means choosing food from different food groups.

***Variety:*** This means including different foods within each food group, e.g. consuming a variety of fruits.

***Moderation:*** This means keeping serving sizes reasonable. This involves self-control. The food guide pyramid provides recommendation for the number of daily servings that should be consumed from each of the food groups.

## COOKING METHODS: MERITS AND DEMERITS

Food preparation is an important step in meeting the nutritional needs of the family. Food has to be pleasing in appearance and taste in order to be consumed. Foods like fruits, vegetables and nuts can be eaten raw but most foods are cooked to bring about desirable changes. The process of subjecting food to the action of heat is termed as cooking.

### Objectives of Cooking

- ***Cooking sterilizes food:*** Above 40°C the growth of bacteria decreases rapidly. Hence food is made safe for consumption.
- Cooking softens the connective tissues of meat and the coarse fiber of cereals, pulses and vegetables so that the digestive period is shortened and the gastrointestinal tract is less subjected to irritation.
- ***Palatability and food quality is improved by cooking:*** Appearance, flavor, texture and taste of food are enhanced while cooking.
- ***Introduces variety:*** Different dishes can be prepared with the same ingredients, e.g. rice can be made into biriyani and kheer.
- ***Increases food consumption:*** Cooking brings about improvement in texture and flavor thereby increasing consumption of food.
- ***Increases availability of nutrients:*** Example in raw egg, avidin binds biotin making it unavailable to the body.

By cooking, avidin gets denatured and biotin is made available.

### Cooking Methods

Heat is transferred to the food during cooking by conduction, convection, radiation or microwave energy.

Cooking takes place by moist and dry heat. Moist heat involves water and steam. Air or fat are used in dry heat.

### Moist Heat Methods

#### *Boiling*

Boiling is a method of cooking foods by just immersing them in water at 100°C and maintaining the water at that temperature till the food is tender. Rice, egg, dhal, meat, roots and tubers are cooked by boiling.

*Merits*

- ***Simple method:*** It does not require special skill and equipment.
- Uniform cooking can be achieved.

*Demerits*

- Continuous excessive boiling leads to damage in the structure and texture of food.
- Loss of heat labile nutrients such as B and C vitamins if the water is discarded.
- ***Time consuming:*** Boiling takes more time to cook food and fuel may be wasted.
- ***Loss of color:*** Water-soluble pigments may be lost.

#### *Stewing*

It refers to the simmering of food in a pan with a tight-fitting lid using small quantities of liquid to cover only half the food. This is a slow method of cooking. The liquid is brought to boiling point and the heat is reduced to maintain simmering temperatures (82–90°C). The food above the liquid is cooked by the steam generated within the pan. Apple, meat along with roots, vegetables and legumes are usually stewed.

*Merits*

- Loss of nutrients is avoided as water used for cooking is not discarded.
- Flavor is retained.

*Demerits*

The process is time-consuming and there is wastage of fuel.

#### *Steaming*

It is a method of cooking food in steam generated from vigorously boiling water in a pan.

The food to be steamed is placed in a container and is not in direct contact with the water or liquid. Idli, custard and idiappam are made by steaming. Vegetables can also be steamed.

*Merits*

- Less chance of burning and scorching.
- Texture of food is better as it becomes light and fluffy, e.g. idli.
- Cooking time is less and fuel wastage is less.
- Steamed foods like idli and idiappam contain less fat and are easily digested and are good for children, aged and for therapeutic diets.
- Nutrient loss is minimized.

*Demerits*

- Steaming equipment is required.
- This method is limited to the preparation of selected foods.

#### *Pressure Cooking*

When steam under pressure is used the method is known as pressure cooking and the equipment used is the pressure cooker. In this method the temperature of boiling water can be raised above 100°C. Rice, dhal, meat, roots and tubers are usually pressure cooked.

*Merits*

- Cooking time is less compared to other methods.
- Nutrient and flavor loss is minimized.
- Conserves fuel and time as different items can be cooked at the same time.
- Less chance for burning and scorching.
- Constant attention is not necessary.

*Demerits*

- The initial investment may not be affordable to everybody.
- Knowledge of the usage, care and maintenance of cooker is required to prevent accidents.
- Careful watch on the cooking time is required to prevent overcooking.

#### *Poaching*

This involves cooking in the minimum amount of liquid at temperatures of 80–85°C that is below the boiling point. Egg and fish can be poached.

*Merits*

- No special equipment is needed.
- Quick method of cooking and therefore saves fuel.
- Poached foods are easily digested since no fat is added.

*Demerits*

- Poached foods may not appeal to everybody as they are bland in taste.
- Food can be scorched if water evaporates due to careless monitoring.
- Water-soluble nutrients may be leached into the water.

### Blanching

In meal preparation, it is often necessary only to peel off the skin of fruits and vegetables without making them tender. This can be achieved by blanching. In this method, food is dipped in boiling water for 5 sec. to 2 min. depending on the texture of the food. This helps to remove the skin or peel without softening food.

Blanching can also be done by pouring enough boiling water on the food to immerse it for some time or subjecting foods to boiling temperatures for short periods and then immediately immersing in cold water. The process causes the skin to become loose and can be peeled off easily.

*Merits*

- Peels can easily be removed to improve digestibility.
- Destroys enzymes that bring about spoilage.
- Texture can be maintained while improving the color and flavor of food.

*Demerit*

Loss of nutrients if cooking water is discarded.

## Dry Heat Methods

### Roasting

In this method food is cooked in a heated metal or frying pan without covering it, e.g. groundnut.

*Merits*

- Quick method of cooking.
- It improves the appearance, flavor and texture of the food.
- Spices are easily powdered if they are first roasted.

*Demerits*

- Food can be scorched due to carelessness.
- Roasting denatures proteins reducing their availability.

### Grilling

Grilling or broiling refers to the cooking of food by exposing it to direct heat. In this method food is placed above or in between a red hot surface. Papads, corn, phulkas, chicken can be prepared by this method.

*Merits*

- Enhances flavor, appearance and taste of the product.
- It requires less time to cook.
- Minimum fat is used.

*Demerits*

Constant attention is required to prevent charring.

### Toasting

This is a method where food is kept between two heated elements to facilitate browning on both sides. Bread slices are cooked by toasting.

*Merits*

- Easy and quick method.
- Flavor improved.

*Demerits*

- Special equipment required.
- Careful monitoring is needed to prevent charring.

### Baking

In this method, the food gets cooked in an oven or ovenlike appliance by dry heat. The temperature range maintained in an oven is 120–260°C.

The food is usually kept uncovered in a container greased with a fat coated paper. Bread, cake, biscuits, pastries and meat are prepared by this method.

*Merits*

- Baking lends a unique baked flavor to foods.
- Foods become light and fluffy—cakes, custards, bread.
- Certain foods can be prepared only by this method—bread, cakes.
- Uniform and bulk cooking can be achieved, e.g. bun, bread.
- Flavor and texture are improved.
- Variety of dishes can be made.

*Demerits*

- Special equipment like oven is required.
- Baking skills are necessary to obtain a product with ideal texture, flavor and color characteristics.
- Careful monitoring needed to prevent scorching.

### Sauteing

It is a method in which food is lightly tossed in little oil just enough to cover the base of the pan. The pan is covered with a lid and the flame or intensity of heat is reduced. The food is allowed to cook till tender in its own steam.

The food is tossed occasionally, or turned with a spatula to enable all the pieces to come in contact with the oil and get cooked evenly.

The product obtained by this method is slightly moist and tender but without any liquid or gravy. Foods cooked by sauteing are generally vegetables which are used as side dishes in a menu. Sauteing can be combined with other methods to produce variety in meals.

*Merits*

- Takes less time.
- Simple technique.
- Minimum oil is used.

*Demerit*

Constant attention is needed as there is chance of scorching or burning.

### Frying

In this method, the food to be cooked is brought into contact with larger amount of hot fat. When food is totally immersed in hot oil, it is called deep fat frying. Samosa, chips, pakoda are examples of deep fat fried foods. In shallow fat frying, only a little fat is used and the food is turned in order that both sides are browned, e.g. ommlette, cutlets, parathas.

*Merits*

- Very quick method of cooking.
- The calorific values of food is increased since fat is used as the cooking media.
- Frying lends a delicious flavor and attractive appearance to foods.
- Taste and texture are improved.

*Demerits*

- Careful monitoring is required as food easily gets charred when the smoking temperature is not properly maintained.
- The food may become soggy due to too much oil absorption.
- Fried foods are not easily digested.
- Repeated use of heated oils will have ill effects on health.

### Combination of Cooking Methods

***Braising:*** It is a combined method of roasting and stewing in a pan with a tight fitting lid. Flavorings and seasonings are added and food is allowed to cook gently. Food preparations prepared by combination methods are:

***Upma:*** Roasting and boiling.

***Cutlet:*** Boiling and deep frying.

***Vermicilli payasam:*** Roasting and simmering.

### Microwave Cooking

Microwaves are electromagnetic waves of radiant energy with wavelengths in the range of 250 × 106 to 7.5 × 109 angstroms.

The most commonly used type of microwave generator is an electronic device called a magnetron which generates radiant energy of high frequency. A simple microwave oven consists of a metal cabinet into which the magnetron is inserted. The cabinet is equipped with a metal fan that distributes the microwave throughout the cabinet. Food placed in the oven is heated by microwaves from all directions.

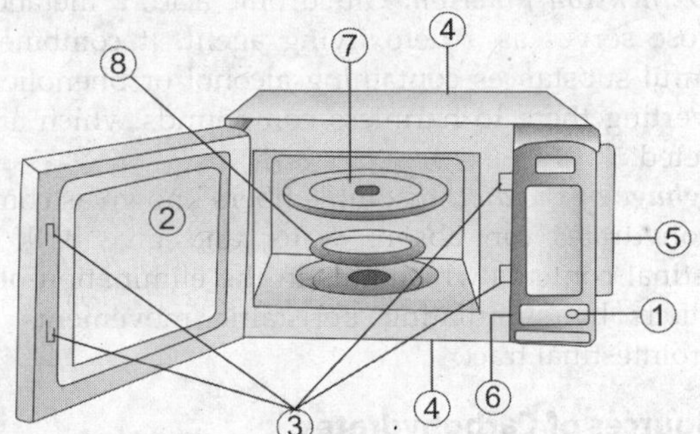


**Microwave oven**

**1.** Door release button, **2.** See–through window, **3.** Door safety lock system, **4.** External air vents, **5.** Control panel, **6.** Identification plate, **7.** Glass tray, **8.** Roller ring

Moist foods and liquid foods can be rapidly heated in such ovens. Food should be kept in containers made of plastic, glass or china ware which do not contain metallic substances.

These containers are used because they transmit the microwaves but do not absorb or reflect them.

### Merits

- ***Quick method:*** 10 times faster than conventional method. So loss of nutrients can be minimized.
- Only the food gets heated and the oven does not get heated.
- Food gets cooked uniformly.
- Leftovers can be reheated without changing the flavor and texture of the product.
- Microwave cooking enhances the flavor of food because it cooks quickly with little or no water.

### Demerits

- Baked products do not get a brown surface.
- Microwave cooking cannot be used for simmering, stewing or deep frying.
- Flavor of all ingredients do not blend well as the cooking time is too short.

### Solar Cooking

Solar cooking is a very simple technique that makes use of sunlight or solar energy which is a nonconventional source of energy. Solar cooker consists of a well-insulated box which is painted black on the inside and covered with one or more transparent covers.

The purpose of these transparent covers is to trap heat inside the solar cooker. These covers allow the radiation from the sun to come inside the box but do not allow the heat from the hot black absorbing plate to come out of the box. Because of this, temperature upto 140°C can be obtained which is adequate for cooking.

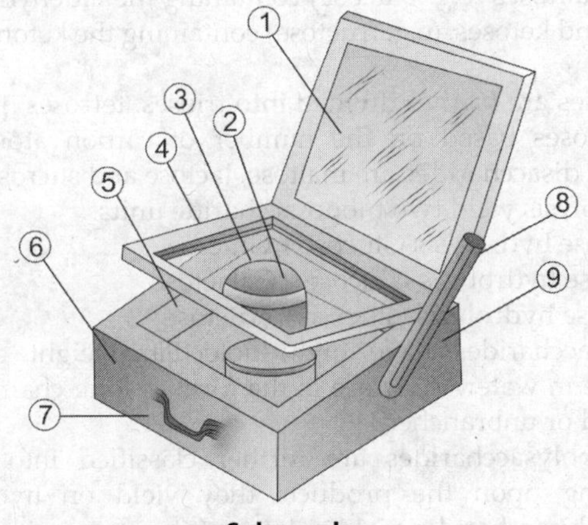


**Solar cooker**

**1.** Solar plane mirror, **2.** Cooking container, **3.** Glass sheet, **4.** Cover, **5.** Insulation material glass, **6.** Outer box, **7.** Handle, **8.** Mirror support, **9.** Hinged adjuster and guide

### Merits

- Simple technique – requires no special skill.
- Cost effective as natural sunlight is the form of energy.

- Original flavor of food is retained.
- There is no danger of scorching or burning.
- Loss of nutrients is minimum as only little amounts of water is used in cooking.

### *Demerits*

- Special equipment is needed.
- Slow cooking process.
- Cannot be used in the absence of sunlight – rainy season, late evening and night.

## CARBOHYDRATES

Energy that is needed to move, perform work and live is chiefly consumed in the form of carbohydrates. Carbohydrates, primarily starches, are least expensive, easily obtained and readily digested form of fuel.

### Composition

Carbohydrates are organic compounds composed of carbon, hydrogen and oxygen, with the later elements in the ratio of 2:1. The general formula is $C_nH_{2n}O_n$. They are viewed as hydrated carbon atoms.

### Classification: Simple and Complex

Carbohydrates are classified, depending on the number of sugar units they contain, as simple carbohydrates and complex carbohydrates.

Monosaccharides and disaccharides make up simple carbohydrates, called simple sugars containing one and two sugar units respectively. Polysaccharides called complex carbohydrates are structurally larger and more complex than simple sugars. They include starch, dietary fiber and glycogen.

There are two main classes of monosaccharides based on the carbonyl group present in them. They are aldoses and ketoses, aldoses (e.g. glucose) containing the aldehyde group (CHO) and ketoses, (e.g. fructose) containing the ketone group (C=O).

Aldoses are further divided into trioses, tetroses, pentoses and hexoses based on the number of carbon atoms. The common disaccharides are maltose, lactose and sucrose which on hydrolysis yield two monosaccharide units.

Maltose hydrolysis Glucose + Glucose
Lactose hydrolysis Glucose + Galactose
Sucrose hydrolysis Glucose + Fructose

Polysaccharides have high molecular weight and are insoluble in water. They are in the form of long chains either branched or unbranched.

The polysaccharides are further classified into groups depending upon the products they yield on hydrolysis. Homopolysaccharides yield only one type of monosaccharide units on hydrolysis, e.g. starch, dextrin, cellulose, glycogen.

Heteropolysaccharides yield more than one type of monosaccharide units on hydrolysis, e.g. heparin, hyaluronic acid. Heparin is an anticoagulant found in the liver, spleen, lungs and blood. Hyaluronic acid is found in the umbilical cord, synovial fluid and vitreous humor. It has a lubricating action. In tissues it forms an important part of the cementing ground substance. The sugars are also classified as reducing and nonreducing sugar. The reducing property is attributed to the free aldehyde or keto group.

### Functions and Food Sources

Carbohydrates perform the following functions:

- ***Energy:*** The principal function of carbohydrates is to serve as a major source of energy for the body. Each gram of carbohydrate yields 4 kcal of energy regardless of its source. In Indian diets 60–80% of energy is derived from carbohydrate.
- ***Glucose:*** It is indispensable for the maintenance of the functional integrity of the nervous tissue and is the sole source of energy for the proper functioning of the brain. Prolonged lack of glucose may cause irreversible damage to the brain.
- ***Protein sparing action:*** Carbohydrates exert a protein sparing action. If sufficient amounts of carbohydrates are not available in the diet, the body will convert protein to glucose in order to supply energy.
  Hence to spare proteins for tissue building, carbohydrates must be supplied in optimum amounts in the diet. This is called the protein sparing action of carbohydrates.
- ***Fat metabolism:*** Carbohydrates are essential to maintain normal fat metabolism.
  Insufficient carbohydrates in the diet results in larger amounts of fat being used for energy than the body is equipped to handle. This leads to accumulation of acidic intermediate products called ketone bodies.
- ***Synthesis of body substances:*** Carbohydrates aid in the synthesis of nonessential amino acids, glycoproteins (which function as antibodies) and glycolipids (which form a part of cell membrane in body tissues especially brain and nervous system).
  Lactose remains in the intestine longer than other disaccharides and thus encourages growth of beneficial bacteria.
- ***Precursors of nucleic acid:*** Carbohydrates and products derived from them, serve as precursors of compounds like nucleic acids, connective tissue matrix and galactosides of nervous tissue.
- ***Detoxification function:*** Glucuronic acid, a metabolite of glucose serves as a detoxifying agent. It combines with harmful substances containing alcohol or phenolic group converting them to harmless compounds which are later excreted.
- ***Roughage of the diet:*** Insoluble fibers known as composite carbohydrates can absorb water and give bulk to the intestinal contents which aids in the elimination of waste products by stimulating peristaltic movements of the gastrointestinal tract.

### Food Sources of Carbohydrates

Cereal grains, roots and tubers are the major sources of starch. Fruits and vegetables contain varying amounts of monosaccharides and disaccharides. Sugar is obtained from sugarcane.

- *Monosaccharides:* Glucose, fructose, galactose, maltose, fruits, honey, corn-syrup. These do not occur in free form in foods.
- *Disaccharides:* Sucrose, lactose, maltose, cane and beet sugar.
  Milk and milk products.
  Malt and cereal products.
- *Polysaccharides:*
  *Digestible:* Starch and dextrin
  Glycogen.
  *Indigestible:* Cellulose
  Pectins, gums.

Grains, vegetables especially roots and tubers and legumes meat products and seafoods, stalks and leaves of vegetables, outer coat of seeds, fruits, plant secretions and seeds.

## Digestion, Absorption and Utilization

### Digestion

The first stage of digestion of carbohydrate takes place in the mouth. Chewing breaks up food and exposes starch and sugars to the action of enzymes. Saliva contains salivary amylase (ptyalin). It converts starch to maltose but time limits the action of salivary amylase, because as food enters the stomach, the acid present in the stomach blocks the action of salivary amylase.

In the stomach the acid causes hydrolysis of sucrose. In the small intestine pancreatic amylase and intestinal amylase digest starch up to the stage of maltose.

Starch salivary, pancreatic maltose + isomaltose and intestinal amylase. Glycogen is also broken by these enzymes to disaccharides. Enzymes maltase, sucrase and lactase present in the brush borders of the columnar cells of small intestine convert disaccharides to monosaccharides.

Maltose > Maltase > Glucose + Glucose
Lactose > Lactase > Glucose + Galactose
Sucrose > Sucrase > Glucose + Fructose

Cellulose and other polysaccharides are not digested by enzymes, so undigested material passes to large intestine forming bulk which contributes to feces.

The end products of carbohydrate digestion are monosaccharides—glucose, galactose and fructose.

They are absorbed by process of active absorption by the mucosa of the small intestine.

### Metabolism

Metabolism occurs inside the various cells of the body. There are two types of metabolism; anabolism (building up) and catabolism (breaking down).

The major carbohydrate anabolic pathways are conversion of glucose into glycogen (glycogenesis) in the liver and muscles.

The conversion of glucose into fat (lipogenesis) in the liver and adipose tissue.

Carbohydrates follow two major catabolic pathways:

The breakdown of glucose releasing energy (glycolysis) and converting it into usable energy (ATP) and the conversion of glycogen to glucose (glycogenolysis).

After digestion and absorption of glucose into the bloodstream it is utilized directly by the tissues for energy.

When the absorbed glucose exceeds the body's need for energy it is stored as glycogen in the liver and muscle and excess glucose is converted to triglycerides and stored as fat in adipose tissue.

## Requirements

As carbohydrate is utilized as main source of energy, at least 40% of the total energy in the food should come from carbohydrates.

In our country 60–80% of a day's energy needs are met from carbohydrates in the form of starch furnished by cereals and pulses.

In developed countries only 30–40% of day's energy needs are met from carbohydrates.

## Dietary Fiber

Dietary fiber is defined as that portion of plant material ingested in the diet that is resistant to digestion by gastrointestinal secretions. It consists of hemicellulose, cellulose, lignins, oligosaccharides, pectins, gums and waxes.

Some bacteria in the large intestine can degrade some components of fiber releasing products, that can be absorbed into the body and used as energy source. Two categories of fiber are found in food. Crude fiber is defined as the residue remaining after the treatment with hot sulfuric acid, alkali and alcohol. The major component of crude fiber is a polysaccharide called cellulose. Crude fiber is a component of dietary fiber. Several other carbohydrate and related compounds called pectins, hemicellulose and lignins are the second category found in plant foods and are also resistant to digestion. These together with cellulose are collectively known as dietary fiber.

### Types of Fiber

There are two types of fiber: i. soluble and ii. insoluble fibers.

1. *Soluble fibers:* Gums, pectins, mucilages.
   *Major food sources:* Citrus fruits, apple, oats, barley, legumes.
   *Actions in the body:*
   - Delay gastrointestinal transit
   - Delay glucose absorption
   - Lower blood cholesterol
2. *Insoluble fibers:* Cellulose, hemicelluloses, lignin.

*Major food sources:* Whole wheat products, wheat bran, whole grain breads, cereals and vegetables like green peas, beans, cabbage. Skin of vegetables and fruits, grains.

**Actions in the body:**

- Accelerate gastrointestinal transit
- Increase fecal weight
- Slow starch hydrolysis
- Delay glucose absorption.

## PROTEIN

One-fifth of an adult's total body weight is protein. Protein is found in every cell of our body.

All the tissues in our body such as muscle, blood, bone, skin and hair are made up of proteins.

Many hormones and enzymes are either protein or protein-derivatives. The nucleic acids in the cell nucleus occur in combination with proteins as nucleoproteins. Protein is thus essential to maintain cellular integrity and function and for health and reproduction.

## Composition

Proteins contain carbon, hydrogen, oxygen and nitrogen.

They are distinguished from carbohydrates and fats by the presence of nitrogen. Protein is synthesized from basic units called amino acids. Protein molecules, which contain up to hundred amino acids are much larger than carbohydrates or lipid molecule. Chemically amino acids are composed of a carbon atom to which is attached a carboxyl (COOH) group, a hydrogen atom (H), an amino group ($NH_2$) and an amino acid radical (R) as shown below.

### *Structure of an Amino Acid*

```
     COOH
      |
  H — C — R
      |
     NH2
```

The carboxyl group, the amino group and the hydrogen atom are the same for all amino acids.

The R group however distinguishes one amino acid from another. R varies from a single hydrogen atom as found in glycine, to longer chain of up to 7 carbon atoms. A protein molecule is made upon of chains of amino acids joined to each other by a peptide linkage. The amino group of one amino acid is linked to the carboxyl group of another amino acid by removal of water.

Thus two amino àcids form dipeptide and three form tripeptide. Proteins consist of hundreds of such linkages hence called polypeptides.

## Essential and Nonessential Amino Acids

***Amino acids are classified into two groups:*** Essential (indispensable) and nonessential (dispensable). An essential amino acid is one that cannot be synthesized by the body to meet the physiological needs and hence should be supplied by the diet. The essential amino acids are histidine, isoleucine, leucine, lysine, methionine, phenylalanine, threonine, tryptophan and valine. Non-essential amino acids are those that the body can synthesize. They are alanine, arginine, asparagine, asparatic acid, cysteine, glutamic acid, glutamine, glycine, proline, serine and tyrosine.

## Biological Value of Protein

Biological value of protein is the percentage of a protein nitrogen that is absorbed and available for use by the body for growth and maintenance.

Proteins are functionally divided into complete, partially complete and incomplete proteins. A complete protein contains all essential amino acids in relatively the same amounts as human beings require to promote and maintain normal growth, e.g. protein derived from animal foods. A partially complete protein contains sufficient amounts of amino acids to maintain life but fail to promote growth, e.g. gliadin in wheat.

Incomplete proteins are incapable of replacing or building new tissue and cannot support life or growth, e.g. protein in wheat germ.

The quality of a protein is determined by the kind and proportion of amino acid it contains. Proteins that contain all essential amino acids in proportions capable of promoting growth are described as complete protein, good quality protein, or proteins of high biological value.

A good quality protein is digested and utilized well. Egg protein is a complete protein and is considered as a reference protein with the highest biological value. The quality of other proteins is determined based on their comparison with egg protein as in figure.

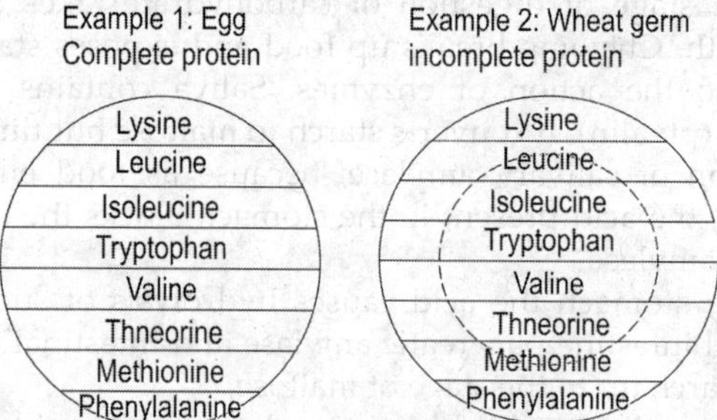


The eight essential amino acids (EAA) must be present in a protein in specific ratios. Egg protein has all eight in the correct proportions used most efficiently and completely by the body.

Wheat germ is an incomplete protein because it is deficient in tryptophan (incomplete circle). As a result of this deficiency only less of the total protein can be used (as represented by the inner dotted circle).

The protein of animal foods like milk, meat, and fish generally compare well with egg in the essential amino acid composition and are categorized as good quality proteins.

Plant proteins are of poor quality, since the essential amino acid composition is not well- balanced. The amino acid, which is not present in sufficient amount in food protein, is called the limiting amino acid of that food, e.g. lysine in cereal protein, tryptophan in wheat germ.

## Functions of Protein

Proteins form a major part of total body structures and they participate in many activities in our body. The major functions of protein in our body can be listed as below:

- ***Build and repair body tissues:*** Proteins form integral parts of most body structure such as skin, tendon, membranes, muscles, organs and bones. They support the growth and repair of body tissues.
- ***Enzymes:*** Lipase helps to breakdown fat and sucrase breaks down sugar.
- ***Hormones:*** Regulate body process.

- ***Antibodies:*** Inactivate foreign invaders thus protecting the body against disease.
- ***Fluid and electrolyte balance:*** Proteins help to maintain the volume and composition of body fluids.
- ***Acid-base balance:*** Proteins help to maintain the acid-base balance of the body fluids by acting as buffers.
- ***Energy:*** Proteins provide fuel for the body's energy needs [4 kcal/g].
- ***Storage:*** Proteins help to store iron and copper.
- ***Homeostasis:*** Proteins maintain normal osmotic balance among body fluids.
- ***Transport proteins:*** Hemoglobin, lipoprotein. These type of proteins carry nutrients to the tissues, e.g. lipoprotein carry lipids, hemoglobin transports oxygen.
- ***Contribute to sensory and physical properties of food:*** Proteins impart color, flavor, odor and texture to foods.

## Digestion, Absorption and Utilization of Proteins

Proteins taken in the diet are digested to amino acids in the stomach and small intestine. Gastric juice contains enzymes pepsin which digests protein in acid medium. It hydrolyses proteins to polypeptides. In the small intestine, pancreatic and intestinal juices contain proteolytic enzymes. Pancreatic juice contains trypsin, chymotrypsin and carboxyl peptidase. They hydrolyse large protein molecule to smaller polypeptide.

Intestinal juices contains polypeptidases and dipeptidases which hydrolyse polypeptide and dipeptide to individual amino acids. There are several peptidases acting on different proteins.

When undigested protein enter large intestines, bacteria causes nitrification of proteins leading to foul smelling flatus. Proteins are mainly absorbed in the form of amino acids. Amino acids are absorbed by active transport mechanism in the intestinal cells. Sometimes whole protein may be absorbed by the mechanism of pinocytosis.

Absorbed amino acids pass into the portal blood and reach liver where they are converted to proteins. Other amino acids are transported through general circulation and are utilized for protein synthesis in the tissues.

### *Utilization of Proteins in the Body*

The amino acids from digested proteins are absorbed rapidly into the blood and passed onto different tissues to meet their needs.

Some nonessential amino acids are synthesized in the liver and also released into the circulation. The amino acids released by hydrolysis of tissue proteins are also added to the amino acid pool in the body.

The protein metabolism of mammals is in a dynamic state and the synthesis and breakdown of tissue protein takes place constantly.

The unwanted amino acids are oxidized in the liver to yield energy and urea. The dynamic aspects of protein metabolism are represented as follows:

## Effects of Deficiency

Deficiency of energy and protein commonly occur in developing countries like India. This is manifested as marasmus and kwashiorkor. Proteine-energy malnutrition (PEM) is a term used to describe clinical disorders resulting from varying degrees of protein and energy deficiency.

Kwashiorkor is due to quantitative and qualitative deficiency of protein in diet in which energy intake is adequate. Marasmus is due to continued restriction of energy intake.

PEM is prevalent in all parts of the world and in all ages. It is primarily a disease that occurs in young children who live in poverty. In India PEM is the most widespread form of malnutrition among preschool children. A majority of them suffer from varying grades of malnutrition.

As many as 43.8% of preschool children suffer from moderate degrees of PEM and 8.7% suffer from extreme forms of malnutrition. The paths leading from early weaning to nutritional marasmus and from protracted breastfeeding to kwashiorkor is depicted below.

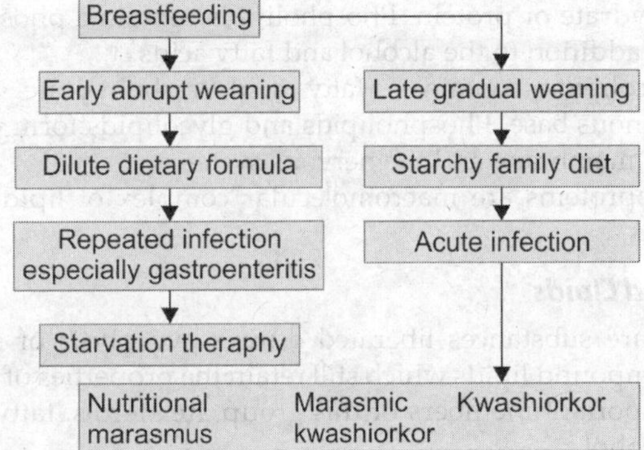


### *Nutrition and Dietetics*

**Clinical symptoms of protein-energy malnutrition:**

- Failure to grow accompanied by thinning, weakening and wasting of muscles.
- Behavioral changes ranging from the irritability of kwashiorkor to the apathy of marasmus.
- Edema which is the accumulation of fluid in the tissues making them soft and spongy.
- Skin changes including changes in color, lack of color, peeling and ulceration.
- Changes in hair which becomes dry and sparse and takes on a characteristic red color (Flags syndrome).
- Loss of appetite, vomitting, diarrhea resulting in dehydration.
- Enlargement of the liver.
- Anemia
- Increased susceptibility to infection and fever.

## LIPID

Lipids—more commonly known as fats and oil, are integral part of our food. They are insoluble in water but soluble in organic solvents. They occur in both plant and animals.

Lipids are a concentrated source of energy.

## Classification

Lipids are classified into simple, compound and derived lipids which are further subdivided as follows.

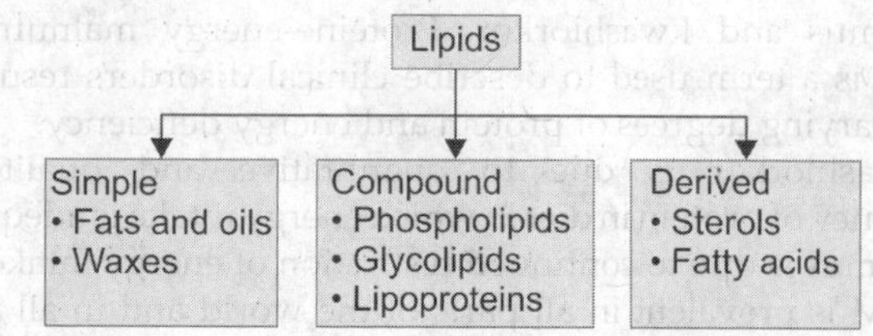


## Simple Lipids

Fats and oils are included in this type. At room temperature, oils are liquids and fats are solids. Fats and oils contain esters of fatty acid and glycerol, a form in which lipids are present in food.

## Compound Lipids

They are esters of fatty acids containing phosphorus, carbohydrate or protein. Phospholipids contain a phosphoric acid in addition to the alcohol and fatty acids.

Glycolipids contain a fatty acid, carbohydrate and a nitrogenous base. Phospholipids and glycolipids form part of the cell membrane and the nervous system.

Lipoproteins are macromolecular complex of lipids with proteins.

## Derived Lipids

These are substances liberated during hydrolysis of simple and compound lipids which still retain the properties of lipids. The important members of this group are sterols, fatty acids and alcohol.

### *Sterols*

Sterols are solid alcohols and form esters with fatty acids. In nature they occur in the free state in the form of esters. Based on their origin sterols are classified as cholesterol (animal origin) and phytosterol (in plants).

Cholesterol is a complex type of lipid that is regularly synthesized by and stored in the liver. It is present in all animal products.

### *Fatty Acids*

Fatty acids are the main building blocks of fat. They have a methyl group (CH3) at one end and a carboxyl group (COOH) at the other end with a chain of carbon and hydrogen atom in the middle. They have a basic formula CH3(CH2)n COOH. Where 'n' denotes the number of carbon atoms which may vary from 2 to 2l.

Fatty acids can be classified into saturated fatty acids (SFA) and unsaturated fatty acids (UFA).

### *Saturated Fatty Acids*

Saturated fatty acids are those that are unable to absorb more hydrogen. They are usually stiff and hard fats, e.g. ghee, butter.

### *Unsaturated Fatty Acids*

Unsaturated fatty acids have one or more double bond in their molecule and are thus not saturated with hydrogen. They are liquid at room temperature, e.g. sunflower oil.

Unsaturated fatty acids may be monounsaturated or polyunsaturated depending on the number of double bonds.

### *Monounsaturated Fatty Acids (MUFA)*

MUFA have only one double bond in their molecule, e.g. oleic acid found in olive oil, peanut oil.

### *Polyunsaturated Fatty Acids (PUFA)*

PUFA have 2 or more double bonds in their molecule, e.g. linoleic acid, linolenic acid. They are present in corn, safflower, soyabean, sunflower oils and fish oils.

Monounsaturated and polyunsaturated fats are usually soft or liquid at room temperature.

## Triglycerides

Fatty acids combine with glycerol to form a glyceride. When only one fatty acid combines with glycerol, it forms a monoglyceride, diglycerides have two fatty acids and triglycerides have three fatty acids attached to glycerol.

Most of the fatty acids present in the body and absorbed from foods occur in the form of triglycerides.

During digestion triglycerides are hydrolyzed to form free fatty acid, monoglycerides and glycerol which are absorbed by the intestinal wall and the majority of these are rebuilt as triglycerides.

### *Long and Short Chain Fatty Acid*

The number of carbon atom in fatty acids decides the chain length. Thus short chain fatty acids contain 4 to 6 carbon atoms, medium chain 8 to 12 carbon atoms and long chain fatty acid have 14 to 18 carbon atoms.

### *Essential Fatty Acid*

Essential fatty acid (EFA) are those which cannot be synthesized by the body and need to be supplied through diet.

Linolenic acid and arachidonic acid are essential fatty acids.

### *Nonessential Fatty Acids*

Nonessential fatty acids are those which can be synthesized by the body and which need not be supplied through the diet. Palmitic acid, oleic acid and butyric acid are examples of nonessential fatty acids.

## Composition

Fat is a complex molecule constituting a mixture of fatty acids and an alcohol, generally glycerol.

It contains carbon, hydrogen and oxygen but differs from carbohydrates in that it contains more carbon and hydrogen and less oxygen.

When one gram of fat is oxidized it yields nine kilocalories.

## Functions of Lipids

**Lipids perform several important functions:**

- They are the concentrated fuel reserve of the body.
- Lipids are the constituents of cell membrane structure and regulate the membrane permeability.
- They are essential for the digestion, absorption and utilization of fat-soluble vitamins like vitamin A, D, E and K.
- Lipids are important as cellular metabolic regulators (steroid hormones and prostaglandin).

- Lipids protect the internal organs serving as insulating materials.
- As compounds of the mitochondria membranes, lipids (phospholipids) participate in electron transport chain.
- Fat imparts palatability to the diet and slows stomach emptying time, thus giving a feeling of fullness. This delay of onset of hunger is called 'satiety value' of fats.
- The calories in fat spare the proteins from being oxidized for energy.
- Fat deposited in the adipose tissue serve as reserve source of energy during starvation. It acts as an insulator conserving the body heat.

Essential fatty acids which are derived lipids perform important functions in our body.

### *Functions of Essential Fatty Acids*

- Maintenance of the function and integrity of cellular and subcellular membrane.
- Regulation of cholesterol metabolism by transporting it between the blood and body tissues.
- Acts as precursor of hormone like—prostaglandin which aid in regulating vascular function and help relieving pain and inflammation.
- Delays blood clotting time.

## Digestion Absorption and Utilization

### *Digestion*

**In the mouth:** Fat digestion starts in the mouth with hard fats beginning to melt when they reach body temperature.

The salivary glands at the base of the tongue release a lipase enzyme which digest fat to a less extent in adults.

**In the stomach:** In the stomach fat floats as a layer above the others components of swallowed food. As a result little fat digestion takes place.

**In the small intestine:** When fat enters the small intestine, the hormone cholecystokinin signals the gallbladder to release bile. Bile emulsifies fat and also provides an alkaline medium for the action of pancreatic lipase and intestinal lipase.

The triglycerides are acted upon by these lipases and hydrolyzed to monoglycerides and fatty acids.

The cholesterol esters are hydrolyzed to give cholesterol and fatty acids.

Triglycerides monoglyceride + fatty acids

Cholesterol esters cholesterol + fatty acids

### *Absorption and Utilization*

Small molecules of digested triglycerides (glycerol, short and medium chain fatty acids) can diffuse into intestinal cells and are absorbed directly into the blood stream.

Larger molecules (monoglycerides, long chain fatty acids) merge into spherical complexes known as micelles. The lipid contents of the micelles diffuse into the intestinal cells. Once inside the monoglycerides and long chain fatty acids are reassembled to new triglycerides.

Within the intestinal cells the new triglycerides and larger lipids like cholesterol and phospholipids are placed into transport vehicle called chylomicrons.

The intestinal cells then release chylomicrons into the lymphatic system. The lymph circulation empties into the thoracic duct which inturn enter the subclavian vein and subsequently into the bloodstream. The blood transport lipids to the rest of the body and cells absorb them and utilize for energy. This breakdown of fat to yield energy is called lipolysis. Majority of lipids enter via the lymph to the liver where the protein and lipid (cholesterol, triglycerides) are bound together to form lipoproteins.

There are four types of lipoproteins, they are:

1. Chylomicrons,
2. Very low density lipoprotein (VLDL)
3. Low density lipoprotein (LDL)
4. High density lipoproteins (HDL).

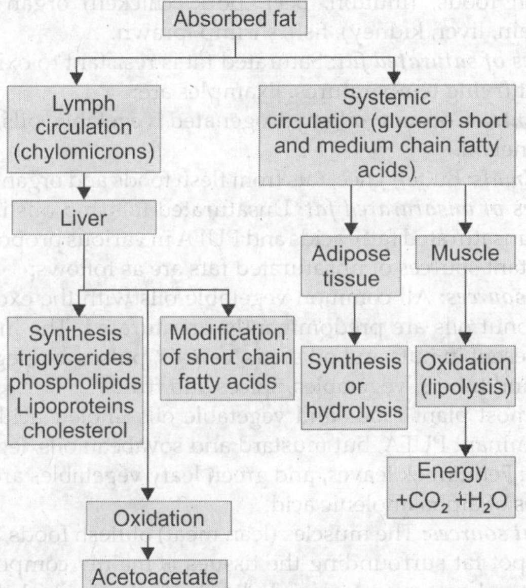


Chylomicrons, VLDL and LDL serve to transport and deposit lipids from the intestine and liver to the tissues for absorption. Low-density lipoprotein which has the highest cholesterol fraction favors lipid deposition in tissues including blood vessels and hence termed 'bad cholesterol'. HDL cholesterol removes the lipids from the tissues and transports it back to liver for disposal, hence it is termed as 'good cholesterol'. High levels of LDL cholesterol indicates a high risk of cardiovascular disease.

Apart from lipoproteins, triglycerides, cholesterol and phospholipids are synthesized in the liver. This is called lipogenesis. It can be represented as follows:

## Food Sources

Foods in general contain two types of fat namely:

1. Visible fats
2. Invisible or hidden fats.

### *Visible Fats*

Visible fats are fats extracted from the following sources.

- ***Oil seeds:*** Coconut, corn, cornseed, groundnut, mustard, palm, rice bran, safflower, seasame, soyabean, sunflower and hydrogenated vegetable oils (vanaspati).

- *Animal fats:* Butter and ghee.
- *Fish oils:* Shark and cod liver oils.

### Invisible or Hidden Fats

Invisible or hidden fats are those which form an integral part of foods and are therefore not visible. It includes the fats present in the cells and cell walls and cell membranes of both plant and animal tissues.

Almost everything we eat as listed below carries some invisible fats.

- *Plant food:* Cereals, millets, vegetables, spices, nuts and oil seeds, coconut, avacado.
- *Animal food:* Milk and milk products (curd, cream, cheese), flesh foods, (mutton, beef, pork, chicken) organ meats (brain, liver, kidney), fish, shrimp, prawn.

*Sources of saturated fat:* Saturated fat is resistant to oxidation even at frying temperatures. Examples are:

- *Plants:* Coconut oil, hydrogenated vegetable oils, palm kernel oil.
- *Animals:* Butter, ghee, fats from flesh foods and organ meats.

*Sources of unsaturated fat:* Unsaturated fats and oils include monounsaturated fatty acids and PUFA in various proportions. Important sources of unsaturated fats are as follows:

*Plant sources:* All common vegetable oils with the exception of coconut oils are predominantly unsaturated. The invisible fats present in nuts and oil seeds, cereals, pulses and legumes, roots and tubers, vegetables, spices and fruits.

In most plant foods and vegetable oils linoleic acid is the predominant PUFA, but mustard and soyabean oils, legumes/pulses. Fenugreek leaves, and green leafy vegetables are good sources of alpha linolenic acid.

*Animal sources:* The muscles (lean meat) of flesh foods, unlike the depot fat surrounding the tissues is mainly composed of cholesterol esters and phospholipids, both of which have a high proportion of long chain n-6 PUFA which are otherwise formed in the body from linolenic acid.

Arachidonic acid is found in animal and human cells.

Fish and fish oils provide long chain n-3 PUFA.

### Hydrogenation

Hydrogenation (addition of hydrogen at double bonds) converts liquid oils into semisolid or solid fats. During hydrogenation, linoleic and alpha linolenic acid present in the oils are converted to trans fatty acids and saturated fatty acids.

Also, the monounsaturated fatty acids are converted to saturated fatty acids.

Hydrogenated fats were designed to imitate ghee. It is used to prepare processed foods like biscuits and cakes.

Vanaspati is produced in India by hydrogenation of vegetable oils.

### Cholesterol

Cholesterol is a constituent of animal foods but is absent in plants. Vegetable oils do not have cholesterol. In human diets, cholesterol is obtained from ghee, butter, cheese, milk, curd, egg, flesh foods, organ meats, fish and prawns. Most animal foods are good sources of both cholesterol and fatty acids.

### Effects of Deficiency

Deficiency of fat in the diet causes the deficiency of essential fatty acids. Deficiency of essential fatty acids leads to cessation of growth.

It also results in flaky skin, development of itchy sores on the scalp. The common disorder in adults and children in India is phrynoderma or toad skin.

The condition is characterized by the presence of horny eruptions on the posterior and lateral aspects of the limbs on the back and buttocks.

Phrynoderma is cured rapidly by the administration of linseed or safflower seed oil rich in EFA.

Infants fed on a EFA deficient diet develop irritation and changes in the skin within a few weeks. The skin changes appear as dryness and desquamation with oozing in the folds.

Diarrhea may also occur, supplementation of the diet with linoleic acid helps to restore the skin to normal condition.

## ENERGY

Energy is the capacity to do work. The energy to perform work is derived from the carbohydrate, fat and protein in the diet. The source of energy in diets varies depending on agricultural, cultural, social and economic factors.

The body needs energy for maintaining body temperature, metabolic activity, supporting growth, for physical work, to maintain constant body weight and good health.

The body's storage energy or potential energy is continuously available in the body from the glycogen in muscle and liver. This stored energy is transformed to other forms to accomplish the work of the body. Examples are:

- *Osmotic energy:* Maintain transport of nutrients.
- *Electrical energy:* Transmission of nerve impulse.
- *Chemical energy:* Synthesis of new compounds.
- *Thermal energy:* Heat regulation.

Whenever one form of energy is produced another form is reduced by exactly the same amount as stated by the law of conservation of energy.

This law states that energy can neither be created or destroyed it can only be transformed from one form to another.

### Units of Energy: Calorie and Joule

The unit of energy, kilocalorie (kcal) was used for a long time. Recently the International Union of Sciences and International Union of Nutritional Science (IUNS) have adopted ' Joule' as the unit of energy in place of kcal. These units are defined as follows:

A Joule is defined as the energy required to move 1 kg mass by 1 meter by a force of 1 Newton acting on it.

One Newton is the force needed to accelerate 1 kg mass by less than a second.

Kcal is defined as the heat required to raise the temperature of 1 kg of water by 1°C.

(From 14.5–15.5°C)

1 kcal = 4.184 KJ (Kilo Joules)

1000 kcal = 4184 = 4.18 MJ (mega joules)

1 KJ = 0.239 kcal.

## Energy Value of Foods

The energy in various foods is measured by calorimetry. Calorimetry is the measurement of heat loss. An instrument for measuring heat output of the body or the energy value of foods is called a Calorimeter. In measuring the calorie value of foods, bomb calorimeter is used. The maximum amount of energy that the sample is capable of yielding when it is completely burnt or oxidized is the energy value of that food, also known as heat of combustion.

The energy measured using a bomb calorimeter is as follows:

1 g of carbohydrate—4.1 kcal
1 g of fat—9.45 kcal
1 g of protein—5.65 kcal

When samples of carbohydrate, fat, protein are burned, the amount of heat produced is always the same for each of these nutrients.

In the bomb calorimeter carbohydrates, fats and proteins are completely oxidized whereas in the human body the process of digestion and absorption does not proceed with 100% efficiency. The extent of digestion varies from one nutrient to another.

The coefficient of digestibility is used to express the proportion of an ingested nutrient that ultimately becomes available to the body cells.

The coefficient of digestibility for carbohydrate, fat and protein are 0.98, 0.95 and 0.92 respectively. It is observed that carbohydrate and fat are metabolized almost completely, whereas protein metabolism is incomplete due to the presence of nitrogen. The physiological energy value of carbohydrate, fat and protein are 4, 9 and 4. These values are known as Atwater Bryant factors or physiological fuel values as given in table.

**Physiological fuel value of carbohydrate, fat and protein**

| | Heat of combustion kcal | Coefficient of digestibility | Digestibility % | Physiological fuel value kcal |
|---|---|---|---|---|
| Carbo-hydrate | 4.1 | 0.98 | 98 | 4.0 |
| Fat | 9.45 | 0.95 | 95 | 9.0 |
| Protein | 5.65 | 0.92 | 92 | 4.0 |

## Basal Metabolism

Basal metabolism is the minimum amount of energy needed by the body for maintenance of life when the person is at postabsorptive state, physical and emotional rest.

Basal metabolic rate (BMR) is a measure of the energy required by the activities of resting tissue.

The BMR can be measured directly from the heat produced (using a respiration calorimeter and metabolic chamber) or indirectly from $O_2$ intake and $CO_2$ expenditure when the subject is at rest.

### *Factors Affecting Basal Metabolic Rate (BMR)*

The factors affecting BMR are listed in table.

| Factor | Effect on BMR |
|---|---|
| Body of composition | The more lean body mass higher is the BMR. This is due to greater metabolic activity in these tissues when compared to bones and fat. Men with a high proportion of muscle mass or lean body mass have a higher BMR than women |
| Fever | Fever raises the BMR. There is a 7% increase in BMR for each degree rise in temperature in Fahrenheit |
| Stress | Stress raises BMR |
| Smoking and caffeine | Increases the BMR |
| Hyperthyroidism (oversecretion of thyroxine) | The BMR is elevated as much as 50–70% |
| Growth | In children and pregnant women the BMR is higher |
| Pregnancy | During the last trimester of pregnancy BMR is increased by 15–25% as there is a increase in muscle mass of uterus, size of mammary gland, fetal mass and placenta, cardiac work and respiratory rate |
| Fasting/starvation | Lowers BMR |
| Hypothyroidism (under secretion of thyroxine) | The BMR is decreased by 30% |
| Age | Lean body mass diminishes with age slowing the BMR. In tall people the BMR is higher |
| Undernutrition | Prolonged undernutrition lowers the BMR |

## Energy Cost of Physical Activities

Next to basal metabolism it is the physical activity, which accounts for the largest energy expenditure. There is a wide variation from individual-to-individual in occupational activity.

The energy required for the actual physical activity varies depending on the type of occupation of an individual.

For computing energy requirements, the occupations have been classified as sedentary, moderate and heavy. The ICMR classification of activities based on occupation is given in table.

**Classification of activities based on occupation**

| Sex | Sedentary (80–180 kcal/hr) | Moderate (170–240 kcal/hr) | Heavy (250–350 kcal/hr) |
|---|---|---|---|
| Male | 1. Teacher<br>2. Tailor<br>3. Executive | 1. Fisherman<br>2. Potter | 1. Stone cutter<br>2. Mine worker<br>3. Wood cutter |
| Female | 1. Teacher<br>2. Executive<br>3. Nurse | 1. Servant maid<br>2. Weaver | 1. Stone cutter |

*Source:* ICMR 2002 nutrient requirements and recommended dietary allowances for Indians, NIN

The energy cost of physical activities is expressed in terms of BMR units.

### *BMR Unit*

The energy cost of rest and physical activity is expressed as multiples of BMR which is called the physical activity ratio (PAR).

The PAR expresses the energy cost of an individual activity per minute as ratio of the cost of BMR per minute. Hence it is advantageous to express the energy expenditure in terms of BMR units.

**Energy cost of some common activities in terms of BMR units**

| Activity | Energy cost of activities in BMR units |
|---|---|
| Sitting quietly | 1.2 |
| Standing quietly | 1.4 |
| Sitting at desk | 1.3 |
| Walking (3MPH) | 3.7 |

*Source:* ICMR 2002 nutrient requirements and recommended dietary allowances for Indians, NIN

Using factorial method the WHO/FAO expert committee has derived the BMR factors for Indian men and women as 1.6, 1.9 and 2.5 respectively for the three categories of activities namely, sedentary, moderate and heavy as given in table.

**Energy requirements of Indian Adults in terms of BMR units**

| Activity | Duration (hrs) | Rate of energy expenditure in terms of BMR units | | |
|---|---|---|---|---|
| | | Sedentary | Moderate | Heavy |
| Sleep | 8 | 1.0 | 1.0 | 1.0 |
| Occupational activity | 8 | 1.7 | 2.8 | 4.5 |
| Nonoccupational activity | 8 | 2.2 | 2 | – |
| Average for 24 hr | | 1.6 | 1.9 | **2.5** |

*Source:* ICMR 2002 nutrient requirements and recommended dietary allowances for Indians, NIN

### Thermic Effect of Food

Food ingestion stimulates metabolism and requires energy to meet the multiple activities of digestion, absorption and transport of nutrients.

This overall stimulating effect of food is called dietary thermogenesis or thermic effect of food (formerly called as specific dynamic action (SDA). The increase in energy cost because of thermogenesis is 10%.

### Estimation of Total Energy Needs

The energy requirement of an individual is the level of energy intake from food that will balance energy expenditure when the individual has a body size and composition and level of physical activity, consistent with long-term good health, and that will allow for maintenance of economically necessary and socially desirable activity. In children, pregnant and lactating women, the energy requirement includes the energy needs associated with the deposition of tissues or the secretion of milk at rates consistent with good health. (WHO). Energy requirements are best determined by measurements of energy expenditure. Energy expenditure from a physiological point of view is made up of three major components:

1. BMR
2. Dietary thermogenesis
3. Physical activity.

For all practical purposes, the component of energy expenditure related to regulatory energy output or dietary thermogenesis are known to merge into measurements related to the cost of physical activity. Hence energy expenditure has only two principal component i. BMR and ii. physical activity.

Calculation of energy requirements.

- ***Predicting BMR:*** Equations for predicting BMR (kcal/24 hr) as proposed by the ICMR expert committee for Indians is given in table.

| Sex | Age (yr) | Prediction equation |
|---|---|---|
| Male | 18–30<br>30–60<br>> 60 | 14.5 × BW (kg) + 645<br>10.9 × BW (kg) + 833<br>12.8 × BW (kg) + 463 |
| Female | 18–30<br>30–60<br>> 60 | 14.0 × BW (kg) + 471<br>8.3 × BW (kg) + 788<br>10.0 × BW (kg) + 565 |

*Source:* ICMR 2002 nutrient requirements and recommended dietary allowances for Indians, NIN

- ***Calculating daily energy requirement:*** Using the computed BMR from body weights and recommended BMR factor for Indians for different levels of physical activity (which is 1.6, 1.9 and 2.5 for sedentary, moderate and heavy activity respectively) the energy requirements are arrived at.

*For example:*

For an Indian adult man 29 years of age, weighing 60 kg and doing moderate activity, the energy requirement is calculated as follows.

- BMR = 14.5 × 60 + 645 = 1515 kcal/24 hr
- Energy requirement = predicted BMR × BMR units for activity = 1515 × 1.9 = 2878.5 kcal/day.

### Energy Balance

To maintain daily energy balance the total energy requirement of an individual is the number of kcal necessary to replace daily basal metabolic loss in addition to loss from exercise and other physical activities. Obesity represents an energy imbalance resulting from an excess of energy input over energy output (expenditure).

Extreme weight loss is a state of energy imbalance resulting from a deficit energy input over energy output.

## MINERALS AND VITAMINS

Until the middle of the nineteenth century, the importance of minerals and vitamins was not known. It was observed that carbohydrate, fat, protein alone were incapable of promoting and sustaining growth.

Hence scientists attempted to find out the 'missing elements', namely minerals and vitamins which are essential for growth and maintenance.

Essential minerals which are inorganic substances are classified as macro and micronutrients based on the amount needed by humans per day.

Macrominerals are those which are vital to health and that are required in the diet by more than 100 mg per day and those required in the diet less than 20 mg per day are called microminerals or trace minerals.

The essential microminerals are calcium, phosphorus, magnesium, sulfur, potassium and chloride. Important microminerals of relevance in human nutrition are iron, zinc, copper, sodium, cobalt, fluoride, manganese, chromium, iodine and molybdenum.

## Functions, Food Sources, Requirements and Effects of Deficiency

### *Calcium and Phosphorus*

Calcium is an essential element required for several life processes. The requirements of calcium and phosphorus are considered together as their function and requirement are closely linked.

Over 99% of the calcium and phosphorus is present in the bones and the remaining 1% in the body fluids.

The calcium and phosphorus are present in the ratio of 2:1 in our body. In the skeletal system calcium and phosphorus is present in the form of hydroxyapatite crystals.

Hydroxyapatite is a compound made up of calcium and phosphate that is deposited into the bone matrix to give it strength and rigidity.

*Functions*

- ***Bone formation:*** The major mineral ions of the bone are calcium, phosphorus and magnesium. For proper calcification of bones, (deposition of minerals on the bone matrix) which occurs during the growing years, adequate supply of these minerals is essential.
- ***Tooth formation:*** Calcium and phosphorus together as a compound is essential for the formation of dentin and enamel.
- ***Physiological Process:***
  - Calcium is essential for the clotting of blood as it is required for prothrombin activation.
  - Calcium regulates the permeability of the capillary walls and ion transport across the cell membranes.
  - It is essential for the contraction of the heart and skeletal muscle.
  - Calcium regulates the excitability of the nerve fibers.
  - Calcium acts as an activator for enzymes such as rennin and pancreatic lipase.
- Phosphorus is essential for the storage and release of adenosine triphosphate (ATP) molecules.
- Phosphates plays an important role as buffers to prevent changes in acidity of the body fluids.
- Phospholipids are major components of cell membrane and intracellular organelles.
- In the DNA and RNA phosphate is an essential part of the nucleic acids.

*Food Sources*

Among cereals ragi contains large amounts of calcium.

Bengal gram whole, gingelly seeds, cumin seeds, poppy seeds, agathi, amaranth, drumstick leaves are good sources of calcium.

Milk and milk products are good sources of calcium and phosphorus. Only 20–30% of the calcium in the diet is absorbed, which is facilitated by vitamin D. All foods contain significant amounts of phosphorus.

*Requirements*

The recommended dietary allowances for calcium, as suggested by the ICMR is given in table.

**ICMR recommended dietary allowances for calcium**

| | Age group | RDA for calcium mg/day |
|---|---|---|
| Infant | 0–12 month | 500 |
| Children | 1–9 year | 400 |
| Children | 10–15 year | 600 |
| Adolescent | 16–18 year | 500 |
| Adult | | 400 |
| Pregnant women | | 1000 |
| Lactating women | | 1000 |

*Deficiency*

Calcium-related health problems occur due to inadequate intake, improper absorption or utilization of calcium.

***Osteoporosis:*** It is a condition found primarily among middle-aged and elderly woman, where the bone mass of the skeleton is diminished.

It is a condition of multiple origin. It results due to the following reasons:

- Prolonged dietary inadequacy
- Poor absorption and utilization of calcium
- Immobility
- Decreased levels of estrogen in post– menopausal women
- Hyperparathyroidism
- Vitamin D deficiency

***Osteomalacia:*** It is a condition in which the quality but not the quantity of bone is reduced. This condition is discussed in detail under deficiency of vitamin D.

### *Tetany*

Tetany occurs when calcium in the blood drops below the critical level. There is a change in the stimulation of nerve cells resulting in increased excitability of the nerve and uncontrolled contraction of the muscle tissue. Hence, calcium and phosphorus ratio in the diet should be maintained at 1:1 for proper utilization of calcium in the body.

### *Microminerals*

Microminerals are also known as trace elements. The microminerals are iron, iodine, zinc, copper, fluoride, selenium, chromium, manganese, cobalt and molybdenum.

However, only the deficiency of few of these elements is observed in humans. Iron and iodine deficiencies are widespread while deficiency of copper, zinc, chromium and selenium have been reported in recent years.

### *Iron*

The total body iron is 4 g in adults. Iron exists in a complex form in our body. It is present as:

- ***Iron porphyrin compounds:*** Hemoglobin in RBC, myoglobin in muscle.
- ***Enzymes:*** For examples, peroxidases, succinase dehydrogenase and cytochrome oxidase.
- ***Transport and storage forms:*** For examples, transferrin and ferritin.

*Functions*

The chief functions of iron in the body are:

- Iron forms a part of the protein—hemoglobin which carries oxygen to different parts of the body.
- It forms a part of the myoglobin in muscles which makes oxygen available for muscle contraction.
- Iron is necessary for the utilization of energy as part of the cells metabolic machinery.
- As part of enzymes iron catalizes many important reactions in the body. Examples are:
  - Conversion of beta carotene to active form of vitamin A
  - Synthesis of carnitine, purines, collagen and neurotransmitters.
  - Detoxification of drugs in the liver.

*Food Sources*

The iron present in food can be as heme and nonheme iron depending upon the source from which it is obtained. Heme iron is obtained from animal tissues, nonheme iron is obtained from plant foods.

Sources of nonheme iron are ragi, green leafy vegetables, dried fruits and jaggery. Liver, fish, poultry, meat, eggs dates are good sources of heme iron.

Heme iron is absorbed and utilized better than the nonheme iron. Iron absorption from Indian diets is only 3% as it is mainly cereal- based diet.

*Requirement*

Iron requirements for various age groups is listed in table.

**ICMR recommended dietary allowances for iron**

| Group | Iron requirement (mg/day) |
|---|---|
| Birth–1 year | 1 |
| 1–5 year | 15–20 |
| 6–12 year | 15–20 |
| 13–18 year | |
| Boys | 25 |
| Girls | 35 |
| Man | 20 |
| Woman | 30 |
| Pregnancy | 40 |
| Lactation | 30 |

*Deficiency*

Dietary iron deficiency leads to nutritional anemia. Nutritional anemia is defined as the condition that results from the inability of the erythropoietic tissue to maintain a normal hemoglobin concentration. Anemia occurs when the hemoglobin level falls below 12 g/dL in adult man and woman. During pregnancy hemoglobin level below 11 g/dL is termed anemia. Nutritional anemia is the common form of anemia affecting women in reproductive years, infants and children which is mainly due to poor intake and absorption.

Iron deficiency anemia is widespread in our country. The prevalence varying from 45% in men and 70% in women and children. The major cause of anemia in India is because of iron and folic acid deficiency.

**Nutritional anemia is manifested as:**

- Reduced hemoglobin level. (less than 12g/dL)
- Defects in the structure, function of the epithelial tissues
- Paleness of skin and the inside of the lower eyelid is pale pink
- Finger nails becoming thin and flat and eventually (spoon-shaped nails) koilonychia develops.
- Progressive untreated anemia results in cardiovascular and respiratory changes leading to cardiac failure. The general symptoms include lassitude, fatigue, breathlessness on exertion, palpitations, dizziness, sleeplessness, dimness of vision, and increased susceptibility to infection.

## Iodine

Iodine is an essential constituent of the thyroid hormone produced by the thyroid glands. It occurs as free iodide ions or as protein bound iodine in our body. About 15–23 mg of iodine is present in the adult human body.

The body store of iodine is predominantly present in thyroid gland and also in salivary gland, mammary glands, gastric glands and in kidneys to a certain extent.

*Function*

Iodine is essential for the synthesis of the thyroid hormones $T_3$ and $T_4$.

*Sources*

The richest source of iodine are sea foods like sea fishes and common salt from sea water. Iodine content of vegetables, fruits and cereals depends upon the iodine content of the soil in which they grow. The soil of mountainous regions contains less iodine.

*Requirement*

The ICMR recommended dietary allowance for iodine is 150 μg/day.

*Deficiency*

Iodine deficiency in the diet, causes enlargement of the thyroid gland called as 'goiter'. Goiter occurs in people staying in hilly regions where the iodine content of water and soil is comparatively less. In India goiter is common in hilly districts of Himalaya. Goiter can be treated by administration of iodine. If treatment is given in early stages goiter can be corrected.

Severe iodine deficiency in children leads to hypothyroidism resulting in retarded physical and mental growth. This condition is known as cretinism.

Goitrogens are substances present in foods which cause goiter. These substances react with iodine present in the food making it unavailable for absorption. Foods like cabbage, cauliflower, raddish contain goitrogens.

## Zinc

Zinc is primarily intracellular substance. Its total quantity in the body is 2.3 g. The largest stores of zinc is present in the bones. Zinc forms a constituent of the blood. Zinc is an important element performing a range of function in the body as it is a cofactor for a number of enzymes.

*Functions*

- Zinc is a constituent of enzymes such as carbonic anhydrase, alkaline phosphatase, lactic dehydrogenase.
- It is a constitent of the hormone insulin.
- It plays a major role in the synthesis of DNA and proteins.

*Sources*

Meat, unmilled cereals and legumes are good sources. Fruits and vegetables are poor sources.

*Requirements*

The daily requirement of zinc in adults is 15.5 mg/day as recommended by the ICMR expert group.

Apart from iron, iodine, zinc, copper, selenium and fluorine are essential trace elements. Copper is essential element in iron absorption.

Selenium is an essential element along with vitamin E for maintaining integrity of the liver cells. Fluorine is required in minimum amounts to prevent dental caries. Excessive consumption leads to mottling of teeth.

## Vitamins

Vitamins are organic substances present in small amounts in food, they are required for carrying out vital functions of the body. They are involved in the utilization of the major nutrients like proteins, fats and carbohydrates.

Though needed in small amounts, they are essential for health and wellbeing of the body. When these vitamins were discovered on the basis of their functions and before their chemical nature were elucidated, they were designated as A, B, C, D or in terms of their major functions like, antineuritic, antirichitic vitamins. Vitamins are classified based on their solubility as fat-soluble and water-soluble vitamins.

**Classification of vitamins**

Vitamins
- Fat-soluble vitamin A, D, E, K,
- Water-soluble vitamin $B_1$, $B_2$, $B_6$, $B_{12}$ (niacin) nicotinic acid folic acid and vitamin C

Water-soluble vitamins are not accumulated in the body, but are readily excreted while fat- soluble vitamins are stored in the body. For this reason excessive intake of fat-soluble vitamins, especially vitamin A and D can prove toxic. Excessive intake leads to the condition called hypervitaminosis.

**Functions, food sources, requirements and effects of deficiency fat-soluble vitamins:**

### Vitamin A

Vitamin A was the first fat-soluble vitamin to be recognized. Three forms of vitamin A are active in the body. These are: i. retinol, ii. retinal and iii. retinoic acid. They are collectively called as retinoids.

Beta carotene is the provitamin of vitamin A.

Provitamins are substances that are chemically related to a vitamin but must be changed by the body into the active form of the vitamin. Vitamin A in the diet comes in two forms. i. retinoids (preformed vitamin A) and ii. carotenoids. Vitamin A is present in vegetable foods which contain yellow pigment called carotenes. It was isolated from carrots hence called carotenoids which are provitamins of vitamin A.

*Functions*

- A well-understood function of retinol is in the visual process. The retina of the human eye contains two distinct photoreceptors of which one is sensitive to light intensities. Vitamin A is essential for the formation of rhodopsin and normal functioning of the retina for clear vision in dim light. Lack of vitamin A leads to impaired adaptation to darkness.
- Participates in protein synthesis and cell differentiation and thereby maintaining the health of the epithelial tissues and skin.
- Supports reproduction and growth.
- Vitamin A regulates the antibodies and cellular immune response. It is essential for maintaining the epithelial tissue which is the first line of defence against invading microorganism.
- Beta carotene acts as an antioxidant capable of protecting the body against disease like cancer, cardiovascular diseases and cataract.

*Sources*

Vitamin A in the human diet exist as retinol or as retinal or beta carotene which has to be converted to vitamin A. Foods of animal origin contain retinol.

Plant sources are rich in beta carotene. Only one-third of the dietary beta carotene is absorbed.

Beta carotene from green leafy vegetables is well-utilized than from carrots and papayas.

Good sources of vitamin A are sheep liver, butter, ghee, egg, milk, curds, liver oils of shark and halibut.

Good sources of beta carotene are agathi, amaranth, drumstick leaves, green leafy vegetables, mango, papaya, carrot and jack fruit.

*Requirements*

The ICMR recommended dietary allowance for retinol is given in table.

**ICMR recommended dietary allowances for retinol**

| Group | Retinol µg/day |
|---|---|
| Men | 600 |
| Women | 600 |
| Pregnant women | 600 |
| Lactation | 950 |
| Infants | 350 |
| Children | 400–600 |

*Effects of Deficiency*

Deficiency of vitamin A is manifested as nutritional blindness and increased susceptibility to infection. Nutritional blindness is an important public health problem among young children in India.

Night blindness is an early symptom of vitamin A deficiency. The individual cannot see in dim light. This can be corrected with adequate supply of vitamin A. In the absence of adequate vitamin A intake the outer lining of the eyeball loses its usual moist, white appearance and becomes dry and wrinkled called xerosis.

This condition is followed by raised muddy dry triangular patches on the conjunctiva called the Bitot's spots.

Redness and inflammation of the eye and gradual loss of vision may follow. The central portion of the eye loses its transparency and becomes opaque and soft if not treated and leads to total blindness termed xerophthalmia. Xerophthalmia encompasses all ocular manifestations of vitamin A deficiency.

Increased susceptibility to infection occurs because the mucous membrane lining becomes dry and rough which is easily invaded by the microorganism.

*Hypervitaminosis*

Intake of large amount of vitamin A for prolonged periods can lead to toxic symptoms which include irritability, headache, nausea and vomiting.

### Vitamin D

Vitamin D can be synthesized in the body in adequate amounts by simple exposure to sunlight, even for 5 minutes per day is sufficient. It is essential for bone growth and calcium metabolism.

It acts as a hormone in the body by facilitating calcium absorption and deposition in the bone.

*Functions*

- Vitamin D helps in the absorption of calcium and phosphorus by increasing the synthesis of calcium binding protein.
- Vitamin D helps to maintain the calcium and phosphorus levels in the body by stimulating:
  - Absorption in the gastrointestinal tract.
  - Retention by the kidney
- Vitamin D helps in deposition of calcium in the bones.

The bones grow denser and stronger.

*Food Sources*

The vitamin D content of food sources from animals varies with the diet, breed and exposure to sunlight of the animal. The good sources of vitamin D are cod liver oil, shrimp, liver, butter, yolk, cheese, milk, spinach and cabbage.

*Requirements*

The expert group of ICMR has not recommended dietary intake of vitamin D for Indians.

Only in those cases where the vitamin D requirement is not met due to inadequate exposure to sunlight the ICMR recommends 400 μg/day of vitamin D.

*Deficiency*

Deficiency of vitamin D leads to decreased absorption of calcium which is manifested as muscular tetany, rickets in children and osteomalacia in adults.

Due to faulty calcification of bones the following derfomities is manifested in children which is called rickets. It is a disease in which there is weakness and abnormalities in bone formation. Rickets primarily affects children.

*Manifestations*

- Faulty deposition of calcium on the bones.
- Bowing of legs
- Enlargement of ends of long bones
- Deformities of ribs – beading of ribs
- Delayed closing of fontanelle
- Slow eruption of teeth.
- Malformed, decay-prone teeth.

*Osteomalacia in Adults*

Osteomalacia is a condition where the quality of the bone is reduced. It occurs in women who are not exposed to sunshine and who have depleted mineral reserves resulting from successive pregnancies and prolonged lactation.

Osteomalacia is associated with low phosphorus level but low blood calcium level is the most frequent cause.

The following symptoms occur:

- Softening of the bones
- Deformities of the limbs, spine, thorax and pelvis
- Demineralization of the bones
- Pain in pelvis, lower back and legs
- Frequent bone fractures.

*Hypervitaminosis*

As in the case of vitamin A intake of excessive amounts of vitamin D leads to toxic symptoms which include irritability, nausea, vomiting and constipation.

### Vitamin E

Vitamin E is known as antisterility vitamin because it is required for normal reproduction in animals and men.

*Functions*

- Vitamin E is the primary antioxidant in the body and serves to protect polyunsaturated fatty acids (PUFA) from oxidation in cells and maintain integrity of the cell membrane. It also prevents the oxidation of beta carotene and vitamin A. Vitamin E helps to maintain cell membrane integrity and protect RBC against hemolysis.
- Vitamin E reduces platelet aggregation.
- Vitamin E is essential for the iron metabolism and the maintenance of nervous tissues and immune function.
- Vitamin E is promoted as an antiaging vitamin, because as cells age they accumulate lipid breakdown products. Vitamin E prevents this accumulation in maintaining cell health.

*Food Sources*

Vitamin E is widely distributed in foods. It is present in high concentration in vegetable oils and in cereal grains. Wheat gum, sunflower seeds, almonds, safflower oil, eggs, butter are good sources.

Meat, fruits and vegetables contain small amounts.
Sesame oil and mustard oil are good sources of vitamin E.

*Requirement*

The requirement of vitamin E is linked to that of essential fatty acids (linoleic and linolenic acids). The requirement of vitamin E is 0.8 mg/g of essential fatty acid.

*Deficiency*

- Prolonged intake of vitamin E deficient diets produces uncoordinated movement, weakness and sensory disturbances.
- It causes hemolytic anemia in low birth weight infants.
- Defective functioning of the retina leading to permanent blindness in premature infants occurs.
- It leads to reproductive failure in humans.
- Vitamin E deficiency is associated with decreased ability of the lymphocytes.

## Vitamin K

Vitamin K is recognized as the antihemorrhagic factor owing to its vital role in blood clotting mechanism.

*Functions*

Synthesis of blood clotting proteins. Vitamin K is essential for the activation of prothrombin. This gets converted to thrombin, which in turn activates fibrinogen to form fibrin.

The process of blood clotting occurs as follows:

Injured tissue releases thromboplastin, which catalyses prothrombin formation. Vitamin K catalyses, conversion of prothrombin to thrombin. This in turn causes conversion of fibrinogen to fibrin which forms the clot.

*Food Sources*

Dark green leafy vegetables are good sources of vitamin K.

Fruits, tubers, seeds, dairy and meat products contain vitamin K.

*Requirements*

The ICMR committee considered that no recommendation is needed for this vitamin, as the synthesis of vitamin K occurs in the lower intestine by the colonic bacteria and present widely in foods.

*Effects of Deficiency*

Primary deficiency arises in infants resulting in delayed blood clotting and hemorrhage. This is because the newborn babies have a sterile intestinal tract thus lack in the colonic bacterial colonies which produces vitamin K. Vitamin K deficiency does not occur in adults.

## Water-soluble Vitamins

**Vitamin C (ascorbic acid):** The chemical name for vitamin C is ascorbic acid. It was discovered in 1747 by the British physician Lind and demonstrated that citrus fruit juices prevented and cured scurvy.

*Functions*

- Ascorbic acid is essential for formation of cement substances and collagen which is found in blood vessels teeth and bones.
- It helps in the biosynthesis of nonessential amino acids, e.g. hydroxy proline, tyrosin.
- It is required for absorption of iron as it reduces ferric to ferrous form which is easily absorbed.
- Vitamin C is essential for the formation of collagen a major structural protein of connective tissues.
- It is required for normal wound healing because it helps in the formation of connective tissue.
- Vitamin C is required for carnitine synthesis which aids in the transport of fatty acids in the cell.
- Vitamin C is essential for the synthesis of norepinephrine a neurotransmitter.
- It activates hormones, e.g. growth hormone, gastrin releasing peptide, calcitonin, gastrin oxytocin.
- Drug detoxifying metabolic systems in the body require vitamin C for its optimal activity.
- Vitamin C is an excellent antioxidant. It combines with free radicals oxidizing them to harmless substances that can be excreted.

*Food Sources*

Amla, drumstick leaves, guava, cashew fruit, agathi, cabbage, bitter gourd, orange, tomato are good sources of ascorbic acid. Cereals and pulses are poor sources. Vitamin C content of pulses increases on germination.

*Requirements*

The recommended dietary allowances of ICMR for ascorbic acid is as given in table.

**ICMR recommended dietary allowances for vitamin C**

| Group | Requirement mg/day |
|---|---|
| Adult | 40 |
| Pregnant women | 40 |
| Lactation | 80 |
| Infants | 25 |
| Children | 40 |

*Effects of Deficiency*

Prolonged deficiency of ascorbic acid produces a disease condition called as 'scurvy' in both infants and adults.

*Infantile Scurvy*

There is loss of appetite, failure to gain weight, irritability, palor, defective growth of bones. Hemorrhage occurs under the skin. There is defective formation of teeth and gums are swollen. The ends of the ribs become prominent resulting in beaded appearance called scorbutic rosary.

*Adult Scurvy*

- General manifestation are fever, susceptibility to infection, and delayed wound healing.
- ***Anemia:*** Microcytic hypochromic anemia develops due to failure of absorption of iron.
- Gums become spongy and bleed easily. Gums become swollen and ulcerated.
- The blood vessels become fragile and porous due to defective formation of collagen. Joints become swollen and tender.

- Clinical symptoms appear when total body pool of ascorbic acid decreases. Skin becomes rough and dry. There are small petechial hemorrhages around hair follicles.

### Thiamine

Thiamine is known as vitamin $B_1$. Deficiency of thiamine leads to beriberi. This condition is widely prevalent among population whose diet contains more of polished cereals.

*Functions*

- Thiamine is converted to thiamine pyrophosphate (TPP), which is an important coenzyme in the carbohydrate metabolism.
- It is involved in transmission of nerve impulses across the cells.
- Thiamine as TPP is an essential cofactor for the conversion of amino acid tryptophan to niacin.

*Sources*

Yeast, whole wheat, millets, hand pounded rice, parboiled rice are good sources of thiamine. The bran contains most of the thiamine in the cereals. Gingelly seeds, groundnut, soyabean, cashew nuts, organ meats, pork, liver and eggs supply thiamine.

*Requirements*

Thiamine is involved in the carbohydrate metabolism. Its requirement is related to energy derived from carbohydrate. The ICMR expert group recommends an allowance of 0.5 mg per 1000 kcal for adults and for infants 0.3 mg/1000 kcal is suggested. The recommended dietary allowance per day is given in table.

**ICMR recommended dietary allowances for thiamine per day**

| Group | Thiamine requirement mg/day |
|---|---|
| Men | |
| Sedentary | 1.2 |
| Moderate | 1.4 |
| Heavy work | 1.6 |
| Women | |
| Sedentary | 0.9 |
| Moderate | 1.1 |
| Heavy work | 1.2 |
| Pregnant women | +0.3 |
| Lactation | +0.3 – +0.2 |
| Infants | 55 μg/kg–50 μg/kg |
| Children (1–9 years) | 0.6–1.2 |
| Boys (10–18 years) | 1.1–1.3 |
| Girls (10–18 years) | 1.0 |

*Effects of Deficiency*

Deficiency of thiamine is associated with low calorie intake. Severe deficiency of thiamine produces a disease known as beri-beri.

It is manifested as:

- ***Dry beriberi:*** There is loss of appetite, tingling numbness and burning sensation in hands and feet. Calf muscles are tender. Knee and ankle jerks are sluggish. In later stages complete loss of sensation in hands and legs occur. It is characterized by foot and waist drop. Mental depression and confusion occurs.
- ***Wet beriberi:*** In this case there is enlargement of heart and the cardiac output is high. Edema or accumulation of fluid in legs, face and trunk is observed. Palpitations are marked.
- ***Infantile beriberi:*** It occurs in first few months of life if the diet of the mother is deficient in thiamine. Symptoms are restlessness, sleeplessness, constipation, enlargement of the heart and breathlessness.

### Riboflavin

Riboflavin or vitamin $B_2$ is the yellow enzyme which is heat stable unlike other B vitamins. Riboflavin in the combined form with proteins form flavoproteins or yellow enzymes.

This enzyme is of two types: i. FAD—Flavin-di-nucleotide. ii. FMN—Flavin mononucleotide.

- These substances act as coenzymes in many biological reactions primarily in oxidation–reduction, and dehydrogenation reaction.
  - Release of energy from glucose, fatty acids and amino acids.
  - Conversion of vitamin $B_6$ and folate to active coenzymes.
- It is essential for the formation of red blood cells.
- It is required for the synthesis of glycogen.

*Food Sources*

Rich sources are liver, dried yeast, egg, milk, meat, fish, whole cereals, legumes, and green leafy vegetables.

*Requirements*

Riboflavin requirement is related to energy intake—0.6 mg/1000 kcal. The ICMR recommends the following requirement per day as given in table.

**ICMR recommended dietary allowance for riboflavin**

| Group | Riboflavin mg/day |
|---|---|
| Men | |
| Sedentary | 1.4 |
| Moderate | 1.6 |
| Heavy work | 1.9 |
| Women | |
| Sedentary | 1.1 |
| Moderate | 1.3 |
| Heavy work | 1.5 |
| Pregnant women | +0.2 |
| Lactation | +0.3 |
| Infants | 65 μg/kg–60 μg/kg |
| Children (1–9 years) | 0.7–1.2 |
| Boys (10–18 years) | 1.3–1.6 |
| Girls (10–18 years) | 1.2 |

*Effects of Deficiency*

Riboflavin deficiency is prevalent mainly among the low-income groups particularly the vulnerable group and the elderly adults. Riboflavin deficiency is characterized by:

- Soreness and burning of the mouth and tongue.
- Lesions at the angles of the mouth called angular stomatitis.
- The inflammation of the tongue called glossitis.
- Dry chapped appearance of the lip with ulcers termed cheilosis.
- The skin becomes dry and results in seborrheic dermatitis.
- Photophobia, lacrimation, burning sensation of the eyes and visual fatigue.
- Decreased motor coordination.
- Normocytic anemia.

## Niacin

Niacin or nicotinamide (amide form) is required by all the cells of our body.

Like thiamine and riboflavin it plays a vital role in the release of energy from carbohydrates, protein, fat and alcohol.

*Functions*

- Nicotinamide is essential for tissue metabolism. The active forms of nicotinamide are NAD—Nicotinamide adenine dinucleotide and NADP—Nicotinamide adenine dinucleotide phosphate.
- NAD and NADP are involved as coenzymes in large number of reversible oxidation reduction reactions.
- Nicotinic acid enhances stomach secretion.
- NAD is involved in catabolic reactions and NADP is involved in anabolic reaction in our body.

*Food Sources*

Dried yeast, liver, rice polishing, peanut, whole cereals, legumes, meat, fish are good sources.

Tryptophan present in dietary protein is converted to niacin in humans. 60 mg of tryptophan yields 1 mg of niacin.

*Requirements*

ICMR recommended dietary allowance of niacin per day is given in table.

**ICMR recommended dietary allowance for niacin**

| Group | Niacin requirement mg/day |
|---|---|
| Men | 16–21 |
| Women | 12–16 |
| Pregnant women | +2 |
| Lactation | +4 |
| Infants | 710 μg/kg – 650 μg/kg |
| Children (1–9 years) | 8–13 |
| Boys (10–18 years) | 15–17 |
| Girls (10–18 years) | 13–14 |

*Effects of Deficiency*

Deficiency of nicotinic acid causes a disease known as pellagra. It is characterized by three D's → Dermatitis, Diarrhea and Dementia.

1. ***Dermatitis:*** Name pellagra comes from pelle–skin and agra–rough. Marked changes occur in the skin especially in the skin exposed to sun and friction areas like elbows, surfaces of arms, knees. Lesions are symmetrically distributed in the affected parts. At first there is reddening, thickening and pigmentation of the skin. Later on there is exfoliation leading to ultimately parchment of skin–butterfly like appearance.
2. ***Diarrhea:*** Diarrhea enhances the deficiency state. There are structural and absorptive defects in the small intestine. Tongue appears raw, and mucous membrane of the tongue is inflamed.
3. ***Dementia:*** There is irritability, depression, poor concentration and loss of memory. Delirium is a common mental disturbance.

## Folic Acid

Folic acid was first extracted from dark green leafy vegetables. It forms yellow crystals and is a conjugated substance made up of three acids namely i. pteroic, ii. para aminobenzoic acid, and iii. glutamic acid.

*Functions*

- Folic acid coenzyme is essential in bringing about transferring single carbon units for many interconversions. A number of key compounds are formed by these reactions like.
  - Purines which are essential constituents of living cells.
  - Thymine—this essential compound forms a key part of DNA.
  - The formation of heme group of hemoglobin.
- The conversion of phenylalanine into tyrosin.

*Food Sources*

Green leafy vegetables, liver, kidney, gingelly seeds, cluster beans are rich sources of folic acid.

*Requirements*

The recommended dietary allowances of folic acid by ICMR are given in table.

**ICMR recommended dietary allowance for folic acid**

| Group | Folic acid mg/day |
|---|---|
| Men | 100 |
| Women | 100 |
| Pregnant women | 400 |
| Lactation | 150 |
| Infants | 25 |
| Children (1–9 year) | 30–60 |
| Boys and girls (10–18 year) | 70–100 |

*Deficiency*

- Simple folate deficiency results in the bone marrow producing immature cells (megaloblasts cells) and few matured red blood cells. This results in reduced oxygen-carrying capacity causing anemia termed megaloblastic anemia.
- Folate deficiency during pregnancy causes neural tube disorders of the fetus.
- Folate deficiency impairs the ability of the immune system to fight infection.

### Pyridoxine ($B_6$)

Pyridoxine is unique among B-complex vitamins in that it functions primarily in protein metabolism.

Pyridoxine denotes related substances such as pyridoxine, pyridoxal and pyridoxamine are three forms in which it is present in our body.

*Functions*

Vitamin $B_6$ in the form of pyridoxal phosphate functions as a coenzyme in many biological reactions.

- Pyridoxine is essential for the process of:
  - ***Transamination:*** Transfer of amino group from one amino acid to another.
  - ***Deamination:*** Removal of the amino group.
  - ***Decarboxylation:*** Removal of the carboxyl group.
- Vitamin $B_6$ is involved in several biochemical steps for the conversion of the amino acid tryptophan to niacin.
- It aids in the formation of elastin, synthesis of messenger RNA and heme part of hemoglobin.
- It aids in the conversion of linoleic acid to arachidonic acid.
- In the carbohydrate metabolism it aids in the release of glycogen from liver and muscle.

*Food Sources*

Meat, pulses and wheat are rich sources. Other Cereals are fair sources of this vitamin. Fruits and vegetables are poor sources. Cooking and processing of food causes loss of this vitamin.

*Requirement*

The ICMR recommended dietary allowance for pyridoxine is given in table.

**The ICMR recommended dietary allowance for pyridoxine**

| Group | Pyridoxine mg/day |
|---|---|
| Adults | 2.0 |
| Pregnant women | 2.5 |
| Lactation | 2.5 |
| Infants | 0.1–0.4 |
| Children (1–9 year) | 0.9–1.6 |
| Boys and girls (10–18 year) | 1.6–2.0 |

*Deficiency*

Vitamin $B_6$ deficiency leads to abnormalities in protein metabolism which is manifested as poor growth, convulsions, anemia, decreased antibody formation and skin lesions. Severe deficiency leads to microcytic hypochromic anemia.

Symptoms such as weakness, nervousness, irritability, insomnia and difficulty in walking is predominant.

### Cyanocobalamin ($B_{12}$)

Until 1926, pernicious anemia was a fatal disease of unknown origin with an unknown cure. In 1926 Minot and Murphy found that pernicious anemia could be cured by feeding a patient at least 0.3 kg of raw liver per day.

Also in 1926 Castle noted that patients with pernicious anemia had a low level of gastric secretion. He suggested that the antipernicious anemia factor had two components: i. An 'extrinsic factor' found in food and ii. An 'intrinsic factor' within normal gastric secretions. The extrinsic factor is now known as vitamin $B_{12}$ or cobalamine.

*Functions*

Vitamin $B_{12}$ is necessary for normal growth and maintenance of healthy nervous tissue and normal blood formation.

Vitamin $B_{12}$ is involved in DNA synthesis and thus in cell replication.

In the bone marrow the vitamin $B_{12}$ co-enzymes are essential for the formation of red blood cells.

It facilitates the formation of folate co-enzymes needed for nucleic acid synthesis.

Vitamin $B_{12}$ is also required for the synthesis of myelin sheath that surrounds the nerve fiber.

*Food Sources*

Vitamin $B_{12}$ is present only in foods of animal origin.

Liver sheep, shrimp, mutton, egg, milk are good sources of vitamin $B_{12}$. Vitamin $B_{12}$ is synthesized by the colonic bacteria.

*Requirements*

The recommended dietary allowance prescribed by ICMR for $B_{12}$ are given in table.

**The ICMR recommended dietary allowance for vitamin $B_{12}$**

| Group | Vitamin $B_{12}$ mg/per day |
|---|---|
| Men | 1.0 |
| Women | 1.0 |
| Pregnancy | 1.0 |
| Lactation | 1.5 |
| Infants | 0.2 |
| Children, boys and girls | 0.2–1.0 |

*Deficiency*

Pernicious anemia is the major problem arising from an inadequate amount of vitamin $B_{12}$.

Pernicious anemia is a condition characterized by very large, immature red blood cells with normal amounts of hemoglobin.

## WATER

Water is vital for human existence. We can live without food for extended periods of time, but without water will result in death.

Water is colorless, calorie less compound of hydrogen and oxygen that virtually every cell in the body needs to survive. Water is closer being a universal solvent than any other compound.

Water is the largest single compound of the body and it is distributed as follows:

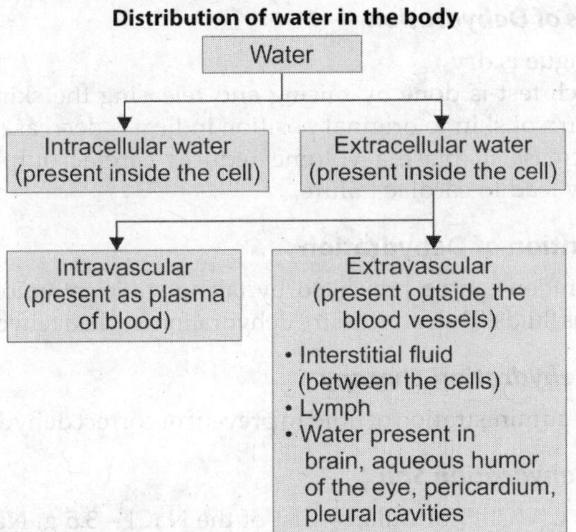


Total body water content is mainly determined by total amount of salt in the body. Salt and water concentration in the body is controlled by the kidneys.

## Functions of Water

- It is an essential constituent of all the cells of the body and the internal environment.
- Serves as a transport medium by which most of the nutrients pass into the cells and removes excretory products.
- Water is a medium for most biochemical reactions within the body and sometimes a reactant.
- It is a valuable solvent in which various substances such as electrolytes, non-electrolytes, hormones, enzymes, vitamins are carried from one place to another.
- Plays a vital role in the maintenance of body temperature. Heat is produced when food is burnt for energy. Body temperature must be kept at 80–108°F for higher or lower body temperature will cause death. Body heat is lost through the skin, lungs, urine and feces.
- It forms a part of fluids in body tissues, e.g. the amniotic fluid surrounds and protects the fetus during pregnancy.
- Saliva is about 99.5% water. In healthy individuals it makes swallowing easier by moistening the food.
- Water helps in maintaining the form and texture of the tissues.
- Water is essential for the maintenance of acid base and electrolyte balance. It should be noted that pure water consists of hydrogen ion ($H^+$) and hydroxyl ion ($OH^-$).

Substances dissolve in water as ions with positive and negative charge. They are called electrolytes. The common electrolytes in our body are sodium, potassium and chloride.

Changes in electrolyte balance causes accumulation or depletion of water in intracellular and extracellular fluid.

The balance between the positively and negatively charged ions is essential for water flow and maintain osmolarity between the cells. This is called electrolyte balance.

Acid-base balance is the dynamic state of equilibrium of hydrogen ion concentration. When pH falls below 7 it is termed acidity and when it increases above 7 it is termed alkalinity.

Extremes of both cases results in death. The pH of the body should be maintained near neutrality. Enzymatic action depends on the pH. The digestion, absorption and utilization of nutrients are dependent on pH. Most body fluids are near neutral with the exception of gastric juice.

The pH value of some solutions are given below:

**Acid**

0 – Hydrochloric acid
1
2 – Gastric juice
3 – Vinegar, orange juice
4 – Grapes
5 – Bread, coffee, neutral
6 – Urine
7 – Pure water, eggs, blood
8 – Sea water
14 – Sodium hydroxide alkali

Water forms good source of macrominerals like calcium, magnesium, fluoride, iron and iodine.

## Requirements

Requirements of water varies with climate, dietary constituents, activities and surface area of the body. As a rule a person should take enough water to excrete about 1200–1500 mL of urine per day. In tropics because of greater water loss through perspiration increased water intake is required to maintain urine volume. Normal intake of water ranges between 8–10 glasses per day.

### *Daily Water Input*

In tropical countries like India the daily water input amounts to 2400–3000 mL of water through food, as fluid drinks and as metabolic water.

| | | |
|---|---|---|
| 1 | As fluid drinks—water, tea, coffee, milk soups | 1500–1750 mL |
| 2 | Water intake through solid food | 600–900 mL |
| 3 | Oxidation of carbohydrate, fat, proteins (metabolic water) | 300–350 mL |
| | **Total** | **2400–3000 mL** |

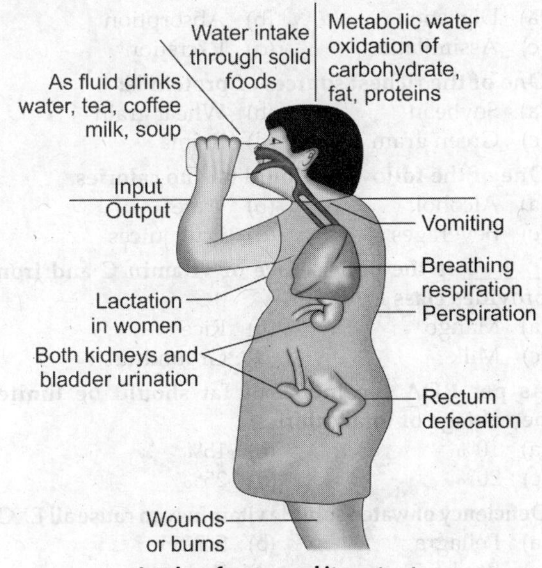


**Intake of water and its output**

**Daily Output of Water**

| | | | |
|---|---|---|---|
| 1 | Urine | 1200–1500 mL | → (Kidney) |
| 2 | Perspiration | 700–900 mL | → (Skin) |
| 3 | Respiration | 400 mL | → (Lung) |
| 4 | Feces | 100–200 mL | → (Intestine) |
| | **Total** | **2400–3000 mL** | |

Therefore the water intake and output is fairly kept constant. This is called water balance. The average adult metabolizes 2.5–3.00 L of water and a constant balance is maintained between intake and output. Inadequate water intake disturbs water equilibrium resulting in decreased urinary output, thereby causing changes in extracellular fluid (ECF) and intracellular fluid (ICF). The water equilibrium is maintained by kidneys, lungs, intestine and pituitary gland. The water balance coordinates with both electrolyte and acid-base balance.

## Causes and Effects of Dehydration

### *Causes*

When water is constantly lost from the body as in severe vomiting, diarrhea, excessive sweating or excessive urine formation due to treatment with diuretics, the total water content of the body is reduced. Extracellular and intracellular fluid decreases leading to dehydration.

### *Effects of Dehydration*

- Tongue is dry
- Pinch test is done by raising and releasing the skin. Slow return of skin to original position indicates decreased ECF.
- Decrease in plasma volume reduces cardiac output and may lead to cardiac failure.

### Prevention of Dehydration

Dehydration can be prevented by taking sufficient amounts of water as fluids. The correction of dehydration is called rehydration.

### *Oral Rehydration Therapy*

It is the administration of fluid to prevent or correct dehydration.

### *Oral Rehydration Salt*

WHO, UNICEF formula consist of the NaCl – 3.5 g, $NaHCO_3$ – 2.5 g, KCl – 1.5 g and glucose – 20 g to be dissolved in 1 L of potable drinking water.

The glucose present aids in the absorption of sodium chloride and potassium chloride apart from giving energy. This mixture is administered through the oral route at frequent intervals until the normal state is attained.

Potable water is that water which is safe and wholesome. It should be:

- Free from pathogenic agents
- Free from harmful chemical substance
- Pleasant to taste; free from color and odor
- Usable for domestic purpose.

## MULTIPLE CHOICE QUESTIONS

**1. Nutrients are obtained from the food by the process of metabolism that takes place in all the following steps EXCEPT:**
(a) Digestion (b) Absorption
(c) Assimilation (d) Excretion

**2. One of the richest sources of protein is:**
(a) Soybean (b) Wheat grain
(c) Green gram (d) Rajma

**3. One of the following liquid has no calories:**
(a) Alcohol (b) Water
(c) Beverages (d) Fruit juices

**4. ______ is the poor source of vitamin C and iron but provides class I protein.**
(a) Mango (b) Rice
(c) Milk (d) Groundnut

**5. As per RDA the intake of fat should be limited to percentage of total calories:**
(a) 10% (b) 15%
(c) 20% (d) 25%

**6. Deficiency of water-soluble vitamins can cause all EXCEPT:**
(a) Pellagra (b) Scurvy
(c) Beriberi (d) Rickets

**7. Beta carotene is precursor of:**
(a) Vitamin D (b) Vitamin C
(c) Vitamin A (d) Vitamin E

**8. In five food group fish, poultry and meat are grouped under:**
(a) Body building food
(b) Protective food
(c) Energy food
(d) Other food

**9. Edema is present in case of:**
(a) Marasmus (b) Kwashiorkor
(c) Rickets (d) Goiter

**10. Table sugar is:**
(a) Maltose (b) Lactose
(c) Sucrose (d) Fructose

**11. Megaloblastic anemia is caused due to deficiency of:**
(a) Folic acid (b) Pyridoxine
(c) Ascorbic acid (d) Thiamine

**12. Minimum number of exchange of fruits that must be included daily in diet of normal adult:**
(a) At least 2 (b) 4–5
(c) 6–8 (d) 8–10

13. **The primary structure of protein is formed by _____ bond.**
(a) Hydrogen (b) Peptide
(c) Disulfide (d) Ketoacid

14. **Tetany can occur in _____**
(a) Hypocalcemia (b) Hyperglycemia
(c) Hypoglycemia (d) Hypercalcemia

15. **Which of the following food stuff has higher fiber content?**
(a) A slice of bread (b) Chapati
(c) Vermicelli kheer (d) Slice of cake

16. **Earliest sign of vitamin A deficiency is:**
(a) Night blindness (b) Keratomalacia
(c) Bitot spot (d) Corneal ulcer

17. **Baking and roasting are _____ method of cooking.**
(a) Moist heat (b) Hot air
(c) Frying (d) Dry heat

18. **The RDA of energy for a man weighing 55 kg and working heavily is _____ cal/ day.**
(a) 2400 (b) 2800
(c) 3200 (d) 3900

19. **The vegetarian people who consume plant food along with eggs, milk and milk products are known as _____.**
(a) Lacto vegetarian (b) Ovolactovegetarian
(c) Pure vegetarian (d) Fruitarian

20. **Out of the following the mineral required for clotting of blood is:**
(a) Na (b) Ca
(c) K (d) Mg

21. **The apparatus used to determine the energy requirement during work**
(a) Calorimeter
(b) Bomb calorimeter
(c) Max Plank Respirometer
(d) Spirometer

22. **Which of the following is mono- unsaturated fatty acid?**
(a) Oleic acid (b) Linoleic acid
(c) Linolenic acid (d) Stearic acid

23. **One of the following is not the principal feature of marasmus.**
(a) Muscle wasting
(b) Loss of subcutaneous fat
(c) Moon face
(d) Usually good appetite

24. **The precursor of vitamin A found in all yellow chlorophyll containing compound food:**
(a) Retinal (b) Retinoic acid
(c) Beta carotene (d) Retinine

25. **One of the following is not macronutrient:**
(a) Vitamin (b) Protein
(c) Fat (d) Carbohydrate

26. **Ragi is the richest source of:**
(a) Iron (b) Calcium
(c) Magnesium (d) Selenium

27. **One of the following is not nutritional deficiency disorder:**
(a) Diabetes mellitus (b) Anemia
(c) Goiter (d) Osteomalacia

28. **Which of the following nutrient provides 4 kcal energy per gram?**
(a) Fat
(b) Vitamin
(c) Protein and carbohydrates
(d) Mineral

29. **This vitamin is lost by discarding cooking water:**
(a) A (b) $B_6$
(c) D (d) E

30. **National Mid Day Meal Programme was initiated in year:**
(a) 1995 (b) 1964
(c) 1978 (d) 1975

31. **ICDS programme provides a package of services to control**
(a) Economic problem
(b) Environmental problem
(c) Political problem
(d) Nutritional problem

32. **Absorption of iron is enhanced by the presence of _____ in diet.**
(a) Fiber (b) Protein
(c) Mineral (d) Vitamin C

33. **Factors affecting RDA are all EXCEPT:**
(a) Age and sex (b) Body size
(c) Physiological state (d) Political state

34. **An amino acid which cannot be synthesized in adequate amount in body and muscle be supplied in diet.**
(a) Essential amino acid
(b) Semiessential amino acid
(c) Nonessential amino acid
(d) Dispensable amino acid

35. **One of the following is not a major mineral.**
(a) Na (b) K
(c) Zn (d) Mg

36. **Water content of bone is:**
(a) 10–15% (b) 20–25%
(c) 30–35% (d) 40–45%

37. **Pernicious anemia is a deficiency disease of:**
(a) Vitamin $B_6$ (b) Iron
(c) Vitamin $B_{12}$ (d) Pantothenic acid

38. **One of the following is millet:**
(a) Rice (b) Wheat
(c) Ragi (d) Legumes

39. **Lathyrism is caused due to consumption of:**
(a) Red gram (b) Bengal gram
(c) Kesari dal (d) Green gram

40. **In food industry, _____ is used as an ingredient of jam and jelly.**
(a) Hemicelluloses (b) Pectin
(c) Pentosan (d) Fructosan

**41. Forming free fatty acid when fat is hydrolyzed by lipase is:**
(a) Hydrolytic rancidity
(b) Oxidative rancidity
(c) Hydrogenated rancidity
(d) Oxygenated rancidity

**42. The cheapest natural source of complete protein is:**
(a) Egg (b) Milk
(c) Chicken (d) Fish

**43. The cheapest natural source of calcium is:**
(a) Ragi (b) Milk
(c) Cheese (d) Green leafy vegetables

**44. Protein requirement for a child with protein-energy malnutrition is:**
(a) 7–9 g/kg (b) 5–7 g/kg
(c) 3–5 g/kg (d) 2–3 g/kg

**45. It is used for the treatment of pernicious anemia:**
(a) Folic acid (b) Vitamin $B_{12}$
(c) Vitamin $B_6$ (d) Vitamin $B_1$

**46. 1 kcal is equal to:**
(a) 4.184 joule (b) 4.184 millijoule
(c) 4.184 millijoule (d) 4.184 kilojoule

**47. In keratomalacia, the corneal epithelium becomes:**
(a) Dull and hazy
(b) Wrinkled and pigmented
(c) Dry and pigmented
(d) Opaque and ulcerated

**48. _____ is essential for normal reproduction in animal and man.**
(a) Vitamin K (b) Vitamin E
(c) Vitamin D (d) Vitamin C

**49. Mid Day Meal Programme provides protein per child per day is:**
(a) 2–5 g (b) 5–8 g
(c) 8–12 g (d) 12–15 g

**50. The richest source of vitamin A is:**
(a) Spinach (b) Cucumber
(c) Almond (d) Ash ground

**51. Deficiency of vitamin C leads to:**
(a) Rickets (b) Beriberi
(c) Night blindness (d) Scurvy

**52. Pasteurization destroys 20–30% of:**
(a) Vitamin B (b) Vitamin C
(c) Vitamin D (d) Vitamin K

**53. Loss of ascorbic acid during cooking occurs by:**
(a) Oxidation due to exposure to air
(b) Leaching in water
(c) Contamination with copper
(d) All the above

**54. Sucrose, lactose and maltose are example of:**
(a) Monosaccharide
(b) Disaccharide
(c) Polysaccharide
(d) Complex polysaccharide

**55. Craniotabes of skull and bending of osteochondral junction of ribs is classic feature of:**
(a) Rickets (b) Pellagra
(c) Scurvy (d) Beriberi

**56. Loss of thiamine and riboflavin occurs by adding to dal_______during cooking:**
(a) Sodium chloride (b) Sodium fluoride
(c) Sodium iodide (d) Sodium bicarbonate

**57. Which of the following will be unsuitable for a person on low-protein diet?**
(a) Fruit salad
(b) Baked potatoes
(c) Egg and cheese sandwich
(d) Cabbage and salad

**58. Thiamine deficiency causes disease**
(a) Scurvy (b) Marasmus
(c) Beriberi (d) Tetany

**59. Vitamin K is required for the formation of:**
(a) Prothrombin (b) Thrombin
(c) Albumin (d) Hemoglobin

**60. The richest source of vitamin C is:**
(a) Amla (b) Guava
(c) Lemon juice (d) Tomato

**61. Burning feet syndrome is related to deficiency of:**
(a) Protein (b) Pantothenic acid
(c) Riboflavin (d) Vitamin A

**62. Which of the following mineral is constituent of insulin?**
(a) Mg (b) K
(c) Na (d) Zn

**63. Intrinsic factor is required for absorption of:**
(a) Na (b) K
(c) Vit $B_{12}$ (d) Glucose

**64. 1 g of fat provides _____kcal of energy.**
(a) 10 (b) 9
(c) 8 (d) 7

**65. Following food stuff are called first class protein:**
(a) Milk, egg, meat, fish
(b) Cereal, root, tubers
(c) Oil, ghee, oil seed
(d) Green leafy vegetables and fruits

**66. Fat serve as vehicle for absorption of:**
(a) B complex
(b) Vitamin C
(c) Mineral water and electrolytes
(d) Fat-soluble vitamins

**67. During pregnancy folate requirement is:**
(a) 600 μg/day
(b) 700 μg/day
(c) 800 μg/day
(d) 900 μg/day

**68. Daily intake of Vitamin A recommended by ICMR for adult is**
(a) 550 μg (b) 650 μg
(c) 750 μg (d) 850 μg

**69. The richest source of vitamin K is:**
(a) Human milk (b) Goat milk
(c) Buffalo milk (d) Cow milk

**70. The main source for iron absorption is:**
(a) Stomach (b) Pylorus
(c) Large intestine (d) Duodenum

**71. Deficiency of this leads to dental caries in children:**
(a) Vitamin C (b) Fluoride
(c) Vitamin D (d) Ca

**72. Fat contain:**
(a) Only carbon
(b) Carbon and water
(c) Carbon, hydrogen and oxygen
(d) Carbon, hydrogen, nitrogen

**73. Dietary source of polysaccharide is:**
(a) Glucose
(b) Biscuit
(c) Sago
(d) Dietary fibers such as vegetables, fruits, grain

**74. Monosaccharide such glycogen are stored in:**
(a) Stomach (b) Pancreas
(c) Liver and muscle (d) Spleen and kidney

**75. Sodium benzoate added to tomato sauce as:**
(a) Nutrient (b) Preservative
(c) Colorant (d) Antioxidant

**76. Which of the following is NOT an essential fatty acid?**
(a) Linoleic acid (b) Linolenic acid
(c) Oleic acid (d) Pantothenic acid

**77. Dental caries can be prevented by adding:**
(a) Chloride to water (b) Fluoride to water
(c) Bromide to water (d) Iodide to water

**78. Proteolytic enzyme present in gastric juices is called:**
(a) Pectin (b) Ptyalin
(c) Trypsin (d) Pepsin

**79. Methylene blue reduction test is done for estimating:**
(a) Activity of bacteria in milk
(b) Fat content in milk
(c) Protein content in milk
(d) Fecal contamination in milk

**80. Organic acid used in food preparation are:**
(a) Citric acid, tartaric acid, hydrochloric acid
(b) Citric acid, acetic acid, hydrochloric acid
(c) Citric acid, acetic acid, tartaric acid
(d) Acetic acid, tartaric acid and hydrochloric acid

**81. Disease caused by food intoxication are all EXCEPT:**
(a) Lathyrism (b) Endemic ascitis
(c) Pellagra (d) Epidemic dropsy

**82. Beriberi is predominantly rice eating communities can be prevented by:**
(a) Milling (b) Polishing
(c) Steeping (d) Parboiling

**83. The best source of vitamin K is:**
(a) Cabbage (b) Carrot
(c) Potato (d) Milk

**84. The richest dietary source of tocopherol is:**
(a) Cod liver oil (b) Soybean oil
(c) Coconut oil (d) Butter

**85. Energy requirement per kg bodyweight is highest in the age group:**
(a) Birth to 1 year (b) 4 to 6 year
(c) 10 to 12 year (d) 16 to 18 year

**86. Fortification of food mean:**
(a) Making food taste better
(b) Adding micronutrients to food
(c) Making food available throughout the year
(d) Adding substances to food

**87. Calcium requirement in pregnancy is:**
(a) 1 g/day (b) 0.5 g/day
(c) 2 g/day (d) 2.5 g/day

**88. The average loss of CHO during digestion is:**
(a) 20% (b) 2%
(c) 5% (d) 8%

**89. Cod liver oil is a good source of:**
(a) Vitamin D (b) Vitamin C
(c) Vitamin K (d) Vitamin $B_{12}$

**90. The main nutrient required for the formation of blood is:**
(a) Iron (b) Calcium
(c) Iodine (d) Sodium

**91. The iron deficiency anemia occurs more commonly among:**
(a) Children (b) Old age
(c) Women (d) Men

**92. Egg is a rich source of:**
(a) Protein (b) Vitamin
(c) Mineral (d) Carbohydrate

**93. Bitot spot occurs due to deficiency of:**
(a) Vitamin K (b) Vitamin E
(c) Vitamin D (d) Vitamin A

**94. After digestion, one gram of protein supplies:**
(a) 2 kcal (b) 3 kcal
(c) 4 kcal (d) 5 kcal

**95. Milk contain sugar______.**
(a) Maltose (b) Lactose
(c) Cellulose (d) Fructose

**96. Methionine is**
(a) A fatty acid
(b) Essential amino acid
(c) Nonessential amino acid
(d) Semiessential amino acid

**97. Bile helps in digestion of_____.**
(a) Fat (b) Protein
(c) Carbohydrate (d) Mineral

**98. Folic acid deficiency anemia also called as:**
(a) Pernicious anemia
(b) Megaloblastic anemia
(c) Hypochromic anemia
(d) Microcytic anemia

**99. Primary source of energy for man is:**
(a) Oxygen (b) Food
(c) Air (d) Water

**100. One gram of carbohydrate gives:**
(a) 3 kcal (b) 4 kcal
(c) 7 kcal (d) 9 kcal

**101. Premature infant is sensitive to lack of this vitamin:**
(a) Vitamin $B_1$ (b) Vitamin D
(c) Vitamin K (d) Vitamin E

**102. Protein requirement recommended by ICMR is:**
(a) 1.5 g/kg body weight
(b) 1 g/kg body weight
(c) 2 g/kg body weight
(d) 0.5 g/kg body weight

**103. Milk is poor in:**
(a) Cholesterol (b) Retinol
(c) Calcium (d) Iron

**104. The energy contained in a specific amount of food is measured:**
(a) Grams (b) Pounds
(c) Kilograms (d) Kilocalories

**105. Kwashiorkor baby is otherwise called as ______.**
(a) Red head (b) Weak and tired
(c) Hungry baby (d) Red boy

**106. One calorie is equal to:**
(a) 48 Joules (b) 3.5 Joules
(c) 4 Joules (d) 4.2 Joules

**107. The other name of vitamin E is ________.**
(a) Thiamine
(b) Ascorbic acid
(c) Tocopherol
(d) Folic acid

**108. Patient with thyroid problem should be evaluated for the following potential mineral imbalance:**
(a) Magnesium (b) Iodine
(c) Zinc (d) Manganese

**109. Polyneuritis is the deficiency of:**
(a) Riboflavin (b) Nicotine
(c) Niacin (d) Thiamine

**110. The ORS fluid:**
(a) Stops diarrhea
(b) Reduces fever
(c) Replaces lost fluid
(d) Corrects pH balance

**111. Peanut is a good source of:**
(a) Ph (b) Zn
(c) Fe (d) Ca

**112. Fruit rich in sodium is:**
(a) Oranges (b) Plum
(c) Papaya (d) Muskmelon

**113. Fats are essential as they carry:**
(a) Water-soluble vitamin
(b) Bile
(c) Fatty acid
(d) Plaque

**114. The following statements are correct for cellulose EXCEPT:**
(a) Provides bulk in diet
(b) Reduces cholesterol
(c) Contribute satiety
(d) It is soluble and digestible polysaccharide

**115. The following include anthropometric measurements EXCEPT:**
(a) Height (b) Weight
(c) Skin fold thickness (d) Hemoglobin estimation

**116. Ragi is the staple food of:**
(a) Karnataka (b) Madras
(c) Kerala (d) Uttar Pradesh

**117. Good source of vitamin C are:**
(a) Meat (b) Milk and milk product
(c) Bread and cereals (d) Citrus food

**118. Adding vanaspati to ghee is an example of:**
(a) Food fortification (b) Food adulteration
(c) Food intoxication (d) Food additives

**119. Pyridoxine is other name for:**
(a) Vitamin $B_6$ (b) Vitamin $B_{12}$
(c) Niacin (d) Riboflavin

**120. Absorption of calcium is facilitated by all EXCEPT:**
(a) Low intestinal pH
(b) Vitamin D
(c) Increased Ca content of diet
(d) Green leafy vegetables

**121. The only form of carbohydrate that the brain uses for energy:**
(a) Glycogen (b) Galactose
(c) Glucose (d) Glucagon

**122. The symptoms of hyperkalemia are all EXCEPT:**
(a) Anorexia
(b) Mental disorientation
(c) Diminished tendon reflex
(d) Weakness of muscle

**123. The protein content of soybean:**
(a) 43% (b) 60%
(c) 70% (d) 20%

**124. Iron is necessary component of:**
(a) Thyroxine (b) Adipose tissue
(c) Hemoglobin (d) Amino acid

**125. Which of the following food is rich in potassium?**
(a) Milk and ice cream
(b) Beef and lamb
(c) Whole grain bread and cereal
(d) Banana and oranges

**126. Goiter prevalent states in India is:**
(a) Kashmir (b) Andhra Pradesh
(c) Kerala (d) Rajasthan

**127. The nutritional problem which more drastically affects the children is:**
(a) Anemia
(b) Marasmus
(c) Protein-energy malnutrition
(d) Kwashiorkor

**128. The highest percentage of total body weight in man attributes to:**
(a) Protein (b) Fat
(c) Carbohydrates (d) Minerals

**129. Patient receiving INH drug, an anti-TB are often provided with the supplement of:**
(a) Riboflavin (b) Pyridoxine
(c) Niacin (d) Thiamine

**130. Protein differs from fat and carbohydrates in the respect that it contains:**
(a) Nitrogen (b) Oxygen
(c) Hydrogen (d) Carbon

**131. Glycolic aldehyde is an example of:**
(a) Polysaccharides (b) Monosaccharide
(c) Oligosaccharide (d) Complex polysaccharide

**132. Glucose can be obtains from:**
(a) Milk (b) Starch
(c) Fruits (d) Legumes

**133. Obesity can be caused by:**
(a) Proteins (b) Fats
(c) Carbohydrates (d) Minerals

**134. Cooking methods do not easily destroy:**
(a) Vitamin A (b) Vitamin $B_1$
(c) Vitamin $B_6$ (d) Vitamin C

**135. Oils and fats are example of:**
(a) Compound lipids (b) Simple lipids
(c) Derived lipids (d) Waxes

**136. Chronic alcoholic suffer from deficiency of:**
(a) Folic acid (b) Thiamine
(c) Iron (d) Calcium

**137. One cup of buffalo's milk supplies:**
(a) 50 calories (b) 100 calories
(c) 150 calories (d) 200 calories

**138. One of the example of protective food:**
(a) Green leafy vegetable
(b) Milk
(c) Egg
(d) Pulses

**139. Vanaspati ghee is fortified with:**
(a) Vitamin A and D (b) Vitamin E and C
(c) Vitamin A and B (d) Vitamin $B_{12}$ and $B_6$

**140. The daily requirement of vitamin D for an infant and a preschool child is:**
(a) 5 μg (b) 10 μg
(c) 20 μg (d) 25 μg

**141. Percentage of total calories provided by the fat in balance diet is:**
(a) 10–30% (b) 20–30%
(c) 25–30% (d) 15–35%

**142. ICDS services are delivered through:**
(a) PHC (b) Subcenters
(c) Balwadi (d) Anganwadi

**143. Following provides calories EXCEPT:**
(a) Proteins (b) Carbohydrates
(c) Vitamins (d) Fats

**144. The most essential minerals for bone are:**
(a) Fe and Ca (b) Ca and Ph
(c) I and Fe (d) Ca and I

**145. Breastfeeding is beneficial for mothers because:**
(a) Protects child
(b) Decreases the risk of carcinoma
(c) Helps to develop emotional bonding
(d) All the above

**146. Nutrients primarily used as the source of energy by the body are:**
(a) Proteins (b) Carbohydrates and fats
(c) Minerals (d) Vitamins

**147. Diet in heart disease is:**
(a) High protein diet (b) Low fat diet and salt free
(c) Liquid diet (d) Low sugar diet

**148. Carbohydrates constitutes_____ % of total body weight.**
(a) 17 (b) 70
(c) 90 (d) 25

**149. Most abundant intracellular mineral is:**
(a) Na (b) Ca
(c) K (d) Cu

**150. Reference protein is:**
(a) Cow milk (b) Hens egg
(c) Meat (d) Fish

**151. Mid Day Meal Programme is sponsored by:**
(a) Health ministry (b) Educational ministry
(c) UNICEF (d) Ministry of social welfare

**152. The enzyme pepsin is secreted by:**
(a) Salivary glands (b) Stomach
(c) Small intestine (d) Pancreas

**153. Nitrogen content of 1 g of good protein is:**
(a) 8 (b) 32
(c) 16 (d) 48

**154. Fat is stored in:**
(a) Connective tissue
(b) Skeletal tissue
(c) Adipose tissue
(d) Muscle

**155. Animal fat is also known as:**
(a) Glucose (b) Galactose
(c) Lactose (d) Glycogen

**156. Which of the following are fat-soluble vitamin?**
(a) A,B,C (b) B,C,D
(c) B,C,K (d) A,D,E

**157. 3 g of fat provides __________ calories.**
(a) 27 (b) 21
(c) 12 (d) 16

**158. Excessive intake of fats leads to:**
(a) Marasmus
(b) PEM
(c) Bitot spots
(d) Coronary artery disease

**159. Carbohydrates help in oxidation of:**
(a) Protein (b) Fat
(c) Mineral (d) Vitamin

## ANSWERS

| 1. | (d) | 31. | (d) | 61. | (c) | 91. | (c) | 121. | (c) | 151. | (b) |
|---|---|---|---|---|---|---|---|---|---|---|---|
| 2. | (a) | 32. | (d) | 62. | (a) | 92. | (a) | 122. | (b) | 152. | (b) |
| 3. | (b) | 33. | (d) | 63. | (c) | 93. | (d) | 123. | (a) | 153. | (c) |
| 4. | (c) | 34. | (a) | 64. | (b) | 94. | (b) | 124. | (c) | 154. | (c) |
| 5. | (d) | 35. | (c) | 65. | (a) | 95. | (b) | 125. | (d) | 155. | (d) |
| 6. | (d) | 36. | (a) | 66. | (d) | 96. | (b) | 126. | (a) | 156. | (d) |
| 7. | (c) | 37. | (c) | 67. | (a) | 97. | (a) | 127. | (c) | 157. | (a) |
| 8. | (a) | 38. | (c) | 68. | (d) | 98. | (b) | 128. | (a) | 158. | (d) |
| 9. | (a) | 39. | (c) | 69. | (d) | 99. | (b) | 129. | (b) | 159. | (b) |
| 10. | (c) | 40. | (b) | 70. | (d) | 100. | (b) | 130. | (a) | | |
| 11. | (a) | 41. | (a) | 71. | (b) | 101. | (b) | 131. | (b) | | |
| 12. | (a) | 42. | (a) | 72. | (c) | 102. | (b) | 132. | (b) | | |
| 13. | (b) | 43. | (c) | 73. | (d) | 103. | (d) | 133. | (c) | | |
| 14. | (a) | 44. | (d) | 74. | (c) | 104. | (d) | 134. | (a) | | |
| 15. | (c) | 45. | (b) | 75. | (b) | 105. | (b) | 135. | (b) | | |
| 16. | (a) | 46. | (d) | 76. | (c) | 106. | (d) | 136. | (b) | | |
| 17. | (d) | 47. | (d) | 77. | (b) | 107. | (c) | 137. | (d) | | |
| 18. | (d) | 48. | (b) | 78. | (d) | 108. | (b) | 138. | (a) | | |
| 19. | (b) | 49. | (c) | 79. | (b) | 109. | (d) | 139. | (a) | | |
| 20. | (b) | 50. | (a) | 80. | (a) | 110. | (c) | 140. | (b) | | |
| 21. | (a) | 51. | (d) | 81. | (c) | 111. | (a) | 141. | (c) | | |
| 22. | (a) | 52. | (b) | 82. | (b) | 112. | (c) | 142. | (d) | | |
| 23. | (d) | 53. | (a) | 83. | (a) | 113. | (c) | 143. | (c) | | |
| 24. | (c) | 54. | (b) | 84. | (a) | 114. | (d) | 144. | (b) | | |
| 25. | (a) | 55. | (a) | 85. | (a) | 115. | (d) | 145. | (d) | | |
| 26. | (b) | 56. | (d) | 86. | (b) | 116. | (a) | 146. | (b) | | |
| 27. | (a) | 57. | (c) | 87. | (a) | 117. | (d) | 147. | (b) | | |
| 28. | (c) | 58. | (c) | 88. | (d) | 118. | (b) | 148. | (d) | | |
| 29. | (b) | 59. | (a) | 89. | (a) | 119. | (a) | 149. | (c) | | |
| 30. | (a) | 60. | (a) | 90. | (a) | 120. | (b) | 150. | (a) | | |

# QUICK REVIEW

## Biochemistry Review and Multiple Choice Questions

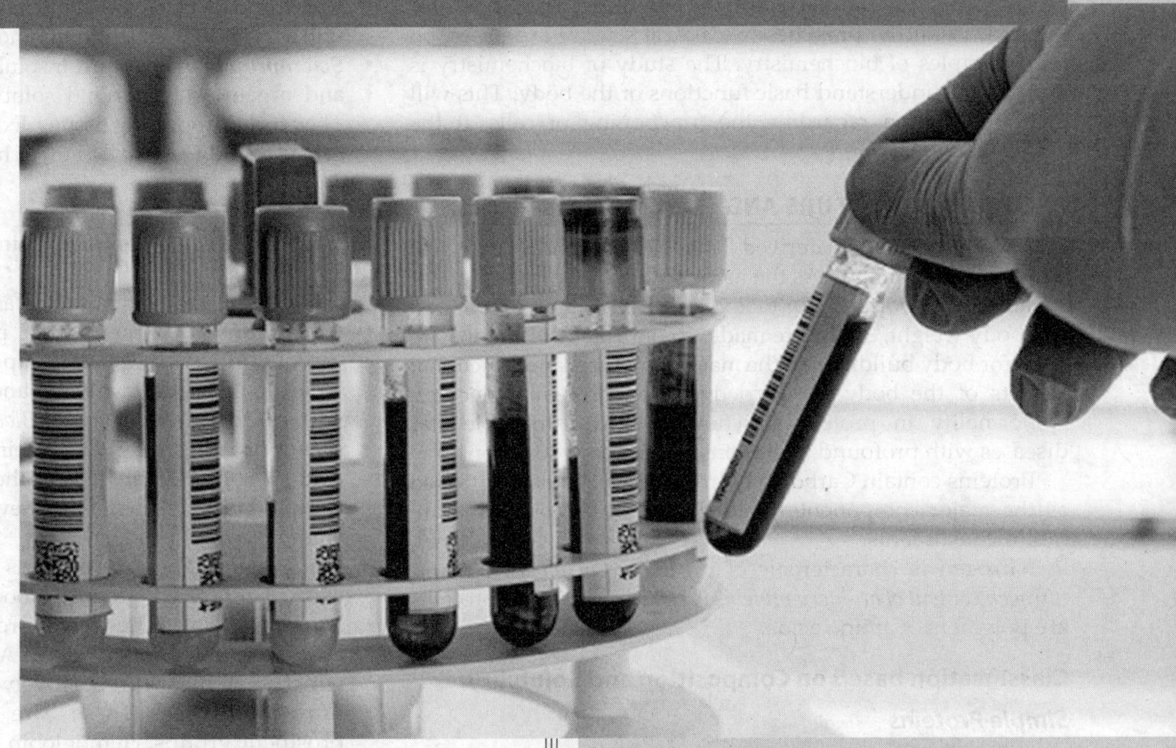

### HIGHLIGHTS

- Proteins: Structure and Function
- General Amino Acid Metabolism
- Urea Cycle
- Chemistry of Carbohydrates
- Glycolysis (Embden-Meyerhof Pathway)
- Gluconeogenesis
- Chemistry of Lipids
- Metabolism of Ketone Bodies
- Enzymology: General Concepts and Enzyme Kinetics
- Fat Soluble Vitamins (A, D, E and K)
- Water Soluble Vitamins
- Multiple Choice Questions

# Biochemistry

Biochemistry is the language of biology. The tools for research in all the branches of medical science are based on the principles of biochemistry. The study of biochemistry is essential to understand basic functions of the body. This will give information regarding the functioning of cells at the molecular level.

## PROTEINS: STRUCTURE AND FUNCTION

The word protein is derived from Greek word, 'proteios' which means primary. As the name shows, the proteins are of paramount importance for biological systems. Out of the total dry body weight, 3/4ths are made up of proteins. Proteins are used for body building; all the major structural and functional aspects of the body are carried out by protein molecules. Abnormality in protein structure will lead to molecular diseases with profound alterations in metabolic functions.

Proteins contain Carbon, Hydrogen, Oxygen and Nitrogen as the major components while Sulfur and Phosphorus are minor constituents.

Nitrogen is characteristic of proteins. *On an average, the nitrogen content of ordinary proteins is 16% by weight.* All proteins are polymers of amino acids.

### Classification based on Composition and Solubility

#### Simple Proteins

According to definition, they contain only amino acids.

- ***Albumins:*** They are *soluble in water* and coagulated by heat. Human serum albumin has a molecular weight of 69,000. Other examples are lactalbumin of milk and egg albumin.
- ***Globulins:*** These are insoluble in pure water, but soluble in *dilute salt solutions*. They are also coagulated by heat. Examples are egg globulin, serum globulins, legumin of peas.
- ***Protamines:*** These are soluble in water, *dilute acids and alkalies*. They are not coagulated by heating. They contain large number of arginine and lysine residues, and so are strongly basic. Hence, they can combine with other acidic proteins. Protamine zinc insulinate is a common commercial preparation of insulin.
- ***Prolamins:*** They are soluble in 70–80% *alcohol*, but insoluble in pure water. They are rich in proline but lack in lysine. Examples are zein from corn, gliadin of wheat, hordein of barley.
- ***Lectins:*** Lectins are precipitated by 30–60% *ammonium sulfate*. They are proteins having high affinity to sugar groups. Lectin from *Dolichos biflorus* will agglutinate human blood group A1 RBCs. Phytohemagglutinin (PHA), a lectin from *Phaseolus vulgaris* (red kidney bean) agglutinates all RBCs and WBCs. Concanavalin-A (ConA) from legumes will specifically attach to mannose and glucose.
- ***Scleroproteins:*** They are insoluble in water, salt solutions and organic solvents and soluble only in *hot strong acids*. They form supporting tissues. Examples are collagen of bone, cartilage and tendon; keratin of hair, horn, nail and hoof.

#### Conjugated Proteins

They are combinations of protein with a non-protein part, called *prosthetic group*.

Conjugated proteins may be classified as follows:

- ***Glycoproteins:*** These are proteins combined with carbohydrates. Hydroxyl groups of serine or threonine and amide groups of asparagine and glutamine form linkages with carbohydrate residues. *Blood group antigens* and many serum proteins are glycoproteins. When the carbohydrate content is more than 10% of the molecule, the viscosity is correspondingly increased they are sometimes known as *mucoproteins* or proteoglycans.
- ***Lipoproteins:*** These are proteins loosely combined with lipid components. They occur in blood and on cell membranes.
- ***Nucleoproteins:*** These are proteins attached to nucleic acids, e.g. Histones. The DNA carries negative charges, which combines with positively charged proteins.
- ***Chromoproteins:*** These are proteins with colored prosthetic groups. Hemoglobin (Heme, red), Flavoproteins (Riboflavin, yellow), Visual purple (Vitamin A, purple) are some examples of chromoproteins.
- ***Phosphoproteins:*** These contain phosphorus. *Casein* of milk and *vitellin* of egg yolk are examples. The phosphoric acid is esterified to the hydroxyl groups of serine and threonine residues of proteins.
- ***Metalloproteins:*** They contain metal ions. Examples are Hemoglobin (Iron), Cytochrome (Iron), Tyrosinase (Copper) and Carbonic anhydrase (Zinc).

#### Derived Proteins

They are degradation products of native proteins. Progressive hydrolysis of protein results in smaller and smaller chains: Protein $\rightarrow$ peptones $\rightarrow$ peptides $\rightarrow$ amino acids.

### Classification based on Nutritional Value

#### Nutritionally Rich Proteins

They are also called as *complete proteins or first class proteins*. They contain all the essential amino acids in the required proportion. On supplying these proteins in the diet, children will grow satisfactorily. A good example is *casein* of milk.

### Incomplete Proteins

They *lack one essential amino acid.* They cannot promote body growth in children; but may be able to sustain the body weight in adults. Proteins from *pulses are deficient in methionine,* while proteins of *cereals lack in lysine*. If both of them are combined in the diet, adequate growth may be obtained.

### Poor Proteins

They *lack in many essential amino acids* and a diet based on these proteins will not even sustain the original body weight. Zein from corn lacks tryptophan and lysine.

## GENERAL AMINO ACID METABOLISM

The main role of amino acids is in the *synthesis of structural and functional proteins.* Unlike carbohydrates and fats, there is no storage form of proteins in the body. A 70 kg man has an average protein turnover rate of 400 g per day (same amount synthesized and same amount broken down). The non-essential amino acids are either derived from the diet or synthesized in the body. The *essential amino acids are obtained from the diet.* Even if one is deficient, protein synthesis cannot take place. The body amino acid pool is always in a dynamic steady state. In an adult, the rate of synthesis of proteins balances the rate of degradation, so that nitrogen balance is maintained.

## DIGESTION OF PROTEINS

The dietary proteins are denatured on cooking and therefore more easily digested. All these enzymes are hydrolases (class 3 enzymes) in nature. Proteolytic enzymes are secreted as inactive *zymogens* which are converted to their active form in the intestinal lumen. This would prevent autodigestion of the secretory acini. The proteolytic enzymes include:

- ***Endopeptidases:*** They act on peptide bonds inside the protein molecule, so that the protein becomes successively smaller and smaller units. This group includes Pepsin, Trypsin, Chymotrypsin, and Elastase.
- ***Exopeptidases:*** Which act at the peptide bond only at the end region of the chain. This group includes:
  - ***Carboxypeptidase*** acts on the peptide bond only at the carboxy terminal end on the chain.
  - ***Aminopeptidase,*** which acts on the peptide bond only at the amino terminal end on the chain.

The digestion of protein is effected by enzymes in:

- Stomach
- Pancreas and
- Intestinal cells

### Gastric Digestion of Proteins

In the stomach, hydrochloric acid is secreted. It makes the pH optimum for the action of pepsin and also activates pepsin. The acid also denatures the proteins.

### Rennin

Rennin otherwise called *Chymosin,* is active in infants and is involved in the curdling of milk. It is absent in adults. Milk protein, casein is converted to paracasein by the action of rennin. This denatured protein is easily digested further by pepsin.

### Pepsin

It is secreted by the chief cells of stomach as inactive *pepsinogen*. The conversion of pepsinogen to pepsin is brought about by removal of 44 amino acids from the N-terminal end, by the hydrochloric acid. The optimum pH for activity of pepsin is *around* 2. Pepsin is an endopeptidase. Pepsin catalyses hydrolysis of the bonds formed by carboxyl groups of Phe, Tyr, Trp and Met. By the action of pepsin, proteins are broken into proteoses and peptones.

### Pancreatic Digestion of Proteins

The optimum pH for the activity of pancreatic enzymes (pH 8) is provided by the alkaline bile and pancreatic juice. The secretion of pancreatic juice is stimulated by the peptide hormones, *Cholecystokinin* and *Pancreozymin*. Pancreatic juice contains the important endopeptidases, namely *Trypsin, Chymotrypsin, Elastase* and *Carboxypeptidase.*

These enzymes are also secreted as zymogens (trypsinogen, chymotrypsinogen and pro-elastase), so that the pancreatic acinar cells are not autolysed. All the three are serine proteases, i.e. the active centers of these enzymes contain serine residues.

### Trypsin

Trypsinogen is activated by *enterokinase* (enteropeptidase) present on the intestinal microvillus membranes. Once activated, the trypsin activates other enzyme molecules. Trypsin is activated by the removal of a hexapeptide from N-terminal end.

Trypsin catalyzes hydrolysis of the bonds formed by carboxyl groups of Arg and Lys.

***Acute pancreatitis:*** Premature activation of trypsinogen inside the pancreas itself will result in the autodigestion of pancreatic cells. The result is acute pancreatitis. It is a life-threatening condition.

### Chymotrypsin

Trypsin will act on chymotrypsinogen, in such a manner that A , B and C peptides are formed. These 3 segments are approximated, so that the active site is formed. Thus, selective proteolysis produces the catalytic site.

### Carboxypeptidases

Trypsin and chymotrypsin degrade the proteins into small peptides these are further hydrolyzed into dipeptides and tripeptides by *carboxypeptidases* present in the pancreatic juice. The procarboxy peptidase is activated by trypsin. They are metalloenzymes requiring zinc.

### Intestinal Digestion of Proteins

Complete digestion of the small peptides to the level of amino acids is brought about by enzymes present in intestinal juice (**succus entericus**). The luminal surface of intestinal epithelial cell contains the following enzymes:

### *Leucine Aminopeptidase*

It releases the N-terminal basic amino acids and glycine.

### *Proline Amino Peptidase*

It removes proline from the end of polypeptides.

### *Dipeptidases and Tripeptidases*

They will bring about the complete digestion of proteins.

## ABSORPTION OF AMINO ACIDS

The absorption of amino acids occurs mainly in the small intestine. It is an energy requiring process. These transport systems are carrier mediated and or ATP sodium dependent symport systems.

There are *5 different carriers* for amino acids:

1. Neutral amino acids (Alanine, Valine, Leucine, Methionine, Phenylalanine, Tyrosine, Isoleucine)
2. Basic amino acids (Lys, Arg) and Cysteine
3. Amino acids and Glycine
4. Acidic amino acids (Asp, Glu)
5. Beta amino acids (beta alanine).

### Inter-organ Transport of Amino Acids

In plasma, all amino acids are seen at a level roughly of 1 mg/dl, except glutamic acid and glutamine, which are present in higher concentrations (each about 10 mg/dl). Breakdown of muscle protein is the source of amino acids for tissues while liver is the site of disposal.

### *In Fasting State*

The muscle releases mainly alanine and glutamine of which **alanine is taken up by liver** and glutamine by kidneys. Liver removes the amino group and converts it to urea and the carbon skeleton is used for **gluconeogenesis**. The brain predominantly takes up branched chain amino acids.

### *In the Fed State*

Amino acids absorbed from the diet are taken up by different tissues. Both muscle and brain take up branched chain amino acids, and release glutamine and alanine. The glutamine is delivered to kidneys to aid in regulation of acid–base balance while alanine is taken up by liver.

## GENERAL METABOLISM OF AMINO ACIDS

- The *anabolic reactions* where proteins are synthesized.
- *Synthesis* of specialized products such as heme, creatine, purines and pyrimidines.
- The *catabolic reactions* where dietary proteins and body proteins are broken down to amino acids.
- *Transamination:* amino group is removed to produce the carbon skeleton (keto acid). The amino group liberated as ammonia is detoxified and excreted as *urea.*
- The carbon skeleton is used for synthesis of *nonessential* amino acids.
- It is also used for *gluconeogenesis* or for complete oxidation.
- Other minor metabolic functions like conjugation, methylation, amidation, etc.

## FORMATION OF AMMONIA

The first step in the catabolism of amino acids is to remove the amino group as *ammonia.*

This is the major source of ammonia. However, small quantities of ammonia may also be formed from catabolism of purine and pyrimidine bases.

Ammonia is *highly toxic* especially to the nervous system. Detoxification of ammonia is by conversion to urea and excretion through urine.

### Transamination

- Transamination is the exchange of the alpha amino group between one alpha amino acid and another alpha keto acid, forming a new alpha amino acid.
  amino acid 1 + keto acid 2 $\rightarrow$ amino acid 2 + keto acid 1
- As an example, amino group is interchanged between alanine and glutamic acid. In almost all cases, the amino group is accepted by *alpha ketoglutaric acid* so that glutamic acid is formed.
- The enzymes catalyzing the reaction as a group are known as *amino transferases*. These enzymes have *pyridoxal phosphate* as prosthetic group. The reaction is readily reversible.

### *Biological Significance of Transamination*

- *First step of catabolism:* In this first step, *ammonia* is removed, and the carbon skeleton of the amino acid enters into catabolic pathway.
- *Synthesis of nonessential amino acids:* By means of transamination, all nonessential amino acids can be synthesized by the body from keto acids available from other sources. For example, *pyruvate* can be transaminated to synthesize *alanine*. Similarly oxaloacetate produces aspartic acid. Alpha keto glutarate is transaminated to form glutamic acid. Those amino acids, which cannot be synthesized in this manner, are therefore essential; they should be made available in the food.
- *Interconversion of amino acids:* If amino acid no. 1 is high and no. 2 is low, the amino group from no. 1 may be transferred to a keto acid to give amino acid no. 2 to equalize the quantity of both. This is called *equalization* of quantities of nonessential amino acids.

### *Exceptions*

Lysine, threonine and proline are not transaminated. They follow direct degradative pathways.

### *Clinical Significance of Transamination*

Aspartate aminotransferase (**AST**) and Alanine aminotransferase (**ALT**) are induced by glucocorticoids which favor gluconeogenesis. AST and ALT are markers of *liver* injury.

### Trans-deamination

- The amino group of most of the amino acids is released by a coupled reaction, transdeamination, that is *transamination followed by oxidative deamination.*

- Transamination takes place in the cytoplasm of all the cells of the body; the amino group is transported to liver as *glutamic acid* which is finally oxidatively deaminated in the mitochondria of hepatocytes.
- Thus, the two components of the reaction are physically far away, but physiologically they are coupled. Hence, the term trans-deamination.

### *Oxidative Deamination of Glutamate*

Only *liver* mitochondria contain *glutamate dehydrogenase (GDH)* which deaminates glutamate to alpha keto glutarate plus ammonia. So, all amino acids are first transaminated to glutamate, which is then finally deaminated *(transdeamination)*.

Amino acids are deaminated at the rate of about 50–70 g per day. During the transamination reaction the amino group of all other amino acids is funnelled into glutamate. Hence, the glutamate dehydrogenase reaction is the final reaction which removes the amino group of all amino acids. It needs NAD+ as coenzyme. (NADP can also act as a coenzyme).

It is an allosteric enzyme; it is activated by ADP and inhibited by GTP.

The hydrolysis of glutamine also yields $NH_3$ but this occurs mainly in the kidney where the $NH_4^+$ excretion is required for acid base regulation.

## DISPOSAL/DETOXIFICATION OF AMMONIA

### First line of Defense (Trapping of Ammonia)

Being highly toxic, ammonia should be eliminated or detoxified, as and when it is formed. Even very minute quantity of ammonia may produce toxicity in central nervous system. But, ammonia is always produced by almost all cells, including neurons. The intracellular ammonia is immediately trapped by glutamic acid to form *glutamine*, especially in brain cells. The glutamine is then transported to liver, where the reaction is reversed by the enzyme *glutaminase*. The ammonia thus generated is immediately detoxified into urea.

Aspartic acid may also undergo similar reaction to form *asparagine*.

### Transportation of Ammonia

Inside the cells of almost all tissues, the transamination of amino acids produce glutamic acid.

However, glutamate dehydrogenase is available only in the liver. Therefore, the final deamination and production of ammonia is taking place in the liver. Thus, *glutamic acid* acts as the link between amino groups of amino acids and ammonia. The concentration of glutamic acid in blood is 10 times more than other amino acids.

***Glutamine*** is the transport form of ammonia from brain and intestine to liver; while alanine is the transport form from muscle.

### Final Disposal

The ammonia from all over the body thus reaches liver. It is then *detoxified to urea by liver* cells, and then excreted through kidneys. *Urea is the end product of protein metabolism.*

Since mammals including human beings excrete amino nitrogen mainly as urea, they are referred to as ureotelic. Fishes excrete ammonia as such (ammonotelic) while birds and reptiles as uric acid (uricotelic).

Although ammonia is toxic and has to be immediately detoxified, in kidney cells, ammonia is purposely generated from glutamine with the help of glutaminase. This is for buffering the acids, and maintaining acid-base balance.

## UREA CYCLE

In 1773, Rouelle isolated urea from urine. Frederic Wohler in 1828 obtained urea by boiling an aqueous solution of ammonium cyanate. The urea cycle is the first metabolic pathway to be elucidated (1932). The cycle is known as *Krebs–Henseleit* urea cycle. As ornithine is the first member of the reaction, it is also called as *Ornithine cycle*.

The two nitrogen atoms of urea are derived from two different sources, one from ammonia and the other directly from the alpha amino group of aspartic acid.

***Step 1. Formation of Carbamoyl Phosphate:*** One molecule of ammonia condenses with $CO_2$ in the presence of *two molecules of ATP* to form carbamoyl phosphate. The reaction is catalyzed by the mitochondrial enzyme *carbamoyl phosphate synthetase-I (CPS-I)*. An entirely different cytoplasmic enzyme, carbamoyl phosphate synthetase-II, (CPS-II) is involved in pyrimidine nucleotide synthesis. CPS-I reaction is the *rate-limiting step* in urea formation. It is irreversible and allosterically regulated.

***Step 2. Formation of Citrulline:*** The second reaction is also *mitochondrial*. The carbamoyl group is transferred to the $NH_2$ group of ornithine by *ornithine transcarbamoylase* (OTC). The citrulline leaves the mitochondria and further reactions are taking place in cytoplasm. Citrulline is neither present in tissue proteins nor in blood; but it is *present in milk*.

***Step 3. Formation of Argininosuccinate:*** One molecule of aspartic acid adds to citrulline forming a carbon to nitrogen bond which provides the 2nd nitrogen atom of urea. *Argininosuccinate synthetase* catalyzes the reaction. This needs hydrolysis of ATP to AMP level, so *two high energy phosphate bonds* are utilized. The PPi is an inhibitor of this step.

***Step 4. Formation of Arginine:*** Argininosuccinate is cleaved by *argininosuccinate lyase* (argininosuccinase) to arginine and fumarate. The enzyme is inhibited by fumarate, but this is avoided by the cytoplasmic localization of the enzyme. The fumarate formed may be funnelled into TCA cycle to be converted to malate and then to oxaloacetate to be transaminated to aspartate. Thus the urea cycle is linked to TCA cycle through fumarate. The 3rd and 4th steps taken together may be summarized as:

Citrulline + aspartate $\rightarrow$ Arginine + fumarate A similar reaction of donation of amino group by aspartate takes place in purine nucleotide synthesis also.

***Step 5. Formation of Urea:*** The final reaction of the cycle is the hydrolysis of arginine to urea and ornithine by arginase. The ornithine returns to the mitochondria to react with another molecule of carbamoyl phosphate so that the cycle will proceed. Thus, ornithine may be considered as a catalyst which enters the reaction and is regenerated.

### Energetics of Urea Cycle

The overall reaction may be summarized as:

$NH_3 + CO_2$ + Aspartate → Urea + fumarate

During these reactions, 2 ATPs are used in the 1st reaction. Another ATP is converted to AMP + PPi in the 3rd step, which is equivalent to 2 ATPs.

The urea cycle consumes *4 high energy phosphate bonds.* However, fumarate formed in the 4th step may be converted to malate. Malate when oxidised to oxaloacetate produces 1 NADH equivalent to 2.5 ATP. So *net energy expenditure is only 1.5 high energy phosphates*. The urea cycle and TCA cycle are interlinked, and so, it is called as *'urea bicycle'*.

### Regulation of the Urea Cycle

- ***Coarse Regulation:*** The enzyme levels change with the protein content of diet. During starvation, the activity of urea cycle enzymes is elevated to meet the increased rate of protein catabolism.
- ***Fine Regulation:*** The major regulatory step is catalyzed by CPS-I where the positive effector is *N-acetyl glutamate* (NAG). It is formed from glutamate and acetyl CoA. Arginine is an activator of NAG synthase.
- ***Compartmentalization:*** The urea cycle enzymes are located in such a way that the first two enzymes are in the mitochondrial matrix. The inhibitory effect of fumarate on its own formation is minimized because argininosuccinate lyase is in the cytoplasm, while fumarase is in mitochondria fluids results in toxic symptoms. Nowadays, defects in enzymes of urea cycle are detected in neonatal blood by tandem mass spectrometry.

***Brain is very sensitive to ammonia:*** Child may be put on a low protein diet and frequent small feeds are given. Attempts may be made to eliminate the amino nitrogen in other forms, e.g. as hippuric acid (Benzoyl conjugate of glycine) or phenyl acetyl glutamine. Gene therapy is in experimental stage for treating urea cycle disorders.

Since *Citrulline* is present in significant quantities in milk, breast milk is to be avoided in citrullinemia.

### Hepatic Coma (Acquired Hyperammonemia)

In diseases of the liver, hepatic failure can finally lead to hepatic coma and death. Hyperammonemia is the characteristic feature of liver failure. The condition is also known as portal systemic encephalopathy. Normally the ammonia and other toxic compounds produced by intestinal bacterial metabolism are transported to liver by portal circulation and detoxified by the liver. But when there is portal systemic shunting of blood, the toxins bypass the liver and their concentration in systemic circulation rises.

The signs and symptoms are mainly pertaining to CNS dysfunction (altered sensorium, convulsions), or manifestations of failure of liver function (ascites, jaundice, hepatomegaly, edema, hemorrhage, spider naevi). The management of the condition is difficult. A low protein diet and intestinal disinfection (bowel clearing and antibiotics), withholding hepatotoxic drugs and maintenance of electrolyte and acid base balance are the main lines of management.

### Urea Level in Blood

In clinical practice, blood urea level is taken as an *indicator of renal function*. The normal urea level in plasma is from *20 to 40 mg/dl*. Blood urea level is increased where renal function is inadequate. Urea level in blood may be theoretically increased when protein intake is very high. However in usual conditions, this will be only within the upper limit of the normal values. Urinary excretion of urea is 15 to 30 g/day (6–15 g nitrogen/day). This corresponds to the breakdown of 40 to 80 g of proteins per day. Urea constitutes 80% of urinary organic solids.

## CHEMISTRY OF CARBOHYDRATES

### Functions of Carbohydrates

- Carbohydrates are the main sources of *energy* in the body. Brain cells and RBCs are almost wholly dependent on carbohydrates as the energy source. Energy production from carbohydrates will be 4 k calories/g (16 k Joules/g).
- Storage form of energy (starch and glycogen).
- Excess carbohydrate is converted to fat.
- Glycoproteins and glycolipids are components of cell membranes and receptors.
- Structural basis of many organisms: Cellulose of plants; exoskeleton of insects, cell wall of microorganisms, mucopolysaccharides as ground substance in higher organisms.

The general molecular formula of carbohydrate is $C_n(H_2O)_n$. For example, glucose has the molecular formula $C_6H_{12}O_6$. Carbohydrates are *polyhydroxy aldehydes or ketones* or compounds which yield these on hydrolysis.

#### *Nomenclature*

Molecules having only one actual or potential sugar group are called *monosaccharides* (Greek, mono = one; saccharide = sugar). They cannot be further hydrolyzed into smaller units. When two monosaccharides are combined together with elimination of a water molecule, it is called a *disaccharide* (e.g. $C_{12}H_{22}O_{11}$). *Trisaccharides* contain three sugar groups. Further addition of sugar groups will correspondingly produce tetrasaccharides, pentasaccharides and so on, commonly known as *oligosaccharides* (Greek, oligo = a few). When more than 10 sugar units are combined, they are generally named as *polysaccharides* (Greek, poly = many). Polysaccharides having only one type of monosaccharide units are called *homopolysaccharides* and those having different monosaccharide units are *heteropolysaccharides*.

Sugars having aldehyde group are called *aldoses* and sugars with keto group are *ketoses*. Depending on the number of carbon atoms, the monosaccharides are named as triose (C3), tetrose (C4), pentose (C5), hexose (C6), heptose (C7) and so on.

#### *Stereoisomers*

Compounds having same structural formula, but differing in spatial configuration are known as stereoisomers. While writing the molecular formula of monosaccharides, the spatial arrangements of H and OH groups are important, since they contain asymmetric carbon atoms. Asymmetric carbon means that four different groups are attached to the same carbon. The reference molecule is glyceraldehyde (glycerose) which has a single asymmetric carbon atom. The number of possible stereoisomers depends on the number of asymmetric carbon atoms by the formula 2n where n is the number of asymmetric carbon atoms.

## Reference Carbon Atom of Sugars

The configuration of H and OH groups at the second carbon atom of glyceraldehydes may be noticed. The two mirror forms are denoted as D- and L-varieties. All monosaccharides can be considered as molecules derived from glyceraldehydes by successive addition of carbon atoms.

Therefore, *penultimate carbon atom is the reference carbon atom* for naming the mirror images. This is also referred to as absolute configuration.

### *D and L Isomerism of Glucose*

With reference to the penultimate carbon atom (i.e. C5 in the case of glucose), the configuration of H and OH groups is changed and two mirror images are produced. It may be noted that in D and L varieties, the groups in 2nd, 3rd, 4th and 5th carbon atoms are totally reversed, so as to produce the mirror images. These two forms are also stereoisomers.

*D sugars are naturally occurring* sugars and body can metabolize only D sugars.

## Optical Activity

The presence of asymmetrical carbon atom causes optical activity. When a beam of plane-polarized light is passed through a solution of carbohydrates, it will rotate the light either to right or to left. Please note that the D- and L-notation has no bearing with the optical activity. Depending on the rotation, molecules are called dextrorotatory (+) (d) or levorotatory (–) (l).

Thus *D-glucose is dextrorotatory but D-fructose is levorotatory*. Equimolecular mixture of optical isomers has no net rotation (*racemic mixture*).

Heyrovsky was awarded Nobel prize in 1924 for polarographic analysis of sugars.

### *Diastereoisomers of Glucose*

Configurational changes with regard to C2, C3 and C4 will produce eight different monosaccharides. Out of these, only 3 are seen in human body. They are *Glucose, Galactose and Mannose*.

There are 8 diastereoisomers for aldohexoses. With reference to C5, all of them will have D and L forms. Hence, the molecular formula of hexose ($C_6H_{12}O_6$) represents 16 different monosaccharides, due to spatial arrangement of constituent groups.

*Glucose* is the most predominant sugar in human body. It is the major source of energy. It is present in blood. D-glucose is dextrorotatory.

In clinical practice, it is often called as *dextrose*. *Galactose* is a constituent of lactose (milk sugar) and glycoproteins. Galactose is epimerized to glucose in liver and then utilized as a fuel. The term galactose is derived from Greek word gala, meaning milk.

*Mannose* is a constituent of many glycoproteins. Mannose was isolated from plant mannans; hence the name.

### *Epimerism of Aldoses*

When sugars are different from one another, only in configuration *with regard to a single carbon atom, other than the reference carbon atom,* they are called epimers. For example, glucose and mannose are an epimeric pair which differ only with respect to C2. Similarly, galactose is the 4th epimer of glucose. Galactose and mannose are not epimers but diastereoisomers.

### *Anomerism of Sugars*

When D glucose is crystallized at room temperature, and a fresh solution is prepared, its specific rotation of polarized light is +112°, but after 12–18 hours it changes to +52.5°. If initial crystallization is taking place at 98°C and then solubilized, the specific rotation is found to be +19°, which also changes to +52.5° within a few hours. This change in rotation with time is called *mutarotation*.

This is explained by the fact that D-glucose has two anomers, alpha and beta varieties. These anomers are produced by the spatial configuration with reference to the first carbon atom in aldoses and second carbon atom in ketoses. Hence, these carbon atoms are known as anomeric carbon atoms. Thus α-D-glucose has specific rotation of +112° and β-D-glucose has +19°. Both undergo mutarotation and at equilibrium one-third molecules are alpha type and 2/3rd are beta variety to get the specific rotation of +52.5°.

The differences between α and β anomeric forms are dependent on the 1st carbon atom only. In the previous section 16 stereoisomers of glucose are described. Each of them will have 2 anomers; and hence there are a total of 32 isomers for glucose.

## Disaccharides

When two monosaccharides are combined together by glycosidic linkage, a disaccharide is formed. The important disaccharides are:

- Sucrose
- Maltose and isomaltose
- Lactose.

### *Sucrose*

- It is the sweetening agent known as cane sugar. It is present in sugarcane and various fruits.
- Sucrose contains glucose and fructose. Sucrose is **not a reducing sugar**; and it will not form osazone. This is because the linkage involves first carbon of glucose and second carbon of fructose, and free reducing groups are not available.
- When sucrose is hydrolyzed, the products have reducing action. A sugar solution which is originally nonreducing, but becomes reducing after hydrolysis, is identified as sucrose *(specific sucrose test)*.

- Hydrolysis of sucrose (optical rotation +66.5°) will produce one molecule of glucose (+52.5°) and one molecule of fructose (–92°). Therefore the products will change the dextrorotation to levorotation, or the plane of rotation is inverted. Equimolecular mixture of glucose and fructose thus formed is called *invert sugar*. The enzyme producing hydrolysis of sucrose is called *sucrase or invertase*. Honey contains invert sugar. Invert sugar is sweeter than sucrose.

### Lactose

- It is the sugar present in milk. It is a *reducing disaccharide*. On hydrolysis lactose yields glucose and galactose. *Beta glycosidic linkage* is present in lactose.
- The anomeric carbon atom of beta-galactose is attached to the 4th hydroxyl group of glucose through beta-1,4 glycosidic linkage. The lactose may be alpha or beta variety, depending on the configuration of 1st carbon of glucose moiety.
- Lactose forms osazone which resembles 'badminton ball' or '*hedgehog*' or flower of 'touch-me-not'.
- Lactose and lactate should not be confused.

### Maltose

- Maltose contains two glucose residues.
- There is alpha-1,4 linkage, i.e. the anomeric 1st carbon atom of one glucose is combined with 4th hydroxyl group of another glucose through alpha-glycosidic linkage.
- Maltose may be alpha or beta depending on the configuration at the free anomeric carbon atom.
- It is a *reducing disaccharide*. It forms *petal shaped crystals* of maltose-osazone.

## Polysaccharides

These are polymerized products of many monosaccharide units. They may be:

- ***Homoglycans*** are composed of single kind of monosaccharides, e.g. starch, glycogen and cellulose.
- ***Heteroglycans*** are composed of two or more different monosaccharides, e.g. hyaluronic acid, chondroitin sulfate.

### Starch

#### Structure of Starch

- It is the reserve carbohydrate of *plant kingdom*.
- ***Sources:*** Potatoes, tapioca, cereals (rice, wheat) and other food grains.
- Starch is composed of amylose and amylopectin. When starch is treated with boiling water, 10–20% is solubilized; this part is called *amylose*. Amylose is made up of glucose units with *alpha-1,4 glycosidic linkages* to form an unbranched long chain with a molecular weight 400,000 D or more.
- The insoluble part absorbs water and forms paste like gel; this is called *amylopectin*.

Amylopectin is also made up of glucose units, but is highly branched with molecular weight more than 1 million. The branching points are made by *alpha-1,6 linkage*.

#### Hydrolysis of Starch

- Starch will form a *blue colored complex with iodine*; this color disappears on heating and reappears when cooled. This is a sensitive test for starch. Starch is non-reducing because the free sugar groups are negligible in number.
- When starch is hydrolyzed by mild acid, smaller and smaller fragments are produced.
- Thus hydrolysis for a short-time produces *amylodextrin* which gives violet color with iodine and is non-reducing. Further hydrolysis produces *erythrodextrin* which gives red color with iodine and mild reduction of Benedict's solution. Later achrodextrins (no color with iodine, but reducing) and further on, maltose (no color with iodine, but powerfully reducing) are formed on continued hydrolysis.

#### Action of Amylases on Starch

- Salivary amylase and pancreatic amylase are *alpha-amylases*, which act at random on alpha-1,4 glycosidic bonds to split starch into smaller units (dextrins), and finally to *alpha-maltose*.
- ***Beta-amylases*** are of plant origin (almond, germinating seeds, etc.) which split starch to form *beta-maltose*. They act on amylose to split maltose units consecutively. Thus the enzyme starts its action from one end.
- When beta-amylase acts on amylopectin, maltose units are liberated from the ends of the branches of amylopectin, until the action of enzyme is blocked at the 1,6-glycosidic linkage. The action of beta-amylase stops at branching points, leaving a large molecule, called *limit dextrin* or *residual dextrin*.

### Glycogen

- It is the *reserve carbohydrate in animals*. It is stored in *liver and muscle*. About 5% of weight of liver is made up by glycogen. Excess carbohydrates are deposited as glycogen.
- Glycogen is composed of glucose units joined by alpha-1,4 links in the straight chains. It also has alpha-1,6 glycosidic linkages at the branching points. Molecular weight of glycogen is about 5 million. Innermost core of glycogen contains a primer protein, *Glycogenin*. Glycogen is *more branched and more compact* than amylopectin.

### Cellulose

- It is the supporting tissues of plants. Cellulose constitutes 99% of cotton, 50% of wood and is the most abundant organic material in nature.
- It is made up of glucose units combined with *beta-1,4 linkages*. It has a straight line structure, with no branching points. Molecular weight is in the order of 2 to 5 million.
- Beta-1,4 bridges are hydrolyzed by the enzyme *cellobiase*. But this enzyme is absent in animal and human digestive system, and hence cellulose *cannot be digested*.
- Herbivorous animals have large cecum, which harbor bacteria. These bacteria can hydrolyze cellulose, and the glucose produced is utilized by the animal. White ants (termites) also digest cellulose with the help of intestinal bacteria.
- Cellulose has a variety of commercial applications, as it is the starting material to produce fibres, celluloids, nitrocellulose and plastics.

### Inulin

It is a long chain homoglycan composed of *D-fructose* units with repeating beta-1,2 linkages.

It is the reserve carbohydrate present in various bulbs and tubers such as chicory, dahlia, dandelion, onion, garlic. It is clinically used to find *renal clearance* value and glomerular filtration rate.

### Dextrans

These are highly branched homopolymers of glucose units with 1–6, 1–4 and 1–3 linkages. They are produced by microorganisms. They have molecular weight 1 million to 4 millions. Since they will not easily go out of vascular compartment, they are used for intravenous infusion as *plasma volume expander* for treatment of hypovolemic shock. It may be noted that dextrans are different from previously described dextrins.

### Chitin

It is present in exoskeletons of crustacea and insects. It is composed of units of N-acetylglucosamine with beta-1,4 glycosidic linkages.

## Mucopolysaccharides

Mucopolysaccharides or *glycosamino glycans* (GAG) are heteropolysaccharides, containing uronic acid and amino sugars. Acetylated amino groups, sulfate and carboxyl groups are also generally present. Because of the presence of these charged groups, they attract water molecules so they produce viscous solutions. Mucopolysaccharides in combination with proteins form mucoproteins.

Examples of mucopolysaccharides are hyaluronic acid, heparin, chondroitin sulfate, dermatan sulfate and keratan sulfate.

- ***Hyaluronic acid:*** It is present in connective tissues, tendons, synovial fluid and vitreous humor. It serves as a lubricant in joint cavities. It is composed of repeating units of N-Acetyl-glucosamine → beta-1, 4-Glucuronic acid → beta-1-3-N-Acetyl glucosamine and so on.
- ***Heparin:***
  - It is an *anticoagulant* widely used when taking blood *in vitro* for clinical studies. It is also used *in vivo* in suspected thrombo-embolic conditions to prevent intravascular coagulation. It activates antithrombin III, which in turn inactivates thrombin, factor X and factor IX.
  - Heparin is present in liver, lungs, spleen and monocytes. Commercial preparation of heparin is from animal lung tissues.
  - It contains repeating units of sulfated glucosamine → alpha-1, 4-L-iduronic acid → and so on. Idose is the 5th epimer of glucose. Iduronic acid is the oxidized form of idose. Sulfated heparin or *heparan sulfate* is also present in tissues.
- ***Chondroitin sulfate:*** It is present in ground substance of connective tissues widely distributed in cartilage, bone, tendons, cornea and skin. It is composed of repeating units of glucuronic acid → beta-1,3-N-acetyl galactosamine sulfate → beta-1, 4.
- ***Keratan sulfate:*** It is the only GAG which *does not contain any uronic acid*. The repeating units are galactose and N-acetyl glucosamine in beta linkage. It is found in cornea and tendons.
- ***Dermatan Sulfate:*** It contains L-iduronic acid and N-acetyl galactosamine in beta -1, 3 linkages. It is found in skin, blood vessels and heart valves.

## Metabolic Pathways of Glucose

### Digestion of Carbohydrates

- In the diet carbohydrates are present as complex polysaccharides (starch, glycogen), and to a minor extent, as disaccharides (sucrose and lactose). They are hydrolyzed to monosaccharide units in the gastrointestinal tract. Cooking makes the digestion process easier.
- This process of digestion starts in mouth by the *salivary alpha-amylase*. However, the time available for digestion in the mouth is limited, because the gastric hydrochloric acid will inhibit the action of salivary amylase.
- In the *pancreatic* juice another *alpha-amylase* is available which will hydrolyze the alpha-1,4 glycosidic linkages randomly, so as to produce smaller subunits like maltose, isomaltose, dextrins and branched or unbranched oligosaccharides.
- The cells of brush border of intestine contain the enzymes, *sucrase, maltase, isomaltase* and *lactase*. They hydrolyze the corresponding disaccharides into component monosaccharides which are then absorbed.

*Clinical Application; Lactose Intolerance*

- Lactase hydrolyzes lactose to glucose and galactose. *Lactase* is present in the brush border of enterocytes.
- ***Deficiency of lactase*** leads to lactose intolerance. In this condition, lactose accumulates in the gut. Irritant diarrhea and flatulence are seen.
- There may be congenital (primary) or acquired (secondary) causes. As age advances, lactase enzyme will be lost. Another reason for acquired lactose intolerance may be sudden change into a milk based diet. Lactase is an *inducible* enzyme. If milk is withdrawn temporarily, the diarrhea will be limited. Curd is also an effective treatment, because the lactobacilli present in curd contains the enzyme lactase. Lactase is abundantly seen in yeast, which could also be used in treatment.

### Absorption of Carbohydrates

Only monosaccharides are absorbed by the intestine. Absorption rate is maximum for galactose; moderate for glucose; and minimum for fructose.

### Absorption of Glucose

Glucose has specific transporters, which are transmembrane proteins.

*Co-transport from Lumen to Intestinal Cell*

- This process is mediated by *Sodium Dependent Glucose Transporter-1 (SGluT-1)*. Absorption from intestinal lumen into intestinal cell is by co-transport mechanism (secondary active transport).

- A membrane bound *carrier protein* is involved, which carries glucose, along with sodium. This sodium is later expelled by the *sodium pump* with utilization of energy. So energy is needed indirectly.
- The transporter in intestine is named as *SGluT-1* and the transporter in the kidney is called *SGluT-2*. The first one is involved in glucosegalactose malabsorption. The SGluT-2 is defective in congenital renal glycosuria.
- ***Clinical application:*** Common treatment for diarrhea is *oral rehydration fluid*. It contains glucose and sodium. Presence of glucose in oral rehydration fluid allows uptake of sodium to replenish body sodium chloride.

*Another Uniport System Releases Glucose into Blood*

- The same intestinal epithelial cells have a different transport mechanism on the membrane facing capillaries. Intestinal cells release glucose into blood stream by the carrier mechanism called *Glucose Transporter Type 2 (GluT2)*.
- This transporter is not dependent on sodium. It is a *uniport, facilitated diffusion* system.
- Glucose binds to the transporter on one side of the membrane. When fixed, the complex changes configuration. This leads to the closure of the first binding site. At the same time, the binding site is now exposed on the inner side of the membrane, releasing the glucose. The process is called ping-pong mechanism.
- GluT2 *(facilitated transport)* is involved in absorption of glucose from blood stream to cells. GluT2 is present in intestinal epithelial cells, liver cells, beta cells of pancreas and kidney.
- Since GluT2 has a high Km for glucose, its presence in beta cells is ideally suited for sensing a high glucose level and releasing insulin. So this mechanism enables the pancreas to *monitor the glucose level* and adjust the rate of insulin secretion.

*Glucose Transporter 4*

- GluT4 is the major glucose transporter in *skeletal muscle and adipose tissue.*
- GluT4 is under the control of *insulin*. But other glucose transporters are not under the control of insulin.
- ***Clinical application:*** Insulin induces the movement of intracellular GluT4 molecules to the cell surface and thus increases glucose uptake. In Type 2 *diabetes mellitus*, membrane GluT4 is reduced, leading to insulin resistance in muscle and fat cells. In diabetes, entry of glucose into muscle is only half of normal cells.

### *Glucose Metabolism*

Abbate Spallanzani (1768) showed that living tissues take up oxygen and give off carbon dioxide. In 1860, Louis Pastueur demonstrated the fermentation process of glucose to alcohol by yeast. Fick (1882) indicated that chemical energy in muscle is converted to contraction of muscle. Gad (1893) found out that lactic acid is formed during muscle contraction. In 1902, Sir Walter Fletcher established that this lactic acid is derived from glycogen. In 1914, Gustav George Embden (1874–1933) studied the lactic acid formation from pyruvate. In 1919, Otto Fritz Meyerhof (1884–1951) enunciated most of the steps of the glycolytic pathway (Nobel prize, 1922). Hexokinase enzyme was first identified by von Euler-Chelpin in 1915 (Nobel prize, 1922). Other enzymes in the glycolytic pathway were then identified rapidly; pyruvate decarboxylase by Neuberg in 1911, phospho fructo kinase by sir Arthur Harden in 1920 (Nobel prize, 1929); phospho hexose isomerase by Lohmann in 1933; pyruvate kinase by Parnas in 1934; enolase by Meyerhof in 1935; phospho gluco mutase by Leloir in 1938 (Nobel prize, 1970); glyceraldehyde phosphate dehydrogenase by Warburg in 1939; phosphoglyceromutase by Sutherland in 1942 (Nobel prize, 1971). Between 1935 and 1943, all enzymes of glycolytic pathway were crystallized and characterized by Warburg. He was awarded Nobel prize in 1931 for his earlier work on cellular respiration. He was awarded Nobel prize for second time in 1944 for his contributions in glycolysis; but Hitler did not permit him to receive it.

*Clinical Importance of Glucose*

- Glucose is the preferred source of energy for most of the body tissues. Brain cells derive the energy mainly from glucose.
- When glucose metabolism is deranged, life-threatening conditions may occur. A minimum amount of glucose is always required for normal functioning.
- ***Normal fasting plasma glucose level is 70 to 110 mg/dl.*** After a heavy carbohydrate meal, it rises; but in a normal person, this level is below 150 mg/dl.

## GLYCOLYSIS (EMBDEN-MEYERHOF PATHWAY)

**Definition:** In the pathway of glycolysis, glucose is split into two 3-carbon *pyruvate* molecules under aerobic conditions; or *lactate* under anaerobic conditions, along with production of a small quantity of energy. Glycolysis is derived from the Greek words, glykys = sweet; and lysis = splitting.

***Site of reactions:*** All the reaction steps take place in the cytoplasm.

### Significance of the Glycolysis Pathway

- It is the only pathway that is taking place in all the cells of the body.
- Glycolysis is the only source of energy in erythrocytes.
- In strenuous exercise, when muscle tissue lacks enough oxygen, *anaerobic glycolysis forms the major source of energy for muscles.*
- The glycolytic pathway may be considered as the preliminary step before complete oxidation.
- The glycolytic pathway provides carbon skeletons for synthesis of non-essential amino acids as well as glycerol part of fat.
- Most of the reactions of the glycolytic pathway are reversible, which are also used for gluconeogenesis.

### Steps of Glycolytic Pathway

#### *Step 1 of Glycolysis*

- Glucose is phosphorylated to glucose-6-phosphate.
- The enzyme is *hexokinase* (HK), which splits the ATP into ADP, and the Pi is added on to the glucose. The energy

released by the hydrolysis of ATP is utilized for the forward reaction.

- Hexokinase is a *key glycolytic enzyme.* Hexokinase catalyzes a regulatory step in glycolysis that is *irreversible.* But this irreversibility is circumvented by another enzyme glucose-6-phosphatase.
- Hexokinase and glucokinase may be considered as iso-enzymes. Glucokinase is under the influence of insulin, but hexokinase is not.
- The phosphorylation of glucose traps it within the cells. Once phosphorylated, glucose-6-phosphate is trapped within the cell and has to be metabolized.

### Step 2 of Glycolysis

Glucose-6-phosphate is isomerized to fructose-6-phosphate by phosphohexose *isomerase.* This is readily reversible.

### Step 3 of Glycolysis

- Fructose-6-phosphate is further phosphorylated to fructose1,6-bisphosphate. The enzyme is *phosphofructokinase.*
- PFK is an allosteric, inducible, regulatory enzyme. It is an important *key enzyme* of this pathway. This is again an activation process, the energy being derived by hydrolysis of yet another molecule of ATP. This *irreversible* step is the rate limiting reaction in glycolysis. However, during gluconeogenesis, this step is circumvented by fructose-1,6-bisphosphatase.
- The steps 1, 2 and 3 together are called as the *preparatory phase.*

### Step 4 of Glycolysis

The 6 carbon fructose-1, 6-bisphosphate is cleaved into two 3 carbon units; one glyceraldehyde-3-phosphate and another molecule of dihydroxy acetone phosphate (DHAP). Since the backward reaction is an aldol condensation, the enzyme is called *aldolase.* This reaction is reversible.

#### Step 4-A of Glycolysis

Dihydroxy acetone phosphate is isomerized to glyceraldehyde-3-phosphate by the enzyme phosphotriose *isomerase.* Thus net result is that glucose is now cleaved into 2 molecules of glyceraldehyde-3-phosphate. The steps 4 and 4-A are together called the *splitting phase.*

Glycerol portion of the neutral fat can enter into glycolytic or gluconeogenic pathways at this point. Similarly for neutral fat synthesis, glycerol is required which can be derived from glucose through DHAP.

### Step 5 of Glycolysis

Glyceraldehyde-3-phosphate is dehydrogenated and simultaneously phosphorylated to 1,3-bisphospho glycerate (1,3-BPG) with the help of NAD+. The enzyme is *glyceraldehyde-3- phosphate dehydrogenase.* The product contains a *high energy bond.* This is a reversible reaction.

The oxidation of the aldehyde is an exergonic reaction that drives the synthesis of the high energy compound, 1,3 bisphosphoglycerate with high phosphoryl group transfer potential. The enzyme has a cysteinyl SH group at the active center and is inhibited by iodoacetate. During this reaction, NAD+ is reduced to NADH.

### Step 6 of Glycolysis

- The energy of 1,3-BPG is trapped to synthesize one ATP molecule with the help of *bisphospho glycerate* kinase.
- This is an example of *substrate level phosphorylation,* where energy is trapped directly from the substrate, without the help of the complicated electron transport chain reactions.
- When energy is trapped by oxidation of reducing equivalents such as NADH, it is called *oxidative phosphorylation. Step 6 is reversible.*

### Step 7 of Glycolysis

3-phosphoglycerate is isomerized to 2-phosphoglycerate by shifting the phosphate group from 3rd to 2nd carbon atom. The enzyme is *phosphogluco mutase.* This is a readily reversible reaction.

### Step 8 of Glycolysis

- 2-phosphoglycerate is converted to phosphoenolpyruvate by the enzyme *enolase*. One water molecule is removed.
- A *high energy phosphate bond* is produced. The reaction is reversible.
- Enolase requires $Mg^{++}$, and by removing magnesium ions, *fluoride* will irreversibly inhibit this enzyme. Thus, fluoride will stop the whole glycolysis. So when taking blood for sugar estimation, fluoride is added to blood. If not, glucose is metabolized by the blood cells, so that lower blood glucose values are obtained.

### Step 9 of Glycolysis

- Phosphoenolpyruvate (PEP) is dephosphorylated to pyruvate, by *pyruvate kinase.* First PEP is made into a transient intermediary of enol pyruvate which is spontaneously isomerized into keto pyruvate, the stable form of pyruvate.
- One mole of ATP is generated during this reaction. This is again an example of *substrate level phosphorylation.*
- The pyruvate kinase is a *key glycolytic enzyme.* This step is *irreversible.* The reversal, however, can be brought about in the body with the help of two enzymes (pyruvate kinase and phosphoenol pyruvate carboxy kinase) and hydrolysis of 2 ATP molecules (see gluconeogenesis).

### Step 10 of Glycolysis

In anaerobic condition, pyruvate is reduced to lactate by lactate dehydrogenase (LDH).

- A *high energy phosphate bond* is produced. (an=not, aer=air, bios=life). LDH has 5 iso-enzymes.

The cardiac iso-enzyme of LDH will be increased in myocardial infarcts. In aerobic conditions, the pyruvate enters the citric acid cycle for complete oxidation. The end product of anaerobic glycolysis is lactate which enters the Cori's cycle.

#### Energy Yield from Glycolysis

- During *anaerobic* (oxygen deficient) condition, when one molecule of glucose is converted to 2 molecules of lactate, there is a net yield of 2 molecules of ATP.

- 4 molecules of ATP are synthesized by the 2 substrate level phosphorylations (steps 6 and 9). But 2 molecules of ATP are used in the steps 1 and 3, hence the *net yield is only 2 ATP*.
- The whole reaction is summarized as
  Glucose + 2 Pi + 2 ADP → 2 Lactate + 2 ATP
- But when *oxygen is in plenty*, the two NADH molecules, generated in the glyceraldehyde-3-phosphate dehydrogenase reaction (step 5), can enter the mitochondrial electron transport chain for complete oxidation. As each NADH provides 2.5 ATPs, this reaction generates 2.5 × 2 = 5 ATPs. Thus when oxygen is available, the net gain of energy from the glycolysis pathway is *7 ATPs*.
- Hence the ATP yield from glycolysis is different in anaerobic and aerobic conditions.
- Pyruvate is later oxidatively decarboxylated to acetyl CoA, which enters into the citric acid cycle. Complete oxidation of glucose through glycolysis plus citric acid cycle will yield a *net 32 ATPs*.

*Regulation of Glycolysis*

The regulatory enzymes or key enzymes of glycolysis are:
- Glucokinase/Hexokinase, step 1
- Phosphofructokinase, step 3
- Pyruvate kinase, step 9

*Factors Regulating Glycolysis*

- ***Glucokinase/Hexokinase:*** Phosphorylation of glucose by these enzymes is a reaction which is regulated by feedback inhibition (hexokinase by glucose-6-phosphate) and activated by insulin (glucokinase is induced by insulin). Glucokinase that is active mainly in liver has a high Km for glucose and low affinity. Hence, glucokinase can act only when there is adequate glucose supply so that excess can be stored. Hexokinase with low Km and high affinity can phosphorylate glucose even at lower concentrations so that glucose is made available to brain, cardiac and skeletal muscle. Glucokinase can act only when there is plenty of glucose. Thus, when the supply of glucose is limited, glucose is made available to brain and muscles.
- ***Phosphofructokinase (PFK)*** (step 3) is the most important *rate-limiting* enzyme for glycolysis pathway. *ATP* and *citrate* are the most important allosteric inhibitors. AMP acts as an allosteric activator.
- ***Fructose-2,6-bisphosphate (F-2,6-BP)*** increases the activity of phosphofructokinase. F-2,6-BP is formed from fructose-6-phosphate by the action of an enzyme called PFK-2. (It is different from the PFK1). Fructose-2,6-bisphosphate is hydrolyzed to fructose-6-phosphate by fructose-2,6-bisphosphatase. The activities of both the enzymes (PFK2 and fructose-2,6-bisphosphatase) are *reciprocally regulated*. When glucose supply is in plenty, PFK-2 is dephosphorylated and activated so F-2,6-BP concentration increases this in turn, activates PFK. Thus glycolysis is favored.
- ***Pyruvate Kinase*** catalyzes an irreversible step and is a regulatory enzyme of glycolysis. When energy is plenty in the cell, glycolysis is inhibited. Insulin increases its activity where as glucagon inhibits. Pyruvate kinase is inactive in the phosphorylated state.
- ***Insulin*** favors glycolysis by activating the above three key glycolytic enzymes.
- ***Glucagon and glucocorticoids*** inhibit glycolysis and favor gluconeogenesis.

## CORI'S CYCLE OR LACTIC ACID CYCLE

- ***Definition:*** It is a process in which glucose is converted to lactate in the muscle and in the liver this lactate is re-converted into glucose.
- In an actively contracting muscle, pyruvate is reduced to lactic acid which may tend to accumulate in the muscle. The muscle cramps often associated with strenuous muscular exercise are thought to be due to lactate accumulation.
- To prevent the lactate accumulation, body utilizes Cori's cycle.
- This lactic acid from muscle diffuses into the blood. Lactate then reaches liver, where it is oxidized to pyruvate. Thus, it is channeled to gluconeogenesis. Regenerated glucose can enter into blood and then to muscle. This cycle is called Cori's cycle.
- ***Significance of the Cori's cycle:*** The lactate produced in the muscle is efficiently reutilized by the body. But this is an energy-consuming process. During exercise, lactate production is high, which is utilized by liver to produce glucose. This process needs ATP in significant quantities, which is provided by increased metabolism. This leads to increased oxygen consumption. This is the explanation for the **oxygen debt** after vigorous exercise.

### Metabolic Fate of Pyruvate

Under aerobic conditions, pyruvate is converted to acetyl CoA which enters the TCA cycle to be oxidized to $CO_2$. ATP is generated.

Glycolysis is taking place in cytoplasm. So pyruvate is generated in cytoplasm. This is transported into mitochondria by a *pyruvate transporter*.

### *Pyruvate Dehydrogenase Complex*

Inside the mitochondria, pyruvate is *oxidatively decarboxylated* to acetyl CoA by pyruvate dehydrogenase (PDH). It is a multi-enzyme complex with 5 coenzymes and 3 apo-enzymes. The coenzymes needed are:

1. Thiamine pyrophosphate (TPP)
2. Coenzyme A (CoA)
3. FAD
4. NAD+
5. Lipoamide. The lipoic acid, otherwise called thioctic acid has two sulfur atoms and 8 carbon atoms. It can accept or donate hydrogen atoms.
6. The enzyme part of the PDH complex is made up of three component enzymes.

6A. ***Pyruvate Dehydrogenase (Enzyme 1):*** It catalyzes oxidative decarboxylation. TPP is required in this step. So, *Thiamine*, a B-complex group vitamin is essential for utilization of pyruvate. The two-carbon unit remain attached to the enzyme, as hydroxyethyl thiamine pyrophosphate.

6B. ***Dihydrolipoyl Transacetylase (Enzyme 2):*** Then, hydroxyethyl group is oxidized to form an acetyl group and then transferred from TPP to lipoamide to form acetyl lipoamide.

6C. *Dihydrolipoyl Dehydrogenase (Enzyme 3):* The last step is the oxidation of lipoamide. At the end of the reaction the cofactors, namely TPP, Lipoamide and FAD are regenerated.

A similar enzyme complex brings about the oxidative decarboxylation of alpha keto glutarate to succinyl CoA in the TCA cycle.

***Regulation:*** PDH is subject to regulation by allosteric mechanisms and covalent modification. Allosteric inhibitors are the products acetyl CoA and NADH. PDH or E1 is covalently modified by phosphorylation by PDH kinase and dephosphorylated by PDH phosphatase. The dephosphorylated form of the enzyme is active. Hence activators of PDH kinase like ATP, NADH and acetyl CoA inhibit PDH reaction. PDH phosphatase is activated by $Ca^{++}$, $Mg^{++}$ and AMP; this will increase the rate of PDH reaction where as PDH kinase is inhibited by $Ca^{++}$. When there is adequate ATP and acetyl CoA, the enzyme is inhibited.

### *Importance of Pyruvate Dehydrogenase*

- *Completely irreversible process:* There is no pathway available in the body to circumvent this step. Glucose through this step is converted to acetyl CoA from which fatty acids can be synthesized. But the backward reaction is not possible, and so *there is no net synthesis of glucose from fat.*
- Pyruvate may be channeled back to glucose through gluconeogenesis. But when pyruvate becomes acetyl CoA, it cannot go back. Thus, pyruvate dehydrogenase step is the *committed step* towards oxidation of glucose.
- *Energetics:* The NADH generated in this reaction, enters the electron transport chain to produce 2.5 ATP molecules.
- Pyruvate dehydrogenase is regulated by *end product inhibition* as well as by *covalent modification*. Phosphorylation of the enzyme by a kinase decreases the activity of the enzyme. Dephosphorylation activates the enzyme.

### *Pyruvate as a Junction Point*

Pyruvate occupies an important junction between various metabolic pathways. It may be decarboxylated to *acetyl CoA* which enters the TCA cycle, or may be utilized for fatty acid synthesis. Pyruvate may be carboxylated to *oxaloacetate* which is used for gluconeogenesis.

## GLUCONEOGENESIS

### Definition

It is the process by which glucose molecules are produced from non-carbohydrate precursors. These include lactate, glucogenic amino acids, glycerol part of fat and propionyl CoA derived from odd chain fatty acids.

### Site

Gluconeogenesis occurs mainly in the liver, and to a lesser extent in the renal cortex. The pathway is partly mitochondrial and partly cytoplasmic.

### Key Gluconeogenic Enzymes

- Pyruvate carboxylase
- Phosphoenolpyruvate carboxykinase
- Fructose-1-6-bisphosphatase
- Glucose-6-phosphatase

Gluconeogenesis involves several enzymes of glycolysis, but *it is not a reversal* of glycolysis. The irreversible steps in glycolysis are circumvented by four enzymes which are designated as the key enzymes of gluconeogenesis.

### *Pyruvate Carboxylase Reaction*

Pyruvate in the cytoplasm enters the mitochondria. Then, carboxylation of pyruvate to oxaloacetate is catalyzed by a mitochondrial enzyme, pyruvate carboxylase. It needs the coenzymes *biotin* and ATP.

#### *Malate Aspartate Shuttle*

The carboxylation of pyruvate (previous reaction) takes place in mitochondria. So, oxaloacetate is generated inside the mitochondria. This oxaloacetate has to be transported from mitochondria to cytosol, because further reactions of gluconeogenesis are taking place in cytosol. This is achieved by the *malate aspartate shuttle.* Oxaloacetate is first converted to malate, which traverses the membrane and reaches cytoplasm. Malate is then re-converted to oxaloacetate. Malate dehydrogenase is present in both mitochondria and cytoplasm. Oxaloacetate may also be transported as aspartate formed by transamination of oxaloacetate.

When alanine is the substrate for gluconeogenesis, the malate shuttle predominantly operates, because NADH is also required in the cytoplasm for the gluconeogenesis to continue. When lactate is the substrate for gluconeogenesis, the aspartate shuttle operates, because sufficient NADH is available in the cytoplasm by the LDH reaction.

### *Phosphoenolpyruvate Carboxykinase*

In the cytoplasm, PEPCK enzyme then converts oxaloacetate to phosphoenolpyruvate by removing a molecule of $CO_2$. GTP or ITP donates the phosphate. The net effect of these two reactions is the conversion of pyruvate to phosphoenolpyruvate.

This circumvents the irreversible step in glycolysis catalyzed by pyruvate kinase (step 9 of glycolysis).

#### *Partial Reversal of Glycolysis*

The phosphoenolpyruvate undergoes further reactions catalyzed by the glycolytic enzymes to form fructose-1,6-bisphosphate (see glycolysis steps 8, 7, 6, 5 and 4). All these reactions are freely reversible.

### *Fructose 1,6-bisphosphatase*

Fructose 1,6-bisphosphate is then acted upon by fructose 1,6-bisphosphatase to form fructose -6-phosphate. This will bypass the step of PFK reaction (see step 3 of glycolysis).

Fructose 1,6-bisphosphatase

Fructose-1,6- $\longrightarrow$ Fructose-6-bisphosphate phosphate + Pi

Then fructose-6-phosphate is isomerized to glucose-6-phosphate by the freely reversible reaction catalyzed by hexose phosphate isomerase (second step in glycolysis).

### *Glucose-6-phosphatase Reaction*

The glucose 6-phosphate is hydrolyzed to free glucose by glucose-6-phosphatase.

Glucose-6-phosphate + $H_2O \longrightarrow$ Glucose + Pi

It is *active in liver*. It is present in kidney and intestinal mucosa to a lesser extent, but is *absent in muscle*.

## Significance of Gluconeogenesis

- ***Only liver can replenish blood glucose*** through gluconeogenesis, because glucose-6-phosphatase is present mainly in liver. So liver plays the major role in maintaining the blood glucose level.
- ***During starvation*** gluconeogenesis maintains the blood glucose level. The stored glycogen is depleted within the first 12–18 hours of fasting. On prolonged starvation, the gluconeogenesis is speeded up and protein catabolism provides the substrates, namely glucogenic amino acids.
- ***Energy requirement:*** The reactions catalyzed by pyruvate carboxylase, phosphoenolpyruvate carboxykinase and phosphoglycerate kinase require one ATP each, so 3 ATPs are used by 1 pyruvate residue to produce one-half molecule of glucose or 6 ATPs are required to generate one glucose molecule.
  2 pyruvate $\rightarrow$ 2 oxaloacetate = 2 ATP
  2 oxaloacetate $\rightarrow$ 2 phosphoenolpyruvate (2GTP) = 2 ATP
  2 × 3-phosphoglycerate $\rightarrow$ 2 × 1,3-bisphospho, glycerate = 2 ATP
  Total = 6 ATP.

## Substrates for Gluconeogenesis

Lactate and glucogenic amino acids are the most important substrates for gluconeogenesis.

### *Lactate*

The lactate formed in the muscle is transported to the liver. In the liver cell lactate dehydrogenase converts lactate to pyruvate. The pyruvate enters the gluconeogenic pathway to form glucose.

### *Glucogenic Amino Acids*

- When glucose is not readily available (starvation or diabetes mellitus), the glucogenic amino acids are transaminated to corresponding carbon skeletons. These then enter the TCA cycle and form oxaloacetate or pyruvate.
- ***Alanine*** released from the muscle is the major substrate for gluconeogenesis. Muscle wastage seen in uncontrolled diabetes mellitus could be explained by this factor.

#### *Glucose-Alanine Cycle (Cahill Cycle)*

- Alanine is transported to liver, transaminated to pyruvate and converted to glucose. This glucose may again enter the glycolytic pathway to form pyruvate, which in turn, can be transaminated to alanine.
- Glucose-alanine cycle is important in conditions of starvation. Thus net transfer of amino acid (nitrogen) from muscle to liver and corresponding transfer of glucose (energy) from liver to muscle is effected.
- Alanine cycle is intimately related with Cori's cycle.

### *Glycerol*

The glycerol part of fat is phosphorylated in the liver cytosol by ATP to glycerol-3-phosphate. It is then oxidized to dihydroxy acetone phosphate by an NAD+ dependent dehydrogenase.

### *Propionyl CoA*

Propionyl CoA is formed from odd chain fatty acids and carbon skeleton of some amino acids. It is converted to succinyl CoA. It is a minor source for glucose.

***Important:*** Even chain fatty acids cannot be converted to glucose they are not substrates for gluconeogenesis.

## Regulation of Gluconeogenesis

Gluconeogenesis and glycolysis are reciprocally regulated so that one pathway is relatively inactive when the other is active. The regulatory steps are:

- ***Pyruvate carboxylase:*** It is an allosteric enzyme. *Acetyl CoA* is an activator of pyruvate carboxylase so that generation of oxaloacetate is favored when acetyl CoA level is sufficiently high.
- ***Fructose 1,6-bisphosphatase:*** Citrate is an activator while fructose 2,6-bisphosphate and AMP are inhibitors. All these three effectors have an exactly opposite effect on the phosphofructokinase (PFK).
- ***ATP:*** Gluconeogenesis is enhanced by ATP.
- ***Hormonal regulation of gluconeogenesis***
  The hormones *glucagon* and *gluco corticoids* increase gluconeogenesis.
  - Glucocorticoids induce the synthesis of hepatic aminotransferases thereby providing substrate for gluconeogenesis.
  - The high glucagon-insulin ratio also favors induction of synthesis of gluconeogenic enzymes (PEPCK, Fructose-1,6-bisphosphatase and glucose-6-phosphatase).
  - At the same time, synthesis of glycolytic enzymes HK, PFK and PK are depressed.
  - Insulin inhibits the process.

## Glycogen Synthesis (Glycogenesis)

The glycogen synthesis occurs by a pathway distinctly different from the reversal of glycogen break down which would prevent the operation of futile cycles. The steps are:

### *Activation of Glucose*

UDP glucose is formed from glucose-1-phosphate and UTP (uridine triphosphate) by the enzyme *UDP glucose pyrophosphorylase*.

UDP-glucosepyrophosphorylase
Glucose-1 $\longrightarrow$ UDP-glucose
Phosphate + UTP + PPi.

### *Glycogen Synthase*

The glucose moiety from UDP-glucose is transferred to a glycogen primer *(glycogenin)* molecule. The primer is essential to accept the glucosyl unit. The primer is made up of a protein-carbohydrate complex. It is a dimeric protein, having two identical monomers. An oligosaccharide chain of 7 glucose units is added to each monomer.

Glycogen synthase
Glycogen primer (n) ⟶ Glycogen (n + 1)
+ UDP-glucose + UDP.

In the next step, activated glucose units are sequentially added by the enzyme glycogen synthase. The glucose unit is added to the non-reducing (outer) end of the glycogen primer to form an alpha-1,4 glycosidic linkage and UDP is liberated.

### *Branching Enzyme*

- The glycogen synthase can add glucose units only in alpha-1,4 linkage. A branching enzyme is needed to create the alpha-1,6 linkages.
- When the chain is lengthened to 11–12 glucose residues, the branching enzyme will transfer a block of 6 to 8 glucose residues from this chain to another site on the growing molecule. The enzyme amylo-[1,4]→[1,6]-transglucosidase *(branching enzyme)* forms this alpha-1,6 linkage.
  To this newly created branch, further glucose units can be added in alpha-1,4 linkage by glycogen synthase.

## Regulation of Glycogen Metabolism

- The synthetic and degradative pathways are reciprocally regulated *to prevent futile cycles.*
- The phosphorylated form of glycogen phosphorylase is active but glycogen synthase becomes inactive on phosphorylation. The covalently modified phosphorylase is active even without AMP. Active (dephosphorylated) glycogen synthase is responsive to the action of glucose-6-phosphate. Covalent modification modulates the effect of allosteric regulators. The hormonal control by covalent modification and allosteric regulation are interrelated.
- These hormones act through a second messenger, cyclic AMP (cAMP).
- The covalent modification of glycogen phosphorylase and synthase is by a cyclic AMP mediated cascade. Specific protein kinases bring about phosphorylation and protein phosphatases cause dephosphorylation.

### *Generation of Cyclic AMP (cAMP)*

- Both liver and muscle phosphorylases are activated by a *cyclic AMP mediated activation cascade* triggered by the hormonal signal.
- The hormones epinephrine and glucagon can activate liver glycogen phosphorylase but glucagon has no effect on the muscle.
- When the hormone binds to a specific receptor on the plasma membrane, the enzyme adenyl cyclase is activated which converts ATP to cyclic AMP (cAMP).
- When level of cyclic AMP rises, it will activate a protein kinase.

#### *Protein Kinase Activation*

The protein kinase is inactive when the catalytic (C) and regulatory (R) subunits are associated with each other.

Earl Sutherland (Nobel Prize, 1971) studied the role of cyclic AMP as the second messenger in glycogenolysis. In 1992, Nobel prizes were awarded to Edwin Krebs and Edmond Fisher for their work on protein kinase, phosphorylase kinase and phosphorylase phosphatase.

The cAMP combines with the R subunit so that the C subunit is free to have its catalytic activity. PKA is an enzyme that can phosphorylate serine and threonine residues of several enzyme proteins and is activated by cAMP which combines with the regulatory subunit of PKA. In the absence of cAMP, PKA is an inactive tetramer.

$$R_2C_2 + 4\ cAMP \rightarrow 2C + R_2\ (cAMP)_2$$

The intracellular concentration of cAMP therefore decides the level of active PKA and cAMP level depends on the activity of adenylate cyclase and phospho diesterase. Cyclic AMP level is increased by glucagon and decreased by insulin.

Adenylate cyclase PDE
ATP ⟶ cAMP ⟶ 5′AMP
+ Glucagon + Insulin.

#### *Phosphorylase Kinase Activation*

The active protein kinase can now convert the phosphorylase kinase to an active phosphorylated form, which converts phosphorylase-b to phosphorylase-a. Phosphorylase kinase itself is a tetrameric enzyme (alpha, beta, gamma, delta). Of these the gamma subunit has the catalytic site and the other 3 subunits have regulatory effects. Phosphorylase kinase is activated by $Ca^{++}$ and phosphorylation of alpha and beta subunits by PKA. Phosphorylation of alpha and beta subunits relieves autoinhibition of catalytic activity of gamma subunit. Binding of $Ca^{++}$ to the delta subunit which is identical to calmodulin (CaM) is also necessary for full activity of delta subunit since it also has a role in dysregulating the gamma subunit. Calcium triggers muscle contraction as well as glycogen breakdown through the action of phosphorylase kinase. The rate of glycogenolysis is linked to rate of muscle contraction.

The dephosphorylation of the active form by PP1 involves removal of phosphate group from phosphorylase a and alpha and beta subunits of phosphorylase kinase. The activity of *protein phosphatase 1* (PP1) is controlled differently in liver and muscle. The catalytic subunit of PP1 in muscle is active only when it is bound to glycogen through the glycogen binding GM subunit. The phosphorylation of PP1 by an insulin stimulated protein kinase (site1) activates the enzyme where as phosphorylation at site 2 by PKA makes its action ineffective.

When cAMP level is high, PP1 is inhibited by inhibitor 1 which is activated by phosphorylation by PKA. The effect of cyclic AMP is not only by increasing the phosphorylation of enzymes but also by decreasing dephosphorylation.

### *Glycogen Phosphorylase in Liver and Muscle*

- *Liver:* The liver phosphorylase-b is the inactive form. It becomes *active on phosphorylation*.
  The active enzyme is denoted as *phosphorylse-a*. The enzyme is inhibited by ATP and glucose-6-phosphate In the liver the PP1 is regulated differently through the intermediary of *glycogen binding subunit* (GL).
  GL complex can bind to R and T forms of phosphorylase a, but the phosphate group attached to ser14 is exposed only in the T state, so that PP1 can convert phosphorylase a to phosphorylase b. Glucose is an allosteric inhibitor of

phosphorylase a. Insulin favors this effect by promoting the uptake and phosphorylation of glucose.

- *Muscle:* Skeletal muscle glycogen is degraded only when the demand for ATP is high. The regulation of glycogenolysis in skeletal muscle is by epinephrine. Glucagon has no effect on muscle glycogenolysis. AMP formed by degradation of ATP during muscle contraction is an allosteric activator of phosphorylase b.

The active form of phosphorylase is referred to as 'a' (active, phosphorylated) and the relatively inactive dephosphorylated form as 'b'. On the other hand, the active glycogen synthase (a) is dephosphorylated and phosphorylated (b) is relatively inactive.

Glycogen phosphorylase is activated by phosphorylation by phosphorylase kinase that adds phosphate group to a specific serine residue of phosphorylase b (ser14). This phosphorylase kinase, in turn, is activated by protein kinase A or cyclic AMP dependent protein kinase. Phosphoprotein phosphatase I dephosphorylates both phosphorylase kinase and phosphorylase b. Phosphorylase b is sensitive to allosteric effectors but phosphorylase a is not sensitive. High concentration of ATP and Glucose-6-phosphate in the cell will inhibit phosphorylase b.

### *Glycogen Synthase*

- Glycogen synthase and phosphorylase activities are *reciprocally regulated.*
- The same protein kinase, which phosphorylates the phosphorylase kinase would also phosphorylate glycogen synthase.
- The activity of the glycogen synthase is markedly decreased on phosphorylation.

Insulin promotes glycogen synthesis by favoring dephosphorylation.

Glycogen synthase is active in the dephosphorylated state. Phosphorylase kinase can phosphorylate glycogen synthase and inactivate the enzyme.

PKA can also inactivate the enzyme by phosphorylation.

$Ca^{++}$ and calcium dependent kinase can also phosphorylate the enzyme.

Relative rates of glycogen synthesis and breakdown are therefore controlled by the action of PKA, phosphorylase kinase and PP1. PP1 can activate glycogen synthase only after dephosphorylating and inactivating phosphorylase a. The regulation of glycogen phosphorylase and synthase is a typical example of multisite phosphorylation (primary and secondary sites) for metabolic regulation.

Control by allosteric effectors is superimposed on covalent modification. Glucose-6-phosphate can activate glycogen synthesis. Insulin activates PP1 and PDE which decreases cAMP level and increases G6P level to promote glycogen synthesis.

The reciprocal regulation of glycogenolysis and glycogenesis is by covalent modification (phosphorylation and dephosphorylation). Insulin and glucagon are the major regulatory hormones, although epinephrine has stimulatory effect on glycogenolysis in both liver and muscle. They bring about alterations in the activity of protein kinases and phosphatases by varying the level of cAMP.

### *Summary of Regulation*

- The key enzyme for glycogenolysis is phosphorylase, which is activated by glucagon and adrenaline, under the stimulus of hypoglycemia.
- The key enzyme for glycogen synthesis is glycogen synthase, the activity of which is decreased by adrenaline but is enhanced by insulin, under the stimulus of hyperglycemia.

Glycogen metabolism is regulated by coordinated regulation of glycogen synthase and glycogen phosphorylase. The regulatory mechanisms include allosteric control, as well as hormonal control by covalent modification of enzymes. The allosteric effectors are ATP, Glucose-6-phosphate and AMP.

### Glycogen Storage Diseases

These are inborn-errors of metabolism. That phrase was coined by Sir Archibald Garrod.

### *Glycogen Storage Disease Type-I*

- It is also called *Von Gierke's Disease.* Most common type of glycogen storage disease is type I.
- Incidence is 1 in 100,000 live births.
- *Glucose-6-phosphatase* is deficient.
- *Fasting hypoglycemia that does not respond into stimulation by adrenaline.* The glucose cannot be released from liver during over night fasting.
- Hyperlipidemia, *lactic acidosis and ketosis.*
- Glucose-6-phosphate is accumulated so it is channeled to HMP shunt pathway producing more ribose and more nucleotides.
- Purines are then catabolized to uric acid, leading to *hyperuricemia.*
- Glycogen gets deposited in liver. Massive liver enlargement may lead to *cirrhosis.*
- Children usually die in early childhood.
- Treatment is to give small quantity of food at frequent intervals.

## CITRIC ACID CYCLE

### Functions of the Citric Acid Cycle

- It is the final common oxidative pathway that oxidizes acetyl CoA to $CO_2$.
- It is the source of reduced coenzymes that provide the substrate for the respiratory chain.
- It acts as a link between catabolic and anabolic pathways (amphibolic role).
- It provides precursors for synthesis of amino acids and nucleotides.
- Components of the cycle have a direct or indirect controlling effect on key enzymes of other pathways.

### Reactions of the Cycle

### *Preparatory Steps*

Acetyl CoA enters the cycle, and is completely oxidized. During this process, energy is trapped.

*Pyruvate* derived from glycolysis is oxidatively decarboxylated to acetyl CoA by *pyruvate dehydrogenase.* This is the link between the TCA cycle and glycolysis. The pyruvate dehydrogenase reaction occurs in the mitochondria. Pyruvate with the help of a carrier can enter the mitochondria from the cytoplasm.

The acetyl CoA derived from beta oxidation is formed in the mitochondria itself. All the enzymes of citric acid cycle are located inside the *mitochondria*.

*1st Step: Formation of Citric Acid*

The 4 carbon, *oxaloacetate* condenses with 2 carbon, *acetyl CoA* to form 6 carbon compound, the citrate (a tricarboxylic acid). The enzyme is *citrate synthase* (step 1). The hydrolysis of the thioester bond in acetyl CoA drives the reaction forward. This is an irreversible step. However, body can reverse this step by another enzyme, ATP-citrate lyase.

*2nd Step: Formation of Isocitrate*

Citrate is isomerized to isocitrate by *aconitase* (Step 2). This reaction is a two-step process. At first, one water molecule is removed from citrate forming *cis aconitate*; a *transient* compound with a very short half-life. Immediately, one water molecule is added to aconitate to form isocitrate. Thus the position of the hydroxyl group is shifted.

*3rd Step: Formation of Alpha Ketoglutarate*

- This reaction is a two-step process, both catalyzed by the same enzyme, *isocitrate dehydrogenase* (Step 3). In the first part of the reaction, isocitrate is dehyrogenated to form *oxalosuccinate*. It is an unstable compound which undergoes spontaneous decarboxylation to form alpha ketoglutarate.
- The *NADH generated* in this step is later oxidized in electron transport chain (ETC) to generate *ATPs*.
- Isocitrate (6 carbons) undergoes *oxidative decarboxylation* to form alpha ketoglutarate (5 carbons). In this reaction, one molecule of $CO_2$ *is liberated*.
- The isocitrate dehydrogenase has isoenzymes; the mitochondrial form utilizes NAD+, while cytoplasmic enzyme is NADP+ dependent.

*4th Step: Formation of Succinyl CoA*

- Next, alpha ketoglutarate is *oxidatively decarboxylated* to form succinyl CoA by the enzyme *alpha ketoglutarate dehydrogenase* (step 4).
- The *NADH* thus generated enters into ETC to generate *ATPs*.
- Another molecule of $CO_2$ *is removed* in this step.
- This is the *irreversible step* in the whole reaction cycle.
- The enzyme alpha keto glutarate dehydrogenase is a *multi-enzyme complex* having 3 enzyme proteins and 5 coenzymes. This is similar to the pyruvate dehydrogenase reaction.

The first two enzyme activities are similar to the corresponding components of pyruvate dehydrogenase complex and the 3rd enzyme is the same in both complexes.

*5th Step: Generation of Succinate*

The next reaction involves a *substrate level phosphorylation* whereby a high energy phosphate is generated from the energy trapped in the thioester bond of succinyl CoA. The enzyme is *succinate thiokinase* (step 5). A molecule of GDP is phosphorylated to *GTP* and succinate is formed. The GTP can be converted to ATP by reacting with an ADP molecule:

GTP + ADP → GDP + ATP

*6th Step: Formation of Fumarate*

Succinate is dehydrogenated to fumarate, an unsaturated dicarboxylic acid, by *succinate dehydrogenase* (step 6). The hydrogen atoms are accepted by FAD. The *$FADH_2$* then enters into ETC to generate *ATPs*. The enzyme is a flavoprotein. The succinate dehydrogenase is competitively inhibited by malonate.

*7th Step: Formation of Malate*

The formation of malate from fumarate is catalyzed by *fumarase* (step 7). The reaction involves the addition of a water molecule. Only L-malate is formed.

*8th Step: Regeneration of Oxaloacetate*

Finally malate is oxidized to oxaloacetate by *malate dehydrogenase* (Step 8). The coenzyme is NAD+. The *NADH* is generated in this step, which enters the electron transport chain, when *ATPs* are produced. The oxaloacetate can further condense with another acetyl CoA molecule and the cycle continues.

### Oxaloacetate as a Junction Point

- Oxaloacetate may be viewed as a **catalyst**, which enters into the reaction, causes complete oxidation of acetyl CoA and comes out of it without any change.
- Oxaloacetate is an important junction point in metabolism.

## Significance

### Complete Oxidation of Acetyl CoA $CO_2$ Removal Steps

During the citric acid cycle, two carbon dioxide molecules are removed in the following reactions:

A. ***Step 3,*** isocitrate (oxalosuccinate) to alpha ketoglutarate.
B. ***Step 4,*** alpha ketoglutarate to succinyl CoA. Acetyl CoA contains 2 carbon atoms. These two carbon atoms are now removed as $CO_2$ in steps 3 and 4. Net result is that *acetyl CoA is completely oxidized during one turn of cycle.*

### ATP Generating Steps in TCA Cycle

There are 3 NADH molecules generated during one cycle, each of them will give rise to 2 ½ ATPs on oxidation by electron transport chain (ETC); so altogether they will give 3 × 2 ½ = 7 ½ (7.5) high energy phosphates. The $FADH_2$ will generate 1½ molecules of ATP. In addition, one molecule of GTP (equivalent to one molecule of ATP) is formed by *substrate level* phosphorylation. Hence, per turn of the cycle, *10 high energy* phosphates are produced.

***Note:*** Recent work shows that in the electron transport chain, NADH produces only 2.5 ATPs and FADH only 1.5 ATPs.

Alpha ketoglutarate dehydrogenase reaction is the only one *irreversible step* in the cycle. The free energy changes of the reactions of the cycle are such that the cycle will operate spontaneously in the clockwise direction.

Only about 33% of energy liberated is trapped as ATP. The rest is used to keep the body temperature at a higher level than the environment.

### Final Common Oxidative Pathway

Citric acid cycle may be considered as the final common oxidative pathway of all foodstuffs. All the major ingredients of foodstuffs are finally oxidized through the TCA cycle. Almost all the biochemical processes use ATP for meeting energy needs—muscle contraction, active transport, biosynthetic reactions, etc. A thermodynamically unfavorable reaction when coupled with hydrolysis of ATP becomes favorable.

### *Integration of Major Metabolic Pathways*

- **Carbohydrates** are metabolized through glycolytic pathway to pyruvate, then converted to acetyl CoA, which enters the citric acid cycle.
- ***Fatty acids*** through beta oxidation, are broken down to acetyl CoA and then enter this cycle.
- ***Glucogenic amino acids*** after transamination enter at some points in this cycle. Ketogenic amino acids are converted into acetyl CoA.
- The integration of metabolism is achieved at junction points by key metabolites. Ketogenic amino acids are converted into acetyl CoA. Several pathways can converge at this point with the result that carbon atoms from one source can be used for synthesis of another.

Important intermediates are *acetyl CoA* and *oxaloacetate*.

### *Fat is Burned on the Wick of Carbohydrates*

The oil in a lamp by itself cannot be lighted; the flame needs a wick. Similarly in the body, oxidation of fat (acetyl CoA) needs the help of oxaloacetate.

One passage of cycle oxidizes acetyl CoA into two $CO_2$ molecules. Here oxaloacetate acts as a true catalyst; it enters the cycle and is regenerated in the end. The major source of oxaloacetate is pyruvate (carbohydrate). Hence carbohydrates are absolutely required for oxidation of fats, or *fats are burned in the fire of carbohydrates*.

### *Excess Carbohydrates are Converted to Neutral Fat*

Excess calories are deposited as fat in adipose tissue. The pathway is glucose to pyruvate to acetyl CoA to fatty acid. However, *fat cannot be converted to glucose* because pyruvate dehydrogenase reaction (pyruvate to acetyl CoA) is an *absolutely irreversible* step.

### *No Net Synthesis of Carbohydrates from Fat*

Acetyl CoA entering in the cycle is completely oxidized to $CO_2$ by the time the cycle reaches succinyl CoA. So, acetyl CoA is completely broken down in the cycle. Thus acetyl CoA cannot be used for gluconeogenesis.

Therefore, there is no net synthesis of carbohydrates from fat.

### *Amino Acids Finally Enter the TCA Cycle*

Some amino acids, such as leucine, catabolized to acetyl CoA; *are not converted to glucose*, because *pyruvate to acetyl CoA reaction is irreversible*. The acetyl CoA molecules either enter the TCA cycle and are completely oxidized, or are channeled to ketone body formation. Hence they are called as *ketogenic amino acids*.

Glucogenic amino acids also get converted to intermediates of TCA cycle.

### *Amphibolic Pathway*

All other pathways such as beta oxidation of fat or glycogen synthesis are either catabolic or anabolic. But TCA cycle is truly amphibolic (*both catabolic and anabolic*) in nature. (Greek, amphi = both). There is a continuous influx (pouring into) and a continuous efflux (removal) of 4-carbon units from the TCA cycle. In a traffic circle, many roads converge and traffic flows toward one direction. Since various compounds enter into or leave from TCA cycle, it is sometimes called as *'metabolic traffic circle'*. Important anabolic reactions related with citric acid cycle are:

- Oxaloacetate is the precursor of aspartate
- Alpha ketoglutarate can be made into glutamate
- Succinyl CoA is used for synthesis of heme
- Mitochondrial citrate is transported to cytoplasm, where it is cleaved into acetyl CoA, which then is the starting point of fatty acid synthesis.

### *Anaplerotic Role of TCA Cycle*

The citric acid cycle acts as a source of precursors of biosynthetic pathways, e.g. heme is synthesized from succinyl CoA and aspartate from oxaloacetate.

To counterbalance such losses, and to keep the concentrations of the 4-carbon units in the cell, anaplerotic reactions are essential. This is called anaplerotic role of TCA cycle (Greek word, ana = up; plerotikos = to fill). Anaplerotic reactions are *'filling up'* reactions or 'influx' reactions or *'replenishing'* reactions which supply 4-carbon units to the TCA cycle. The important anaplerotic reactions are:

- Pyruvate to oxaloacetate by pyruvate carboxylase enzyme. It needs ATP.
- Glutamate is transaminated to alpha keto–glutarate; and aspartate to oxaloacetate.
- Pyruvate can be carboxylated to malate by NADP+ dependent malic enzyme.

### Regulation of the Citric Acid Cycle

- ***Citrate and citrate synthase:*** The formation of citrate from oxaloacetate and acetyl CoA is an important part of control (step 1). *ATP acts as an allosteric inhibitor of citrate synthase.* Citrate allosterically inhibits PFK, the key enzyme of glycolysis; stimulates fructose-1,6-bisphosphatase, a key enzyme of gluconeogenesis and activates acetyl CoA carboxylase, key enzyme of fatty acid synthesis.
- ***Availability and cellular need of ATP:*** When the energy charge of the cell is low, the cycle operates at a faster rate. *The cycle is tightly coupled to the respiratory chain providing ATP.* The Krebs cycle is the largest generator of ATP among metabolic pathways.

  *Anaerobiasis* (hypoxia) will inhibit ETC, when NADH and $FADH_2$ are accumulated, which, in turn, will cause inhibition of TCA cycle.
- ***Isocitrate dehydrogenase:*** Step 3. ADP acts as a positive modifier enhancing the binding of substrate. NADH is an inhibitor.
- ***Alpha ketoglutarate dehydrogenase:*** It is inhibited by succinyl CoA and NADH.

### Inhibitors of TCA Cycle

The above-said mechanisms are physiological and regulatory in nature. But the following are toxic or poisonous (non-physiological) agents which inhibit the reactions.

- ***Aconitase*** (citrate to aconitate) is inhibited by fluoro-acetate. This is non-competitive inhibition.
- ***Alpha ketoglutarate dehydrogenase*** (alpha ketoglutarate to succinyl CoA) is inhibited by Arsenite. This again is non-competitive inhibition.
- ***Succinate dehydrogenase*** (succinate to fumarate) is inhibited by malonate, this is competitive inhibition.

## CHEMISTRY OF LIPIDS

Lipids constitute a heterogeneous group of compounds of biochemical importance. Lipids may be *defined as* compounds which are relatively insoluble in water, but freely soluble in nonpolar organic solvents like benzene, chloroform, ether, hot alcohol, acetone, etc.

### Classification of Lipids

Based on the chemical nature, lipids are classified as:

- *Lipids:* They are esters of fatty acids with glycerol or other higher alcohols
- *Compound lipids:* They are fatty acids esterified with alcohol; but in addition they contain other groups. Depending on these extra groups, they are subclassified
  - Phospholipids, containing phosphoric acid
  - Non-phosphorylated lipids.
- *Derived lipids:* They are compounds which are derived from lipids or precursors of lipids, e.g. fatty acids, steroids
- Lipids complexed to other compounds.

### Fatty Acids

Fatty acids are included in the group of derived lipids. It is the most common component of lipids in the body. They are generally found in ester linkage in different classes of lipids. In the human body, free fatty acids are formed only during metabolism.

Fatty acids are *aliphatic carboxylic acids* and have the general formula, R—CO—OH, where COOH (carboxylic group) represents the functional group. Depending on the R group (the hydrocarbon chain), the physical properties of fatty acids may vary.

### Classification of Lipids

#### *Simple Lipids*

- Triacyl glycerol or Triglycerides or neutral fat
- Waxes

#### *Compound Lipids*

*Phospholipids, Containing Phosphoric Acid*

- ***Nitrogen containing glycerophosphatides:***
  - Lecithin (phosphatidylcholine)
  - Cephalin (phosphatidylethanolamine)
  - Phosphatidyl serine
- ***Non-nitrogen glycerophosphatides:***
  - Phosphatidyl inositol
  - Phosphatidyl glycerol
  - Diphosphatidyl glycerol (cardiolipin)
- ***Plasmalogens, having long chain alcohol:***
  - Choline plasmalogen
  - Ethanolamine plasmalogen
- ***Phospho sphingosides with sphingosine:*** Sphingomyelin.

*Non-phosphorylated Lipids*

- ***Glycosphingolipids (carbohydrate):***
  - Cerebrosides (ceramide monohexosides)
  - Globosides (ceramide oligosaccharides)
  - Gangliosides (ceramide + oligosaccharides + N-acetyl neuraminic acid)
- ***Sulfolipids or sulfatides:***
  - Sulfated cerebrosides
  - Sulfated globosides
  - Sulfated gangliosides.

#### *Derived Lipids*

Fatty acids, steroids, prostaglandins, leukotrienes, terpenes, dolichols, etc.

### *Lipids Complexed to Other Compounds*

Proteolipids and lipoproteins.

*Lung Surfactants*

Normal lung function depends on a constant supply of lung surfactants. It is produced by epithelial cells.

It decreases surface tension of the aqueous layer of lung and prevents collapse of lung alveoli. Constituents of surfactants are *dipalmitoyl lecithin*, phosphatidyl glycerol, cholesterol and surfactant proteins A, B and C. During fetal life, the lung synthesizes sphingomyelin before 28th week of gestation. But as fetus matures, more lecithin is synthesized. The lecithin-sphingomyelin (LS) ratio of amniotic fluid is an index of fetal maturity. A ratio of 2 indicates full lung maturity. Low levels of surfactant leads to respiratory distress syndrome (RDS), which is a common cause of neonatal morbidity.

*Respiratory Distress Syndrome (RDS)*

It is due to a defect in the biosynthesis of dipalmitoyl lecithin (DPL), the main pulmonary surfactant.

Premature infants have a higher incidence of RDS because the immature lungs do not synthesize enough DPL.

### Digestion of Lipids

The major dietary lipids are triacylglycerol, cholesterol and phospholipids. The average normal Indian diet contains about 20–30 g of lipids per day.

Western diet generally contains two or three times more than this quantity.

### *Digestion in Stomach*

The *lingual lipase* from the mouth enters stomach along with the food. It has an optimum pH of 2.5–5.

The enzyme, therefore, continues to be active in the stomach. It acts on short chain triglycerides (SCT). SCTs are present in milk, butter and ghee.

The action of lingual lipase is observed to be more significant in the newborn infants. *Gastric lipase* is acid stable, with an optimum pH around 5.4. It is secreted by chief cells, the secretion is stimulated by gastrin. Upto 30% digestion of triglycerides occurs in stomach.

### Digestion in Intestines

***Emulsification*** is a prerequisite for digestion of lipids. The lipids are dispersed into smaller droplets, surface tension is reduced and surface area of droplets is increased. This process is favored by:

- Bile salts (detergent action)
- Peristalsis (mechanical mixing)
- Phospholipids.

*Bile Salts are Important for Digestion of Lipids*

The bile salts present in the bile (sodium glycocholate and sodium taurocholate) *lower surface tension.* They emulsify the fat droplets. The emulsification increases the surface area of the particles for enhanced activity of enzymes.

*Lipolytic Enzymes in Intestines*

- ***Pancreatic lipase*** with Colipase
- Cholesterol esterase
- Phospholipase A2.

The bile (pH 7.7) entering the duodenum serves to neutralize the acid chyme from the stomach and provides a pH favorable for the action of pancreatic enzymes.

*Digestion of Triglycerides*

- ***Pancreatic lipase*** can easily hydrolyze the fatty acids esterified to the 1st and 3rd carbon atoms of glycerol forming 2-monoacylglycerol and two molecules of fatty acid.
- Then an *isomerase* shifts the ester bond from position 2 to 1. The bond in the 1st position is then hydrolyzed by the *lipase* to form free glycerol and fatty acid.
- The major end products of the digestion of TAG are 2-MAG (78%), 1-MAG (6%), glycerol and fatty acids (14%). Thus digestion of TAG is partial (incomplete).
- ***Cholesterol*** ester may be hydrolyzed to free cholesterol and fatty acid. The action of *phospholipase* A2 produces lysophospholipid and a fatty acid.

*Colipase*

The binding of colipase to the triacyl glycerol molecules at the oil water interface is obligatory for the action of lipase. The colipase is secreted by the pancreas as an inactive zymogen (molecular weight 11,000). It is activated by trypsin.

### Absorption of Lipids

### Absorption of Long Chain Fatty Acids

Long chain fatty acids (chain length more than 14 carbons) are absorbed to the lymph and not directly to the blood. The theory proposed by *Bergstrom* (Nobel Prize, 1982) has the following steps.

*Mixed Micelle Formation*

- The products of digestion, namely 2-monoglycerides, long chain fatty acids, cholesterol, phospholipids and lysophospholipids are incorporated into molecular aggregates to form *mixed micelle.* The micelles are spherical particles with a hydrophilic exterior and hydrophobic interior core. Due to their detergent action, the *bile salts* help to form micellar aggregates.
- Micellar formation is essential for the absorption of fat-soluble vitamins such as vitamin A, D and K.
- The micelles are aligned at the microvillous surface of the *jejunal mucosa.* Fatty acids, 2-MAG and other digested products passively diffuse into the mucosal cell.

*Enterohepatic Circulation of Bile Salts*

The bile salts are left behind which are mostly reabsorbed from the ileum and returned to the liver to be re-excreted (enterohepatic circulation). About 98% of dietary lipids are normally absorbed.

*Re-esterification Inside the Mucosal Cell*

- Once inside the intestinal mucosal cell, the long chain fatty acids are re-esterified to form triglycerides.
- The fatty acids are first activated to fatty acyl CoA by the enzyme, *acyl CoA synthetase* or thiokinase. This needs lysis of two high energy bonds.
- Two such activated fatty acids react with monoacyl glycerol (MAG) to form the triglyceride. Majority of molecules follow this MAG pathway.
- Free *glycerol* absorbed from intestinal lumen directly enters into the bloodstream. So free glycerol is not available for re-esterification. But the cells can convert glucose to glycerol phosphate, and then add 3 molecules of acyl groups to synthesize TAG.

*Chylomicrons*

The TAG, cholesterol ester and phospholipid molecules along with apoproteins B48, and apo-A are incorporated into chylomicrons. The chyle (milky fluid) from the intestinal mucosal cells loaded with chylomicrons are transported through the lacteals into the thoracic duct and then emptied into lymph circulation. The serum may appear milky after a high fat meal (postprandial lipemia) due to the presence of chylomicrons in circulation. Normally the lipemia clears within a few hours by the uptake of chylomicrons by tissues.

*SCFA Absorption is Different*

- *Short chain* fatty acids (SCFA) (seen in milk, butter, ghee) and *medium chain* fatty acids (MCFA) (in coconut oil and mother's milk) do not need re-esterification.
- They can directly enter into blood vessels, then to portal vein, finally to liver where they are immediately utilised for energy.
- Their absorption is rapid. They are better absorbed than long chain fatty acids.

*Abnormalities in Absorption of Lipids*

- ***Defective digestion:*** In steatorrhea, daily excretion of fat in feces is more than 6 g/day. (Greek word, 'stear', means fat). It is due to chronic diseases of pancreas. In such cases, unsplit fat is seen in feces.

- *Defective absorption:* On the other hand, if the absorption alone is defective, most of the fat in feces may be split fat, i.e. fatty acids and monoglycerides. Defective absorption may be due to diseases.
  - *Celiac* disease, sprue, Crohn's disease.
  - *Surgical removal* of intestine.
  - *Obstruction of bile duct:* This may be due to gall stones, tumors of head of pancreas, enlarged lymph glands, etc. The result is deficiency of bile salts. In such cases, triglycerides with short chain and medium chain fatty acids (SCT and MCT) are digested and absorbed properly, because they do not require micellerisation for absorption. Since milk fat and coconut oil are made up of MCT, they are therapeutically useful in malabsorption syndromes.
- *Chyluria:* There is an abnormal connection between the urinary tract and lymphatic drainage system of the intestine. Urine appears milky due to lipid droplets. *Chylothorax* can result from an abnormal connection between the pleural cavity and thoracic duct.

#### Fate of Chylomicrons

- The absorbed (exogenous) triglycerides are transported in blood as *chylomicrons*. They are taken up by adipose tissue and liver.
- Liver synthesizes endogenous triglycerides. These are transported as *VLDL* (very low density lipoproteins) and are deposited in adipose tissue.
- During starvation states, triglycerides in adipose tissue are hydrolyzed to produce *free fatty acids*. In the blood, they are transported, complexed with albumin. These free fatty acids are taken up by the cells, and are then oxidized to get energy.

## Beta Oxidation of Fatty Acids

This process is known as beta oxidation, because the oxidation and splitting of two carbon units occur at the beta-carbon atom. The oxidation of the hydrocarbon chain occurs by a sequential cleavage of two carbon atoms (Fray Knoop, 1904).

## Preparative Steps for Beta Oxidation

The coenzyme A is a complex molecule containing B complex vitamin pantothenic acid and a molecule of beta mercapto ethanolamine; this SH group forms thioester bond in acyl CoA. To emphasize the function of the SH group, the CoA is sometimes written as CoA-SH.

***Preparative Step 1: Activation of Fatty Acids:*** Fatty acids are activated to their coenzyme A (CoA) derivative. This activation is taking place in *cytoplasm*. ATP is hydrolyzed to AMP and PPi and the energy from hydrolysis of PPi drives the reaction forward. Thus *two high energy bonds* are utilized in this reaction.

The enzyme is a *thiokinase* or fatty acyl CoA *synthetase* (step 0).

Three different enzymes, one each for short chain, medium chain and long chain fatty acids have been identified. Small chain fatty acids may also be activated by thiophorase enzyme, using succinyl CoA (see under ketone bodies).

***Preparative Step 2: Role of Carnitine:*** Fatty acids are activated in the cytoplasm; but the *beta oxidation is in mitochondria*. So transport of fatty acids through the mitochondrial membrane is essential. The long chain fatty acyl CoA cannot pass through the inner mitochondrial membrane.

Therefore a transporter, carnitine is involved in transfer of fatty acids. **Carnitine** is beta-hydroxygamma-trimethyl ammonium butyrate, $(CH_3)_3$–$N^+$–$CH_2$–CHOH–$CH_2$–COOH.

It is synthesized from lysine and methionine in liver and kidney.

***Preparative Step 3: Carnitine Acyl Transferase:*** The enzyme carnitine acyl transferase-I (*CAT-I*) will transfer the fatty acyl group to the hydroxyl group of carnitine to form *acyl carnitine*. The reaction occurs on the cytosolic side of inner mitochondrial membrane.

***Preparative Step 4: Translocase:*** A protein *translocase* will carry the acyl carnitine across the membrane to the matrix of mitochondria.

On the matrix side of the membrane another enzyme, carnitine acyl transferase-II (*CAT-II*) will transfer the acyl group back to coenzyme A molecule. Carnitine is returned to the cytosolic side by the translocase.

### Clinical Applications

- Medium chain and short chain fatty acids do not require carnitine for transport across the inner mitochondrial membrane. So medium chain and short chain fatty acids are easily oxidized.
- *Carnitine deficiency* is reported in preterm infants, in whom impaired fatty acid oxidation is noticed. So more glucose is utilized, resulting in episodes of hypoglycemia.
- *Deficiency of translocase:* It leads to defective metabolism of long chain fatty acids. In this condition, muscle cramps are precipitated by fasting, exercise and high fat diet.
- Inherited *CPT-I deficiency* affects only the liver, resulting in reduced fatty acid oxidation and ketogenesis, with hypoglycemia. *CPT-II deficiency* affects primarily skeletal muscle and, when severe, the liver. The sulfonylurea drugs (*glibenclamide* and *tolbutamide*), used in the treatment of type 2 diabetes mellitus, reduce fatty acid oxidation and, therefore, hyperglycemia by inhibiting CPT-I.

## Beta Oxidation Steps

The next 4 reactions are sequentially repeated for complete oxidation of fatty acids. After one round of four metabolic steps, one acetyl CoA unit is split off and acyl CoA with 2 carbon atoms less is generated. This would undergo the same series of reactions again until the fatty acid is completely oxidized.

***Step 1: FAD Linked Dehydrogenase:*** The fatty acyl CoA is dehydrogenated to a trans enoyl CoA with the FAD accepting the hydrogen atoms (step 1). *$FADH_2$* when oxidized in electron transport chain will produce *1.5 ATP* molecules.

***Step 2: Hydration:*** This is catalyzed by an enoyl CoA hydratase (step 2). This step forms a beta-hydroxy fatty acyl CoA. The L isomer alone is formed during the hydration of the trans double bond.

***Step 3: NAD+ Dependent Dehydrogenase:*** The beta-hydroxy fatty acyl CoA is again oxidized to form beta-keto fatty acyl CoA (step 3).

This dehydrogenase acts only on L isomer. The *NADH* when oxidized in electron transport chain will generate *2.5 ATPs*.

*Step 4: Cleavage:* The beta-keto fatty acyl CoA now undergoes thiolytic cleavage, splitting off a molecule of acetyl CoA and leaving behind a fatty acid with 2 carbon atoms less (step 4).

### Further Cycles

The newly formed fatty acyl CoA will sequentially undergo further cycles of steps 1, 2, 3 and 4 of beta-oxidation until the fatty acid is completely converted to acetyl CoA.

### Energetics of Beta Oxidation (ATP Yield)

*Palmitic acid* (16 C) needs 7 cycles of beta oxidation. So, it gives rise to 8 molecules of acetyl CoA. Every molecule of acetyl CoA when oxidized in the TCA cycle gives 10 molecules of ATP. Each molecule of $FADH_2$ produces 1.5 molecules of ATP and each NADH generates 2.5 molecules of ATP, when oxidised in the electron transport chain. Hence the energy yield from one molecule of palmitate may be calculated as:

8 acetyl CoA × 10 = 80 ATP
7 $FADH_2$ × 1.5 = 10.5 ATP
7 NADH × 2.5 = 17.5 ATP
Gross total = 108 ATP
**Net yield = 108 – 2 = 106 ATP.**

In the initial activation reaction, the equivalents of 2 high energy bonds are utilised. The efficiency of beta oxidation is about 33%.

*Important Note:* In the previous editions of this textbook, calculations were made assuming that NADH produces 3 ATPs and FADH generates 2 ATPs. This will amount to a net generation of 129 ATP per palmitate molecule. Recent experiments show that these old values are overestimates, and net generation is only 106 ATPs.

### Regulation of Beta Oxidation

- The availability of free fatty acid (FFA) regulates the net utilization through beta oxidation.
- The level of FFA, in turn, is controlled by glucagon : insulin ratio. Glucagon increases FFA level and insulin has the opposite effect.
- CAT-I is the regulator of entry of fatty acid into mitochondria. Malonyl CoA inhibits CAT-I activity. Thus during *de novo* synthesis of fatty acid, the beta oxidation is inhibited.

### Defects in Beta Oxidation

Abnormalities in transport of fatty acids into mitochondria and defects in oxidation can lead to deficient energy production by oxidation of long chain fatty acids. Common features are hypoketotic hypoglycemia, hyperammonemia, skeletal muscle weakness and liver diseases.

*Acyl carnitine* accumulates when the transferase or translocase is deficient. Dietary supplementation of carnitine has been found to improve the symptoms in some cases.

## Fatty Liver and Lipotropic Factors

Fatty liver refers to the deposition of excess triglycerides in the liver cells. The balance between the factors causing fat deposition in liver versus factors causing removal of fat from liver determines the outcome.

### Causes of Fatty Liver

*Causes of Fat Deposition in Liver*

1. Mobilization of NEFA from adipose tissue.
2. Excess synthesis of fatty acid from glucose.

*Reduced Removal of Fat from Liver*

1. Toxic injury to liver. Secretion of VLDL needs synthesis of apo B-100 and apo C.
2. Decreased oxidation of fat by hepatic cells.

An increase in factors (1) and (2) or a decrease in factors (3) and (4) will cause excessive accumulation, leading to fatty liver.

- *Excessive mobilization of fat:* The capacity of liver to take up the fatty acids from blood far exceeds its capacity for excretion as VLDL. So fatty liver can occur in *diabetes mellitus and starvation* due to increased lipolysis in adipose tissue.
- *Excess calorie intake:* Excess calories, either in the form of carbohydrates or as fats, are deposited as fat. Hence *obesity* may be accompanied by fatty liver.
- *Toxic injury to liver:*
  - In toxic injury to the liver due to **poisoning** by compounds like carbon tetrachloride, arsenic, lead, etc. the capacity to synthesize VLDL is affected leading to fatty infiltration of liver.
  - In *protein calorie malnutrition,* amino acids required to synthesize apoproteins may be lacking. Occurrence of fatty liver in protein energy *malnutrition* (PEM) may be due to defective apoprotein synthesis.
  - ***Hepatitis B virus*** infection reduces the function of hepatic cells.
- *Alcoholism*
  - It is the most common cause of fatty liver and cirrhosis in India.
  - Alcohol is oxidized to acetaldehyde. This reaction produces increased quantities of NADH, which converts oxalo-acetate to malate. As the availability of oxalo-acetate is reduced, the oxidation of acetyl CoA through citric acid cycle is reduced.
  - So fatty acid accumulates leading to TAG deposits in liver.
- *Nonalcoholic Fatty Liver Disease (NAFLD) and Nonalcoholic Steatohepatitis (NASH):* NAFLD is the most common liver disease, where fat is accumulated in hepatocytes. High fat diet and uncontrolled diabetes mellitus are the most common causes. As the disease progresses, inflammatory reaction occurs, which is then termed as NASH.
- *Fatty liver progresses to cirrhosis*
  - Fat molecules infiltrate the cytoplasm of the cell (*fatty infiltration*). These are seen as fat droplets, which are merged together so that most of the cytoplasm becomes laden with fat.
  - The nucleus is pushed to a side of the cell, nucleus disintegrates (*karyorrhexis*), and ultimately the hepatic cell is lysed.

- As a healing process, fibrous tissue is laid down, causing *fibrosis* of liver, otherwise known as *cirrhosis*. *Liver function tests* show abnormal values when chronic liver damage occurs.

### Lipotropic Factors

They are *required for the normal mobilization* of fat from liver. Therefore, deficiency of these factors may result in fatty liver. They can afford protection against the development of fatty liver.

- ***Choline:*** Feeding of choline has been able to reverse fatty changes in animals.
- ***Lecithin and methionine:*** They help in synthesis of apoprotein and choline formation. The deficiency of methyl groups for carnitine synthesis may also hinder fatty acid oxidation.
- ***Vitamin E and selenium*** give protection due to their anti-oxidant effect.
- ***Omega 3 fatty acids*** present in marine oils have a protective effect against fatty liver.

## METABOLISM OF KETONE BODIES

Carbohydrates are essential for the metabolism of fat or *fat is burned under the fire of carbohydrates.*

The acetyl CoA formed from fatty acids can enter and get oxidized in TCA cycle only when carbohydrates are available.

During *starvation and diabetes mellitus,* the acetyl CoA takes the alternate fate of formation of ketone bodies.

### A. Ketogenesis

Acetoacetate is the *primary ketone body* while beta-hydroxy butyrate and acetone are *secondary ketone* bodies. They are synthesized exclusively by the *liver mitochondria.*

***Step 1. Condensation:*** Two molecules of acetyl CoA are condensed to form acetoacetyl CoA.

***Step 2. Production of HMG CoA:*** One more acetyl CoA is added to acetoacetyl CoA to form HMG CoA (beta hydroxy beta methyl glutaryl CoA). The enzyme is HMG CoA synthase.

***Mitochondrial HMG CoA is used for ketogenesis,*** while cytosolic fraction is used for cholesterol synthesis.

***Step 3. Lysis:*** Then HMG CoA is lysed to form acetoacetate.

Acetoacetate may also be formed by the degradation of carbon skeleton of ketogenic amino acids like leucine, lysine, phenylalanine and tyrosine. HMG CoA lyase is present *only in liver.*

***Step 4. Reduction:*** Beta-hydroxy butyrate is formed by reduction of acetoacetate. Ratio between acetoacetate and beta hydroxy butyrate is decided by the cellular NAD : NADH ratio.

***Step 5. Spontaneous decarboxylation:*** Acetone is formed.

### Ketolysis

The ketone bodies are formed in the liver; but they are utilized by *extrahepatic tissues.* The heart muscle and renal cortex prefer the ketone bodies to glucose as fuel. Tissues like skeletal muscle and brain can also utilize the ketone bodies as alternate sources of energy, if glucose is not available.

Acetoacetate is activated to acetoacetyl CoA by *thiophorase* enzyme. Then acetoacetyl CoA enters the beta oxidation pathway to produce energy.

## KETOSIS

- Normally the rate of synthesis of ketone bodies by the liver is such that they can be easily metabolized by the extrahepatic tissues. Hence the blood level of ketone bodies is less than 1 mg/dl and only traces are excreted in urine (not detectable by usual tests).
- But when the rate of synthesis exceeds the ability of extrahepatic tissues to utilize them, there will be accumulation of ketone bodies in blood.
- This leads to *ketonemia,* excretion in urine (*ketonuria*) and smell of *acetone* in breath. All these three together constitute the condition known as *ketosis.*

### Causes for Ketosis

- ***Diabetes Mellitus:*** Uncontrolled diabetes mellitus is the most common cause for ketosis.
  Even though glucose is in plenty, the *deficiency of insulin* causes accelerated lipolysis and more fatty acids are released into circulation. Oxidation of these fatty acids increases the acetyl CoA pool. Enhanced gluconeogenesis restricts the oxidation of acetyl CoA by TCA cycle, since availability of oxaloacetate is less.
- ***Starvation:*** In starvation, the dietary supply of glucose is decreased. Available oxaloacetate is channeled to gluconeogenesis. The increased rate of lipolysis is to provide alternate source of fuel. The excess acetyl CoA is converted to ketone bodies. The high *glucagon* level favors ketogenesis. The brain derives 60–75% of energy from ketone bodies under conditions of prolonged starvation. *Hyperemesis* (vomiting) in early pregnancy may also lead to starvation like condition and may lead to ketosis.

### Explanation for Ketogenesis

- During starvation and diabetes mellitus, the blood level of *glucagon* is increased. Glucagon inhibits glycolysis, activates gluconeogenesis, activates lipolysis, decreases malonyl CoA level and stimulates ketogenesis.
  High glucagon–insulin ratio is potentially ketogenic.
- ***Insulin*** has the opposite effect; it favors glycolysis, inhibits gluconeogenesis, depresses lipolysis, increases malonyl CoA level and decreases ketogenesis.

The ketone body formation is regulated at the following 3 levels:

***Level 1: Lipolysis:*** Free fatty acids are the precursors of ketone bodies. So factors regulating the mobilization of fatty acid from adipose tissue will also control ketogenesis. Insulin inhibits lipolysis, while glucagon favors lipolysis.

***Level 2: Entry of Fatty Acid to Mitochondria:*** The mobilized fatty acid then enters mitochondria for beta oxidation. Carnitine acyl transferase I (CATI) regulates this entry. Malonyl CoA is the major regulator of CAT-I activity. In diabetes and starvation, glucagon is increased, which decreases malonyl CoA and so beta oxidation is stimulated.

*Level 3: Oxidation of Acetyl CoA*

- When the above two steps are increased, more acetyl CoA is produced. Normally, acetyl CoA is completely oxidised in the citric acid cycle. In diabetes and starvation, glucagon insulin ratio is increased, and key gluconeogenic enzymes are activated.
- When *oxaloacetate is diverted for gluconeogenesis*; citric acid cycle cannot function optimally. Thus, on the one hand, acetyl CoA is generated in excess, on the other hand, its utilization is reduced. This excess acetyl CoA is channeled into ketogenic pathway.
- In both diabetes mellitus and starvation, the oxaloacetate is channeled to gluconeogenesis; so the availability of oxaloacetate is decreased. Hence acetyl CoA cannot be fully oxidized in the TCA cycle.

### Salient Features of Ketosis

- *Metabolic acidosis:* Acetoacetate and betahydroxy butyrate are acids, when they accumulate, metabolic acidosis results.
- *Reduced buffers:* The plasma bicarbonate is used up for buffering of these acids.
- *Kussmaul's respiration:* Patients will have typical acidotic breathing due to compensatory hyperventilation.
- *Smell of acetone* in patient's breath.
- *Osmotic diuresis* induced by ketonuria may lead to dehydration.
- *Sodium loss:* The ketone bodies are excreted in urine as their sodium salt, leading to loss of cations from the body.
- *Dehydration:* The sodium loss further aggravates the dehydration.
- *Coma:* Dehydration and acidosis contribute to the lethal effect of ketosis.

### Diagnosis of Ketosis

The presence of ketosis can be established by the detection of ketone bodies in urine by *Rothera's test.* Supportive evidence may be derived from estimation of serum electrolytes, acid-base parameters, glucose and urea estimation.

## ENZYMOLOGY: GENERAL CONCEPTS AND ENZYME KINETICS

### Enzymes are Biocatalysts

Life is possible due to the coordination of numerous metabolic reactions inside the cells. Proteins can be hydrolyzed with hydrochloric acid by boiling for a very long time; but inside the body, with the help of enzymes, proteolysis takes place within a short time at body temperature. Enzyme catalysis is very rapid; usually 1 molecule of an enzyme can act upon about 1000 molecules of the substrate per minute. Lack of enzymes will lead to block in metabolic pathways causing *inborn errors of metabolism*.

The substance upon which an enzyme acts, is called the *substrate.* The enzyme will convert the substrate into the *product* or products.

### Characteristics of Enzymes

- Almost all enzymes are proteins. Enzymes follow the physical and chemical reactions of proteins.
- They are heat labile.
- They are water-soluble.
- They can be precipitated by protein precipitating reagents (ammonium sulfate or trichloroacetic acid).
- They contain 16% weight as nitrogen.

### Classification of Enzymes

When early workers isolated certain enzymes, whimsical names were given. Some of these, such as Pepsin, Trypsin, Chymotrypsin, etc. are still used.

Later, it was agreed to call the enzymes by adding the suffix *'-ase'* to the substrate. Thus, enzyme *Lactase* acts on the substrate lactose, and the products glucose and galactose are formed.

Enzymes that hydrolyze starch (amylose) are termed as amylases, those that dehydrogenate the substrates are called dehydrogenases. These are known as the *trivial names* of the enzymes.

#### *IUBMB System of Classification*

International Union of Biochemistry and Molecular Biology (IUBMB) in 1964, (modified in 1972 and 1978), suggested the IUBMB system of nomenclature of enzymes. It is complex and cumbersome; but unambiguous. As per this system, the name starts with EC (enzyme class) followed by 4 digits.

***First*** digit represents the class

***Second*** digit stands for the subclass

***Third*** digit is the sub-subclass or subgroup

***Fourth*** digit gives the number of the particular enzyme in the list.

The enzymes are grouped into following *six major classes.*

*Class 1: Oxidoreductases*

This group of enzymes will catalyze oxidation of one substrate with simultaneous reduction of another substrate or coenzyme. This may be represented as

$AH_2 + B \longrightarrow A + BH_2$

For example, Alcohol + $NAD^+ \longrightarrow$ Aldehyde + NADH + $H^+$

The enzyme is *Alcohol dehydrogenase*: IUB name is Alcohol-NAD-oxidoreductase; Code number is EC.1.1.1.1. Oxidoreductases may also oxidize substrates by adding oxygen, e.g. oxidases, oxygenases and dehydrogenases.

*Class 2: Transferases*

This class of enzymes *transfers one group* (other than hydrogen) from the substrate to another substrate. This may be represented as

$A - R + B \rightarrow A + B - R$, e.g.

Hexose + ATP $\rightarrow$ Hexose-6-phosphate + ADP

The name of enzyme is *Hexokinase* and systematic name is ATP-Hexose-6-phosphatetransferase.

*Class 3: Hydrolases*

This class of enzymes can hydrolyze ester, ether, peptide or glycosidic bonds by adding water and then breaking the bond.

Acetyl choline + $H_2O \longrightarrow$ Choline + acetate

The enzyme is *Acetyl choline esterase* or Acetyl choline hydrolase (systematic). All digestive enzymes are hydrolases.

*Class 4: Lyases*

These enzymes can remove groups from substrates or break bonds by mechanisms other than hydrolysis. For example,

Fructose-1,6-bisphosphate $\longrightarrow$
Glyceraldehyde-3-phosphate
+ dihydroxy acetone phosphate
The enzyme is *Aldolase.*

*Class 5: Isomerases*

These enzymes can produce optical, geometric or positional isomers of substrates. Racemases, epimerases, cis-trans isomerases are examples.

Glyceraldehyde-3-phosphate $\longrightarrow$
Di-hydroxy-acetone-phosphate
Enzyme is Triose phosphate isomerase.

*Class 6: Ligases*

These enzymes link two substrates together, usually with the simultaneous hydrolysis of ATP, (Latin, Ligare = to bind). For example, Acetyl CoA + $CO_2$ + ATP $\rightarrow$ Malonyl CoA + ADP + Pi

Enzyme is Acetyl CoA carboxylase.

## Coenzymes

- Enzymes may be simple proteins, or complex enzymes, containing a non-protein part, called the *prosthetic group.* The prosthetic group is called the *coenzyme.* It is heat stable.
- The protein part of the enzyme is then named the *apoenzyme.* It is heat labile.
- These two portions combined together is called the *holoenzyme.*
- Coenzymes may be divided into *two groups:*
  a. Those taking part in reactions catalyzed by *oxidoreductases* by donating or accepting hydrogen atoms or electrons.
  b. Those coenzymes taking part in reactions transferring groups *other than hydrogen.*

### First Group of Coenzymes

In the first group, the change occurring in the substrate is counter-balanced by the coenzymes. Therefore, such coenzymes may be considered as *co-substrates* or secondary substrates.

### Nicotinamide Adenine Dinucleotide ($NAD^+$)

- This is a coenzyme synthesized from Nicotinamide, a member of vitamin B complex. The structure of $NAD^+$ is Nicotinamide-Ribose-P-P-Ribose-Adenine. Warburg (Nobel prize, 1931) elucidated the structure of $NAD^+$.
- The reversible reaction of lactate to pyruvate is catalyzed by the enzyme lactate dehydrogenase, but the actual transfer of hydrogen is taking place on the coenzyme, $NAD^+$.
- In this case, two hydrogen atoms are removed from lactate, out of which one hydrogen and two electrons are accepted by the $NAD^+$ to form NADH, and the remaining $H^+$ is released into the surrounding medium. The hydrogen is accepted by the *nicotinamide* group.

### Second Group of Coenzymes

These coenzymes take part in reactions *transferring groups other than hydrogen.* A particular group or radical is transferred from the substrate to another substrate. Most of them belong to vitamin B complex group.

### Adenosine Triphosphate (ATP)

- ATP is considered to be the *energy currency* in the body. Fiske and Subba Row first isolated ATP in 1926 and Lohmann in 1929 showed the importance of ATP in muscle contraction.
- In the ATP molecule, the second and the third phosphate bonds are '*high energy*' bonds.
- During the oxidation of food stuffs, energy is released, a part of which is stored as *chemical energy* in the form of ATP.
- The endergonic reactions are carried out with the help of energy released from hydrolysis of ATP.

### Metallo-enzymes

- These are enzymes which require certain metal ions for their activity.
- In certain cases, e.g. copper in Tyrosinase, the metal is *tightly bound* with the enzyme.
- In other cases, even without the metal ion, enzyme may be active, but when the metal ion is added, the activity is enhanced. They are called *ion-activated enzymes,* e.g. calcium ions will activate pancreatic lipase.

### Cofactors

The term cofactor is used as a collective term to include coenzymes and metal ions. Coenzyme is an organic cofactor.

## Mode of Action of Enzymes

There are a few theories explaining the *mechanism of action of enzymes*. Perhaps each of them tries to view the fact from different perspectives to explain a particular aspect of the action.

### Lowering of Activation Energy

- Enzymes lower the energy of activation.
- Activation energy is defined as the energy required to convert all molecules of a reacting substance from the ground state to the transition state.
- Substrates are remaining in an *energy trough,* and are to be placed at a higher energy level, whereupon spontaneous degradation can occur. Suppose, we want to make a fire; even if we keep a flame, the wood will not burn initially; we have to add kerosene or paper for initial burning. Similarly, the activation energy is to be initially supplied.
- During enzyme substrate binding, weak interactions between enzyme and substrate are optimized. This weak binding interaction between enzyme and substrate provides the major driving force for the enzymatic catalysis.
- ***Enzymes reduce the magnitude of this activation energy***. This can be compared to making a tunnel in a mountain, so that the barrier could be lowered. For example, activation energy for acid hydrolysis of sucrose is 26,000 cal/mol, while the activation energy is only 9,000 cal/mol when hydrolyzed by sucrase.

### Acid Base Catalysis

Protonated form of histidine is an example of a general acid and its conjugate base, the general base. The action of *ribonuclease* is an example of acid-base catalysis. Histidine residues 12 and 119 at the active site of ribonuclease function as acid and base in catalysis. Histidine 12 acts as an acid and donates a proton to form the basic form. Then the 2′–3′ cyclic phosphate is formed. Histidine 112 accepts a proton from the cyclic phosphate and product is released.

In the enzymes of *aspartyl protease family,* catalysis involves two aspartyl residues, which act as acid base catalysts. Catalysis by pepsin, cathepsin and protease of HIV (human immunodeficiency virus) belong to this group of enzymes.

### Substrate Strain

Binding of substrate to a preformed site on the enzyme can induce strain in the substrate. The energy level of the substrate is raised. A combination of substrate strain and acid base catalysis is seen in the action of lysozyme.

The lysozyme substrate has a repeating hexasaccharide unit. Binding of the substrate to the enzyme generates a strained conformation in the enzyme substrate complex. In the transition state, acid catalyzed hydrolysis of the glycosidic linkage by a glutamic acid residue at the active site generates a carbonium ion on the D residue. This relieves the strain generated in the initial enzyme-substrate complex.

This results in the change from transition state to products. The glycosidic bond between N-acetyl glucosamine and N-acetylmuramic acid on the bacterial cell wall is thus hydrolyzed. This accounts for bactericidal action of lysozyme.

Lysozyme was purified and studied by Howard Florey (Nobel prize, 1945).

### Serine Proteases

They are enzymes with a serine residue at the active site and most of the proteolytic enzymes belong to this group, e.g. trypsin, chymotrypsin, clotting factors.

### Action of Chymotrypsin

It is a combination of covalent and acid base catalysis. The peptide bond is hydrolyzed through acid catalyzed nucleophilic attack, utilizing the serine 195 residue of the enzyme. The enzyme substrate complex is formed by the binding of the aromatic amino acid residue with the hydrophilic pocket on the active site on the enzyme. A covalent acyl enzyme intermediate is formed. Cleavage of the peptide bond occurs. Serine 195, Histidine 57 and Aspartate 102 are the catalytic groups.

### Covalent Catalysis

In covalent catalysis, a nucleophilic (negatively charged) or electrophilic (positively charged) group of the enzyme attacks the substrate. This results in covalent binding of the substrate to the enzyme. Similarly, coenzymes often form covalent bonds with the substrates.

### Entropy Effect

Enzymes enhance reaction rates by decreasing entropy. When correctly positioned and bound on the enzyme surface, the substrates are strained to the transition state. This is referred to as the *proximity effect.* Chemical reactions need physical apposition of two reactants. The occurrence of collision between two substrate molecules is determined by statistical probability. Since substrates usually are present in low concentrations, the collision probability is less and hence the reaction velocity is low. But a complex formation between the enzyme and the two substrate molecules can improve the collision probabilities many fold, causing the rapid rate of reaction.

### Product Substrate Orientation Theory

Enzyme has appropriate three dimensional structure to keep the substrates in a specific orientation, such that the reactive groups come in to physical apposition, leading to speedy reactions. It has been shown that the hydroxyl group of the 6th carbon atom of glucose and the terminal phosphate group of ATP are juxtaposed with the help of hexokinase.

## Factors Influencing Enzyme Activity

The various factors which affect enzyme activity:

- Enzyme concentration
- Substrate concentration
- Product concentration
- Temperature
- Hydrogen ion concentration (pH)
- Presence of activators
- Presence of inhibitors
- Presence of repressor or derepressor
- Covalent modification.

*Enzyme Concentration*

- *Rate of a reaction or velocity (V) is directly proportional to the enzyme concentration,* when sufficient substrate is present. Velocity of reaction is increased proportionately with the concentration of enzyme, provided substrate concentration is unlimited.
- Hence, this property is made use of in determining the level of particular enzyme in plasma, serum or tissues.
- Known volume of serum is incubated with substrate for a fixed time, then reaction is stopped and product is quantitated (*end point method*). Since the product formed will be proportional to the enzyme concentration, the latter could be assayed.

*Effect of Substrate Concentration*

In a series of test tubes, equal volume of enzyme solution is taken, but increasing quantity of substrate is added and the rate of reaction is assayed in each tube. The velocity (v) is expressed in micromoles of substrate converted per minute.

If the velocity is plotted against the substrate concentration, a typical curve will be obtained. *As substrate concentration is increased, the velocity is also correspondingly increased in the initial phases; but the curve flattens afterwards.* At lower concentrations of substrate (point A in the curve), some enzyme molecules are remaining idle. As substrate is increased, more and more enzyme molecules are working. At half-maximal velocity, 50% enzymes are attached with substrate (point B in the curve). As more substrate is added, all enzyme molecules are saturated (point C). Further increase in substrate cannot make any effect in the reaction velocity (point D). *The maximum velocity obtained is called Vmax*. It represents the maximum reaction rate attainable in presence of excess substrate (at *substrate saturation level*).

### Effect of Concentration of Products

In a reversible reaction, $S \rightarrow P$, when equilibrium is reached, as per the law of mass action, the reaction rate is slowed down. So, when product concentration is increased, the reaction is slowed, stopped or even reversed. In inborn errors of metabolism, one enzyme of a metabolic pathway is blocked. For example,

E1 E2 E3

A ⟶ B ⟶ C ——||⟶ D

If E3 enzyme is absent, C will accumulate, which in turn, will inhibit E2. Consequently, in course of time, the whole pathway is blocked.

### Effect of Temperature

The velocity of enzyme reaction increases when temperature of the medium is increased; reaches a maximum and then falls (*Bell shaped curve*).

The temperature at which maximum amount of the substrate is converted to the product per unit time is called the *optimum temperature*. As temperature is increased, more molecules get activation energy, or molecules are at increased rate of motion. So their collision probabilities are increased and so the reaction velocity is enhanced.

The *temperature coefficient* (Q10) is the factor by which the rate of catalysis is increased by a rise in 10°C. Generally, the rate of reaction of most enzymes will double by a rise in 10°C.

But when temperature is more than 50°C, heat denaturation and consequent loss of tertiary structure of protein occurs. So activity of the enzyme is decreased. Most human enzymes have the optimum temperature around 37°C. Certain bacteria living in hot springs will have enzymes with optimum temperature near 100°C.

### Effect of pH

Each enzyme has an optimum pH, on both sides of which the velocity will be drastically reduced. The graph will show a *bell shaped curve*.

The pH decides the charge on the amino acid residues at the active site. The net charge on the enzyme protein would influence substrate binding and catalytic activity. *Optimum pH* may vary depending on the temperature, concentration of substrate, presence of ions, etc. Usually enzymes have the optimum pH between 6 and 8. Some important exceptions are *pepsin* (with optimum pH 1–2), *alkaline phosphatase* (optimum pH 9–10) and acid phosphatase (4–5).

### Enzyme Activation

- In presence of certain *inorganic ions*, some enzymes show higher activity. Thus chloride ions activate salivary amylase and calcium activate lipases.
- Another type of activation is the conversion of an inactive *pro-enzyme* or *zymogen* to the active enzyme.
  - By splitting a single peptide bond, and removal of a small polypeptide from *trypsinogen*, the active trypsin is formed. This results in unmasking of the active center.
  - Similarly Trypsin activates chymotrypsinogen, to form active chymotrypsin and two peptides (A and B peptides). As a result, three aminoacid residues, his (57), asp (102) and ser (195) that are far apart in the primary sequence are aligned at the active site and take part in the catalytic process.
  - All the gastrointestinal enzymes are synthesized in the form of pro-enzymes, and only after secretion into the alimentary canal, they are activated. This prevents autolysis of cellular structural proteins.
  - ***Coagulation factors*** are seen in blood as zymogen form, their activation pathways.
  - Similar activation of precursor protein is taking place in the case of *complement components*. These activities are needed only occasionally; but when needed, a large number of molecules are to be produced instantaneously. Hence, the cascade system of *chemical amplification* of such factors.

### Enzyme Inhibition

- ***Competitive inhibition:***
  - Here *inhibitor molecules are competing with the normal substrate* molecules for binding to the active site of the enzyme, because the inhibitor is a structural analog of the substrate.

    E + S → E-S ⟶ E + P

    E + I → E-I
  - Since E-I (enzyme–inhibitor complex) can react only to reform the enzyme and inhibitor, the number of enzyme molecules available for E-S formation is reduced. Suppose 100 molecules of substrate and 100 molecules of inhibitor are competing for 100 molecules of the enzyme. So, half of enzyme molecules are trapped by the inhibitor and only half the molecules are available for catalysis to form the product.
  - Since effective concentration of enzyme is reduced, the reaction *velocity is decreased*.
  - In competitive inhibition, the inhibitor will be a *structural analog* of the substrate. There will be similarity in three dimensional structure between substrate (S) and inhibitor (I). For example, the succinate dehydrogenase reaction is inhibited by malonate.
  - ***Competitive inhibition is usually reversible or excess substrate abolishes the inhibition.***

    In the previous example of 100 moles of E and 100 moles of I, if 900 moles of S are added, only 1/10th of enzyme molecules are attached to inhibitor and 90% are working with substrate.

    Thus 50% inhibition in the first example is now decreased to 10% inhibition.
  - It is obvious that in the case of competitive inhibition, *the Km is increased in presence of competitive inhibitor*. Thus competitive inhibitor apparently increases the Km. In other words, the affinity of the enzyme toward substrate is apparently decreased in presence of the inhibitor.
- ***Non-competitive Inhibition (Irreversible)***
  - A variety of *poisons*, such as iodoacetate, heavy metal ions (lead, mercury) and oxidising agents act as irreversible non-competitive inhibitors. There is no competition between substrate and inhibitor.

- The inhibitor usually binds to a different domain on the enzyme, other than the substrate binding site. Since these inhibitors have no structural resemblance to the substrate, an *increase in the substrate concentration generally does not relieve this inhibition.*
  Examples are:
  ***Cyanide*** inhibits cytochrome oxidase.
  ***Fluoride*** will remove magnesium and manganese ions and so will inhibit the enzyme, enolase, and consequently the glycolysis.
  ***Iodoacetate*** would inhibit enzymes having-SH group in their active centers.
  *BAL* (British Anti Lewisite; dimercaprol) is used as an antidote for heavy metal poisoning. The heavy metals act as enzyme poisons by reacting with the SH group. BAL has several SH groups with which the heavy metal ions can react and thereby their poisonous effects are reduced.
- The inhibitor combines with the enzymes by forming a covalent bond and then the reaction becomes irreversible. The velocity (Vmax) is reduced. But *Km value is not changed,* because the remaining enzyme molecules have the same affinity for the substrate.
- ***Increasing the substrate concentration*** will abolish the competitive inhibition, but *will not abolish non-competitive inhibition.*

## Specificity of Enzymes

### Absolute Specificity

Some enzymes are absolutely specific. For example, hydrolysis of urea to ammonia and carbon dioxide is catalyzed by urease. Urea is the only substrate for *urease.* Thiourea, though structurally similar to urea, will not act as the substrate for urease. Similarly glucose oxidase will oxidise only beta-D-glucose and no other isomeric form. Thus, these enzymes show absolute specificity.

### Bond Specificity

Most of the proteolytic enzymes are showing group (bond) specificity. For example, trypsin can hydrolyze peptide bonds formed by carboxyl groups of arginine or lysine residues in any proteins.

### Group Specificity

One enzyme can catalyze the same reaction on a group of structurally similar compounds, e.g. hexokinase can catalyze phosphorylation of glucose, galactose and mannose.

### Stereospecificity

Human enzymes are specific for L-amino acids and D-carbohydrates. Fumarase will hydrate fumaricacid (trans form) to malic acid, but the corresponding cis form, maleic acid will not be acted upon. Lactate dehydro genase, acting on pyruvate will form only L-lactate, but not the D variety.

## FAT SOLUBLE VITAMINS (A, D, E, AND K)

Vitamins may be defined as organic compounds occurring in small quantities in different natural foods and necessary for growth and maintenance of good health in human beings and in experimental animals. Vitamins are essential food factors, which are required for the proper utilization of the proximate principles of food like carbohydrates, lipids and proteins.

Discovery of vitamins started from observation of deficiency manifestations, e.g. scurvy, rickets, beriberi, etc.

The vitamin theory was suggested by Hopkins in 1912 (Nobel Prize, 1929). The term 'vitamine' was coined from the words vital + amine, since the earlier identified ones had amino groups. Later work showed that most of them did not contain amino groups, so the last letter 'e' was dropped in the modern term of vitamin.

Although vitamins are important nutritionally, their role has been over-emphasized in clinical practice. They are useful to correct deficiencies. But taking higher doses of vitamins will not boost up the health. All the vitamins are usually available in an ordinary Indian diet.

The vitamins are mainly classified into two types:

1. The fat soluble vitamins are A, D, E and K.
2. Water soluble vitamins are named as B complex and C.

In general, deficiency of vitamins may occur due to:

- Reduced intake
- Impaired absorption
- Impaired metabolism
- Additional requirements
- Increased losses.

### Vitamin A

McCollum, Simmonds and Kennedy isolated vitamin A in 1913. Richard Kuhn (Nobel prize, 1938) identified carotenes. Paul Karrer in 1931 elucidated the structure of vitamin A1 (Nobel prize, 1937).

### Chemistry

- Vitamin A is fat soluble. The active form is present only in animal tissues.
- The *pro-vitamin,* beta-carotene is present in plant tissues. *Beta carotene* has two beta ionone rings connected by a polyprenoid chain. One molecule of beta carotene can theoretically give rise to two molecules of vitamin A, but it may produce only one in biological systems.
- All the compounds with vitamin A activity are referred to as *retinoids.* They are polyisoprenoid compounds having a *beta-ionone* ring system.
- Three different compounds with vitamin A activity are *retinol* (vitamin A alcohol), *retinal* (vitamin A aldehyde) and *retinoic acid* (vitamin A acid).
- The retinal may be reduced to retinol by retinal reductase. This reaction is readily reversible. Retinal is oxidized to retinoic acid, which cannot be converted back to the other forms.
- The side chain contains alternate double bonds, and hence many isomers are possible.

The *all-trans* variety of retinal, also called *vitamin A1* is most common.

Vitamin A2 is found in *fish oils* and has an extra double bond in the ring. Biologically important compound is *11-cis-retinal.*

### *Absorption of Vitamin A*

- Beta carotene is cleaved by a di-oxygenase, to form retinal. The retinal is reduced to retinol by an NADH or NADPH dependent retinal reductase present in the intestinal mucosa. Intestine is the major site of absorption.
- The absorption is along with other fats and requires bile salts. In biliary tract obstruction and steatorrhea, vitamin A absorption is reduced.
- Within the mucosal cell, the retinol is reesterified with fatty acids, incorporated into chylomicrons and transported to liver. In the liver stellate cells, vitamin is stored as *retinol palmitate.*

### *Transport from Liver to Tissues*

The vitamin A from liver is transported to peripheral tissues as trans-retinol by the *retinol binding protein* or RBP. One molecule of RBP binds one molecule of retinol. In the case of vitamin A deficiency, the RBP level in blood falls.

### *Uptake by Tissues*

The retinol-RBP complex binds to specific receptors on the retina, skin, gonads and other tissues. The RBP does not enter in the cell. Inside the cytoplasm of cells, vitamin binds to cellular retinoic acid binding protein (CRBP) and finally to hormone responsive elements (HRE) of DNA. Thus, genes are activated.

## Biochemical Role of Vitamin A

### *Wald's Visual Cycle*

*Generation of Nerve Impulse*

- Wald was awarded Nobel Prize in 1967, for identifying the role of vitamin A in vision. *Rhodopsin* (mol. wt. 35,000 Daltons) plays the pivotal role in vision. It is a membrane protein found in the photoreceptor cells of the retina. Rhodopsin is made up of the protein *opsin and 11-cis-retinal.*
- When light falls on the retina, the 11-cisretinal isomerizes to *all-trans-retinal.* A single photon can excite the rod cell. The photon produces immediate conformational change. The unstable intermediates produced are: Rhodopsin → Bathorhodopsin → Lumirhodopsin → Metarhodopsin-I → Metarhodopsin-II → and finally Opsin + all-trans-retinal. Each of these intermediaries has a lifespan of only few picosecond to microseconds. The all-trans-retinal is then released from the protein.
- Visual pigments are G-protein-coupled receptors and 11-cis-retinal locks the receptor protein (opsin) in its inactive form. The isomerization and photo-excitation leads to activation of G-protein and generation of cyclic-GMP. Cyclic GMP acts as the gate for cation specific channels.
  *Transducin* is the G-protein in retina. The nerve impulse thus generated in the retina is transmitted to visual centers in the brain. The signal is terminated by phosphorylation of a serine residue of activated rhodopsin, by an enzyme rhodopsin kinase, so that the inhibitory protein *beta-arrestin* can bind and inactivate rhodopsin.

*Regeneration of 11-cis-retinal*

- After dissociation, opsin remains in retina; but trans-retinal enters the blood circulation. Later cis-retinal is generated, reaches retina. The re-attachment of 11-cis retinal to opsin is critical for shutting off the pigment's catalytic activity.
- The all-trans-retinal is isomerized to 11-cis retinal in the retina itself in the dark by the enzyme *retinal isomerase.* This reaction is taking place in retinal pigment epithelium. The 11-*cis* retinal can recombine with opsin to regenerate rhodopsin.
- Alternatively, all-trans-retinal is transported to liver and then reduced to all-trans-retinol by *alcohol dehydrogenase* (ADH), an NADH dependent enzyme. ADH contains zinc, and, therefore, *zinc* is important in retinol metabolism.

The all-trans-retinol is isomerized to 11-cis-retinol and then oxidized to 11-cis retinal in liver. This is then transported to retina. This completes the Wald's visual cycle.

### *Dark Adaptation Mechanism*

For his work on dark adaptation, Torsten Wiesel was awarded Nobel prize in 1981.

- Bright light depletes stores of rhodopsin in rods. Therefore, when a person shifts suddenly from bright light to a dimly lit area, there is difficulty in seeing, for example, entering a cinema theater. After a few minutes, rhodopsin is resynthesized and vision is improved. This period is called *dark adaptation time.*
- It is increased in vitamin A deficiency. Red light bleaches rhodopsin to a lesser extent; so doctors use red glasses, during fluoroscopic X-ray examination of the patients.

### *Rods are for Vision in Dim Light*

In the retina, there are two types of photosensitive cells, the rods and the cones. Rods are responsible for perception in dim light. Rhodopsin present in rods is made up of 11-cis-retinal + opsin. Deficiency of cis-retinal will lead to increase in dark adaptation time and night blindness. In humans, one eye contains about 120 million rods, each of which carries 120 million molecules of rhodopsin. The number of rods is more in cats, mice and owls.

### *Cones are for Color Vision*

- Cones are responsible for vision in bright light as well as color vision. They contain the photosensitive protein, *conopsin.*
- There are 3 types of cones, each is characterized by a different conopsin, that is maximally sensitive to either blue (*cyanopsin*), green (*iodopsin*) or red (*porphyropsin*).
- In cone proteins also, 11-cis-retinal is the chromophore. Reduction in number of cones or the cone proteins, will lead to *color blindness.* One eye contains about 6 million cones.

### *Other Biochemical Functions of Vitamin A*

- Retinoic acid has a role in the regulation of gene expression and *differentiation* of tissues. All-trans-retinoic acid and 9-cisretinoic acid act like steroid hormones. They bind to nuclear receptors; retinoic acid along with the receptor binds to the response elements of DNA. Retinoic acid receptors (RAR) bind all-trans-retinoic acid, while retinoic x receptors (RXR) bind to 9-cisretinoic acid. RXRs form dimers with vitamin D-receptor also. This explains why deficiency of vitamin A impairs vitamin D function; when there is lack of 9-cis-retinoic acid to form receptor dimers, vitamin D function is not optimal.

- Retinol is necessary for the reproductive system. Retinol acts like a steroid hormone in controlling the expression of certain genes. This may account for the requirement of vitamin A for normal *reproduction*. In vitamin deficiency, miscarriages are noticed in female rats while atrophy of germinal epithelium and sterility are seen in male rats.
- ***Anti-oxidant property:*** There is a correlation between the occurrence of epithelial cancers and vitamin A deficiency. The anticancer activity has been attributed to the natural antioxidant property of *carotenoids*. Fresh vegetables containing carotenoids were shown to reduce the incidence of cancer.
- Beta carotenes may be useful in preventing *heart attacks*. Those who were given beta carotene supplements suffered half as many heart attacks as in the group taking placebo.
- Vitamin A is necessary for the maintenance of normal *epithelium* and skin.

## Deficiency Manifestations of Vitamin A

### Night Blindness or Nyctalopia

Visual acuity is diminished in dim light. The patient cannot read or drive a car in poor light. The dark adaptation time is increased.

### Xerophthalmia

The conjunctiva becomes dry, thick and wrinkled. The conjunctiva gets keratinized and loses its normal transparency. Dryness spreads to cornea.

It becomes glazy and lusterless due to keratinization of corneal epithelium. Infections may supercede.

### Bitot's Spots

These are seen as greyish-white triangular plaques firmly adherent to the conjunctiva. This is due to increased thickness of conjunctiva in certain areas.

All the ocular changes mentioned so far are completely reversible when vitamin is supplemented.

### Keratomalacia

When the xerophthalmia persists for a long time, it progresses to keratomalacia (softening of the cornea). There is degeneration of corneal epithelium which may get vascularized. Later, corneal opacities develop. Bacterial infection leads to corneal ulceration, perforation of cornea and total blindness.

### Preventable Blindness

The deficiency of vitamin A is the most common cause of blindness in Indian children below the age of 5. One-third of the world's blind population are residing in India. About 40% of blindness is preventable. Vitamin A deficiency is a major public health problem. A single dose of vitamin A is given as a prophylactic measure to children below 1 year age.

### Skin and Mucous Membrane Lesions

- Follicular *hyperkeratosis* or phrynoderma results from hyperkeratinization of the epithelium lining the follicles. The skin becomes rough. Keratinizing metaplasia of the epithelium of the respiratory, gastrointestinal and genitourinary tract have been observed. Epithelium is *atrophied*. Keratinization of urinary tract epithelium may lead to *urinary calculi*.
- The alterations in skin may cause increased occurrence of generalized *infections*. Therefore in old literature, vitamin A is referred to as anti-inflammatory vitamin.
- Isoretinone, a synthetic variant of vitamin A is known to reduce the sebaceous secretions, hence it is used to prevent *acne* formation during adolescence.

## Causes for Vitamin A Deficiency

- Decreased intake.
- Obstructive jaundice causing defective absorption.
- Cirrhosis of liver leading to reduced synthesis of RBP.
- Severe malnutrition where amino acids are not available for RBP synthesis.
- Chronic nephrosis, where RBP is excreted through urine.

### Assessment of Deficiency

- Dark adaptation test—it is the time required to adapt the eye to see objects in dim light. It is increased in vitamin A deficiency.
- RBP (retinol-binding protein) level in serum is decreased.
- Vitamin A in serum is decreased. The colorimetric measurement is based on Carr and Price reaction, where retinoids are made to react with antimony trichloride to give a blue color. Vitamin A may be directly measured by spectrophotometry; it has maximum absorption at 325 nm.
- ***Normal blood level*** of vitamin A is 25 to 50 microgram/dl.

## Daily Requirement of Vitamin A

The recommended daily allowance (RDA) for

- Children = 400–600 microgram/day
- Men = 750–1000 microgram/day
- Women = 750 microgram/day
- Pregnancy = 1000 microgram/day.

One international unit = 0.3 mg of retinol. One retinol equivalent = 1 mg of retinol or 6 mg of beta carotene.

### Dietary Sources of Vitamin A

Animal sources include milk, butter, cream, cheese, egg yolk and liver. Fish liver oils (cod liver oil and shark liver oil) are very rich sources of the vitamin.

Vegetable sources contain the yellow pigment beta carotene. Carrot contains significant quantity of beta carotene. Papaya, mango, pumpkins and green leafy vegetables (spinach, amaranth) are other good sources for vitamin A activity. During cooking, the activity is not destroyed.

### Therapeutic Use of Vitamin A

When deficiency of vitamin A is identified, supplementation is given as capsules or injection. Therapeutic dose is generally

20–50 times higher than the RDA. All-trans-retinoic acid is used as adjuvant in the treatment of *promyelocytic leukemia.*

It causes remission due to its effect on differentiation of cells.

### Hypervitaminosis A or Toxicity

Excessive intake can lead to toxicity since the vitamin is stored. It has been reported in children where parents have been overzealous in supplementing the vitamins. Eskimos refrain from eating the liver of polar bear due to its high vitamin A content. Symptoms of toxicity include anorexia, irritability, headache, peeling of skin, drowsiness and vomiting. Some of these signs are due to increased intracranial tension. Sometimes swelling over long bones (bony exostosis) may occur with painful bones. Enlargement of liver is also seen in children. Higher concentration of retinol increases lysosomal enzymes, leading to cellular death.

Hypercarotenemia can result from persistent excessive consumption of foods rich in carotenoids. The skin becomes yellow, but no staining of sclera as in jaundice is observed.

## Vitamin D (Cholecalciferol)

There are reports of symptoms of rickets from historians as early as 2nd century AD. Francis Glisson wrote a classical account of infantile rickets in 1650. Experimental rickets induced by dietary deficiency was produced in rats by McCollum in 1919. Angus and coworkers isolated vitamin D in 1931 and named it as calciferol, which was later identified as Vitamin $D_3$. The structural elucidation was done independently by Otto Diels and Kurt Alder. Both were awarded Nobel prize in 1950.

### Formation of Vitamin D

Vitamin D is derived either from 7-dehydrocholesterol or ergosterol by the action of ultraviolet radiations. *7-dehydrocholesterol*, an intermediate of a minor pathway of cholesterol synthesis, is available in the Malpighian layer of epidermis. In the skin, ultraviolet light (290–315 nm) breaks the bond between position 9 and 10 of the steroid ring. So, the ring B is opened, to form the provitamin, *secosterol.* The cis double bond between 5th and 6th carbon atoms, is then isomerized to a trans double bond (rotation on the 6th carbon atom) to give rise to vitamin $D_3$ or *cholecalciferol*. So, vitamin D is called the *'sun-shine vitamin'*.

Skin is the largest organ in the body. It makes about 16% of body weight. It is kept nourished by a quarter of the body's blood supply. It is the temperature regulator of the body. The production of vitamin D in the skin is directly proportional to the exposure to sunlight and inversely proportional to the pigmentation of skin. An increase in solar zenith angle during November to March shifts the wavelength of UV rays to longer wavelengths which will not produce the vitamin; hence vitamin deficiency is seen in winter. Excessive exposure to sunlight does not result in vitamin D toxicity since excess previtamin $D_3$ and $D_3$ are destroyed by sunlight itself.

Commercially the vitamin is derived from the fungus, ergot. The ergosterol when treated with ultraviolet light, *ergocalciferol* or vitamin $D_2$ is produced. Ergocalciferol differs in having an unsaturation in the side chain and an extra methyl group (C28).

### Activation of Vitamin D

- Vitamin D is a *prohormone.* The cholecalciferol is first transported to *liver,* where hydroxylation at *25th position* occurs, to form 25-hydroxy cholecalciferol (25-HCC). The hepatic 25-hydroxylase is a microsomal monooxygenase. It requires cytochrome P-450 and NADPH. 25-HCC is the major storage form.
- In plasma, 25-HCC is bound to 'vitamin D binding protein' (VDBP), an alpha-2 globulin.
- In the *kidney,* it is further hydroxylated at the *1st position.* The 1-alpha hydroxylase is located in mitochondria of proximal convoluted tubules. It requires cytochrome P-450, NADPH and ferrodoxin (an iron-sulfur protein).

Thus 1,25-dihydroxy cholecalciferol (*DHCC*) is generated. Since it contains three hydroxyl groups at 1, 3 and 25 positions, it is also called *Calcitriol.* The calcitriol thus formed is the *active form* of vitamin; it is a *hormone.* 24, 25-dihydroxy cholecalciferol may be formed by hydroxylation of 25-HCC at the 24th position.

### Biochemical Effects of Vitamin D

The sites of action are:
- Intestinal villi cells
- Bone osteoblasts
- Kidney distal tubular cells.

#### Vitamin D and Absorption of Calcium

Calcitriol promotes the absorption of calcium and phosphorus from the intestine. In the brush-border surface, calcium is absorbed passively. From the intestinal cell to blood, absorption of calcium needs energy. It is either by the sodium-calcium exchange mechanism or by pumping out the calcium-calbindin complex. *Calcitriol* acts like a steroid hormone. It enters the target cell and binds to a cytoplasmic receptor. The hormone-receptor complex interacts with DNA and causes *derepression* and consequent transcription of specific genes that code for *Calbindin.* Due to the increased availability of calcium binding protein, the absorption of calcium is increased.

#### Effect of Vitamin D in Bone

***Mineralization*** of the bone is increased by increasing the activity of osteoblasts. Calcitriol coordinates the remodelling action of osteoclasts and osteoblasts. It produces the differentiation of osteoclast precursors from multinucleated cells of osteoblast lineage. Calcitriol stimulates osteoblasts which secrete alkaline phosphatase. Due to this enzyme, the local concentration of phosphate is increased. The ionic product of calcium and phosphorus increases, leading to mineralization.

#### Effect of Vitamin D in Renal Tubules

Calcitriol increases the reabsorption of calcium and phosphorus by renal tubules, therefore both minerals are conserved (PTH conserves only calcium).

#### Regulation of Calcitriol

The hormonal level of calcitriol is maintained by the feedback control. The rate of production is modulated by serum levels of calcium, phosphorus, PTH and calcitriol itself. The major site of control is on the 1-alpha-hydroxylase of kidney.

Hypercalcemia decreases calcitriol. Low dietary calcium and hypocalcemia increase the rate of production of 1,25-DHCC.

The stimulatory effect of hypocalcemia on 1-alpha-hydroxylase is through PTH. Hypercalcemia decreases calcitriol. The half-life of 1, 25-DHCC is 6-8 hours and is mainly excreted through the bile. The inactivation is by oxidation of the side chain. Hydroxylation at the 24th position by the kidney also lowers the activity. Vitamin D deficient state (low calcium and phosphate) will enhance the action of 1-alpha hydroxylase. When vitamin D status is adequate, or calcium level is high, 24-hydroxylation is favored, forming 24,25-DHCC, which is less active. 1,25-DHCC level directly regulates PTH secretion.

## Deficiency of Vitamin D

The deficiency diseases are *rickets* in children and *osteomalacia* in adults. Hence vitamin D is known as antirachitic vitamin.

*Causes for Vitamin D Deficiency*

- Deficiency of vitamin D can occur in people who are not exposed to sunlight properly, e.g. inhabitants of northern latitudes, in winter months, in people who are bedridden for long periods, or those who cover the whole body *(purdah)*.
- Nutritional deficiency of calcium or phosphate may also produce similar clinical picture.
- Malabsorption of vitamin (obstructive jaundice and steatorrhea). High phytate content in diet may also reduce the absorption of vitamin.
- Abnormality of vitamin D activation. Liver and renal diseases may retard the hydroxylation reactions.
- Deficient renal absorption of phosphates.

*Clinical Features of Rickets*

- Rickets is seen in children. There is insufficient mineralization of bone. Bones become soft and pliable. The bone growth is markedly affected.
- Plasma calcium and phosphorus are low normal with alkaline phosphatase (bone isoenzyme) being markedly elevated. The classical features of rickets are *bone deformities*. Weight bearing bones are bent. Continued action of muscles also cause bone malformations.
- The clinical manifestations include bow legs, knock-knee, rickety rosary, bossing of frontal bones, and pigeon chest.
- An enlargement of the epiphysis at the lower end of ribs and costochondral junction leads to beading of ribs or *rickety rosary*.
- ***Harrison's sulcus*** is a transverse depression passing outwards from the costal cartilage to axilla. This is due to the indentation of lower ribs at the site of the attachment of diaphragm.

*Clinical Features of Osteomalacia*

- The term is derived from Greek *'osteon'* = bone; and *'malakia'* = softness. The bones are softened due to insufficient mineralization and increased osteoporosis. Patients are more prone to get fractures.
- The abnormalities in *biochemical parameters* are a slightly lower serum calcium, and a low serum phosphate.
- It may be noted that vitamin D deficiency never produces severe hypocalcemia. Tetany will not be manifested.
- Serum *alkaline phosphatase,* bone isoenzyme, is markedly increased.

*Different Types of Rickets*

- The classical vitamin D *deficiency* rickets can be cured by giving vitamin D in the diet.
- The *hypophosphatemic* rickets mainly result from defective renal tubular reabsorption of phosphate. Supplementation of vitamin D along with phosphate is found to be useful.
- ***Vitamin D resistant*** rickets is found to be associated with *Fanconi syndrome,* where the renal tubular reabsorption of bicarbonate, phosphate, glucose and amino acids are also deficient.
- ***Renal rickets:*** In kidney diseases, even if vitamin D is available, calcitriol is not synthesized. These cases will respond to administration of calcitriol.
- ***End organ refractoriness*** to 1,25-DHCC will also lead to rickets. Either a decrease in the number of cytosolic receptor or a structurally abnormal receptor is noticed. The bone disease has been found to respond to megadoses of calcitriol (35 mg/day).

## Other Actions of Vitamin D

Recent research has proved that most tissues possess vitamin D receptor and several tissues have the enzymes to generate calcitriol. 1,25-DHCC has been found to have a modulatory effect on immunohematopoietic system. Therapeutic doses given to children with rickets have been found to correct the anemia, hypocellularity of the bone marrow and increased susceptibility to infection. It has also been found to reduce the risk of cancer and coronary vascular disease. Beneficial effects have been observed in patients with AIDS.

## Requirement of Vitamin D

- Children = 10 microgram (400 IU)/day
- Adults = 5 microgram (200 IU)/day
- Pregnancy, lactation = 10 microgram/day
- Above the age of 60 = 600 IU per day.

*Sources of Vitamin D*

Exposure to **sunlight** produces cholecalciferol. Moreover fish liver oil, fish and egg yolk are good sources of the vitamin. Milk contains moderate quantity of the vitamin.

*Hypervitaminosis D*

Doses above 1500 units per day for very long periods may cause toxicity. Symptoms include weakness, polyuria, intense thirst, difficulty in speaking, hypertension and weight loss. Hypercalcemia leads to calcification of soft tissues, (metastatic *calcification*, otherwise called *calcinosis*), especially in vascular and renal tissues.

Although vitamin D is toxic in higher doses, excessive exposure to sunlight does not result in vitamin D toxicity, because excess $D_3$ is destroyed by sunlight itself.

## Vitamin E

The active vitamin was isolated from wheat germ oil and named tocopherol (*tokos* = child birth, *pheros* = to bear, *ol* =

alcohol). Initial studies of induced vitamin E deficiency in laboratory animals resulted in infertility and therefore the vitamin came to be known as anti-infertility vitamin. Now vitamin E is known as the most potent biological antioxidant.

### Chemical Nature

A chromane ring (tocol) system, with an isoprenoid side chain is present in all the eight naturally occurring tocopherols. Of these, *alpha tocopherol* (5, 7, 8-trimethyl tocol) has greatest biological activity. The structure of vitamin E was elucidated by Paul Karrer, who was awarded Nobel prize in 1937.

### Metabolism of Vitamin E

Normal blood level of tocopherol is 0.5–1 mg/dl. It is absorbed along with other fats and needs the help of bile salts.

Tocopherol is absorbed and transported as chylomicrons. It is stored in adipose tissue. During catabolism, the chromane ring and side chain may be oxidized and excreted in bile after conjugation with glucuronic acid.

### Biochemical Role of Vitamin E

- Vitamin E is the *most powerful natural antioxidan.* Free radicals are continuously being generated in living systems. Their prompt inactivation is of great importance. Vitamin E is a known biological antioxidant able to quench the lipid peroxidation chain and to protect the plasma membranes from the attack of free radicals.
- The free radicals would attack bio-membranes. Vitamin E protects RBC from *hemolysis*. By preventing the peroxidation, it keeps the structural and functional integrity of all cells.
- Gradual deterioration of *ageing* process is due to the cumulative effects of free radicals. Vitamin E also boosts immune response.
- It reduces the risk of atherosclerosis by reducing oxidation of LDL.
- Vitamin E can depress leukocyte oxidative bactericidal activity.

### Inter-relationship with Selenium

Selenium is present in *glutathione peroxidase*; an important enzyme that oxidizes and destroys the free radicals. Selenium has been found to decrease the requirement of vitamin E and vice versa. They act synergistically to minimize lipid peroxidation.

### Deficiency Manifestations of Vitamin E

In rats, inability to produce healthy ovum and loss of motility of spermatozoa, hemolysis of red cells, acute hepatic necrosis and muscular dystrophy are observed. In a normal adult, the body vitamin E stores can meet the requirement for several months.

Human deficiency has not been reported. But in volunteers, vitamin E deficiency has been shown to produce increased fragility of RBCs, muscular weakness and creatinuria.

### Recommended Daily Allowance

Males: 10 mg/day
Females: 8 mg/day
Pregnancy: 10 mg/day
Lactation: 12 mg/day.

15 mg of vitamin E is equivalent to 33 international units. The requirement increases with higher intake of PUFA. Pharmacological dose is 200–400 IU per day.

#### Sources of Vitamin E

***Vegetable oils*** are rich sources of vitamin E, e.g. wheat germ oil, sunflower oil, safflower oil, cotton seed oil, etc. Fish liver oils are devoid of vitamin E.

#### Hypervitaminosis E

At doses above 1,000 IU per day, it may cause tendency to hemorrhage, as it is a mild anticoagulant.

## Vitamin K

### Chemistry of Vitamin K

The letter 'K' is the abbreviation of the German word 'koagulation vitamin'. They are *naphthoquinone* derivatives, with a long isoprenoid side chain. The length of side chain will differ. Vitamin $K_1$ has 20C side chain (phylloquinone). Vitamin $K_2$ has a 30C side chain. Yet another structurally similar synthetic compound having vitamin K activity is *Menadione*. It is water soluble synthetic vitamin, widely used in clinical practice. Henrik Dam isolated vitamin $K_1$ in 1929, while Edward Doisy isolated vitamin $K_2$ in 1939.

Both of them were awarded Nobel Prize in 1943.

### Absorption and Storage

Absorption of vitamin K occurs in the intestine along with chylomicrons. Bile salts are required for the normal absorption. The vitamin K may be derived from the diet or intestinal bacterial synthesis. It is stored in the liver and transported in plasma along with beta lipoproteins.

### Biochemical Role of Vitamin K

- Vitamin K is necessary for coagulation. Factors dependent on vitamin K are Factor II (*prothrombin*); Factor VII (SPCA); Factor IX (Christmas factor); Factor X (Stuart Prower factor).
- All these factors are synthesized by the liver as inactive zymogens. They undergo *post-translational* modification; gamma carboxylation of glutamic acid residues. These are the binding sites for calcium ions. The *gamma carboxy glutamic acid* (GCG) synthesis requires vitamin K as a cofactor.
- Vitamin K dependent gamma carboxylation is also necessary for the functional activity of osteocalcin as well as structural proteins of kidney, lung and spleen. *Osteocalcin* is synthesized by osteoblasts and seen only in bone. It is a small protein (40-50 amino acids length) that binds tightly to hydroxy apatite crystals of bone. This binding is dependent on the degree of gamma carboxylation.

Osteocalcin also contains hydroxyproline, so it is dependent on both vitamins K and C. Moreover, vitamin D induces its synthesis.

### Vitamin K Dependent Carboxylase

It is microsomal enzyme. It requires oxygen, $CO_2$, NADPH and reduced vitamin K. In this process, the vitamin passes through a cycle. This process is competitively inhibited by *warfarin* and *dicoumarol*.

### *Causes for Deficiency of Vitamin K*

In normal adults dietary deficiency seldom occurs since the intestinal bacterial synthesis is sufficient to meet the needs of the body. However deficiency can occur in conditions of *malabsorption* of lipids.

This can result from obstructive jaundice, chronic pancreatitis, sprue, etc. Prolonged *antibiotic* therapy and gastrointestinal infections with diarrhea will destroy the bacterial flora and can also lead to vitamin K deficiency.

### *Clinical Manifestations of Deficiency*

- Hemorrhagic disease of the newborn is attributed to vitamin K deficiency. The newborns, especially the *premature infants* have relative vitamin K deficiency. This is due to lack of hepatic stores, limited oral intake (breast milk has very low levels, 15 mg/liter) and absence of intestinal bacterial flora.
- It is often advised that preterm infants be given prophylactic doses of vitamin K (1 mg Menadione).
- In children and adults, Vitamin K deficiency may be manifested as bruising tendency, ecchymotic patches, mucous membrane hemorrhage, post-traumatic *bleeding* and internal bleeding.
- Prolongation of prothrombin time and delayed clotting time are characteristic of vitamin K deficiency.
- Measurement of *prothrombin time* (PT) is taken as an index of liver function. When liver function is considerably lowered, prolongation of PT occurs due to deficient synthesis of the coagulation factors. In such cases, administration of vitamin fails to restore PT to normal levels. Hence before undertaking any surgery on jaundiced patients, PT before and after administration of vitamin K should be done.
- ***Warfarin*** and ***dicoumarol*** will competitively inhibit the gamma carboxylation system due to structural similarity with vitamin K. Hence they are widely used as anticoagulants for therapeutic purposes.
- Treatment of pregnant women with warfarin can lead to fetal bone abnormalities (*fetal warfarin syndrome*).

### *Daily Requirement of Vitamin K*

Recommended daily allowance is 50–100 mg/day. This is usually available in a normal diet.

*Sources of Vitamin K*

***Green leafy vegetables*** are good dietary sources. Even if the diet does not contain the vitamin, intestinal bacterial synthesis will meet the daily requirements, as long as absorption is normal.

*Hypervitaminosis K*

Hemolysis, hyperbilirubinemia, kernicterus and brain damage are the manifestations of toxicity. Administration of large quantities of menadione may result in toxicity. This should be kept in mind in treating premature babies.

## WATER SOLUBLE VITAMINS

**(Thiamine, Riboflavin, Niacin, Pyridoxine, Pantothenic acid, Biotin, Folic acid, Vitamin $B_{12}$ and Ascorbic acid)**

### B Complex Group of Vitamins

These vitamins are chemically not related to one another. They are grouped together because all of them function in the cells as coenzymes. The important members of vitamin B complex group are enumerated as 1 to 8 above. In old literature, a few more members such as Choline, Inositol, Lipoic acid and para amino benzoic acid (PABA) are also included in this group.

Although they have important functions inside the body, they cannot be considered as vitamins, because they are available in plenty. PABA is not a vitamin for higher species, but it is required by bacteria for synthesis of folic acid.

### Thiamine (Vitamin $B_1$)

Thiamine is also called as vitamin $B_1$. In old literature, it is designated as Aneurine (it can relieve neuritis) or antiberiberi factor. In 1900, Christian Eijkman produced beriberi in chicken by feeding polished rice (Nobel Prize, 1929). Adolf Windaus (Nobel prize, 1928) elucidated the structure of the vitamin.

### *Sources*

Aleurone layer of cereals (food grains) is a rich source of thiamine. Therefore, whole wheat, flour and unpolished hand-pound rice have better nutritive value than completely polished refined foods. When the grains are polished, aleurone layer is usually removed. Yeast is also a very good source.

Thiamine is partially destroyed by heat.

### *Structure of Thiamine*

Thiamine contains a substituted *pyrimidine* ring connected to a substituted thiazole ring by means of methylene bridge. The vitamin is then converted to its active coenzyme form by addition of two phosphate groups, with the help of ATP. It is catalyzed by thiamine pyrophosphotransferase.

### *Physiological Role of Thiamine*

- ***Pyruvate dehydrogenase:*** The coenzyme form is *thiamine pyrophosphate* (TPP). It is used in oxidative decarboxylation of alpha keto acids, e.g. pyruvate dehydrogenase catalyzes the breakdown of pyruvate, to acetyl CoA and carbon dioxide.
- ***Alpha ketoglutarate dehydrogenase:*** An analogous biochemical reaction that requires TPP is the oxidative decarboxylation of *alpha ketoglutarate* to succinyl CoA and $CO_2$.
- ***Transketolase:*** The second group of enzymes that use TPP as coenzyme are the transketolases in the hexose monophosphate shunt pathway of glucose.
- The main role of thiamine (TPP) is in *carbohydrate* metabolism. So, the requirement of thiamine is increased along with higher intake of carbohydrates.

### *Deficiency Manifestations of Thiamine*

- ***Beriberi:*** Deficiency of thiamine leads to beriberi. It is a Singhalese word, meaning 'weakness'. The early symptoms are anorexia, dyspepsia, heaviness and weakness. Subjects feel weak and get easily exhausted.
- ***Wet beriberi:*** Here cardiovascular manifestations are prominent. Edema of legs, face, trunk and serous cavities

are the main features. Palpitation, breathlessness and distended neck veins are observed. Death occurs due to heart failure.

- *Dry beriberi:* In this condition, CNS manifestations are the major features. Walking becomes difficult. Peripheral neuritis with sensory disturbance leads to complete paralysis.
- *Infantile beriberi:* It occurs in infants born to mothers suffering from thiamine deficiency. Restlessness and sleeplessness are observed.
- *Wernicke-Korsakoff syndrome:* It is also called as *cerebral beriberi*. Carl Wernicke in 1894 and Sergiei Sergievich Korsakoff in 1887 described the condition. Clinical features are those of encephalopathy (ophthalmoplegia, nystagmus, cerebellar ataxia) plus psychosis. It is seen only when the nutritional status is severely affected.
- *Polyneuritis:* It is common in chronic alcoholics. Alcohol utilization needs large doses of thiamine. Alcohol inhibits intestinal absorption of thiamine, leading to thiamine deficiency.

Polyneuritis may also be associated with pregnancy and old age. Such thiamine deficiency in alcoholism may cause impairment of conversion of pyruvate to acetyl CoA. This results in increased plasma concentration of pyruvate and lactate, leading to *lactic acidosis*.

### Biochemical Parameters

In thiamine deficiency, blood thiamine is reduced, but pyruvate, alpha ketoglutarate and lactate are increased. Erythrocyte *transketolase* activity is reduced, this is the earliest manifestation seen even before clinical disturbances.

### Recommended Daily Allowance of Thiamine

It depends on calorie intake (0.5 mg/1000 calories).

Requirement is 1–1.5 mg/day. Thiamine is useful in the treatment of beriberi, alcoholic polyneuritis, neuritis of pregnancy and neuritis of old age.

## Riboflavin (Vitamin $B_2$)

Lactoflavin (milk), hepatoflavin (liver) and ovoflavin (eggs) are chemically identical to riboflavin. Riboflavin was the first B complex component to be isolated in a pure state. This vitamin is synthesized by green plants and micro-organisms. Warburg (Nobel prize 1931), isolated the 'yellow enzyme' of cellular respiration. Later Axel Theorell (Nobel prize, 1955) isolated riboflavin. In 1935, Paul Karrer (Nobel prize, 1937) determined the structure.

### Structure of Riboflavin

Riboflavin has a dimethyl isoalloxazine ring to which a ribitol is attached. Ribitol is the alcohol of ribose sugar.

Riboflavin is converted to its active coenzyme forms (FMN and FAD) with the help of ATP. Riboflavin is heat stable.

### Coenzyme Activity of Riboflavin

Riboflavin exists in tissues tightly bound (but not covalently) with enzymes. Enzymes containing riboflavin are called *flavoproteins.* The two coenzymes are *FMN* (flavin mono nucleotide) and *FAD* (flavin adenine dinucleotide).

#### *FAD Accepts Hydrogen*

During the oxidation process, FAD accepts two hydrogen atoms from substrate. In turn, FAD is reduced to $FADH_2$. The two nitrogen atoms of isoalloxazine nucleus accept the hydrogen atoms.

#### *FMN-dependent Enzymes*

- During the *amino acid oxidation,* FMN is reduced. It is reoxidized by molecular oxygen to produce hydrogen peroxide.
- In the *respiratory chain,* the NADH dehydrogenase contains FMN. The electrons are transported in the following manner.

#### *FAD-dependent Enzymes*

$FADH_2$ when oxidized in the electron transport chain will generate 1 ½ ATP molecules.

### Riboflavin Deficiency

- *Causes:* Natural deficiency of riboflavin in man is uncommon, because riboflavin is synthesized by the intestinal flora. Riboflavin deficiency usually accompanies other deficiency diseases such as beriberi, pellagra and kwashiorkor.
- *Manifestations:* Symptoms are confined to skin and mucous membranes.
  - ***Glossitis*** (Greek, glossa = tongue).
  - Magenta colored tongue
  - ***Cheilosis*** (Greek, cheilos = lip)
  - ***Angular stomatitis*** (inflammation at the corners of mouth).
  - Circumcorneal vascularization.
  - Proliferation of the bulbar conjunctival capillaries is the earliest sign of riboflavin deficiency.

### Dietary Sources of Riboflavin

Rich sources are liver, dried yeast, egg and whole milk. Good sources are fish, whole cereals, legumes and green leafy vegetables.

### Daily Requirement

Riboflavin is concerned mainly in the metabolism of *carbohydrates* and requirement is related to calorie intake. Adults on sedentary work require about 1.5 mg per day. During pregnancy and old age, additional 0.2 to 0.4 mg/day are required.

## Niacin

Niacin and Nicotinic acid are synonyms. It is also called as Pellagra preventing factor of Goldberger. The term nicotinic acid should not be confused with nicotine. Nicotinic acid is a vitamin; but, nicotine is the potent poison from tobacco.

Niacinamide is the active form of the vitamin, present in tissues. Warburg (Nobel prize, 1931) elucidated the structure of NAD+, and Alexander Todd (Nobel prize, 1957) demonstrated its function. It was originally named as coenzyme-I which was later designated as DPN (diphosphopyridine nucleotide), and finally in 1965 as $NAD^+$.

### Chemistry of Niacin

Niacin is pyridine-3-carboxylic acid. Niacinamide is the acid amide. In $NAD^+$ or $NADP^+$, the reactive site is the carbon atom 4 and the nitrogen atom of the nicotinamide ring. The coenzyme is bound to the apoenzyme.

### Coenzyme Forms of Niacin

Niacin is converted to its coenzyme forms, viz. Nicotinamide adenine dinucleotide (*$NAD^+$*) and Nicotinamide adenine dinucleotide phosphate (*$NADP^+$*). The niacin is attached to a ribose phosphate to form a mononucleotide. It is then attached to AMP to form the dinucleotide.

The nitrogen atom of niacinamide contains *one positive charge.* The structure is abbreviated as $NAD^+$. (The +ve sign is always shown). In the case of $NADP^+$, one more phosphoric acid is attached to the ribose of the AMP.

### One Hydrogen Atom and One Electron

- In the oxidized form, nitrogen of the nicotinamide residue has a positive charge. Hence the oxidized form of coenzyme is usually written as $NAD^+$.
- In the process of reduction, $NAD^+$ accepts one hydrogen atom fully. The other hydrogen is ionized. Only the electron is accepted. See the positive sign in the molecule is removed.

$$2H \longrightarrow H + H^+ + e^-$$

Thus $NAD^+$ accepts one H atom and one e-(electron), to form NADH. The hydrogen ion ($H^+$) is released into the surrounding medium. During the oxidation of NADH, the reaction is reversed.

### $NAD^+$ Dependent Enzymes

They are so many, that an exhaustive listing is not attempted. One NADH molecule is oxidized in the respiratory chain to generate 2½ ATPs. But NADPH is used almost exclusively for reductive biosynthetic reactions.

### NADPH Dependent Reactions

Some enzymes can use either $NAD^+$ or $NADP^+$ as coenzyme, e.g. glutamate dehydrogenase. In addition to this coenzyme role, $NAD^+$ is the source of ADP-ribose for the *ADP-ribosylation* of proteins and poly-ADP-ribosylation of nucleoproteins.

### Niacin Deficiency

*Pellagra*

Deficiency of niacin leads to the clinical condition called pellagra. Pellagra is an Italian word, meaning 'rough skin'. Pellagra is caused by the deficiency of Tryptophan as well as Niacin. Pellagra is seen more in women this may be because tryptophan metabolism is inhibited by estrogen metabolites. The symptoms of pellagra are:

- ***Dermatitis:*** In early stages, bright red erythema occurs, especially in the feet, ankles and face. Increased pigmentation around the neck is known as *Casal's necklace.* The dermatitis is precipitated by exposure to sunlight.
- ***Diarrhea:*** The diarrhea may be mild or severe with blood and mucus. This may lead to weight loss. Nausea and vomiting may also be present.
- ***Dementia:*** It is frequently seen in chronic cases. Delerium is common in acute pellagra. Irritability, inability to concentrate and poor memory are more common in mild cases. Ataxia and spasticity are also seen.

*Niacin is Synthesized from Tryptophan*

Quinolinate phosphoribosyl transferase is the rate limiting enzyme in the conversion of niacin to $NAD^+$. About 60 mg of tryptophan is equivalent to 1 mg of niacin.

*Causes for Niacin Deficiency*

- ***Dietary deficiency of tryptophan:*** Pellagra is seen among people whose staple diet is maize (South and Central America). In *maize,* niacin is present; but it is in a bound form, and is unavailable. Pellagra is also seen when staple diet is *sorghum* (jowar or guinea corn) as in Central and Western India. Sorghum, contains leucine in high quantities. Leucine inhibits the QPRT enzyme, and so niacin cannot be converted to $NAD^+$ (Leucine pellagra).
- ***Deficient synthesis:*** Kynureninase, an important enzyme in the pathway of tryptophan is pyridoxal phosphate dependent. So conversion of tryptophan to niacin is not possible in pyridoxal deficiency.
- ***Isoniazid (INH):*** It is an anti-tuberculous drug, which inhibits pyridoxal phosphate formation. Hence there is block in conversion of tryptophan to $NAD^+$.
- ***Hartnup disease:*** Tryptophan absorption from intestine is defective in this congenital disease. Moreover, tryptophan is excreted in urine in large quantities. This leads to lack of tryptophan and consequently deficiency of nicotinamide.
- ***Carcinoid syndrome:*** The tumor utilizes major portion of available tryptophan for synthesis of serotonin; so tryptophan is unavailable.

### Dietary Sources of Niacin

The richest natural sources of niacin are dried yeast, rice polishing, liver, peanut, whole cereals, legumes, meat and fish. About half of the requirement is met by the conversion of tryptophan to niacin. About 60 mg of tryptophan will yield 1 mg of niacin.

### Recommended Daily Allowance (RDA)

Normal requirement is 20 mg/day. During lactation, additional 5 mg are required.

### Therapeutic Use of Niacin

Nicotinic acid inhibits the flux of free fatty acids from adipose tissue; so acetyl CoA pool is reduced and hence serum *cholesterol* is lowered.

### Toxicity of Niacin

Nicotinic acid when given orally or parenterally produces a transient vasodilatation of the cutaneous vessels and *histamine release.* The reaction is accompanied by itching, burning and tingling. Intake of nicotinic acid in excess of 50 mg/day may lead to liver damage.

## Vitamin $B_6$

### Coenzyme Form

Vitamin $B_6$ is the term applied to a family of 3 related pyridine derivatives; *pyridoxine* (alcohol), *pyridoxal* (aldehyde) and *pyridoxamine*. Active form of pyridoxine is *pyridoxal phosphate (PLP)*. It is synthesized by pyridoxal kinase, utilizing ATP.

Main supply of $B_6$ compounds in food is in the form of pyridoxine which can be readily converted to pyridoxal and pyridoxamine in the body. Richard Kuhn (Nobel prize 1938) did the isolation and structural analysis.

### Functions of Pyridoxal Phosphate

The pyridoxal phosphate (PLP) acts as coenzyme for many reactions in *amino acid* metabolism.

*Transamination*

These reactions are catalyzed by amino transferases (transaminases) which employ PLP as the coenzyme, e.g.

Alanine + Alpha keto glutarate → Pyruvate + Glutamic acid (Enzyme Alanine transaminase).

*Decarboxylation*

All decarboxylation reactions of amino acids require PLP as coenzyme. A few examples are given below:

- Glutamate → GABA (gamma amino butyric acid). GABA is an inhibitory neurotransmitter, and hence in $B_6$ deficiency, especially in children, *convulsions* may occur
- Histidine → histamine, which is the mediator of *allergy* and anaphylaxis
- 5-hydroxy tryptophan → serotonin
- Cysteine → taurine
- Serine → ethanol amine.

*Sulfur Containing Amino Acids*

PLP plays an important role in methionine and cysteine metabolism.

- Homocysteine + Serine → Cystathionine. (Enzyme Cystathionine synthase)
- Cystathionine → Homoserine + Cysteine (Enzyme Cystathionase)

Both these reactions require PLP. Hence in vitamin $B_6$ deficiency *homocysteine* in blood is increased. Homocysteine level is correlated with *myocardial infarction*. Therefore, pyridoxine is used to prevent homocysteinemia.

*Heme Synthesis*

ALA synthase is a PLP dependent enzyme. This is the rate limiting step in heme biosynthesis. So, in $B_6$ deficiency, *anemia* may be seen.

*Production of Niacin*

Pyridoxal phosphate is required for the synthesis of niacin from tryptophan (*one vitamin is necessary for synthesis of another vitamin*). 3-hydroxy kynurenine → 3-hydroxy anthranilic acid (Enzyme Kynureninase).

Kynureninase is a PLP dependent enzyme. Hence in vitamin $B_6$ deficiency niacin production is less.

Moreover kynurenine cannot be converted further, which is metabolized to xanthurenic acid and excreted through urine.

*Glycogenolysis*

***Phosphorylase*** enzyme (glycogen to glucose-1-phosphate) requires PLP. In fact, more than 70% of total PLP content of the body is in muscles, where it is a part of the phosphorylase enzyme.

### Deficiency Manifestations of Pyridoxine

*Neurological Manifestations*

In vitamin $B_6$ deficiency, PLP dependent enzymes function poorly. So, serotonin, epinephrine, noradrenalin and gamma amino butyric acid (GABA) are not produced properly. *Neurological* symptoms are therefore quite common in $B_6$ deficiency. In children, $B_6$ deficiency leads to convulsions due to decreased formation of *GABA*. PLP is involved in the synthesis of sphingolipids; so $B_6$ deficiency leads to demyelination of nerves and consequent *peripheral neuritis*. This is reversible with high doses of $B_6$.

*Dermatological Manifestations*

Deficiency of $B_6$ will also affect tryptophan metabolism. Since niacin is produced from tryptophan, $B_6$ deficiency in turn leads to niacin deficiency which is manifested as *pellagra*.

*Hematological Manifestations*

In adults hypochromic microcytic *anemia* may occur due to the inhibition of heme biosynthesis. Impaired antibody formation is also reported.

The metabolic disorders which respond to vitamin $B_6$ therapy are *xanthurenic* aciduria and *homocystinuria*.

### Assay of Vitamin $B_6$

Vitamin $B_6$ status is assayed by the activation of erythrocyte transaminases by addition of pyridoxal phosphate in the reaction mixture.

### Effect of Drugs on Vitamin $B_6$

- ***INH:*** Isonicotinic acid hydrazide (isoniazid) is an antituberculosis drug. It inhibits pyridoxal kinase; reduces the formation of PLP and causes vitamin $B_6$ deficiency.
- ***Cycloserine:*** It acts as $B_6$ antagonist.
- ***Oral contraceptives:*** Mild vitamin $B_6$ deficiency may be seen in women taking oral contraceptive pills.
- ***Ethanol:*** It is converted to acetaldehyde, which inactivates PLP. Hence $B_6$ deficiency neuritis is quite common in alcoholics.

### Dietary Sources of Vitamin $B_6$

Rich sources are yeast, rice polishing, wheat germs, cereals, legumes (pulses), oil seeds, egg, milk, meat, fish and green leafy vegetables.

### Requirement of $B_6$

Vitamin $B_6$ requirements are related to *protein intake* and not to calorie intake. It is recommended that adults need 1 to 2 mg/day.

During pregnancy and lactation, the requirement is increased to 2.5 mg/day.

### *Toxicity of Vitamin $B_6$*

Doses over 100 mg may lead to *sensory neuropathy*.

Further excess is manifested by imbalance, numbness, muscle weakness and nerve damage.

## Pantothenic Acid

The Greek word *'pantos'* means everywhere. As the name suggests, it is widely distributed in nature. Pantothenic acid contains beta alanine and D-pantoic acid in amide linkage. Lipmann discovered the CoA in 1946 (Nobel prize in 1953).

### *Structure*

Synthesis of the CoA needs the expenditure of 4 high energy bonds. Pantothenic acid and beta mercaptoethanol amine are parts of coenzyme A (CoA). The CoA is a nucleotide.

### *Coenzyme Activity of Pantothenic Acid*

- The beta mercaptoethanol amine ($NH_2$-$CH_2$-$CH_2$-SH) contains one thiol or *sulfhydryl* (-SH) group. It is the active site where acyl groups are carried. Therefore, the coenzyme A is sometimes abbreviated as CoA-SH to denote this active site.
- The thio ester bond in acyl-CoA is a high energy bond. These acyl groups are transferred to other acceptors, for example:
  Acetyl CoA + Choline → Acetyl choline + CoA (enzyme is acetyl choline synthase).
- Acyl groups are also accepted by the CoA molecule during the metabolism of other substrates, for example:
  Pyruvate + CoA + NAD + → Acetyl CoA + $CO_2$ + NADH (Enzyme is pyruvate dehydrogenase).
- The important CoA derivatives are:
  - Acetyl CoA
  - Succinyl CoA
  - HMG CoA
  - Acyl CoA.
- Coenzyme A is an important component of fatty acid synthase complex. The ACP (acyl carrier protein) also contains pantothenic acid.

### *Deficiency of Pantothenic Acid*

Gopalan's *Burning Foot Syndrome* is manifested as paresthesia (burning, lightning pain) in lower extremities, staggering gait due to impaired coordination and sleep disturbances.

These deficiency manifestations are rare in human beings. The syndrome is seen during famine, in prison camps, in chronic alcoholics and in some renal dialysis patients.

In experimental animals, deficiency has resulted in anemia (due to reduced heme synthesis from succinyl CoA), reduced steroidogenesis (due to lack of acetyl CoA), dermatitis, fatty liver and adrenal necrosis.

### *Sources of Pantothenic Acid*

It is widely distributed in plants and animals. Moreover, it is synthesized by the normal bacterial flora in intestines. Therefore, deficiency is very rare. Yeast, liver and eggs are good sources.

### *Requirement of Pantothenic Acid*

RDA is assumed to be about 10 mg/day.

## Biotin

In old literature Biotin was known as anti-egg white injury factor.

Biotin was isolated in 1942 by Vincent du Vigneaud, who was awarded Nobel prize in 1955.

### *Structure of Biotin*

It consists of an imidazole ring fused with a thiophene ring with a valeric acid side chain. The carboxyl group forms an amide linkage with the epsilon nitrogen of a lysine residue in the apoenzyme.

### *Coenzyme Activity of Biotin*

Biotin acts as coenzyme for *carboxylation reactions*. Biotin captures a molecule of $CO_2$ which is attached to nitrogen of the biotin molecule. The energy required for this reaction is provided by ATP. Then the activated carboxyl group is transferred to the substrate.

### *Biotin Requiring $CO_2$ Fixation Reactions*

*Acetyl CoA Carboxylase*

This enzyme adds $CO_2$ to acetyl CoA to form malonyl CoA. This is the rate limiting reaction in biosynthesis of fatty acids.

Acetyl CoA + $CO_2$ + ATP → Malonyl CoA + ADP + Pi

*Propionyl CoA Carboxylase*

Propionyl CoA + $CO_2$ + ATP→
Methyl malonyl CoA + ADP + Pi

*Pyruvate Carboxylase*

Pyruvate + $CO_2$ + ATP → Oxaloacetate + ADP + Pi. This is important in two aspects. One, it provides the oxaloacetate, which is the catalyst for TCA cycle. Second, it is an important enzyme in the gluconeogenic pathway.

### *Biotin-Independent Carboxylation Reactions*

- Carbamoyl phosphate synthetase, which is the stepping stone for urea and pyrimidine synthesis.
- Addition of $CO_2$ to form C6 in purine ring.
- Malic enzyme, converting pyruvate to malate.

### *Biotin Antagonists*

- ***Avidin***, a protein present in *egg white* has great affinity to biotin. Hence intake of raw (unboiled) egg may cause biotin deficiency. Biotin was originally named as anti-egg-white injury-factor.
- Avidin is heat labile, and boiling of egg will neutralize the inhibitory activity. One molecule of avidin can combine with four molecules of biotin. It is curious that egg white contains avidin and egg yolk contains biotin.
- The affinity of avidin to biotin is greater than most of the usual antigen-antibody reactions. Therefore avidin-biotin system is commonly utilized for detection of pathogens in the *ELISA test*.

- DNA is generally labelled by radioactive nucleotides. Recently, biotin labelling of DNA is becoming more popular. Biotin is added to nucleotides, which will be incorporated into the newly synthesized DNA. The fixed biotin can be identified by reaction with avidin.
- ***Streptavidin*** purified from *Streptomyces avidinii*, can bind 4 molecules of biotin.

### Deficiency of Biotin

- Prolonged use of antibacterial drugs.
- Biotin deficiency symptoms include dermatitis, atrophic glossitis, hyperesthesia, muscle pain, anorexia and hallucinations. Injection of biotin 100–300 mg will bring about rapid cure of these symptoms.

### Requirement of Biotin

About 200–300 mg will meet the daily requirements.

### Sources of Biotin

Normal acterial flora of the gut will provide adequate quantities of biotin. Moreover, it is distributed ubiquitously in plant and animal tissues. Liver, yeast, peanut, soybean, milk and egg yolk are rich sources.

## Folic Acid

The name is derived from the Latin word *folium*, which means leaf of vegetable. Folic acid is abundant in vegetables. Angier in 1941 established the chemical structure of folic acid. The name folic acid was assigned by Mitchell, Snell and Williams.

### Chemistry of Folic Acid

The Latin word *folium* means leaf of vegetable.

Folic acid is abundant in vegetables. It is composed of three constituents. The *pteridine* group linked with para amino benzoic acid (*PABA*)) is called *pteroic acid*. It is then attached to *glutamic acid* to form pteroyl glutamic acid or folic acid. In nature, polyglutamates are seen where up to seven glutamate residues are linked to the pteroyl group. Folacin is the generic name for such folic acid related compounds. Folic acid is soluble in water. When exposed to light, it is rapidly destroyed.

### Absorption of Folic Acid

Folic acid is readily absorbed by the *upper part of jejunum*. In the blood, it is transported by beta globulins. It is taken up by the liver where the coenzymes are produced. Folic acid is not stored in tissues. There are different tissue specific *transporters* for folic acid. These high affinity binding proteins are anchored on plasma membrane. Folate-transporter complex is internalized by a nonclathrin mediated endocytosis. The term '*potocytosis*' is used to denote the recycling of transport proteins by vesicular structures, named *caveolae*.

### Coenzyme Functions of Folic Acid

- The folic acid is first reduced to 7,8-dihydrofolic acid and further reduced to 5,6,7,8-*tetrahydrofolic acid* (THFA). Both reactions are catalyzed by *NADPH* dependent folate reductase.
- The THFA is the *carrier of one-carbon* groups.

  One carbon compound is an organic molecule that contains only a single carbon atom. The following groups are one carbon compounds:
  - Formyl (-CHO)
  - Formimino (-CH=NH)
  - Methenyl (-CH=)
  - Methylene ($-CH_2-$)
  - Hydroxymethyl ($-CH_2OH$)
  - Methyl ($-CH_3$).
- These one carbon compounds are attached either to the 5th or to the 10th or to both 5 and 10 nitrogen atoms of THFA.
- Methyl group in N5-methyl THFA is used for synthesis of active methionine, which takes part in transmethylation reactions. Such *transmethylation* reactions are required for synthesis of choline, epinephrine, creatine, etc.

### Causes for Folate Deficiency

Folic acid deficiency is very common in India, and is perhaps the most commonly seen vitamin deficiency.

- ***Pregnancy:*** Folate deficiency is commonly seen in pregnancy where requirement is increased.
- ***Defective absorption:*** In sprue, celiac disease, gluten induced enteropathy, resection of jejunum and short-circuiting of jejunum in gastroileostomy, absorption is defective.
- ***Drugs:*** In the diet, folacins are mainly in polyglutamate form. Gastrointestinal enzymes in the gut remove the glutamate residues and only the mono-glutamate form of folic acid is absorbed. Anticonvulsant drugs (hydantoin, dilantin, phenytoin, phenobarbitone) will inhibit the intestinal enzyme, so that folate absorption is reduced.
- ***Hemolytic anemias:*** As requirement of folic acid becomes more, deficiency is manifested.
- ***Dietary deficiency:*** Absence of vegetables in food for prolonged periods may lead to deficiency.
- ***Folate trap:*** When $B_{12}$ is deficient, this reaction cannot take place, leading to folate deficiency (see under vitamin $B_{12}$).

### Deficiency Manifestations

*Reduced DNA synthesis*

In folate deficiency, THFA is reduced and thymidylate synthase enzyme is inhibited. Hence dUMP is not converted to dTMP. So dTTP is not available for DNA synthesis. Thus cell division is arrested.

Very rapidly dividing cells in bone marrow and intestinal mucosa are therefore most seriously affected.

*Macrocytic Anemia*

- It is the most characteristic feature of folate deficiency. During erythropoiesis, DNA synthesis is delayed, but protein synthesis is continued. Thus hemoglobin accumulates in RBC precursors. This asynchrony or dissociation between the maturity of nucleus and cytoplasm is manifested as *immature looking nucleus* and mature eosinophilic cytoplasm in the bone marrow cells.
- ***Reticulocytosis*** is often seen. These abnormal RBCs are rapidly destroyed in spleen. This *hemolysis* leads to the

reduction of lifespan of RBC. Reduced generation and increased destruction of RBCs result in anemia.

- *Leukopenia* and thrombocytopenia are also manifested.
- The peripheral blood picture in folate deficiency is described as *macrocytic*, and in cobalamin deficiency as *megaloblastic*. In $B_{12}$ deficiency, there are additional neurological symptoms.

*Homocysteinemia*

Folic acid deficiency may cause increased homocysteine levels in blood. Plasma homocysteine levels above 15 micromoles/L is known to increase the risk of *coronary artery diseases*. Providing adequate doses of pyridoxine, $B_{12}$ and folic acid may lower the homocysteine levels.

*Birth Defects*

Folic acid deficiency during pregnancy may lead to homocysteinemia and neural tube defects in the fetus. Folic acid prevents *birth defects* (fetal malformations such as spina bifida). So, supplementation of folic acid from early pregnancy is a must to prevent neural tube defects in the child.

*Cancer*

Folic acid is beneficial in prevention of **cancer**. Folate deficiency contributes to the etiology of bronchial carcinoma and cervical carcinoma.

### Assessment of Folate Deficiency

- ***Blood Level:*** Normal folic acid level in serum is about 20 nanogram/mL and about 200 microgram/mL of packed cells. The level is measured by radio-immuno-assay.
- ***Histidine load test or FIGLU excretion test:*** Histidine is normally metabolized to formimino glutamic acid (FIGLU) from which formimino group is removed by THFA. Therefore in folate deficiency, FIGLU is excreted in urine.
- ***AICAR excretion:*** In the purine nucleotide synthesis, the last step is the addition of C2 with the help of N10-formyl THFA. When this is blocked, the precursor, amino imidazole carboxamide ribosyl-5-phosphate (AICAR) accumulates and is excreted in urine.
- ***Peripheral blood picture.***

### Sources of Folic Acid

Rich sources of folate are yeast, green leafy vegetables. Moderate sources are cereals, pulses, oil seeds and egg. Milk is a poor source for folic acid.

### Recommended Daily Allowance (RDA)

The requirement of free folate is 200 mg/ day. In pregnancy the requirement is increased to 400 mg/day and during lactation to 300 mg/day.

### Folic Acid Therapy

Therapeutic dose is 1 mg of folic acid per day orally.

Folic acid alone should not be given in macrocytic anemia because it may aggravate the neurological manifestation of $B_{12}$ deficiency. So, folic acid and vitamin $B_{12}$ are given in combination to patients.

Regular supplementation of folic acid may reduce the incidence of birth defects, cardiovascular diseases and cancers.

### Toxicity of Folic Acid

Doses over 1 mg may cause aggravation of vitamin $B_{12}$ deficiency and may precipitate nerve damage. Since solubility of folic acid is low, large doses should not be given parenterally, as there is danger of crystallization in kidney tubules leading to renal damage.

### Folate Antagonists

*Sulphonamides*

They have structural similarity with PABA.

Therefore, they competitively inhibit the enzyme responsible for the incorporation of PABA into dihydro pteroic acid, the immediate precursor of folic acid. Bacteria can synthesize folic acid from the components, pteridine, PABA and glutamate. When sulphonamides are given, such microorganisms cannot synthesize folic acid and hence their growth is inhibited. As man cannot synthesize folic acid, the entire molecule has to be supplied in the diet. The preformed folic acid cannot enter into bacteria, but only into mammalian cells. Thus sulphonamides are very good *antibacterial* agents, which do not affect the human cells.

Gerhard Domagk discovered the antibacterial effect of Prontosil (a sulphonamide) in 1932 for which he was awarded Nobel prize in 1939.

*Pyrimethamine*

This antifolate agent is used against plasmodial infections (*antimalarial* drug). Gertrude Elion synthesized pyrimethamine, who got Nobel prize in 1988.

*Aminopterin and Amethopterin*

Aminopterin (4-amino folic acid) and amethopterin (methotrexate) (4-amino, 10-methyl folic acid) are powerful inhibitors of folate reductase and THFA generation. Thus these drugs decrease the DNA formation and cell division. They are widely used as *anticancer* drugs, especially for leukemias and choriocarcinomas. Folinic acid (citrovorum factor) is given to rescue the patient from toxicity of methotrexate.

## Vitamin $B_{12}$

Synonyms are cobalamin, extrinsic factor (EF) of Castle and antipernicious anemia factor. In 1849, Thomas Addison described the pernicious anemia. William Murphy and George Minot showed that liver therapy is very effective to treat pernicious anemia. For this work, they were awarded Nobel prize in 1934. Dorothy Hodgkin suggested the structure by X-ray diffraction studies (Nobel prize, 1964). Later Robert Woodward synthesized $B_{12}$ and proved the structure (Nobel prize, 1965).

### Chemistry

Vitamin $B_{12}$ is water soluble, heat stable and red in color. It contains 4.35% cobalt by weight. It contains one cobalt atom. Four pyrrole rings coordinated with a cobalt atom is called a *Corrin ring*. Note the similarity between the Corrin ring and the porphyrin ring system. The 5th valency of the cobalt is covalently linked to a substituted benzimidazole ring. This is then called *cobalamin*. The 6th valency of the cobalt is satisfied by any of the following groups: cyanide, hydroxyl, adenosyl or methyl.

*Cyanocobalamin*

When cyanide is added at the R position, the molecule is called cyanocobalamin. During the isolation procedure, cyanide is added to get stable crystals. The CN group has no physiological function, it is only a laboratory artefact. Oral preparations are in this form.

*Hydroxy Cobalamin*

When hydroxyl group is attached at the R position, it is called hydroxy cobalamin or vitamin $B_{12a}$. *Injectable preparations* are in this form.

*Adenosyl Cobalamin (Ado-$B_{12}$)*

When taken up by the cells, these groups are removed and deoxy adenosyl cobalamin or Ado-$B_{12}$ is formed. This is the major *storage form* seen in liver.

*Methyl Cobalamin*

When the methyl group replaces adenosyl group, it is known as methyl cobalamin. This is the major form *seen in blood* circulation as well as in cytoplasm of cells. The Ado-$B_{12}$ and methyl $B_{12}$ are the *functional coenzymes* in the body.

## Absorption of Vitamin $B_{12}$

- Absorption of vitamin $B_{12}$ requires two binding proteins. First is the *intrinsic factor* (IF) of Castle. William B Castle described it in 1929. The $B_{12}$ is otherwise known as extrinsic factor (EF), that is, the factor derived from external sources. Intrinsic factor is secreted by the gastric parietal cells. It is a glycoprotein with a molecular weight of 50,000.
- The second factor is *cobalophilin*, secreted in the saliva. Gastric *pepsin* release the vitamin from proteins of the food, and then $B_{12}$ binds with cobalophilin. In duodenum, cobalophilin is hydrolyzed by *trypsin* of pancreatic juice; vitamin is released, and then vitamin binds to intrinsic factor. In pancreatic insufficiency (absence of trypsin), the vitamin may not be released. Then vitamincobalophilin complex is excreted, resulting in vitamin deficiency.
- One molecule of IF can combine with 2 molecules of $B_{12}$. This IF-$B_{12}$ complex is attached with specific receptors on mucosal cells. The whole IF-$B_{12}$ complex is internalized. It may be noted that $B_{12}$ is absorbed from *ileum*, while folic acid is from jejunum.

## Transport and Storage

In the blood, *methyl $B_{12}$* form is predominant. *Transcobalamin*, a glycoprotein, is the specific carrier. It is stored in the liver cells, as *ado-$B_{12}$* form, in combination with *transcorrin*. Generally, B complex vitamins are not stored in the body, $B_{12}$ is an exception. Whole liver contains about 2 mg of $B_{12}$, which is sufficient for the requirement for 2–3 years. So, $B_{12}$ deficiency is seen only years after gastrectomy.

## Functional Role of $B_{12}$

*Methyl Malonyl CoA Isomerase*

D-Methyl malonyl CoA is formed in the body from propionyl CoA. It is then converted to L form by a racemase and then isomerized by methyl malonyl CoA mutase (containing Ado–$B_{12}$) to succinyl CoA, which enters into citric acid cycle.

In $B_{12}$ deficiency, methyl malonyl CoA is excreted in urine (*methyl malonic aciduria*).

The metabolism of odd chain fatty acids, valine, isoleucine, methionine and threonine leads to the production of methyl malonyl CoA.

*Homocysteine Methyl Transferase*

Step 2 is catalyzed by the enzyme methionine synthase or homocysteine methyl transferase.

*Methyl Folate Trap and Folate Deficiency*

The production of methyl THFA is an irreversible step. Therefore, the only way for generation of free THFA is step No. 1. When $B_{12}$ is deficient, this reaction cannot take place. This is called the methyl *folate trap*. This leads to the associated *folic acid scarcity in $B_{12}$ deficiency.*

## Causes of $B_{12}$ Deficiency

- ***Nutritional:*** Nutritional vitamin $B_{12}$ deficiency is very common in India, especially among vegetarians of low socioeconomic group. The only source for $B_{12}$ in vegetarian diet is curd/milk, and lower income group may not be able to afford it.
- ***Decrease in absorption:*** Absorptive surface is reduced by gastrectomy, resection of ileum and malabsorption syndromes.
- ***Addisonian pernicious anemia:*** It is very rare in India, but common in European countries. When it was described in 1849 by Thomas Addison, it was pernicious (fatal), without any known remedy. It is manifested usually in persons over 40 years. It is an autoimmune disease with a strong familial background. Antibodies are generated against IF. So, IF becomes deficient, leading to defective absorption of $B_{12}$.
- ***Gastric atrophy:*** Although true Addisonian pernicious anemia is rare, similar atrophy of gastric epithelium leading to deficiency of IF and decreased $B_{12}$ absorption is common in India. In chronic *iron deficiency* anemia, there is generalized mucosal atrophy. In about 40% cases of iron deficiency anemia, superadded gastric atrophy is seen.
- ***Pregnancy:*** Increased requirement of vitamin in pregnancy is another common cause for vitamin $B_{12}$ deficiency in India.
- ***Fish tapeworm:*** Although not seen in India, the fish tapeworm, *diphillobothrium latum* infection is common in Scandinavian countries where eating live fish is a delicacy. This tapeworm has a special affinity to $B_{12}$ causing reduction in available vitamin.

## Deficiency Manifestations

- ***Folate trap:*** Vitamin $B_{12}$ deficiency causes simultaneous folate deficiency due to the folate trap. Therefore all the manifestations of folate deficiency are also seen (for details see under folic acid).
- ***Megaloblastic anemia:*** In the peripheral blood, megaloblasts and immature RBCs are observed.
- ***Abnormal homocysteine level:*** In vitamin $B_{12}$ deficiency, step No. 2 is blocked, so that homocysteine is accumulated, leading to *homocystinuria.* Homocysteine level in blood has a positive correlation with myocardial infarction. So, $B_{12}$ and folic acid are protective against ischemic heart disease.

- ***Demyelination:*** In vitamin $B_{12}$ deficiency, step 3 is also suppressed due to the non-availability of active methionine. Therefore methylation of phosphatidyl ethanolamine to phosphatidyl choline is not adequate. This leads to deficient formation of myelin sheaths of nerves, demyelination and neurological lesions.
- ***Subacute combined degeneration:*** Damage to nervous system is seen in $B_{12}$ deficiency (but not in folate deficiency). There is *demyelination* affecting cerebral cortex as well as dorsal column and pyramidal tract of spinal cord. Since sensory and motor tracts are affected, it is named as combined degeneration. Symmetrical paresthesia of extremities, alterations of tendon and deep senses and reflexes, loss of position sense, unsteadiness in gait, positive *Romberg's* sign (falling when eyes are closed) and positive *Babinski's* sign (extensor plantar reflex) are seen.
- ***Achlorhydria:*** Absence of acid in gastric juice is associated with vitamin $B_{12}$ deficiency.

### Assessment of $B_{12}$ Deficiency

- ***Serum $B_{12}$:*** It is quantitated by radio-immuno-assay or by ELISA.
- ***Schilling test:*** Radioactive labelled (Cobalt-60) vitamin $B_{12}$, one microgram is given orally. Simultaneously an intramuscular injection of unlabeled vitamin $B_{12}$ is given, in order to saturate tissues with normal vitamin $B_{12}$. So, radioactive vitamin $B_{12}$ will not bind to body tissues.
  Therefore, the entire absorbed radioactivity will pass into the urine. The patient's urine is then collected over the next 24 hours to assess the absorption. In a normal person, the ingested vitamin $B_{12}$ will be absorbed into the body. Since the liver receptors for vitamin $B_{12}$ are saturated by the injection, much of the ingested vitamin $B_{12}$ will be excreted in the urine. In patients with pernicious anemia or with deficiency due to impaired absorption, less than 5% of the radioactivity is detected in urine. If an abnormality is found, the test is repeated, with radioactive vitamin plus intrinsic factor given orally, and urine is collected for 24 hours. In pernicious anemia, there is lack of intrinsic factor, so that the first test is abnormal; but the second test is normal.
- ***Methyl malonic acid:*** It is seen in urine.
- ***FIGLU excretion test:*** (see folic acid).
- ***Peripheral smear:*** Peripheral blood and bone marrow morphology shows megaloblastic anemia.

### Treatment

If megaloblastic anemia is treated with folic acid alone, the anemia may improve, but associated neurological symptoms are aggravated. Hence all macrocytic anemias are generally treated with folate and vitamin $B_{12}$. Therapeutic dose of $B_{12}$ is 500 to 1000 microgram by intramuscular injections.

### Requirement of Vitamin $B_{12}$

Normal daily requirement is 1–2 microgram/day. During pregnancy and lactation, this is increased to 2 mg/day. Those who take folic acid, should also take vitamin $B_{12}$. Elderly people are advised to take $B_{12}$ supplementation.

### Dietary Sources

Vitamin $B_{12}$ is not present in vegetables. Liver is the richest source. Curd is a good source, because lactobacillus can synthesize $B_{12}$.

## Choline

Best and Huntsman (1934) discovered that choline deficiency in the rat produces fatty liver. It plays an active role in transmethylation. Choline is synthesized in the body and therefore it is not a vitamin. But in view of its importance in nutrition, conventionally, it is included as a member of vitamin B complex. Rice polishings, vegetables, milk, egg and liver are good sources. It is synthesized from serine.

### Chemistry

It is hydroxyethyl trimethyl amine, or trimethyl ethanol amine. It is water soluble.

### Biochemical Functions

- ***Phospholipid synthesis:*** Choline is a part of *phospholipids* which are essential constituents of the membranes of all cells.
- ***Myelin sheath:*** It is made by phospholipids. *Demyelination* causes severe diseases of nervous system.
- ***Fatty liver:*** Phospholipids are involved in the transport of fat and cholesterol from the liver. In choline deficiency, neutral fat and cholesterol esters accumulate in liver, leading to fatty liver. Choline is able to prevent fatty liver and cirrhosis.
- ***Transmethylation reactions:*** Choline can donate three methyl groups to the one-carbon pool. Finally, these methyl groups are transferred to homocysteine to produce methionine, which is used for transmethylation reactions.
- ***Acetyl choline (ACh) synthesis:***
  ***Choline acetylase***
  Choline + Acetyl CoA ⟶ Acetyl choline + CoA
  ***Acetyl choline esterase***
  Acetyl choline ⟶ Choline + Acetate

### Acetyl Choline

It is synthesized in the neurons, which reaches the presynaptic region of synaptosomes, where ACh is stored in packets. When a nerve impulse reaches, the ACh is liberated into the synaptosome. At the post-synaptic region, the ACh is picked up by the specific receptors, which produces a nerve impulse.

Thus the nerve impulse is transmitted through the synapses by the chemical messenger, the ACh. As soon as the nerve impulse is generated in the postsynaptic fiber, the ACh is hydrolyzed by the ACh-esterase.

In 1914, Henry Dale isolated Ach. In 1920, Otto Loewi studied the effect of ACh on nerve transmission. Both of them were awarded Nobel prize in 1936. Later work of Bernard Katz on the effect of ACh on neuromuscular end plates earned him the Nobel prize in 1970.

### Clinical Applications

- The post-synaptic receptors for ACh may be competitively blocked by *succinyl choline*, a structural analog of ACh. Then

ACh cannot act, producing muscle relaxation. It is widely used as a *muscle relaxant* during surgery.

- Cholinesterase inhibitors (e.g. *neostigmine*) will allow prolonged action of ACh and therefore nerve impulse is sustained. These drugs are used in *myasthenia gravis*.

  Myasthenia is an autoimmune condition where antibodies are produced against neuromuscular end plate proteins destroying the end plates.
- Pseudocholinesterase is seen in RBCs, more in immature cells.

## Inositol

Inositol is hexahydroxy cyclohexane. Out of the many isomers, *myo-inositol* is seen in tissues. It is seen in yeast, cereals and milk. Inositol deficiency is unknown to man. Therefore it cannot be considered as a vitamin.

### *Biochemical Functions of Inositol*

- Studies in tissue culture have revealed that inositol is required for growth of fibroblasts.
- Inositol is a constituent of certain phospholipids.
- It occurs in large quantities in mammalian heart muscle.
- Hexa phosphate of inositol is called *phytin*. It is found in vegetables, which prevent the absorption of calcium and iron from intestine.
- ***Phosphatidyl inositol*** is an important constituent of cell membranes. In response to extracellular signals, *inositol triphosphate* (IP3) is released from phosphatidyl inositol.IP3 is a second messenger. It may allow calcium inflow into the cells, leading to cellular metabolic activation.
- ***Peripheral neuropathy*** very commonly seen in diabetes mellitus, is associated with inositol metabolism. Decreased inositol in nerve fibers may be the cause for neuropathy.
- It is a *lipotropic factor* and prevents fatty liver.

## Ascorbic Acid (Vitamin C)

A description of scurvy was found in the Ebers papyrus written in 1500 BC in Egypt. During the voyage of Vasco da Gama, around the cape of Good Hope to India in 1498, he lost two-third of the crew due to scurvy. The French explorer, Jacques Cartier, in 1536, during the voyages to discover eastern parts of Canada, was laid up with scurvy. A friendly native gave an extract from the leaves of spruce tree, which produced remarkable cure to scurvy. James Lind published 'Treatise on Scurvy', in 1753. These observations led to compulsory rationing of lime or lemon juice to all the crew of the British Royal Navy from 1795 onwards. So the British sailors were nicknamed as 'Limeys'. However, it helped to eliminate scurvy from the British Navy, while opponents continued to suffer. No wonder, in course of time, Britain had the colonies in which the sun never set. In 1907, Holst and Trochlich produced scurvy in guineapigs. Zilva and associates, in 1928, showed that the antiscorbutic factor present in lemon juice is a reducing substance. The factor was isolated in 1930 and named as 'Hexuronic acid' by Albert Szent-Gyorgi (Nobel prize, 1937). In 1933, Haworth established the molecular structure. He renamed it as ascorbic acid (Nobel prize, 1937).

### *Chemistry of Vitamin C*

It is water soluble and is easily destroyed by heat, alkali and storage. In the process of cooking, 70% of vitamin C is lost.

The structural formula of ascorbic acid closely resembles that of carbohydrates. The strong reducing property of vitamin C depends on the double-bonded (enediol) carbons.

Only L-ascorbic acid and dehydroascorbic acid have antiscorbutic activity. The D-ascorbic acid has no activity.

### *Biosynthesis of Ascorbic Acid in Animals*

Most animals and plants can synthesize ascorbic acid from glucose. *Man, higher primates,* guineapigs and bats are the only species which cannot synthesize ascorbic acid (block in gulono lactone oxidase step). They lack the genes responsible for the synthesis of this enzyme. The vitamin therefore should be supplied in the diet of these species. The staple diet of primates contains fruits and vegetables rich in ascorbic acid, and so the gene deletion will have no deleterious effect in primates. Human beings, of course, carried over this gene deletion.

### *Metabolism of Ascorbic Acid*

- Ascorbic acid is readily absorbed from gastrointestinal tract. The vitamin is excreted in urine. Since vitamin C is a strong reducing agent, the *Benedict's test* will be positive in the urine sample after the vitamin administration.
- Oxidation of ascorbic acid yields dehydro ascorbic acid, which is oxidized further to oxalic acid through diketo-Lgulonic acid. Ascorbic acid is partly excreted unchanged and partly as oxalic acid. Most of the oxalates in urine are derived from ascorbic acid, and the rest from glycine metabolism.
- The ascorbic acid level varies between 0.7 to 1.2 mg/100 mL of plasma and 25 mg/100 cc of WBC. A low level in blood is noted in women taking contraceptive pills and also in chronic alcoholics.
- A very high concentration of vitamin C is observed locally in healing wounds. Vitamin C is essential for wound healing.

### *Biochemical Functions of Vitamin C*

- ***Reversible oxidation-reduction:*** It can change between ascorbic acid and dehydroascorbic acid. Most of the physiological properties of the vitamin could be explained by this redox system.
- ***Hydroxylation of proline and lysine:*** Ascorbic acid is necessary for the post-translational hydroxylation of proline and lysine residues. Hydroxyproline and hydroxylysine are essential for the formation of cross links in the *collagen*, which gives the tensile strength to the fibres. This process is absolutely necessary for the normal production of supporting tissues such as osteoid, collagen and intercellular cement substance of capillaries.
- ***Tryptophan metabolism:*** Ascorbic acid is necessary for the hydroxylation of tryptophan to 5-hydroxy tryptophan. This is required for the formation of serotonin.
- ***Tyrosine metabolism:*** Vitamin C helps in the oxidation of parahydroxy phenyl pyruvate to homogentisic acid.

- ***Iron metabolism:*** Ascorbic acid enhances the iron absorption from the intestine. Ascorbic acid reduces ferric iron to ferrous state, which is preferentially absorbed.
- ***Hemoglobin metabolism:*** It is useful for re-conversion of met-hemoglobin to hemoglobin.
- ***Folic acid metabolism:*** Ascorbic acid is helping the enzyme folate reductase to reduce folic acid to tetrahydrofolic acid. Thus it helps in the maturation of RBC.
- ***Steroid synthesis:*** Large quantities of vitamin C are present in adrenal cortex. The ascorbic acid is depleted by ACTH stimulation. So the vitamin has some role in adrenal steroidogenesis. Vitamin C helps in the synthesis of bile acids from cholesterol. The initial 7-alphahydroxylase step is stimulated by the vitamin.
- ***Phagocytosis:*** Ascorbic acid stimulates phagocytic action of leukocytes and helps in the formation of antibodies.
- ***Anti-oxidant property:*** As an anti-oxidant, it may prevent cancer formation. Aniline dyes are known to induce bladder cancer in factory workers. Daily intake of vitamin C reduces this risk for cancer.
- ***Cataract:*** Vitamin C is concentrated in the lens of eye. Regular intake of ascorbic acid reduces the risk of cataract formation.

### Deficiency Manifestations of Vitamin C

- ***Scurvy:*** Gross deficiency of vitamin C results in scurvy.
- ***Infantile scurvy (Barlow's disease):*** In infants between 6 to 12 months of age, (period in which weaning from breast milk), the diet should be supplemented with vitamin C sources. Otherwise, deficiency of vitamin C is seen.
- ***Hemorrhagic tendency:*** In ascorbic acid deficiency, *collagen is abnormal* and the intercellular cement substance is brittle. So capillaries are fragile, leading to the tendency to bleed even under minor pressure. Subcutaneous hemorrhage may be manifested as *petechiae* in mild deficiency and as *ecchymoses* or even hematoma in severe conditions. If a sphygmomanometer cuff is placed in the forearm, and the pressure is kept for 5 minutes, petechiae may be seen under the skin. This is a useful clinical test.
- ***Internal hemorrhage:*** In severe cases, hemorrhage may occur in the conjunctiva and retina. Internal bleeding may be seen as epistaxis, hematuria or melena.
- ***Oral cavity:*** In severe cases of scurvy, the gum becomes painful, swollen and spongy. The pulp is separated from the dentine and finally teeth are lost. Wound healing may be delayed.
- ***Bones:*** In the bones, the deficiency results in the failure of the osteoblasts to form the intercellular substance, *osteoid*. Without the normal ground substance, the deposition of bone is arrested. The resulting scorbutic *bone is weak* and fractures easily. There may be hemorrhage into joint cavities. Painful swelling of joints may prevent locomotion of the patient.

  Vitamin C and vitamin B are essential nutrients to maintain bone density and bone quality. Recent literature clearly shows that vitamin C and B affect bone quality determinant 'collagen cross-link formation'. Mildly elevated plasma homocysteine levels induced by vitamin B insufficiency and methylenetetrahydrofolate reductase (MTHFR) deteriorate normal collagen cross-link formation.
- ***Anemia:*** In vitamin C deficiency, microcytic, hypochromic *anemia* is seen. Poikilocytosis and anisocytosis are also common in anemia due to deficiency of vitamin C. The reasons for anemia may be:
  - Loss of blood by hemorrhage
  - Decreased iron absorption
  - Decreased tetrahydrofolic acid
  - Accumulation of met-hemoglobin.

### Dietary Sources of Vitamin C

Rich sources are amla (Indian gooseberry) (700 mg/100 g), guava (300 mg/100 g), lime, lemon and green leafy vegetables.

### Requirement of Vitamin C

Recommended daily allowance is 75 mg/day (equal to 50 mL orange juice). During pregnancy, lactation and in aged people requirement may be 100 mg/day.

### Therapeutic Use of Vitamin C

- Vitamin C is used as an adjuvant in infections. Beneficial effect of ascorbic acid is reported in the treatment of tuberculosis, when plasma level is kept near to saturation point. Clinical dose is 500 mg per day.
- Because of its power to *heal wounds,* vitamin C has been recommended for treatment of ulcer, trauma and burns. Except in scurvy and sub-scorbutic conditions the therapeutic use of vitamin is not specific.

### Megadose of Vitamin C

Linus Pauling (Nobel laureate) advocated megadoses (2000–5000 mg) of vitamin to prevent infections. But there is no clear evidence to support this theory. Classical picture of scurvy did not include common cold or respiratory infections as major features. There is experimental evidence in animals that ageing process is prevented by megadoses of vitamin C.

### Toxicity of Vitamin C

Since it is a water soluble substance, excess vitamin C is excreted, and not accumulated in the body. However, more than 2000 mg of vitamin C daily for a long time can cause iron overload, because vitamin C helps in absorption of iron.

## MULTIPLE CHOICE QUESTIONS

1. **Nonessential amino acids:**
(a) Are not seen in tissue protein
(b) Could be synthesized in the body
(c) Have no role in body metabolism
(d) Have aromatic ring structure

2. **Digestive enzymes belong to the class:**
(a) Hydrolases (b) Ligases
(c) Lysases (d) Oxidoreductases

3. **Glucose and Galactose are:**
(a) Anomers b) Constituent of sucrose
(c) Diastereoisomers (d) Epimers

4. **The HMP shunt pathway is important for all the following EXCEPT:**
(a) Generation of ATP
(b) Fatty acid bio –synthesis
(c) Synthesis of reduced glutathione
(d) Synthesis of ribose

5. **Gluconeogenesis can proceed from all the following EXCEPT:**
(a) Pyruvate (b) Palmitic acid
(c) Propionyl CoA (d) Oxaloacetate

6. **Ammonia is traped in brain by:**
(a) Glutamine synthetase reaction
(b) Glutaminase reaction
(c) Urea synthesis cycle
(d) Glutamate dehydrogenase reaction

7. **The Methyl donor in methyl transfer reaction is:**
(a) Methyl cobalamine
(b) Methyl malonyl reaction
(c) S-adenosyl methionine
(d) S-adenosyl homhcystine

8. **Pellagra is a deficiency disorder of following vitamin:**
(a) Thiamine (b) Riboflavin
(c) Pyridoxine (d) Niacin

9. **All of the following are precursor of heme EXCEPT:**
(a) Porphobilinogen (b) Urobilinogen
(c) Uroporphyrinogen (d) Protoporphyrinogen

10. **Normal blood urea level is:**
(a) 3–4 mg (b) 4–8 mg
(c) 8–16 mg (d) 20–40 mg

11. **Serum LDL has been found to be increased in:**
(a) Obstructive jaundice
(b) Hepatitis jaundice
(c) Hemolytic jaundice
(d) Septicemia

12. **In many protein, the hydrogen bonding produces a regular coiled arrangement called:**
(a) Beta helix (b) Alpha helix
(c) Both a and b (d) None of the above

13. **Cellulose is made up of the molecules of:**
(a) Alpha glucose (b) Beta glucose
(c) Both a and b (d) None of the above

14. **The reaction involving succinyl CoA → succinate requires:**
(a) CDP (b) ADP
(c) GDP (d) NADP

15. **Tryptophan give rise to following EXCEPT:**
(a) Niacin (b) Melanin
(c) Alanine (d) Serotonin

16. **Cobalt is a constituent of:**
(a) Folic acid (b) Vitamin $B_{12}$
(c) Niacin (d) Biotin

17. **Lecithin contains a nitrogenous base named as:**
(a) Ethanolamine (b) Choline
(c) Inositol (d) All of the above

18. **Fatty acid synthesis takes place in the presence of coenzyme:**
(a) NAD+ (b) Reduced NAD
(c) NADP+ (d) Reduced NADP+

19. **Most of the coenzyme are derivatives of:**
(a) Water-soluble vitamin
(b) Fat soluble vitamin
(c) Protein
(d) Nucleic acid

20. **Bile acids are derived from:**
(a) Phospholipid (b) Triacylglycerol
(c) Fatty acid (d) Cholesterol

21. **The functionally active form of Vitamin D is:**
(a) Calcitriol (b) Cholecalciferol
(c) Ergocalciferol (d) Dehydrocholestrol

22. **Plasma membrane is made up of:**
(a) Lipid bilayer
(b) Protein bilayer
(c) Carbohydrate bilayer
(d) None of the these

23. **An example of disaccharide is:**
(a) Glucose (b) Fructose
(c) Lactose (d) Mannose

24. **Buffer system present in kidney is:**
(a) Hemoglobin buffer (b) Amino buffer
(c) Bicarbonate buffer (d) Phosphate buffer

25. **An example of Basic amino acid is:**
(a) Glycine (b) Leucine
(c) Lysine (d) Isoleucine

26. **An immunoglobin which can cross the placental barrier is:**
(a) Ig E (b) Ig M
(c) Ig A (d) Ig G

27. **One of the causes of metabolic acidosis is:**
(a) Hyperventilation (b) Hypoventilation
(c) Diabetes mellitus (d) None of the above

28. **Hetropolysaccharide which can be used as an anticoagulant is:**
(a) Chondroitin sulfate (b) Heparan sulfate
(c) Keratin sulfate (d) Heparin

**29. Transamination require coenzyme called:**
(a) Biotin
(b) Pyridoxal phosphate
(c) Acetyl CoA
(d) Tetrahydrofolate

**30. Oxidative deamination is catalyzed by:**
(a) Glutamate dehydrogenase
(b) Glutaminase
(c) Lactate dehydrogenase
(d) Glutamine synthases

**31. Which of the following bio-chemical pathway does not take place in mitochondria?**
(a) Electron transport chain
(b) Glycolysis
(c) TCA cycle
(d) Beta oxidation of fatty acid

**32. Which of the following is not an essential amino acid?**
(a) Tyrosine (b) Tryptophan
(c) Valine (d) Threonine

**33. Uric acid is a catabolic product formed from:**
(a) Puerile (b) Palmitic acid
(c) Adenine (d) Alanine

**34. The iron transport protein present in plasma is:**
(a) Ceruloplasmin (b) Lipoprotein
(c) Ferritin (d) Transferrin

**35. The total number of ATP produced for complete oxidative phosphorylation:**
(a) 96 (b) 110
(c) 131 (d) 36

**36. The triglycerides in plasma are mainly transported as:**
(a) Very low density lipoprotein
(b) High density lipoprotein
(c) Low density lipoprotein
(d) Lipoprotein

**37. The end product of glycolytic pathway under anaerobic condition is mainly:**
(a) Lactate
(b) Citrate
(c) Glyceraldehyde-3 phosphate
(d) Fructose-1,6 Biphosphate

**38. The cholesterol and ketone bodies are synthesized from which common precursor:**
(a) Succinyl CoA (b) Malonyl CoA
(c) Acetyl CoA (d) Oxaloacetate

**39. Hemolysis can occur on administration of certain antimalarial in an individual with deficiency of:**
(a) Glucose-6 – phosphate
(b) Glucose-6 – phosphate dehydrogenase
(c) Glucose-6 – phosphate isomerase
(d) Glyceraldehydes 3-phosphate dehydrogenase

**40. Absence of an essential amino acid from adequate diet will lead to:**
(a) Positive nitrogen balance
(b) Negative nitrogen balance
(c) Nitrogen balance at equilibrium
(d) None of the above

**41. The main function of mitochondria is:**
(a) Electron transfer (b) Fat synthesis
(c) Protein synthesis (d) Oxidation only

**42. Lipotropic factors are all EXCEPT:**
(a) Betaine (b) Pre Beta lipoprotein
(c) Methionine (d) Choline

**43. Before pyruvic acid enter the TCA cycle it must be converted to:**
(a) Citrate (b) Alpha-ketoglutarate
(c) Lactate (d) Acetyl CoA

**44. Cytochrome oxidase is inhibited by:**
(a) Rotenone (b) Cyanide
(c) BAL (d) Selenium

**45. Rate limiting step in cholesterol biosynthesis is:**
(a) Thiokinase
(b) Mevalonate kinase
(c) HMG CoA reductase
(d) HMG CoA synthase

**46. Ketosis is ascribed in part to:**
(a) Slow down in fat metabolism
(b) Overproduction of acetyl CoA
(c) Underproduction of acetyl CoA
(d) Over utilization of glucose

**47. Vitamin functioning as reducing agent:**
(a) Cyanocobalamin (b) Folic acid
(c) Ascorbic acid (d) Thiamine

**48. The major site of urea synthesis:**
(a) Brain (b) Kidney
(c) Liver (d) Muscle

**49. The protein rich in hydroxyproline is:**
(a) Prolamine (b) Procollagen
(c) Collagen (d) Proinsuline

**50. The powerhouse of cell is:**
(a) Golgi apparatus (b) Mitochondria
(c) Ribosome (d) Nucleus

**51. The passage of water and gases through membrane occurs by:**
(a) Facilitated diffusion (b) Active transport
(c) Co-transport (d) Passive diffusion

**52. Deficiency of vitamin C leads to:**
(a) Scurvy
(b) The abnormality of beriberi
(c) Osteomalacia
(d) Pellagra

**53. In children deficiency of vitamin D leads to:**
(a) Xeropthalmia (b) Anemia
(c) Rickets (d) Night blindness

**54. Wilson disease is caused due to abnormality in metabolism of:**
(a) Copper (b) Chromium
(c) Iron (d) Iodine

**55. Storage form of lipid in body is:**
(a) Cholesterol (b) Phospholipid
(c) Triacylglycerol (d) Free fatty acid

56. **Major source of ammonia produced by the kidney:**
(a) Leucine
(b) Glycine
(c) Alamine
(d) Glutamine

57. **Zinc containing enzyme is:**
(a) Carbonic anhydrous
(b) Tyrosinase
(c) Cytochrome oxidase
(d) Peroxidase

58. **At the pH 7.4, the ratio of .............. buffer is 20:1 :**
(a) Bicarbonate buffer
(b) Phosphate buffer
(c) Protein buffer
(d) None of the above

59. **Selenium is an integral component of:**
(a) Alkaline phosphate
(b) Pyruvate carboxylase
(c) Glutathione peroxide
(d) Thiokinase

60. **Site of final stage of protein synthesis:**
(a) Ribosome
(b) Golgi bodies
(c) Peroxisome
(d) Endoplasmic reticulate

61. **The function of nucleus is:**
(a) Transmission of genetic material
(b) Energy release
(c) Storage of protein
(d) Excretion of waste

62. **One of the following is ketose sugar:**
(a) Glucose (b) Galactose
(c) Fructose (d) Ribose

63. **Cholesterol is:**
(a) Simple lipid
(b) Derived lipid
(c) Glycolipid
(d) Phospholipid

64. **Basic protein is:**
(a) Albumin (b) Globulin
(c) Histone (d) Glutelin

65. **Daily requirement of vitamin A:**
(a) 3 IU (b) 30 IU
(c) 300 IU (d) 3000 IU

66. **Biologically active form of vitamin $B_6$:**
(a) Pyridoxine (b) Pyridoxal phosphate
(c) Pyridoxamine (d) Cobalamin

67. **Which of the following conjugate protein contain lipid as prosthetic group?**
(a) Phosphoprotein
(b) Lipoprotein
(c) Nucleoprotein
(d) Chromoprotein

68. **Following cell organelle is rich in hydrolytic enzyme:**
(a) Lysosomes
(b) Ribosomes
(c) Endoplasmic reticulate
(d) Golgi apparatus

69. **The precursor of prostaglandin is:**
(a) Arachidonic acid
(b) Oleic acid
(c) Linoleic acid
(d) Linolenic acid

70. **Enolase is inhibited by fluoride is an example of:**
(a) Competitive inhibition
(b) Non-competitive irreversible inhibition
(c) Allosteric inhibition
(d) Non-competitive reversible inhibition

71. **In hemoglobin, iron is linked to globin by which amino acid.**
(a) Arginine
(b) Lysine
(c) Histidine
(d) Glycine

72. **Which of the following fat soluble vitamin can be synthesized by intrinsic bacteria?**
(a) Vitamin A
(b) Vitamin D
(c) Vitamin E
(d) Vitamin K

73. **Iron is transported in form of:**
(a) Ferritin
(b) Hemosiderin
(c) Siderophillin
(d) Transferring

74. **Glucose enter RBC's by:**
(a) Passive diffusion
(b) Facilitated transport
(c) Active transport
(d) Endocytosis

75. **The principal of electrophoresis is based on:**
(a) Charge
(b) Adsorption
(c) Partition
(d) Solubility

## ANSWERS

| | | | | | | | |
|---|---|---|---|---|---|---|---|
| **1.** | (b) | **21.** | (a) | **41.** | (d) | **61.** | (a) |
| **2.** | (a) | **22.** | (a) | **42.** | (b) | **62.** | (c) |
| **3.** | (c) | **23.** | (c) | **43.** | (d) | **63.** | (b) |
| **4.** | (b) | **24.** | (c) | **44.** | (b) | **64.** | (a) |
| **5.** | (b) | **25.** | (c) | **45.** | (c) | **65.** | (d) |
| **6.** | (d) | **26.** | (d) | **46.** | (b) | **66.** | (b) |
| **7.** | (a) | **27.** | (c) | **47.** | (c) | **67.** | (b) |
| **8.** | (d) | **28.** | (d) | **48.** | (c) | **68.** | (a) |
| **9.** | (a) | **29.** | (b) | **49.** | (c) | **69.** | (a) |
| **10.** | (d) | **30.** | (a) | **50.** | (b) | **70.** | (b) |
| **11.** | (a) | **31.** | (b) | **51.** | (d) | **71.** | (c) |
| **12.** | (c) | **32.** | (a) | **52.** | (a) | **72.** | (d) |
| **13.** | (b) | **33.** | (a) | **53.** | (c) | **73.** | (d) |
| **14.** | (c) | **34.** | (d) | **54.** | (a) | **74.** | (b) |
| **15.** | (a) | **35.** | (d) | **55.** | (c) | **75.** | (d) |
| **16.** | (b) | **36.** | (a) | **56.** | (d) | | |
| **17.** | (a) | **37.** | (a) | **57.** | (a) | | |
| **18.** | (c) | **38.** | (c) | **58.** | (d) | | |
| **19.** | (a) | **39.** | (b) | **59.** | (c) | | |
| **20.** | (d) | **40.** | (b) | **60.** | (a) | | |

# QUICK REVIEW

## Medical-surgical Nursing Review and Multiple Choice Questions

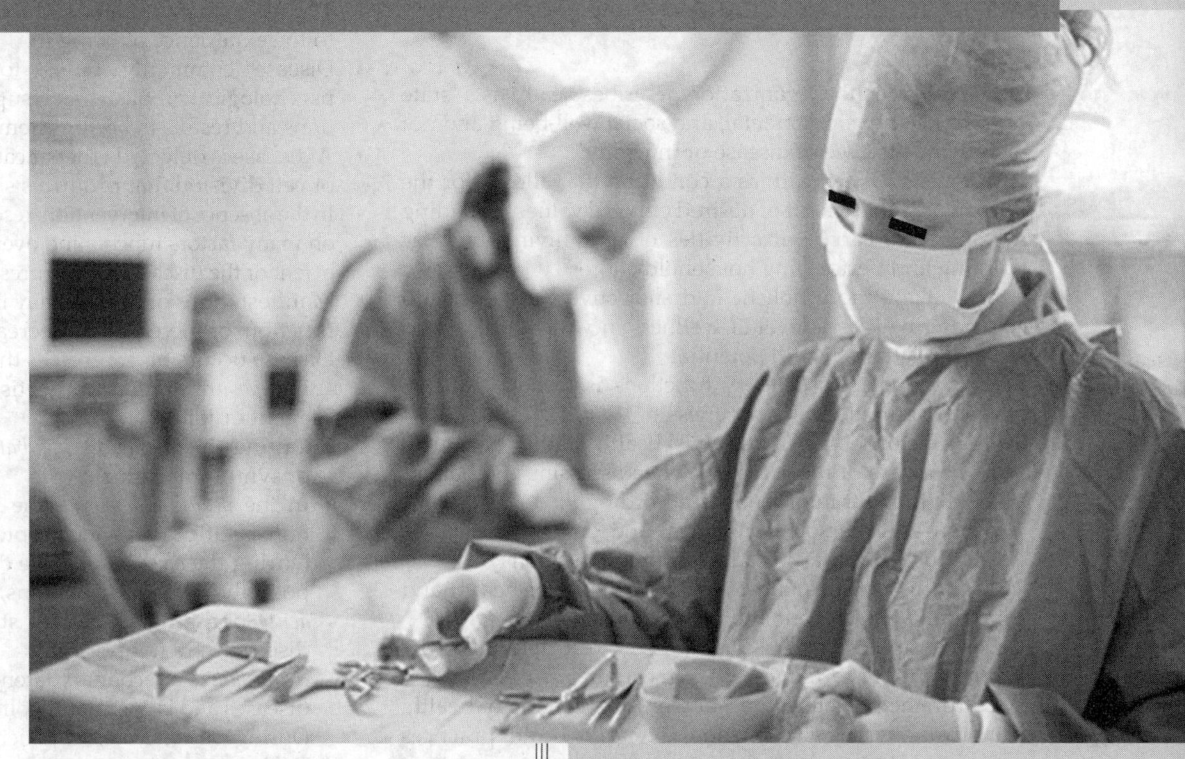

### HIGHLIGHTS

- Health and Wellness Care
- Nursing Process
- Wound Healing and Wound Care
- Disruption of Homeostasis
- Cardiovascular Disorders
- Hematologic Disorders
- Respiratory Disorders
- Gastrointestinal Disorders
- Renal and Urinary Tract Disorders
- Reproductive System Disorders
- Immune System Disorders
- Eye, Ear and Nose Disorders
- Multiple Choice Questions

# Medical-Surgical Nursing

## HEALTH AND WELLNESS CARE

### Health

- The World Health Organization describes health as a 'state of complete physical, mental, and social well-being and not merely the absence of disease or infirmity'
- Sociologists view health as a condition that allows for the pursuit and enjoyment of desired cultural values, including the ability to carry out activities of daily living, such as working and performing household chores
- Others take a more holistic and subjective view of health and describe it as a level of wellness in which a person is striving to attain his full potential
- One of the nurse's primary functions is to help patients reach an optimal level of wellness
- Several factors affect a patient's health status, the nurse must be aware of these factors when assessing the patient and plan to tailor interventions accordingly:
  - Genetics—a person's biological and genetic makeup—can cause illness and lead to chronic conditions
  - Cognitive abilities affect a person's view of health and his ability to seek out and use resources
  - Demographics such as age and sex can determine the prevalence of certain diseases in certain groups
  - Culture helps determine a person's perception of health, motivations to seek care and the types of health practices performed
  - Lifestyle choices and environment such as diet, level of activity and exposure to toxins can influence a patient's health
  - Health beliefs and practices can affect health positively or negatively
  - Previous health experiences can influence a patient's reaction to illness and the decision to seek care
  - Spirituality affects a person's view of illness and health care
  - Support systems affect the degree to which a person adapts and copes with a situation.

### Illness

- Illness can be defined as a sickness or deviation from a healthy state, it is considered a broader concept than disease.
- Illness occurs when a person is no longer in a state of perceived 'normal' health.
- Illness also encompasses how a patient interprets a disease's source and importance, how that disease affects his behavior and relationships with others and how the patient tries to remedy the problem.
- The nurse must understand the meaning a person attaches to the experience of being ill.
- Disease commonly refers to a specific biological or psychological problem that is supported by clinical manifestations and results in body system or organ malfunction.
- A disease is detected when it causes a change in metabolism or cell division that produces signs and symptoms.
- In the absence of intervention, resolution of the disease depends on many factors functioning over a period of time such as the extent of the disease and the presence of other diseases.
- Manifestations of disease may include hypofunction, hyper function, or increased or decreased mechanical function.
- Disease occurs or progresses through stages:
  - In *exposure* or *injury*, target tissue is exposed to a causative agent or injury
  - During the *latency* or *incubation period*, no evident signs or symptoms occur
  - In the *prodromal period*, the patient generally has mild, nonspecific signs and symptoms
  - During the *acute* phase, the disease is at its full intensity, possibly with complications, this is called the *subclinical acute* phase if the patient still functions as though the disease were not present
  - *Remission* is a secondary latency phase that occurs in some diseases and is commonly followed by another acute phase
  - During *convalescence*, the patient progresses toward recovery
  - During *recovery*, the patient returns to health or normal functioning with no remaining signs or symptoms of disease.
- Illness can be acute or chronic
  - *Acute illness* refers to a disease or condition that has a relatively abrupt onset, high intensity and short duration, if no complications occur, most acute illnesses end in full recovery, with a patient returning to his previous or similar level of functioning.
  - *Chronic illness* refers to a condition that typically has a slower onset, less intensity and a longer duration than acute illness, with a patient typically experiencing periods of exacerbation, the nurse's goal is to help the patient regain and maintain the highest possible level of health, although a patient may fail to return to his previous level of functioning.

### Health and Wellness Promotion

- Good health practices have the benefit of fewer illnesses, a longer life span and lower health care costs.
- Health promotion involves teaching people good health practices and finding ways to help them correct their poor health practices.

- *Healthy People 2020* sets forth major comprehensive health goals for the United States with the aim of reducing mortality and morbidity in all ages.
  - Increase the quality and years of life
  - Eliminate health disparities among segments of the population such as those that occur by gender, race, education, disabilities, geographic location and sexual orientation.
- Health indicators used to measure the health of the nation are physical activity, tobacco use, responsible sexual behavior, mental health, being overweight or obese, substance abuse, injury and violence, environmental quality, immunization, and access to health care.
- The components of health promotion are self-responsibility, stress reduction and management, physical fitness, and nutritional awareness.
  - Self-responsibility is based on the theory that the individual has a responsibility to control his life and can make choices to live a healthy lifestyle or not
  - Stress reduction and management recognizes the role stress can play in disease and focuses on the importance of managing stress.
  - Physical fitness has become increasingly important as the nation struggles with obesity.
  - Nutritional awareness involves understanding the importance of a healthy diet and recognizing the role diet can play in disease or wellness.

## NURSING PROCESS

### History of the Nursing Process

- In the 1970s, the American Nurses Association (ANA) mandated that the nursing process be part of nursing practice and instituted a five-step process (assessment, diagnosis, planning, implementation, and evaluation).
- In 1982, the North American Nursing Diagnosis Association, now known as NANDA International (NANDA-I) was established to develop, review and update nursing diagnoses, this organization meets every 2 years.

### Purpose of the Nursing Process

- The nursing process provides a basis for problem-solving, clinical decisions and individualized patient care.
- It uses the scientific method of observation, measurement, data collection and data analysis to evaluate the needs of patients and their families.
- The nursing process provides an organized and universal method of communication for nurses in education, practice and research.
- Through the nursing process, nurses have adopted a body of knowledge that is unique to nursing this knowledge encompasses illness, illness prevention and health maintenance.

### Standards of Practice

- The Standards of Clinical Nursing Practice are directly related to the nursing process.
  - Standard I ('The nurse collects patient health data') relates to step 1 of the nursing process (assessment)
  - Standard II ('The nurse analyzes the assessment data in determining diagnosis') relates to step 2 of the nursing process (diagnosis)
  - Standard III ('The nurse identifies expected outcomes individualized to the patient') and Standard IV ('The nurse develops a care plan that prescribes interventions to attain expected outcomes') relate to step 3 of the nursing process (planning)
  - Standard V ('The nurse implements the interventions in the care plan') relates to step 4 of the nursing process (implementation)
  - Standard VI ('The nurse evaluates the patient's progress toward outcomes') relates to step 5 of the nursing process (evaluation)
- These clinical standards use the steps of the nursing process to help achieve the standards of practice that have been set forth by state nurse practice acts and the ANA standards of professional performance as well as the Academy of Medical-Surgical Nurses Scope and Standards of Nursing Practice
- These varying standards help assure quality nursing care and provide the gauge by which to measure quality.

### Steps of the Nursing Process

- Assessment
  - Assessment is the collection and organization of data
  - Data collection involves the formation of a database from the patient interview, patient history, subjective data (what the patient says or believes), objective data (vital signs, laboratory results), and physical assessment (inspection, palpation, percussion and auscultation)
  - Data organization involves clustering related findings, reviewing the amount and completeness of data and evaluating it through comparison with normal or baseline data
  - Data documentation involves recording all data on the patient's chart and comparing it with research and medical findings.
- Diagnosis
  - Diagnosis is the identification of actual or potential health problems as indicated by the assessment data, it is also defined as the responses to actual or potential health problems
  - The diagnostic statement consists of three parts: identifying the problem or need, identifying the cause of the problem or need ('related to'), and identifying related signs and symptoms ('as evidenced by')
  - A sample diagnostic statement is 'ineffective breathing pattern related to fatigue, as evidenced by shortness of breath, shallow respirations, and tachycardia'
  - Nursing diagnoses are organized in a taxonomy based on human response patterns. They also may be grouped by functional health patterns (health perception–health management, nutritional-metabolic, elimination, activity-exercise, sleep-rest, cognitive-perceptual, self-perception–self-concept, role-relationship, sexuality-reproductive, coping–stress tolerance and value-belief)

- Planning
  - Planning involves determining expected outcomes, setting priorities, establishing goals, selecting appropriate interventions and documenting care.
  - Priorities can be based on Maslow's hierarchy of needs (in which physical needs, such as oxygen and safety, take priority over psychosocial needs, such as self-esteem and self-actualization) or other factors.
  - Goals are established by identifying the desired outcomes, short-term and long-term goals can be defined and are measurable and time-specific.
  - Specific nursing interventions are selected to develop an individualized care plan, interventions should specify times, frequencies and amounts.
  - The care plan is documented so that all health care team members know the patient's individualized plan.
- Implementation
  - Implementation involves providing actual care to the patient.
  - Data collection and assessment continue during this step.
- Evaluation
  - To provide effective care, the goals, outcomes, and appropriateness of interventions must be evaluated on an ongoing basis in relation to the care plan.
  - During evaluation, the care plan is revised as needed in terms of nursing diagnoses, goals, outcomes, and interventions.

## ROLES OF THE NURSE

### General Information

- Nursing's goal is to promote, restore and maintain the health of people who are regarded as holistic beings
- Although the expectations for providing nursing care have expanded and increased, this goal has remained constant.

### Roles

- In adapting to changing health care needs, nurses assume various roles in health care settings
- Each role has specific responsibilities, but some facets of these roles are common to all nursing positions
- Medical-surgical nurses are not only caregivers but also educators, advocates, coordinators, agents of change, discharge planners and researchers
- Medical-surgical nurses as caregivers conduct independent assessments and implement patient care based on knowledge and skills and collaborate with other members of the health care team to implement and evaluate that care.

## PRACTICE ROLES OF THE NURSE

No matter what the practice setting, the medical-surgical nurse assumes various roles.

### Caregiver

- As a caregiver, the nurse assesses the patient, analyzes his needs, develops nursing diagnoses and plans, delivers and evaluates nursing interventions and patient outcomes.

### Advocate

- As an advocate, the nurse helps the patient and his family members interpret information from other health care providers and make decisions about health-related needs.
- The nurse ensures the health, welfare, and safety of the patient.
- The nurse makes every attempt to respect the patient's decisions and to communicate those wishes to other members of the health care team.
- The nurse accepts the patient's decisions, even if they differ from the decisions the nurse would make.

### Educator

- With a greater emphasis on health promotion and illness prevention, the nurse's role as an educator becomes increasingly important.
- As an educator, the nurse assesses learning needs, plans and implements teaching strategies to meet those needs, and evaluates the effectiveness of the teaching.
- The nurse employs interpersonal communication skills and principles of adult learning to provide patient teaching.
- The nurse considers the educational, cultural, and socio-economic background of the patient when planning and providing patient teaching.

### Coordinator

- As a coordinator, the nurse practices leadership and manages time, people, resources and the environment in which the nurse provides care.
- The nurse carries out these tasks by directing, delegating, and coordinating activities.
- The nurse plays an important role in coordinating the efforts of all team members to meet the patient's goals and may conduct team conferences to facilitate communication among team members.

### Discharge Planner

- As a discharge planner, the nurse assesses the patient's needs for discharge starting at the time of admission, including the patient's support systems and living situation.
- The nurse links the patient with available community resources.

### Change Agent

- As a change agent, the nurse works with the patient to address his health concerns and with staff members to address organizational and community concerns.
- The nurse employs a knowledge of change theory, which provides a framework for understanding the dynamics of change, human responses to change and strategies for effecting change.
- The nurse serves as a role model in the community, assisting consumers in bringing about change to improve the environment, work conditions, or other factors that affect health.
- The nurse works to bring about change through legislation by helping to shape and support the laws that mandate the use of safety seats and motorcycle helmets.

### Researcher

- As a researcher, the nurse takes part in nursing research, which promotes growth in the science of nursing and develops a scientific basis for nursing practice and applies research findings to nursing practice.
- Even if not trained in nursing research methods, the nurse participates by remaining alert for nursing problems and asking questions about care practices.
- The nurse improves nursing care by incorporating research findings into nursing practice and by communicating research to others.

## NURSE PRACTICE ACTS

### State Statutes

- Each state has statutes, or Nurse Practice Acts, that define the levels of nursing (for example, advanced practice nurse [nurse practitioner, clinical nurse specialist, certified nurse midwife, certified nurse anesthetist], registered nurse, licensed practical nurse, and nursing assistant), they are the most important laws governing nurses and nursing practice.
  - Most statutes set licensure requirements for each level of nursing
  - They may prescribe minimum educational qualifications for licensure
- Regulatory boards created by the Nurse Practice Acts govern nursing practice in the state.
- Nurse Practice Acts may provide for a board of nursing accreditation and approval of educational programs in the state.

### Disciplinary Actions

- The state board of nursing may take action against a nurse who violates the Nurse Practice Act or the licensing board's regulations
  - A nurse can be disciplined for habitual substance abuse affecting the ability to practice, fraud or deceitin obtaining a nursing license, incompetence, criminal felony conviction and unprofessional conduct
  - Other actions or conditions that would inhibit the nurse's safe and effective nursing practice also are grounds for discipline.
- A licensed nurse has a limited property right to her license
  - The state must follow specific procedures to determine if a nurse's license should be revoked to protect public safety.
  - The licensee must be notified of the complaint must have an opportunity to respond to the complaint and present evidence and must be allowed to have a hearing before an impartial panel and to appeal the panel's decision.

### Possible Sanctions

- The nurse's license may be revoked
- The license may be suspended for a predetermined time
- The license may be suspended for an undetermined time, and the nurse may reapply after completing a course of study or treatment
- Conditions may be placed on the license to limit the nurse's practice
- The nurse may voluntarily surrender the license or enter into a consensual agreement with the nursing board, agreeing to limitations on the license or supervision of practice for a time
- The nurse may receive a disciplinary warning or reprimand.

## LEGAL CONCEPTS OF RESPONSIBILITY

### Individuals

- In the absence of mental or legal incapacity, a person is responsible for his own actions; a nurse, as a professional, is legally accountable for her nursing assessment and care
- Although the nurse may be individually accountable, other people or entities also may be legally responsible for a nurse's negligence.

### Employers and Supervisors

- An employer is automatically liable for its employees' actions within the scope of their employment, the employer is thereby encouraged to hire competent employees
- A nurse in a management or supervisory position may be liable for the actions of a negligent nurse under her supervision, liability can result if the supervisor did not adequately assess the nurse's competence or the assignment's requirements, did not adequately supervise the nurse's performance, or knew the nurse's limitations and did not provide adequate training or staffing.

### Independent Contractors

- An independent contractor is one who contracts with another to do a specific job, in nursing, the private duty nurse who is employed by an agency but hired on a per diem basis by a health care facility is the most common example of an independent contractor.
- The independent contractor's actions are not directly controlled by the employer, the contractor has independent discretion in performing the job.
- The employer may not be liable for the negligent actions of an independent contractor unless the employer knew or should have known of the independent contractor's incompetence.

### Corporations

- A health care facility is obligated to carefully monitor the credentials and competence of employees and independent contractors.
- A health care facility that does not ensure its workers' competence may be liable for injuries caused by the workers' negligence.

## POSSIBLE CIVIL ACTIONS

### Torts

- A tort is a civil action for damages for injury to a person, property or reputation.
- Torts are classified as unintentional or intentional.

### Unintentional Torts

- *Professional negligence* and *professional malpractice* are the most common legal claims against nurses
  - Negligence is the failure to exercise the degree of care that a person of ordinary prudence would exercise under the same circumstances, e.g. if a nurse notices water on the floor of a room and does not wipe it up and the water causes a patient to fall and injure himself, this constitutes negligence
  - The plaintiff in a negligence suit must prove that the nurse's actions caused harm
  - Professional malpractice or professional negligence requires a plaintiff to introduce proof of duty, breach of duty, proximate cause, and damages or harm; proof of the nurse's standard of care is critical to establishing the first three elements
  - Unlike negligence cases, professional negligence cases require expert testimony as to the duty of care, its breach, and its causal relationship to the injury
- A nurse also can be sued for *negligent infliction of emotional distress*
  - In many states, a plaintiff can be awarded damages for severe emotional distress resulting from a nurse's negligent actions
  - Some states require that the plaintiff have physical manifestations of the emotional distress such as palpitations, gastric discomfort, or insomnia.

### Intentional Torts

- *Assault* is an act that places a patient in fear of harmful or offensive touching
- *Battery* is touching a patient without justification or permission
- *Defamation* results when a nurse communicates false information verbally (slander) or in writing (libel) about a patient that damages the patient's reputation or causes the patient to be shunned or avoided by the community
- *Invasion of privacy* occurs when a nurse gives unauthorized access to the patient or information about the patient; taking photographs of a patient without permission is an invasion of privacy
- *Fraud* and *misrepresentation* are false or misleading statements by the nurse that the patient relies on to his detriment
- *False imprisonment* is unjustifiable restriction of patient, movement
- *Intentional infliction of emotional distress* results when a nurse's actions produce distress so severe that no reasonable person could be expected to endure it.

### Contract Actions

- Contract actions are determined by whether the parties performed obligations agreed to in a contract
- A breach of contract results when one party fails to perform as required by the contract
- Nurses are most commonly involved in employment contracts and malpractice insurance contracts.

## POSSIBLE DEFENSES TO A HEALTH CARE NEGLIGENCE SUIT

### Comparative and Contributory Negligence

- With comparative negligence (the more common defense), the jury compares the degree of negligence of the parties or of various defendants and apportions damages (i.e. compensation or indemnification) accordingly
- With contributory negligence, because the plaintiff's conduct contributes to the cause of his injury and falls below the standard by which individuals are expected to conform, he cannot recover damages, even though the defendant violated a duty of care to the plaintiff and would be liable.

### Statutes of Limitation

- A statute of limitation sets a time limit within which the legal action must be brought; a nurse cannot be sued for negligence if the claim is made after the time limit expires
- Statutes of limitation for health care negligence are established by the state legislature
- These statutes may not apply in some cases, such as those involving fraudulent concealment of negligence or later discovery of negligence.

### Good Samaritan Laws

- All states have Good Samaritan laws to protect people who render assistance at the scene of an emergency
- Some statutes protect all citizens; others cover only specified health care providers
- Those protected under Good Samaritan laws are liable only for grossly negligent acts.

### Statutory Defenses

- Many states have statutes that prescribe special procedures for health care negligence cases
- A suit may be dismissed if the statutory requirements are not met.

## PROFESSIONAL LIABILITY INSURANCE FOR NURSES

### Types of Policies

- A *claims-made* policy provides coverage for claims made during the policy period
- An *occurrence policy* provides coverage for negligence that occurs during the policy period.

### Obligations of the Insurer and the Insured

- Insurers must provide and pay for legal counsel to defend the nurse in the lawsuit and must pay damages (within coverage limits) for which the nurse is judged liable
- The nurse must notify the insurer that a claim has been made and must assist as needed in preparing the defense.

## PATIENT'S BILL OF RIGHTS

### Self-determination

- Self-determination is often used synonymously with autonomy

- It means having a form of personal liberty to choose and implement one's own decisions, free from deceit, duress, constraint, or coercion
- It involves the right of patients to decide what will or will not happen to their bodies
- Basic elements of self-determination include the patient's ability to decide, the power to act upon his own decision, and respect for the individual autonomy of others
- Although self-determination is often addressed in relation to death and dying, it concerns all aspects of consent and its refusal
- To practice this right, the individual must be competent to make his own decisions about accepting or refusing treatment
- Some states uphold the patient's in orally expressed desires, provided they are documented, including the patient's awareness of consequences of his actions
- The Patient Self-Determination Act has three basic premises:
  1. Patients who are informed of their rights are more likely to take advantage of them
  2. If patients are more actively involved in decisions about their medical care, then that care will more closely respond to their needs
  3. Patients may choose care that is less costly.

### Informed Consent

- Informed consent is the voluntary authorization by a patient to a care provider to do something to the patient
- Some states accept oral forms of consent as being equally as valid as written consent
- Contents of an informed consent include the procedural information, associated risks and benefits, alternatives to the procedure, and the name of the person who will perform the procedure
- Generally, physicians have the responsibility to obtain informed consents
- Nurses can witness and have the responsibility to advocate for the patient to ensure that all criteria for autonomous decision making are met
- Four exceptions to consents are emergency situations, therapeutic privilege, patient waiver, and prior patient knowledge.

### Living Wills

- Living wills, or health care directives, are directives from competent individuals to medical personnel regarding treatment they wish to receive
- A living will takes effect when the previously competent person becomes sick and can no longer make decisions for himself
- It typically contains information about the conservator or health care agent, the patient's code status, and the patient's desire for organ donation; it may also contain other information
- Because living wills are not typically legally enforced, medical practitioners may choose to abide by them or to ignore them as they see fit
- There is no protection for the practitioner against criminal or civil liabilities for proceeding under a living will's directions.

### Durable Power of Attorney

- Durable (or medical) power of attorney for health care allows competent patients to appoint a surrogate to make decisions for them in the event that they lose competence
- The power includes the right to ask questions, select and remove physicians from the patient's care, assess risks and complications, and select treatments.

## ETHICAL ASPECTS OF NURSING

### General Information

- Ethics is a branch of philosophy that examines values, actions and choices to determine right and wrong
  - Nursing ethics is part of normative ethics, a type of ethics that is based on the criteria by which people make moral judgments
  - As the basis for professional codes of ethics, ethical theories attempt to provide a system of principles and rules for resolving ethical dilemmas
  - The American Nurses Association's 'Code of Ethics for Nurses' provides guidance for carrying out nursing responsibilities consistent with the ethical obligations of the profession
- Morality involves rules of conduct about right and wrong
  - It is based on norms of conduct determined by society
  - Society's moral codes guide what people ought to do, professional codes such as the code of ethics for nurses, communicate the goals and ideals of a profession
- Although *ethics* and *morals* are theoretically distinct terms, they're used interchangeably to describe right and wrong actions.

### Professional Code of Ethics for Nurses

- Nurses have a contract with society to behave in accordance with rules dictated by society and the nursing profession
- Whereas Nurse Practice Acts set the legal standards for safe nursing practice, the code for nurses delineates nursing's moral ideals, provides guidelines for ethically principled behavior, and holds nurses morally accountable for their actions.

### Ethical Theories

- *Deontology* holds that an Act's moral rightness is determined by the inherent duty one has to act in accordance with rules and principles
  - It presumes that the rightness of an Act is determined by the intent to conform with a moral rule, not by the consequences of the Act
  - Immanuel Kant is a principal deontologic theorist
- *Utilitarianism* holds that an Act's moral rightness is determined by its ability to produce good consequences and to avoid harmful ones
  - It presumes that the rightness of an Act is determined by its consequences, not by the person's intent
  - John Stuart Mill and Jeremy Bentham are utilitarian theorists.

### Ethical Principles

- *Autonomy* is a state of being self-regulating, self-defining, and self-reliant
  - Immanuel Kant believed that all people are worthy of unconditional positive regard (Kantian principle of 'respect for persons'); he also introduced the concept of freedom of will
  - John Stuart Mill believed that a person should be respected for his freedom of thought and action
  - The principle of autonomy, that actions and choices should not be restricted by others, has many clinical applications
- A patient's right to informed consent derives from the principle of autonomy
- The principle of 'respect for persons' dictates that a patient has a right to treatment and a right to refuse treatment
- Advance directives, such as living wills and durable powers of attorney for health care, maintain a patient's autonomy
- *Beneficence* is a moral principle that holds that individuals should promote good
  - Based on the duty to help, beneficence requires nurses to act in their patients' best interests
  - This principle may create a duty when the law does not
  - This principle often conflicts with the principle of autonomy—e.g. a nurse may violate the autonomy principle by preventing a patient from acting on suicidal impulses (a beneficent act)
- *Nonmaleficence* mandates that a nurse does not harm others or put them at risk for harm; this principle causes many debates about euthanasia, withholding and withdrawing treatment, and the use of artificial hydration and nutrition
- *Justice* is a moral concept that maintains equals should be treated equally and those who are not equal should be treated according to their differences; it is used when there are scarcities or competition for resources or benefits
- *Veracity* obligates the nurse to be truthful with patients
- *Privacy* requires the nurse to restrict access to the patient appropriately; *confidentiality* requires the nurse to deny access to information about the patient
- *Fidelity* refers to a nurse's faithfulness in keeping a promise; in practice, the nurse makes an implied promise to care for a patient.

### Ethical Dilemmas

- An ethical dilemma arises when a nurse must choose between competing claims or select from equally undesirable alternatives
- When faced with an ethical dilemma, the nurse should apply a rational decision-making process by gathering all the facts, identifying the problem or dilemma, listing possible actions, choosing the most appropriate action, and evaluating the results of the action.

### Code of Ethics for Nurses

The American Nurses Association's 'Code of Ethics for Nurses' provides ethical standards of conduct and guidelines for all aspects of nursing practice.

- The nurse, in all professional relationships, practices with compassion and respect for the inherent dignity, worth, and uniqueness of every individual, unrestricted by considerations of social or economic status, personal attributes, or the nature of health problems.
- The nurse's primary commitment is to the patient, whether an individual, family, group, or community.
- The nurse promotes, advocates for, and strives to project the health, safety, and rights of the patient.
- The nurse is responsible and accountable for individual nursing practice and determines the appropriate delegation of tasks consistent with the nurse's obligation to provide optimum patient care.
- The nurse owes the same duties to self as to others, including the responsibility to preserve integrity and safety, to maintain competence, and to continue personal and professional growth.
- The nurse participates in establishing, maintaining, and improving health care environments and conditions of employment conducive to the provision of quality health care and consistent with the values of the profession through individual and collective action.
- The nurse participates in the advancement of the profession through contributions to practice, education, administration, and knowledge development.
- The nurse collaborates with other health professionals and the public in promoting community, national and international efforts to meet health needs.
- The profession of nursing, as represented by associations and their members, is responsible for articulating nursing values, for maintaining the integrity of the profession and its practice, and for shaping social policy.

## COMMON LEGAL CONCERNS FOR NURSES

Three areas commonly cause legal problems for nurses—confidentiality, consent to treatment, and the right to refuse treatment.

### Confidentiality

Confidential information is any information that the patient communicates to the nurse or practitioner for diagnosis or treatment with the expectation that it won't be disclosed. Nurses have an ethical and legal duty to avoid disclosing such confidential information to unauthorized people who aren't involved in the patient's care and treatment. A nurse who discloses confidential information without the patient's permission may be subject to a lawsuit or disciplinary action for unprofessional conduct. The nurse can be liable for invasion of privacy, defamation, intentional or negligent infliction of emotional distress or breach of an implied contract of secrecy. Some states provide a statutory penalty against health care providers who violate the patient's right to confidentiality. However, confidential information can be disclosed under certain circumstances. For example, the nurse must disclose such information when authorized by a patient (but only to the extent authorized), when a patient is a danger to himself or others, or when required by law for a reportable communicable disease or suspected abuse. In some cases, the court may order disclosure of confidential patient information.

### Consent to Treatment

The law presumes that adults are legally capable of consenting to treatment. To provide a valid consent, a patient must be mentally capable of understanding the nature and consequences of treatment. Expressed consent is obtained orally or in writing; implied consent is obtained by the patient's voluntarily submitting to treatment. Medical treatment performed without a patient's expressed or implied consent may result in legal claims of battery or negligence. Therefore, informed consent should be obtained before a patient undergoes an invasive procedure, receives anesthesia or blood, or undergoes procedures that carry a significant risk of harm. Informed consent requires the health care provider (physician, nurse practitioner, physician assistant, nurse midwife) to provide appropriate information. The adequacy of this information is evaluated by two questions: Did the health care provider provide information that a reasonably competent health care provider in the same situation would provide? Did the patient receive sufficient information such that a reasonable person in the same circumstances could make an informed decision? If a patient receives appropriate information and refuses care or treatment against medical advice, the physician or health care provider is responsible for documenting that the informed consent conversation took place, the general facts discussed, and the patient's decision.

#### *Exceptions to Informed Consent*

Informed consent isn't required if a delay to obtain consent for emergency treatment would cause imminent harm that outweighs the risk of treatment, if the patient would be substantially harmed by disclosing the risks of treatment, if the patient waives the right to consent and asks not to be informed, or if compulsory treatment is mandated by law or a court order.

### Right to Refuse Treatment

Adults are presumed to be legally capable of refusing treatment. In fact, mentally competent patients with terminal conditions can refuse life-sustaining treatment without creating legal liability for their health care providers. The Patient Self-Determination Act of 1990 encourages persons to express their wishes about life-sustaining treatment should they become legally incapacitated. The Act requires health care facilities that participate in Medicare and Medicaid to develop programs to inform patients about advance directives, such as living wills and durable powers of attorney and do-not-resuscitate (DNR) orders. Under this Act, the health care facility must provide patients with written materials explaining their rights under their state laws to make decisions concerning medical care, including the right to accept or refuse treatment and the right to execute an advance directive. A living will expresses a patient's wishes about withholding or withdrawing life-sustaining treatment. A durable power of attorney designates a person to make health care decisions, including termination of life support, for a patient who can no longer do so. A DNR order authorizes health care personnel not to initiate resuscitative measures. The Patient Self-Determination Act specifically prohibits covered health care facilities from conditioning the provision of care or discriminating against an individual based on whether the individual has executed an advance directive. When a patient is no longer mentally capable of making health care decisions, a court order, statute, or law may authorize a surrogate decision maker to accept or refuse medical treatment for the patient based on the patient's prior documentation or expressed wishes.

## WOUND HEALING AND WOUND CARE

### Introduction

- Skin, the body's largest organ and the outer covering of the body, serves as a protective barrier against microorganisms
- The skin is subject to injury from various external and internal factors
  - *External factors* include extremes of heat and cold, mechanical forces such as pressure and shearing, allergens, chemicals, radiation, and excretions and secretions (for instance, from an ostomy or draining wound)
  - *Internal factors* include emaciation, drugs, altered circulation and impaired oxygen transport, altered metabolic state, and infections.

### Definitions

- *Angiogenesis* is the formation of new granulation vessels
- *Cellulitis* is the inflammation of cellular or connective tissue
- *Colonization* refers to the presence of bacteria that cause no local or systemic indications of infection
- *Dehiscence* is the separation of the layers of a surgical wound
- *Eschar* is thick, leathery, necrotic, devitalized tissue
- *Friction* is the mechanical force exerted when skin rubs against a coarse surface such as bed linens
- *Full thickness* describes a wound that involves skin loss with extensive destruction, tissue necrosis, or damage to muscle, bone, or supporting structures
- *Infection* is the invasion and multiplication of microorganisms in body tissue in a sufficient quantity (greater than 1 million organisms per gram of tissue) to overwhelm tissue defenses; an infection can produce purulent exudate, odor, erythema, warmth, tenderness, edema, pain, fever, and an elevated white blood cell (WBC) count
- *Maceration* is the softening of tissue by wetting or soaking; it can produce skin degeneration and disintegration if left uncontrolled
- *Partial thickness* describes a wound that involves damage to epidermal and, possibly, dermal skin layers
- *Sloughing* is the separation of necrotic tissue from viable tissue
- *Shearing* is trauma caused by tissue layers sliding against one another; it results in disruption or strangulation of blood vessels and can result in skin tear injuries
- A *wound* is any disruption to the anatomic or physiologic function of tissue.

## Types of Wounds

- An *acute* wound heals uneventfully within an expected time frame unless underlying systemic conditions interrupt the process; examples include surgical incisions and trauma wounds.
- A wound is *chronic* when underlying pathophysiology causes the wound or interferes with the course of healing; several types exist.

## Wound-Healing Process

A dynamic process that restores anatomic and functional integrity, wound healing works on a continuum from injury to healing.

- In *healing by primary intention,* the wound is surgically closed (such as with sutures, staples, glue, or Steri-Strips), and healing occurs by fibrous adhesion; granulation tissue is not apparent, and there's little or no scar tissue; examples include surgical wounds and superficial traumatic wounds.
- In *healing by secondary intention,* the wound's edges are too far apart to be surgically closed, and there's marked tissue loss; the wound is instead closed naturally by the formation and adhesion of granulation tissue and epithelialization; examples include pressure ulcers, dehisced surgical wounds, and traumatic injuries.
- In *healing by tertiary intention,* also known as *delayed primary closure,* there's a delay in wound closure, resulting in granulation of the wound edges; later surgical closure results in more scar formation; these wounds are sometimes left open for several days to allow edema or infection to resolve or exudate to drain.

### *Wound Healing Consists of Several Phases*

- The *injury* is a break in the skin's integrity
- *Hemostasis* is a brief period of vasoconstriction at the site of injury as the body attempts to prevent excessive bleeding
- The *inflammatory phase* starts right after the injury and lasts from 2 to 6 days; this defensive reaction to tissue injury involves increased blood flow and capillary permeability and aids in phagocytosis or autolytic debridement; it is marked by increased heat, redness, swelling, and pain in the affected area
- During the *proliferative phase,* granulation tissue forms and epithelialization begins
  - Granulation tissue is a pink-to-red, moist tissue that contains new blood vessels, collagen, fibroblasts, and inflammatory cells; the tissue fills the open deep wound and acts as a kind of scaffolding for the eventual migration of epithelial cells
  - During epithelialization, epithelial cells migrate across the wound's surface, forming a layer of new tissue; these cells look silvery and form a perimeter around the granulation tissue
- As *epithelial closure* occurs, the wound contracts and begins to close
- During the final *maturation phase,* collagen reorganizes and strengthens, a process that continues for months and sometimes years; chronic wounds may regain 50% of their original tensile strength after 2 to 3 weeks, but they will ultimately regain only 70 to 75% of their original strength.

## Factors that affect Wound Healing

### *Local Factors*

- Moisture—for instance, from incontinence—leads to skin maceration and edema, making the epidermis more susceptible to abrasion; the chemicals and bacteria in urine and stool also cause tissue break down
- Necrotic debris and other foreign material in a wound interfere with optimal healing and must be removed; by increasing the bacterial count, dead tissue increases the risk of infection
- Infection at a level of more than 1 million organisms per gram of tissue inhibits granulation and epithelialization.

### *Systemic Factors*

- Aging has a profound impact on all body systems; it affects wound healing by decreasing the inflammatory response, delaying angiogenesis, decreasing collagen synthesis and degradation, slowing epithelialization (resulting in a thinner epidermal layer), decreasing cohesion between the epidermal and dermal layers, decreasing the function of sebaceous glands (resulting in dryness), and altering the function of melanocytes (resulting in skin discoloration)
- Malnutrition delays or prevents healing by depriving the body of the nutrients it needs to combat the physiologic stress of infection and to meet the increased metabolic demands of tissue repair, patients with chronic or difficult-to-heal wounds have special dietary needs (see *The role of nutrition in wound healing)*
- Dehydration can hasten debilitation and death, a patient with a large wound can lose far more than 1 L of water per day, the water loss of a healthy adult
- Vascular insufficiency can lead to poor healing and the development of leg ulcers
  - Arterial insufficiency results in an inadequate blood supply, which can lead to tissue hypoxia, infection and death
  - Cardiovascular insufficiency leads to systemic hypoxemia which impedes wound healing
  - Venous insufficiency—impaired flow toward the heart and elevated pressure in the venous system—leads to the leakage of fibrinogen around capillaries into the dermis, this results in formation of a fibrin layer that blocks tissue oxygenation, nutrient exchange, and waste removal.

## Metabolic Factors

- A patient with diabetes mellitus requires strict maintenance of normal blood glucose levels for proper wound healing, particularly for the acute phase of tissue repair, during periods of stress, after surgery, and for combating sepsis; poorly controlled diabetes results in notoriously slow and complicated wound healing for several reasons.
  - Impaired circulation caused by thickening of the capillary basement membrane results in reduced local blood flow
  - Reduced sensation from diabetic neuropathy significantly reduces sensation in the lower extremities, making patients less aware of injuries and serious infections

- Hyperglycemia impairs the inflammatory response and collagen synthesis and produces leukocyte dysfunction, which increases the risk of infection
- Renal failure or insufficiency increases the risk of infection and wound dehiscence and delays granulation
- A newly recognized disorder, reperfusion injury is thought to result from the uncontrolled release of free radicals (superoxide anion, hydroxyl radicals, and hydrogen peroxide) when ischemic tissue is reperfused or reoxygenated; oxygen-free radicals can cause damage to cell membranes, lipids, proteins, blood vessels, and deoxyribonucleic acid and can trigger the inflammatory process.

### Neurologic Factors

- The absence of pain sensation can lead to significant tissue damage from pressure or trauma; a patient who does not feel pain cannot respond to alleviate the pain
- Immobility and impaired sensory perception contribute to pressure ulcer development and delayed healing.

### Psychological Factors

- Stress, depression, and sleep disorders can alter the immune response
- A stressed, depressed, or sleep-deprived patient is less likely to participate in self-care, including wound care
- The sleep deprivation that can result from many psychological disorders interferes with the restorative properties of rest and sleep
- Some patients with severe psychiatric disorders may deliberately injure themselves or interfere with wound care measures.

### Immunologic Deficiencies

- Immunologic deficiencies impair many aspects of the inflammatory phase of healing
- Such deficiencies also predispose patients to infection.

### Clotting Disorders

- Clotting disorders interfere with the coagulation cascade critical in wound healing
- Platelet aggregation normally initiates hemostasis and the release of chemotactic and growth-promoting substances, but clotting factor deficiencies (for instance, from hemophilia, malnutrition, or hepatic disease), thrombocytopenia and anticoagulation therapy can prolong bleeding into a wound and delay healing.

### Other Factors

- Glucocorticoid therapy (for instance, with prednisone or hydrocortisone) can interfere with healing by suppressing the inflammatory response, preventing macrophages from migrating into the wound, reducing fibroblast and endothelial cell activity and delaying contraction and epithelialization
- Medications including anti-inflammatory drugs, cancer-fighting agents, anticoagulants, and anti-prostaglandins, interfere with the normal healing process.

## Nursing Assessment

### General Assessment

- Determine the patient's age
- Ask about urinary and fecal incontinence
- Note any chronic illnesses that can interfere with wound healing, including diabetes mellitus, chronic obstructive pulmonary disease and arteriosclerotic heart disease
- Assess the patient's nutritional status, including general appearance and skin turgor, and hydration status; look for signs of weight loss
- Make sure the patient's laboratory values fall within the normal range: serum albumin level, 3.5 to 5 g/dL, serum transferrin level, 200 to 400 mg/dL; total lymphocyte count, 1,800 to 3,000 mL and thyroxine-binding prealbumin level, 15.7 to 29.6 mg/dL
- Assess the patient's oxygenation and circulation status, noting indications of respiratory and circulatory impairment and peripheral vascular disease, ask if he smokes
- Assess the patient's immune status, ask about corticosteroid use, and ask if the patient has been diagnosed with cancer and is undergoing chemotherapy, determine whether he tests positive for the human immunodeficiency virus
- Ask about use of medications, including steroids, nonsteroidal antiinflammatories, immunosuppressants, antineoplastics, anticoagulants and antiprostaglandins
- Determine the patient's stress level, asking about family support and community resources.

### Wound Assessment

- Determine the wound's cause
- Note the wound's location
- Measure the wound's length, width, and depth in centimeters
- Determine the wound's stage
- Observe the wound margins, looking for undermining, tunneling, and sinus tracts
- Look for exudate in the wound, observing the amount and type (serous, serosanguineous, sanguineous, or purulent); note any odor
- Assess the tissue in the wound bed
  - Granulation tissue will look beefy red
  - Epithelial tissue will look pearly pink
  - Sloughing necrotic or devitalized tissue will look soft and yellow-gray, eschar necrotic tissue will look thick and black
- Note signs of infection, including induration, fever, erythema, edema, an elevated WBC count, and purulent drainage.

## Management

### Prevention of Pressure Ulcers

- Identify patients at risk, including bedridden and chair-bound patients and patients who have difficulty repositioning themselves
- Using a valid risk assessment tool, assess at-risk patients for pressure ulcers on admission and at regular intervals; document your assessment on the Braden or Norton scale (see *Norton Scale*)

| Norton scale | | | | | | | | | | | |
|---|---|---|---|---|---|---|---|---|---|---|---|
| Total the numbers from each category that describes your patient. A score of 14 or less indicates a risk of developing pressure ulcers | **Physical condition** | | **Mental condition** | | **Activity** | | **Mobility** | | **Incontinence** | | |
| | Good | 4 | Alert | 4 | Ambulatory | 4 | Full | 4 | None | 4 | |
| | Fair | 3 | Apathetic | 3 | Walk/help | 3 | Slightly limited | 3 | Occasional | 3 | |
| | Poor | 2 | Confused | 2 | Chairbound | 2 | Very limited | 2 | Usually-urine | 2 | |
| | Very bad | 1 | Stuporous | 1 | Bedridden | 1 | Immobile | 1 | Urine/feces | 1 | **Total score** |
| Name Date | | | | | | | | | | | |
| Name Date | | | | | | | | | | | |
| Name Date | | | | | | | | | | | |

*Source:* Norton, D, et al. (1962) An investigation of geriatric nursing problems in the hospital. London National Corporation for the care of Older People (now the centre for Policy on Ageing). Used with permission of the publisher.

- Identify risk factors that contribute to skin breakdown, including immobility, incontinence, nutritional deficiencies, and an altered level of consciousness.

### *Prevention of Vascular Ulcers*

- Identify patients at risk, including those with chronic diseases such as diabetes mellitus, and cardiovascular, renal and neurologic disease
- Identify risk factors that can contribute to vascular ulcers, including aging, malnutrition and therapy with such drugs as glucocorticoids, anti-inflammatories, antineoplastics, anticoagulants and antiprostaglandins.

### *Prevention of Skin Tear Injuries*

- Identify patients at risk, especially elderly patients and those with a history of skin tears
- Use a valid skin integrity risk assessment tool and a classification system such as Payne-Martin.

### *Early Intervention*

- Treat the underlying disorder—for example, monitor blood glucose levels, administer insulin or an oral antidiabetic, and teach proper nutrition to the patient with diabetes
- Minimize skin exposure to moisture from incontinence, perspiration, or wound drainage
- Clean skin as soon as it becomes wet, and bathe the patient regularly
  - Avoid soap that dries the skin
  - Use warm, not hot, water
  - Use cream on dry, scaly skin
  - Do not rub reddened areas over bony prominences
- Use topical moisture barriers to protect skin from urine and feces
- Make sure the patient receives adequate protein, calories, vitamins and minerals
- Encourage daily activity and if possible, exercise
- If the patient is bedridden, take steps to minimize pressure on vulnerable skin areas
  - Reposition the patient—from back to side, to opposite side, to back—at least every 2 hours
  - When the patient is on his side, make sure he is not lying directly on the trochanter
  - Use pillows or foam wedges to keep bony prominences from direct contact with the bed
  - Avoid massaging the skin over bony prominences
  - Take steps to reduce shearing and friction
- Use the sheet to lift or reposition the patient in bed; do not drag the patient up in bed
- Have an overhead trapeze bar installed for a patient who has enough strength in his upper extremities to reposition himself
- Use a slide board for transferring the patient from a bed to a stretcher
- Place sheepskin directly under the patient (unless he is incontinent)
- Elevate the head of the bed to no more than 30 degrees, unless contraindicated
  - Lift the patient's heels off the bed, or use a device that totally relieves pressure on the heels
  - Consider using a pressure-reducing or pressure-relieving mattress for a patient who is at high risk for developing pressure ulcers
- If the patient is chair bound, take steps to minimize pressure on vulnerable skin areas
  - Make sure the patient shifts his weight frequently
  - Seat the patient on a 4′ pressure-reducing, high-density foam pad—not a doughnut-type device
  - Consider postural alignment, distribution of weight, balance and stability, and pressure relief when positioning a patient in a chair or wheelchair
  - Use elbow and heel pads to protect skin and minimize friction.

### Treatment

- Protect the wound from further trauma
  - Use pressure-reducing devices
  - Reduce friction and shear
- Elevate the head of the bed no more than 30 degrees
- Use a sheet to reposition the patient in bed
- Remove dressings gently
  - Use nonadhering dressings or those with minimal adherent
  - Use wraps, such as a stockinette or soft gauze, to protect areas at high risk of skin tearing
- Prevent infection and promote a clean wound base
  - Cover the wound to protect it from infection
  - Remove or debride any necrotic tissue
- *Mechanical debridement* is the manual removal of devitalized tissue using physical forces, such as whirl pooling, wet-to-dry gauze dressings, and wound irrigation
- *Sharp debridement* is the removal of foreign material or devitalized tissue with a sharp instrument, such as a scalpel or scissors
- *Autolytic debridement* uses synthetic dressings to cover the wound; this allows the enzymes naturally present in the wound fluid to digest devitalized tissue
- *Chemical* or *enzymatic debridement* involves the topical application of a proteolytic substance (such as enzymes) to break down devitalized tissue
  - Use pressurized irrigation (a 35-mL syringe with a 18 needle or angiocatheter) to clean the wound surface or cavity; use a noncytotoxic agent such as normal saline solution
  - Absorb excess exudate with collagen or calcium alginates or absorbent powders, beads, or paste
  - Pack dead space with collagen or calcium alginates or moistened saline nonwoven gauze dressings
- Use a moisture-retentive dressing that keeps the wound bed moist but leaves the surrounding skin dry
  - Use one of the following dressings for a wound with light to moderate exudate
- A *transparent film* is a clear, adherent, nonabsorptive, polymer-based dressing that is permeable to oxygen and water vapor but not to water; it is used to treat partial-thickness wounds and wounds with eschar (to promote autolysis)
- A *hydrogel* is a nonadherent dressing composed of water and a polymer that has some absorptive properties; it is used to treat partial- to full-thickness wounds, dry wounds, wounds with minimal drainage, wounds with necrosis or slough and infected wounds
- A *foam dressing* is made up of a sponge like polymer; it can be adherent and has some absorptive properties, and is used to treat partial- to full-thickness wounds and wounds with minimal to heavy drainage (including around tubes)
- A *hydrocolloid* is an adhesive, moldable wafer made of a carbohydrate-based material, usually with a backing that's impermeable to oxygen, water, and water vapor, the thin version has some absorptive properties; it is used to treat partial- to full-thickness wounds, wounds with minimal to moderate drainage, and wounds with necrosis or slough
  - For a wound with moderate to heavy exudate, use a foam dressing, a collagen or calcium alginate dressing (a nonwoven, absorptive dressing made from seaweed), or a hydrocolloid dressing, which is more absorbent than the thin dressing
- Take steps to improve the patient's overall condition
  - Provide nutritional support
- Arrange for a nutritional consultation
- Provide nutritional supplements as needed
- Make sure the patient is hydrated
  - Maintain the patient's oxygenation and circulation
- If the patient experiences venous insufficiency, use compression to optimize venous return
- If the patient is diabetic, take steps to control his blood glucose level
- Institute measures to optimize the patient's arterial blood supply and avoid circulatory impairment
  - Help the patient reduce his stress level by involving him and his family in his care, contact the appropriate community resources
- Minimize the patient's pain
  - Provide sufficient analgesia before, during, and after dressing changes
  - Choose dressings that maximize the time between dressing changes and that cause minimal tissue trauma
  - Teach the patient relaxation techniques and guided imagery to help control pain and maximize the effects of pain medication.

## DISRUPTION OF HOMEOSTASIS

### Stress

### General Information

- Stress is the body's response to stressors or stimuli that are perceived as threatening
- Stressors can be *biophysical* (such as disease, trauma, and overexertion), *chemical* (such as pollution, drugs, and alcohol), *psychosocial* (such as job loss, divorce, and bankruptcy), or *cultural* (such as traveling, being separated from family members during hospitalization, and delegating decision making to health care providers)
- The body responds to stress physiologically and psychologically.

### Selye's Stress Theory

- Hans Selye's theory describes a general adaptation syndrome that consists of three stages of a hormonally controlled stress response
  - The first stage is the alarm reaction, in which the person is alerted to the presence of a stressor and the need to act
  - The second stage is resistance
- In this stage, the pituitary gland secretes corticotropin
- Corticotropin stimulates the production of glucocorticoids and mineralocorticoids, which promote and inhibit inflammation, allowing the body to protect or surrender tissue
  - If resistance continues and the body does not adapt, the third stage is exhaustion, which can lead to disease or death

- According to Selye, stress can result from positive or negative events.

### Physiologic Stress Responses

- Physiologic responses to stress involve the central nervous system, hypothalamus, sympathetic nervous system, anterior and posterior pituitary gland, adrenal medulla, and adrenal cortex
  - Hormones and catecholamines are secreted or stimulated by these organs in response to a stressor
  - Their release results in the body's fight-or-flight response to stress
- The initial reaction to stress is increased alertness in preparation for fight or flight
- Blood vessels dilate, heart rate increases, the rate and depth of respirations increase, and bronchodilation occurs, these reactions increase the oxygen supply to organs and muscles
- The arterioles in the skin, kidneys, and abdominal viscera constrict; blood is shunted from the GI tract and periphery to the brain, heart and major muscles
- Gluconeogenesis increases, decreased insulin secretion and increased fatty acid metabolism increase the amount of glucose available for energy
- Localized sweat production increases, and muscles become tense
- Pain tolerance increases as endorphins (endogenous opiates) are released
- Repeated physiologic stress responses can damage the body, resulting in problems such as kidney failure, gastric ulcers, and exacerbation of an existing disorder
- The body's level of physiologic response to stress varies according to the stimuli, most physiologic stress responses aren't helpful in coping with the daily stresses of life.

### Psychological Stress Responses

- Psychological stress responses result when the body's ability to adapt to change is exceeded; a person adapts to psychological stress through coping strategies, such as problem solving, reappraising stressors, and rehearsing responses to stress.
- The body's psychological response to stress varies according to the stressor's intensity and duration and the perceived control over the stressor.
  - Psychological stress can cause physical manifestations, such as hypertension and digestive disorders, and psychological manifestations, such as anxiety attacks and eating disorders
  - When psychological stress exceeds a person's coping abilities, crisis (extreme psychological disequilibrium) may occur.

### Nursing Assessment of Stress

- The nurse should identify the source and duration of the stress, the patient's resources and coping strategies, and the effects of the stress on the patient and family members
- Sources of stress include illness and hospitalization
  - Stressors related to illness include pain, fear of loss of a body part or function, fear of prognosis, and fear of disfigurement
  - Stressors related to hospitalization or treatment include perceived loss of control, increased dependence, change in environment, loss of roles as worker and provider for family, change in routine, and lack of trust in the caregivers
- The duration of the stress depends on the stressor, which can be acute or chronic, intermittent or continuous
- External resources include family members and significant others, internal resources include past experiences with illness or hospitalization, education, and spirituality
- Coping strategies consist of past methods that have been effective for the patient such as information seeking, relaxation techniques, prayer, counseling, physical or mental activity, meditation, discussion of options and review of events or event rehearsal
- Repeated stress responses can have physical effects
  - Immediate responses include rapid speech, restlessness, rapid heart rate, light-headedness, and palpitations
  - Long-term responses include headaches, neck and stomach aches, muscle cramps, and changes in eating, elimination, and sleep patterns
- Repeated stress responses can cause psychosocial symptoms, including changes in family or working relationships, denial or anger, hopelessness, silence, or the inability to make decisions
- The nurse can use life-event questionnaires to measure stressors in a patient's life and hardiness scales to determine a patient's ability to cope with or adapt to stress.

### Nursing Interventions

- Physical interventions reduce tension and support organ function
- Massage, heat application, warm baths, stretching exercises, and physical activity can reduce muscle tension, serve as distractions, and increase the ability to put stressors in perspective
  - Activities to protect organ function include monitoring for complications such as ileus and GI bleeding, checking urine output and assessing glucose levels
- Educational interventions include teaching the patient or family about stress and the body's response to it and rehearsing events to prepare the patient for stress-producing events
  - Teaching plans should include what to expect from the stress-producing situation
  - Event rehearsal helps the patient to review an expected sequence of events and deal with anxiety-producing situations in a controlled environment before the actual event occurs
- Emotional support can be given through counseling, encouraging discussions, sharing feelings, verbalizing difficulties, and supporting family problem solving; helping patients to separate themselves from the issue can help maintain their self-esteem
- Social support activities include evaluating financial status, assisting with insurance forms, providing referrals for home health care assistance, and evaluating spirituality needs (with appropriate referrals to clergy).

## Shock

### General Information

- Shock is an acute state of reduced perfusion of all body tissues
- Inadequate circulating blood volume results in decreased delivery of oxygen to tissues and decreased gas exchange in the capillaries
- Inadequate oxygenation leads to impaired cellular metabolism and an inability to excrete metabolic waste products.

### Pathogenesis of Shock

- Initial stage
  - Decrease in cardiac output leads to decrease in mean arterial pressure
  - Sympathetic nervous system is stimulated, leading to initiation of stress response
  - Signs and symptoms include normal to slightly increased heart rate, normal to slightly decreased blood pressure, thirst, and pale, cool, moist skin over the face
- Compensatory stage
  - Decrease in mean arterial pressure stimulates the sympathetic nervous system to release epinephrine and norepinephrine to try to achieve homeostasis
  - Stimulation of alpha1-adrenergic fibers causes vasoconstriction of vessels in the skin, GI organs, kidneys, muscles, and lungs, shunting blood to the heart and brain
  - Stimulation of beta-adrenergic fibers causes vasodilation of coronary and cerebral arteries, increases heart rate, and increases force of myocardial contractions, resulting in increased cardiac output
  - Reduced renal blood flow leads to release of renin and production of angiotensin, resulting in vasoconstriction and stimulation of the adrenal cortex to release aldosterone, increasing renal sodium reabsorption
  - Increased serum osmolarity stimulates the release of antidiuretic hormone, resulting in increased water reabsorption by the kidneys and increased venous blood return to the heart and ultimately increased cardiac output
  - Signs and symptoms include restlessness, normal or decreasing blood pressure, bounding or thready pulse, tachycardia, tachypnea, normal or hypoactive bowel sounds, slightly decreased urine output, and pale, cool skin (flushed and warm in septic shock)
- Progressive stage
  - Compensatory mechanisms become ineffective and possibly even counter productive
  - Falling cardiac output and vasoconstriction cause cellular hypoxia and anaerobic metabolism; metabolic acidosis occurs as lactic acid levels rise
  - Renal ischemia stimulates the renin-angiotensin-aldosterone system, causing further vasoconstriction
  - Fluid shifts from intravascular to interstitial space
  - Signs and symptoms include falling blood pressure; narrowed pulse pressure; cold, clammy skin, rapid, shallow respirations, tachycardia, weak, thready, or absent pulses, arrhythmias, absent bowel sounds, anuria; and subnormal body temperature (subnormal or elevated in septic shock)
- Irreversible stage
  - Compensatory mechanisms are ineffective
  - Lactic acid continues to accumulate, and capillary permeability dilation increases, resulting in loss of intravascular volume and tachycardia, this further aggravates falling blood pressure and cardiac output
  - Coronary and cerebral perfusion decline, and organ systems fail
  - Signs and symptoms include unresponsiveness; areflexia, severe hypotension, slow, irregular heart rate, absent pulses, slow, shallow, irregular respirations, Cheyne-Stokes respirations and respiratory and cardiac arrest.

### Types of Shock

- *Cardiogenic shock* results from an inadequate pumping function that causes decreased cardiac output and stroke volume, leading to inadequate tissue perfusion and a precipitous drop in blood pressure and urine output; it results from such occurrences as acute myocardial infarction (MI), acute mitral insufficiency, right ventricular infarction, arrhythmias, heart failure, myocarditis, cardiac tamponade and cardiac surgery
- *Hypovolemic shock* results from decreased intravascular volume in relation to the vascular bed's size; loss of blood plasma into the tissues leads to decreased circulating blood volume and venous return, reduced cardiac output, and inadequate tissue perfusion
  - This type of shock is classified by the amount of blood loss: class I is an acute loss of up to 15% of blood volume, class II, 16 to 30%, class III, 31 to 40% and class IV, more than 40%
  - Absolute, or measurable, external fluid losses can be caused by hemorrhage, burns, trauma, surgery, dehydration, intestinal obstruction, diabetes mellitus, diabetes insipidus, diuretic therapy, peritonitis, pancreatitis, cirrhosis, hemothorax, and hemoperitoneum
  - Relative, or immeasurable, internal fluid losses in the intravascular space can be caused by venous or arterial pooling and in the extravascular space, by capillary leakage
- *Distributive shock* results from poor distribution of blood to the tissues, which is caused by acute vasodilation without simultaneous expansion of the intravascular volume; anaphylactic, neurogenic, and septic shock are types of distributive shock
  - *Anaphylactic shock* results from an antigen-antibody reaction that releases histamine into the bloodstream, which causes widespread dilation of arterioles and capillary beds and bronchial hypersensitivity; it can be caused by allergic reactions to contrast media used in diagnostic tests, drugs, foods, animal and insect bites, and blood
  - *Neurogenic shock* results from decreased vasomotor tone with generalized vasodilation, it can result from

general or spinal anesthesia, epidural block, spinal cord injury, vasovagal syncope, barbiturate or phenothiazine ingestion, and insulin shock
- *Septic shock* results from a systemic response to microorganisms in the blood, causing vasodilation with selective vasoconstriction and poor distribution of blood; it commonly stems from overt infection, localized infection that spreads to the systemic circulation, urinary tract infection, postabortion or postpartal infection, or immunosuppressant therapy
- *Obstructive shock* results from a physical obstruction that reduces cardiac output despite normal contractility and intravascular volume; it is caused by pulmonary embolism, dissecting aortic aneurysm, atrial myxoma, cardiac tamponade and tension pneumothorax.

### Complications of Shock

- Myocardial depression may be caused by decreased coronary blood flow and acidosis and can lead to arrhythmias, MI and cardiac failure
- Acute respiratory distress syndrome, also known as shock lung, may result from decreased perfusion to pulmonary capillaries
- Renal failure may occur when prolonged renal hypoperfusion causes acute tubular necrosis
- Hepatic insufficiency may stem from poor perfusion to the liver and can lead to recirculation of bacteria and cellular debris
- Disseminated intravascular coagulation may occur because shock causes excessive consumption of clotting factors
- GI ulcerations may occur when reduced blood flow increases acid production.

### Nursing Interventions

- Ensure an adequate airway
  - Encourage coughing and deep breathing; administer medications for pain as needed to ensure deep breathing, suction as needed and position the patient to maintain a patent airway and maximum ventilation
  - Turn the patient frequently, and elevate the head of the bed, unless contraindicated
  - Administer oxygen as prescribed
  - Perform postural drainage and chest physiotherapy to mobilize secretions
  - Evaluate breath sounds for crackles and wheezes
- Maintain hemodynamic stability
  - Assess pulse rate and rhythm
  - Assess blood pressure for changes, using a Doppler ultrasound transducer if a sphygmomanometer does not provide an audible blood pressure
- Maintain a normal temperature
  - Prevent hypothermia (core temperature less than 95°F [35°C]) by setting the room thermostat higher, warming the room with infrared lights, covering the patient with warmed blankets, using a warming mat as prescribed, warming lavage solutions, and using a fluid warmer when infusing IV solutions or blood
  - Prevent hyperthermia (increase in body temperature and metabolic rate) by removing excess blankets, administering medications as prescribed to decrease temperature, giving a tepid sponge bath, and using a cooling mat as prescribed
- Maintain normal volume status to prevent fluid imbalance
  - Assess skin turgor for signs and symptoms of dehydration
  - Note signs of extreme thirst
  - Monitor urine output (amount, color, and specific gravity)
  - Monitor drainage (wound, gastric and chest tube drainage)
  - Check for abnormal breath sounds
  - Assess the patient for weight gain or loss
  - Infuse fluids as prescribed
  - Assess blood loss, if possible
- Prevent complications of shock
  - Assess nutritional status to ensure adequate caloric intake to meet metabolic demands
  - Watch for signs of decreased tissue perfusion, such as changes in skin color and temperature, level of consciousness (LOC), peripheral pulses, and urine output
  - Prepare for transfer to the critical care unit if the patient's status deteriorates
- Reduce patient and family anxiety
  - Explain all procedures in understandable terms
  - Medicate the patient for pain to ensure patient comfort
  - Teach the patient relaxation techniques used to reduce anxiety
  - Give family members time to ask questions and express concerns
- Follow infection control policies.

## Inflammation and Infection

### Inflammation

- The inflammatory process is a defense mechanism that is activated in response to localized injury or infection; also called the local adaptation syndrome, this process acts to limit the spread of infection and promote wound healing.
- The inflammatory process occurs in three phases:
  - In the first phase, blood vessels at the injury site constrict to control bleeding, vasoconstriction is followed by the release of histamines and increased capillary permeability to encourage blood flow and attract white blood cells (WBCs) to the area
  - In the second phase, exudate is produced, the amount of which depends on the wound's size, location, and severity, exudate is composed of cells and fluid that have escaped from blood vessels and may be serous, sanguineous, purulent, or a combination of the three
  - In the final stage, damaged cells are repaired by regeneration or formation of scar tissue.

### Infection

- The infectious process results from a combination of several factors:
  - A causative agent (pathogen) must be present
  - A reservoir must be available for the pathogen

- The reservoir must have a means of exit, such as the nares, feces, or wound drainage
- The pathogen must be transmitted directly or indirectly to the new host; direct transmission requires contact between the reservoir and the new host, whereas indirect transmission usually occurs when an inanimate object carries the pathogen
- The pathogen must enter the host through a portal of entry, such as the GI tract, respiratory tract, or a wound
- The pathogen's virulence and the host's susceptibility also affect the infection process

- Signs and symptoms of systemic and localized infections
  - *Systemic infections* are generalized and produce symptoms in multiple body systems
- Prodromal symptoms, which may be vague, include malaise, weakness, fatigue, aches and anorexia
- Progression of infection is evidenced by symptoms such as fever, tachycardia, leukocytosis with a shift in differential and lymphadenopathy
- Severe untreated systemic infections can produce altered mental status, seizures, and shock
  - *Localized infections* are limited to a specific body region and produce symptoms in only one or two body systems
- Presenting signs and symptoms include pain, warmth, swelling, erythema, and itching at the affected site
- Progression of infection is evidenced by increasing redness and induration and the development of exudate
- Diagnostic findings for both types of infection include elevated WBC counts and positive aerobic or anaerobic cultures
- Medical treatments for infections include antibiotic therapy, surgery to remove an infected body part, dead tissue debridement, and abscess drainage; these procedures remove the infection or reduce the number of organisms to be eliminated
- Nursing interventions for a patient with an infection consist primarily of monitoring and teaching
  - Monitor the progression of infection
- Take the patient's vital signs
- Measure the extent of induration or visible erythema
- Assess the patient's LOC
- Administer oral, parenteral, or topical antibiotics
- Apply heat to localized infections
- Apply sterile dressings to draining or open wounds
- Monitor drainage for amount, color, and odor
- Maintain standard precautions
- Document infection progression, treatments performed, and patient response
- Encourage adequate nutrition for wound healing
  - Teach the patient to prevent future infections
- Instruct the patient to protect intact skin and mucus membranes by using precautions to prevent breakdown
- Stress the importance of hand washing
- Encourage nutritional maintenance of immune system responses
- Discuss avoidance of pathogens transmitted by way of the respiratory or GI tract
- Promote good hygiene
- Teach about wound care and antibiotic therapy.

## Fluid Imbalances

### *General information*

- Water accounts for 60% of the total body weight in adults and 80% in infants, the leaner the person, the greater the proportion of water to total body weight.
- The *intracellular fluid (ICF) compartment* includes water in the cells; this compartment accounts for 70% of total body water, or about 25 L of fluid in an adult
- The *extracellular fluid (ECF) compartment* includes water outside the cells; this compartment accounts for 30% of total body water, or about 15 L of fluid (including 5 L of blood)
- Additional fluids are contained in other body compartments
  - Interstitial fluid is found in the spaces between cells
  - Plasma, an intravascular fluid, is found within arteries, veins, and capillaries
  - Cerebrospinal fluid and intraocular fluid are found in the spinal cord and eyes, respectively
- Alterations in the amount or composition of body fluids can cause complications; a 10% fluid loss (4 L) is serious, and a 20% loss (8 L) is fatal
- Body fluids transport nutrients to and remove wastes from cells.

### *Fluid Movement*

- Body compartments are separated by semipermeable membranes that control fluid movement through filtration, hydrostatic pressure and osmosis
  - *Filtration* is the passage of water and solutes across a semipermeable membrane
  - *Hydrostatic pressure* is pressure caused by a fluid column in an enclosed area such as a blood vessel wall
  - *Osmosis* is the passage of water through a semipermeable membrane from an area of low solute concentration to an area of high solute concentration
- A solution's osmolality, which is determined by the number of dissolved particles in the fluid, also influences fluid movement
  - In an *isotonic solution*, the dissolved particle concentration equals that of ICF, causing no net water movement
  - In a *hypertonic solution*, the dissolved particle concentration exceeds that of ICF, causing water to move out of the cell to the area of greater concentration; this movement causes cell shriveling
  - In a *hypotonic solution*, the dissolved particle concentration is less than that of ICF, causing water to move into the cell; this movement causes cell swelling.

### *Organs that Regulate Fluid Movement*

- The kidneys filter 180 L of plasma daily and excrete 1.5 L of urine daily (1 mL/kg/hour)
  - They regulate ECF volume, osmolality, and electrolyte levels by selective retention and excretion of fluids and electrolytes

- They regulate the pH of ECF by influencing hydrogen ion excretion or retention and the excretion of metabolic wastes and toxic substances
- The heart and blood vessels affect fluid movement because adequate cardiac output is needed to maintain the renal perfusion pressure required for kidney function; decreased cardiac output decreases renal perfusion pressure
  - Decreased renal perfusion pressure stimulates the stretch receptors in the atria and blood vessels to increase perfusion
  - It also stimulates the release of aldosterone, which increases fluid retention
- The lungs expel water vapor at the rate of 300 to 400 mL/day
  - Increased respiratory rate or depth increases vapor loss
  - Vapor loss is considered insensible water loss because the actual loss cannot be observed or measured
- Skin affects fluid movement by means of sweat (visible fluid loss) and evaporation
  - The rate of fluid loss by means of sweat, which ranges from 0 to 1,000 mL/hour, is affected by body temperature; temperatures exceeding 101°F (38.3°C) increase the rate of loss, whereas temperatures below 101°F decrease the rate of loss
  - Sweat is considered a sensible water loss because the actual loss can be observed and measured
  - Evaporation of fluid from the skin also accounts for a water loss of 600 mL/day, it occurs as insensible perspiration
- The GI tract normally loses 100 to 200 mL of fluid daily, diarrhea and fistulas greatly increase this fluid loss.

### *Hormonal Influence*

- Antidiuretic hormone (ADH), or vasopressin, is a hormone synthesized in the hypothalamus and released by the posterior pituitary; it affects fluid balance by increasing water reabsorption in the renal tubules
  - Increased osmolality and water deficiency stimulate ADH release
  - Decreased osmolality and excess water intake inhibit ADH release
- Aldosterone is a mineralocorticoid secreted by the adrenal cortex
  - Increased aldosterone levels increase sodium retention, thereby increasing water retention
  - Decreased sodium levels stimulate aldosterone secretion
  - Increased sodium levels inhibit aldosterone secretion.

### Thirst

- The thirst center is located in the anterior hypothalamus; intracellular dehydration stimulates hypothalamus cells, causing a sensation of thirst
- Thirst leads to increased water intake, which restores ECF volume.

### *Fluid Volume Deficit*

- Description
  - Fluid volume deficit (FVD) results from loss of body fluids, isosmolar FVD occurs when equal proportions of water and sodium are lost, hyperosmolar FVD occurs when more water than sodium is lost, resulting in hypovolemia and hypernatremia
  - Isosmolar FVD can result from traumatic injury, rapid blood loss, and decreased fluid intake from nausea, anorexia, fatigue, depression, confusion, neurologic deficits that alter the ability to swallow or detect thirst, and oral or pharyngeal pain
  - Hyperosmolar FVD can result from loss of GI fluids through vomiting, diarrhea, GI suctioning, fistulas, drains, third-space fluid loss, and excessive use of tap water enemas, it also can result from polyuria or excessive urine formation, which is associated with diabetic ketoacidosis, hyperosmolar hyperglycemic nonketotic syndrome, nephritis and diuretic use
  - Fever can increase fluid loss through diaphoresis and increased respiratory rate; a temperature more than 101°F (38.3°C) requires an extra 500 mL of fluid daily, and more than 103°F (39.4°C) requires an extra 1,000 mL of fluid daily
  - Sweating can contribute to FVD
- Signs and symptoms
  - Weight loss may be rapid (1L of fluid equals 2 lb)
  - Skin turgor and elasticity may be decreased
  - The oral cavity may be dry and have a smaller than normal tongue lined with visible longitudinal furrows
  - Urine output may be decreased (less than 30 mL/hour for an adult), but specific gravity may be increased
  - Altered vital signs may include a subnormal body temperature, orthostatic hypotension, and increased heart rate
  - Signs of decreased volume may include decreased central venous pressure (CVP), flattened jugular veins, and slow-filling hand veins
  - Altered sensorium and cold extremities also may occur
  - Laboratory data may include elevated hematocrit, elevated blood urea nitrogen (BUN) level in relation to creatinine level, and serum sodium level greater than 150 mEq/L
- Medical management
  - Replace fluid loss orally, if possible, or by IV infusion
  - Correct the deficit's cause
- Nursing Interventions
  - Encourage fluid intake, as appropriate, by providing adequate pain control, relieving nausea, offering fluids, performing frequent skin and mouth care, and consulting the practitioner if the patient cannot ingest fluids orally
  - Maintain accurate input and output records to evaluate the effectiveness of interventions
  - Administer parenteral therapy as prescribed, and assess for complications
  - Teach the patient and family about preventing, recognizing, and treating FVD.

### *Fluid Volume Excess*

- Description
  - Fluid volume excess (FVE) is the abnormal retention of water

- When accompanied by altered sodium levels, the condition is referred to as hyperosmolar FVE
- When water and sodium are retained in equal proportions, the condition is referred to as isosmolar FVE
  - FVE results from compromised regulatory mechanisms, such as those seen in heart failure, renal failure, cirrhosis, and steroid excess
  - It also can result from excessive administration of parenteral fluids (especially those with a high sodium content) and excessive ingestion of sodium chloride or sodium salts
- Signs and symptoms
  - Rapid weight gain that may be accompanied by peripheral edema
  - Distended neck or peripheral veins and increased CVP
  - Changes in breath sounds, pulmonary edema, ascites, and pleural effusion
  - Bounding pulses
  - Increased urine output
  - Vital signs changes that may include increased pulse rate and blood pressure
  - Shortness of breath and orthopnea
  - Laboratory data that may include a decreased BUN level, decreased hematocrit, and a serum sodium level less than 135 mEq/L
- Medical management
  - Reduce sodium intake through diet changes
  - Reevaluate the need for IV therapy and the type of IV fluids administered
- Nursing interventions
  - Monitor daily intake and output
  - Encourage strict adherence to diet and fluid orders
  - Administer a diuretic as prescribed, and prepare the patient for possible dialysis
  - Assess the patient's need for an indwelling urinary catheter during diuresis
  - Monitor the patient for complications of diuretic therapy such as alterations in potassium levels
  - Check weight daily; weight gain may reflect volume gain
  - Check for signs of pitting edema in the extremities, and assess the patient for neck vein distention
  - Monitor arterial blood gas (ABG) studies for respiratory alkalosis
  - Monitor breath sounds for changes such as crackles, and administer a diuretic as ordered
  - Encourage rest periods to relieve shortness of breath and fatigue
  - Protect the patient's skin from breakdown caused by the pressure of pitting edema
  - Encourage use of the semi-Fowler position to increase lung capacity
  - Educate the patient and family about preventing, recognizing, and treating FVE.

### *Third-space Fluid Shift*

- Description
  - Third-space fluid shift occurs when body fluids move into the interstitial space from which these fluids aren't exchanged readily with ECF
  - It can result from acute intestinal obstruction, ascites, acute peritonitis, pancreatitis, acute gastric dilation, postoperative complications, fistulas, trauma, burns, fractures, hypoalbuminemia, lymphatic system blockage, and declamping phenomenon (which occurs when a clamp on the aorta is released during surgery)
- Phases of third-space fluid shift
  - In the *fluid accumulation phase,* fluid shifts from the intravascular space to the interstitial space
- The clinical presentation is similar to that of FVD, fluid is lost from the intravascular space, thus decreasing perfusion
- Fluid losses cannot be observed or measured
  - In the *fluid shifting phase,* interstitial fluid shifts back to the intravascular space; the clinical presentation is similar to that of FVE when fluid enters the intravascular space and enters the circulation
- Medical management
  - Correct the fluid shift's cause
  - Treat the patient for symptoms of FVD or FVE as appropriate
- Nursing Interventions
  - For a patient with signs of FVD, see 'Fluid volume deficit: Nursing interventions.
  - For a patient with signs of FVE, see 'Fluid volume excess: Nursing interventions.

## Electrolyte Imbalances

### *General Information*

- Electrolytes are substances that dissociate in solution and conduct a weak electrical current
- Intracellular electrolytes include potassium, magnesium, and phosphate
  - *Potassium* is the principal intracellular cation, it controls cellular osmotic pressure, influences skeletal and cardiac muscle activity, and is dramatically affected by acid–base imbalance
  - *Magnesium* which also is an intracellular cation, is contained mostly in bone, it activates intracellular enzymes, contributes to carbohydrate and protein metabolism, and acts to dilate vessels, decrease blood pressure, imbalances can trigger ventricular arrhythmias and cardiac arrest
  - *Phosphate* is the principal intracellular anion; it is essential for muscle, red blood cell (RBC), and nervous system functioning, and it plays a role in carbohydrate, protein and fat metabolism
- Extracellular electrolytes include sodium, calcium, bicarbonate and chloride
  - *Sodium* is the principal extracellular cation, it is responsible for the osmotic pressure of ECF and it does not readily cross the cell membrane
  - *Calcium,* an extracellular cation, is concentrated in the skeletal system; it acts as cell cement, has a sedative effect on nerve cells, regulates muscle contraction and relaxation (including heartbeat), activates enzymes that stimulate chemical reactions, and plays a role in blood coagulation

- *Bicarbonate,* an extracellular anion, plays a role in acid–base balance; it serves as a buffer to keep serum pH within normal limits and is regulated primarily by the kidneys
- *Chloride* is the principal extracellular anion; it helps maintain acid-base balance and works with sodium to help maintain osmotic pressure
• When the body cannot maintain the normal level of an electrolyte, an imbalance can result.

### *Electrolyte Movement*

• Electrolytes move in and out of cells through diffusion, osmosis, active transport, filtration, and plasma colloid osmotic pressure
• *Diffusion* is the movement of particles from an area of higher concentration to an area of lower concentration across a semipermeable membrane
- The number of particles diffused depends on permeability, or the relative size of cell membrane pores in relation to the particle's size
- The greater the difference in particle concentration, the greater the diffusion rate
- Cell membrane pores are lined with positively charged ions that repel other positive ions and attract negative ions
- The difference in electric potential helps diffusion occur even without a concentration difference
- The pressure increase intensifies the molecular forces striking the membrane which increases the amount of diffusion
• *Osmosis* is the passive movement of fluid across a membrane from a region of low solute concentration to a region of high solute concentration in an effort to maintain homeostasis
- Osmolality refers to the specific gravity of body fluids; the higher the specific gravity, the greater the osmotic pressure, which attracts more water to the area
- Osmolality measures the number of dissolved particles per unit of water; normal osmolality of plasma is 280 to 294 mOsm/kg
• *Active transport* occurs when the cell membrane must move molecules against their concentration gradient; it requires energy (from cellular chemical reactions) and a carrier substance such as sodium
• *Filtration* is the movement of fluid through a permeable membrane from a region of high pressure to a region of low pressure
• *Plasma colloid osmotic pressure* is the osmotic pressure caused by plasma proteins; it results from the selective retention of colloids in plasma, which lowers the concentration of water and electrolytes.

## Acid–base Imbalances

### *General Information*

• An acid is any substance that can donate a hydrogen ion; a base is any substance that can accept or combine with a hydrogen ion
• Acid–base balance optimizes enzymatic function, nerve conduction, synaptic transmission and muscle contraction
• Acids are generated by cellular metabolism of fats and carbohydrates to maintain acid-base balance, acids must be excreted by the lungs and kidneys at the same rate they are generated
• Acidemia is a condition in which the blood is too acidic (has a pH below 7.35), acidosis causes acidemia
• Alkalemia is a condition in which the blood is too alkaline (has a pH above 7.45), alkalosis causes alkalemia.

### *Regulation of Acid-base Balance*

• Most of the 12,000 to 20,000 mEq of carbon dioxide produced daily is excreted by the lungs
- Carbon dioxide is carried from peripheral tissues to the lungs by RBCs, plasma proteins and plasma (as carbonic acid and bicarbonate)
- The acid-base balance is regulated by adjustments in ventilation
• In acidosis, an increased arterial carbon dioxide content or a decreased pH (below 7.35) stimulates hyperventilation, less carbon dioxide results in less carbonic acid and hydrogen ion in the blood, increasing the blood pH
• In alkalosis, a decreased arterial carbon dioxide content or an increased pH leads to hypoventilation; carbon dioxide retention increases the acid load, thus decreasing the blood pH
• The kidneys usually excrete 70 mEq of acid daily
- Renal tubular excretion occurs in several ways
• Hydrogen ions are directly excreted in exchange for sodium ions
• Hydrogen ions are indirectly excreted with urine buffers.
• Hydrogen ions are indirectly excreted with the ammonia produced in the distal tubular cells
- Sodium and bicarbonate are absorbed, and hydrogen is secreted in the proximal tubule
- Carbonic acid is dissociated into hydrogen ions and bicarbonate in the distal tubule; hydrogen ions are excreted, and bicarbonate moves into the bloodstream
- Renal compensation for imbalances can take hours to days in acidosis, the kidneys excrete hydrogen ions and conserve bicarbonate ions, but in alkalosis, the kidneys retain hydrogen ions and excrete bicarbonate ions.

### *Buffering*

• Buffering is a mechanism that corrects acid–base imbalances by removing or releasing hydrogen
• Buffers prevent significant pH changes when an acid or a base is added to a solution; they rapidly react with a strong acid or base by replacing it with a relatively weak acid or base
- Bicarbonate is a buffer for blood and interstitial fluid
• The normal ratio of bicarbonate to carbonic acid is 20 to 1
• Carbon dioxide mixed with water becomes carbonic acid
- Hemoglobin is a buffer for carbon dioxide
- Phosphates and plasma proteins are intracellular buffers.

### *Evaluation of ABG Studies*

• Potential of hydrogen (pH) is a measure of the acid–base balance in terms of the concentration of free hydrogen ions,

the greater the concentration of hydrogen, the more acidic the solution, and the lower the pH
- A pH of 6.8 to 7.0 indicates severe, life-threatening acidosis
- A pH of 7.0 to 7.35 indicates acidosis
- A pH of 7.35 to 7.45 is normal
- A pH of 7.45 to 7.7 indicates alkalosis
- A pH of 7.7 to 7.8 indicates severe, life-threatening alkalosis

- *$PaCO_2$*, or the partial pressure of carbon dioxide in arterial blood, is the best measure of adequate alveolar ventilation.
  - A $PaCO_2$ of 34 to 44 mm Hg is normal
  - A $PaCO_2$ above 44 mm Hg indicates hypercapnia resulting from hypoventilation; a $PaCO_2$ below 34 mm Hg indicates hypocapnia resulting from hyperventilation
- *$PaO_2$*, or the partial pressure of oxygen in arterial blood is a measure of the blood's oxygen content
  - A $PaO_2$ of 80 to 100 mm Hg is normal
  - A $PaO_2$ of 70 to 80 mm Hg is borderline hypoxemia, a $PaO_2$ of 50 to 70 mm Hg indicates hypoxemia, a $PaO_2$ below 50 mm Hg indicates severe hypoxemia
- $HCO_3^-$ is the level of the buffer bicarbonate
  - An $HCO_3^-$ of 24 mEq/L is normal
  - An $HCO_3^-$ above 26 mEq/L indicates excess bicarbonate; an $HCO_3^-$ below 22 mEq/L indicates inadequate bicarbonate.

### Compensation

- Compensation is the return of an abnormal pH to a normal pH
- The unaffected system (metabolic or respiratory) is responsible for returning the pH to normal
  - In respiratory acidosis with a high $PaCO_2$, the kidneys compensate by retaining bicarbonate, which changes the $HCO_3^-/PaCO_2$ ratio and returns the pH to normal
  - In respiratory alkalosis with a low $PaCO_2$, the kidneys compensate by excreting bicarbonate, which changes the $HCO_3^-/PaCO_2$ ratio and returns the pH to normal
  - In metabolic acidosis with a low $HCO_3^-$ or base excess, the lungs compensate through hyperventilation, which lowers $PaCO_2$ and returns the pH to normal
  - In metabolic alkalosis with high $HCO_3^-$, the lungs compensate through hypoventilation, which increases $PaCO_2$ and returns the pH to normal
- Compensation can be assessed by examining the ABG values
  - Look at the primary system affected ($PaCO_2$ or $HCO_3^-$)
  - Look at the system not affected ($PaCO_2$ or $HCO_3^-$)
  - If the ABGs in the unaffected system are moving in the same direction as those in the primary system, compensation is occurring (see Interpreting arterial blood gas levels).

## Pain

### General Information

- Pain is a complex phenomenon that involves biological, psychological, cultural and social factors, it is a primarily subjective experience
- Margo McCaffery, a pain researcher, defines *pain* as 'whatever the experiencing person says it is, existing whenever the experiencing person says it does'
- The International Association on Pain defines *pain* as unpleasant sensory and emotional experiences related to actual or potential tissue damage.

### Pain Theories

- All current pain-control theories are hypothetical none completely explain the pain experience and all its components
- The *specificity theory* holds that highly specific structures and pathways exist for pain transmission; this biologically oriented theory does not explain pain tolerance and ignores social, cultural, and empirical factors that influence pain
- The *pattern theory* holds that rapid and slow conduction pathways exist, which relay pain information through the spinal cord to the brain although this theory addresses the brain's ability to determine the amount, intensity, and type of sensory input, it does not address nonbiological influences on pain perception and transmission
- The *gate control theory* describes a hypothetical gate mechanism in the spinal cord that allows nerve fibers to receive pain sensations; the gate can be closed to pain sensation by occupying the receptor sites with other stimuli
  - This theory has encouraged a holistic approach to pain control and research by considering nonbiological components of pain
  - Pain management techniques, such as cutaneous stimulation, distraction and acupuncture are partly based on this theory.

### Anatomic and Physiologic Basis of Pain

- Stimulation of pain receptors in skin and soft tissues typically causes defined, localized pain
- Stimulation of pain receptors in deep tissues causes dull, poorly localized pain
- Stimulation of pain receptors in the viscera or organs causes diffuse, sometimes referred pain
- Pain can be stimulated by mechanical sources such as sharp objects, thermal sources such as fire or chemical sources, such as stomach acids and battery acid
- Pain travels from the periphery to the spinal cord to the brain by way of a pathway composed of A (delta) fibers (intense pain) and C fibers (dull, aching pain)
- Pain is processed in the thalamus, midbrain, and cortex
- Certain neurotransmitters such as histamine, serotonin, and prostaglandins, enhance pain impulse transmission
- Other neurotransmitters, such as endogenous opiates, endorphins and enkephalins, inhibit pain impulse transmission, chronic pain syndrome may be related to a deficiency of these inhibitory neurotransmitters.

### Factors that Affect Pain Response

- Pain is primarily a physical problem that has psychological effects
- The physical and psychological sources of pain are often complex and intertwined, with causative factors difficult to isolate

- *Psychogenic pain* is pain without a physiologic basis, this term is not helpful because all physical causes of pain cannot be diagnosed and all pain is real to the patient
- *Pain threshold* is the point at which a patient experiences pain
- *Pain tolerance* is affected by individual, psychosocial, cultural, religious, and environmental factors, it influences pain duration and intensity.

## Pain Assessment

### General Information

- Pain can be assessed with a subjective pain assessment tool
  - *0 to 10 rating scale:* The patient is asked to rate pain on a scale of 0 to 10, with 0 being no pain and 10 being the worst pain imaginable
  - *Face rating scale:* The patient is shown illustrations of five or more faces demonstrating varying levels of emotion, from happy to sad; by selecting the face that most closely approximates the pain sensation, the patient helps the nurse gauge the effectiveness of interventions
  - *Visual analog scale:* The patient places a mark on the scale, ranging from no pain to pain as bad as it can be, to indicate his current level of pain
  - *Body diagram:* The patient draws the location and radiation of pain on a paper illustration of the body
  - *Questionnaire:* The patient answers questions about the pain's location, intensity, quality, onset, and relieving and aggravating factors
  - *Pain flowchart:* The nurse documents variations in pain, vital signs and LOC in response to treatments, these forms are particularly useful for monitoring patient response to epidural opioid infusions and for titrating dosages
- Pain also can be assessed by observing for objective signs, such as facial grimacing; elevated blood pressure and increased pulse and respiratory rates, muscle tension, restlessness or an inability to concentrate, decreased interest in surroundings and increased focus on pain, perspiration and pallor, crying, moaning, or verbalizations of pain, and guarding the painful body part.

### Pain Classification

- *Acute pain* is mild to severe pain that's rapid in onset and lasts less than 6 months, it can be intermittent or recurrent as in migraine and sinus headaches and gallbladder colic.
- *Chronic pain* lasts beyond the expected healing time and may be difficult to relate to the original injury or tissue damage; it can be further classified as chronic benign pain (as in lower back pain), chronic cancer pain, or pain with ongoing peripheral pathology.

### Pharmacologic Management of Pain

- Nonopioid drugs, such as nonsteroidal anti-inflammatory drugs (NSAIDs) and acetaminophen, are used to treat acute pain caused by inflammation or tissue destruction and mild to moderate pain; they are useful adjuncts to opioid analgesics for controlling severe, acute pain
- Opioid analgesics such as narcotic agonist-antagonists relieve pain by occupying opioid receptor sites in the brain and spinal cord, they are used to treat moderate to severe acute pain (postoperative pain and fractures), recurrent acute pain (sickle cell crisis, angina, and renal colic), prolonged time-limited pain (cancer and burns), and pain that requires rapid, short-term relief (procedures such as bone marrow biopsy and thoracentesis)
- Sometimes small doses of antidepressants are used as adjuncts to pain control; they affect pain perception and reduce the accompanying anxiety
- The oral route of administration is the least expensive, easiest for patients to manage, and most widely accepted by patients; most NSAIDs and some opioids can be administered orally
- Parenteral routes (subcutaneous [Subcut], IM, and IV) are widely used to administer opioids
- Intraspinal (epidural) routes are used for short-term acute pain, such as that caused by abdominal surgery; the opioid's systemic effect is reduced with the intraspinal route compared with other parenteral routes
- Topical patches, such as those containing fentanyl, are useful during the transition from epidural to oral opioids
- Rectal administration of opioids may be indicated when a patient cannot tolerate oral medications temporarily because of nausea and vomiting
- Patient-controlled analgesia is the IV, Subcut, or intraspinal administration of opioids by means of an electronic controller that is programmed to respond with small doses when the patient requests medication
- Scheduled dosing is preferred to 'as needed'; around-the-clock dosing controls pain by avoiding the major peaks and valleys of the pain experience.

### Nonpharmacologic Management of Pain

- *Cutaneous stimulation* is a low-risk, inexpensive, noninvasive, readily available pain management technique that requires little skill to implement; examples include heat application, cold application, massage, pressure, vibration, and transcutaneous electrical nerve stimulation (the application of electric current through skin patches connected to a portable electrical source)
- *Therapeutic touch* unblocks congested areas of energy in the body; in this technique, the practitioner redirects energy by using touch to promote comfort, relaxation, healing, and a sense of well-being
- *Acupuncture* is the use of needles of various sizes to stimulate parts of the body to produce analgesia; this centuries-old technique originated in China and is gaining acceptance in Western medicine
- *Cognitive and behavioral pain management* uses imagery, distraction, relaxation techniques, and humor to help patients manage pain
- *Biofeedback* teaches patients to control involuntary body mechanisms, such as heart rate, muscle spasms, and circulation.

### Surgical Management of Pain

- Surgery seldom is used as a primary treatment for pain but can be considered to manage pain when pharmacologic therapies fail

- *Nerve blocks* involve the injection of phenol or alcohol to destroy nerve endings in a specific area
- *Rhizotomy* is the surgical destruction of sensory nerve roots where they enter the spinal cord; *chordotomy* is the transection of spinal cord nerves at the spinal cord's midline portion
- *Neurectomy* is the resection or partial or total excision of a spinal or cranial nerve
- *Cryoanalgesia* deactivates a nerve using a cooled probe that causes temporary nerve injury
- *Radio-frequency lesioning* may affect the nerve from the heat generated, the magnetic field created by the radio waves, or both
- *Percutaneous electrical nerve stimulation* uses implanted leads and a surface stimulator or implanted generator to block pain impulses by delivering electric charges to a nerve root
- Spinal nerve blocks, rhizotomy, and chordotomy can impair bladder, bowel, and sexual functioning.

### Nursing Care of the Patient in Pain

- Assess the pain's location, and ask the patient to rate the pain using a pain scale
- Ask the patient to describe the pain's quality and pattern, including any precipitating or relieving factors
- Monitor vital signs and note subjective responses to pain, such as facial grimacing and guarding of a body part
- Administer pain medication around the clock as ordered
- Provide comfort measures, such as back massage, positioning, linen changes, and oral or skin care
- Teach the patient noninvasive techniques to control pain, such as relaxation, guided imagery, distraction and cutaneous stimulation
- Teach the importance of taking prescribed analgesics before the pain becomes severe
- Instruct the patient on the need for adequate rest periods and sleep.

### Referral to a Pain Clinic or Hospice

- Patients with chronic benign pain that cannot be controlled by nonpharmacologic interventions may benefit from treatment at a pain clinic
- The clinic's interdisciplinary staff works with the patient to assess the pain and develops a pain control regimen that helps the patient regain or maintain an acceptable level of functioning
- Hospice programs give care and support to dying patients and their families; pain control—one of the primary goals—provides the patient with adequate pain relief at home.

## CARDIOVASCULAR DISORDERS

### Introduction

- Proper functioning of the cardiovascular system ensures the adequate delivery of nutrients to and the removal of wastes from body cells
- Disruptions in the cardiovascular system can lead to alterations in organ function, disability, and death.

### Nursing History

- The nurse asks the patient about his *chief complaint*
  - The patient with a cardiovascular problem will likely cite a specific complaint, including chest, jaw, arm, or neck pain; irregular heartbeat or palpitations; shortness of breath on exertion, lying down, or at night; cough; cyanosis or pallor; weakness; fatigue; unexplained weight change; swelling of the extremities; dizziness; high or low blood pressure
  - The patient with a cardiovascular problem may also report peripheral skin changes, such as decreased hair distribution, skin color changes, or a thin, shiny appearance to the skin; and pain in the extremities, such as leg pain or cramps
- The nurse then questions the patient about his *present illness*
  - Ask the patient about his symptom, including when it started, associated signs and symptoms, location, radiation, intensity, duration, frequency, and precipitating and alleviating factors; if pain is the symptom, ask him to rate it on a scale of 0 to 10 (with 0 being no pain and 10 worst pain experienced)
  - Ask about the use of prescription and over-the-counter drugs, herbal remedies, vitamin and nutritional supplements, and alternative or complementary therapies used
- The nurse asks about *medical history*
  - Question the patient about other cardiac and related disorders, such as hypertension, diabetes mellitus, hyperlipidemia, stroke, scarlet fever, rheumatic fever, strep throat, anemia, syncope, and congenital heart defects
  - Ask the female patient about the use of oral contraceptives and hormones and whether she's premenopausal or postmenopausal
- The nurse then assesses the *family history*
  - Ask about a family history of hypertension, coronary artery disease (CAD), vascular disease, congenital heart disease, or hyperlipidemia
  - Also ask the patient if he has a family history of diabetes mellitus
- The nurse obtains a *social history*
  - Ask about work, exercise, diet, caffeine intake, use of recreational drugs, alcohol use, and hobbies
  - Also ask about stress, support systems, coping mechanisms, and his cultural and religious background.

### Physical Assessment

- The nurse begins with *inspection*
  - Observe the patient's general appearance: Is he/she thin, cachectic, or obese? Is he/she alert or anxious? What is his/her respiratory rate and breathing pattern? Check his/her hair distribution
  - Note the skin color: Is it pink, pale, or cyanotic?
  - Note any clubbing, edema, and skin lesions
  - Observe the chest and thorax: The lateral diameter should be twice the anteroposterior diameter; note any deviations from the typical chest shape

- Inspect the neck for visible pulsations and jugular vein distention
- Look for pulsations, symmetry of movement, retractions, or heaves; note the location of the apical impulse
- Next, the nurse uses *palpation*
  - Palpate the precordium for heaves, thrills, and the point of maximum impulse; also palpate the sternoclavicular, aortic, pulmonic, tricuspid, and epigastric areas
  - Palpate pulses in the extremities and neck for strength, rhythm, and equality
  - Palpate the extremities for skin temperature, edema, capillary refill time, and turgor
- Then the nurse *percusses* the heart
  - Percuss the left border of the heart, noting the sound change from resonance to dullness
  - Try to percuss the right border of the heart; in most people, it is under the sternum and cannot be percussed
- The nurse continues by *auscultating* the heart and vessels
  - Use the diaphragm of the stethoscope to listen over the mitral or apical area for 1 minute; note heart rate and rhythm
  - Proceed sequentially through the auscultatory landmarks and listen for first and second heart sounds (S1 and S2)
  - Listen for extra sounds, such as a third and fourth heart sound (S3 and S4), murmurs, clicks, snaps, and rubs
  - Repeat the sequence, using the bell of the stethoscope
  - An S3 (ventricular gallop) is low pitched and best heard over, the apex of the heart; the rhythm is similar to a horse gallop, and the cadence sounds like 'Kentucky'
  - An S4 occurs during atrial contraction, just before S1; its cadence sounds like 'Tennessee'
  - The S3 and S4 sounds are best heard with the bell of the stethoscope placed at the apical area while the patient is supine or lying on his left side
  - Auscultate for bruits over the abdominal aorta and the carotid and femoral arteries.

## Acute Coronary Syndrome

### Description

- Acute coronary syndrome (ACS) includes three major thrombotic effects of CAD and the resulting myocardial ischemia (see *Acute coronary syndromes*)
  - Unstable angina
  - Non-ST-segment elevation myocardial infarction (non-STEMI)
  - STEMI
- ACS results when a rupture or erosion of plaque occurs in one or more coronary arteries, resulting in platelet adhesions, activation of thrombin, and clot formation, reducing myocardial blood flow
- ACS requires prompt evaluation to differentiate noncardiac pain from cardiac pain, so proper treatment can be quickly initiated
- Complications of myocardial infarction (MI) may include heart failure, mitral valve insufficiency, cardiogenic shock, arrhythmias, and death.

## Arrhythmias

### Description

- During a cardiac arrhythmia, abnormal electrical conduction or automaticity changes heart rate and rhythm
- Arrhythmias vary in severity, from mild and asymptomatic ones that require no treatment (such as sinus arrhythmia, in which heart rate increases and decreases with respirations) to catastrophic ventricular fibrillation, which necessitates immediate resuscitation
- Arrhythmias are generally classified according to their origin (atrial or ventricular); their effect on cardiac output and blood pressure, partially influenced by the site of origin, determines their clinical significance (see *The 8-step method of rhythm strip analysis*)
- Causes of arrhythmias include congenital heart disease, degeneration of the conduction system, drug effects or toxicity, heart disease, myocardial ischemia, stress, alcohol, electrolyte imbalance, acid-base imbalances, cellular hypoxia, and conditions such as anemia, anorexia, thyroid dysfunction, adrenal insufficiency, and pulmonary disease (see cardiac arrhythmias).

### Signs and Symptoms

- The patient with an arrhythmia may be asymptomatic or may report palpitations, chest pain, dizziness, weakness, fatigue, and feelings of impending doom
- Other signs and symptoms include an irregular heart rhythm, bradycardia or tachycardia, hypotension, syncope, reduced level of consciousness, diaphoresis, pallor, nausea, vomiting, and cold, clammy skin
- Life-threatening arrhythmias may result in pulselessness, absence of respirations, and no palpable blood pressure.

### Nursing Interventions

- Monitor the pulse for an irregular pattern or an abnormally rapid or slow rate; if the patient is receiving continuous cardiac monitoring, observe him for arrhythmias
- Assess the patient for signs and symptoms of hemodynamic compromise
- If the patient has an arrhythmia, promptly assess his airway, breathing, and circulation
- Initiate basic life support measures if indicated, until other advanced cardiac life support measures are available and successful
- Perform defibrillation early for ventricular tachycardia and ventricular fibrillation
- Administer medications as needed, and prepare for medical procedures (for example, cardioversion or pacemaker insertion) if indicated
- Monitor the patient for fluid and electrolyte imbalance and signs of drug toxicity, especially digoxin; correct the underlying cause and adjust medications as needed
- Provide adequate oxygen and reduce the heart's workload, while carefully maintaining metabolic, neurologic, respiratory, and hemodynamic status.

| Acute coronary syndromes | | | | | |
|---|---|---|---|---|---|
| Thrombotic effect | Description | Signs and symptoms | Diagnosis | Treatment | Nursing consideration |
| • Unstable angina | • Angina increasing in frequency and severity from patient's baseline<br>• Easily induced<br>• Lasts 5 to 15 minutes | • Burning squeezing substernal or retrosternal pain spreading across chest; may radiate to inside of arm neck, jaw or shoulder blade<br>• Possible associated symptoms shortness of breath, dizziness, nausea, palpitations, weakness, and cold sweats<br>• Possible associated signs: hypertension or hypotension, tachycardia or bradycardia<br>• Most often occurs with physical activity<br>• Often relieved by rest or nitrates | • Electrocardiogram (ECG) may be normal or may show ischemla with transient T wave or ST-segment changes<br>• Cardiac biomarkers usually remain within normal limits | • Rest<br>• Nitrates to reduce myocardial oxygen consumption<br>• Beta-drenergic blockers to reduce the workload and oxygen demand<br>• Calcium channel blockers if caused by coronary artery spasm<br>• Oxygen to increase oxygenation of the blood<br>• Antiplatelet drugs to minimize platelet aggregation<br>• Coronary angiography to determine stenosis or obstruction with possible angioplasty or stent placement | • During acute anginal episode, monitor blood pressure and heart rate<br>• Obtain an ECG before administering nitrates<br>• Record duration of pain, amount of medication required to relieve pain, and accompanying symptoms<br>• Obtain cardiac enzyme levels<br>• Administer oxygen<br>• Administer oxygen<br>• Administer medications as ordered |
| • Non-ST-segment elevation myocardial infarction (MI) | • MI that usually occurs due to occlusion of coronary vessel<br>• Occlusion may be complete or partial | • Burning squeezing substernal or retrosternal pain spreading across chest; may radiate to inside of arm neck jaw, or shoulder blade; pain more intense than that of angina<br>• Associated symptoms: Shortness of breath, dizziness, nausea, palpitations, weakness, and cold sweats<br>• Associated signs: Hypertension or hypotension, tachycardia or badycardia<br>• Pain not relieved with rest<br>• Difficult to distinguish from angina<br>• $S_1$ and $S_4$ may be present | • Positive cardiac markers<br>• ECG shows ST-segment depression or may be normal<br>• ECG may have ST-segment elevation for less than 20 minutes | • Oxygen to increase oxygenation of the blood<br>• Nonenteric-coated aspirin for antiplatelet effect<br>• Beta-adrenergic blockers to reduce the workload and oxygen demand<br>• Angiotensin-converting enzyme (ACE) inhibitor to reduce afterload and preload | • Adminster oxygen<br>• Administer medications as ordered<br>• Monitor ECG, vital signs, and level of consciousness (LOC)<br>• Obtain cardiac markers.<br>• Monitor cardiopulmonary status frequently and notify practitioner of changes. |
| • ST-segment elevation (MI) | • MI that usually occurs due to complete occlusion of coronary vessel | • Burning squeezing substernal or retrosternal pain spreading across chest may radiate to inside of arm neck, jaw, or shoulder blade, pain more intense than that of angina<br>• Associated symptoms: Shortness of breath, dizziness, nausea, palpitations, weakness and cold sweats<br>• Associated signs: Hypertension or hypotension, tachycardia or bradycardia<br>• Pain not relieved with rest<br>• $S_1$ and $S_4$ may be present | • Positive cardiac markers<br>• ECG shows ST-segment elevation or new left bundle-branch block in leads associated with occluded artery<br>• Nuclear imaging studies show areas of ischemia | • Oxygen to increase oxygenation of the blood<br>• Nonenteric-coated aspririn for antiplatelet effect<br>• Fibrinolytic therapy for eligible patients<br>• Coronary angioplasty with percutaneous coronary intervention<br>• Beta-adrenergic blockers to reduce the workload and oxygen demand<br>• ACE inhibitor to reduce afterload and preload | • Administer oxygen<br>• Administer medications as ordered<br>• Monitor ECG, vital signs, and LOC<br>• Obtain cardiac markers as ordered<br>• If patient received fibrinolytic, monitor for bleeding<br>• Monitor cardiopulmonary status frequently and notify practitioner of changes |

## The 8-step method of rhythm strip analysis

Rhythm strip analysis requires a sequential and systematic approach. The following eight steps provide a good outline for you to follow:

### Step 1: Determine rhythm

To determine the hearts atrial and ventricular rhythms, use either the pen-and-pencil method or the caliper method.

To determine the atrial rhythm, measure the P-P intervals, the intervals between consecutive P waves. These intervals should occur regularly, with only small variations associated with respirations. Then compare the P-P intervals indicate regular atrial rhythm; dissimilar P-P intervals indicate irregular atrial rhythm.

To determine the ventricular rhythm, measure the intervals between two consecutive R waves in the QRS complexes. If an R wave is not present, use either Q waves or S waves of consecutive QRS complexes. The R-R intervals should occur regularly. Then compare the R-R intervals in several cycles. As with atrial rhythms, consistently similar intervals mean a regular rhythm; dissimilar intervals point to an irregular rhythm.

After completing your measurements ask yourself:

- Is the rhythm regular or irregular? Consider a rhythm with only slight variations up to 0.04 second to be regular.
- If the rhythm is irregular, is it slightly irregular or markedly irregular? Does the irregularity occur in pattern (a regularly irregular pattern?)

### Step 2: Calculate rate

You can use one of the three methods to determine the atrial and ventricular heart rates from an electrocardiogram (ECG) waveform. Although these methods can provide accurate information, you shouldn't rely solely on them when assessing your patient keep in mind that the ECG waveform represents electrical not mechanical, activity.

Therefore, although an ECG can show that ventricular depolarization has occurred, it does not mean that ventricular contraction has occurred. To determine this, you must assess the patient's pulse.

- *Times-ten method:* The simplest quickest and most common way to calculate rate is the times-ten method especially if the rhythm is irregular ECG paper is marked in increments of 3 seconds or 15 large boxes. To calculate the atrial rate obtain a 6-second strip count the number of P waves that appear on it and multiply this number by 10. Ten 6-second strips equal 1 minute. Calculate the ventricular rate the same way using the R waves.
- *1,500 method:* If the heart rhythm is regular, use the 1,500 method, so named because 1,500 small squares equal 1 minute. Count the number of small squares between identical points on two consecutive P waves, and then divide 1,500 by that number to determine the atrial rate. To obtain the ventricular rate, use the same method with two consecutive R waves.
- *Sequence method:* The third method of estimating heart rate is the sequence method, which requires memorizing a sequence of numbers. For the atrial rate find a P wave that peaks on a heavy black line. Estimate the ventricular rate the same way, using the R wave.

**Step 3: Evaluate P waves**

When examining a rhythm strip for P wave ask yourself:
- Are P waves present?
- Do the P waves have a normal configuration?
- Do all of the P waves have a similar size and shape?
- Is there one P wave for every QRS complex?

**Step 4: Determine PR interval duration**

To measure the PR interval count the small squares between the start of the P wave and the start of the QRS complex; then multiply the number of squares by 0.04 second. After you perform this calculation, ask yourself:

- Does the duration of the PR interval fall within normal limits 0.12 to 0.20 second (or 3 to 5 small squares)?
- Is the PR interval constant?

**Step 5: Determine QRS complex duration**

When determining QRS complex duration, make sure to measure straight across from the end of the PR interval to the end of the S wave, not just to the peak. Remember the QRS complex has no horizontal components. To calculate duration count the number of small squares between the beginning and the end of the QRS complex, and multiply this number by 0.04 second. Then ask yourself the following questions:
- Does the duration of the QRS complex fall within normal limits, 0.06 to 0.10 second?
- Are all QRS complexes the same size and shape? (If not measure each one and describe them individually)
- Does a QRS complex appear after every P wave?

**Step 6: Evaluate T wave**

Examine the T waves on the ECG strip. Then ask yourself:
- Are T waves present?
- Do all of the T waves have a normal shape?
- Could a P wave be hidden in a T wave?
- Do all of the T waves have a normal amplitude?
- Do the T waves have the same deflection as the QRS complexes?

**Step 7: Determine QT interval duration**

Count the number of small squares between the beginning of the QRS complex and the end of the T wave, where the T wave returns to the baseline. Multiply this number by 0.04 second ask yourself:
- Does the duration of the QT interval fall within normal limits, 0.36 to 0.44 second?

**Step 8: Evaluate other components**

Note the presence of ectopic or aberrantly conducted beats or other abnormalities. Also check the ST segment for abnormalities and look for the presence of a U wave.

Next, interpret your findings by classifying the rhythm strip according to one or all of the following features:
- *Site of origin of the rhythm:* For example, sinus node, atria, atrioventricular node, or ventricles.
- *Rate:* Normal (60 to 100 beats/minute), bradycardia (less than 60 beats/minute), or tachycardia (greater than 100 beats/minutes).
- *Rhythm:* Normal or abnormal, for example, flutter fibriliation, heart block, escape rhythm or other arrhythmias.

## Cardiac arrhythmias

**Normal Sinus Rhythm**

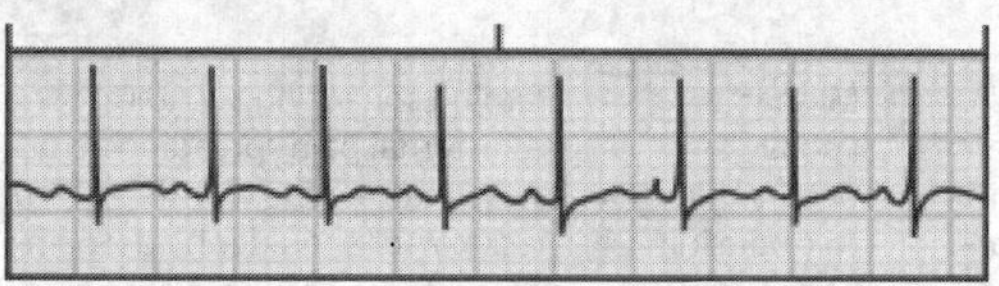

- Ventricular and atrial rates of 60 to 100 beats/minute (BPM)
- QRS complexes and P waves regular and uniform
- PR interval 0.12 to 0.2 second
- Duration of QRS complex < 0.12 second
- Identical atrial and ventricular rates, with constant PR interval

**Sinus Tachycardia**

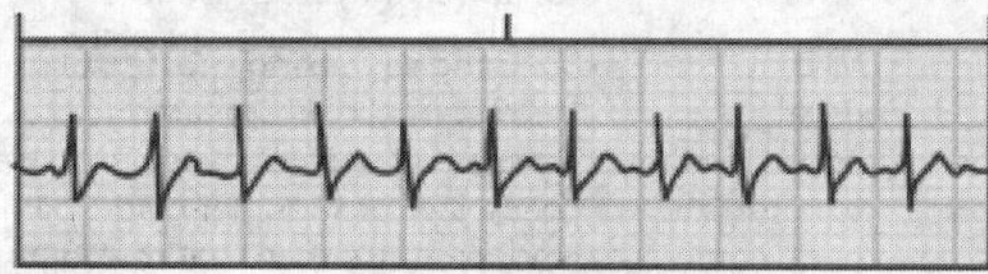

***Description***
- Rate > 100 BPM: rarely > 160 BPM
- Every QRS complex follows a P wave

***Treatment***
- Correction of underlying cause; a beta-adrenergic blocker or channel blocker if symptomatic or cardiac related

**Sinus Bradycardia**

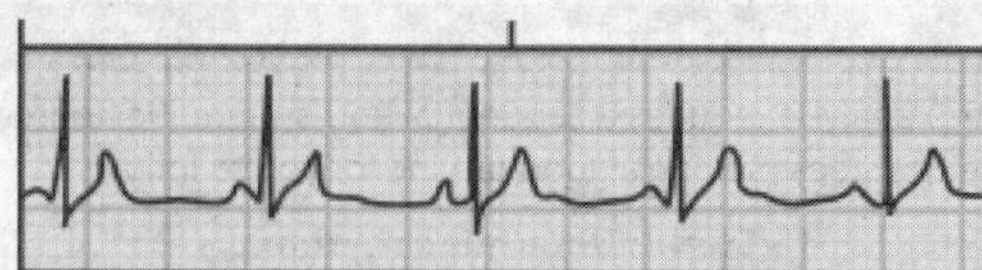

***Description***
- Rate < 60 BPM
- QRS complex follows each P wave

***Treatment***
- For low cardiac output, dizziness, weakness, altered level of consciousness, or low blood pressure, advanced cardiac life support (ACLS) protocol for administration of atropine IV

- Dopamine, epinephrine, if atropine fails
- Transcutaneous pacemaker (TCP)

**Paroxysmal Atrial Tachycardia or Paroxysmal Supraventricular Tachycardia**

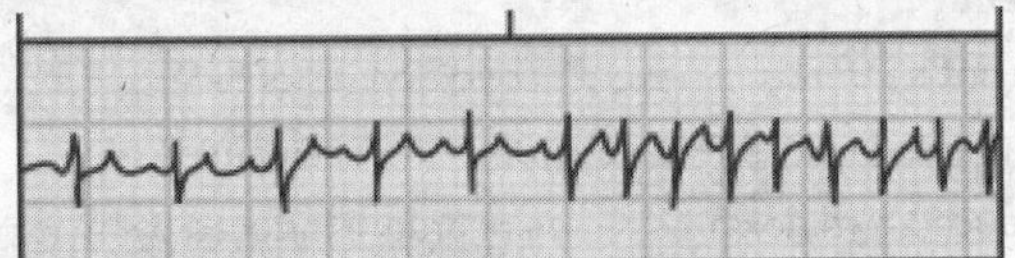

***Description***

- Heart rate > 140 BPM rarely exceeds 250 BPM
- P waves regular but aberrant; difficult to differentiate from preceding T wave
- Sudden onset and termination of arrhythmia
- May cause palpitations and light headedness

***Treatment***

- Vagal maneuvers
- Adenosine by rapid IV push
- Other treatments: Beta-adrenergic blockers, verapamil, diltiazem, and digoxin (If it is not the cause of arrhythmia) to alter atrioventricular (AV) node conduction
- Elective cardioversion, if patient symptomatic and unresponsive to drugs
- Radiofrequency catheter ablation

**Atrial flutter**

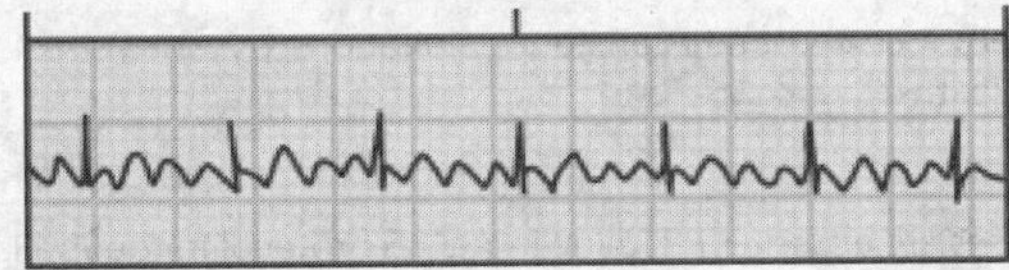

***Description***

- Ventricular rate depends on degree of AV block (may be 60 to 100 BPM; however, 150 BPM; is not uncommon)
- Atrial rate 250 to 400 BPM and regular
- QRS complexes uniform in shape, but typically irregular in rate
- P waves may have sawtooth configuration (F waves)

***Treatment***

- If patient is stable, ACLS protocol for cardloversion and drug therapy including calcium channel blockers beta-adrenergic blockers, or antiarrhythmics
- If patient is unstable with a ventricular rate > 150 BPM, immediate cardioversion
- Radiofrequency ablation to control rhythm
- Possible anticoagulation therapy

**Atrial Fibrillation**

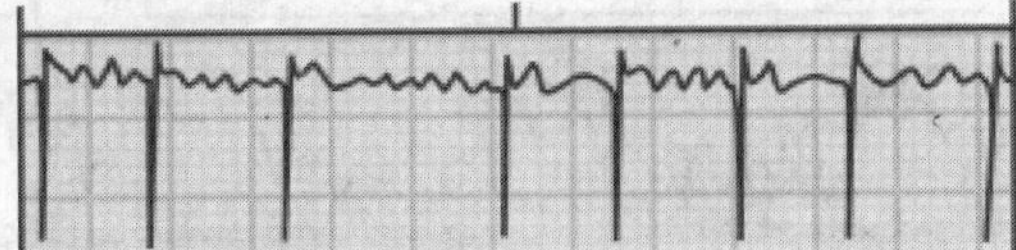

***Description***

- Atrial rate > 400 BPM; ventricular rate varies
- QRS complexes uniform in shape but at irregular intervals
- PR interval indiscernible
- No P waves or P waves appear as erratic, irregular baseline F waves

***Treatment***

- If patient is unstable with a ventricular rate > 150 BPM, immediate cardioversion
- If patient is stable, ACLS protocol and drug therapy including calcium channel blockers, beta-adrenergic blockers, or antiarrhythmics
- In some patients uncontrolled by drugs, radiofrequency ablation
- Anticoagulation therapy to reduce risk of thromboemboli

**AV Junctional Rhythm (Nodal Rhythm)**

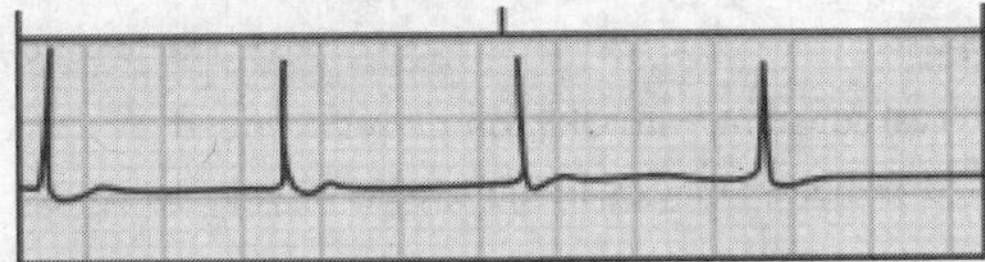

***Description***

- Ventricular rate usually 40 to 60 BPM (60 to 100 BPM is accelerated junctional rhythm)
- P waves may precede, be hidden within, or follow a QRS complex; if visible, they're altered
- Duration of QRS complex normal except in aberrant conduction
- Patient may be asymptomatic unless ventricular rate very slow

***Treatment***

- Correction of underlying cause
- Atropine or pacemaker for slow rate
- If patient taking digoxin, it is discontinued

**First-degree AV block**

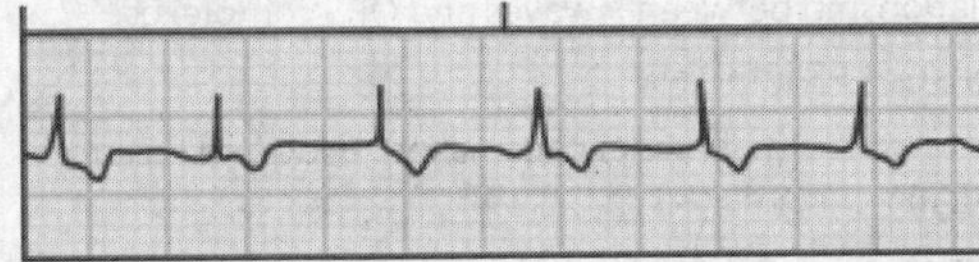

***Description***

- PR interval prolonged > 0.20 second
- QRS complex normal

***Treatment***

- Digoxin (cautiously)
- Correction of underlying cause; otherwise, monitoring for increasing block
- Possibly atropine, if severe symptomatic bradycardia develops

**Second-degree AV Block Mobitz Type I (Wenckebach)**

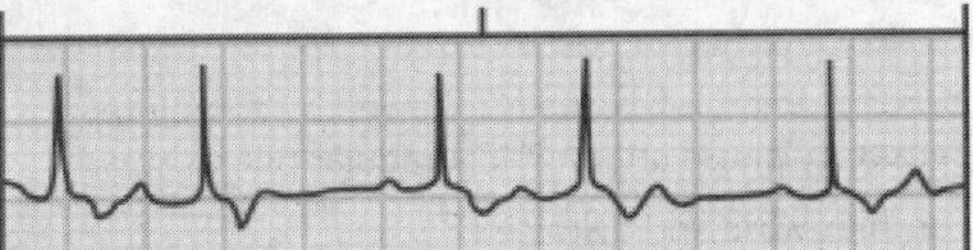

***Description***

- PR interval becomes progressively longer with each cycle until QRS complex disappears (dropped beat); after a dropped beat, PR interval shorter
- Ventricular rate irregular; atrial rhythm regular

***Treatment***

- Atropine, if patient symptomatic
- May discontinue digoxin
- Temporary pacing, if ventricular rate slow

**Second-degree AV Block Mobitz Type II**

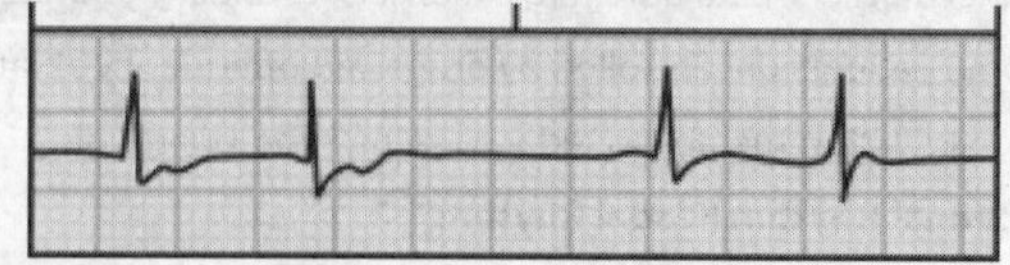

***Description***

- PR interval constant, with QRS complexes dropped
- Ventricular rhythm may be irregular with varying degree of block
- Atrial rate regular

***Treatment***

- Temporary pacemaker sometimes followed by permanent pacemaker
- If patient taking digoxin, it is discontinued
- Atropine, dopamine, or epinephrine for symptomatic bradycardia

**Third-degree AV Block (Complete Heart Block)**

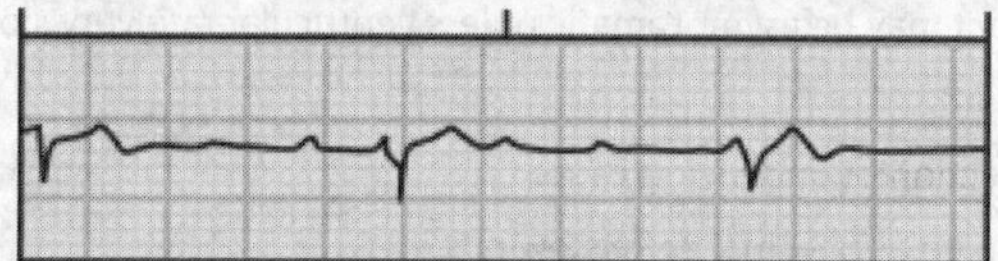

***Description***

- Atrial rate regular; ventricular rate slow and regular
- No relationship between P waves and QRS complexes
- No constant PR interval
- QRS interval normal (nodal pacemaker); wide and bizarre (ventricular pacemaker)

***Treatment***

- Usually requires TCP, followed by permanent pacemaker
- Dopamine and epinephrine to maintain blood pressure
- Atropine for symptomatic bradycardia
- Cardiopulmonary resuscitation (CPR) until pacing initiated

**Premature Ventricular Contraction (PVC)**

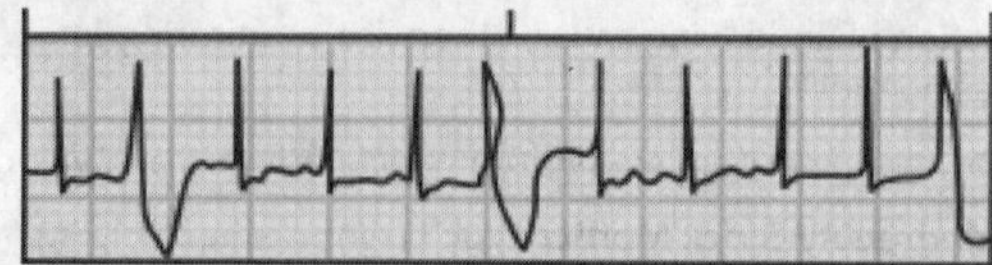

***Description***

- Beat occur prematurely, usually followed by complete compensatory pause after a PVC; irregular pulse
- QRS complex wide and distorted
- Can occur singly in pairs or in threes; can alternate with normal beats; focus can be from one or more sites
- PVCs most ominous when clustered, multifocal and with R wave on T pattern

***Treatment***

- May not be treated if patient's condition is stable
- If warranted lidocaine amiodarone, or procainamide IV
- If induced by digoxin, cessation of drug; if induced by hypokalemia, potassium chloride IV; if induced by hypomagnesemia, magnesium sulfate IV
- An oral type III agent (such as amiodarone or sotalol), if maintenance therapy necessary

**Ventricular Tachycardia**

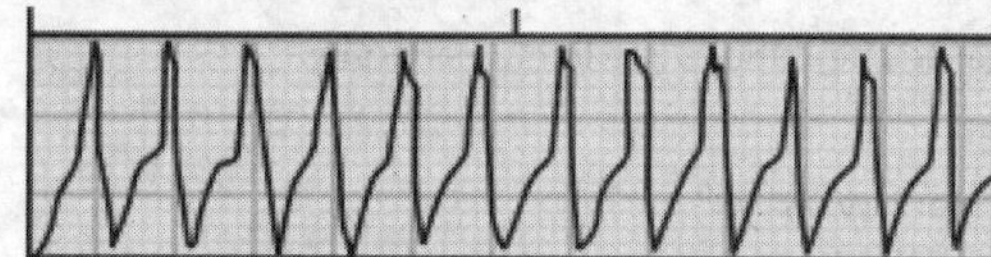

***Description***

- Ventricular rate 100 to 220 BPM; may be regular
- Three or more PVCs in a row
- QRS complexes wide, bizarre, and independent of P wave
- QRS complexes may be monomorphic (look alike) or polymorphic (look different)
- Usually no visible P waves
- Can produce chest pain, anxiety, palpitations, dyspnea shock, coma and death

***Treatment***

- If pulses are absent, CPR following ACLS protocol for defibrillation and administration of epinephrine IV or vasopressin, followed by amniodarone, lidocaine, magnesium or procainamide
- If pulse present with polymorphic QRS complexes and normal QT interval, beta-adrenergic blockers, lidocaine, amiodarone, procainamide, or sotalol (following ACLS protocol); if drug unsuccessful, cardioversion
- If pulse present with polymorphic QRS and prolonged QT interval magnesium IV, then overdrive pacing if rhythm persists
- If pulse present and patient's condition stable with monomorphic QRS complexes, procainamide sotalol, amiodarone, or lidocaine (follow ACLS protocol); if drugs ineffective, cardioversion
- Correction of underlying cause
- Maintenance therapy with drugs, such as amiodarone and sotalol
- Implanted cardiovert tachycardia defibrillator if recurrent ventricular tachycardia

**Ventricular Fibrillation**

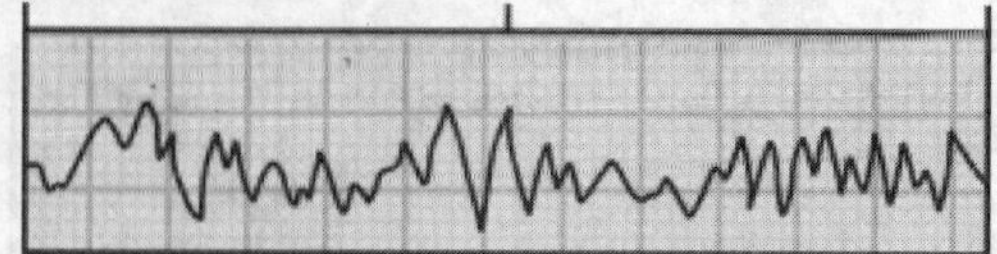

| Description |
|---|
| • Ventricular rhythm rapid and chaotic |
| • No QRS complexes; no visible P waves |
| • Loss of consciousness, with no peripheral pulses, blood pressure, or respirations: possible seizures; sudden death |
| **Treatment** |
| • CPR, following ACLS protocol for defibrillation and administration of epinephrine, vasopressin, amiodarone or lidocaine and if ineffective, magnesium sulfate or procainamide |
| • Implanted cardioverter defibrillator if risk for recurrent ventricular fibrillation |

**Pulseless Electrical Activity (Electromechanical Dissociation)**

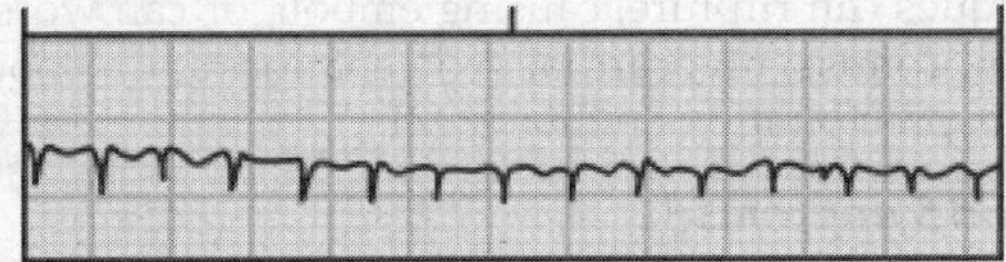

| Description |
|---|
| • Organized electrical activity without pulse or other evidence of effective myocardial contraction |
| • Any rhythm possible |
| **Treatment** |
| • CPR |
| • Epinephrine |
| • Atropine for bradycardia |
| • Correction of underlying cause |

**Ventricular Standstill (Asystole)**

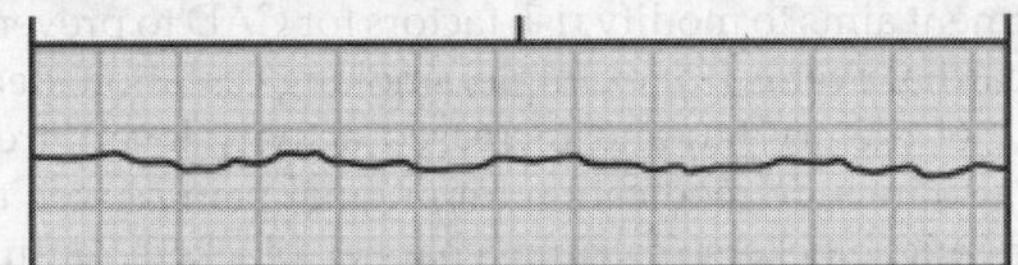

| Description |
|---|
| • *Primary ventricular standstill:* Regular P waves, no QRS complexes |
| • *Secondary ventricular standstill:* QRS complexes wide and slurred, occurring at irregular intervals; agonal heart rhythm |
| • Loss of consciousness, no peripheral pulses, blood pressure, or respirations |
| **Treatment** |
| • CPR |
| • ACLS protocol for endotracheal intubation, TCP, and epinephrine and atropine administration |

## Buerger's Disease

### Description

- Buerger's disease, also called thromboangiitis obliterans, is an inflammatory, nonatheromatous occlusive condition that causes segmental lesions and subsequent thrombus formation in the small and medium arteries (and sometimes the veins), resulting in decreased blood flow to the feet and legs
- It usually occurs in men between ages 20 and 30 and in heavy smokers.

### Signs and Symptoms

- Buerger's disease typically causes intermittent claudication of the instep or legs, which is aggravated by exercise and relieved by rest
- Pulses are diminished or absent, and the patient may experience coldness, numbness, tingling, or burning in the affected extremity
- As the disease progresses, redness, heat, tingling, or cyanosis may appear when the extremity is in a dependent position, and ulcers and gangrene may appear.

### Diagnosis and Treatment

- Diagnostic tests may include Doppler ultrasonography, plethysmography, arteriography, venography, and digital subtraction angiography
- For patients with severe disease, lumbar sympathectomy may improve blood flow through vasodilation
- Amputation may be necessary for nonhealing ulcers, intractable pain, or gangrene
- Vasodilator therapy hasn't proved to be effective, but pentoxifylline (Pentoxil), calcium channel blockers, and thromboxane inhibitors may be helpful, especially if vasospasm is present.

### Nursing Interventions

- Warn the patient that he/she must stop smoking to avoid worsening of his/her symptoms
- Tell him to avoid excessive cold temperatures to reduce vasoconstriction
- Avoid the use of vasoconstricting medications
- Teach the patient to take measures to protect the extremities from trauma and infection
- Encourage the patient to participate in progressive exercise.

## Cardiomyopathy

### Description

- Cardiomyopathy is a disease of the heart muscle, reducing cardiac output and eventually resulting in heart failure
- Cardiomyopathy is classified according to the structural and functional abnormalities of the heart muscle; types include dilated, or congestive (most common form; dilated cardiac chambers contract poorly, causing blood to pool and thrombi to form); hypertrophic obstructive (hypertrophied left ventricle is small, unable to relax and fill properly); restrictive (rare form; stiff ventricles are resistant to filling); arrhythmogenic right ventricular; and unclassified
- Causes of dilated cardiomyopathy include chronic alcoholism, viral or bacterial infection, metabolic and immunologic disorders, and pregnancy and postpartum disorders; causes of hypertrophic cardiomyopathy include congenital disorders and hypertension; restrictive cardiomyopathy may be idiopathic, or it may stem from amyloidosis, cancer, or heart transplant; arrhythmogenic right ventricular cardiomyopathy most likely has a genetic

cause and results from the infiltration of fibrous and adipose tissue into the myocardium; unclassified cardiomyopathy does not fit into other categories and can have various causes.

### Signs and Symptoms

- Signs and symptoms of heart failure are present, including tachycardia, S3 and S4 heart sounds, exertional dyspnea, paroxysmal nocturnal dyspnea, cough, fatigue, jugular venous distention, dependent pitting edema, peripheral cyanosis, and hepatomegaly
- Heart murmurs and arrhythmias may also occur.

### Diagnosis and Treatment

- Diagnostic tests include electrocardiogram (ECG), echocardiogram, cardiac catheterization, radionuclide studies, and chest X-ray
- Medications for dilated cardiomyopathy include an angiotensin-converting enzyme (ACE) inhibitor or hydralazine plus a nitrate (the mainstay of therapy), a beta-adrenergic blocker, digoxin, a diuretic, and an anticoagulant
- Medications for hypertrophic cardiomyopathy include a beta-adrenergic blocker and a calcium channel blocker
- No specific medications are used to treat restrictive cardiomyopathy; however, diuretics, digoxin, nitrates, and other vasodilators can worsen the condition and should be avoided
- An antiarrhythmic, a pacemaker, or an implantable cardiac defibrillator may be necessary to control arrhythmias
- Surgery, such as heart transplantation or cardiomyoplasty (for dilated cardiomyopathy) or ventricular myotomy or myectomy (for hypertrophic obstructive cardiomyopathy) may be indicated if medications fail.

### Nursing Interventions

- Monitor ECG results, cardiovascular status, vital signs, and hemodynamic variables to detect heart failure and arrhythmias and assess the patient's response to medications
- If the patient is receiving a diuretic, monitor his serum electrolyte levels to detect abnormalities such as hypokalemia
- Administer oxygen and keep the patient in semi-Fowler's position to promote oxygenation
- Make sure the patient restricts activity if necessary to reduce oxygen demands on the heart
- Teach the patient the signs and symptoms of heart failure he should report to the practitioner
- Explain the importance of checking his weight daily and reporting an increase of 3 lb (1.4 kg) or more (1 liter of fluid equals 1 kg or 2.2 lb)
- Encourage the patient to express his feelings such as a fear of dying.

## Coronary Artery Disease

### Description

- In CAD, plaques partially or totally occlude the coronary artery vasculature; it is the leading cause of death and disease in the United States
- Some risk factors for CAD cannot be modified: old age, male gender, and family history of heart disease
- Other risk factors can be modified: Increased levels of triglycerides, low-density lipoprotein, and very-low-density lipoprotein; high-fat diet; hypertension; obesity; diabetes; cigarette smoking; sedentary lifestyle; and high stress level
- CAD begins when endothelial cells in the arterial lining are injured, making them permeable to lipoproteins
  - Clot-forming platelets adhere to the injury site, and lipoproteins build up around smooth-muscle cells, causing fatty streaks
  - Fibrofatty plaques form from repeated injury to the endothelial cells; as the process is repeated, the vessel progressively narrows
  - Plaques can rupture, causing emboli, or can worsen and compromise myocardial oxygenation and blood flow, thus precipitating angina or MI.

### Signs and Symptoms

- Anginal pain is a classic symptom of CAD
- Others include the secondary effects of CAD, such as MI, heart failure, sudden cardiac death, cardiomegaly, valvular insufficiencies, cardiogenic shock, and stroke.

### Diagnosis and Treatment

- Diagnostic tests may include ECG, exercise ECG (stress test), cardiac catheterization, coronary angiography, intravascular ultrasound, myocardial perfusion imaging, and echocardiography
- Laboratory tests for cardiac isoenzymes (CK-MB and LD1), troponin, myoglobin, cholesterol, lipoproteins, and triglycerides also may be performed
- Treatment aims to modify risk factors for CAD to prevent acute myocardial events (for example, smoking cessation, decreased intake of dietary fat, and increased activity level); treatment may also include medication for anginal pain as well as beta-adrenergic blockers, calcium channel blockers, antiplatelet, antilipemic, antihypertensive drugs, and oxygen therapy
- Surgical treatment, such as angioplasty, rotational atherectomy or stent placement, percutaneous transluminal coronary angioplasty, or coronary artery bypass grafting (CABG), may be required to prevent progression to MI.

### Nursing Interventions

- Increase the patient's knowledge of the relationship between risk factors and the development of CAD
- Teach the patient and family how to modify risk factors
- Encourage the patient to establish healthful habits, such as regular exercise and a low-fat diet
- Encourage participation in a smoking cessation program
- Emphasize the importance of prevention in treating heart disease
- Administer medication for anginal pain as ordered.

## Heart Failure

### Description

- Heart failure is a condition in which the heart can no longer pump enough blood to meet the body's demands

- Left-sided heart failure may be caused by anterior MI, ventricular septal defect, cardiomyopathy, cardiac tamponade, constrictive pericarditis, increased circulating blood volume, aortic stenosis and insufficiency, or mitral stenosis and insufficiency
- Right-sided heart failure may be caused by left-sided heart failure, a right ventricular MI, atrial septal defect, fluid overload and sodium retention, mitral stenosis, pulmonary embolism, pulmonary outflow stenosis, chronic obstructive pulmonary disease, pulmonary hypertension (cor pulmonale), or thyrotoxicosis
- With left-sided heart failure, the diseased left ventricle cannot pump effectively because of decreased cardiac output, decreased contractility, increased volume, and increased left ventricular pressure
  - The left atrium cannot empty into the left ventricle, causing increased pressure in the left atrium; this pressure increase affects the lungs, causing pulmonary congestion that leads to decreased oxygenation
  - Increased pressure in the lungs causes increased right-sided heart pressure; the right ventricle cannot relieve the pressure by emptying into the lungs, which impairs venous return to the right side of the heart
  - As systemic pressure builds, body organs become congested with venous blood
- Heart failure may also be classified as systolic or diastolic dysfunction
  - With systolic dysfunction, poor ventricular contraction results in inadequate emptying of the ventricle
  - With diastolic dysfunction, reduced ventricular compliance results in increased resistance to ventricular filling
- High-output failure may occur in high-output states, such as anemia, pregnancy, thyrotoxicosis, beriberi, and arteriovenous fistula
  - High-output failure results in high cardiac output and leads to ventricular dysfunction
  - Despite increased cardiac output, the heart is unable to meet the body's increased metabolic needs.

### Signs and Symptoms

- Both right- and left-sided heart failure may cause chest discomfort, shortness of breath, paroxysmal nocturnal dyspnea, bloating, edema in the extremities, jugular venous distention, and decreased urine output
- Left-sided heart failure also may produce anxiety, orthopnea, dyspnea on exertion and at night, Cheyne-Stokes respirations, cough with frothy sputum, diaphoresis, crackles, rhonchi, cyanosis of extremities, respiratory acidosis, hypoxia, increased pulmonary artery pressures (determined with a pulmonary artery catheter), mental confusion, abnormal heart sounds (S3 and S4), fatigue, lethargy, mitral insufficiency murmur, oliguria, edema, anoxia, and nausea
- Right-sided heart failure also may produce hepatomegaly, anorexia, nausea, splenomegaly, dependent edema, hepatojugular reflex, bounding peripheral pulses, oliguria, arrhythmias, increased right and left-sided heart pressures (determined with a pulmonary artery catheter), Kussmaul's respirations, abnormal heart sounds (S3 and S4), fatigue, lethargy, abdominal pain, and weight gain.

### Diagnosis and Treatment

- Diagnostic tests may include ECG, chest X-ray, echocardiography, pulmonary artery catheter insertion, and arterial blood gas studies
- Laboratory tests may include a CBC; liver function tests; serum creatinine, BUN, electrolyte, glucose; albumin levels (patients with atrial fibrillation should have thyroid function tests performed); and B-type natriuretic peptide
- The goals of treatment are to decrease cardiac workload, increase cardiac output and contractility, decrease fluid and sodium retention, and decrease venous congestion
- Activity is restricted to decrease cardiac workload
- Oxygen may be administered to counteract desaturation
- Drug therapy includes an ACE inhibitor (the cornerstone of therapy) to decrease afterload; a diuretic to decrease preload and afterload; digoxin to increase contractility and cardiac efficiency and decrease heart rate; and a beta-adrenergic blocker to reduce heart rate and myocardial oxygen consumption
  - Diuretics and vasodilators should be avoided in patients with diastolic dysfunction because they may not be able to tolerate reduced blood pressure or reduced volume
  - Other drugs that may be useful in treating heart failure include vasodilators (such as hydralazine) combined with a nitrate (such as isosorbide), angiotensin II receptor blockers in patients who cannot tolerate ACE inhibitors, or nesiritide (a human B-type natriuretic peptide) to augment diuresis and decrease afterload
  - Patients with acute pulmonary edema may also be treated with nitroglycerin IV, morphine sulfate, oxygen, and mechanical ventilation
- If the patient has high-output failure, correct the underlying cause.

### Nursing Interventions

- Monitor the patient for common signs and symptoms of heart failure, such as chest discomfort, shortness of breath, and paroxysmal nocturnal dyspnea
- Also watch for signs and symptoms of left-sided heart failure, such as anxiety, orthopnea, and abnormal breath sounds
- Monitor for signs and symptoms of right-sided heart failure, such as jugular venous distension, hepatomegaly, splenomegaly, peripheral edema, and bounding peripheral pulses
- Encourage bed rest in semi-Fowler's position for ease of breathing
- Provide rest intervals between periods of activity
- Restrict fluids as prescribed
- Administer medications as prescribed, and monitor for their therapeutic and adverse effects.
- Monitor fluid intake and output

- Administer oxygen as prescribed
- Monitor vital signs carefully, especially when administering vasoactive drugs
- Check the patient's weight daily
- Frequently assess for cardiac and respiratory signs of heart failure
- Note changes that suggest worsening of heart failure or fluid imbalance
- Explain procedures and provide reassurance to decrease patient and family anxiety
- Teach the patient and family about medications and the importance of careful management of fluids, sodium intake, and weight.

## Hypertension

### Description

- Hypertension is persistent high blood pressure, usually defined as a systolic pressure above 140 mm Hg or a diastolic pressure above 90 mm Hg based on two or more consecutive readings over a 2-week period
- Three types of hypertension exist: Essential or idiopathic (elevated blood pressure of unknown cause); secondary (elevated blood pressure of known cause, such as renovascular disease, pregnancy, and coarctation of the aorta); and malignant (severe, fulminant form with a diastolic pressure above 140 mm Hg)
- Hypertension may result from renovascular disease, toxemia of pregnancy, pheochromocytoma, pituitary tumor, coarctation of the aorta, adrenocortical hyperfunction, Cushing's syndrome, polycythemia, atherosclerosis, and some medications; a genetic predisposition, smoking, diabetes, stress, sedentary lifestyle, and obesity increase the risk of developing hypertension.

### Signs and Symptoms

- The cardinal sign is consistently elevated blood pressure although there may be no other symptoms or physical findings
- Related signs and symptoms may include headache (usually in the morning), dizziness, bruits, flushed face, epistaxis, blurred vision, retinopathy, retinal hemorrhages, restlessness, crackles, and dyspnea (if the lungs are involved).

### Diagnosis and Treatment

- Diagnostic tests depend on the suspected cause or effects of hypertension
  - For example, kidney function tests, such as urinalysis and creatinine and BUN levels, may be performed because renal damage can cause hypertension
  - ECG, chest X-ray, and echocardiography may be done to determine if hypertension has affected cardiac function
  - Ophthalmic examination may reflect retinal damage
- Diet, exercise, and lifestyle modifications (such as smoking cessation, reducing alcohol intake, stress management, and weight reduction) are recommended first
- If nonpharmacologic measures fail to maintain blood pressure within normal limits, antihypertensives, such as diuretics, ACE inhibitors, beta-adrenergic blockers, calcium channel blockers, angiotensin II receptor blockers, alpha-adrenergic blockers, and combined alpha-and beta-adrenergic blockers, are prescribed.

### Nursing Interventions

- Monitor the patient's blood pressure regularly, and assess for other signs and symptoms of hypertension, such as headache and retinal hemorrhages
- Provide a calm, quiet environment
- Teach the patient and family about weight control, stress reduction, and smoking cessation
- Discuss the importance of a low-sodium diet; include the dietitian in teaching low-sodium recipes and recipe modification for the patient and the person who does the cooking
- Teach the patient how to take his blood pressure.

## Thrombophlebitis

### Description

- Thrombophlebitis is marked by inflammation of the venous wall and thrombus formation of the deep or superficial veins
- Deep vein thrombophlebitis may lead to occlusion of the vessels or systemic embolization such as pulmonary embolism
- Several conditions may lead to thrombophlebitis, including hypercoagulability (such as from cancer, blood dyscrasias, or oral contraceptives); injury to the venous wall (such as from IV injections, fractures, antibiotics, or infection); and venous stasis (such as from varicose veins, pregnancy, heart failure, or prolonged bed rest).

### Signs and Symptoms

- Deep vein thrombophlebitis will sometimes cause no clinical symptoms or physicial findings; when they do occur, they may include cramping pain, edema, positive Homans' sign, tenderness to touch, fever, chills, and malaise
- Superficial thrombophlebitis produces visible and palpable signs, such as heat, pain, swelling, rubor, tenderness, and induration along the affected vein's length.

### Diagnosis and Treatment

- Diagnostic tests may include photoplethysmography, Doppler ultrasonography, and venography; laboratory tests include a CBC
- Superficial thrombophlebitis may require no specific therapy other than treatment for symptoms
- An anticoagulant (initially IV heparin or low-molecular-weight heparin followed by oral warfarin [Coumadin]) is administered to prolong clotting time
- Thrombolytic therapy (such as streptokinase [Streptase]) is indicated for acute, extensive deep vein thrombophlebitis
- Embolectomy, venous ligation, or insertion of a vena caval umbrella or filter may also be indicated.

### Nursing Interventions

- If the patient is receiving a thrombolytic, heparin, or warfarin (Coumadin), monitor him for signs and symptoms of bleeding

- If the patient is receiving heparin, measure partial thromboplastin time (PTT) regularly; if the patient is receiving warfarin, measure prothrombin time (PT) and international normalized ratio (INR) (therapeutic values for PTT and PT are 1½ to 2 times control values; for INR, between 2 and 3)
- Assess the patient for signs and symptoms of pulmonary embolism, such as crackles, dyspnea, tachypnea, hemoptysis, tachycardia, and chest pain
- Make sure the patient maintains bed rest and elevates the affected extremity
- Apply moist, warm compresses to improve circulation to the affected area and relieve pain
- Tell the patient to avoid prolonged sitting and standing to help prevent recurrence
- Teach the patient how to properly apply and use antiembolism stockings
- To prevent thrombophlebitis in high-risk patients, perform range-of-motion exercises while the patient is on bed rest, use intermittent pneumatic calf massage during lengthy surgical or diagnostic procedures, apply antiembolism stockings or pneumatic compression devices postoperatively, and encourage early ambulation.

## Valvular Heart Disease

### Description

- Three types of mechanical disruption can occur in patients with valvular heart disease: narrowing (stenosis) of the valve opening, incomplete closure of the valve (insufficiency), or prolapse of the valve
- Valvular heart disease may result from conditions such as endocarditis (most common), rheumatic fever, congenital defects, or inflammation and can lead to heart failure
- The most common forms of valvular heart disease include mitral stenosis, mitral insufficiency, mitral valve prolapse, aortic stenosis, aortic insufficiency, and tricuspid insufficiency.

| Types of valvular heart disease | | |
|---|---|---|
| **Causes and incidence** | **Clinical features** | **Diagnostic measures** |
| **Aortic Insufficiency** | | |
| • Results from rheumatic fever, syphilis hypertension, or endocarditis, or may be idiopathic<br>• Associated with Marfan syndrome<br>• Most common in males<br>• Associated with ventricular septal defect, even after surgical closure | • Dyspnea, cough fatigue, palpitations angina, syncope<br>• Pulmonary vein congestion heart failure pulmonary edema (left-sided heart failure), pulsating nail beds (Quincke's sign)<br>• Rapidly rising and collapsing pulses (pulsus biferlens), cardiac arrhythmias, wide pulse pressure in severe insufficiency<br>• Auscultation reveals a third heart sound ($S_2$) and diastolic blowing murmur at left sternal border<br>• Palpation and visualization of apical impulse in chronic disease | • Cardiac catheterization: Reduction in arterial diastolic pressures, aortic insufficiency, other valvular abnormalities, and increased left ventricular end-diastolic pressure<br>• X-ray: Left ventricular enlargement pulmonary vein congestion<br>• Echocardiography: Left ventricular enlargement, alterations in mitral valve disease and mitral thickening<br>• Electrocardiography (ECG): Sinus tachycardia, left ventricular hypertrophy and left atrial hypertrophy in severe disease |
| **Aortic Stenosis** | | |
| • Results from congenital aortic bicuspid valve (associated with coarctation of the aorta), congenital stenosis of valve cusps, degenerative calcifications caused by mechanical stress diabetes mellitus, hypercholesterolemia, or hypertension<br>• Most common in males | • Exertional dyspnea paroxysmal noctumal dyspnea, fatigue syncope, angina, palpitations<br>• Pulmonary vein congestion, heart failure, pulmonary edema<br>• Diminished carotid pulses, decreased cardiac output cardiac arrhythmias; may have pulsus altemans<br>• Auscultation reveals systolic murmur at base or in carotids and possibly, a fourth heart sound ($S_4$) | • Cardiac catheterization: Pressure gradient across valve (indicating obstruction) increased left ventricular end-diastolic pressures<br>• X-ray: Valvular calcification, left ventricular enlargement, and pulmonary venous congestion<br>• Echocardiograpy: Thickened aortic valve and left ventricular wall<br>• ECG: Left ventricular hypertrophy |
| **Mitral Insufficiency** | | |
| • Results from rheumatic fever, hypertrophic cardiomyopathy, mitral valve prolapse, myocardial infarction, severe left-sided heart failure or ruptured chordae tendineae<br>• Associated with other congenital anomalies such as transposition of the great arteries<br>• Rare in children without other congenital anomalies | • Orthopnea, dyspnea, fatigue angina, palpitations<br>• Peripheral edema, jugular vein distention, hepatomegaly (right-sided heart failure)<br>• Tachycardia, crackles, pulmonary edema<br>• Auscultation reveals a holosystolic murmur at apex, possible split second heart sound ($S_2$ and $S_1$) | • Cardiac catheterization: Mitral insufficiency with increased left ventricular end-diastolic volume and pressure, increased atrial pressure and decreased cardiac output<br>• X-ray: Left atrial and ventricular enlargement, pulmonary venous congestion<br>• Echocardiography: Abnormal valve leaflet motion, left atrial enlargement<br>• ECG: May show left atrial and ventricular hypertrophy, sinus tachycardia, and atrial fibrillation |

*Contd...*

*Contd...*

| Types of valvular heart disease | | |
|---|---|---|
| **Causes and incidence** | **Clinical features** | **Diagnostic measures** |
| **Mitral Stenosis** | | |
| • Results from rheumatic fever (most common cause), atrial myxoma or endocarditis<br>• Most common in females<br>• May be associated with other congenital anomalies | • Exertional dyspnea, paroxysmal nocturnal dyspnea, orthopnea, weakness, fatigue, palpitations<br>• Peripheral edema, jugular vein distention, ascites, hepatomegaly (right-sided heart failure in severe pulmonary hypertension)<br>• Crackles, cardiac arrhythmias (atrial fibrillation), signs of systemic emboli<br>• Auscultation reveals a loud first heart sound ($S_1$) or opening snap and a diastolic murmur at the apex | • Cardiac catheterization: Diastolic pressure gradient across valve; elevated left atrial pressure and PAWP with severe pulmonary hypertension and pulmonary artery pressures; elevated right-sided heart pressure, decreased cardiac output; and abnormal contraction of the left ventricle<br>• X-ray: Left atrial and ventricular enlargement, enlarged pulmonary arteries and mitral valve calcification<br>• Echocardiography: Thickened mitral valve leaflets, left atrial enlargement<br>• ECG: Left atrial hypertrophy, atrial fibrillation, right ventricular hypertrophy and right axis deviation |
| **Mitral Valve Prolapse Syndrome** | | |
| • Cause unknown; researchers speculate that metabolic or neuroendocrine factors cause constellation of signs and symptoms<br>• Most commonly affects young women but may occur in both sexes and in all age-groups | • May produce no signs or may produce signs and symptoms of mitral insufficiency<br>• Chest pain, palpitations, headache, fatigue, exercise intolerance, dyspnea, syncope, light-headedness, mood swings, anxiety panic attacks<br>• Auscultation typically reveals a mobile, midsystolic click, with or without a mid-to-late systolic murmur | • Two-dimensional echocardiograpy: Prolapse of mitral valve leaflets into left atrium<br>• Color-flow Doppler studies: Mitral insufficiency<br>• Resting ECG: ST-segment changes biphasic or inverted T waves in leads II, III, or A,<br>• Exercise ECG: Evaluates chest pain and arrhythmias |
| **Pulmonic Insufficiency** | | |
| • May be congenital or may result from pulmonary hypertension<br>• May rarely result from prolonged use of pressure monitoring catheter in the pulmonary artery | • Dyspnea, weakness, fatigue, chest pain<br>• Peripheral edema, jugular vein distention, hepatomegaly (right-sided heart failure)<br>• Auscultation reveals diastolic murmur in pulmonic area | • Cardiac catheterization: Pulmonic insufficiency increased right ventricular pressure, and associated cardiac defects<br>• X-ray: Right ventricular and pulmonary arterial enlargement<br>• ECG: Right ventricular or right atrial enlargement |
| **Pulmonic Stenosis** | | |
| • Results from congenital stenosis of valve cusp or rheumatic heart disease (infrequent)<br>• Associated with other congenital heart defects such as tetralogy of Fallot | • Asymptomatic or symptomatic with exertional dyspnea, fatigue, chest pain, syncope<br>• May lead to peripheral edema, jugular vein distention, hepatomegaly (right-sided heart failure)<br>• Auscultation reveals a systolic murmur at the left sternal border, a split $S_2$ with a delayed or absent pulmonic component | • Cardiac catheterization: Increased right ventricular pressure, decreased pulmonary artery pressure, and abnormal valve orifice<br>• ECG: May show right ventricular hypertrophy, right axis deviation right atrial hypertrophy, and atrial fibrillation |
| **Tricuspid Insufficiency** | | |
| • Results from right-sided heart failure, rheumatic fever and rarely, trauma and endocarditis<br>• Associated with congenital disorders | • Dyspnea and fatigue<br>• May lead to peripheral edema, jugular vein distention, hepatomegaly, ascites (right-sided heart failure)<br>• Auscultation reveals possible $S_1$ and systolic murmur at lower left sternal border that increases with inspiration | • Right-sided heart catheterization: High atrial pressure, tricuspid insufficiency, and decreased or normal cardiac output<br>• X-ray: Right atrial dilation, right ventricular enlargement<br>• Echocardiography: Shows systolic prolapse of tricuspid valve, right atrial enlargement<br>• ECG: Right atrial or right ventricular hypertrophy, atrial fibrillation |

*Contd...*

*Contd...*

| Types of valvular heart disease | | |
|---|---|---|
| **Causes and incidence** | **Clinical features** | **Diagnostic measures** |
| **Tricuspid Stenosis** | | |
| • Results from rheumatic fever<br>• May be congenital<br>• Associated with mitral or aortic valve disease<br>• Most common in females | • May be symptomatic with dyspnea, fatigue, syncope<br>• Possibly peripheral edema jugular vein distention, hepatomegaly, ascites (right-sided heart failure)<br>• Auscultation reveals diastolic murmur at lower left sternal border that increases with inspiration | • Cardiac catheterization: Increased pressure gradient across valve increased right atrial pressure, and decreased right atrial pressure, and decreased cardiac output<br>• X-ray: Right atrial enlargement<br>• Echocardiography: Leaflet abnormality, right atrial enlargement<br>• ECG: right atrial hypertrophy, right or left ventricular hypertrophy, and atrial fibrillation |

### *Treatment*

- Medications are administered to treat heart failure and arrhythmias
- An anticoagulant may be prescribed to prevent thrombus formation around diseased or replaced valves
- Surgery to repair or replace valves is indicated when medical management can no longer control symptoms.

### *Nursing Interventions*

- Offer a low-sodium diet, and maintain fluid restrictions
- Place the patient in an upright position to relieve dyspnea
- Instruct the patient on the use of anticoagulants, including signs and symptoms of bleeding to report, the need for frequent monitoring, and precautions to take while taking the drug
- Explain that he/she will need to take a prophylactic antibiotic if he/she undergoes dental work, surgery, or another invasive procedure

## HEMATOLOGIC DISORDERS

### Introduction

- Blood circulates in the cardiovascular system, carrying oxygen to the cells and removing wastes from them
- The continuous movement of blood also provides a defense against infection and injury, which are more likely to occur with stasis
- The cellular components of red blood cells (RBCs), white blood cells (WBCs), and platelets are subject to pathologic alterations that can cause severe disruptions in homeostasis.

### *Nursing History*

- The nurse asks the patient about his *chief complaint*
- A patient with a hematologic disorder may report any of the following signs or symptoms: A ching bones, anorexia, bleeding gums, bruising, dyspnea, fatigue, infection, lethargy, malaise, nausea, nosebleeds, numbness, paresthesia, swollen and tender lymph nodes, tarry stools, tingling, vomiting, and in women, heavy menses
- The nurse then questions the patient about his *present illness*
  - Ask the patient about his symptoms, including when they started, associated symptoms, location, radiation, intensity, duration, and frequency
  - Question the patient about what factors make the symptoms feel better or worse
- The nurse asks about *medical history*
  - Ask about the present and past use of prescription and over-the-counter drugs, herbal remedies, and vitamin and nutritional supplements because many of these products can interfere with hematologic function
  - Ask the patient about previous problems, such as anemia, leukemia, enlarged lymph nodes, malabsorption, and spleen or liver disorders
  - Ask about previous treatments, such as blood transfusions and radiation treatments
  - Question him about his diet, and look for deficiencies—for example, in folic acid, iron, or vitamin B12
- The nurse then assesses the *family history*
  - Ask about a family history of blood and lymph disorders, acquired and genetic
  - Ask about a family history of cancers involving the blood or lymph systems
- The nurse obtains a *social history*
  - Ask about ethnic background and race
  - Question the patient about use of cigarettes, alcohol, and recreational drugs
  - Ask him about occupational or household exposure to radiation or chemicals.

### *Physical Assessment*

- The nurse begins with *inspection*
  - Observe the patient's general appearance; does he appear alert, confused, tired, or irritable?
  - Note the patient's skin color; look for bruising, diaphoresis, dyspnea, lesions, petechiae, and swelling of the lymph nodes
  - Note the size and color of his tongue
  - Ask the patient whether his abdominal girth is enlarged
- The nurse uses *auscultation*
  - Listen to heart sounds, noting abnormal sounds, rhythms, or tachycardia
  - Auscultate the abdomen, noting bowel sounds, bruits, friction rubs, or venous hums
- Next, the nurse uses *palpation*

- Palpate the lymph nodes, noting consistency, mobility, shape, size, and tenderness; compare nodes on one side of the body with those on the other side
- Palpate the abdomen, noting ascites, enlarged organs, or tenderness
- The nurse then uses *percussion*
  - Percuss the liver and spleen to estimate size
  - Note the size and location of other abdominal organs.

## Anemias

- Anemia exists when the number of RBCs in a designated volume of blood is less than normal
- Anemias include those from blood loss or hemolysis and aplastic, iron deficiency, and megaloblastic anemias.

### *Types of Anemia*

The chart given here summarizes the etiology, signs and symptoms, medical management, and nursing for each type of anemia which is defined as a decreased number of red blood cells (RBCs).

## Disseminated Intravascular Coagulation

### *Description*

- Disseminated intravascular coagulation (DIC) is a serious blood coagulation disorder that occurs as a complication of conditions that accelerate blood clotting.
- It is characterized by suppression of the fibrinolytic system and the development of small clots in the microcirculation, which consumes clotting factors, resulting in excessive bleeding.

| Description and etiology | Signs and symptoms | Medical management | Nursing interventions |
|---|---|---|---|
| **Anemia from blood loss anemia resulting from the loss of more than 500 mL of blood** | | | |
| • Acute blood loss as in trauma or surgery<br>• Chronic blood loss as in menstrual or GI bleeding | • RBC indices below normal on serurn blood tests<br>• With acute blood loss: Sudden onset of symptoms such as hypovolemia, hypotension, hypoxemia, irrirabiltiy, stupor, weakness, tachycardia and cool moist skin<br>• With chronic blood loss: Gradual and vague symptoms, such as exertional dyspnea, increased fatigue and pallor | • The source of the bleeding is identified and controlled through medical or surgical means<br>• Transfusion and iron supplementation may be needed. Whole blood is transfused if the total blood volume has dropped, packed RBCs are transfused if it has not dropped<br>• Shock must be treated if it occurs | • Help determine the cause of bleeding by testing stool, urine, vomitus or sputum for blood.<br>• Help control blood loss by applying pressure to obvious bleeding sites, assessing the patient for internal bleeding and performing dressing changes as needed to assess blood loss |
| **Aplastic anemia: Anemia characterized by a decreased hemoglobin level and pancytopenia** | | | |
| • Unknown etiology or an autoimmune disturbance (50% of cases)<br>• Drug therapy with a chemotherapeutic drug, chloramphenicol, mephenytoin, phenylbutazone, or a sulfonamide<br>• Exposure to environmental or occupational hazards, such as benzene, insecticides, or raditation<br>• Infection, such as cytomegalovirus, Epstein-Barr virus, hepatitis, or miliary tuberculosis<br>• Congenital causes | • Exertional dyspnea, fatigue infection, pallor and palpitation<br>• Hemorrhage—for example bleeding (nasal oral, rectal or vaginal) ecchymosis, petechiae, or purpura<br>• Low platelet, RBC, and white blood cell counts<br>• Dry bone marrow (on aspiration) | • Initial treatment involves the causative agent, if possible and administering transfusions<br>• Medication such as antithymocyte globulin (ATG), cyclosporine, granulocyte colony- stimulating factors, and granulocyte-monocyte colony-stimulating factor may be administered<br>• Treat the idiopathic form of the disease with steroids<br>• If the anemia cannot be reversed or if it result from an autoimmune disturbance, bone marrow transplantation is recommended; this treatment is more effective if the patient does not receive blood products first and is younger than age 30 | • Help identify the causative agent<br>• Assist a weak patient with daily activities<br>• If the patient has pancytopenia , take safety precautions and steps to control infection because his ability to fight infection and sustain clotting are decreased<br>• Help the patient and family cope with the severity of the illness and its prognosis (Death may result from infection or hemorrhage)<br>• If the patient is receiving antithymocyte globulin (ATG) perform skin testing and monitor him for allergic reaction |

Contd...

*Contd...*

| Description and etiology | Signs and symptoms | Medical management | Nursing interventions |
|---|---|---|---|
| **Congential hemolytic anemia: Sickle cell anemia characterized by RBC destruction beyond the bone marrow's ability to produce these cells and misshapen hemoglobin and RBCs** | | | |
| • Inherited (primarily affects blacks) | • Painful vaso-occlusive events in the extremities or affected organs (Sickle cell crisis)<br>• Other symptoms similar to other chronic anemias | • No cure or prevention is available<br>• Supportive interventions are used to prevent infection, relieve pain and provide fluid and oxygen during a sickle cell crisis, which can cause massive organ damage | • If the patient has sickle cell anemia, provide genetic counseling and possible gene replacement therapy<br>• Teach the patient to avoid factors that may precipitate sickle cell crisis, such as cold exposure, dehydration, excessive exercise, high altitudes and smoking |
| **Congenital hemolytic anemia: Thalassemia anemia characterized by RBC destruction beyond the bone marrow's ability to produce these cell and mutated hemoglobin** | | | |
| • Inherited (primarily affects blacks, Asians and people of Mediterranean origin) | • Cardiac problems such as cardiomegaly heart failure and murmurs<br>• Excessive hematopoiesis and iron overload<br>• Other symptoms similar to other chronic anemias | • Transfusions are the primary treatment. Chelating agents are used to remove excess iron from the blood after multiple transfusions have been administered<br>• Splenectomy may be required for severe thalassemia<br>• Bone marrow transplant also is an option | • If the patient has thalassemia, provide genetic counseling |
| **Iron-deficiency anemia: Anemia caused by inadequate iron supplies** | | | |
| • Chronic blood loss without iron replacement<br>• Poor nutrition<br>• Decreased iron absorption from the intestines<br>• Increased need for iron, such as during childhood or pregnancy | • Possibly asymptomatic<br>• Possibly sense of being cold due to iron's role in regulating body temperature<br>• Brittle, spoon-shaped nails with longitudinal ridges; cheilosis (painful mouth cracks or sores); exertional dyspnea; insidious development of fatigue; and red, shiny tongue<br>• Hypochromic, microcytic anemia (on blood smears); low serum iron level; and elevated serum iron-binding capcacities | • The cause of blood loss or nutritional deficits is identified and corrected.<br>• An oral iron supplement may be prescribed. If the patient is unable to tolerate it, a parenteral iron formulation may be adminstered IM via the Z-track method or IV | • Help determine the cause of bleeding by testing stool, urine, vomitus and sputum for blood<br>• Teach the patient how to take oral iron. Advise the patient to take iron pills with meals to reduce GI irritation and to continue therapy until the underlying problem is corrected<br>• Teach the patient about adverse reaction to oral iron therapy such as black stools constipation or diarrhea and GI disturbances<br>• Educate the patient about nutrition, including the need for iron rich food and adequate vitamin C to enchance iron absorption |
| **Megaloblastic anemia: Anemia characterized by a predominance of megaloblasts and a relative lack of normoblastic: Includes pernicious vitamin B12 deficiency and folic acid deficiency anemias** | | | |
| • Gastric surgery pernicious of the terminal ileum where vitamin B12 is absorbed strict vegetarian diets; and prolonged exposure to nitrous oxide<br>• Aging and long-term gastritis (pernicious anemia)<br>• Alcoholic malnutrition and malabsorption (folic acid deficienty anemia) | • Epithelial atrophy loss of coordination, neuropathy and paresthesia of the extremities<br>• Gastritis glossitis (red beefy tongue), and malabsorption with anorexia and weight loss<br>• Decreased RBC and platelet counts | • Monthly administration of parenteral vitamin B12 typically is required for pernicious and vitamin B12 deficiency anemias.<br>• An oral folic acid supplement and dietary improvement typically are required for a patient with folic acid deficiency which commonly result from nutritional deficits | • Provide care for oral mucus membranes to help relieve glossitis<br>• Teach the patient how to Increase dietary intake of folic acid and vitamin B12<br>• Refer the patient with anemia related to alcohol abuse to an alcohol rehabilitation clinic<br>• If the patient has a vitamin B12 deficiency teach him about long-term treatment with an oral or parenteral vitamin B12 supplement treatment typically calls for monthly LM administration of cyanocobalamin. |

- The disorder can result from septicemia; obstetric complications, such as abruptio placenta and amniotic fluid embolism; cancer; blood transfusion reactions; and cirrhosis
- Tissue hypoxia and multiple organ failure can occur; the mortality rate can exceed 80%.

### *Signs and Symptoms*

- The main sign is abnormal bleeding, evidenced by cutaneous oozing, petechiae, ecchymoses, hematomas, GI bleeding, and bleeding from wounds and IV sites
- Signs of organ compromise include dyspnea, oliguria, and muscle or abdominal pain; shock can also occur.

### *Diagnosis and Treatment*

- Laboratory tests show a steadily decreasing platelet count, elevated prothrombin time (PT) and partial thromboplastin time (PTT), elevated fibrin degradation products, and decreased hemoglobin and hematocrit
- Medical management aims to identify and treat the underlying disorder, promote oxygenation, replace fluids and electrolytes, and provide hemodynamic support
- Treatments include clotting factor and blood replacement and IV heparin.

### *Nursing Interventions*

- Early recognition of the onset of DIC improves patient outcomes, so closely monitor patients at risk, watching for signs and symptoms
- For a patient with DIC, avoid trauma to skin or wounds to minimize bleeding, protect the patient from injury, and avoid dislodging clots
- Apply pressure to puncture sites until bleeding stops
- Monitor the patient's vital signs, and administer IV fluids and blood products as ordered
- Monitor the patient's intake and output carefully and record blood loss
- Watch for signs of tissue ischemia and failure
- Provide emotional support to the patient and family.

## Hemophilia

### *Description*

- Hemophilia is a hereditary bleeding disorder that results from the lack of specific clotting factors
- Two main forms exist: Hemophilia A, called 'classic hemophilia,' results from deficiency of factor VIII and is seen in 80% of cases, and hemophilia B, called 'Christmas disease,' results from deficiency of factor IX and is seen in 15% of cases; the two types are clinically indistinguishable
- Hemophilia A and B are X-linked recessive traits; female carriers have a 50% chance of transmitting the gene to each child; sons who receive the gene have the disease, whereas daughters who receive the gene are carriers; patients with the disease are usually identified in childhood
- Hemophilia produces bleeding, with the degree of bleeding varying depending on the degree of clotting factor deficiency
  - Mild hemophilia usually causes bleeding only during major surgery or trauma
  - Moderate hemophilia occasionally causes spontaneous bleeding in addition to bleeding during surgery and from trauma
  - Severe hemophilia causes spontaneous bleeding; bleeding from minor trauma may be severe.

### *Signs and Symptoms*

- Signs of hemophilia include excessive bleeding from wound and puncture sites, hematomas, spontaneous bleeding (such as nosebleeds), and GI bleeding
- Joint pain results from bleeding into joints a common occurrence
- A change in the level of consciousness can be obtained by signal intracranial bleeding.

### *Diagnosis and Treatment*

- Laboratory tests include abnormal clotting factor assays, which confirm diagnosis; prolonged PTT with normal PT and normal platelet count may also occur
- Treatment typically consists of replacement of deficient clotting factors (VIII or IX); however, patients can develop antibodies to factor concentrates, which reduces their effectiveness
- Aminocaproic acid inhibits fibrinolysis and can be used to stabilize clots
- Desmopressin (DDAVP) can be used to induce a transient rise in factor VIII.

### *Nursing Interventions*

- During bleeding episodes, administer the deficient clotting factors or plasma as ordered
- Prevent trauma, and limit activity when bleeding occurs
- Minimize injections and apply pressure for at least 10 minutes to puncture sites
- Monitor vital signs and be alert for hemodynamic changes
- Administer analgesics and cold packs for joint pain; promote joint mobility when bleeding is controlled
- Teach the patient and family about the disease process, monitoring, treatment and genetic testing.

## Hodgkin's Disease

### *Description*

- Hodgkin's disease is a malignant B lymphocyte cell line disease of the lymph system that primarily affects those between ages 15 and 30 and those older than age 55
- The malignant cell associated with Hodgkin's disease is the Reed-Sternberg cell, a giant, morphologically unique cell, i.e. most likely of immature lymphoid origin
- Although the cause is unknown, this cancer is associated with viral infections and sustained immunosuppression; a genetic and environmental association may also exist
- It is among the most treatable of adult cancers and has a better prognosis than malignant, or non-Hodgkin's disease.

### *Signs and Symptoms*

- This cancer is characterized by greatly enlarged, painless, movable lymph nodes in the cervical or supraclavicular area
- The patient may also experience fever, malaise, night sweats, pruritus, and weight loss

- Symptoms resulting from compression by the enlarged lymph nodes depend on the area involved.

### *Diagnosis and Treatment*

- Lymph node biopsy showing Reed-Sternberg cells supports the diagnosis
- Staging is done after the initial diagnosis of Hodgkin's disease is confirmed
  - The stage of disease is determined by biopsies of distant lymph nodes, bilateral bone marrow biopsies, lymphangiography, computed tomography scan or magnetic resonance imaging (MRI) of the thorax and abdomen, gallium scan, positron emission tomography (PET), chest X-ray, a complete blood count (CBC), and serum alkaline phosphatase
  - A splenectomy is traditionally done during staging
- Hodgkin's disease has four stages
- Early stages of Hodgkin's disease are treated with external radiation of the affected lymph nodes
- More advanced stages require a combination of chemotherapy and radiation therapy
- Autologus bone marrow transplantation or autologus peripheral blood sternal transfusions and immunotherapy are used for disease resistant to standard treatment.

### *Nursing Interventions*

- Provide supportive care related to the adverse effects of radiation therapy and chemotherapy
- Provide psychological support to help the patient cope with the diagnosis, treatment, and effects of treatment
- Provide education to the patient and his family regarding the diagnosis of Hodgkin's disease and its treatment.

## Leukemia

### *Description*

- Leukemia is a group of malignant disorders of the hematopoietic system that involves the bone marrow and lymph nodes and is characterized by the uncontrolled proliferation of immature WBCs.
- Leukemias are classified by onset and severity of symptoms (acute or chronic) and by the precursor cell (myeloid or lymphoid) involved in the formation of the abnormal cells.
- Although the cause of leukemia is unknown, it has been linked to genetic damage to cells, which transforms normal cells into malignant cells; it is associated with Down's syndrome and other chromosomal abnormalities, chronic exposure to chemicals such as benzene, use of drugs that cause aplastic anemia, radiation exposure, and chemotherapy
- In leukemia, WBC (leukocyte) proliferation interferes with the production of other cells, leading to thrombocytopenia and anemia; the immature leukocytes decrease immuno competence and increase susceptibility to infection.

### *Signs and Symptoms*

- A patient with either acute or chronic leukemia may report vague signs and symptoms, such as fatigue, malaise, petechiae, night sweats, bone or joint pain, and weight loss
- Acute leukemia produces anemia, bleeding, and symptoms of infection such as sudden onset of high fever; hepatosplenomegaly and lymphadenopathy may also be present
- Chronic leukemia causes milder anemia and splenomegaly; however, many patients are asymptomatic at the time of diagnosis
- Additional signs and symptoms depend on the organ or tissue involved, e.g. central nervous system involvement may cause headache and vomiting.

### *Diagnosis and Treatment*

- Diagnosis is usually based on bone marrow examination that reveals leukemic blast cells and on a CBC
- Chemotherapy, with or without stem cell transplantation, is standard treatment for leukemia
- Patients with low-risk chronic lymphocytic leukemia may not receive treatment if they are asymptomatic
- Stem cell transplantation is used to treat leukemia
  - In *allogenic transplantation,* donor stem cells are transplanted into the patient
- Before transplantation, the patient undergoes chemotherapy and total body radiation to eliminate the leukemic cells; these procedures destroy all the patient's bone marrow in preparation for grafting from the donor
- The principal complication of this type of transplantation is graft-versus-host disease (GVHD), a type of organ rejection in which the transplanted cells reject the patient
  - An alternative method is to harvest the patient's own stem cells during remission, treat the cells to remove residual tumor cells, and reinfuse them after the patient undergoes immunosuppressant chemotherapy and radiation therapy; this method, called *autologous stem cell transplantation,* avoids GVHD because the patient receives his own cells
- Transfusion therapy may be necessary to treat severe thrombocytopenia, leukopenia, and anemia resulting from the disease process or from treatment
  - Most RBC transfusions involve 250 to 300 mL/unit of packed RBCs; whole blood is seldom transfused to treat leukemia
- The blood must be refrigerated until it is used
- The nurse must take baseline vital signs before transfusion, monitor cardiac status before and during transfusion, confirm blood product compatibility with the patient's blood type, administer blood through a filter (only with normal saline solution), check the blood according to facility policy with another professional nurse, infuse it slowly (2 to 4 hours/unit), observe for reactions, and record vital signs at least hourly and at the end of the transfusion
  - Platelet transfusions may be prescribed; a 6-unit IV bolus of platelets should be infused over 20 to 30 minutes
- Platelets should not be refrigerated
- The nurse must take baseline vital signs before transfusion, premedicate with steroids or antihistamines, as prescribed, to prevent reactions, and administer platelets through a filter (only with normal saline solution)

- WBC transfusions must be infused within 24 hours of collection; the process for WBC transfusions is similar to that for RBC transfusions.

### *Nursing Interventions*

- Follow infection-control procedures if the WBC count is low, e.g. place a severely neutropenic patient in a private room, with no flowers, plants, or fresh fruits; avoid unnecessary invasive procedures; limit patient contact with infected personnel or visitors; and teach hand hygiene techniques to the patient, family, and visitors
- If the patient has a low platelet count, monitor blood counts and take precautions to prevent bleeding, e.g. avoid parenteral injections, limit the number of venipunctures, and advise the patient to use an electric razor for shaving
- Prevent or manage stomatitis by inspecting the oral cavity daily and encouraging oral care with peroxide or saline solution on a regular basis
- Teach the patient how to care for an indwelling vascular access device and how to detect signs of infection
- Educate patients undergoing chemotherapy about the effects, adverse effects, and length of treatment
- Provide supplemental feedings as prescribed
- Conserve the patient's energy, but promote his independence
- Provide emotional support to the patient and his family, and encourage the patient and his family to verbalize feelings.

## Non-Hodgkin's Lymphoma

### *Description*

- Non-Hodgkin's lymphoma describes a group of malignant neoplasms arising from abnormal lymphocytes that affect the immune system; this disease is usually disseminated when diagnosed and produces systemic symptoms
- It may be associated with viral infection, congenital immunodeficiency, or immunosuppression after organ transplantation
- The prognosis is poor but depends on the histologic type and progression of the disease.

### *Signs and Symptoms*

- Non-Hodgkin's lymphoma can affect any organ or tissue and produces a wide range of symptoms
- Signs and symptoms resemble those of Hodgkin's disease
- Fever, painless lymphadenopathy, profuse sweating (especially at night), severe pruritus, abdominal pain or swelling, and weight loss are common signs and symptoms.

### *Diagnosis and Treatment*

- Diagnostic procedures are similar to those for Hodgkin's disease; however, no Reed-Sternberg cells are present
- Staging is similar to Hodgkin's disease
- Radiation therapy, chemotherapy, and stem cell transplantation are the principal treatments
- Biological response modifiers, such as interferon and monoclonal antibodies, also may be used to change the tumor-host relationship
- Radioimmunotherapy may also be used.

### *Nursing Interventions*

- Educate the patient and his family about transfusions, chemotherapy, and stem cell transplantation
- Initiate interventions similar to those for leukemia
- Prevent infection
- Support nutritional status.

## Polycythemia Vera

### *Description*

- Polycythemia vera is a proliferative disorder of myeloid stem cells that results in elevated levels of RBCs, WBCs, and platelets in the circulating blood
- In the early phase and for 10 or more years, hematocrit is elevated; in later stages, the bone marrow becomes fibrotic, with the resultant inability to produce as many cells, while the spleen resumes its embryonic function of hematopoiesis and enlarges
- The disease eventually progresses into myeloid metaplasia with myelofibrosis or acute myelogenous leukemia (AML)
- The median age at onset is 65, and the median survival is 10 years after diagnosis
- Death results from thrombosis, hemorrhage, or complications of AML.

### *Signs and Symptoms*

- Patients typically have a ruddy complexion and splenomegaly
- Symptoms of an increased blood volume or increased blood viscosity includes headache, dizziness, tinnitus, fatigue, paresthesias, blurred vision, angina, claudication, dyspnea, thrombophlebitis, and hypertension
- Pruritus, gout, and burning in the fingers and toes may also occur
- Complications include stroke, myocardial infarction (MI), thrombotic events, and bleeding from dysfunctional platelets.

### *Diagnosis and Treatment*

- Laboratory tests include hematocrit, which can initially exceed 60%; leukocyte and platelet counts are elevated, and uric acid levels are often increased
- Treatment aims to reduce the high blood cell mass; regular phlebotomy is performed to keep Hematocrit below 45%
- Drug therapy may include chemotherapeutics agents to suppress bone marrow function as well as platelet inhibitors.

### *Nursing Interventions*

- Be alert for thrombotic complications such as deep vein thrombosis, and observe for excessive bleeding
- Control pruritus with warm or cool baths and antihistamines as ordered
- Teach the patient and family about the disease process and how to prevent complications
- Provide emotional support.

## Thrombocytopenia

### *Description*

- Thrombocytopenia is an abnormally low level of circulating platelets (less than 100,000/mm$^3$) due to decreased

production, decreased survival, increased destruction, or increased sequestration of platelets in the spleen
- It may result from antibody production (idiopathic thrombocytopenic purpura [ITP]), bone marrow radiation, excessive alcohol use, or a disease, such as aplastic anemia or leukemia, DIC, hypothermia, or an autoimmune disorder
- It also may result from drug therapy with an analgesic, an antibiotic (resulting in ITP, a chemotherapeutic drug, an anti-inflammatory, or a thiazide diuretic; although the platelet count may return to normal 1 to 2 weeks after the drug is withdrawn, more than 90% of adults do not go into spontaneous remission.

### *Signs and Symptoms*

- Ecchymoses, petechiae and purpura may affect the skin
- Epistaxis, gingival bleeding, severe hemorrhage and menorrhagia also may occur.

### *Diagnosis and Treatment*

- The diagnosis is made by examining the platelet count, blood smear, bleeding time, and bone marrow to determine whether the platelet loss is caused by lack of production or increased destruction
- Treatment focuses on correcting the underlying cause
- For ITP, the principal treatment is corticosteroid therapy; for severe or resistant cases, immunosuppressant therapy or splenectomy may be used; platelet transfusions are not helpful because of continued platelet destruction
- For other types of thrombocytopenias, platelet transfusions are indicated and can increase the platelet count for 1 to 3 days.

### *Nursing Interventions*

- Monitor platelet counts; the patient is more susceptible to injury and bleeding when the platelet count falls below 60,000/mm$^3$ and may develop spontaneous hemorrhage, particularly cerebral hemorrhage when the platelet count drops below 20,000/mm$^3$.
- Test all stools and urine for blood
- Avoid taking the patient's temperature rectally and giving IM injections
- Apply pressure to venipuncture and arterial puncture sites
- Provide meticulous oral care to prevent stomatitis
- Tell the patient to use only electric shavers and to avoid contact sports, elective surgery, tooth extraction, and the use of aspirin and ibuprofen.

## RESPIRATORY DISORDERS

### Introduction

- The function of the respiratory system is to exchange gases (oxygen and carbon dioxide) with the external environment; the respiratory system maintains the level of these gases within a narrow range, regardless of the demand for oxygen
- Respiration, which the central nervous system controls, is regulated by metabolic demands and cardiac output.

### *Nursing History*

- The nurse asks the patient about his *chief complaint*
  - A patient with a respiratory disorder may report the following signs or symptoms: chest pain, cough, dyspnea, orthopnea, shortness of breath, or wheezing
  - The patient may also report hemoptysis, increased sputum production, or a change in the characteristics of his sputum
- The nurse then questions the patient about his *present illness*
  - Ask the patient about his symptoms, including when it is started, associated symptoms, location, duration, frequency, and precipitating and alleviating factors
  - If the patient has dyspnea, ask him to rate it on a scale of 0 to 10, in which 0 means no dyspnea and 10 means the worst dyspnea experienced
  - If the patient has orthopnea, ask him how many pillows he uses to sleep
  - Ask if the patient's cough is productive or non-productive. Is the cough recent? If not recent, how long has he experienced it? Has it changed recently?
  - When a patient produces sputum, ask him to estimate the amount produced in teaspoons or another common measurement; ask him at what time of day he coughs the most; question him about the color and consistency of his sputum; ask whether its character has changed recently. If so, how? Does he cough up blood?
  - If a patient wheezes, ask when the wheezing occurs. What makes the patient wheeze? Does he wheeze loudly enough for others to hear it? What helps to stop the wheezing?
  - If the patient has chest pain, ask him where the pain is located, what it feels like, what characteristics it has, whether it moves or radiates, how long it lasts, what causes it to occur, and what makes it better; have him rate the pain on a scale of 0 to 10 (with 0 being no pain and 10 worst pain experienced)
  - Ask about the use of prescription and over-the-counter drugs, herbal remedies, vitamin and nutritional supplements, and alternative or complementary therapies used
- The nurse asks the patient about *medical history*
  - Ask the patient about other respiratory disorders—such as allergies, asthma, cystic fibrosis, pneumonia, tuberculosis, and upper respiratory tract infections
  - Ask the patient if he has undergone chest or lung surgery
- The nurse then assesses the *family history*
  - Ask about a family history of chronic obstructive pulmonary disease (COPD), pneumonia, or tuberculosis
  - Determine if there's a family history of lung cancer
- The nurse obtains a *social history*
  - Ask about smoking habits and environmental exposure to irritants such as asbestos
  - Ask the patient about his tolerance for exercise.

### *Physical Assessment*

- The nurse begins with *inspection*
  - Observe the patient's general appearance; note the patient's position. Is he sitting upright? Leaning forward? In a tripod position?

- Take note of his level of awareness and general appearance. Does he appear relaxed? Anxious? Uncomfortable? Is he having trouble breathing?
- Note deformities, masses, or scars of the chest; look for chest wall symmetry at rest and with inspiration; note the anterior-posterior chest diameter; observe chest wall movement. Is it paradoxical, or uneven?
- Note tracheal deviation; look for spinal abnormalities such as kyphosis; note whether the costal angle is enlarged
- Observe the patient's respirations, noting rate, depth, rhythm, and inspiratory-expiratory ratio; look for the use of accessory muscles with breathing, pursed lip breathing (PLB), nostril flaring, and retracting
- Observe the color of the patient's skin, lips, mucus membranes, and nail beds; check nails for clubbing

- Next, the nurse uses *palpation*
  - Palpate the chest for temperature, dryness, crepitus, pain, and tactile fremitus
  - Check for respiratory excursion
- Then the nurse *percusses* the heart
  - Percusses the anterior and posterior chest, noting lung boundaries and movement of the diaphragm
  - Also note percussion sounds; describe any abnormal ones, including the location and size of the area
- The nurse continues with *auscultation*
  - Auscultate the anterior, posterior, and lateral chest, comparing breath sounds
  - Classify each sound according to its intensity, location, pitch, duration, and characteristic; note whether the sound occurs during inhalation, exhalation, or both
  - Auscultate for vocal fremitus, noting bronchophony, egophony, and whispered pectoriloquy.

## Acute Respiratory Distress Syndrome

### *Description*

- Acute respiratory distress syndrome (ARDS), a severe form of lung injury, occurs when the lungs cannot maintain the oxygen–carbon dioxide balance
- Although its exact cause is unknown, ARDS occurs as a result of diffuse alveolar damage; its mortality rate is 50% or higher; death is usually due to a multisystem failure or an infection
- Risk factors for ARDS include aspiration pneumonia, drug overdose, fat or amniotic emboli, head injury, hemorrhagic shock, massive blood transfusions or transfusion reactions, near drowning, pulmonary contusion, sepsis, smoke inhalation, and trauma
- With ARDS, capillaries leak, causing interstitial edema; this decreases blood flow to the lungs and causes platelet aggregation
  - The respiratory membrane becomes inflammed; alveolar edema develops, leading to pulmonary edema
  - Lung compliance decreases, and patches of atelectasis develop; the patient hyperventilates, thereby causing hypocapnia and hypoxemia and leading to multisystem organ dysfunction syndrome
  - A ventilation-perfusion mismatch occurs.

### *Signs and Symptoms*

- Vital sign measurement reveals an increased blood pressure, tachycardia, and tachypnea (along with increased respiratory effort and accessory muscle use)
- Other signs and symptoms may include barotrauma symptoms, bibasilar crackles, crepitus, cyanosis, decreased breath sounds, diaphoresis, dyspnea, progressive hypoxemia despite oxygen therapy, restlessness, and thick, frothy sputum.

### *Diagnosis and Treatment*

- Early diagnosis and prompt treatment allow for successful management of ARDS
- Arterial blood gas (ABG) studies reveal decreased partial pressure of arterial oxygen ($PaO_2$) unresponsive to supplemental oxygen
- A pulmonary artery (PA) catheter inserted to measure pressures reveals pulmonary artery wedge pressure (PAWP) of less than 18 mm Hg
- Chest X-ray shows bilateral infiltrates (in early stages) and lung fields with ground-glass appearance, irreversible hypoxemia, and massive consolidation seen as 'white lung' (in later stages)
- Mechanical ventilation may be necessary
  - Raising the fraction of inspired oxygen ($FiO_2$) with a ventilator helps to reverse hypoxemia but may increase the risk of oxygen toxicity and pulmonary fibrosis
  - Supplementing mechanical ventilation with positive end–expiratory pressure (PEEP) provides a constant pressure that prevents the alveoli from collapsing
  - PEEP allows the use of a lower $FiO_2$ to obtain an adequate $PaO_2$
  - Pressure control ventilation that prevents overdistention of the alveoli and inverse ratio ventilation in which inspiration is longer than expiration may also be used
- A diuretic may be administered to reduce pulmonary edema
- An antibiotic is used to treat any respiratory tract infection or underlying systemic infection
- Pharmacologic paralysis is used to decrease oxygen consumption; the patient must be sedated for this treatment
- Vasopressors are given to maintain blood pressure
- Electrolyte and acid-base imbalances are corrected to maintain cellular integrity.

### *Nursing Interventions*

- Make sure the patient maintains bed rest in semi-Fowler's or the prone position, if possible, to improve oxygenation
- Provide oxygen therapy (and mechanical ventilation, if indicated) to maintain $PaO_2$ above 60 mm Hg; this will maintain oxygenation and help to reverse hypoxemia
- Implement chest physiotherapy to loosen secretions
- If the patient is not on mechanical ventilation, teach him effective coughing and deep-breathing exercises to maximize lung expansion and reexpand collapsed alveoli
- Suction the patient's airway as needed to maintain patency and to clear secretions; sterile technique prevents bacterial contamination of lower airways
- Administer drugs to relieve pain and discomfort as needed

- If the patient is on mechanical ventilation, administer a paralyzant and a sedative as necessary
- Monitor fluid intake and output to determine the effectiveness of diuretic therapy
- Frequently reposition the patient to prevent complications of immobility, help to loosen secretions, and promote lung perfusion
- Provide 2,500 calories daily to prevent weakness and an increase immune response; use enteral or parenteral feeding if needed
- Teach relaxation techniques, and encourage the patient not to fight the ventilator
- Because a mechanically ventilated patient cannot speak, provide communication alternatives, such as letter and picture boards.

## Acute Respiratory Failure

### *Description*

- In acute respiratory failure, the lungs' inability to adequately maintain arterial oxygenation or eliminate carbon dioxide results in inadequate ventilation
- The disorder is classified as hypoxemic (type I) or hypercapnic (type II)
- Primarily hypercapnic respiratory failure results from inadequate alveolar ventilation caused by a ventilation-perfusion (V/Q) mismatch and shunting
- Primarily hypoxemic respiratory failure results from inadequate oxygen exchange between the alveoli and capillaries
- The disorder also commonly occurs as a combination of hypercapnic and hypoxemic respiratory failure
- Causes include accumulated secretions secondary to cough suppression; airway irritants; any condition that increases the work of breathing and decreases the respiratory drive of patients with COPD; bronchospasm; central nervous system depression; disorders of the peripheral nervous system, respiratory muscles, and chest wall; endocrine or metabolic disorders; gas exchange failure; heart failure; myocardial infarction (MI); and pulmonary embolism.

### *Signs and Symptoms*

- Signs include changes in mental status, such as confusion, somnolence, and cyanosis of the oral mucosa, lips, and nail beds
- Assessment may reveal absent breath sounds, wheezes, rhonchi, and crackles in the lung fields
- Other signs and symptoms include yawning and use of accessory muscles, pursed-lip breathing, nasal flaring, ashen skin, and tachypnea.

### *Diagnosis and Treatment*

- ABG analysis reveals hypercapnia (partial pressure of arterial carbon dioxide [$PaCO_2$] greater than 50 mm Hg) and hypoxemia ($PaO_2$ less than 60 mm Hg) on room air
- If a bacterial infection is involved, laboratory tests show an increased serum white blood cell (WBC) count; blood cultures, gram stain, and sputum cultures reveal the pathogen
- Serum hemoglobin and hematocrit show decreased oxygen-carrying capacity
- Chest X-rays may reveal underlying pulmonary diseases or conditions, such as emphysema, atelectasis, lesions, pneumothorax, infiltrates, and effusions
- Electrocardiography (ECG) may show arrhythmias, cor pulmonale, or myocardial ischemia
- Pulse oximetry may show decreased arterial oxygen saturation
- Treatment may include mechanical ventilation with an endotracheal or a tracheostomy tube
- If the underlying cause is heart failure, the patient will need fluid restriction
- Initially, the patient is maintained on bed rest, progressing to activity as tolerated
- Oxygen therapy increases the pressure of arterial oxygen
- Antibiotics treat any underlying infection
- Bronchodilators, such as terbutaline, albuterol, theophylline, and ipratropium bromide, alleviate obstruction and bronchospasm
- Corticosteroids reduce inflammation
- Positive inotropic agents, such as dopamine or dobutamine, maintain perfusion
- Nitrates, such as nitroglycerin or nitroprusside, reduce myocardial oxygen demand
- Morphine serves as an adjunct treatment for acute pulmonary edema
- Diuretics alleviate heart failure.

### *Nursing Interventions*

- Monitor the patient's vital signs, pulse oximetry readings, and ECG
- Administer prescribed drugs as indicated (via inhalation, the oral route, nebulization, or IV, as appropriate)
- Orient the patient frequently
- Administer humidified, supplemental oxygen as ordered
- Maintain a patent airway
- Help to clear the patient's secretions with postural drainage and chest physiotherapy; also suction as necessary
- Encourage pursed-lip breathing
- Encourage the use of an incentive spirometer to promote lung expansion
- Reposition the patient every 1 to 2 hours to help in mobilize secretions
- Perform or assist with oral hygiene
- Position the patient for comfort, with the head of the bed elevated, if appropriate, to promote optimal gas exchange
- Maintain a normal body temperature with antipyretics
- Cluster nursing activities and schedule care to provide frequent rest periods
- Prepare for intubation and mechanical ventilation if needed
- Provide sedation as necessary
- Provide education and emotional support to the patient and family.

## Asthma

### *Description*

- Asthma is a chronic reactive airway disorder that involves episodic, reversible airway obstruction resulting from bronchospasms, increased mucus secretions, and mucosal edema

- It is characterized by airway inflammation, intermittent airflow obstruction, and bronchial hyperresponsiveness
- Asthma can result from several types of triggers
  - exposure to tobacco or wood smoke
  - breathing polluted air
  - inhaling other respiratory irritants, such as perfumes or cleaning products
  - exposure to airway irritants at the workplace
  - breathing in allergy-causing substances (allergens), such as molds, dust, or animal dander
  - upper respiratory tract infection, such as a cold, influenza, sinusitis, or bronchitis
  - exposure to cold
  - dry weather
  - emotional excitement or stress
  - physical exertion or exercise (exercise-induced asthma)
  - reflux of stomach acid (gastroesophageal reflux disease, or GERD)
  - ingestion of sulfites, an additive found in some foods and wine
- Comorbidities include GERD, drug-induced asthma, and other allergic reactions, such as eczema, rashes, and temporary edema.

### Signs and Symptoms

- Overall signs and symptoms of asthma range from mild wheezing and dyspnea to life-threatening respiratory failure; signs and symptoms of bronchial airway obstruction may persist between acute episodes
- An asthma attack may begin dramatically, with simultaneous onset of severe, multiple signs and symptoms, or insidiously, with gradually increasing respiratory distress
- Exposure to a particular allergen is followed by a sudden onset of dyspnea and wheezing and by tightness in the chest accompanied by a cough that produces thick, clear, or yellow sputum (cough, dyspnea, and wheezing are the three most common signs and symptoms of asthma)
- An attack often starts during the night or in the early morning
- Physical findings may include visible dyspnea, use of accessory respiratory muscles, complaints of chest tightness, diaphoresis, increased anteroposterior thoracic diameter, and hyperresonance
- Tachycardia, tachypnea, mild systolic hypertension, and pulsus paradoxus may occur as the exacerbation progresses
- Inspiratory and expiratory wheezes may occur, along with wheezing and coughing (which may be exercise-induced), a prolonged expiratory phase of respiration, and diminished breath sounds
- The occurrence of cyanosis, confusion, and lethargy indicate the onset of life-threatening status asthmaticus and respiratory failure.

### Diagnosis and Treatment

- ABG analysis provides the best indication of an attack's severity and may reveal hypoxemia during an acute attack; in acutely severe asthma, $PaO_2$ is less than 60 mm Hg, $PaO_2$ is 40 mm Hg or more, and pH is usually decreased; normal $PaO_2$ during an acute attack may signal impending respiratory failure
- Radioallergosorbent (RAST) testing shows an increased serum immunoglobulin E levels as a result of an allergic reaction
- A complete blood count (CBC) including WBC count and differential shows an increased eosinophil count in acute phases
- Chest X-rays may show hyperinflation, flattened diaphragms, areas of focal atelectasis, pneumothorax, or pneumomediastinum
- Pulmonary function tests commonly show decreased peak flow rates and forced expiratory volume in 1 second, low-normal or decreased vital capacity, and increased total lung and residual capacities, although results may be normal between attacks
- Skin testing may identify specific allergens
- Bronchial challenge testing shows the clinical significance of allergens identified by skin testing
- Pulse oximetry measurements may show decreased oxygen saturation
- Peak flow monitoring reveals a result of less than 80% of personal best; a reading below 50% of personal best indicates a severe exacerbation
- Treatment involves identifying and avoiding precipitating factors and desensitizing the patient to specific antigens
- Generally, asthma medications are divided into two categories: quick relief for relief of immediate symptoms and long-acting medications to control the underlying inflammation
  - Quick-relief bronchodilators include an albuterol sulfate inhaler used as needed
  - Quick-relief anticholinergics for bronchospasms include ipratropium bromide
  - Corticosteroids, such as systemic methylprednisolone, prednisolone, and prednisone, prevent exacerbation and progression during moderate or severe exacerbations
  - Corticosteroids for persistent asthma include inhaled corticosteroid of fluticasone (Flovent), beclomethasone (QVAR), budesonide inhaled (Pulmicort Turbuhaler), and mometasone inhaled (Asmanex)
  - Long-acting beta-agonist or combination of drugs include salmeterol inhaled (Serevent), formoterol inhaled (Foradil), fluticasone and salmeterol inhaled (Advair), and budesonide and formoterol inhaled (Symbicort)
  - Leukotriene antagonists (antileukotrienes) include montelukast (Singulair)
  - Anticholinergic bronchodilators include tiotropium inhaled (Spiriva)
  - Monoclonal antibodies such as omalizumab (Xolair) and anti-inflammatory agents such as nedocromil sodium (Tilade) inhaled before exercise reduce bronchospasm.

### Nursing Interventions

- Give prescribed inhalers and asthma medications
- Place the patient in high Fowler's position
- Encourage pursed-lip and diaphragmatic breathing

- Administer prescribed humidified oxygen
- Adjust oxygen according to the patient's vital signs and ABG values
- Assist with intubation and mechanical ventilation, if appropriate
- Perform postural drainage and chest percussion, if tolerated
- If the patient is intubated, suction as needed
- Treat the patient's dehydration with IV or oral fluids as tolerated
- Keep the room temperature comfortable
- Use an air conditioner or a fan in hot, humid weather
- Monitor the patient's vital signs, intake and output, response to treatment, signs and symptoms of theophylline toxicity, breath sounds, ABG results, pulmonary function test results, pulse oximetry, complications of corticosteroid treatment, and anxiety level.

## Atelectasis

### *Description*

- Atelectasis is the partial or total collapse of the functioning alveoli
- Airway obstruction, COPD, ascites, and lung compression resulting from hemothorax, pneumothorax, or tumor can cause atelectasis; atelectasis also is a common complication of thoracic and upper abdominal surgery that can occur 24 to 48 hours postoperatively
- General anesthesia, immobility, lung disease, obesity, opioid use, pain, and smoking increase the risk of atelectasis
- A patient with atelectasis has decreased ventilation because the collapsed alveoli cannot exchange gases; this decreased ventilation leads to hypoxemia
- Stasis of mucus leads to bacterial growth and pneumonia.

### *Signs and Symptoms*

- Vital sign assessment typically reveals fever (which may occur 24 to 48 hours postoperatively), tachycardia, and tachypnea
- Auscultation may reveal crackles and decreased breath sounds over the affected area
- Other effects may include cyanosis, dyspnea, and increased sputum production.

### *Diagnosis and Treatment*

- The patient should undergo ABG studies, chest X-ray, and sputum culture
- A bronchodilator is administered to dilate bronchioles and promote secretion removal
- An antibiotic is administered to treat infection
- If present, tumors are removed surgically or treated with radiation therapy
- A chest tube is inserted for a patient with hemothorax (to drain blood) or pneumothorax (to reinflate the lung).

### *Nursing Interventions*

- Encourage the patient to cough and breathe deeply to maximize lung expansion and re-expand collapsed alveoli; use an incentive spirometer hourly after surgery
- Provide adequate hydration to liquefy secretions; thin secretions are easier to expectorate
- Implement chest physiotherapy to help clear secretions; postural drainage uses gravity to clear secretions, whereas percussion and vibration loosen secretions, making them easier to cough up
- Suction the patient's airway to maintain patency and to clear secretions
- Provide oxygen therapy to improve $PaO_2$ and maintain adequate oxygenation
- Medicate for pain or discomfort as needed, which will allow the patient to cough and deep-breathe effectively
- Teach the patient to use a pillow to splint abdominal and chest incisions during coughing exercises
- Encourage early ambulation and frequent position changes to prevent complications of immobility and promote lung expansion.

## Chronic Obstructive Pulmonary Disease

### *Description*

- COPD is the term used for preventable and treatable disorders that block the normal flow of air through the lungs, thereby trapping air in the alveoli
- Chronic bronchitis, and emphysema are types of COPD; asthma once classified as a type of COPD, is now considered a distinct restrictive rather than obstructive disorder.

### *Chronic Bronchitis*

- Chronic bronchitis affects the lung parenchyma; it is characterized by a productive cough for at least 3 months a year for 2 or more consecutive years
- It results from lung irritants, such as air pollution and smoking, as well as from genetic factors
- With chronic bronchitis, increased bronchial mucus gland production and goblet cell hyperplasia result in an increased sputum production; ciliary damage and epithelial metaplasia may occur
- Bronchial irritants or infection may cause bronchial edema, bronchospasm, impaired mucociliary clearance, impaired ventilation (especially during expiration), increased secretions, and small-airway blockage
- Impaired diffusion is caused by decreased airflow, mucus plugs, and secondary infection; cyanosis and polycythemia develop as a result of hypoxemia
- Signs of emphysema may be present, and as the disease progresses, cor pulmonale and pulmonary hypertension may develop.

### *Emphysema*

- Emphysema is a disease of the lung parenchyma characterized by changes in the alveolar wall and enlarged alveoli distal to the non-respiratory bronchioles
- It results from alpha1-antitrypsin deficiency and is associated with smoking and air pollution
- Emphysema impairs ventilation by decreasing lung elasticity, collapsing small airways during exhalation, trapping air, and causing poor gas exchange in the alveoli

- It impairs diffusion by enlarging distal air spaces (which increases the distance for diffusion) and causing loss of capillary membranes and pulmonary vasoconstriction
- It impairs perfusion by causing loss of pulmonary vasculature, pulmonary hypertension, and cor Pulmonale.

## Cor Pulmonale

### Description

- In cor pulmonale, hypertrophy and dilation of the right ventricle secondary to disease affect the structure or function of the lungs or their vasculature, resulting in right-sided heart failure
- The disorder can occur at the end stage of various chronic disorders of the lungs, pulmonary vessels, chest wall, and respiratory control center
- Pulmonary hypertension increases the heart's workload
- To compensate, the right ventricle hypertrophies to force blood through the lungs
- In response to hypoxia, the bone marrow produces more red blood cells, causing polycythemia; the resulting increased viscosity further aggravates pulmonary hypertension and increases right ventricular workload
- Causes include primary pulmonary hypertension, pulmonary embolism, asthma, connective tissue disorders, COPD (the cause in more than half of all cases), chronic severe tricuspid regurgitation, disorders affecting the pulmonary parenchyma, and neuromuscular disease
- Cor pulmonale accounts for approximately 6 to 8% of all types of heart disease in adults in the United States
- Patients with cor pulmonale are typically older than age 45; males are more likely to be affected than females.

### Signs and Symptoms

- Signs and symptoms include a hisory of dyspnea, chronic productive cough, fatigue, and weakness
- Other signs and symptoms include tachypnea, wheezing, chest wall retractions, hemoptysis, pitting edema in the extremities, distended jugular veins, an enlarged liver, and tachycardia with pansystolic murmur at the lower left sternal border.

### Diagnosis and Treatment

- ABG analysis reveals decreased $PaO_2$ (usually less than 70 mm Hg and rarely more than 90 mm Hg), hypercapnia, and hypoxia
- Hematocrit is typically over 50%
- Serum liver enzyme levels may show an elevated level of aspartate aminotransferase
- Brain natriuretic peptide level may be elevated
- Chest X-ray, echocardiography, angiography, and magnetic resonance imaging (MRI) demonstrate right ventricular enlargement
- An ECG shows arrhythmias and may show atrial fibrillation (AF) and right bundle-branch block (RBBB)
- Pulmonary function studies reflect the underlying pulmonary disease
- A hemodynamic profile shows an increased pulmonary vascular resistance
- The key to treatment is correcting the underlying problem
- Oxygen therapy improves oxygenation
- Phlebotomy is indicated for patients with COPD with a hematocrit of 55% or more
- Continuous positive airway pressure or biphasic positive air pressure is indicated for sleep apnea
- The patient should be on moderate sodium restriction and diuretics
- Patients should limit activity as tolerated; during the acute phase, patients should be on bed rest
- Beta selective agonists, such as epoprostenol (Flolan), treprostinil (Remodulin), and iloprost (Ventavis), are used to treat primary pulmonary hypertension
- Bronchodilators administered by nebulizer include ipratropium (Atrovent), metaproterenol, and albuterol (Accuneb)
- For patients with persistent disease, vasodilators include hydralazine, nifedipine (Procardia), diltiazem (Cardizem), and prazosin (Minipress)
- The endothelin-1 receptor antagonists bosentan can help patients with pulmonary hypertension and severe symptoms to improve exertional tolerance and an increase in walking distance
- Antibiotics treat acute respiratory infections
- Anticoagulants help to prevent thromboembolism.

### Nursing Interventions

- Monitor the patient's vital signs, and pay attention to his cardiac and respiratory status
- Reposition the patient often; elevate the head of the bed to increase thoracic expansion and ease the work of breathing
- Administer oxygen as ordered based on oxygen saturation levels obtained with pulse oximetry and ABG results
- Give prescribed drugs; if the patient will receive IV diuretics, ensure patent IV access
- Encourage the patient to take slow, deep breaths when using nebulized medications, as appropriate
- Provide frequent rest periods; cluster nursing activities to minimize oxygen and metabolic demands
- Teach the patient and family about the disorder, the patient's diagnosis, the underlying cause and its relationship to the patient's current condition, treatment, and follow-up care.

## Hemothorax

### Description

- Hemothorax is the presence of blood in the pleural cavity; it typically accompanies pneumothorax
- It may result from chest trauma, lacerated liver, penetrating trauma, perforated blood vessels, perforated diaphragm, pleural damage that causes bleeding, or rib fracture
- In hemothorax, blood collects in the pleural layer, compressing the lung on the affected side; this lung compression compromises gas exchange.

### Signs and Symptoms

- Chest pain, cyanosis, dyspnea, and tachypnea commonly occur

- With marked blood loss, hypertension and shock may occur
- Asymmetrical lung expansion is accompanied by decreased breath sounds on the affected side.

### Diagnosis and Treatment

- Chest X-ray, CBC, and ABG studies are commonly prescribed
- A chest tube is inserted, and a water seal or suction is used to facilitate drainage
- Thoracotomy may be indicated if blood loss is severe
- If total blood loss is severe, the patient is treated with IV fluids and transfusion.

### Nursing Interventions

- Administer oxygen to maintain adequate oxygenation, improve $PaO_2$ and reverse hypoxemia
- Teach techniques for effective coughing and deep breathing to prevent atelectasis and promote lung expansion
- Maintain the integrity of the chest tube system to facilitate blood drainage from around the lung and promote lung expansion
- Check the chest tube insertion site for crepitus, which indicates air leakage into tissue and may indicate a leak in the chest tube system
  - An air leak in the system may indicate that the lung is damaged, causing air to leak from the lung into the pleural space
  - If the air leak is outside the chest cavity (such as from the chest tube), air entering the system may increase air accumulation in the pleural space
- Encourage frequent position changes to prevent complications of immobility and promote lung expansion
- Provide an analgesic as needed to reduce an anxiety, relieve pain, and ease coughing and deep breathing.

## Influenza

### Description

- Influenza is an infectious disease caused by ribonucleic acid (RNA) viruses that can affect humans, birds, and other mammals
- Influenza A, Influenza B, and Influenza C can all infect humans
- H1N1 is a subtypes of Influenza A; strains are endemic in pigs (swine) and in birds (avian).

### Avian Influenza

- Infected migratory and domestic birds shed the virus in their saliva, nasal secretions, and feces
- The strain is known as H5N1.
- Transmission has been limited to people, and some animals such as cats, in contact with infected birds
- Should this virus become more easily transmissible person-to-person, it may lead to a pandemic.

### Signs and Symptoms

- Symptoms range from typical human Influenza-like symptoms, such as fever, cough, sore throat, and muscle aches, to eye infections, pneumonia, and acute respiratory distress
- Diarrhea, vomiting, and abdominal pain may occur.

### Diagnosis and Treatment

- Chest X-ray may show pneumonia, infi ltrates, or consolidations
- Sputum gram stains and culture isolate the virus
- Neuraminidase inhibitor class drugs, such as oseltamivir (Tamiflu) and zanamivir (Relenza), can reduce the severity and duration of illness caused by seasonal Influenza; efficacy depends on early administration
- M2 inhibitors amantadine and rimantadine could possibly be used for pandemic infuenza, but resistance to these drugs may develop
- The patient may require treatment to maintain fluid and electrolyte balance
- The patient may need mechanical ventilation for acute respiratory distress.

### Nursing Interventions

- Follow standard and contact precautions, wear a fit-tested ventilator, and perform frequent hand hygeine
- Wear eye protection within 3 feet of the patient
- Maintain a patent airway, suctioning the patient when necessary
- Notify the National Respiratory and Enteric Virus Surveillance System.

## Pleural Effusion

### Description

- Pleural effusion is an accumulation of fluid in the pleural space (the thin space between the visceral and parietal pleura); although it is not a disease itself, it occurs secondary to other disease states
- Empyema is the accumulation of pus and necrotic tissue in the pleural space; blood (hemothorax) and chyle (chylothorax) may also collect in this space
- A pleural effusion can be classified either as exudative (caused by inflammation of the pleura) or transudative (caused by excessive hydrostatic pressure or decreased osmotic pressure)
  - Common causes of exudative effusions are bacterial or fungal empyema or pneumonitis, chest trauma, collagen disease, malignancy, myxedema, pancreatitis, pulmonary embolism, subphrenic abscess, and tuberculosis
  - Common causes of transudative effusions are heart failure, hepatic disease with ascites, hypoalbuminemia, and peritoneal dialysis.

### Signs and Symptoms

- The most common symptoms are pleuritic pain and dyspnea
- Physical examination may reveal decreased chest wall movement, decreased breath sounds over the affected area, and dullness on percussion
- Infection from empyema may produce cough, fever, and night sweats.

### *Diagnosis and Treatment*

- Chest X-ray can diagnose pleural effusion; other tests that may be prescribed include CT scan of the chest, bronchoscopy, pleurocentesis, and ultrasonography
- The underlying cause should be treated if it can be identified
- Thoracentesis is performed to remove fluid; chest tubes may be placed for continued drainage
- Thoracotomy may be needed if thoracentesis is not effective
- An antibiotic is prescribed to treat empyema; the specific antibiotic used to depend on the causative organism.

### *Nursing Interventions*

- Explain thoracentesis to the patient, and support him during the procedure
- Watch for respiratory distress or pneumothorax after thoracentesis
- Administer oxygen to improve oxygenation
- Encourage deep-breathing exercises and incentive spirometry to promote lung expansion
- Maintain the integrity of the chest tube drainage system; monitor the amount, color, and consistency of drainage; and check for air leaks.

## Pneumonia

### *Description*

- Pneumonia is an acute lung infection with inflammation accompanied by accumulation of exudate in the alveoli
- The risk of pneumonia increases with aspiration, central nervous system depression, chronic illness, COPD, dehydration, existence of a tracheostomy opening, immobility, immunosuppression, intubation, pain in the thoracic cavity, and use of general anesthesia
- It may result from a bacterial, fungal, or viral infection or from exposure to a chemical irritant, through aspiration or gas inhalation
- Pneumonia remains a major cause of morbidity and mortality among elderly and chronically ill people.

### *Signs and Symptoms*

- Dyspnea or tachypnea, fatigue, and fever commonly occur
- Signs of cyanosis or hypoxia may occur in those with advanced disease
- Irritability or restlessness may signal cerebral hypoxia
- Sputum may vary in amount, color, and consistency, depending on the causative agent.
- Lung auscultation may reveal crackles, rhonchi, bronchial breath sounds over areas of consolidation, or wheezes over the affected areas; breath sounds may be decreased in those with advanced disease.

### *Diagnosis and Treatment*

- Chest X-ray, ABG studies, sputum culture (for bacterial infection), and serologic testing (for viral infection) may be prescribed
- Needle or open biopsy may obtain lung tissue specimens (for fungal infection), and cold agglutinins may reveal antibodies associated with *Mycoplasma pneumoniae* infection
- Pneumonia is treated with antibiotics to eradicate the infecting organism
- A bronchodilator is used to open narrowed airways.

### *Nursing Interventions*

- Teach effective coughing and deep breathing to improve airway clearance
- Provide adequate hydration to liquefy secretions; thin secretions are easier to expectorate
- Implement chest physiotherapy; postural drainage uses gravity to clear secretions, and percussion and vibration loosen secretions, making them easier to cough up
- Administer oxygen to aid ventilation, improve $PaO_2$, and preserve oxygenation
- Suction the patient's airway as needed to maintain patency and to clear secretions
- Advise the patient to limit activity and to rest for long periods to decrease oxygen consumption
- Provide pain medication as needed to allow effective coughing and deep breathing
- Maintain adequate nutrition to offset the increased use of calories secondary to infection
- Teach the patient how to contain secretions to reduce the risk of spreading infection
- Practice good hand hygiene techniques to reduce the risk of spreading infection
- Teach relaxation and stress-reduction techniques; anxiety can compromise the immune system and increase the risk of infection.

## Pulmonary Edema

### *Description*

- Pulmonary edema is the collection of fluid in the interstitium and alveoli of the lungs as pressure rises in the pulmonary vessels
- It can result from ARDS, fluid overload, left-sided heart failure, mitral stenosis, MI, or pulmonary emboli
- With pulmonary edema, the left ventricle cannot effectively pump blood from the heart
  - With an increased resistence to left ventricular filling, fluid backs up into the lungs
  - Surface tension increases, the alveoli shrink, and the lungs become stiff, making breathing more difficult
  - Hypoxemia and an altered V/Q ratio develop
  - Fluid moves into the larger airways, where it is coughed up as pink, frothy sputum.

### *Signs and Symptoms*

- Tachycardia and tachypnea may be accompanied by narrowed pulse pressures and hypotension; third and fourth heart sounds may be present; skin may be cold and clammy
- Dyspnea, increased respiratory rate, orthopnea, and pulmonary hypertension may occur
- Jugular veins may be distended, and PAWP may be elevated
- Coughing may produce blood-tinged or pink, frothy sputum

- Lung auscultation may reveal dependent crackles
- Other signs and symptoms may include confusion, decreased urine output, diaphoresis, drowsiness, lethargy, and restlessness.

### *Diagnosis and Treatment*

- Chest X-ray, pulse oximetry, and ABG studies typically are prescribed
- A PA catheter is inserted to measure pressures
- A diuretic is administered to decrease edema
- Other drugs that may be administered include an inotropic drug to increase myocardial contractility, nitroglycerin to reduce preload and after load, IV nitroprusside to reduce preload and after load, and a vasopressor to maintain blood pressure.
- Intubation and mechanical ventilation may be necessary to treat respiratory distress
- Morphine is administered to decrease preload, respiratory rate, and anxiety
- Patients who do not respond to drug therapy may be treated with an intra-aortic balloon pump, which temporarily assists the failed left ventricle, or with surgery (such as angioplasty, coronary artery bypass grafting, or valvular repair), depending on the underlying heart condition.

### *Nursing Interventions*

- Administer oxygen to aid ventilation, improve $PaO_2$ and reverse hypoxemia
- Place the patient in semi-Fowler's position to maximize oxygenation and increase comfort
- Carefully monitor fluid intake and output to assess the effectiveness of diuretic therapy and prevent sudden increase in venous return caused by oral and IV intake
- Medicate for pain as needed to reduce anxiety and increase in comfort
- Frequently change the patient's position to prevent pressure ulcers and encourage lung expansion.

## Pulmonary Embolism

### *Description*

- Pulmonary embolism is a blockage in the pulmonary vasculature
- Risk factors include atrial fibrillation; COPD; a family history of pulmonary embolism; oral contraceptive use; prior thromboembolic disease; venous injury caused by abdominal, pelvic, or thoracicsurgery or leg or pelvic trauma; and venous stasis caused by age (older than age 55), burns, obesity, pregnancy, or prolonged immobility
- Pulmonary embolism is commonly caused by dislodged thrombi from deep veins in the pelvis or legs or from any systemic veins
- In this disorder, an embolism lodges in a branch of the pulmonary vasculature; the embolism may consist of bone, air, fat, amniotic fluid, a thrombus, or a foreign object
  - The area of the lung below the embolism is not perfused, causing altered V/Q ratio, which can cause alveolar collapse and led to atelectasis and hypoxemia
  - Pulmonary infarction may occur, destroying lung tissue
  - A massive pulmonary embolism can cause pulmonary hypertension as a result of increased vascular resistance, right-sided heart failure as a result of increased right ventricular workload, or ventricular hypertrophy as a result of increased right ventricular workload.

### *Signs and Symptoms*

- Dyspnea may occur suddenly, accompanied by chest pain
- Pleuritic chest pain may indicate pulmonary infarction
- Cough may produce hemoptysis
- Anxiety, increased restlessness, hypotension, and tachycardia may occur
- Lung auscultation may reveal crackles, pleural friction rub, and wheezes
- Low-grade fever and tachypnea may occur
- Signs of Cor Pulmonale and right-sided heart failure may develop
- If the patient has a massive pulmonary embolism, he may experience arrhythmias, cyanosis, or diaphoresis
- If the patient has a fat embolism, he may experience confusion, dyspnea, or petechiae on his chest and axillae
- The patient's legs may have signs and symptoms of deep vein thrombosis, such as edema, redness, tenderness, and warmth.

### *Diagnosis and Treatment*

- Several tests are used to diagnose pulmonary embolism: ABG studies, chest X-ray, electrocardiography, lung scintigraphy, MRI, pulmonary angiography, and V/Q lung scanning
- Several tests are used to diagnose deep vein thrombosis, which can lead to pulmonary embolism: contrast venography, doppler ultrasonography, impedance plethysmography, and leg scan after injection of fibrinogen
- After an initial IV bolus of heparin, a therapeutic heparin infusion is given to inhibit clot formation, prevent emboli development, and maintain the partial thromboplastin time (PTT) between 1.5 and 2 times the control (60 to 70 seconds)
- If the patient needs long-term therapy, warfarin (Coumadin) is administered to maintain the prothrombin time (PT) between 1.5 and 2 times the control (11 to 12 seconds) or the International Normalized Ratio (INR) between 2 and 3; once the therapeutic dose of warfarin is achieved, the heparin infusion may be discontinued
- If the patient has a life-threatening embolism, a thrombolytic is administered, or a surgical embolectomy is performed
- If the patient cannot tolerate anticoagulant therapy or continues to develop clots despite taking these drugs, surgical insertion of a vena caval filter may be needed
- A diuretic may be prescribed for a patient with a fat embolism; an antibiotic, for a patient with a septic embolism
- An antiarrhythmic may be used to correct heart rhythm disturbances caused by ischemia.

### *Nursing Interventions*

- Administer oxygen to improve $PaO_2$, reverse hypoxemia, and promote lung expansion

- If the patient requires mechanical ventilation, assist as needed
- Teach effective coughing and deep breathing to help clear secretions and prevent atelectasis
- Provide adequate hydration to liquefy secretions; thin secretions are easier to expectorate
- Encourage early ambulation to prevent clot formation in deep veins; encourage range-of-motion (ROM) exercises or perform passive ROM exercises if the patient cannot walk
- Use antiembolism stockings or a compression device to divert blood flow to the large veins, prevent emboli formation, and to promote venous return
- Do not raise the patient's knees; this obstructs venous flow and increases the risk of deep vein thrombosis
- Elevate the patient's legs to prevent venous stasis
- Maintain the heparin infusion, and monitor the PTT
- Administer warfarin daily, as prescribed, and monitor the PT or INR
- Test all stool for blood caused by anticoagulant-induced GI bleeding
- Provide analgesia and comfort measures to reduce anxiety
- Teach the patient about anticoagulant therapy to reduce the risk of bleeding, and help the patient to maintain therapeutic PT or INR
- Have the family or home health nurse check the home for hazards, especially those that may cause falls; a safe environment is necessary because a patient receiving an anticoagulant has an increased tendency to bleed
- Instruct the patient not to cross his legs, sit for long periods, or wear restrictive clothing; these activities inhibit venous return and promote clot formation.

## Severe Acute Respiratory Syndrome

### *Description*

- Severe acute respiratory syndrome (SARS) is a life-threatening viral infection believed to be coronavirus
- A theory suggests that coronavirus may have mutated from pigs, birds, and other animals, allowing transmission to and infection of humans
- The incubation period is estimated to range from 2 to 7 days (average is 3 to 5 days)
- Risk factors include close contact with an infected person, contact with exhaled droplets and bodily secretions from an infected person, or travel to endemic areas.

### *Signs and Symptoms*

- In early stages, signs and symptoms include non-productive cough, rash, high fever, headache, body aches, and pneumonia
- Shortness of breath and respiratory distress occur in later stages.

### *Diagnosis and Treatment*

- Serum electrophoresis detects antibodies to the coronavirus
- Sputum Gram stain and culture isolates the coronavirus
- SARS-specific polymerase chain reaction tests detect SARS-CoV RNA
- Isolation (strict respiratory and mucosal barrier) prevents the spread of disease
- Antivirals treat viral infection, and a combination of corticosteroids and antimicrobials treat inflammation and infection
- Mechanical ventilation treats respiratory failure.

### *Nursing Interventions*

- Maintain isolation for the patient
- Practice good hygiene to prevent further transmission
- Maintain a patent airway through suctioning if the patient requires mechanical ventilation
- Monitor the patient's vital signs and nutritional fluid and respiratory status.

## Tuberculosis

### *Description*

- Tuberculosis (TB) is an infectious disease that commonly affects the lungs; it typically occurs only after repeated, close contact with a person infected with *Mycobacterium tuberculosis*
- Risk factors for TB include alcoholism, immunosuppression, low economic status, and malnutrition; elderly people, populations in crowded areas (for example, shelters and prisons), and immigrants from areas with high incidences of TB (such as Africa, Southeast Asia, and the Caribbean islands) are also more susceptible
- The incidence of TB has increased in proportion to the increase in patients who are infected with the human immunodeficiency virus
- *M. tuberculosis* is spread by way of infected airborne droplets; after infected droplets are inhaled into the terminal bronchioles, localized pneumonia develops, initiating an inflammatory response
  - Bacilli are phagocytized by macrophages but remain viable within the phagocyte
  - Tubercles form and grow in the lungs
  - The lesion center forms a yellow, cheesy mass called caseous necrosis
  - Healing begins, walling off the initial infection, and adenopathy occurs
  - Systemic infection may develop in the absence of appropriate treatment.
- Within 6 weeks of exposure to the infected droplets, cellular immunity occurs, and skin test results become positive
- Latent TB infection can become active TB disease years after exposure, when resistance is lowered.

### *Signs and Symptoms*

- Anorexia, weight loss, chills, fever, chest pain, coughing up blood or sputum, and night sweats may occur in patients with active TB disease
- Lung ausculation may reveal crackles, pleural effusions, and rhonchi.

### *Diagnosis and Treatment*

- The Mantoux TB skin test or the Quanti FERON - TB Gold test, a gamma interferon blood test for TB, can be used to test for *M. tuberculosis* infection

- Abnormalities seen during a chest X-ray may suggest TB, but cannot be used to diagnose TB
- The presence of acid-fast bacilli on a sputum smear or other specimen after indicates disease
- A positive culture for *M tuberculosis* confirms the diagnosis of active TB disease
- Preventive treatment with isoniazid for 9 to 12 months is recommended for other members of the patient's household, those with recently converted positive skin tests, and those with positive skin tests (depending on medical history)
- If the patient has active TB disease, an antituberculotic is used for 6 to 9 months; isoniazid with rifampin usually is the first choice; other antituberculotics include ethambutol, and pyrazinamide.

### Nursing Interventions

- Teach the patient how to contain airborne droplets and secretions to reduce the risk of spreading the infection
- Practice of good hand hygiene techniques to reduce the risk of spreading the infection
- Explain disease transmission to the patient and the need for prolonged therapy help to increase his compliance with the treatment plan
- Teach the patient about the prescribed drugs, including how to recognize adverse reactions (especially the symptoms of hepatotoxicity)
- Encourage the patient to maintain adequate dietary intake to maintain nutritional status, build strength, and improve the body's defense mechanisms weigh the patient daily to assess nutritional status.

## GASTROINTESTINAL DISORDERS

### Introduction

- The GI, or digestive, system breaks down food and prepares it for absorption by the body's cells; nonabsorbable ingested substances pass through the system and are eliminated as solid waste
- Although not part of the alimentary canal, the liver, gallbladder, and pancreas are essential for accessory components of the GI system.

### Nursing History

The nurse asks the patient about his *chief complaint.*

- The patient with a GI problem may report a change in appetite, heartburn, nausea, pain, or vomiting
- The patient may also report a change in bowel habits, such as constipation, diarrhea, or stool characteristics.

The nurse then questions the patient about his *present illness.*

- Ask the patient about his symptom, includes—associated symptoms, location, radiation, intensity, duration, frequency, and precipitating and alleviating factors
- Ask about the use of prescription and over-the-counter drugs, herbal remedies, and vitamin and nutritional supplements; ask about the use of laxatives
- If the patient's chief complaint is diarrhea, find out if he recently traveled abroad
- Ask the patient about changes in appetite and in bowel habits (e.g. a change in the amount, appearance, or color of his stool or the appearance of blood in it) and difficulty eating or chewing.

The nurse asks about *medical history*

- Question the patient about other GI disorders, such as gallbladder disease, GI bleeding, inflammatory bowel disease, or ulcers
- Also, ask about previous abdominal surgery or trauma.

The nurse then assesses the *family history*

- Ask about a family history of diseases with a hereditary link, such as alcoholism, colon cancer, Crohn's disease, stomach ulcers, and ulcerative colitis
- Also, question the patient about a family history of chronic diseases.

The nurse obtains a *social history*

- Ask about work, exercise, diet, use of recreational drugs and alcohol, caffeine intake, and hobbies
- Also ask about stress, support systems, and coping mechanisms.

### Physical Assessment

- When assessing the abdomen, use this sequence: inspection, auscultation, percussion, and palpation; palpating or percussing the abdomen before you auscultate can change the character of the patient's bowel sounds and lead to an inaccurate assessment
- The nurse begins with *inspection*
  - Observe the patient's general appearance, and note his behavior
  - Inspect the skin for turgor, color, and texture; note abnormalities such as bruising, decreased axillary or pubic hair, edema, petechiae, scars, spider angiomas, and stretch marks
  - Observe the patient's head for color of the sclera, sunken eyes, dentures, caries, lesions, breath odor, and tongue color, swelling, or dryness
  - Check the size and shape of the abdomen, noting distention, peristalsis, pulsations, contour, visible masses, and protrusions
  - Observe the rectal area for abnormalities
- The nurse continues by using *auscultation*
  - Note the character and quality of bowel sounds in each quadrant
  - Auscultate the abdomen for vascular sounds
- Then the nurse *percusses* the abdomen
  - Percuss the abdomen to detect the size and location of the abdominal organs
  - Note the presence of air or fluid
- Next, the nurse uses *palpation*
  - Palpate the abdomen to determine the size, shape, position, and tenderness of major abdominal organs and to detect masses and fluid accumulation
  - Note abdominal muscle tone and tenderness
  - Palpate the rectum, noting any abnormalities.

## Appendicitis

### Description

- Appendicitis is an inflammation of the vermiform appendix; it results when mucosal ulceration triggers inflammation, which temporarily obstructs the appendix
- In this disorder, bacteria multiply and inflammation and pressure increase, restricting blood flow and causing thrombus and abdominal pain
- Causes include fecal mass (fecalith), foreign body obstruction, barium ingestion, neoplasm, stricture, and infection
- Appendicitis is the most common major abdominal surgical disease
- If left untreated, it can be fatal; gangrene and perforation can develop within 36 hours with resulting peritonitis and sepsis.

### Signs and Symptoms

- Appendicitis causes abdominal periumbilical pain that's initially generalized and then localizes in the right lower abdomen (McBurney's point)
- The patient feels right lower quadrant and rebound tenderness; he may continually adjust his posture to relieve pain and exhibits guarding
- The patient may display the Rovsing sign (pain in the right lower quadrant that occurs with palpation of left lower quadrant), psoas sign (abdominal pain that occurs when flexing the hip when pressure is applied to the knee), or obturator sign (abdominal pain that occurs when the hip is rotated)
- A patient with a retrocele or pelvic appendix may not have abdominal or flank tenderness
- Other signs and symptoms include anorexia, nausea, and vomiting; low-grade fever; and tachycardia.

### Diagnosis and Treatment

- White blood cell (WBC) count may be elevated, with an increase in immature cells
- Ultrasonography of the abdomen can help diagnose a nonperforated appendix; a computed tomography (CT) scan can also be useful
- Appendectomy is only effective treatment.

### Nursing Interventions

- Place the patient in Fowler's position to minimize pain
- Before surgery, administer analgesics judiciously because they may mask pain or perforation
- Prepare the patient for appendectomy; initiate nothing-by-mouth status and establish IV access; administer IV fluids to prevent dehydration
- After appendectomy, watch for surgical complications, including wound infection, intestinal obstruction, peritonitis, and abdominal abscess
- Administer pain medication as needed
- If the patient has developed peritonitis, administer antibiotics and maintain a nasogastric (NG) tube
- Monitor the patient's vital signs closely
- Increase the patient's activity and advance his diet as tolerated.

## Cholecystitis

### Description

- Cholecystitis is an acute or a chronic inflammation of the gallbladder; it is commonly associated with cholelithiasis (presence of gallstones)
- In most cases, cholecystitis is caused by gallstones; bacterial infection plays a minor role in acute cholecystitis; secondary, bacterial infection occurs in approximately 50% of cases.

### Signs and Symptoms

- Sharp abdominal pain may affect the right upper quadrant of the abdomen, especially after ingestion of fatty foods, and may be referred to the right shoulder area
- Other GI effects include abdominal tenderness and muscle rigidity on palpation, eructation, flatulence, nausea, and vomiting
- Fever may result from acute infection
- Positive Murphy's sign (painful inspiration due to severe tenderness) may be present
- Jaundice may occur if gallstones obstruct the common bile duct.

### Diagnosis and Treatment

- Diagnosis is based on ultrasonography of the upper abdomen and oral cholecystography that shows an enlarged gallbladder and gallstones
- Percutaneous transhepatic cholangiography supports the diagnosis of obstructive jaundice and reveals calculi in the ducts
- Levels of serum alkaline phosphate, lactate dehydrogenase, aspartate aminotransferase, cholesterol, and total bilirubin are elevated
- The patient is placed on a low-fat diet
- An anticholinergic, such as propantheline or dicyclomine, is given to decrease spasms of the common bile duct
- An analgesic is prescribed for pain
- An antibiotic may be given to prevent or treat infection
- Chenodeoxycholic acid or ursodeoxycholic acid may be administered to dissolve gallstones; it must be taken for 6 to 12 months to be effective
- If pain persists, the gallbladder and gallstones are surgically removed by means of laparoscopic microsurgery or abdominal laparotomy; lithotripsy may also be performed to break up gallstones using ultrasonic waves.

### Preoperative Nursing Interventions

- Monitor the patient for abdominal pain in the right upper quadrant that may radiate to the right shoulder
- Check the skin and conjunctiva for jaundice.

### Postoperative Nursing Interventions

- Monitor vital signs every 1 to 2 hours for 4 to 8 hours and then every 4 hours to detect fluid imbalances, hemorrhage, or shock

- Monitor bowel sounds every 4 hours and bowel output to determine return of GI functions
- Check the wound area for signs of bleeding and inflammation
- Change the wound dressing as needed; the wound may be left uncovered if no drainage is present
- Monitor drainage from the T tube, if present; a T tube is used if gallstones were in the common bile duct because it lets bile pass into the small intestine and decreases duct inflammation
- Administer an opioid analgesic every 4 hours as needed and IV antibiotics every 6 to 8 hours as prescribed to maintain comfort and prevent infection
- Make sure the patient maintains nothing-by-mouth status as prescribed; administer IV fluids (up to 3,000 mL daily) to maintain fluid balance, also monitor fluid intake and output every 8 hours
- Start giving the patient clear liquids, then progress to a regular diet as prescribed; fat restrictions may be lifted because gallbladder removal increases the patient's tolerance to fatty foods
- Help the patient sit on the bed or in a chair and ambulate as prescribed to promote recovery from the surgery
- Record pertinent data in the patient's chart for continuity of care.

## Cirrhosis of the Liver

### *Description*

- Cirrhosis is a chronic, progressive disease that causes extensive degeneration and destruction of parenchymal liver cells; it is twice as common in men as in women, and most patients are between ages 40 and 60
- Common types of cirrhosis include *micronodular* (Laënnec's), which is caused by excessive alcohol intake; *macronodular* (postnecrotic, toxin-induced), which is caused by chemicals, bacteria, and viruses; *biliary,* which is caused by irritating biliary products; *pigment,* which is caused by hemochromatosis; and *cardiac,* which is caused by right-sided heart failure and chronic liver disease.

### *Signs and Symptoms*

- GI effects include anorexia, constipation or diarrhea, dull abdominal pain and heaviness, marked flatulence, nausea, vomiting, and weight loss
- The liver may be enlarged and have nodules; jaundice and hepatic encephalopathy may occur
- Hematologic effects may include anemia and thrombocytopenia
- Fever and malaise may be present
- Ascites, esophageal varices, and peripheral edema may occur
- Skin lesions may include petechiae, purpura, and spider angiomas; dry skin and pruritus also may occur
- Asterixis (liver flap, a hand-flapping tremor commonly seen in patients with hepatic coma), lethargy, mental changes, slurred speech, and peripheral neuropathies may occur.
- Endocrine effects may include gynecomastia and impotence in men and amenorrhea in women.

### *Diagnosis and Treatment*

- Diagnosis is based on patient history (especially excessive alcohol intake or hepatitis), physical examination, liver biopsy and liver function studies, ultrasonography, CT scan, magnetic resonance imaging (MRI), and serologic studies, including complete blood count (CBC), serum electrolyte levels, and prothrombin time (PT)
- Paracentesis may be used to remove ascitic fluid
- For intractable chronic ascites, a peritoneovenous shunt may be inserted to transfer ascitic fluid into the venous system for eventual excretion in the urine
- A potassium-sparing diuretic is used to decrease ascites and peripheral edema
- An antiemetic is used to reduce nausea and vomiting
- Vitamin K is used to reduce bleeding tendencies stemming from hypothrombinemia
- Lactulose is used to treat hepatic encephalopathy; lactulose decreases the pH of the colon, which inhibits the diffusion of ammonia from the colon into the blood
- Bleeding esophageal varices are treated by administering vasopressin and a beta-adrenergic blocker; performing endoscopic sclerosis; and inserting a Sengstaken-Blakemore tube or various surgical shunts (such as a portacaval shunt)
- Blood transfusions may be required for massive hemorrhage; IV therapy using colloid volume expanders or crystalloids may be given for volume expansion
- The recommended diet is typically high in calories and has moderate to high protein, moderate to low fat, and low sodium content; fluids are restricted; protein is restricted if encephalopathy develops.

### *Nursing Interventions*

- Make sure the patient maintains bed rest; reposition him every 2 hours to help keep the skin intact and prevent pressure ulcers
- Encourage active range-of-motion exercises, and use special mattresses to relieve pressure
- Encourage deep breathing, and listen for breath sounds in all lung lobes
- Observe closely for changes in behavior or personality, such as stupor, lethargy, hallucinations, or neuromuscular dysfunction
- Administer an antiemetic as prescribed to control nausea and vomiting
- Administer a diuretic as prescribed; weigh the patient daily, and measure fluid intake and output; note signs of hypokalemia
- Measure abdominal girth, and note the changes
- Check the patient's level of consciousness, neurologic status, and vital signs to detect encephalopathy or developing infection
- Monitor the patient for bleeding by checking vomitus and stool for blood; apply pressure to injection sites to prevent bleeding
- Monitor the results of laboratory tests and other studies; report abnormal findings to the practitioner

- Consult the dietitian regarding a low-sodium, fluid-restricted diet; provide four to six small meals daily, including foods that the patient likes, when possible
- Perform oral hygiene before meals and as needed to prevent stomatitis and remove characteristic fetid or ammonia-like mouth odor; have the patient use a soft toothbrush
- Provide meticulous skin care to prevent excoriation; check for edema, jaundice, petechiae, pruritus, purpura, spider angiomas, and ulcerations
- Tell the patient to avoid straining when turning, moving in bed, or defecating to lessen pressure on varices or hemorrhoids
- Explain upcoming diagnostic tests or treatments as needed
- Instruct the patient to avoid spicy or irritating foods, nonsteroidal anti-inflammatory drugs (NSAIDs), and aspirin
- Discuss patient concerns about the disease and lifestyle or body image change; provide a psychological referral, if needed
- Encourage the use of community agencies or services to help the patient control alcohol intake; stress the importance of abstaining from alcohol
- Record all data in the patient's chart for continuity of care.

## Gastroesophageal Reflux Disease

### Description

- GERD is the backflow of gastric contents or duodenal contents, or both, past the lower esophageal sphincter (LES) into the esophagus without associated belching or vomiting
- The disorder occurs when the LES pressure is deficient or pressure in the stomach exceeds LES pressure
- The degree of mucosal injury is based on the amount and concentration of refluxed gastric acid, proteolytic enzymes, and bile acids
- Causes include anything that lowers LES pressure, such as alcohol, smoking, hiatal hernia, increased an abdominal pressure with obesity or pregnancy, medications (such as morphine, diazepam, calcium channel blockers, meperidine, or anticholenergic), NG intubation for more than 4 days, and weakened esophageal sphincter.

### Signs and Symptoms

- Burning pain in the epigastric area, possibly radiating to the arms and chest, results from reflux of gastric contents into the esophagus
- Pain, usually after a meal or when lying down, occurs secondary to increased an abdominal pressure, causing reflux
- Feeling of fluid accumulation occurs in the throat without a sour or bitter taste because of hypersecretion of saliva.

### Diagnosis and Treatment

- Diagnosis is based on a patient history that reveals heartburn, physical examination, esophagoscopy, barium swallow, an upper GI series, esophageal acidity testing, and an acid perfusion test
- Abdominal pressure may be reduced by eating small, frequent meals and not eating before bedtime
- Patient positioning may be helpful in reducing abdominal pressure and preventing reflux, e.g. sitting up during and after meal times or sleeping with the head of the bed elevated)
- Antacids may help to neutralize the acidic content of the stomach
- Histamine-2 receptor antagonists may be given to inhibit gastric acid secretion
- Proton pump inhibitors may be prescribed to reduce gastric acidity
- Cholinergic agents may be given to increase LES pressure
- Smoking cessation is recommended.

### Nursing Interventions

- Teach the patient about the causes and symptoms of GERD
- Tell the patient how to avoid reflux with an antireflux regimen that includes diet, positioning, and antacids.

### Factors Affecting LES Pressure

Various dietary and lifestyle factor can increase or decrease lowers esophageal sphincter (LES) pressure. Take these factors into account when you plan the patient's treatment program.

| Factors that increase LES pressure | Factors that decrease LES pressure |
|---|---|
| • Protein | • Fat |
| • Carbohydrates | • Whole milk |
| • Non-fat milk | • Orange juice |
| • Low-dose ethnol | • Tomatoes |
| | • Antiflatulent (simethicone) |
| | • Chocolate |
| | • High-dose ethanol |
| | • Cigarette smoking |
| | • Lying on the right or left side |
| | • Sitting |
| | • Caffeine |

## Gastrointestinal Bleeding

### Description

- Acute GI bleeding can range from minor to severe
- About 85% of GI bleeding involves the upper GI tract
- Bleeding may be caused by a disrupted mucosal-epithelial barrier or by a ruptured artery or vein.
- Common conditions leading to GI bleeding include peptic ulcer disease, esophageal varices, diverticular disease, tumors, and ulcerative colitis signs and symptoms
- The patient may vomit blood or have coffee-ground vomitus
- Stools may appear bloody, maroon-colored, or black and tarry
- Abdominal cramping may occur

- The patient with chronic bleeding may have symptoms of anemia
- Signs of hypovolemic shock include cold, clammy skin; hypotension; reduced urine output; and tachycardia.

### Diagnosis and Treatment

- Diagnosis is based on physical examination and patient history, including previous bleeding abnormalities, current medications, recent illnesses, and alcohol use
- Colonoscopy and esophagogastroduodenoscopy can detect the source of the bleeding
- Blood tests, such as CBC, coagulation studies, and liver function tests, are also helpful
- Treatment depends on the location and cause of GI bleeding
- Blood or blood component replacement may be indicated
- An NG tube may be inserted and the stomach lavaged with room-temperature fluid to remove blood and clots from the stomach
- A Sengstaken-Blakemore tube may be indicated for the treatment of esophageal varices
- Bleeding blood vessels may be treated with cauterization or endoscopic injection sclerotherapy
- A transjugular intrahepatic portosystemic shunt may be indicated to connect the portal and hepatic veins
- Commonly administered drugs include antacids, histamine blockers, sucralfate, proton pump inhibitors, and antibiotics for the treatment of *H pylori*; vasopressin may be administered to produce vasoconstriction.

### Nursing Interventions

- Monitor vital signs and other hemodynamic parameters for early detection of bleeding and hypovolemic shock; monitor hourly intake and output; maintain nothing by mouth status until bleeding is controlled
- Initiate two large-bore IV lines for fluid, drug, and blood administration
- Ensure patency and proper placement of the NG tube
- If the patient has a Sengstaken-Blakemore tube, make sure it is properly positioned and secured; the balloon should not be inflated for more than 72 hours because of the high risk of tissue damage; keep scissors at the bedside to cut the airway lumens for immediate tube removal or airway obstruction occur
- During vasopressin administration, continuously monitor electrocardiogram results blood pressure
- Teach the patient how to prevent recurrence of GI bleeding by avoiding aspirin, aspirin-containing products, and NSAIDs.

## Hepatitis

### Description

- Hepatitis is an acute or a chronic inflammation of the liver
- It is caused by viruses, bacteria, trauma, immune disorders, exposure to chemicals such as vinyl chloride and hydrocarbons, and toxins
- Five major types of viral hepatitis exist: hepatitis A, B, C, D, and E (see *Characteristics of viral hepatitis*); of the 60,000 annual cases of viral hepatitis in the United States, about one-half are hepatitis B; hepatitis G is a newly identified virus thought to be blood-borne, with transmission similar to that of hepatitis C.

### Signs and Symptoms

- The *prodromal* or *preicteric phase,* which lasts 1 to 2 days, can cause arthralgia, anorexia, aversion to cigarettes (among smokers), constipation or diarrhea, decreased senses of taste and smell, dislike of dietary protein, elevated serologic test results, headache, hepatomegaly, low-grade fever, lymphadenopathy, malaise, nausea, right upper quadrant pain or discomfort, splenomegaly, urticaria with or without rash, vomiting, and weight loss
- The *clinical phase,* which lasts 1 to 2 weeks, may produce bilirubinuria, dark urine, fatigue, hepatomegaly, jaundice, light-colored stools, lymphadenopathy, pruritus, right upper quadrant tenderness, and weight loss
- The *posticteric* or *recovery phase,* which averages 2 to 12 weeks, may result in easy fatigability, hepatomegaly, malaise, resolving jaundice (early in this phase), and resolving liver tenderness and enlargement.

### Diagnosis and Treatment

- Diagnosis may rely on patient history; physical examination that reveals hepatomegaly, liver tenderness, and jaundice; serologic liver function tests (such as bilirubin and protein levels and PT); and antibody tests for surface or cellular antigens in serum (Serologic assays for hepatitis G are being developed.)
- Rest is prescribed, including bed rest if hepatomegaly is severe
- Supplements of vitamins B, C, and K are administered
- The recommended diet is high in calories and carbohydrates and has moderate to high protein and moderate fat
- If the patient has hepatitis B, C, or D, antiviral therapy may be used for the treatment of chronic disease.

### Nursing Interventions

- Use standard precautions to avoid spreading the disease and to protect the patient from other diseases
- Balance rest and activity to reduce metabolic demands on the liver
- Monitor the patient for changes in signs and symptoms—especially dark-colored urine, fatigue, fever, jaundice, and liver function—to assess the disease's status
- Monitor fluid intake and output; correct fluid and electrolyte imbalances as prescribed
- Administer immune serum globulin (ISG) as prescribed to modify the effects of hepatitis A and B in people who have been exposed
- Consult a dietitian about the prescribed diet; discuss the patient's food preferences, and intervene to increase the patient's appetite and food retention to ensure adequate calorie and protein intake
- Discuss the dangers of self-medication, and encourage the patient to use only prescribed medications; an inflamed liver cannot metabolize drugs well, and some drugs—especially acetaminophen—may exacerbate inflammation

| Characteristics of viral hepatitis | | | | | |
|---|---|---|---|---|---|
| **Characteristics** | **Hepatitis A** | **Hepatitis B** | **Hepatitis C** | **Hepatitis D** | **Hepatitis E** |
| Incubation period | 15 to 45 days | 28 to 180 days | 15 to 60 days | 28 to 180 days | 14 to 63 days |
| Mode of transmission | Fecal-oral route | Parenteral serum of infected persons; saliva, semen and vaginal secretions | Parenteral (Serum of infected persons) | Parenteral (Serum of infected persons); saliva semen and vaginal secretions | Fecal-oral route |
| Sources of infection | Poor sanitation and personal hygiene; contaminated food milk water raw or steamed shellfish, persons with subclinical infections | Contaminated needles syringes blood products and other instruments sexual intercourse; kissing asymptomatic carries | Needles syringes blood and blood products | Contaminated needles syringes blood products and other instruments sexual intercourse kissing asymptomatic carriers | Poor sanitation contaminated water |
| Virus in feces | 3 to 4 weeks before jaundice | Degraded by enzymes if present | Not identified in feces | Not applicable | Probably present in feces |
| Virus in serum | Briefly | Hepatitis B | | | |
| Hepatitis B immune globulin (HBIG) or ISG within 2 weeks of exposure | Possible (some trials with immunoglobulin) | Avoidance of infection with hepatitis B (must be present for hepatitis D to develop) | Questionable protection with previous inoculation with immunoglobuin | | |
| Hepatitis B surface antigen specific antigen in serum | Hepatitis A antigen | Hepatitis B surface antigen (HBsAg) Hepatitis B antigen (HBeAg) | Hepatitis C virus | Hepatitis D virus | Not applicable |
| Specific antibody in serum | Anti-hepatitis A virus | HBsAg antibody hepatitis B core antigen (HBcAg), anti-hepatitis E | Anti-hepatitis D virus | Anti-hepatitis D virus | Not applicable |
| Vaccine | Available | Available | None | None specification for hepatitis D; vaccine for hepatitis B should be given | None |
| Prognosis | Complete recovery common infection does not recur | Persistence in chronic or fulminant form id possible; possible precursor to a malignant liver tumor | Mild or severe and fulminant many will have chronic infection | Increased mortality | Similar to hepatitis A expect very severe in pregnant women |

- Follow preventive measures for hepatitis A: proper hand hygiene, good personal hygiene, environmental sanitation, screening and control of food handlers, enteric precautions, and ISG administration for exposure prophylaxis
- Follow preventive measures for hepatitis B: proper hand hygiene, screening of blood donors for hepatitis B surface antigen, use of disposable needles and syringes, registration of carriers, passive immunization with ISG and hepatitis B immune globulin for exposure to mucus secretions or needle-stick exposure, and active immunization with hepatitis B vaccine for high-risk populations such as health care providers
- Follow the same preventive measures for hepatitis C as for hepatitis B
- Follow standard precautions for hepatitis A: use gloves and a gown if touching soiled or infective material (feces) is likely; place the patient who has poor personal hygiene in a private room, and follow precautions for 7 days after jaundice appears
- Follow standard precautions for hepatitis B: use gloves and a gown if touching soiled or infective materials (blood, body fluids, or feces if patient has GI bleeding) is likely
- Follow standard precautions for hepatitis C; use gloves and a gown if touching soiled or infective materials (blood or body fluids) is likely
- Provide a referral to a community nurse for continuity of care as needed.

## Large-and Small-Bowel Obstruction

### *Description*

- Large-bowel obstruction can occur in the ascending, transverse, or descending colon; the rectum; or several areas simultaneously
- Small-bowel obstruction can occur in any area of the duodenum, jejunum, or ileum or in several areas simultaneously
- Small- and large-bowel obstructions may result from infection, tumor, or intestinal ulcerations with scar formation

that lead to obstruction, volvulus, intussusception, adhesions, or paralytic ileus
- Complications of small or large-bowel obstruction include hypovolemic shock, peritonitis, rupture, septicemia and death.

### Signs and Symptoms

- Abdominal pain and distention may be mild to severe
- Anorexia and nausea may be accompanied by severe vomiting with a fecal odor
- Bowel sounds may be high-pitched or absent
- Constipation or obstipation may be present, or diarrhea may occur as liquid intestinal secretions and feces move around the obstruction; blood, mucus, or undigested food may appear in stool
- Abdominal girth may increase due to distention
- Vital sign changes may include fever and signs of shock, such as hypotension, tachycardia, and tachypnea
- Other effects may include anxiety, dehydration, dry skin, fatigue, malaise, and weight loss

### Diagnosis and Treatment

- Diagnosis may require patient history, physical examination, abdominal X-rays (such as flat plate of the abdomen, barium enema, and GI series), serologic studies, endoscopy, gastric analysis, stool examination, colonoscopy, and proctoscopy
- Maintain nothing-by-mouth status, and administer IV therapy to restore fluid balance
- An NG or intestinal tube is inserted to relieve abdominal distention and vomiting
- An opioid analgesic is used to relieve pain
- An antibiotic is administered to treat possible infection
- Abdominal girth is measured every 2 to 4 hours
- Bowel output is monitored, and stools are checked for occult blood
- Surgery may be used to correct the obstruction; exploratory laparotomy can determine the cause, small- or large-bowel resection can remove diseased portions, ileostomy or colostomy may be done to permit waste discharge, and total ablation (removal) of the large and most of small intestine may be used if the obstruction is caused by mesenteric artery thrombosis.

### Nursing Interventions

- Monitor vital signs, particularly noting signs of shock (increased pulse and respiratory rates and decreased blood pressure) and peritonitis or other infection (increased temperature)
- Administer prescribed medications promptly to maintain therapeutic blood levels
- Maintain IV therapy to ensure proper hydration because the patient must maintain nothing-bymouth status
- Monitor fluid intake and output (including vomitus and diarrhea) carefully; excessive fluid loss can lead to shock and dehydration
- Monitor, measure, and record drainage from the NG or intestinal tube; check drainage for blood and odor, irrigate the tube as prescribed to maintain patency, and turn the patient as prescribed to facilitate tube passage to the obstruction site
- Measure abdominal girth every 2 to 4 hours to assess distention
- Auscultate and characterize bowel sounds; high-pitched sounds indicate anoxia resulting from marked distention or obstruction, whereas absent sounds indicate ileus or obstruction
- Monitor eructation (a sign of continuing obstruction) or flatus passage (a sign of resolving obstruction)
- Monitor the patient for abdominal pain or tenderness, noting its location; pain may be related to distention or inflammation
- Encourage the patient to perform deep-breathing exercises every 2 hours; abdominal distention may elevate the diaphragm and decrease deep breathing
- Prepare the patient for surgery, if indicated
- Keep the patient and family appraised of the situation.

## Pancreatitis

### Description

- Pancreatitis is an inflammation of the pancreas accompanied by the release of digestive enzymes into the gland, resulting in autodigestion of the organ
- Pancreatitis may be acute or chronic
- Causes of pancreatitis include alcohol abuse, trauma, infection, drug toxicity, and obstruction of the biliary tract.

### Signs and Symptoms

- Pancreatitis is characterized by severe epigastric pain that worsens after meals and may radiate to the shoulder, substernal area, back, and flank
- Fever and malaise may be present
- The patient may experience abdominal tenderness and distention, nausea, and vomiting; he may lie in a knee-chest or fetal position or lean forward for comfort
- Bulky, fatty, foul-smelling stool may occur
- Signs of hypovolemic shock may be present.

### Diagnosis and Treatment

- Diagnosis is based on patient history, including alcohol intake and use of prescription and nonprescription drugs
- Laboratory tests include increased serum amylase, spartate aminotransferase, bilirubin, glucose, and lipase levels; increased WBC count; and decreased serum calcium levels
- Other diagnostic tools include abdominal and chest X-rays, ultrasound, CT scan, MRI, and endoscopic retrograde cholangiopancreatography
- Cullen's sign (bruising of the subcutaneous tissue near the umbilicus) and Grey Turner's sign (bruising of the flanks of the abdomen) are positive
- The patient maintains nothing-by-mouth status, and an NG tube is inserted; total parenteral nutrition may be indicated
- IV fluids are administered, and electrolytes are replaced as indicated
- An analgesic and an antibiotic may be prescribed; elevated glucose levels are controlled

- Surgical intervention is used to treat the underlying cause, if appropriate.

### *Nursing Interventions*

- Make sure the patient maintains nothing-by-mouth status during the acute phase; then begin to introduce bland, low-fat, high-protein diet of small, frequent meals with restricted caffeine and gasforming foods
- Monitor for symptoms of calcium deficiency (such as tetany, cramps, carpopedal spasm, and seizures)
- Provide mouth, nares, and skin care
- Check the NG tube for patency, and correct placement each shift
- Monitor intake and output and vital signs, and obtain daily weights
- Administer an analgesic (usually meperidine) as needed
- Advise the patient to avoid alcohol, caffeine, and spices
- Explain the importance of a quiet, restful environment to conserve energy and decrease metabolic demands.

## Peptic Ulcer Disease

### *Description*

- Peptic ulcer disease is characterized by ulcerations in the esophagus, stomach (gastric), or small intestine (duodenal); approximately 80% are duodenal
- Peptic ulcer disease is caused by erosion of the lining cells of the stomach or duodenum; factors such as *H pylori* infection and NSAIDs disrupt the normal mucosal defense, making the mucosa more susceptible to the effects of gastric acid.

### *Signs and Symptoms*

- Gastric and duodenal ulcers have different signs and symptoms (see *Common signs and symptoms of peptic ulcer disease*)
- Other effects may include anorexia, dizziness, eructation, and light-headedness or syncope
- The patient may have a family history of peptic ulcer disease; medication history of aspirin or other anti-inflammatory drug use; or a personal history of cigarette, alcohol, or caffeine use or of stressful conditions at home or on the job.

### *Diagnosis and Treatment*

- Diagnosis may be based on patient history, physical examination, gastric endoscopy, barium test, upper-GI series, gastric analysis, gastric cytology, serologic studies, testing for *H pylori,* and stool tests for occult blood
- A histamine blocker—such as cimetidine (Tagamet), famotidine (Pepcid), nizatidine (Axid), or ranitidine (Zantac)—is used to decrease gastric acid production; an antacid is also prescribed to neutralize hydrochloric acid
- A proton pump inhibitor, such as esomeprazole (Nexium) or lansoprazole (Prevacid), may be used to suppress acid production by halting the mechanism that pumps acid into the stomach
- Sucralfate, a cytoprotective drug, may be prescribed; it works by forming a protective barrier over the ulcer's surface
- Misoprostol (Cytotec), a synthetic prostaglandin analogue, may be prescribed to prevent ulcers from forming in patients who take high doses of an NSAID by protecting the gastric mucus; an antibiotic may be prescribed to treat *H pylori* infections; bismuth is also used as adjunct therapy against *H pylori*
- Stress-reduction techniques are recommended to prevent development of a stress ulcer or worsening of peptic ulcers
- Smoking cessation is recommended
- If drug therapy is ineffective, surgical repair may include laser cauterization of a bleeding site, partial gastrectomy with gastroduodenostomy (Billroth I), partial gastrectomy with gastrojejunostomy (Billroth II), or vagotomy with pyloroplasty (rare).

**Common sign and symptoms of peptic ulcer disease**

| Symptoms | Gastic ulcer | Duodenal ulcer |
|---|---|---|
| Pain type | Gnawing, burning aching heartburn | Gnawing burning cramping heartburn at times |
| Duration | Constant unless relieved by food or drugs | Intermittent and relieved by food or drugs (steady pain may be related to a perforated ulcer of the postertor wall of the duodenum) |
| Site | Upper epigastrium with localization to left of umbilicus | Right epigastric area to right of umbilicus radiation of pain to right upper quadrant may be due to a perforated ulcer of the postertor wall of the duodenum |
| Time of day | At night and when stomach is empty | At night and when duodenum is empty |
| Cause | Presence of hydrochloric acid in stomach | High acid content of chyme moving into duodenum |
| Periodicity | Recurs daily for a period of time then disappears for month only to recur | Recurs daily for a period of time then disappears for months only to recur |
| Nausea | Intermittent | Intermittent |
| Vomiting | Occasional (more often than with duodenal ulcers) | Occasional |
| Feeling of fullness | Present at times eructation common | Present at times |
| Bleeding | Detected in vomitus unless hemorhage occurs | Detected in stools through stool gualac test unless hemorrhage occurs |

### *Nursing Interventions*

- Administer prescribed medications
- Help the patient to identify and eliminate foods that cause distress
- Teach the patient about the disease, its treatment, and stress-reduction techniques, if needed
- Encourage the patient to stop smoking to eliminate the effects of nicotine on ulcers
- Provide postoperative care as needed
  - Verify placement and maintain patency of the NG tube
  - Make sure the patient maintains nothing-by-mouth status as prescribed; administer IV fluids to maintain fluid and electrolyte balance

- To help control pain, encourage the patient to use patient-controlled analgesia, or administer an opioid analgesic every 3 to 4 hours
- Measure abdominal girth to assess abdominal distention or ileus
- Auscultate bowel sounds to detect the return of peristalsis
- Help the patient perform deep-breathing exercises every 2 hours and use an incentive spirometer every 2 hours to prevent pulmonary complications
- Help the patient ambulate as prescribed
- Take steps to avoid dumping syndrome (a rapid gastric emptying produced by a bolus of food, causing distention of the dodenum or jejunum)
- Start giving the patient clear liquids when prescribed; observe him for nausea or vomiting, assess his tolerance of intake, and increase to small, frequent meals
- Monitor for flatus or bowel movements to determine bowel functions
- Before discharge, teach the patient about rest, activity restrictions, diet, medications, smoking cessation, and stress control.

## Regional Enteritis and Ulcerative Colitis

### Description

- *Regional enteritis,* also known as Crohn's disease, is an inflammatory disease of the small bowel that may also affect the large intestine; it typically begins in the ileum but can affect all areas of the small intestine and even the esophagus
- *Ulcerative colitis* is a chronic inflammatory disease of the large intestine, commonly in the sigmoid and rectal areas.

### Signs and Symptoms

- Regional enteritis and ulcerative colitis produce different signs and symptoms (see *Comparing regional enteritis and ulcerative colitis*)
- The stool of a patient with ulcerative colitis may appear liquid, with blood, pus, and mucus; the patient with regional enteritis typically has diarrhea without visible blood.

### Diagnosis and Treatment

- Regional enteritis and ulcerative colitis are diagnosed and managed similarly; regional enteritis is diagnosed by small bowel X-ray, barium study of the upper GI tract, barium enema, and intestinal biopsy; ulcerative colitis is diagnosed by biopsy with colonoscopy, barium enema, and abdominal X-ray
- Tailored to the patient's specific needs, the diet typically restricts raw fruits and vegetables as well as fatty and spicy foods; debilitated patients may require total parenteral nutrition
- An anticholinergic is used to manage intestinal spasms; an antidiarrheal to control diarrhea; an anti-inflammatory such as sulfasalazine to reduce inflammation; an antimicrobial to prevent infection; a corticosteroid to decrease inflammation, and an immunosuppressant to decrease antigen-antibody reactions
- Surgery is indicated for fistula formation, intestinal obstruction, bowel perforation, hemorrhage, and intractable disease (if ulcerative colitis persists for more than 10 years, cancer may develop)
  - Intestinal resections may need to be performed repeatedly
  - Ileostomy is curative; ileorectal anastomosis may be performed.

### Nursing Interventions

- Make sure the patient understands the purpose, therapeutic effects, and adverse effects of prescribed medications
- Provide postoperative care for a patient undergoing surgery
- Maintain patency of the NG tube, if present, by irrigating with normal saline solution every 2 hours as needed
- Encourage the patient to use patient-controlled analgesia, or administer an opioid analgesic to relieve pain; administer a steroid to prevent adrenal insufficiency and an antibiotic to prevent infection
- Monitor vital signs every 1 to 2 hours for 4 to 8 hours and then every 4 hours
- Make sure the patient maintains nothing-by-mouth status as prescribed; monitor IV fluids every 1 to 2 hours; upto 3,000 mL of fluid daily is needed
- Check wound sites for drainage and signs of inflammation, infection, and healing; use aseptic technique to prevent infection
- Monitor bowel sounds every 2 to 4 hours to detect the return of peristalsis or, possibly, ileus
- Monitor bowel output to determine return of bowel function
- Help the patient ambulate as prescribed
- Encourage the patient to perform deep-breathing exercises and use an incentive spirometer every 2 hours to prevent pulmonary complications
- Start giving the patient clear liquids when prescribed; the diet initially may be a low-residue one, gradually increasing to a regular diet as tolerated
- Provide care for a patient with an ileostomy or a colostomy (see *Comparing colostomy and ileostomy*)
  - Change bags if they start leaking to prevent skin excoriation; the patient may change bags on a regular schedule to prevent leaking
  - Make sure the opening of the bag around the stoma is no larger than 1/8' (3 mm) to prevent skin excoriation
  - Refer the patient to an enterostomal nurse therapist for care of the stoma and colostomy and psychosocial adjustment
- Provide opportunities for the patient to discuss feelings about the disease and its treatment
- Teach the patient how to care for the incision or the colostomy or ileostomy
- Refer the patient for continued nursing monitoring or assistance after discharge for continuity of care and support with new self-care procedures.

### Table of Contents Entries Found

| Comparing regional enteritis and ulcerative colitis | | |
|---|---|---|
| The following chart compares some key characteristics of regional enteritis (Crohn's disease) and ulcerative colitis | | |
| **Characteristics** | **Regional enteritis** | **Ulcerative colitis** |
| Areas affected | All layers of the bowel in various areas of the bowel at the same time | Only the mucosal and submucosal layers |
| Lesion | Skip or discontinuous lesions edematous redish-purple area with granulomas (scaring) | Continous diffuse lesion that do not skip segments ulceration with erosion and bleeding |
| Incidence | Slightly more common in women than men primarily between age 20 and 50 more common in jews and non-whites | More common in women than men primarily those between ages 20 and 40 more common in jews and non-whites |
| Cause | Unknown but may be genetic or immunologic may be exacerbated by stress | Unknown but may be genetic immunologic or infectious |
| Signs and symptoms | • Abdominal distention<br>• Anemia<br>• Arthralgia<br>• Cramping abdominal pain and tenderness<br>• Dehydration and fluid and electrolyte imbalances<br>• Flatuence<br>• Low-grade fever<br>• Nauses and vomiting<br>• Three to four semisoft stools daily with no blood expect in patients with advanced disease, some fat is present and stools may be foul-smelling<br>• Weight loss | • Abdominal distention<br>• Abdominal rigidity at times<br>• Anemia<br>• Bowel distention<br>• Cramping abdominal pain typically in lower left quadrant<br>• Dehydration and fluid and electrolyte imbalances<br>• Diarrhea (Pronounced 5 to 25 stools daily with blood mucus and pus but no fat)<br>• Fever<br>• Nausea and vomiting<br>• Rectal bleeding<br>• Weight loss |
| Diagnostic tests | • Barium enema<br>• Proctosigmoidoscopy<br>• Stool analysis for occult blood and culture<br>• X-ray of small bowel | • Barium enema<br>• Biopsy of rectal cells<br>• Fiberoptic colonoscopy<br>• Sigmoidoscopy<br>• Stool analysis |

## RENAL AND URINARY TRACT DISORDERS

### Introduction

The urinary system forms and stores urine, regulates body fluids and electrolytes, and controls urine elimination.

Urinary tract infections (UTIs) and obstructions may cause permanent loss of renal function.

Acute and chronic renal failure are both serious and potentially life-threatening conditions.

- In a patient with *renal impairment* or *diminished renal reserve*, the healthier kidney compensates for the impaired kidney and continues to clear metabolic waste unless it meets with increased demand or unusual stress; as a result, the patient is asymptomatic, and specific concentration and dilution tests are needed to detect reduced renal function
- In a patient with *renal insufficiency*, compensation begins to fail, and metabolic wastes build up; the degree of insufficiency can be mild, moderate, or severe and is measured by the decreasing glomerular filtration rate (GFR)
- In a patient with *end-stage renal disease*, the kidneys cannot perform their normal homeostatic functions or meet normal body demands
  - Excess nitrogenous wastes build up in the blood
  - Fluid, electrolyte, and acid–base abnormalities occur
  - Dialysis or kidney transplantation is necessary to sustain life.

### *Nursing History*

- The nurse asks the patient about the *chief complaint*
  - A patient with a renal or urinary tract disorder may be experiencing output changes, such as polyuria, oliguria, or anuria; he may also note voiding pattern changes, such as hesitancy, frequency, urgency, nocturia, or incontinence; urine color changes; or pain
  - The patient may also see changes in voiding pattern, such as hesitancy, frequency, urgency, nocturia, or incontinence; urine color changes; or pain
- The nurse then questions the patient about his *present illness*
  - Ask the patient about his symptom, including when it started, associated symptoms, location, radiation, intensity, duration, frequency, and precipitating and alleviating factors
  - Ask about the use of prescription and over-the-counter drugs, herbal remedies, and vitamin and nutritional supplements
- The nurse asks about *medical history*
  - Question the patient about other renal and urinary disorders, such as UTIs, kidney trauma, and kidney stones
  - Ask about a history of other chronic illnesses that may affect the renal system, such as diabetes mellitus or hypertension

- The nurse then assesses the *family history*
  - Ask about a family history of chronic illnesses that can affect the renal system, such as hypertension, diabetes mellitus, coronary artery disease, vascular disease, or hyperlipidemia
  - Determine whether the family history suggests a genetic predisposition to certain renal diseases such as polycystic kidney disease.
- The nurse obtains a *social history*
  - Ask about work, exercise, diet, use of recreational drugs and alcohol, and hobbies
  - Also ask about stress, support systems, and coping mechanisms.

### Physical Assessment

- Nurse begins with *inspection*
  - Observe the patient's overall appearance; note his mental status and behavior
  - Examine his skin for color, turgor, intactness, edema, and texture
  - Inspect his abdomen for size and shape, noting any abnormal markings
- Next, the nurse uses *palpation*
  - Palpate the bladder for distention
  - Note any areas of tenderness
- Then the nurse uses *percussion*
  - Percuss for costovertebral tenderness
  - Percuss the bladder to elicit tympany or dullness
- The nurse then uses *auscultation*
  - Listen for renal artery bruits
  - Note any bruits over the aorta, iliac, and femoral arteries.

## Acute Renal Failure

### Description

- Acute renal failure is a sudden and almost complete loss of kidney function characterized by rising levels of blood urea nitrogen (BUN) and serum creatinine and an inability of the kidneys to regulate fluid and electrolyte balance; it occurs over several hours to several days
- Acute renal failure may be reversible or it may lead to death
- *Prerenal failure*, or prerenal azotemia, occurs when blood flow to the kidneys is disrupted, which causes ischemia and nephron damage
  - It can result from a condition that decreases blood flow and kidney perfusion, such as hypovolemia, hemorrhage, or burns; a condition that decreases cardiac output, such as a myocardial infarction (MI) or an arrhythmia; vascular failure related to sepsis, anaphylaxis, or severe acidosis; or an occlusion that obstructs renal arteries
  - It generally can be reversed by treating the cause and restoring normal intravascular volume
- *Intrarenal failure* occurs when the renal parenchyma is damaged; when this occurs, the kidneys cannot concentrate urine or excrete nitrogenous wastes
  - Intrarenal failure can be caused by nephron damage resulting from acute tubular necrosis, acute glomerulonephritis, or a related disorder or from exposure to a nephrotoxic drug or chemical, such as certain antibiotics, an antineoplastic, a fluorinated anesthetic, a heavy metal, or a radiographic contrast dye
  - Other causes include trauma, neoplasms, hypertension, systemic lupus erythematosus, toxemia of pregnancy, and hypercalcemia
- *Postrenal failure*, or postrenal azotemia, occurs when urine flow from the collecting ducts in the kidney to the external urethral orifi ce is obstructed or when venous blood flow from the kidney is obstructed
  - Renal calculi, tumors, clots, benign prostatic hyperplasia, strictures, trauma, bilateral renal vein thrombosis, and congenital malformation can all cause urinary obstruction
  - Postrenal failure is usually reversible
- Acute renal failure can lead to hyperkalemia or can cause uremia that compromises the immune system.

### Signs and Symptoms

- Acute renal failure typically progresses through three phases: an oliguric or anuric phase, a diuretic phase, and a recovery phase; signs and symptoms vary from phase to phase
- The oliguric phase produces a BUN level of 25 to 30 mg/dL, a serum creatinine level of 1.5 to 2 mg, sudden oliguria (urine output less than 400 mL daily) or anuria (rare), and reduced GFR
- The diuretic phase causes a gradual return of renal function; normal or high urine output (1 to 5 L daily); potentially life-threatening loss of sodium, potassium, and magnesium; and increased azotemia (elevated BUN and serum creatinine levels)
- The recovery phase is associated with decreasing BUN and serum creatinine levels; it continues until normal renal tubular function is established
- High-output renal failure, a type of acute nonoliguric renal failure, occasionally occurs; it commonly results from the use of a nephrotoxic antibiotic
  - Although symptoms of acute renal failure may develop, fluid overload generally is not a problem
  - If high-output renal failure is recognized early and the antibiotic is discontinued, normal renal function gradually returns.

### Diagnosis and Treatment

- Diagnosis of acute renal failure is based on patient history and abnormal laboratory findings, assessment of fluid balance, preexisting disorders, precipitating events, and current health status
- Other diagnostic tests may include abdominal X-ray, ultrasonography, or computed tomography (CT); excretory urography or cystoscopy with retrograde pyelography; renal angiography; and renal biopsy
- Laboratory tests include serum creatinine and BUN levels (the normal ratio of BUN to creatinine ranges from 10:1 to 15:1), electrolyte and hemoglobin levels, hematocrit, urinalysis, and creatinine clearance; laboratory changes can help differentiate among prerenal, intrarenal, and postrenal acute renal failure

- With prerenal acute renal failure, the BUN-creatinine ratio is greater than 15:1; urine specific gravity and osmolarity are increased, and the urine sodium level is decreased
- With intrarenal acute renal failure, urine specific gravity and osmolarity fall to levels similar to those in serum or plasma, and the urine sodium level may exceed 30 mEq/L
- With postrenal acute renal failure, urine osmolarity and sodium levels may be normal; if the condition is not quickly diagnosed and treated, the patient may develop urinary system changes similar to those of intrarenal acute renal failure.

- Treatment aims to identify and eliminate or control the underlying cause, restore normal fluid and electrolyte balance, and prevent uremic complications while the kidneys repair themselves
- Reduced intravascular volume is treated early with aggressive fluid therapy to restore urine output and prevent acute tubular necrosis
  - A therapeutic fluid challenge (500 mL over 30 minutes) may be used to differentiate prerenal from intrarenal causes of oliguria
  - If urine output improves after the fluid challenge, IV fluids are continued at a rate that maintains adequate hourly urine volume
  - If the fluid challenge is unsuccessful, a diuretic—such as mannitol (Osmitrol), bumetanide, furosemide (Lasix), or ethacrynic acid (Edecrin)—may be used to restore urine output
- A patient with hypervolemia and fluid overload, hyperkalemia, metabolic acidosis, severe hyponatremia, encephalopathy, or pericarditis may require dialysis
- Hyperkalemia is aggressively treated with IV hypertonic glucose and insulin (to shift extracellular potassium into cells), oral or rectal administration of the cation-exchange resin sodium polystyrene sulfonate (to exchange sodium for potassium ions in the GI tract), and dialysis (to maintain normal potassium levels); hyperkalemic patients with electrocardiogram changes are commonly treated with IV calcium gluconate to prevent arrhythmias
- Hypotension is commonly treated with volume replacement, although a vasopressor may be needed
- Hypertension is treated with restriction of fluid intake to prevent fluid overload, restriction of dietary sodium, and antihypertensive therapy
- Diet therapy helps manage acute renal failure; the recommended diet is high in calories and carbohydrates, is low in potassium, and may restrict protein (depending on the degree of azotemia and the frequency of dialysis); protein in the diet must provide essential amino acids while minimizing the degree of nitrogenous waste products.

### *Nursing Interventions*

- Monitor for signs of acute renal failure and its complications
- Monitor fluid intake and output, weigh the patient daily, and administer fluids carefully; monitor electrolyte levels, and maintain proper electrolyte balance
- Prevent infection by frequently washing your hands; using aseptic technique with incisions, wound care, and care of IV and central venous catheters; assisting the patient with hygiene, including oral hygiene; frequently turning and positioning him; encouraging deep breathing, coughing, and ambulation (if possible); and avoiding use of an indwelling urinary catheter
- Monitor the patient for signs of infection, such as fever, local redness, swelling, heat, drainage, and elevated white blood cell (WBC) count; watch for signs and symptoms of pericarditis, including pleuritic chest pain, tachycardia, and pericardial friction rub
- Provide a diet high in calories and low in potassium, protein, and sodium
- Monitor the patient's response to medications; because many drugs are excreted by the kidneys, the type of drug, dosage, or administration interval may need to be adjusted, based on the patient's renal function (as evidenced by GFR and other indicators)
- Teach the patient and family the reasons for interventions and the importance of infection-prevention measures; because the patient may be acutely ill and have a decreased level of consciousness, information should be given verbally (briefly) and in writing
- Encourage the patient and family to express their concerns.

## Chronic Renal Failure

### *Description*

- Chronic renal failure is a slow, insidious, irreversible deterioration in renal function
- It typically progresses through four stages:
  - Reduced renal reserve: GFR of 60 to 89% of normal
  - Renal insufficiency: GFR of 30 to 59% of normal
  - Renal failure: GFR of 15 to 29% of normal
  - End-stage renal disease: GFR less than 15% of normal.
- Diseases that contribute to chronic renal failure include diabetic, gouty and hypertensive nephropathies; chronic glomerulonephritis, pyelonephritis, urinary tract obstruction; cystic kidney disease; renal cell carcinoma, renovascular disease; lupus nephritis; multiple myeloma, amyloidosis, chronic hypercalcemia and hypokalemia, renal tuberculosis and sarcoidosis
- Chronic renal failure begins with a functional loss of nephrons, i.e. asymptomatic, except for decreased urinary creatinine clearance; creatinine clearance normally ranges from 85 to 135 mL/minute; in patients with mild renal failure, it ranges from 50 to 84 mL/minute; in patients with moderate renal failure, from 10 to 49 mL/minute; and in patients with severe renal failure, 10 mL/minute or less
- Next, renal insufficiency occurs as more nephrons cease to function; insufficiency may be mild, moderate, or severe
  - At first, the patient experiences no physical limitations in daily activity, although laboratory changes—such as azotemia, anemia, and loss of the ability to concentrate urine—are detectable
  - As renal deterioration continues, the kidneys' ability to function under stress (e.g. during dehydration, salt

- depletion, or heart failure) is impaired; renal insufficiency may progress to renal failure during periods of stress
- Once renal failure develops, the patient must limit daily activities; he will eventually develop overt signs of renal failure and uremia, beginning with fluid, electrolyte, and metabolic abnormalities (including azotemia, anemia, metabolic acidosis, hypertension, and hypocalcemia)
- End-stage renal disease occurs when most of the nephrons have been irreversibly damaged; the GFR falls below 100 mL/minute, and the patient requires long-term dialysis or kidney transplantation.

### *Signs and Symptoms*

- Altered fluid, electrolyte, and acid–base balances may include dehydration (early) or overhydration (later in the disease), hypocalcemia and hyperkalemia, and metabolic acidosis (as evidenced by low arterial blood pH and decreased bicarbonate levels)
- Skin changes may include gray-bronze or yellow skin color related to uremia or pallor related to anemia, dry skin, uremic frost (white, dustlike deposits of urea and phosphate crystals on the face, nose, forehead, and upper trunk), pruritus, excoriations, ecchymosis, purpura, or infections; related changes may include thin, brittle nails and a whitened proximal section with a darker distal edge and nail ridges
- Cardiovascular effects may include hypertension, acceleration of atherosclerosis, increased risk of MI and stroke, left ventricular hypertrophy, heart failure, pericarditis (which may cause a fever and pericardial friction rub and, rarely, chest pain and hypotension), pericardial effusion (which causes disappearance of any friction rub and appearance of a paradoxical pulse), cardiac tamponade (which causes hypotension, muffled heart sounds, narrowed pulse pressure, weak peripheral pulses, and bulging neck veins), life-threatening cardiac arrhythmias, and cardiac arrest
- Respiratory effects may include thick, tenacious sputum and a depressed cough reflex, which increases the risk of pulmonary infections and complications; Kussmaul's respirations; uremic breath odor; increased incidence of infections, including tuberculosis; pulmonary edema; pleural effusion; and uremic pneumonitis
- Hematologic effects may include normochromic, normocytic anemia (which causes fatigue, weakness, pallor, exertional dyspnea, and intolerance of activity and cold); platelet dysfunction (which causes prolonged bleeding time, clotting abnormalities, easy bruising, purpura, and bleeding from mucus membranes and other body parts); and changes in the immune system and granulocytic function (which decrease cellular and humoral immunity and the inflammatory response)
- GI effects may include a metallic or ammonia-like taste in the mouth, stomatitis, ammonia or fishy breath odor, an increased incidence of oral infections and tooth decay, anorexia (especially for highprotein foods), nausea, vomiting, GI bleeding, increased gastric acid production, diarrhea or constipation, fecal impaction, and an increased incidence of diverticulosis
- The patient may develop hepatitis.
- Metabolic dysfunction may include carbohydrate intolerance (with abnormal glucose clearance), accumulation of end products of protein metabolism (which causes lethargy, headache, fatigue, irritability, and depression), and hyperlipidemia
- Central nervous system effects may include decreased attention span, memory problems, inability to think clearly (progressing to actual confusion), flattened affect, depression, irritability, lability, stupor, coma, and seizures
- Peripheral nervous system effects may include peripheral neuropathies (numbness, tingling, or pain of the feet and hands; weakness of the feet; and atrophy of leg muscles), footdrop, loss of motor function, and 'burning feet' syndrome (swelling, redness, and extreme tenderness of the soles and dorsum of the feet)
- Autonomic nervous system effects may include loss of the ability to compensate for a change in blood pressure through reflex tachycardia or bradycardia, which leads to poor blood pressure control
- Musculoskeletal effects may include impaired physical mobility, loss of muscle mass and muscle strength, osteomalacia, osteoporosis, and osteitis fibrosa cystica
- Reproductive effects may include impotence in men, amenorrhea and infertility in women, and markedly decreased libido in both sexes.

### *Diagnosis and Treatment*

- Laboratory tests, X-rays, and other diagnostic tests for chronic renal failure are the same as those for acute renal failure; renal biopsy establishes the percentage of functioning nephrons
- Treatment has several goals: to preserve current renal function and prevent or delay further deterioration of function, to treat symptoms of uremia, to postpone or eliminate the need for long-term dialysis or kidney transplantation, to prevent complications of uremia, and to promote comfort and improve the patient's quality of life
- Most patients with chronic renal failure can be managed successfully with diet and fluid therapy; long-term dialysis or kidney transplantation is unnecessary until the GFR falls to 10% to 15% of the normal rate
- Strict adherence to a low-protein diet can delay progression to end-stage renal disease
  - A high-protein load causes the kidneys to dilate from increased blood flow and increased GFR in an attempt to clear the by-products of protein metabolism; this increased vasodilation accelerates the deterioration of renal function
  - For adult patients, a protein intake of about 50 g daily appears to have a therapeutic effect without contributing to malnutrition; most of the protein must be of high biological value to supply sufficient essential amino acids; protein of low biological value increases the waste load to the kidneys

- Depending on the stage of the disease and on fluid and electrolyte alterations, fluid intake may need to be restricted
  - If urine output is decreased, and fluid overload becomes a problem, fluid intake typically is restricted to the previous day's urine output plus 500 mL for insensible loss
  - If excessive fluid is lost, e.g. because of fever, vomiting, or diarrhea—fluid requirements may increase
- Sodium, potassium, and phosphorus also may be restricted
  - Sodium restriction may be warranted if the patient develops hypertension, edema, or heart failure
  - Dietary potassium generally is not restricted if the urine output exceeds 1,000 mL daily; it is restricted if the serum potassium level exceeds 5.5 mEq/L
- Supplements of B-complex vitamins, folic acid, and vitamin C may be needed to compensate for deficiencies that result from a restrictive diet or dialysis; iron and zinc supplements also may be prescribed
- Once long-term dialysis begins, a more liberal protein intake is allowed, and the fluid intake is controlled to allow a weight gain of 2 to 2.5 lb (0.9 to 1.1 kg) between dialysis treatments
- Despite anorexia, nausea, and taste changes, the patient must consume sufficient calories to prevent catabolism and muscle breakdown
- Disturbances in calcium metabolism may be managed with calcium supplements, dietary restriction of phosphorus, and phosphate binders, such as aluminum hydroxide gels (Amphojel), which are given at mealtimes; a patient receiving hemodialysis may receive calcium carbonate instead of a phosphate binder, which can exacerbate bone disease and promote faulty mineralization
- When end-stage renal disease develops, and diet, fluid restrictions, and drugs are no longer effective, the patient may undergo long-term dialysis (peritoneal dialysis or hemodialysis) or kidney transplantation; peritoneal dialysis and hemodialysis achieve the same results but in different ways.

### *Nursing Interventions*

- Monitor physiologic changes and fluid and electrolyte changes
- Consult the dietitian about ways to ensure that the patient consumes sufficient calories while adhering to dietary restrictions
- Teach the patient how to relieve uremic skin symptoms; dry, itchy skin contributes to discomfort, irritability, restlessness, and frustration, and scratching increases the risk of infection
  - Use tepid water and avoid soap (hot water and soap can worsen dryness and itching); use emollients, creams, and bath oils liberally to control dryness
  - Administer antihistamines and antipruritics as needed to control itching
  - Keep the patient's nails clean and trimmed short to reduce the risk of infection from scratching; tell the patient to use a soft washcloth, not fingernails, to scratch
  - Keep the patient's hair clean and moisturized but avoid frequent shampooing to prevent dryness
- Teach the patient how to perform oral care; decreased salivary flow and fluid restrictions can contribute to problems in the oral mucosa
  - Encourage frequent and gentle brushing with a soft toothbrush to decrease oral bacteria, prevent stomatitis, improve taste, and eliminate mouth odors
  - Encourage the patient to use mouthwash and to suck on hard candy to treat dry mouth, alleviate thirst, and improve taste
- Teach the patient how to prevent constipation by encouraging increased intake of dietary fiber, use of stool softeners, and increased activity; advise him to avoid laxatives that contain magnesium because of the risk of magnesium toxicity
- Help the patient increase mobility and activity as tolerated to help him plan activities to avoid fatigue, teach him how to use ambulatory aids, and refer him to a physical therapist if needed
- Help prevent pulmonary complications by teaching the patient how to deep-breathe, cough, and use an incentive spirometer to prevent atelectasis and infection and by preventing and treating fluid overload
- Teach the patient and family about the disease, its complications, and measures that can prevent further renal deterioration; refer the patient to the National Kidney Foundation
- Make sure the following areas are discussed with the patient and family: monitoring of fluid intake and output; signs of fluid overload and common electrolyte imbalances; therapeutic and adverse effects of prescribed drugs; methods of promoting skin integrity; methods of preventing infection, pulmonary complications, hyperkalemia, constipation, and fecal impaction; importance of controlling blood pressure; methods of maintaining mobility; need for phosphate-binders to prevent bone disease; need for dietary modifications; advantages and disadvantages of peritoneal dialysis and hemodialysis; and home dialysis.

## Glomerulonephritis

### *Description*

- Glomerulonephritis is an inflammation of the glomeruli
- Acute glomerulonephritis follows a streptococcal infection of the respiratory tract or, less commonly, a skin infection, such as impetigo, immunoglobulin A nephropathy (Berger's disease) or lipid nephrosis; most people fully recover, but others may progress to chronic renal failure
- Chronic glomerulonephritis is a slowly progressive disease that results in sclerosis, scarring and eventually, renal failure.

### *Signs and Symptoms*

- The patient with acute glomerulonephritis may experience azotemia, dyspnea, edema, fatigue, hematuria, mild to severe hypertension, oliguria, and proteinuria
- Chronic glomerulonephritis develops insidiously and without symptoms, typically over many years; when it

becomes suddenly aggressive, the patient may have edema and hypertension; in later stages, the patient may complain of nausea, vomiting, pruritus, dyspnea, malaise, fatigue, and mild to severe edema.

### Diagnosis and Treatment

- Urinalysis typically reveals proteinuria, hematuria, WBCs, and casts
- A 24-hour urine sample shows low creatinine clearance and impaired glomerular filtration
- Blood studies reveal rising BUN and serum creatinine levels in those with advanced renal insufficiency as well as a decrease in hemoglobin levels
- Renal biopsy can confirm the diagnosis and identify underlying disease
- Elevated antistreptolysin-O titers, elevated streptozyme and anti-Dnase B titers, and low serum complement levels verify recent streptococcal infection
- Treatment depends on the cause; the goals are to correct fluid overload, hypertension, and uremia
  - Antibiotics are given to treat streptococcal infections
  - Antihypertensives are given to control hypertension
  - Diuretics may be given to reduce fluid overload
  - Sodium, potassium, protein, and fluid restrictions may be instituted
  - Dialysis may be necessary to correct fluid and electrolyte imbalances
  - Dialysis or kidney transplantation for chronic glomerulonephritis may be needed.

### Nursing Interventions

- Check vital signs and electrolyte levels, monitor fluid intake and output and daily weight, assess renal function daily through serum creatinine and BUN levels and urine creatinine clearance, and watch for signs of acute renal failure, including oliguria, azotemia, and acidosis
- Consult the dietitian to provide a diet high in calories and low in protein, sodium, potassium, and fluids
- Provide bed rest during the acute period of the disease
- Provide emotional support for the patient and family; if the patient is receiving dialysis, explain the procedure
- Teach the patient to report signs and symptoms of infection to the practitioner and the importance of follow-up examinations
- Explain any dietary restrictions to the patient and family.

## Nephrotic Syndrome

### Description

- Nephrotic syndrome is a type of renal failure characterized by an increased glomerular permeability, marked proteinuria, hypoalbuminemia, and edema
- Prognosis varies depending on the underlying cause; some forms progress to end-stage renal failure
- Nephrotic syndrome can result from many intrinsic renal and systemic diseases that cause glomerular damage; causes include glomerulonephritis; certain neoplastic diseases such as multiple myeloma; bronchogenic, breast, and colon cancer; lymphomas; leukemias; circulatory diseases; and diabetes mellitus.

### Signs and Symptoms

- Edema is the major manifestation; it is typically soft and pitting and commonly occurs around the eyes, in dependent areas, and on the abdomen
- Other signs and symptoms include weight gain, dyspnea, orthostatic hypotension, hypertension, ascites, pleural effusion, irritability, malaise, and decreased urination.

### Diagnosis and Treatment

- Proteinuria that exceeds 35 g/day is a hallmark of the disorder
- Urinalysis reveals an increased number of hyaline, granular, waxy, fatty casts; oval fat bodies; and consistent, heavy proteinuria (levels greater than 30 mg/dL for 24 hours)
- Serum cholesterol, phospholipid, and triglyceride levels are elevated, and the serum albumin level is decreased
- A needle biopsy of the kidney can confirm the diagnosis
- Treatment focuses on treating the underlying disease state responsible for proteinuria and relieving symptoms
- Drug treatment includes diuretics, angiotensin- converting enzyme inhibitors, and anti-lipid agents; the patient should also follow a high-protein, low-sodium diet.

### Nursing Interventions

- Teach the patient and family about the disease and its treatment; provide support
- Weigh the patient and measure his abdominal girth daily
- Monitor the patient's fluid and electrolyte status
- Administer medications as ordered, and note the patient's response
- Provide a low-cholesterol, no-added-salt diet with adequate protein; if appropriate, encourage the patient to consume foods high in potassium
- Obtain urine specimens for testing to evaluate the degree of proteinuria
- Teach the patient about follow-up care, and tell him to report any exacerbation of his symptoms.

## Neurogenic Bladder

### Description

- Neurogenic bladder refers to all types of bladder dysfunction caused by an interruption of normal bladder innervation
- Subsequent complications include incontinence, residual urine retention, UTI, stone formation, and renal failure
- A neurogenic bladder may be described as spastic (resulting from an upper motor neuron lesion) or flaccid (resulting from a lower motor neuron lesion)
- Neurogenic bladder may result from an acute infectious disease; a cerebral disorder; chronic alcoholism; a collagen disease; a peripheral innervation disorder; distant effects of cancer, such as primary oat cell carcinoma of the lung; heavy metal toxicity; herpes zoster; a metabolic disturbance; sacral agenesis; spinal cord disease or trauma; a vascular disease, such as atherosclerosis; or another condition.

### Signs and Symptoms

- A patient with flaccid neurogenic bladder may experience overflow incontinence, diminished anal sphincter tone, and a distended bladder
- A patient with spastic neurogenic bladder may experience spontaneous spasms of the arms and legs, involuntary or frequent scanty urination without a feeling of bladder fullness, and increased anal sphincter tone
- Other signs and symptoms may include altered micturition, hydronephrosis, incontinence, and vesicoureteral reflux (passage of urine from the bladder back into a ureter)
- The patient may also have symptoms of a UTI or kidney stones.

### Diagnosis and Treatment

- Voiding cystourethrography evaluates bladder neck function, vesicoureteral reflux, and continence
- Urodynamic studies—which consist of cystometry, uroflowmetry, urethral pressure profiles, and sphincter electromyography—help evaluate how urine is stored in the bladder, how well the bladder empties, and how quickly urine moves out of the bladder during voiding
- Techniques for bladder elimination include Valsalva's maneuver, indwelling urinary catheter insertion, intermittent self-catheterization, and Crede's maneuver (pressing on the suprapubic area with a downward motion to express urine from the bladder)
- Drug therapy may include terazosin, doxazosin, and phenoxybenzamine to facilitate bladder emptying and propantheline, flavoxate, dicyclomine, imipramine, and pseudoephedrine to aid urine storage
- When conservative treatment fails, surgery may be used to correct the structural impairment through transurethral resection of the bladder neck, urethral dilation, external sphincterotomy, or urinary diversion; implantation of an artificial urinary sphincter may be necessary if permanent incontinence follows surgery.

### Nursing Interventions

- Use strict aseptic technique during insertion and maintenance of an indwelling urinary catheter; do not interrupt the closed drainage system for any reason; keep the drainage bag below the level of the bladder
- Assess the patient for signs and symptoms of infection
- Teach the patient to report signs and symptoms of infection and how to prevent UTI; encourage him to increase his fluid intake
- Teach dietary measures to prevent kidney stone formation
- Keep the patient as mobile as possible; perform range-of-motion exercises, if necessary
- Teach the patient techniques, such as Crede's maneuver and intermittent self-catheterization
- If a urinary diversion procedure is to be performed, arrange for consultation with an enterostomal therapist.

## Urinary Calculi

### Description

- Urinary calculi (stones) are the most common urologic problem in adults; *nephrolithiasis* is the presence of calculi in the renal parenchyma, *urolithiasis* is the presence of calculi in the urinary tract, and *ureterolithiasis* is the presence of calculi in the ureters
- Calculi vary in size, from the size of a grain of sand to the size of a baseball; they are more common in men than in women, more common in hot summer months, and often recur
- Urinary calculi vary in type and composition
- Urinary calculi may be caused by infection, urine retention, urinary stasis, immobility, dehydration, sedentary lifestyle, or persistently low urine output
- The exact mechanism of stone formation is unknown; it may be related to changes in urine pH, volume depletion, or use of diuretics or other drugs
- Calculi formed in the kidney may pass into the ureter, occlude the flow of urine, and cause urine to flow back to the kidney; this can lead to ureteral spasm, hematuria, urinary stasis, UTI, impaired renal function and, eventually, hydronephrosis (kidney enlargement).

### Signs and Symptoms

- Symptoms vary with the location of the calculi and the presence of obstruction, infection, and edema
- Small or large nonobstructing stones in the renal calyces or renal pelvis may cause no symptoms
- Obstructing stones in the renal calyces or renal pelvis can cause recurrent infection, flank pain (described as a constant, intense, deep, dull ache), hematuria, and hydronephrosis; pyelonephritis and gram-negative septicemia may occur
- Renal calculi that pass into the ureter or become lodged at the ureteropelvic junction result in severe, sometimes excruciating, colicky pain in the lumbar area; microscopic or gross hematuria occurs
- Extremely small renal calculi may pass through the urinary system without causing noticeable symptoms
- Bladder calculi usually cause irritation and inflammation or, if they obstruct the urethra, urine retention and urinary obstruction
- Diarrhea, nausea, vomiting, and costovertebral tenderness commonly accompany colicky pain.

### Diagnosis and Treatment

- Abdominal X-ray or X-ray of the kidneys, ureters, and bladder can detect calculi; ultrasonography, nephrotomography, and excretory urography also may be used
- Other diagnostic tests may include urinalysis and urine culture; serum calcium, phosphorus, creatinine,uric acid, and electrolyte levels; urine pH; and tests for hypercalciuria, hyperuricuria, urinary oxalate, citrate, and cystine (using a 24-hour urine specimen)
- Because the causes and treatment of urinary calculi are based on their chemical composition, recovered stones are usually analyzed
- The main goals of treatment are to relieve pain, prevent nephron destruction, eliminate calculi, and prevent recurrence

- Opioids, such as morphine sulfate and meperidine, and antispasmodics, such as oxybutynin chloride (Ditropan) and propantheline bromide, are used to control severe pain; antiemetics are used when pain is accompanied by nausea and vomiting
- Nephron destruction is prevented by controlling infection and by removing obstructions to urine flow to prevent back flow; urosepsis (septicemia related to UTI) is prevented with prophylactic antibiotic therapy
- Because almost 90% of urinary calculi pass spontaneously, calculi that are not causing renal damage, obstruction, or infection are left in place for several months in the hope that they will pass spontaneously
- Depending on the underlying causes and chemical composition of the calculi, dietary modifications and drug therapy may be used to help prevent recurrence; a fluid intake of 3 to 4 qt (3 to 4 L) daily is recommended, regardless of the type of calculi.

- Procedures to remove renal calculi include extracorporeal shock-wave lithotripsy, ureteroscopic stone removal, and percutaneous nephrolithotomy
  - Extracorporeal shock-wave lithotripsy is the most commonly used procedure to treat urinary calculi
- In this procedure, ultrasonic shock waves pulverize the calculi into many small fragments that pass through the urinary tract over several months
- The procedure has reduced the need for surgery and endoscopy to treat urinary calculi
  - Percutaneous nephrolithotomy is used for removing large or inaccessible stones
- A nephroscope is inserted through an incision to the kidney, where the stone is removed
- Ultrasound may be needed to break up larger stones
  - Ureteroscopic stone removal may be used for stones in the ureters
- A fiber-optic ureteroscope is passed through the urethra and bladder into the ureters
- The calculi is then removed or treated with shock waves.

### *Nursing Interventions*

- Promote comfort for the patient with renal calculi
  - Administer opioid analgesics, antispasmodics, and antiemetics, as prescribed
  - Give hot baths or apply warm, moist packs to promote relaxation
  - Administer 3 to 4 qt (3 to 4 L) of fluids daily to help calculi passage; use IV fluids if the patient cannot tolerate oral fluids
  - Encourage the patient to participate in usual activities and to ambulate frequently; these actions promote calculi passage
- Prevent urinary obstruction and infection
  - Teach the patient the importance of monitoring urine output for changes in voiding pattern or amount and for cloudiness, foul odor, and blood
  - Tell the patient to promptly report signs of UTI and flank, lumbar, and abdominal pain to the practitioner
  - Teach the patient the importance of completing the full course of antibiotic therapy and the need to maintain fluid intake at 2 to 3 qt (2 to 3 L) daily to promote dilution and rapid drug excretion
  - Encourage the patient to increase daily fluid intake to 3 qt (3 L) or more to promote urine flow, dilute crystalloids in the urine, and prevent precipitation of crystalloids into stones
  - Encourage the patient with calcium-containing calculi to increase fluid intake 2 to 4 hours after meals, during heavy physical activity and dehydration, and at night; urine is more likely to be saturated with calcium at these times
- Prevent urinary calculi from recurring
  - Encourage increased fluid intake to prevent urinary stasis and calculi development
  - Instruct the patient to strain the urine to recover the calculi
  - Teach the patient about predisposing factors, such as dehydration, low urine output, prolonged immobilization, and UTI
  - Teach the patient with phosphate or uric acid stones how to monitor urine pH and alkalinize or acidify his urine
  - Provide instructions about diet and prescribed drugs for a patient with calcium calculi
- Reduce dietary intake of calcium and vitamin D, which prevents parathyroid hormone production
- Restrict sodium intake to reduce intestinal absorption of calcium
- Limit refined carbohydrates and animal protein to decrease hypercalciuria
- Encourage the intake of high-fiber foods to help bind calcium
- Suggest the use of orthophosphates to decrease the incidence of recurrent calculi formation in patients with hypercalciuria
- Administer thiazide diuretics, as prescribed, to increase calcium reabsorption in the kidneys and reduce calcium excretion
- Administer sodium cellulose phosphate, which binds calcium in the intestinal tract, to lower the urinary calcium level
  - If the patient has phosphate calculi, provide instructions about diet and prescribed drugs
- Because phosphate stones develop in alkaline urine, encourage the intake of ascorbic acid, cranberry and prune juices, plums, meats, eggs, and fish to maintain acid urine
- Use an aluminum hydroxide gel, which combines with excess phosphorus and increases phosphorus excretion through the intestines
  - If the patient has oxalate calculi, provide instructions about diet and prescribed drugs
- Restrict the intake of oxalate-rich foods and drinks, including apples, asparagus, beans, beer, chocolate, citrus fruits, colas, cranberries, grapes, green leafy vegetables (such as spinach and cabbage), instant coffee, peanut butter, peanuts, rhubarb, and tea

- Make sure the patient's urine remains diluted to prevent more calculi from developing
- Administer an antacid that contains aluminum to help bind oxalate and prevent urinary excretion
  - If the patient has uric acid calculi, provide instructions about diet and prescribed drugs
- Recommend a low-purine diet that avoids fish (including shellfish), red wine, and rich foods, such as organ meats and foods with heavy sauces
- If the patient has gout, restrict dietary intake of protein
- Because uric acid stones are less likely to form in alkaline urine, encourage the use of sodium bicarbonate or sodium citrate solutions to maintain alkaline urine
  - If the patient has struvite calculi, provide instructions about diet and prescribed drugs
- Make sure that the patient receives prompt treatment for UTIs and that measures are taken to reduce the incidence of infection
- Administer acetohydroxamic acid to inhibit the chemical reaction caused by bacteria, which may help prevent struvite calculi
  - If the patient has cystine calculi, provide instructions about diet and prescribed drugs
- Restrict dietary protein intake, and encourage the use of measures to alkalinize the urine
- Use penicillamine to reduce cystine in the urine.

## Urinary Tract Infection

### Description

- *Urinary tract infection* is a general term used to describe infections of the upper or lower urinary tract; upper UTIs affect the kidneys, whereas lower UTIs affect the urinary bladder (cystitis) and urethra (urethritis)
- UTIs are the most common bacterial infections in all patients and are a significant source of morbidity; they are more common in women than in men, and they increase in frequency with age
- Factors that increase the risk of developing a UTI include female sex, increased sexual activity, pregnancy, structural and functional urinary tract abnormalities (such as strictures), obstructed urine flow, impaired bladder innervation, urinary stasis, incomplete bladder emptying, chronic health problems that alter renal tissue structure and function, urinary tract instrumentation (such as bladder catheterization and cystoscopy), and age
- UTIs in men and women typically develop as an ascending infection from the urethra; other pathways for infection—such as hematogenous spread, lymphatic spread, and direct extension from other organs—are rare
- A shorter urethra and its anatomic closeness to the vagina and rectum predispose women to ascending UTIs; besides anatomic differences that help protect men against UTIs, prostatic fluid provides an antibacterial effect
- Infection of the kidney by bacteria usually occurs secondary to ascending infection from the bladder; infection commonly results from ureterovesical reflux in which an incompetent valve allows urine to flow back into the ureters during voiding
- Gram-negative bacteria cause most bacterial UTIs; gram-negative and gram-positive bacteria may occasionally cause pyelonephritis (an infectious inflammation of the renal pelvis, tubules, and interstitial tissue that can be acute or chronic and may affect one or both kidneys)
  - Acute pyelonephritis is seldom associated with permanent renal damage
  - Chronic pyelonephritis is commonly associated with structural abnormalities and other conditions (such as calculi and diabetes) that contribute to repeated infection; it is more likely than acute pyelonephritis to cause permanent kidney damage and dysfunction from repeated inflammation and scarring.

### Signs and Symptoms

- Symptoms of UTIs vary; some UTIs are asymptomatic and are diagnosed when routine urine testing detects bacteriuria
- Cystitis commonly causes urinary frequency, urinary urgency, and dysuria (pain and burning on urination); it also may produce microscopic to gross hematuria, urinary tenesmus (persistent desire to urinate small amounts), suprapubic and bladder spasms, and cloudy, foul-smelling urine
- Acute pyelonephritis typically manifests with an abrupt onset of shaking chills and moderate to high fever (101.3° to 104°F [38.5° to 40°C]), tachycardia, flank pain, malaise, nausea, vomiting, and costovertebral angle tenderness
  - These signs and symptoms may be accompanied by symptoms of lower urinary tract involvement (dysuria and urinary frequency and urgency)
  - Chills, fever, and signs of toxicity (such as falling blood pressure, tachycardia, and skin color changes) suggest deeper infection of the kidney
- Chronic pyelonephritis develops slowly and may progress to chronic renal failure.

### Diagnosis and Treatment

- Diagnosis is usually based on the initial clinical presentation
- Urine culture may reveal at least 105 (100,000) colonies of bacteria per milliliter from a clean-catch midstream or catheterized urine specimen
  - Urinalysis shows WBCs, casts, bacteria and, possibly, red blood cells
  - Suprapubic needle aspiration of the bladder (if done) shows bacteria in the specimen
- Patients with recurrent or complicated UTIs may undergo additional diagnostic studies—such as abdominal ultrasonography, excretory urography, cystography, cystoscopy with retrograde pyelography and voiding urography, and abdominal CT—to rule out calculi or structural abnormalities of the urinary tract as the cause of recurrent infections
- Treatment of UTI and acute pyelonephritis has two goals: sterilizing the urine with antibacterial, antimicrobial, or urinary antiseptic drug therapy and identifying any illness or urinary tract abnormality that may be contributing to the infection

- Increased urine output dilutes the urine, which relieves urethral irritation and burning; a continual urine flow also discourages urinary stasis and organism growth
- Acute UTI symptoms may be relieved temporarily with urinary analgesics (such as a phenazopyridine, anticholinergics, or antispasmodics).

### *Nursing Interventions*

- If the patient has a lower UTI, administer antimicrobials, urinary analgesics, or antispasmodics, as prescribed; increase fluid intake up to 3 qt (3 L) daily to help dilute the urine; and give the patient a warm sitz bath two or three times a day for 10 to 20 minutes to relieve local symptoms
- If the patient has pyelonephritis, administer antimicrobials, analgesics, antipyretics, and antiemetics, as prescribed, and maintain adequate fluid intake and output
- Emphasize to the patient the importance of taking antimicrobial medication for the full course of therapy, even if symptoms improve
- Teach the patient how to prevent urinary stasis by drinking 2 to 3 qt (2 to 3 L) of fluid daily, voiding every 2 to 3 hours, and emptying the bladder completely
- Stress to the patient the importance of emptying the bladder as soon as the urge to urinate occurs; delayed urination encourages UTI by promoting urinary stasis
- Encourage women whose UTIs are related to sexual activity to empty their bladders before and after sexual intercourse.
- Teach female patients how to reduce the number of pathogens in the perineal area by wiping from front to back after urination or defecation and cleaning the perineal and perineal area after each bowel movement.

## REPRODUCTIVE SYSTEM DISORDERS

### Introduction

- The chief function of the reproductive system is procreation and the manufacture of sex hormones.
- Alterations in the reproductive system affect the ability to procreate and alter human social and emotional health.

### *Nursing History*

- The nurse asks the patient about the *chief complaint*
  - The female with a reproductive disorder may be experiencing pain, vaginal discharge, abnormal uterine bleeding, pruritus, or infertility
  - The male with a reproductive disorder may be experiencing penile discharge, impotence, infertility, or scrotal or inguinal masses, pain, or tenderness
- The nurse then questions the patient about the *present illness*
  - Ask the patient about his symptoms, including when they started, associated symptoms, location, radiation, intensity, duration, frequency, and precipitating and alleviating factors
  - Ask about the use of prescription and over-the-counter drugs; herbal remedies; vitamin and nutritional supplements, including oral contraceptives and hormones; and use of any alternative therapies
- The nurse asks about the *medical history*
  - Question the female patient about her reproductive history, endocrine disorders, human immunodeficiency virus (HIV) status, infection or cancer of the reproductive organs, and sexually transmitted disease (STD)
  - Question the male patient about his medical history, including diabetes, hypertension, mumps, HIV status, STD, endocrine disorders, and infection or cancer of the reproductive organs
- The nurse then assesses the *family history*
  - Ask about a family history of diabetes and hypertension
  - Also question the patient about a family history of cancer of the reproductive organs, diethylstilbestrol exposure, and other reproductive disorders
- The nurse obtains a *social history*
  - Ask about work, exercise, diet, use of recreational drugs and alcohol, and hobbies
  - Also ask about stress, support systems, and coping mechanisms
  - Question the patient about the use of birth control, safe sex practices, sexual preference, number of sexual partners, and satisfaction.

### *Physical Assessment*

- The nurse begins with *inspection*
  - Observe the patient's general appearance, noting behaviors and mental status
  - Inspect the external genitalia and pubic hair, noting any swelling, lumps, discharge, rashes, lesions, lice, or odors
  - Observe the size and shape of the breasts, noting any nipple discharge
  - Inspect the female patient's internal genitalia using a speculum
  - Assess the male patient for inguinal and femoral hernias during Valsalva's maneuver and while coughing
- Next, the nurse uses *palpation*
  - Palpate the external genitalia, noting any areas of swelling, tenderness, or hardness
  - Palpate the breasts for lumps and nipple discharge
  - Palpate the male patient's scrotal sac, noting the size and shape of the testicles and the presence of masses or tenderness
  - If the patient is a male, palpate the inguinal area, and check for hernias.

### Benign Prostatic Hyperplasia

### *Description*

- Benign prostatic hyperplasia is prostate gland enlargement; about 50% of men older than age 50 and 75% of men older than age 70 have symptoms of such enlargement
- The cause is unknown but may be linked to hormonal changes
- As the prostate enlarges, the urethral opening narrows and obstructs or interferes with urine flow, causing urine retention or incomplete emptying; eventually, the ureters and kidneys dilate, and urinary tract infections (UTIs) result from urinary stasis

- Progressive bladder distention may cause a pouch to form in the bladder that retains urine when the rest of the bladder empties.

### Signs and Symptoms

- Signs and symptoms include urinary frequency; nocturia; smaller, less-forceful urine stream; urinary hesitancy; dribbling after urination; bladder distention; cystitis; and acute urine retention
- Hematuria, bladder calculi, impaired renal function, fatigue, nausea, vomiting, anorexia, and abdominal discomfort also may occur.

### Diagnosis and Treatment

- Digital rectal examination can detect the enlarged lateral lobes of the prostate; cystoscopy, urethrography, excretory urography, and hematologic and kidney function studies may be performed; prostatespecific antigen (PSA) can help to rule out prostatic carcinoma; and postvoid residual urine test and transrectal ultrasonography may also be performed
- Conservative treatment may include finasteride (Proscar) to decrease the size of the prostate and alpha-adrenergic blockers, such as prazos in (Minipress), doxazosin (Cardura), tamsulosin (Flomax), and terazosin (Hytrin), to relax the muscles and promote urination
- For acute cases, a urologist may insert a urinary catheter; a stylet may be needed to pass through the obstruction, or a suprapubic cystostomy (incision and catheter placement in the bladder through the abdomen wall) may be needed
- When a urinary obstruction is present, prostatectomy (surgical removal of soft tissue from the prostate) by one of four techniques is commonly performed
- Newer treatments include balloon urethroplasty, laser therapy, and intraurethral stents
- Other minimally invasive surgical techniques include:
  - Transurethral needle ablation to burn away well-defined regions of the prostate, thereby improving urine flow with less risk
  - Transurethral microwave treatment to destroy portions of the prostate with heat.

### Preoperative Nursing Interventions

- Explain the surgical procedure, perioperative experience, and expected postoperative course to help decrease the patient's anxiety
- Allow the patient to discuss fears and concerns about postoperative urinary incontinence and impotence, but assure him that they are not common after prostate surgery, only after radical perineal resection.

### Postoperative Nursing Interventions

- Evaluate the patient's pain and response to analgesia
  - Explain to the patient that after transurethral resection of the prostate (TURP), bladder spasms are typical; explain to him that the sensation of needing to void is normal and that avoiding straining may decrease the frequency and intensity of bladder spasms
  - Observe and maintain the patency of the three-way irrigation system; clots can obstruct the system and cause pain and bladder spasms; if clots form, increase the flow of saline solution to dilute the urine and allow the clots to flow out
  - Check for pain at the incision site, penile inflammation at the catheter site, and pain in the flank area caused by UTI
  - Administer opioids for pain as prescribed; belladonna and opium suppositories may be prescribed for bladder spasms
- Monitor the patient for potential complications
  - Watch for hemorrhage and shock, which can occur postoperatively because the prostate is a highly vascular gland
- Check urinary drainage, which initially should be reddish pink with a few small clots and then lighter pink during the first 24 hours after surgery; bright red drainage with clots indicates arterial bleeding and typically requires surgical intervention
- Check for hemodynamic alterations (such as tachycardia, increased respiratory rate, and decreased blood pressure) and other signs of hemorrhage, including restlessness, pallor, and cold, clammy skin
  - Monitor the patient's fluid and electrolyte status
  - Make sure that the catheter drains well; catheter obstruction by clots can cause prostatic capsule or bladder distention and hemorrhage
- Assess the patient for bladder distention by palpating for a rounded swelling above the pubis
- Using aseptic technique, perform manual irrigation when needed with 50 mL of sterile normal saline solution to remove clots
- Carefully record the intake of irrigating solution and the output of urine and irrigating solution
  - Observe the patient for signs of cerebral edema, such as confusion and agitation; water intoxication can result when the irrigating solution is absorbed into the vascular system during surgery
  - Check for and take precautions to prevent wound infection, UTI, and epididymitis
- Use aseptic technique when performing catheter care and changing dressings and irrigation solution containers
- Avoid taking rectal temperatures and administering enemas to prevent trauma to the operative area
- Monitor the patient for signs of infection, such as fever, redness, swelling, and drainage from the incision site
- Change wet dressings frequently to prevent skin maceration
  - After a suprapubic, perineal, or retropubic prostatectomy, monitor the patient for and take steps to prevent deep vein thrombosis (DVT) and pulmonary embolism
  - Monitor the patient for postoperative respiratory complications
- Assess urinary continence after the catheter is removed
  - Monitor urine output, and observe the patient for urine retention
  - Explain that incontinence is normal after prostate surgery, that it is transient and will gradually improve, except after radical perineal surgery

- Encourage perineal exercises and voluntary interruption of the urine stream to expedite the return of bladder control
- Prepare the patient for discharge
  - Encourage the patient to discuss his feelings about sexual activity
- Discuss with the surgeon when the patient can resume sexual activity (usually within 3 to 8 weeks)
- Advise the patient about retrograde ejaculation to the bladder (urine may appear milky)
- Refer a patient who has had a radical prostatectomy for counseling because physiologic impotence may occur
  - Tell the patient to avoid prolonged sitting, vigorous exercise, heavy lifting, and straining to decrease pressure on the operative area and help prevent bleeding
  - Discuss ways to avoid constipation; provide dietary suggestions to promote soft stools and enhance wound healing
  - Advise the patient to drink 2½ qt (2.5 L) of fluid daily to keep stools soft and prevent urinary stasis and UTI (unless contraindicated); discourage the intake of caffeine-containing beverages, which can irritate the urinary system; and encourage decreased fluid intake in the evening to minimize nocturia
  - Alert a patient who has undergone TURP about the possibility of secondary hemorrhage 2 weeks after the operation
  - Instruct the patient to call the surgeon immediately if bleeding, decreased urinary stream, or signs of infection develop.

## Breast Cancer

### *Description*

- Breast cancer is the most common cancer in women and the second leading cause of cancer deaths in women; it affects one of eight women in the United States, and its incidence increases with age; 1% of all breast cancer occurs in men
- The cause of breast cancer is unknown, but risk factors include a family history of breast cancer, inherited gene factors BRCA1 and BRCA2, obesity, hypertension, diabetes, exposure to ionizing radiation or chemical carcinogens, nulliparity or low parity, lack of breastfeeding, use of estrogen replacement therapy for menopausal symptoms, a high-fat diet, and the onset of menarche before age 12, menopause after age 55, and first pregnancy after age 30
- The lifetime risk of breast cancer for women with BRCA1 mutation is 50 to 85%, compared with a risk of 11% for women without this gene mutation.
- The prognosis depends on the type of cancer and the stage of the disease at the time of treatment; early detection and treatment result in a more favorable prognosis
- Breast cancer commonly begins as atypical cells, progresses to ductal or lobular carcinoma in situ, and then enters an invasive stage; in the invasive stage, the cancer can spread quickly to regional lymph nodes and the systemic circulation
- Common metastatic sites include the lungs, bone, liver, brain, pelvis, and abdomen.

### *Signs and Symptoms*

- A small, nontender, palpable, movable mass in the breast is an early sign of breast cancer, although it may go undetected until later signs develop; the common site for such a mass is the upper outer quadrant of the breast
- Late signs of breast cancer include skin dimpling or puckering, skin color changes over the lesion, nipple retraction, breast contour changes, serous or bloody nipple discharge, palpable axillary or other lymph nodes, breast asymmetry, erythema, ridging, and a prominent venous pattern
- Inflammatory carcinoma is a rare form of breast cancer that produces a tender, enlarged, reddened, hot breast; in advanced cases, the breast may become ulcerated, infected, and necrotic.

### *Diagnosis and Treatment*

- About 90% of breast cancers are discovered by breast self-examination (BSE); BSE and annual breast examination by a health care professional may detect early disease; however, micrometastases may have disseminated by the time the tumor is palpable
- The American Cancer Society guidelines state that women over age 40 should have a mammogram annually and a clinical examination at least annually and all women should perform breast self examination monthly
- Mammography can detect early lesions before they are palpable; xeroradiography, ultrasonography, magnetic resonance imaging (MRI), and positron emission tomography also may be used
- The diagnosis of breast cancer is made by fine-needle aspiration and excisional biopsy of the tumor; the biopsied tissue is analyzed to determine whether the tumor is hormone-dependent, a factor that influences treatment
  - Newer biopsy techniques include mammotone biopsy, minimally invasive breast biopsy, and advanced breast biopsy instrument
  - Ductal lavage may also be performed to detect malignant cells
  - Sentinel lymph node mapping, in which a radioactive substance or blue dye is injected around the biopsy site, may be performed before surgery; the sentinel node (the one most likely to contain malignant cells) is the one that contains the most radioactivity and blue dye, which then will be biopsied
- Treatment depends on the tumor's histopathology and aggressiveness, hormonal factors (the patient's menopausal status and the tumor's hormone dependency), extent of disease, and the patient's overall health and treatment preferences
- Surgery is the primary treatment for breast cancer; breast reconstruction surgery may be performed immediately after surgery or later; laser ablation is an alternative to lumpectomy in women with tumors that are smaller than ¾″ (2 cm)
- Radiation therapy is the primary treatment for patients who cannot tolerate anesthesia or surgery or who have inflammatory carcinoma

- Primary radiation therapy with 'boost' to the tumor site (application of additional radiation by external beam or placement of iridium needles in the former tumor site) may be used in early stages of breast cancer as a supplement to surgery and primary radiation
- Radiation therapy to the breast and lymph nodes followed by 'boost' to the tumor site is used after breast-preserving surgery (such as lumpectomy, quadrantectomy, and simple mastectomy)

• Adjuvant chemotherapy is recommended after primary treatment and typically involves a combination of doxorubicin (Doxil), cyclophosphamide (Cytoxan), paclitaxel (Abraxane), methotrexate, tamoxifen, and fluorouracil (Floururацil); metastatic breast cancer is usually treated with fluorouracil, paclitaxel, or docetaxel (Taxotere), capecitabine (Xeloda), vinorelbine (Navelbine), or gemcitabine (Gemzar)
• Hormone therapy or surgery is indicated for patients with hormone-dependent breast cancer; antiestrogen drugs such as tamoxifen may be prescribed, and adrenalectomy, oophorectomy, or hypophysectomymay be considered
• Monoclonal antibodies such as trastuzumab may be used to treat metastatic breast cancer in women who have an excess amount of breast cancer cell antigen HER2
• Bone marrow or blood stem cell transplantation may be used to restore stem cells.

### Nursing Interventions for a Patient with Early Breast Cancer

• Assess the patient's and family's understanding of the disease, diagnostic tests, and treatments, and intervene accordingly
• Encourage the patient to discuss her fears and concerns about the disease, diagnostic tests, treatments, and sexuality; clarify misconceptions, and be aware that breast cancer treatment can change the patient's body image and self-concept
• Evaluate the patient's support systems, and refer her to clergy members, home health care services, hospices, or support groups (such as Reach to Recovery, a group of volunteers who provide emotional and educational support during the preoperative and postoperative periods).

### Nursing Interventions for a Patient Undergoing Mastectomy

• Monitor the patient for complications of general anesthesia and surgery, such as hemorrhage, wound infection, and altered respiratory status
  - During the initial postoperative period, frequently check the dressing and Hemovac drains for excessive bleeding
  - Check the patency of the Hemovac drains, and empty drains when half full to maintain suction and prevent fluid accumulation; drains are typically removed after 3 to 5 days
  - Use strict aseptic technique for dressing changes
  - Encourage the patient to perform deep-breathing and coughing exercises; administer analgesics to prevent respiratory splinting
  - Evaluate the patient's nutritional status, and promote adequate nutritional intake to foster wound healing
• Evaluate the patient's level of pain and response to analgesia and comfort measures
  - Promote comfort by elevating the head of the bed and positioning the patient on the unaffected side supported by pillows (lying on the affected side can cause severe pain)
  - Position the affected arm on pillows to provide support and enhance circulation
  - Encourage the patient to use her unaffected arm to help change position or get out of bed
• Monitor the patient for lymphedema, and take steps to prevent it
  - Never perform blood pressure readings, venipuncture, or injections on the affected arm
  - Check for edema in the affected arm; diuretics may be prescribed in the acute phase, and an elastic sleeve may be used during the chronic phase
  - Elevate, massage, and exercise the affected arm to improve circulation and prevent edema; teach the patient to do this at home
  - Teach the patient other techniques for preventing lymphedema, such as avoiding sun exposure, applying cream several times a day, using a thimble while sewing, using gloves while cleaning or gardening, wearing medical identification at all times, avoiding restrictive jewelery and clothing, not carrying heavy objects with the affected arm, and elevating the arm above the right atrium to promote circulatory and lymphatic flow
• Teach the patient arm exercises to prevent muscle shortening, stiffening, and contracture and to preserve muscle tone
• Encourage early and frequent ambulation; help the patient from her unaffected side, and help her maintain posture
• Provide rest periods between activities to avoid tiring the patient
• Prepare the patient for discharge by providing verbal and written instructions about pain medications, activity restrictions, arm exercises, lymphedema prevention, follow-up treatments, referrals to postdischarge support services, and information about prostheses; also provide an opportunity to discuss the effect of surgery on sexuality.

### Nursing Interventions for a Patient Receiving Chemotherapy after a Mastectomy

• Monitor for and teach the patient about the adverse effects and toxicity of chemotherapeutic agents
• Follow guidelines for handling chemotherapeutic agents to prevent personal risks associated with repeated exposure to these drugs
• Monitor the patient for adverse effects of hormone therapy such as fluid retention.

### Nursing Interventions for a Patient Receiving Breast-Preserving Surgery and Radiation Therapy

• Follow postoperative nursing interventions for a patient undergoing mastectomy
• Monitor the patient for complications of radiation therapy, such as nausea, dyspepsia, esophagitis, transient

pneumonitis, cough, fatigue, depression, and altered skin integrity at the surgical site and iridium needle site

- Provide emotional support to the patient and family during 'boost' therapy with an internal interstitial implant because radiation precautions require a private room and restricted visitation while the implant is in place (about 2 days) because of gamma ray emissions.

### Nursing Interventions for a Patient with Advanced Breast Cancer

- Develop an individualized plan of care based on the patient's treatment: radiation therapy, chemotherapy, hormone therapy, oophorectomy, adrenalectomy, or hypophysectomy
- Evaluate the patient's pain and response to pain-control and comfort measures; inform the practitioner and other health care team members if pain-control measures are ineffective
- Promote comfort by positioning the patient, applying heat or cold, using massage, providing pillows and a firm mattress, and teaching the patient relaxation techniques and guided imagery
- Promote adequate nutritional intake, particularly protein
  - Collaborate with the dietitian to improve nutrition; assess the need for supplements
  - Administer antiemetics as prescribed, and provide meticulous oral hygiene to improve the patient's ability and desire to eat
- Prevent alterations in skin integrity
  - Observe the patient's skin and mucus membranes for signs of impaired skin integrity; radiation therapy, chemotherapy, inadequate nutrition, and impaired mobility can lead to skin breakdown and mucus membrane irritation
  - Provide oral and skin care; applying lip gloss or petroleum jelly to the lips may be helpful
  - Promote activity and position changes to prevent prolonged pressure and tissue necrosis
  - Ensure adequate nutrition.

## Erectile Dysfunction

### Description

- Erectile dysfunction is the inability to attain or maintain penile erection long enough to complete intercourse
- The disorder is classified as primary or secondary
  - In *primary impotence*, the patient never achieves sufficient erection
  - In *secondary impotence*, the patient has achieved erection and completed intercourse in the past
  - In most cases, erectile dysfunction has an organic cause, such as vascular insufficiency or venoocclusive dysfunction
- Other causes include certain medications, such as antihypertensives and diuretics, and alcohol and drug abuse
- Some cases may be psychogenic
- All age groups may be affected, although the incidence increases with age.

### Signs and Symptoms

- Onset may occur suddenly, or the patient may experience a gradual decline in sexual function
- A history of medical disorders, drug therapy, or psychological trauma may accompany the disorder.

### Diagnosis and Treatment

- Laboratory findings may include a decrease in serum testosterone levels
- Glycosylated hemoglobin level may be elevated, indicating uncontrolled diabetes mellitus
- Urinalysis results may be abnormal, indicating kidney damage or diabetes mellitus
- Lipid profiles may be increased, indicating atherosclerosis
- Blood glucose levels may be increased, a sign of diabetes mellitus
- Serum creatinine levels may be elevated, resulting from kidney damage
- PSA results help rule out prostate cancer
- Ultrasonography evaluates vascular function; angiography evaluates vaso-occlusive disease
- Direct injection of alprostadil (Caverject) into the corpora evaluates the quality of erection
- Nocturnal penile tumescence testing helps to distinguish psychogenic impotence from organic impotence
- For erectile dysfunction that stems from an organic cause, treatment aims to correct the underlying cause
- For dysfunction that results from a psychogenic cause, psychological counseling and sex therapy may help
- An external vacuum device may allow the patient to achieve a temporary erection
- Phosphodiesterase type 5 (PDE5) inhibitors, such as sildenafil, vardenafil, and tadalafil, are the first line of drug treatment
- The patient may benefit from a surgically inserted inflatable or semi-rigid penile prosthesis.

### Nursing Interventions

- Teach the patient and his partner about the disorder and treatment options
- Encourage the patient to discuss his concerns, and provide support; include the patient's partner in your care
- Assist with measures to determine a possible underlying organic cause
- Provide postoperative care after penile prosthesis surgery; monitor the patient for bleeding, swelling, and infection
- Teach the patient to avoid alcohol before engaging in sexual activity; teach about the proper use of medications to treat erectile dysfunction
- Refer the patient to a practitioner, nurse, psychologist, social worker, or counselor trained in sex therapy as needed.

## Pelvic Inflammatory Disease

### Description

- Pelvic inflammatory disease (PID) refers to any acute, subacute, recurrent, or chronic infection of the oviducts and ovaries with adjacent tissue involvement

- PID includes inflammation of the cervix (cervicitis), uterus (endometritis), fallopian tubes (salpingitis), and ovaries (oophoritis)
- The inflammation may extend to connective tissue that lies between the broad ligaments (parametritis)
- PID is typically caused by bacteria–usually gonorrheal and chlamydial organisms–but it may also result from a virus
- Normally, the cervical mucus and cervicovaginal flora serve as a protective barrier; when this barrier is altered or destroyed–for instance, from sexual activity or instrumentation–bacteria can enter the vagina and cervix and ascend and enter the uterine cavity, causing inflammation of various structures; retrograde menstrual flow may help promote the ascent of such organisms
- Risk factors for PID include multiple sexual partners, a history of STIs, uterine infection after pregnancy, and IUD insertion
- Complications include infertility, septicemia, pulmonary embolus, peritonitis, and shock.

### Signs and Symptoms

- PID may be asymptomatic; if signs and symptoms do occur, they may include low-grade fever, malaise, lower abdominal pain that worsens with intercourse, irregular vaginal bleeding, and purulent vaginal discharge
- Other signs and symptoms include pain during cervical examination and possibly a palpable adnexal mass.

### Diagnosis and Treatment

- Culture and sensitivity testing and Gram stain of endocervix or cul-de-sac secretions show the causative agent; urethral and rectal secretions can also show the causative agent
- The patient's C-reactive protein level, white blood cell count, and erythrocyte sedimentation rate are elevated
- Transvaginal ultrasonography may show the presence of thickened, fluid-filled fallopian tubes
- CT scan may show complex tubo-ovarian abscesses, and MRI may show images of soft tissue; these tests are useful not only for establishing the diagnosis of PID but also for detecting other processes responsible for symptoms
- Diagnostic laparoscopy identifies cul-de-sac fluid, tubal distention, and masses in a pelvic abscess
- Treatment aims to eradicate the underlying infection with antibiotics
- Laparoscopy allows for drainage of pelvic abscesses, pelvic lavage, or lysis of adhesions
- If the patient develops a ruptured pelvic abscess–a life-threatening situation–she may require a total hysterectomy with bilateral salpingo-oophorectomy.

### Nursing Interventions

- Teach the patient about the disorder, including treatment options and how to prevent future infections
- Administer prescribed antibiotics and analgesics; if IV antibiotics are ordered, initiate IV access and ensure its patency
- Provide frequent perineal care; inspect the patient's perineal pads, noting the color and characteristics of drainage
- Use meticulous hand hygiene technique
- Encourage the patient to discuss her feelings about her condition and sexuality; offer emotional support
- Help her to develop effective coping strategies
- Palpate the patient's abdomen for pain and tenderness, noting any distention or rigidity; auscultate bowel sounds for changes
- Be alert for signs of peritonitis
- Prepare the patient and her family for possible surgery if an abscess develops or ruptures
- Provide appropriate postoperative care
- Before discharge, teach the patient to report any fever, increased vaginal discharge, or increases in pelvic pain to her practitioner
- Emphasize the importance of completing the full course of antibiotics to ensure complete eradication of the infection.

## Sexually Transmitted Diseases

### Description

- STDs are the most common infections in the United States; acquired immunodeficiency syndrome (AIDS), herpes, gonorrhea, and hepatitis are considered epidemic.
- These contagious diseases are usually transmitted through intimate sexual contact with an infected person; some are transmitted to an infant during pregnancy or childbirth
- People younger than age 25, those with multiple sex partners, and those with a history of STDs are at higher risk for infection; the incidence of STDs is higher among prostitutes and people having sexual contact with prostitutes, drug abusers, or prison inmates
- Morbidity and mortality depend on the type and stage of STD; many STDs are easy to treat when detected early
- STDs can be prevented by educating the public, identifying and treating partners and contacts of infected people, and identifying and treating symptomatic or asymptomatic infected patients; barrier methods of contraception, such as a condom and a diaphragm with spermicide, reduce the risk of certain infections
- More than 21 diseases are classified as STDs; they are caused by bacteria, viruses, protozoans, fungi, and ectoparasites.

### Signs and Symptoms

- The chief signs of STDs are vaginitis, recurrent vaginitis, epididymitis, lower abdominal pain, pharyngitis, proctitis, and skin or mucus membrane lesions
- Many STDs are asymptomatic, especially in women; by the time the STD is detected, the woman may have severe complications, such as PID, infertility, ectopic pregnancy, or chronic pelvic pain.

### Diagnosis and Treatment

- The diagnosis of a specific STD is made by physical examination, patient history, and laboratory tests to determine the causative organism
- Treatment is based on the specific causative organism; treatment guidelines for each STD are available from the Centers for Disease Control and Prevention (CDC)

- The CDC recommends that specific resources be available for patients with STDs: medical evaluation and treatment facilities for patients with HIV infection; hospitalization facilities for patients with complicated STDs, such as PID and disseminated gonococcal infection; referrals for medical, pediatric, infectious disease, dermatologic, and gynecologic-obstetric services; family-planning services; and substance abuse treatment programs.

### Nursing Interventions

- Develop a therapeutic relationship with the patient that fosters trust and preserves the patient's dignity; ensure privacy and confidentiality, and avoid judging the patient's lifestyle and making assumptions about his sexual preference
- Provide emotional support, and encourage the patient to discuss feelings; he may be anxious and fearful and may experience altered self-esteem and self-image
- Teach the patient about the STD and its treatment
  - Discuss disease transmission, signs and symptoms, the length of the infectious period, infection prevention, and cure (if the STD can be cured)
  - Discuss the health consequences of improper treatment, and emphasize that the patient's partner is also at risk
  - Clarify common misconceptions and promote understanding of healthful sexual practices
- Inform the patient that washing his hands and genital area before and after sexual contact does not prevent STDs
- Encourage the patient to urinate after intercourse
- Advise women to avoid douching because it can alter the normal vaginal flora
- Tell the patient that condoms and a diaphragm with spermicide may provide some protection against certain STDs, but IUDs and birth control pills do not
  - Encourage a sexually active patient who has multiple partners and no STD symptoms to have an STD examination twice a year
  - Tell the patient to seek immediate treatment if STD symptoms develop
  - Inform the patient that treatment does not provide immunity from the same or a different STD
  - Advise the patient to abstain from sexual activity until the posttreatment follow-up verifies a cure
  - Discuss modifications of sexual activity to prevent recurrence: reducing the number of sex partners, avoiding partners who have multiple partners, and questioning partners about their STD history
- Teach the patient about the prescribed medication and its dosing schedule and adverse effects; stress the importance of completing the medication regimen, even if symptoms disappear; advise the patient to return if he develops any adverse reactions so that another drug can be prescribed
- Teach the patient about lesion care, including soaking in a tub two to three times a day, keeping lesions clean and dry between baths, wearing cotton underwear, avoiding panty hose and restrictive clothing, and avoiding creams, lotions, and ointments except those specifically prescribed
- Refer the patient to other social and health services as needed
- Report the STD according to local health department or state health board requirements.

## Testicular Cancer

### Description

- Testicular cancer is the most common type of cancer in men between ages 15 and 35; it is the third leading cause of death in these men but has an overall cure rate of 95% when detected early
- Although the cause of testicular cancer is unknown, incidence is higher in men with cryptorchidism; the disease is also associated with scrotal trauma, heredity, infection, hormonal abnormalities, and orchiopexy (surgical repair of undescended testis)
- Testicular tumors are histologically classified as seminomas or nonseminomas
  - Seminomas typically are localized and highly sensitive to radiation therapy; the prognosis is good with early treatment
  - Nonseminomas are faster growing and more diffuse; they require more aggressive treatment with surgery and chemotherapy
- Educating men to perform testicular self-examination facilitates earlier detection and intervention; however, many patients do not seek treatment for 3 to 6 months after detecting a tumor.

### Signs and Symptoms

- Most patients with testicular cancer report unilateral testicular enlargement, a 'dragging' sensation in the lower abdomen, and heaviness in the scrotum; 70% to 90% of patients do not report pain as an early symptom
- A patient with a palpable tumor that does not transluminate may have testicular cancer
- A patient with metastasis to retroperitoneal lymph nodes may report lower back pain, lymphadenopathy, fatigue, weight loss, and anorexia; the next most common site of metastasis is the lungs
- The patient also may experience breast enlargement and tenderness.

### Diagnosis and Treatment

- Diagnosis of suspected testicular cancer is based on the patient's symptoms and history, testicular examination, urine estrogen and testosterone levels, scrotal illumination, and scrotal ultrasonography; radioimmunoassay studies, which measure antigens produced by malignant cells, aid in diagnosis
- Excretory urography may be used to evaluate renal function and structure; chest X-ray, CT, and MRI are used to evaluate metastasis
- The histologic diagnosis is made by inguinal orchiectomy; testicular biopsy is not done because it can promote the spread of tumor cells
- Testicular cancer is treated with radiation therapy, chemotherapy, and surgery; one, two, or all three of these treatments may be used, depending on the stage of the disease and the type of tumor.

### Nursing Interventions for a Patient in the Early Stages of Testicular Cancer

- Assess the patient's and family's understanding of the disease, diagnostic tests, and treatments, and intervene accordingly
- Encourage the patient to discuss his fears and concerns; clarify misconceptions, and be aware that orchiectomy can change the patient's body image and self-concept; discuss the possibility of joining a sperm bank if sterility is a concern.

### Nursing Interventions for a Patient Undergoing Orchiectomy

- Monitor the patient for complications of anesthesia and hemorrhage immediately after surgery
- Prepare the patient for discharge
  - Teach the patient and family about wound care at home
  - Provide verbal and written instructions about pain medications, activity restrictions (including sexual activity), and follow-up care.

### Nursing Interventions for a Patient Undergoing Retroperitoneal Lymph Node Dissection

- Observe the patient for postoperative complications, such as hemorrhage, fluid and electrolyte imbalances, atelectasis, paralytic ileus, DVT, and wound infection
- Monitor hemodynamics and fluid and electrolyte status
- Initiate leg and breathing exercises and early ambulation to prevent circulatory, respiratory, and GI complications
- Assess the patient's pain and response to analgesia; patient-controlled analgesia is an effective way of administering opioids
- Prepare the patient for discharge
  - Provide verbal and written instructions about pain medications, activity restrictions, and follow-up care
  - Tell the patient to avoid lifting and straining until after he returns to the practitioner for his 6 week postoperative visit
  - Inform the patient that sexual activity generally can be resumed in 4 to 6 weeks.

### Nursing Interventions for a Patient Receiving Chemotherapy

- Be fully knowledgeable about the prescribed chemotherapeutic agents, including their administration protocols, therapeutic and adverse effects and specific nursing considerations; handle chemotherapeutic agents according to federal safety guidelines
- Monitor and treat the patient for complications of chemotherapy
- Prepare the patient for discharge
  - Provide verbal and written instructions about pain medications, wound care, activity restrictions (including sexual activity), and follow-up care
  - Make sure the patient understands how to manage the adverse effects of chemotherapy
  - Teach the patient how to perform testicular self-examination; patients who have had testicular cancer are at higher risk for developing another tumor than those who have not had the disease
  - Tell the patient about the need for follow-up visits; recurrence is most common in the first year after treatment.

### Nursing Interventions for a Patient Receiving Radiation Therapy

- Observe the patient for complications of treatment; common systemic adverse reactions include nausea, vomiting, headache, skin reactions, fatigue, and malaise
- Check for alterations in skin integrity.

## IMMUNE SYSTEM DISORDERS

### Introduction

- The immune system is a complex organization of highly specialized cells and tissue that protect the body from various foreign organisms
- The bone marrow and thymus manufacture the immune cells, which work together with lymphoid tissue to destroy foreign organisms that enter the body; B lymphocytes and T lymphocytes are the primary cells of the immune system.

### Nursing History

- The nurse asks the patient about his *chief complaint*
  - The patient with an immunologic disorder reports vague signs and symptoms, such as lack of energy, light-headedness, frequent infections or bruising, and slow wound healing
- The nurse then questions the patient about his *present illness*
  - Ask the patient about his symptom, including when it started, associated symptoms, location, radiation, intensity, duration, frequency, and precipitating and alleviating factors
  - Ask about the use of prescription and over-the-counter (OTC) drugs, herbal remedies, vitamin and nutritional supplements, and alternative therapies
- The nurse asks about the *medical history*
  - Question the patient about changes in overall health, allergies, childhood diseases, recurrent infections, and immunizations
  - Ask about unexplained rashes, visual disturbances, fever, and changes in elimination patterns
  - Question the patient about a history of immune disorders
  - Ask the female patient about changes in menstrual patterns
- The nurse then assesses the *family history*
  - Ask about a family history of immune disorders
  - Also ask about a family history of recurrent infections, allergies, and cancer
- The nurse obtains a *social history*
  - Ask about work, exercise, diet, use of recreational drugs and alcohol, and hobbies
  - Also ask about stress, support systems, and coping mechanisms

- Question the patient about exposure to chemicals and pathogens.

### Physical Assessment

- The nurse begins with *inspection*
  - Inspect the patient's appearance, and note signs of acute and chronic illness, pain, fatigue, and malnutrition
  - Observe the patient's movements, posture, gait, coordination, balance, range of motion (ROM) and strength
  - Inspect the skin, noting color, rashes, and lesions; evaluate skin integrity
  - Note hair growth, including texture, distribution, color, and amount
  - Check the nose for evidence of chronic allergies; observe mucus membranes for ulcers, patches, and plaques; and observe the eyes for redness, infection, and hydration
  - Inspect the extremities for blanching, cyanosis, pallor, edema, and reddening
  - Assess level of consciousness and mental status, noting behavior, emotional stability, and cognition
- Next, the nurse performs *palpation* and *percussion*
  - Take the patient's vital signs
  - Feel the lymph nodes, noting any enlargement or tenderness
  - Palpate and percuss various organs, noting enlargement, inflammation, masses, or tenderness
  - Assess musculoskeletal integrity and ROM, particularly in the hands, wrists, and knees
  - Palpate the joints to detect nodules, swelling, tenderness, and pain
- Then the nurse performs *auscultation*
  - Listen to the lungs, noting abnormal breath sounds
  - Auscultate the heart, listening for abnormal sounds, rhythm, and rate
  - Listen for bowel sounds in all abdominal quadrants.

## The Immune Response

### General Information

- The primary function of the immune system is to protect the body against pathogenic microorganisms and malignant cells
- The immune response is a complex sequence of events triggered by a stimulus (antigen) and culminating in the elimination of the foreign substance; the process requires the differentiation of intrinsic organisms from foreign organisms
  - Antigens (immunogens) are any substances recognized as foreign that stimulate an immune response; viruses, bacteria, fungi, and parasites are antigens
  - Antibodies (immunoglobulins) are proteins that are formed in response to exposure to an antigen
- The following factors can decrease the immune response: genetics, age extremes, protein-calorie malnutrition, vitamin or mineral deficiency, certain drugs, radiation, and stress.

### Natural Immunity

- Natural, innate immunity is the body's first line of defense against invading pathogens; this nonspecific mechanism can differentiate intrinsic from foreign organisms but cannot identify the specific pathogen
- Types of natural immunity include *physical barriers,* such as intact skin and mucus membranes; *chemical barriers,* such as gastric acidity and enzymes in the saliva; and *inflammation,* which is the sequence of vascular and cellular responses to tissue injury and immunologic stimuli.

### Acquired Immunity

- Adaptive, acquired immunity is the body's second line of defense; it is gained through exposure to pathogens, distinguishes intrinsic from foreign organisms, identifies the specific pathogen, and responds to previously encountered pathogens
- Four types of acquired immunity exist
  - *Passive immunity* occurs when antibodies, such as immunoglobulin, of an infectious agent are supplied to the host's body, providing temporary immunity; antibodies may be obtained by injection, or they may be transferred from mother to neonate
  - *Active immunity* results from direct exposure to an antigen by immunization (such as by tetanus toxoid) or exposure to disease
  - *Humoral immunity,* primarily mediated by B cells, is the body's ability to respond to antigens by forming specific antibodies; the term *humoral* indicates that immunity is transferable by serum
  - *Cell-mediated immunity* is primarily mediated by T cells and macrophages, which are responsible for antigen destruction and delayed hypersensitivity; unlike humoral immunity, cell-mediated immunity is not readily transferred to another person by serum.

### Hypersensitivity and Allergic Reactions

- Hypersensitivity and allergic reactions are destructive immune responses that occur after reexposure to an antigen; they can produce various symptoms within minutes to several days
- Hypersensitivity reactions may be humoral or cell mediated.

## Acquired Immunodeficiency Syndrome

### Description

- Acquired immunodeficiency syndrome (AIDS) is characterized by a progressive compromise of the immune system
- To provide statistical data for public health purposes, the Centers for Disease Control and Prevention (CDC) has developed a case definition for AIDS, based on laboratory evidence of human immunodeficiency virus (HIV) infection and indicator diseases (a seropositive HIV test and laboratory confirmation of one of the indicator diseases supports a diagnosis of AIDS)
- The CDC also has developed a classification method that covers the spectrum of the progression of HIV infection
- AIDS is caused by infection with HIV type 1 (HIV-1) or HIV type 2 (HIV-2); HIV is a retrovirus that selectively infects cells with a CD4+ surface marker, usually T4 lymphocytes

- HIV is transmitted primarily through sexual intercourse, during which blood, semen, and vaginal secretions are shared
- HIV is also transmitted through contaminated blood that enters the body by way of parenteral or percutaneous routes or by way of mucus membranes or open wounds; such transmission can result from sharing or accidental injection with a contaminated needle, transfusion of contaminated blood, or perinatal transfer in the womb, during birth, or through breast milk
- HIV infection reduces cell-mediated immunity by destroying T4 lymphocytes
  - This decreases the ratio of helper T cells to suppressor T cells, which normally is 2:1 (CD4+ – CD8+ ratio)
  - It also increases the patient's susceptibility to opportunistic infections and certain cancers
- HIV infection also affects humoral immunity by producing more non-specific antibodies that are ineffective and by altering the function of monocytes and macrophages; these cells may be responsible for transporting the virus to other organs, such as the brain and lungs.

### *Signs and Symptoms*

- HIV infection may be asymptomatic or cause a mononucleosis-like syndrome associated with seroconversion; symptoms include headache, rash, malaise, and swollen lymph nodes and last about 2 weeks
  - Persistent generalized lymphadenopathy at two or more extrainguinal sites may persist for more than 3 months in the absence of concurrent illness
  - The infected patient also may display signs of opportunistic infections and other diseases
- HIV can produce central nervous system effects
  - AIDS dementia complex, also called HIV encephalopathy, causes cognitive changes, such as confusion, impaired concentration, and memory loss; motor disturbances, such as ataxia, leg weakness, and diminished fine motor movements; and behavioral changes, such as apathy, depression, reduced spontaneity, social withdrawal, anxiety, agitation, and personality changes
  - Atypical aseptic meningitis causes headache, fever, and signs of meningeal infection
  - Vacuolar myelopathy (spinal cord degeneration) may produce leg weakness, incontinence, and ataxia
- HIV wasting syndrome may occur as a complication of advanced HIV infection; it is associated with involuntary weight loss of more than 10% of body weight and diarrhea, recurrent or sustained fevers, and chronic weakness for more than 1 month in the absence of a causative illness, such as cancer or tuberculosis.

### *Diagnosis and Treatment*

- The enzyme-linked immunosorbent assay (ELISA) detects the presence of HIV-1 antibodies; if a patient's blood has a positive reaction on two ELISA tests, the Western blot test is used to confirm the results
- The Western blot test detects the presence of HIV antibodies and determines their type
- HIV infection is characterized by a progressive decline of the CD4+ T-cell count over months to years
- A CD4+ T-cell count of less than 200 cells/mL is diagnostic of AIDS and indicates that the patient is at risk for an opportunistic infection
- Polymerase chain reaction may detect viral genetic material (HIV ribonucleic acid [HIV RNA]) in patients for whom antibodies have not yet developed
- Other laboratory tests may include hematocrit (below 30%, indicating anemia), white blood cell (WBC) count (below 2,500/cm$^3$, indicating leukopenia), the ratio of helper T cells to suppressor T cells (decreased to 1:2), and platelet count (below 100,000/mm$^3$)
- Because many opportunistic infections are reactivations of previous infections, the patient may also be tested for syphilis, hepatitis B, tuberculosis, and toxoplasmosis
- Drug therapy for HIV infection includes six types of antiretrovirals
  - Protease inhibitors, such as ritonavir (Kaletra), indinavir (Crixivan), nelfinavir (Viracept), fosamprenavir (Lexiva), and saquinavir (Invirase)
  - Nucleoside and nucleotide reverse transcriptase inhibitors, such as zidovudine (Retrovir), didanosine (Videx), lamivudine (Epivir), abacavir (Ziagen) and tenofovir (Viread)
  - Nonnucleoside reverse transcriptase inhibitors, such as nevirapine (Viramune), efavirenz (Sustiva), and etravirine (Intelence)
  - Integrase inhibitors such as raltegravir (Isentress)
  - CCR5 co-receptor antagonist such as maraviroc (Selzentry)
  - Fusion inhibitors, such as enfuviritide, which interfere with the virus' ability to fuse with the cellular membrane, thereby blocking entry into the host cell
  - These antiretrovirals are used in various combinations to inhibit HIV viral replication; this is called highly active antiretroviral therapy HAART
  - Treatment protocols combine two or more drugs in an effort to gain the maximum benefit with the fewest adverse reactions
  - Combination therapy helps to inhibit the production of resistant, mutant strains
  - Combination agents that combine two or three drugs in one dose are available and help improve compliance
- Different treatments are required for AIDS indicator diseases.

### *Nursing Interventions*

- Provide respiratory care
- Encourage activity, as tolerated, to prevent fatigue and dyspnea
  - Administer medications, as prescribed, to relieve symptoms and prevent or treat infection
  - Monitor vital signs and laboratory values (arterial blood gas levels, oxygen saturation by pulse oximetry, sputum cultures, CD4+ count, and complete blood count [CBC]) to determine the effectiveness of treatment
  - Provide pulmonary hygiene (including coughing and deep breathing every 2 hours), splinting while coughing,

and suctioning to prevent atelectasis and clear airway secretions; maintain adequate hydration to thin mucus secretions
- Provide throat lozenges and warm saline gargles to soothe an irritated throat
- Administer antitussives and expectorants, as prescribed, for cough
- If appropriate, help the patient to decrease or stop smoking
- Perform GI care
  - Monitor fluid intake and output, weight, urine specific gravity, serum electrolyte levels, and skin turgor to evaluate hydration
  - Obtain stool cultures to identify enteric pathogens
  - Encourage the patient to drink at least 3 qt (3 L) of fluid daily; administer IV therapy, as prescribed, to maintain hydration
  - Administer antibiotics and antivirals to treat infectious diarrhea and antidiarrheals to lessen the severity of diarrhea
- Promote good nutrition
  - Offer small, frequent meals to reduce fatigue
  - Engage the patient in menu planning, and invite the patient's family and friends to meals to encourage eating
- Allowing the patient to include personal food preferences gives him some control over the diet
- Eating with others may improve appetite
  - Encourage the patient to eat meals sitting up and out of bed; sitting up aids digestion and decreases the risk of aspiration
  - Provide a low-residue, high-protein, high-potassium, high-calorie, lactose-free diet to minimize diarrhea and maximize caloric, electrolyte, and fluid intake
  - Use oral dietary supplements, such as Vivonex TEN; initiate and monitor tube feedings or total parenteral nutrition as prescribed
  - Avoid serving rare meats and raw vegetables, which may harbor living microbes
  - Monitor daily weight and laboratory values—including serum protein, albumin, blood urea nitrogen, hemoglobin, and serum electrolyte levels and hematocrit—to evaluate nutrition
  - Provide mouth care, using viscous oral lidocaine (Xylocaine) before meals to relieve mouth, pharyngeal, and esophageal pain; use saline rinses after meals to prevent exacerbation of infection
- Perform skin care
  - Use pressure-relieving devices (convoluted foam mattress, pressure mattress, or pressure pads), and turn the patient every 2 hours to prevent skin deterioration caused by pressure and inadequate circulation
  - Apply A + D Original Ointment or other skin barrier to the perianal area to prevent further maceration of the anal mucosa
  - Maintain wound and skin precautions to prevent further spread of infection
- Prevent and control infection
  - Restrict the patient's contact with visitors, staff members, and other patients who have infections, such as cold or flu
  - Make sure that staff members and visitors adhere to hand hygiene procedures before approaching the patient
  - Use reverse isolation if the patient is immunocompromised
  - Consider moving the patient to a private room and leaving equipment—such as a thermometer, blood pressure cuff, and stethoscope—in the room to minimize pathogen exposure
  - Follow standard precautions to reduce pathogen transfer
  - Inspect the skin, IV sites, vascular access devices, and invasive cardiovascular monitoring lines; loss of skin integrity is a potential source of infection
  - Monitor antimicrobial therapies; antibiotics can increase the likelihood of superinfection and the development of resistant organisms
  - Encourage and maintain adequate nutritional intake, which promotes healing and prevents infection
- Provide neuropsychiatric care
  - Encourage the patient to discuss emotional issues; mood swings may be related to an inability to cope with the illness
  - Identify resources for patient and family support
  - Use reminder devices, such as pictures and appointment books, to help orient the patient
  - Arrange for continuity of caregivers, and avoid frequent room changes to prevent patient confusion
  - Consult occupational and physical therapists; the patient may need special devices, such as a cane or walker, and physical therapy to maintain or prevent further loss of function
- Promote health maintenance
  - Teach the patient, family, significant others, and caregivers about the diagnosis, treatments, modes of transmission, and symptoms to report
  - Explain medications to the patient, including dose, frequency, and adverse effects; reinforce the importance of compliance to help to suppress the virus and to prevent the development of drug- resistant strains
  - Discuss the importance of avoiding high-risk behaviors and reducing the risk of transmission to others
  - Make appropriate referrals—for home care, pain management, legal services, support groups, financial support, and hospice care.

## Anaphylaxis

### *Description*

- Anaphylaxis is a clinical response to an immediate immunologic reaction between a specific antigen and an antibody
- Its onset is sudden, dramatic, and characterized by rapid progression; in severe instances, it can be life-threatening because of vascular collapse and shock
- After the initial exposure to an antigen, the immune system produces specific immunoglobulin (Ig) antibodies in the lymph nodes; helper T cells enhance the process

- The IgE antibodies then bind to membrane receptors located on mast cells and basophils
- After the body re-encounters the antigen, the IgE antibodies, or cross-linked IgE receptors, recognize the antigen as foreign; this activates the release of powerful chemical mediators, which cause an increase in vascular permeability, bronchoconstriction, urticaria, and hypotension
- Substances that most commonly cause anaphylaxis include foods; certain medications, such as antibiotics, radiocontrast dyes, and anesthetic agents; insect stings; and latex
- Some cases have no identifiable cause.

### Signs and Symptoms

- Signs and symptoms range from mild to severe
- A mild reaction consists of peripheral tingling, a sensation of warmth, a feeling of fullness in the throat, pruritus, nasal congestion, and tearing; the reaction occurs within 2 hours of exposure
- A moderate reaction includes more pronounced flushing, warmth, anxiety, and itching
- A severe reaction typically occurs immediately after exposure
  - Signs and symptoms include complaints of a feeling of impending doom or fright and a display of apprehension and restlessness
  - The patient develops cyanosis; cool, clammy skin; erythema; edema; tachypnea; weakness; sweating; sneezing; dyspnea; nasal pruritus; and urticaria
  - The patient feels a 'lump' in his throat, has difficulty swallowing, and complains of chest tightness
  - The reaction can progress to shock and cardiac arrest

### Diagnosis and Treatment

- Diagnosis is based on the patient's history and signs and symptoms
- Skin testing can identify a specific allergen
- Treatment aims to control the patient's reaction
- A patent airway must be maintained, using endotracheal intubation or a tracheotomy, if necessary
- The patient may require immediate administration of epinephrine 1:1,000 aqueous solution, 0.3 to 0.5 mL given subcutaneously every 20 to 30 minutes for up to three doses, or 5 mL of a 1:10,000 solution given by slow IV infusion every 5 to 10 minutes as needed; if IV administration is not possible, endotracheal or intraosseous administration may be used
- Drug treatment may also include corticosteroids, such as hydrocortisone, prednisone, and methylprednisolone, and diphenhydramine (Benadryl) given IV, IM, or by mouth
- The patient may also need oxygen therapy and cardiovascular support with fluids and pressors.

### Nursing Interventions

- Provide supplemental oxygen, and prepare to assist with insertion of an endotracheal tube, if necessary
- Insert a peripheral IV line and maintain patent IV access if necessary
- Continually reassure the patient, and explain all tests and treatments
- If the patient undergoes skin or scratch testing, monitor him for signs of a serious allergic response; keep emergency resuscitation equipment readily available
- Administer prescribed drugs; be aware that epinephrine is considered a first-line agent for treatment
- Give inhaled beta-2 agonists as ordered, typically 10 mg/hour via continuous nebulization or 25 mg every 15 to 20 minutes via nebulization
- Expect to administer oral antihistamines and steroids for 72 hours
- Monitor the patient's vital signs and respiratory status, and note his response to treatment
- If a specific allergen is identified, teach the patient and family about the type of allergy or allergen responsible for the patient's signs and symptoms
- Teach the patient and family about the signs and symptoms of a reaction and the importance of carrying and becoming familiar with an anaphylaxis kit; make sure they learn how to use the kit before the need arises, and teach them about the need for medical identification jewellery to identify the allergy.

## Rheumatoid Arthritis

### Description

- Rheumatoid arthritis is a chronic, systemic inflammatory disease that affects the small joints of the hands and wrists and the surrounding muscles, tendons, ligaments, and blood vessels; it may progress to other joints and body tissues, including the heart, lungs, kidneys, and skin
- This autoimmune disease has no known cause; it affects three times as many women as men between ages 30 and 50 and becomes more evident during the winter.

### Signs and Symptoms

- Edema and stiffness may affect one or more joints, symmetrically and bilaterally, especially on arising and in the morning
- Other signs and symptoms may include malaise; fever; anemia; rheumatoid nodules near joints; dull, aching joint pain; and joint deformity
- Rheumatoid arthritis may be associated with pericarditis and pneumonitis

### Diagnosis and Treatment

- Diagnosis is based on patient history, physical examination, and serologic blood tests, including rheumatoid factor, CBC, erythrocyte sedimentation rate (ESR), serum complement, and C-reactive protein; 75% to 80% of patients with a positive rheumatoid factors test have the disease
- Other diagnostic tests may include immunologic studies, synovial biopsy, X-rays, and magnetic resonance imaging
- Treatment aims to reduce inflammation and maintain or increase joint mobility
- Affected joints are rested, and splints may be used to help maintain functional positions

- Physical therapy exercises are recommended to maintain joint motion
- A paraffin 'glove' may be applied to the affected joints; the patient dips his hands into melted paraffin to form a 1/8″-thick glove, which draws blood to the areas to resolve the inflammation
- Use of ice or cold compresses alternating with the paraffin glove reduces edema and inflammation
- Disease-modifying anti-rheumatic drugs (DMARDs) slow the progression of rheumatoid arthritis (RA) and decrease the risk of permanent damage to the joints and surrounding tissue; DMARDS include methotrexate, sulfasalazine (Azulfidine), and minocycline (Arestin)
- Immunosuppressants act to suppress the immune system; they include azathioprine (Azasan), and cyclosporine (Gengraf)
- Tumor necrosis factor alpha inhibitors, used to inhibit the inflammatory response, include etanercept (Enbrel), infliximab (Remicade), and adalimumab (Humira)
- Various anti-inflammatories are prescribed: salicylates (primarily aspirin), low-dose steroids (primarily prednisone), and nonsteroidal anti-inflammatory drugs (NSAIDs), including ibuprofen, naproxen, flurbiprofen, indomethacin, sulindac, tolmetin, piroxicam, diclofenac and misoprostol may be given to prevent NSAID-induced gastric ulcers
- Gold compounds also may be prescribed to reduce inflammation; opioid analgesics may be used to relieve pain; antimalarials (primarily chloroquine and hydroxychloroquine), immunosuppressants (such as azathioprine), and cytotoxic agents (such as methotrexate) may be used to decrease synovial inflammation; and sulfasalazine may be used to reduce inflammation in patients who have responded inadequately to salicylates or NSAIDs
- Surgical interventions include joint repair or prosthetic replacement and synovectomy (removal of the synovium)
- Lymphapheresis or plasmapheresis may be used for some patients.

### *Nursing Interventions*

- Explain the treatment regimen and the involvement of each member of the health care team to the patient
- Administer drugs as prescribed, and monitor for therapeutic and adverse reactions; drug therapy may need to be changed if adverse reactions are intolerable or therapeutic effects do not occur
- Monitor the patient for relief of pain, stiffness, and soreness; patients have periods of remission and 'flare' when symptoms increase
- Help the patient with self-care, including ROM exercises, splint application, and ambulatory aid use
- Provide modified utensils and equipment suggested by the occupational therapist to help to conserve small-joint and muscle function
- Provide rest periods in the morning and evening, with the patient lying supine in bed to maintain strength while preventing flexion contractures; teach the patient not to overexert
- Provide a quiet environment for night-time sleep; patients with acute rheumatoid arthritis require 8 to 10 hours of sleep
- Discuss home maintenance activities recommended by the occupational therapist to ensure that the patient understands the needed changes
- Prepare the patient for surgery if indicated
- Provide postoperative care appropriate for the surgery
- Encourage compliance with treatments to achieve optimal results
- Teach the patient about medications and adverse effects, activity restrictions, rest periods, and relaxation techniques
- Encourage the patient to verbalize concerns about body image and changes in quality of life.

## EYE, EAR AND NOSE DISORDERS

### Introduction

- Disorders of the eye, ear and nose can be particularly disruptive to activities of daily living (ADLs)
- Full visual function requires normal brain function, an intact retina, a clear lens, and normal intraocular pressure
- Common vision disorders result from alterations in acuity, trauma, and high intraocular pressure; patients with impaired vision are frightened and anxious and require special nursing care
- Hearing loss is a common disability that affects millions of people and causes significant alterations in ADLs; sclerotic disorders and vestibular dysfunction can be especially upsetting
- Although the nose is the primary organ of smell, nasal disorders can affect taste and the smooth passage of air during respirations.

### *Nursing history*

- The nurse asks the patient about his *chief complaint*
  - A patient with an eye disorder may report having diplopia, visual floaters, iridescent vision, vision loss, eye pain, or photophobia
  - The patient may also report decreased visual acuity or clarity, defects in color vision, and difficulty seeing at night
  - A patient with an ear disorder may experience hearing loss, tinnitus, pain, discharge, or dizziness
  - A patient with a nose disorder may experience nasal stuffiness, nasal discharge, or epistaxis
- The nurse then questions the patient about his *present illness*
  - Ask the patient about his symptoms, includes—associated symptoms, location, radiation, intensity, duration, frequency, and precipitating and alleviating factors
  - Ask about the use of glasses or contact lenses
  - Ask about the use of prescription and over-the-counter (OTC) drugs, herbal remedies, and vitamin and nutritional supplements

- The nurse asks about the *medical history*
  - Question the patient about a history of allergies, hypertension, diabetes, cerebrovascular accident, multiple sclerosis, syphilis, human immunodeficiency virus, or sleep apnea
  - Ask about corrective eye surgery
  - Ask the patient about previous ear problems or injuries, frequent colds, hay fever, headaches, nose or head trauma, and sinus trouble
- The nurse then assesses the *family history*
  - Ask about a family history of eye disorders, such as cataracts, glaucoma, or blindness
  - Question the patient about a family history of diabetes and hypertension
  - Question the patient about a family history of eye, ear, and nose problems
- The nurse obtains a *social history*
  - Ask about work, exercise, diet, use of recreational drugs and alcohol, and hobbies
  - Also ask about stress, support systems, and coping mechanisms
  - Question the patient about exposure to chemicals, flying debris, noise, fumes, or infectious agents; ask about the use of protective eyewear
  - Ask the visually impaired patient how well he can manage ADLs.

### Physical Assessment

- Nurse begins with *inspection*
  - Observe the patient's eye movements and ability to focus
  - Note the appearance of the eyelids, eyeballs, and lacrimal apparatus
  - Examine the conjunctiva, sclera, iris, anterior chamber, and cornea
  - Check both pupils for equality of size and shape, pupillary reaction to light, and accommodation
  - Test visual acuity using a Snellen chart and near-vision chart
  - Test extraocular muscles by assessing the corneal light reflex and cardinal positions of gaze
  - Examine intraocular structures using an ophthalmoscope
  - Observe the ears for position and symmetry; inspect the auricles for lesions, nodules, or redness; check the ear canal for hair, foreign bodies, and cerumen
  - Examine the auditory canal, tympanic membrane, and malleus with an otoscope
  - Assess hearing using Weber's and Rinne's tests and pure tone audiometry
  - Observe the nose for position, symmetry, swelling, deformity, and color; note any nasal discharge or flaring
  - Inspect the nasal cavity for septal deviation or perforation; examine the vestibule and turbinates for redness, softness, and discharge
  - Assess the patient's sense of smell
  - Examine the nostrils using a nasal speculum; note color, patency, and the presence of exudate
- Next, the nurse uses *palpation*
  - Gently palpate the eyelids, noting any swelling or complaints of tenderness; eyeballs should feel equally firm, but not hard or rigid
  - Palpate the lacrimal sac while observing the punctum for excessive tearing or drainage
  - Palpate the mastoid area and ear for tenderness, redness, or warmth
  - Palpate the nose for pain, tenderness, swelling, and deformity
  - Palpate the sinuses for tenderness.

## Age-related Macular Degeneration

### Description

- Age-related macular degeneration (AMD) is characterized by small clusters of yellowish debris (called drusen) beneath the retina
- When drusen are located in the macular area, they cause visual loss
- Central vision is most often affected
- Two types of AMD exist: dry type and wet type
  - *Dry type AMD* is nonexudative and is responsible for 85% to 90% of cases; in this type of AMD, the outer layers of the retina slowly break down
  - *Wet type AMD* is exudative and may have an abrupt onset; symptoms result from the proliferation of abnormal vessels under the retina
- Although the cause of AMD is unknown, genetic factors may contribute to its development
- AMD is the most common cause of visual loss in people age 60 and older.

### Signs and Symptoms

- In dry type AMD, drusen can be seen beneath the retina; atrophy of the retinal pigment epithelium also occurs
- In wet type AMD, the patient has subretinal fluid accumulation or hemorrhage with a yellow-green discoloration, i.e. sometimes surrounded by a pigment ring; in the advanced stage, exudates and fibrovascular scarring occur
- Grayness, haziness, or a blind spot may appear in the area of central vision; words may look blurred on a page, straight lines may appear to have kinks in them, and colors may seem dimmer
- The disorder may also cause difficulty with night vision and changing light conditions.

### Diagnosis and Treatment

- Indirect ophthalmoscopy may show changes in the macular region of the fundus
- The Amsler grid test may detect visual distortion
- Fluorescein angiography may show leaking vessels (choroidal neovascular membranes) in the subretinal neovascular net
- Indocyanine green videoangiography identifies hidden or occult choroidal neovascular membranes
- Optical coherence tomography may help to identify choroidal neovascular membranes, subretinal fluid, and retinal thickening

- Although no known cure exists for dry type AMD, some evidence indicates that a diet high in betacarotene, zinc, and vitamins A, C, and E may slow the progression of the disease
- For wet type AMD, treatment targets the development and progression of angiogenesis; laser treatments may be used
- Drug therapy may include a vascular endothelial growth factor antagonist or the monoclonal antibody bevacizumab (Avastin)
- Vitrectomy removes subretinal blood
- Macular translocation shifts the macula away from the choroidal neovascular membranes
- Photodynamic therapy may also be helpful.

### *Nursing Interventions*

- Teach the patient and family about the disorder, including treatment and follow-up care
- Determine the extent of the patient's vision loss
- Help the patient obtain optical aids such as magnifiers
- Assist the patient with adaptations to accommodate his vision changes; promote safely
- Encourage the patient to increase his consumption of vitamins A, C, and E as well as beta-carotene and zinc
- Urge the patient to use eye protection such as glasses or sunglasses that block ultraviolet light to protect his eyes from ultraviolet light
- Offer emotional support
- Encourage the patient to express his fears and concerns, especially those related to vision loss and its impact on his ability to function
- Refer the patient to local support organizations as appropriate.

## Cataracts

### *Description*

- Cataracts, which come in several forms, cause a loss of transparency of the lens of the eye or its capsule
- It is a common cause of gradual vision loss that usually affects both eyes.

### *Signs and Symptoms*

- Gradual painless blurring eventually leads to poor reading vision, reduced vision at night and in bright sunlight, and vision loss
- Other effects may include halos around lights, milky pupils, and unpleasant glares.

### *Diagnosis and Treatment*

- Indirect ophthalmoscopy or slit-lamp examination confirms the diagnosis
- Cataracts are treated surgically by extracapsular extraction, which removes the anterior capsule and its contents; intracapsular extraction, which removes the entire lens in the capsule; or phacoemulsification, which uses ultrasonic vibration to fragment the lens
- Corrective lenses may be prescribed to improve vision
  - A plastic intraocular lens implant may be inserted in the eye as part of the surgical procedure
  - Cataract glasses (glasses with magnifying lenses) or contact lenses may be prescribed 6 to 8 weeks after surgery.

### *Types of Cataracts*

These are several form of cataracts. They occur at various point in the life cycle, but the treatment for each is the same.

| Types of cataract | Description |
|---|---|
| Complicated | Develop as secondary effect in patients with uvettis, glaucoma, retinitis pigmentosa, or retinal detachment or with systemic disease such as diabetes, hypoparthyroidism or atopic dermatitis also develop after exposure to ionizing radiation or infrared rays. |
| Congenital | Develop in utero at the anterior or posterior ocular pole associated with heredity or maternal rubella infection in the first trimester |
| Senile | Occur after age 50 as part of aging the nuclear portion of the lens become increasingly dense transparency decrease and light rays strike the opaque lens and scatter |
| Toxic | Result from drug or chemical toxicity with dinitrophenol ergot naphthalene or phenothiazines |
| Traumatic | Can occur at any age and are caused by mechanical trauma or exposure to chemicals radiation or toxic substances the capsule ruptures, swelling occurs, and opacity increased, usually unilateral |

### *Preoperative Nursing Interventions*

- Explain the importance of compliance in a preadmission interview
- Make sure that someone can drive the patient to and from the day surgery center
- Tell the patient to tilt his head backward when shampooing to prevent jarring the eye and increasing intraocular pressure.
- Administer a preoperative laxative to prevent straining during defecation, which increases intraocular pressure
- Explain preoperative and postoperative care to decrease the patient's anxiety
- Answer questions and encourage the patient to discuss concerns.

### *Postoperative Nursing Interventions*

- Review postoperative instructions to improve compliance and prevent complications; the patient may have difficulty reading instructions because of impaired vision
- Tell the patient not to bend, strain, lift, cough, sneeze, or rub the eye postoperatively; these actions can increase intraocular pressure, which can lead to complications, such as bleeding, vitreous herniation, vision loss, pain, and wound dehiscence; rubbing also increases the chance of infection
- Tell the patient not to make quick movements or read, which could irritate the patched eye or dislodge an implanted lens

- Teach the patient or family member how to administer eye medications properly; tell the patient to avoid using OTC eyedrops
- Teach the patient how to clean the eye to prevent infection
- Have the patient wear an eye shield and patch to protect the eye from injury; tell him to keep the eye patch dry and to wear an eye shield while sleeping
- Tell the patient to call the practitioner if any of these signs or symptoms occur: eye pain that is not relieved with analgesics, yellow or green discharge, temperature above 100°F (37.8°C), blurred vision, nausea and vomiting, and seeing halos around lights.
- Explain postoperative activity restrictions
  - The patient may walk, climb stairs, watch television, and perform ADLs but should avoid engaging in strenuous physical activity and lifting more than 10 lb (4.5 kg)
  - The patient may bathe or shower but should avoid getting water on the eye patch by tilting his head back when shampooing
  - The patient should avoid bending from the waist and hanging the head forward; a long-handled grabber may be used to pick up objects
- Make sure the patient is cared for by a family member or friend after surgery
- Advise the patient to refrain from sexual activity until he receives his practitioner's approval.

## Glaucoma

### Description

- This group of disorders is characterized by high intraocular pressure (IOP) and optic nerve damage that affects peripheral vision
- There are two main forms of glaucoma:
  - *Open-angle* (also known as *chronic, simple,* or *wide angle*) glaucoma begins insidiously and progresses slowly
  - *Angle-closure* (also known as *acute* or *narrow angle*) glaucoma occurs suddenly and can cause permanent vision loss in 48 to 72 hours.

### Signs and Symptoms

- Open-angle glaucoma may cause no symptoms, or it may cause a dull morning headache, mild aching in the eyes, loss of peripheral vision, halos around lights, and reduced visual acuity (especially at night), i.e. uncorrected by glasses
- Angle-closure glaucoma causes the rapid onset of pain and pressure over the eye, blurred vision, decreased visual acuity, halos around lights, and nausea and vomiting.

### Diagnosis and Treatment

- Tonometry measurements reveal increased IOP; perimetry or visual field tests measure loss of peripheral vision
- Ophthalmoscopy shows the effects of glaucoma on the optic disk (called cupping), whereas gonioscopy measures the angle of the anterior chamber of the eye
- Other diagnostic tests may include slit-lamp examination and fundus photography
- Drugs that may be used to treat glaucoma include topical adrenergic agonists, cholinergic agonists, beta-adrenergic blockers, and topical or oral carbonic anhydrase inhibitors that reduce IOP by decreasing the production of aqueous humor
- Surgery or laser treatments may be peformed for patients who are unresponsive to drug therapy
- Bed rest is recommended for patients with acute angle-closure glaucoma.

### Nursing Interventions

- Encourage patient compliance by teaching the patient about the disease process and treatment
- Postoperatively, give medications, as ordered, to dilate the pupil and topical corticosteroids to rest the pupil and protect the affected eye
- Administer pain medication, antiemetics, and stool softeners, as ordered
- Encourage the patient to be ambulatory immediately after surgery
- Teach the patient to avoid activities that can increase IOP such as straining during bowel movements.

## Otitis Externa

### Description

- Otitis externa is an acute or chronic inflammation of the external auditory canal
- Causes include water in the ear canal (swimmer's ear), trauma to the skin of the ear and resulting infection, vitamin deficiencies, and endocrine disorders such as diabetes mellitus
- *Staphylococcus aureus* and *Pseudomonas* are the most common types of bacteria that cause otitis externa. *Aspergillus* is the most common fungus that causes the disorder
- Risk factors include swimming in contaminated water, cleaning the ear canal with cotton-tipped applicators, using ear phones or ear plugs, and chronic drainage from a perforated tympanic membrane.

### Signs and Symptoms

- Signs and symptoms include mild to severe ear itching or pain, i.e. aggravated by jaw motion, teeth clenching, opening the mouth, or chewing
- Other signs and symptoms include a feeling of the ear being plugged; a swollen, inflamed ear canal; foul-smelling, yellow-to-green ear discharge; thick, red epithelium in ear canal (in chronic otitis externa); and periauricular adenitis
- Fungal otitis externa may not produce any symptoms.

### Diagnosis and Treatment

- Microscopic examination reveals the causative organism
- Audiometric testing may reveal a partial hearing loss
- Otoscopy shows a swollen external ear canal, periauricular lymphadenopathy and, occasionally, regional cellulitis
- Treatment includes cleaning debris from the ear canal under direct visualization

- With mild, chronic otitis externa, the patient may need specially fitted earplugs for showering or swimming
- Analgesics help to control pain
- Other medications include antibiotic/corticosteroid eardrops, such as neomycin/polymyxin B/hydrocortisone, betamethasone, ciprofloxacin/dexamethasone, and gentamicin/betamethasone; antifungal eardrops include clotrimazole
- If the patient has lymphadenopathy or a severe infection, he may need oral antibiotics
- Excision and abscess drainage is performed as needed.

### Nursing Interventions

- Clean and dry the patient's ear gently and thoroughly
- Use wet soaks on infected skin
- Give prescribed drugs; use a foam or gauze wick, as indicated, to administer otic medications
- To prevent recurrence, tell the patient to avoid potential irritants, such as hair care products and earrings
- Tell the patient to wear earplugs or to keep his head above water when swimming and to instill two or three drops of 42% acetic acid solution in 70% alcohol (diluted 50/50) into the ears after swimming to toughen the skin of the external ear canal
- Warn against cleaning the ears with cotton-tipped applicators or other objects.

## Otitis Media

### Description

- Otitis media is an inflammation of the middle ear associated with fluid accumulation; it most commonly results from poorly functioning eustachian tubes
- The disorder may be acute, chronic, serous, or suppurative
  - Acute otitis media occurs when a bacterial or viral infection of the fluid of the middle ear occurs, which causes production of fluid or pus
  - Chronic otitis media occurs when the eustachian tube becomes blocked repeatedly due to allergies, multiple infections, ear trauma, or swelling of the adenoids
  - Chronic serous otitis media is a middle ear infection with effusion without perforation
  - Chronic suppurative otitis media is a perforated tympanic membrane with persistent drainage from the middle ear
- The pathogens that most commonly cause otitis media include *Streptococcus pneumoniae, Haemophilus Influenzae,* and *Moraxella catarrhalis*
- Complications of otitis media include rupture of the tympanic membrane, hearing loss, vertigo, meningitis, and septicemia.

### Signs and Symptoms

- Otitis media causes severe, deep, throbbing pain in the ear along with fever, dizziness, nausea, and vomiting
- The patient may also experience a sensation of fullness in the ear as well as popping or crackling sounds when swallowing or chewing
- Other signs and symptoms may include purulent discharge from the ear, evidence of hearing loss and, if tympanic membrane ruptures, pain that abruptly ceases.

### Diagnosis and Treatment

- The patient's history may include upper respiratory infection or allergies
- Otoscopic examination shows fluid behind the tympanic membrane; in chronic otitis media, it reveals thickening or scarring of the tissue
- Culture and sensitivity testing of the exudate shows the causative organism
- A complete blood count shows leukocytosis (if acute otitis media results from bacteria)
- Radiographic studies demonstrate mastoid involvement
- In acute secretory otitis media, Valsalva's maneuver performed several times a day may be the only treatment required
- Treatment aims to eradicate the underlying cause–for instance, eliminating eustachian tube obstruction
- Medications include antibiotics; first-line agents include amoxicillin or, if the patient is allergic to penicillin, azithromycin; second-line agents include cefdinir, cefpodoxime, cefuroxime, amoxicillinclavulanate, ceftriaxone, clarithromycin, erythromycin and trimethoprim-sulfamethoxazole
- Analgesics and antipyretics include acetaminophen; analgesic eardrops include antipyrine/benzocaine
- Surgical procedures include myringotomy and aspiration of middle ear fluid, followed by insertion of a polyethylene tube into the tympanic membrane
- Other procedures may include myringoplasty, tympanoplasty, and mastoidectomy.

### Nursing Interventions

- Teach the patient and his family about the disorder, including treatment and follow-up care
- Administer analgesics, antipyretics, and antibiotics as ordered; institute measures to reduce fever
- Allow the patient and his family to verbalize their feelings and concerns; answer all questions and provide emotional support
- When appropriate, offer reassurance that hearing loss caused by serous otitis media is temporary
- Provide clear, concise explanations
- Prepare the patient and his family for possible surgery; provide appropriate postoperative care
- Teach the patient how to recognize upper respiratory tract infections, and encourage early treatment
- If appropriate, teach the patient to promote eustachian tube patency by performing Valsalva's maneuver several times a day, especially during airplane travel
- After tympanoplasty, advise the patient not to blow his nose or get his ear wet when bathing.

## Otosclerosis

### Description

- Otosclerosis (or hardening of the ear) is an overgrowth of bone that impedes normal ossicular motion and can fix the stapes to the oval window

- It is the most common cause of progressive conductive hearing loss in adults with normal tympanic membranes
- The disease has a familial tendency and usually occurs between ages 15 and 50; twice as many women are affected as men
- Pregnancy may trigger the onset in women.

### Signs and Symptoms

- Progressive hearing loss, which may be unilateral at first and may become bilateral, typically begins at an early age
- Vertigo also can occur
- The patient may report hearing his own voice better than the voices of others.

### Diagnosis and Treatment

- Diagnostic tests may include audiometry; electronystagmography; caloric testing; magnetic resonance imaging or computed tomography; Weber's, Rinne's, and Romberg's tests; and facial nerve testing
- Hearing aids are recommended to improve hearing
- Stapedectomy (surgical removal of the stapes) may be done, and the stapes may be replaced by a prosthesis; complications of this procedure, which is typically performed under local anesthesia, include continued hearing loss, granuloma, oval window rupture that causes perilymph fistula, inflammation, infection, prosthesis displacement, and temporary taste changes.

### Preoperative Nursing Interventions

- Use alternative communication methods as needed; a patient with severe hearing loss may need written instructions or a signing oral interpreter
- Discuss preoperative tests and postoperative care to reduce anxiety and promote compliance
- Encourage the patient to discuss anxieties and expectations; clarify misconceptions, and inform him that his hearing won't improve until 6 weeks after surgery because of edema and packing.

### Postoperative Nursing Interventions

- Elevate the head of the patient's bed 30 degrees; position him according to the practitioner's orders on the unaffected side to prevent graft displacement or on the affected side to facilitate drainage
- Monitor vital signs, and check dressings for bleeding; attempt to quantify bleeding
- Check for headache, stiff neck, fever, and vertigo, which are signs and symptoms of complications
- Observe the patient for edema, meningitis, labyrinthitis, and infection
- Keep dressings intact; when removed, observe the site for bleeding, redness, drainage, and edema
- Clean the suture line as directed; use aseptic technique to prevent infection, and watch for signs of infection
- Keep packing intact; it is absorbable, and it should not be removed
- Assess facial nerve functioning twice daily to detect nerve compromise
- Administer pain medications, as needed, to allow the patient to participate in care
- Help the patient get out of bed to prevent falls
- Remind the patient to avoid rapid head movements, which can cause the dizziness that commonly occurs after surgery
- Tell the patient not to blow his nose and to keep his mouth wide open when coughing or sneezing; Valsalva's maneuver can displace the graft over the oval window and could introduce bacteria to the middle ear by way of the eustachian tube.

### Discharge Nursing Interventions

- Provide written instructions to increase compliance
- Tell the patient to avoid strenuous activity for 1 to 3 weeks but to return to work after 1 week as prescribed; strenuous activity can result in perilymph fistula and may dislodge the prosthesis
- Instruct the patient to keep the ear dry for 6 weeks; he can shampoo his hair after 1 week; to avoid getting water in the affected ear while bathing, he should plug the ear with a cotton ball coated with petroleum jelly
- Tell the patient not to travel by air for 2 to 3 weeks to prevent barotrauma
- Tell the patient to avoid people with colds or upper respiratory tract infections for 4 to 6 weeks; these infections can spread to the middle ear by way of the eustachian tube
- Instruct the patient to report drainage, fever, otalgia (ear pain), vertigo, redness, and tenderness of the incision site
- Tell the patient to change the cotton ball covering the ear canal daily and as needed but not to disturb the packing in the ear canal
- Show the patient how to perform daily incision care.

## Retinal Detachment

### Description

- Retinal detachment is the separation of the sensory layers of the retina from the underlying retinal pigment epithelium; without treatment, the entire retina may detach, causing severe vision impairment and possible blindness
- It may be caused by degenerative changes in the retina or vitreous gel, intraocular inflammation, or mechanical trauma
- In this disorder, vitreous body traction causes retinal tears or holes, which allow vitreous fluid to leak behind the retina and cause it to separate
- Retinal detachment may be primary or secondary; a primary detachment occurs spontaneously due to a change in the retina or vitreous; a secondary detachment results from another problem, such as inflammation or trauma.

### Signs and Symptoms

- Signs and symptoms may occur slowly or suddenly
- They may include dark or irregular vitreous floaters, flashes of light, and progressive loss of vision in one area (as though a curtain is being pulled before the eye).

***Diagnosis and Treatment***

- Diagnosis depends on ophthalmoscopy (both direct and indirect) after full pupil dilation; fluorescein angiography, visual field examination, and ultrasonography may also be useful
- Treatment requires bed rest, with the affected eye patched and the patient's head positioned so that the retinal hole is at the lowest point of the eye
- One of several types of surgery may be performed to find and seal retinal holes or tears
  - *Diathermy* uses extreme heat to seal the hole
  - *Laser photocoagulation* uses laser-generated heat to injure the tissue and cause scars, which create a fibrous adhesion to seal the hole
  - *Cryotherapy* uses nitrous oxide (also known as laughing gas) or carbon dioxide to injure the tissue by freezing it; the injury leaves a scar, which seals the retinal hole
  - *Scleral buckling* places a band around the globe of the eye to bring the choroid into contact with the retina and hold it in place until adhesion occurs.

***Preoperative Nursing Interventions***

- Place the patient on bed rest, patch the eye as prescribed, and position the patient's head so that the retinal tear or hole is at the lowest point of the eye (if the detachment is toward the outer side of the head, have the patient lie on the affected side with the bed flat); these interventions help prevent further detachment
- Provide emotional support to the patient who may be distraught at the potential loss of vision
- Prepare the patient for surgery by cleaning his face and giving him antibiotics and eyedrops, as ordered
- Teach the patient about the role of the retina and why floaters, flashes of light, and decreased vision occur
- Allow the patient and family to discuss their concerns
- Explain the preoperative routines and the surgical procedure.

***Postoperative Nursing Interventions***

- Position the patient as directed; the position varies according to the surgical procedure
- Tell the patient to avoid activities that increase IOP, such as sneezing, coughing, vomiting, lifting, straining during defecation, bending from the waist, and rapidly moving the head; increased IOP may cause more fluid to flow behind the retina before healing is complete
- Administer eyedrops, antiemetics, analgesics, and antibiotics, as ordered; to reduce corneal edema and discomfort, apply ice packs as ordered
- Tell the patient to notify the practitioner if he experiences floaters, flashes of light, blurred vision, or pain that is not relieved with analgesics; these symptoms indicate recurrence of detachment
- Teach the patient to recognize and report the signs and symptoms of infection, such as temperature above 100°F (37.8°C), yellow or green discharge, increased redness or pulling of the eye or lid, and vision loss
- Show the patient how to administer eye medications and change dressings using sterile technique to decrease the risk of infection
- Tell the patient to wear the eye shield at night or when napping to prevent accidental injury to the eye
- Discuss when the patient can return to work, resume ADLs, and drive or perform strenuous activities.

## MULTIPLE CHOICE QUESTIONS

**1. The registered nurse has an unlicensed assistant working with her for the shift. When delegating tasks, the nurse understands that the unlicensed assistant:**
(a) Interprets clinical data
(b) Collects clinical data
(c) Is trained in the nursing process
(d) Can function independently

**2. When performing an assessment, the nurse identifies the following signs and symptoms: impaired coordination, decreased muscle strength, limited range of motion, and reluctance to move. These signs and symptoms indicate which nursing diagnosis?**
(a) Health-seeking behaviors
(b) Impaired physical mobility
(c) Disturbed sensory perception
(d) Deficient knowledge

**3. When prioritizing a patient's care plan based on Maslow's hierarchy of needs, the nurse's first priority would be:**
(a) Allowing the family to see a newly admitted patient
(b) Ambulating the patient in the hallway
(c) Administering pain medication
(d) Using two nurses to transfer the patient

**4. When a nurse asks another nurse for advice on handling a particular patient problem, she is seeking what type of consultation?**
(a) Patient-centered case consultation
(b) Consultee-centered case consultation
(c) Program-centered administrative consultation
(d) Consultee-centered administrative consultation

**5. When implementing an evidence-based nursing program to decrease the incidence of pressure ulcers on a medical-surgical unit, which of the following is the most important to ensure its success?**
(a) Obtaining support from management, administration, and physicians
(b) Determining and documenting patient outcomes
(c) Identifying a significant problem that needs to be addressed
(d) Evaluating research based on its validity and reliability

6. **When planning the implementation of evidence-based practices to prevent falls, which of the following steps should the nurse take first?**
(a) Identify the common causes of falls
(b) Gather and review currently existing literature and guidelines for the prevention of falls
(c) Identify fall prevention practices that are applicable to the patient care setting
(d) Gather data to identify the effectiveness of the new practice guidelines

7. **Which measure most effectively reduces the risk of health care–associated infections?**
(a) Keeping employee health records up-to-date
(b) Performing hand hygiene
(c) Providing annual influenza vaccinations
(d) Always wearing a mask when caring for patients

8. **Which action should the nurse take when receiving a telephone order from a physician?**
(a) Inform the physician that telephone orders are not permitted
(b) Write the order in the patient's medical record immediately
(c) Write down the order and then read back the complete order to the physician
(d) Immediately carry out the order

9. **A secondary latency phase that occurs in some diseases that is commonly followed by another acute phase is referred to as:**
(a) Remission
(b) Convalescence
(c) The acute phase
(d) The subclinical acute phase

10. **Qualitative research emphasizes developing new insights, theories, and knowledge. Which term in qualitative research describes the researcher laying aside what is known about the experience being studied?**
(a) Bracketing (b) Saturation
(c) Intuiting (d) Theoretical sampling

11. **The nurse leaves a patient who is elderly and confused to find someone to assist with transferring the patient to bed. While the nurse is gone, the patient falls and hurts herself. The nurse is at fault because she has not:**
(a) Properly educated the patient about safety measures
(b) Restrained the patient
(c) Documented that she left the patient
(d) Arranged for continual care of the patient

12. **The nurse is caring for a patient admitted to the emergency department after a motor vehicle accident. Under the law, the nurse must obtain informed consent before treatment unless the patient:**
(a) Is mentally ill
(b) Refuses to give informed consent
(c) Is in an emergency situation
(d) Asks the nurse to give substituted consent

13. **Which of the following acts committed by a nurse is an intentional tort?**
(a) Battery
(b) Breach of confidentiality
(c) Negligence
(d) Abandonment

14. **OSHA is responsible for:**
(a) Compensating workers injured in the workplace
(b) Providing rehabilitation for workers injured in the workplace
(c) Inspecting high-hazard workplaces for compliance with protective standards
(d) Disciplining workers injured in the workplace

15. **A patient became seriously ill after a nurse gave him the wrong medication. After his recovery, he filed a lawsuit. Who is most likely to be held liable?**
(a) No one because it was an accident
(b) The hospital
(c) The nurse
(d) The nurse and the hospital

16. **Which of the following is incorrect about informed consent?**
(a) It can be revoked by the state, especially when the benefits outweigh the risks
(b) A person has to be mentally competent to sign an informed consent
(c) Physicians can waive informed consents in emergency situations
(d) The name of the procedure, its risks and benefits and other alternative procedures make up all the essential elements of informed consent

17. **Which of the following is considered identifiable health information?**
(a) A photograph of a patient's leg showing a unique tattoo
(b) A patient's chart listing his history of a stroke last year
(c) A blank menu for a regular diet on the patient's over-bed table
(d) A laboratory report with the patient's name, address, social security number, date of birth, and room number deleted

18. **In a negligence suit against a nurse, what must the plaintiff prove?**
(a) The nurse intended to cause harm
(b) The nurse's actions caused harm
(c) The nurse knew she caused harm
(d) The nurse was sorry for causing harm

19. **A nurse failed to administer a medication to a patient according to accepted standards. Consequently, the patient suffered adverse effects. Failure to provide patient care and to follow appropriate standards is called:**
(a) Breach of duty
(b) Breach of contract
(c) Battery
(d) Tort

**20. The belief that one's own cultural values and beliefs are superior or the only correct values and beliefs is:**
(a) Cultural competency
(b) Cultural diversity
(c) Ethnocentrism
(d) Cultural sensitivity

**21. The nurse is assessing pain in a patient with appendicitis. Which initial statement or question will be most effective in eliciting information?**
(a) 'Tell me how you feel'
(b) 'Point to where you are feeling pain'
(c) 'Does your pain medication relieve your pain?'
(d) 'Coughing makes your pain worse, does not it?'

**22. When performing an abdominal assessment, the nurse should follow which examination sequence?**
(a) Auscultation, inspection, percussion, palpation
(b) Inspection, auscultation, percussion, palpation
(c) Palpation, auscultation, percussion, inspection
(d) Percussion, palpation, auscultation, inspection

**23. To maintain a therapeutic environment with a patient and his family, the nurse can use communication techniques such as clarification. An example of clarification is:**
(a) 'How is it going?'
(b) 'You say you are not concerned, but you have asked me many questions on this same subject.'
(c) 'What do you mean when you say…?'
(d) 'For now, I would like to concentrate on…'

**24. In the stages of death and dying as defined by Elizabeth Kübler-Ross, loss, grief and intense sadness are symptoms of:**
(a) Depression
(b) Denial
(c) Anger
(d) Acceptance

**25. In the levels of basic human needs as defined by Abraham Maslow, which of the following levels is most basic?**
(a) Physiologic
(b) Safety and security
(c) Love, affection, and belonging
(d) Esteem

**26. According to the stages of development, what conflict does the older adult experience?**
(a) Intimacy versus isolation
(b) Generativity versus stagnation
(c) Identity versus role confusion
(d) Integrity versus despair

**27. The nurse is caring for a patient who has just been diagnosed with a terminal illness. The patient says to her, 'I cannot believe this! I feel…' and pauses. The nurse allows the patient time to gather his thoughts. What type of therapeutic communication is this?**
(a) Clarification
(b) Empathy
(c) Reflection
(d) Silence

**28. A patient becomes angry attending a treatment group and complains about it to the nurse. Which response could the nurse give that would best demonstrate clarification?**
(a) 'Can you tell me what about the treatment group made you angry?'
(b) 'Why are you upset? Attending the treatment group will help you get well.'
(c) 'It sounds like group today was pretty upsetting.'
(d) 'Treatment groups have been carefully planned by the staff to help patients.'

**29. Which of Piaget's cognitive developmental stages takes place from ages 7 to 11?**
(a) Formal operations (b) Concrete operations
(c) Preoperational (d) Sensorimotor

**30. Which interaction style describes a nurse who cannot clearly separate her own emotional responses from the patient's needs and wants?**
(a) Holistic (b) Defensive
(c) Sympathetic (d) Silence

**31. A patient with an arterial ulcer over the left lateral malleolus complains of pain at the ulcer site. The nurse caring for this patient understands that the pain is caused most commonly by which of the following?**
(a) Infection (b) Exudate
(c) Ischemia (d) Edema

**32. A patient, age 54, is admitted with a diagnosis of venous ulceration unresponsive to treatment. Which of the following is the nurse most likely to find during an assessment of a patient with venous ulceration?**
(a) Gangrene (b) Heavy exudate
(c) Deep wound bed (d) Pale wound bed

**33. The nurse is providing care for a patient who has a sacral pressure ulcer with a wet-to-dry dressing. Which guideline is appropriate when caring for a patient with a wet-to-dry dressing?**
(a) The wound should remain moist from the dressing
(b) The wet-to-dry dressing should be tightly packed into the wound
(c) The dressing should be allowed to dry before it is removed
(d) A plastic sheet-type dressing should cover the wet dressing

**34. The nurse is assessing the laboratory values of a patient with an abdominal wound healing by secondary intention. Which of the following laboratory values indicates that the patient is receiving adequate nutrition?**
(a) Serum albumin level of 2.5 g/dL
(b) Prealbumin level of 12 mg/dL
(c) Transferrin level of 190 mg/dL
(d) Total lymphocyte count of 1,900 mL

**35. What term describes the softening of tissue by wetting or soaking?**
(a) Eschar (b) Maceration
(c) Sloughing (d) Angiogenesis

**36. After assessing a patient's pressure ulcer, you note that subcutaneous fat is visible but that bone, tendon and muscle are not exposed. You observe slough, but it does not obscure the depth of tissue loss. You also note some undermining and tunneling. What stage pressure ulcer is this?**
(a) Stage II
(b) Suspected deep tissue injury
(c) Stage III
(d) Stage IV

**37. During which stage of healing does granulation tissue form and epithelialization occur?**
(a) The maturation phase
(b) The epithelial closure phase
(c) The inflammatory phase
(d) The proliferative phase

**38. Which of the following are external factors that subject the skin to injury?**
(a) Emaciation and infections
(b) Allergens and radiation
(c) Radiation and emaciation
(d) Allergens and infections

**39. Where is a venous ulcer typically found on a patient?**
(a) The medial lower leg and ankle
(b) The plantar aspect of foot
(c) On a bony prominence
(d) Under the heels

**40. Which substance enables the transport of oxygen during wound healing?**
(a) Zinc (b) Vitamin B6
(c) Folate (d) Vitamin C

**41. The nurse is teaching a group of patient care attendants about infection control measures. The nurse tells the group that the first line of intervention for preventing the spread of infection is:**
(a) Wearing gloves
(b) Administering antibiotics
(c) Hand hygiene
(d) Assigning private rooms for patients

**42. The nurse is caring for a patient who was given pain medication before leaving the recovery room. Upon returning to his room, the patient states that he is still experiencing pain and requests more pain medication. Of the following actions, which is the first for the nurse to take?**
(a) Tell the patient that he must wait 4 hours for more pain medication
(b) Give half of the ordered as-needed dose
(c) Document the patient's pain
(d) Notify the practitioner that the patient is still experiencing pain

**43. A patient is admitted to the health care facility with a possible electrolyte imbalance. The patient is disoriented and weak, has an irregular pulse, and takes hydrochlorothiazide. The patient most likely suffers from:**
(a) Hypernatremia (b) Hyponatremia
(c) Hyperkalemia (d) Hypokalemia

**44. The nurse is assessing a patient who may be in the early stages of dehydration. Early signs and symptoms of dehydration include:**
(a) Coma and seizures
(b) Sunken eyeballs and poor skin turgor
(c) Increased heart rate with hypotension
(d) Thirst and confusion

**45. The nurse is evaluating a postoperative patient for infection. Which sign or symptom would be most indicative of infection?**
(a) Presence of an indwelling urinary catheter
(b) Rectal temperature of 100°F (37.8°C)
(c) Redness, warmth, and tenderness at the incision site
(d) WBC count of 8,000/MI

**46. When planning the postoperative care of a patient who underwent surgery for repair of a lacerated spleen after an alcohol-related motor vehicle accident, what intervention should take priority in the immediate postoperative period?**
(a) Monitoring the patient for signs and symptoms of alcohol withdrawal
(b) Encouraging early ambulation
(c) Splinting the abdomen for coughing and deep-breathing exercise
(d) Monitoring the patient's renal function

**47. Which diet would be most appropriate for a patient with ulcerative colitis?**
(a) A low-fat diet (b) A low-residue diet
(c) A high-calorie diet (d) A high-fiber diet

**48. The nurse performs a nutritional assessment on a patient with lung cancer who is in the postoperative period after a lobectomy. Which of the following could be an early sign of malnutrition?**
(a) A retinal-binding protein level of 2.0 mg/dL
(b) Dry, flaky, discolored skin and brittle nails
(c) A body mass index (BMI) of 20
(d) An albumin level of 3.0 g/dL

**49. The two types of surgery primarily used to promote weight loss are restrictive and mal absorptive-restrictive. Which of the following is an example of restrictive weight-loss surgery?**
(a) Gastric bypass (b) Adjustable gastric banding
(c) Roux-en-Y (d) Biliopancreatic diversion

**50. In what type of electrolyte imbalance would the nurse observe tall, tented T waves; a widened QRS complex; and a prolonged PR interval on the patient's ECG?**
(a) Hypokalemia (b) Hypocalcemia
(c) Hypercalcemi (d) Hyperkalemia

**51. While auscultating the heart sounds of a patient with mitral insufficiency, the nurse hears an extra heart sound immediately after the second heart sound (S2). The nurse should document this extra heart sound as:**
(a) A first heart sound (S1)
(b) A third heart sound (S3)
(c) A fourth heart sound (S4)
(d) A mitral murmur

**52. A 55-year-old black male is found to have a blood pressure of 150/90 mm Hg during a work site health screening. What should the nurse do?**
(a) Consider this to be a normal finding for his age and race
(b) Recommend he have his blood pressure rechecked in 1 year
(c) Recommend he have his blood pressure rechecked within 2 weeks
(d) Recommend he go to the emergency department for further evaluation

**53. The nurse is administering warfarin (Coumadin) to a patient with deep vein thrombophlebitis. Which laboratory value indicates warfarin is at therapeutic levels?**
(a) PTT 1½ to 2 times the control
(b) PT 1½ to 2 times the control
(c) INR of 3 to 4
(d) Hematocrit of 32%

**54. A patient is receiving captopril for heart failure. The nurse should notify the practitioner that the medication therapy is ineffective if an assessment reveals:**
(a) A skin rash (b) Peripheral edema
(c) A dry cough (d) Postural hypotension

**55. A 60-year-old male patient is suspected of having coronary artery disease. Which noninvasive diagnostic method would the nurse expect to be ordered to evaluate cardiac changes?**
(a) Cardiac biopsy
(b) Cardiac catheterization
(c) MRI
(d) Pericardiocentesis

**56. When evaluating an ECG strip of a patient on a telemetry unit, the nurse notices the patient is having premature ventricular contractions (PVCs). What criterion on the ECG strip does the nurse use to evaluate the presence of PVCs?**
(a) An indiscernible PR interval
(b) P waves that appear erratic
(c) P waves that have a sawtooth configuration
(d) A QRS complex followed by a compensatory pause

**57. When locating Erb's point to hear aortic and pulmonic sounds, the nurse should place the stethoscope at the:**
(a) Fifth intercostal space near the midclavicular line
(b) Fifth intercostal space along the left sternal border
(c) Second intercostal space at the left sternal border
(d) Third intercostal space at the left sternal border

**58. When caring for a patient with arterial occlusive disease, which of the following home health care instructions is most appropriate for the nurse to give to the patient?**
(a) 'You should massage your legs to relieve pain.'
(b) 'It is best to sit and rest for several hours a day.'
(c) 'Make sure the head of your bed is slightly elevated when sleeping.'
(d) 'It is best to wear tight socks instead of no socks.'

**59. The nurse prepares to administer an ACE inhibitor to a patient with an acute MI for which reason?**
(a) To minimize platelet aggregation
(b) To reduce preload and after load
(c) To reduce myocardial oxygen consumption
(d) To decrease myocardial oxygen demand

**60. Which of the following conditions can cause right-sided heart failure?**
(a) A ventricular septal defect
(b) An anterior MI
(c) An atrial septal defect
(d) Constrictive pericarditis

**61. When assessing a patient with anemia from acute blood loss, the nurse would expect to find which of the following?**
(a) Sudden onset of symptoms, hypotension and tachycardia
(b) Exertional dyspnea, poor nutrition, and hypotension
(c) Sudden onset of symptoms, glossitis, and tachycardia
(d) Fatigue, neuropathy, and tachycardia

**62. When teaching safety precautions to a patient with thrombocytopenia, the nurse should include which of the following directives?**
(a) Eat foods high in iron
(b) Avoid products that contain aspirin
(c) Avoid people with respiratory tract infections
(d) Eat only cooked vegetables

**63. When assessing the patient, the nurse knows that the body system least affected by multiple myeloma is the:**
(a) Skeletal system
(b) Renal system
(c) Nervous system
(d) Cardiovascular system

**64. The nurse is reviewing assessment data for a patient with a diagnosis of stage III Hodgkin's disease. This diagnosis is most strongly supported by lymphatic involvement on both sides of the:**
(a) Blood–brain barrier
(b) Diaphragm
(c) Descending aorta
(d) Spinal column

**65. A 50-year-old male with a diagnosis of leukemia is responding poorly to treatment. He is tearful and trying to express his feelings, but he is having difficulty. The nurse should first:**
(a) Tell him that she will leave for now but she will be back
(b) Offer to call pastoral care
(c) Ask if he would like her to sit with him while he collects his thoughts
(d) Tell him that she can understand how he is feeling

**66. A patient with blood type B can receive a transfusion of what type of RBCs?**
(a) Type A or type O
(b) Type B or type O
(c) Type AB or type O
(d) Type A or type B

**67. Which type of anemia results from deficiency of all the blood's formed elements, caused by failure of the bone marrow to generate enough new cells?**
(a) Sickle cell anemia
(b) Folic acid deficiency anemia
(c) Aplastic anemia
(d) Iron deficiency anemia

**68. Which disorder results from a deficiency of circulating platelets?**
(a) Hemophilia
(b) Sickle cell anemia
(c) Von Willebrand's disease
(d) Thrombocytopenia

**69. A patient with Hodgkin's disease has lymph node involvement on both sides of the diaphragm and involvement of the spleen. According to the Ann Harbor classification system, what stage lymphoma does this patient have?**
(a) Stage I (b) Stage II
(c) Stage III (d) Stage IV

**70. A patient with anemia from acute blood loss has been admitted to the medical-surgical unit. What assessment findings would the nurse expect to find?**
(a) Night sweats, weight loss and diarrhea
(b) Dyspnea, tachycardia and pallor
(c) Nausea, vomiting and anorexia
(d) Itching, rash and jaundice

**71. A patient with pneumonia in the right lower lobe is prescribed percussion and postural drainage. When performing percussion and postural drainage, the nurse should position him:**
(a) In semi-Fowler's position with his knees bent
(b) In a right side-lying position with the foot of his bed elevated
(c) In a prone or supine position with the foot of his bed elevated higher than his head
(d) Bent at the waist leaning slightly forward

**72. A patient with acquired immunodeficiency syndrome (AIDS) develops *P. jiroveci* pneumonia. Which nursing diagnosis has the highest priority for this patient?**
(a) Impaired gas exchange
(b) Impaired oral mucus membranes
(c) Imbalanced nutrition: Less than body requirements
(d) Activity intolerance

**73. A patient has chronic bronchitis. The nurse is teaching him breathing exercises. Which point should the nurse include in her teaching?**
(a) Make inhalation longer than exhalation
(b) Exhale through an open mouth
(c) Use diaphragmatic breathing
(d) Use chest breathing

**74. A patient with ARDS is intubated and placed on mechanical ventilation. His $PaO_2$ is 60 mm Hg on 1.0 $FiO_2$. To improve his $PaO_2$ without raising the $FiO_2$, the patient will most likely be placed on:**
(a) Time-cycled ventilation
(b) Volume-cycled ventilation
(c) Pressure support
(d) PEEP

**75. When auscultating the chest of a patient with pneumonia, the nurse should expect to hear which type of sounds over areas of consolidation?**
(a) Bronchial (b) Bronchovesicular
(c) Tubular (d) Vesicular

**76. A patient's history reveals that he suffers from daytime symptoms of asthma that occur 3 to 6 days a week. How would his asthma severity be described?**
(a) Mild intermittent
(b) Mild persistent
(c) Moderate persistent
(d) Severe persistent

**77. A 66-year-old patient has marked dyspnea at rest, is thin, and uses accessory muscles to breathe. He is tachypnic, with a prolonged expiratory phase. He has no cough. He leans forward with his arms braced on his knees to support his chest and shoulders for breathing. This patient has signs and symptoms of which respiratory disorder?**
(a) ARDS
(b) Asthma
(c) Chronic obstructive bronchitis
(d) Emphysema

**78. A nurse is preparing to reinforce the teaching plan for a patient who has recently been diagnosed with squamous cell carcinoma of the left lung. Which statement by the nurse is correct?**
(a) 'You have a slow-growing cancer that rarely spreads'
(b) 'In terms of prognosis, you may have only a few months to live'
(c) 'Squamous cell cancer is a very rapidly growing cancer'
(d) 'The cancer has generally metastasized by the time diagnosis is made'

**79. Which respiratory disorder is most common in the first 24 to 48 hours after surgery?**
(a) Atelectasis (b) Bronchitis
(c) Pneumonia (d) Pneumothorax

**80. A patient with acute asthma showing inspiratory and expiratory wheezes and a decreased forced expiratory volume should be treated immediately with which class of medication?**
(a) Beta-adrenergic blockers
(b) Bronchodilators
(c) Inhaled steroids
(d) Oral steroids

**81. The nurse is caring for a patient with a C7 spinal cord injury who develops bradycardia, hypertension, and sweating. Which intervention should the nurse perform first?**
(a) Palpating the patient's bladder
(b) Lying the patient flat in bed
(c) Covering the patient with a blanket
(d) Performing a rectal examination

**82. The nurse is caring for a comatose patient who has suffered a closed head injury. Which intervention should the nurse implement to prevent increases in ICP?**
(a) Suctioning the airway every hour and as needed
(b) Elevating the head of the bed 30 to 45 degrees
(c) Turning the patient and changing his position every 2 hours
(d) Maintaining a well-lit room

**83. The nurse is teaching the patient with multiple sclerosis. When teaching the patient how to reduce fatigue, the nurse should tell the patient to:**
(a) Take a hot bath
(b) Rest in an air-conditioned room
(c) Increase the dose of his muscle relaxant
(d) Avoid naps during the day

**84. To encourage adequate nutritional intake for a patient with Alzheimer's disease, the nurse should:**
(a) Stay with the patient, and encourage him to eat
(b) Help the patient fill out his menu
(c) Give the patient privacy during meals
(d) Fill out the menu for the patient

**85. The nurse is teaching a patient and his family about dietary practices related to Parkinson's disease. A priority for the nurse to address is risk of:**
(a) Fluid overload and drooling
(b) Aspiration and anorexia
(c) Choking and diarrhea
(d) Dysphagia and constipation

**86. An elderly patient has just suffered a stroke that has left him with amnesia. Amnesia is a symptom associated with damage to which vessel?**
(a) Carotid artery
(b) Anterior cerebral arteries
(c) Vertebrobasilar artery
(d) Middle cerebral artery

**87. Which condition places a patient at risk for an embolic stroke?**
(a) Atrial fibrillation
(b) Bradycardia
(c) Deep vein thrombosis
(d) A history of MI

**88. After a patient experiences a brain stem infarction, the nurse should observe for which condition?**
(a) Aphasia
(b) Bradypnea
(c) Contralateral hemiplegia
(d) Numbness and tingling to the face or arm

**89. In a patient with meningitis, irritation to which CN could cause photophobia?**
(a) III (b) IV
(c) V (d) VI

**90. A patient with a subdural hematoma becomes restless and confused, with dilation of the ipsilateral pupil. The physician orders mannitol for which reason?**
(a) To reduce intraocular pressure
(b) To prevent acute tubular necrosis
(c) To promote osmotic diuresis to decrease ICP
(d) To draw water into the vascular system to increase blood pressure

**91. A patient in balanced suspension traction for a fractured femur needs to be repositioned toward the head of the bed. During repositioning, the nurse should:**
(a) Place slight additional tension on the traction cords.
(b) Release the weights, and replace them immediately after positioning.
(c) Lift the traction and the patient during repositioning.
(d) Maintain the same degree of traction tension.

**92. A patient undergoes cast placement for a fractured left radius. The nurse should suspect compartment syndrome if the patient experiences pain that:**
(a) Intensifies with the elevation of the left arm
(b) Disappears with the flexion of the left arm
(c) Increases with the arm in a dependent position
(d) Radiates up the arm to the left scapula

**93. A patient received a right hip prosthesis after a fall. In the immediate postoperative period, the nurse should:**
(a) Maintain the leg in an adducted position
(b) Maintain the leg in an abducted position
(c) Maintain the leg in a neutral position
(d) Maintain the leg with the hip flexed greater than 90°

**94. A 78-year-old patient has a history of osteoarthritis. Which signs and symptoms would the nurse expect to find on physical assessment?**
(a) Joint pain, crepitus, Heberden's nodes
(b) Hot, inflamed joints; crepitus; joint pain
(c) Tophi, enlarged joints, Bouchard's nodes
(d) Swelling, joint pain, tenderness on palpation

**95. The nurse is caring for an elderly female patient who has osteoporosis. When teaching her, the nurse should include information about which major complication?**
(a) Bone fracture (b) Loss of estrogen
(c) Scoliosis (d) Negative calcium balance

**96. Conservative treatment of a herniated nucleus pulposus would include which measures?**
(a) Surgery
(b) Spinal fusion
(c) Bed rest, pain medication, and physiotherapy
(d) Strenuous exercise, pain medication and physiotherapy

**97. Which areas should be included in a neurovascular assessment?**
(a) Orientation, movement, pulses, and warmth
(b) Capillary refill time, movement, pulses, and warmth
(c) Orientation, pupillary response, temperature, and pulses
(d) Respiratory pattern, orientation, pulses, and temperature

**98. Which of the following are considered signs and symptoms of a fracture?**
(a) Tingling, coolness, and loss of pulses
(b) Loss of sensation, redness, and coolness
(c) Coolness, redness, and a new pain site
(d) Discoloration, deformity and pain at the site of injury

**99. What diagnostic test would be used to evaluate the presence of rhabdomyolysis?**
(a) Glycosylated hemoglobin
(b) Serum troponin
(c) Serum myoglobin
(d) Bone biopsy

**100. What complication should the nurse be alert for in a diabetic patient who has been placed in skeletal traction after a motor vehicle collision?**
(a) Osteoarthritis (b) Osteomyelitis
(c) Osteoporosis (d) Osteosarcoma

**101. A patient with peptic ulcer disease secondary to chronic NSAID use is prescribed misoprostol (Cytotec). The nurse would be most accurate in informing the patient that the drug:**
(a) Reduces the stomach's volume of hydrochloric acid
(b) Increases the speed of gastric emptying
(c) Protects the stomach's lining
(d) Increases LES pressure

**102. The nurse is caring for a patient with active upper-GI bleeding. What is the appropriate diet for this patient during the first 24 hours after admission?**
(a) Regular diet
(b) Skim milk
(c) Nothing by mouth
(d) Clear liquids

**103. A patient is scheduled to have a descending colostomy. He is anxious and has many questions concerning the surgery, the care of a stoma, and lifestyle changes. It would be most appropriate for the nurse to refer the patient to which member of the health care team?**
(a) Social worker
(b) Registered dietitian
(c) Occupational therapist
(d) Enterostomal nurse therapist

**104. The nurse is planning care for a female patient with acute hepatitis A. What is the primary mode of transmission for hepatitis A?**
(a) Fecal contamination and oral ingestion
(b) Exposure to contaminated blood
(c) Sexual activity with an infected partner
(d) Sharing a contaminated needle or syringe

**105. A patient experiences an exacerbation of ulcerative colitis. Test results reveal elevated serum osmolality and urine specific gravity. What is the most likely explanation for these test results?**
(a) Renal insufficiency
(b) Hypoaldosteronism
(c) Diabetes insipidus
(d) Deficient fluid volume

**106. A patient has just had a surgical revision of his intestinal tract. What type of procedure would the patient have undergone if his stools are formed?**
(a) Continent ileostomy
(b) Conventional ileostomy
(c) Double-barrel and loop colostomy
(d) Single-barrel, or end, colostomy

**107. Which nursing intervention should take priority when caring for a patient with appendicitis?**
(a) Assessing for pain
(b) Encouraging oral intake of clear fluids
(c) Providing discharge teaching
(d) Assessing for signs and symptoms of peritonitis

**108. When teaching a patient about GERD, the nurse describes the disorder as:**
(a) Erosion of the gastric mucosa
(b) Inflammation of a diverticulum
(c) Inflammation of the gastric mucosa
(d) Reflux of stomach acid into the esophagus

**109. Which type of diet is implicated in the development of diverticulosis?**
(a) A low-fiber diet (b) A high-fiber diet
(c) A high-protein diet (d) A low-carbohydrate diet

**110. Crohn's disease can be described as a chronic relapsing disease. Which area of the GI system may be involved with this disease?**
(a) The entire length of the large colon
(b) Only the sigmoid area
(c) The entire large colon through the layers of mucosa and submucosa
(d) The small intestine and colon, affecting the entire thickness of the bowel

**111. The nurse is teaching a patient diagnosed with basal cell carcinoma. The most common cause of basal cell carcinoma is:**
(a) Immunosuppression
(b) Radiation exposure
(c) Sun exposure
(d) Burns

**112. A patient received burns to his entire back and left arm. Using the Rule of Nines, the nurse can calculate that he has sustained burns on what percentage of his body?**
(a) 9% (b) 18%
(c) 27% (d) 36%

**113. A patient is admitted to a burn intensive care unit with extensive full-thickness burns. The nurse is most concerned about the patient's:**
(a) Fluid and electrolyte status
(b) Risk of infection
(c) Body image
(d) Level of pain

**114. A patient undergoes a biopsy to confirm a diagnosis of skin cancer. Immediately following the procedure, the nurse should observe the site for:**
(a) Infection (b) Dehiscence
(c) Hemorrhage (d) Swelling

**115. The nurse is caring for a patient with malignant melanoma. The nurse explains that the first and most important treatment for malignant melanoma is:**
(a) Chemotherapy
(b) Immunotherapy
(c) Radiation therapy
(d) Wide excision

**116. A 19-year-old patient comes to the clinic with dark red lesions on her hands, wrist, and waistline. She has scratched several of the lesions so that they are open and bleeding. The nurse instructs the patient to try pressing on the itchy lesions. What is the rationale for this intervention?**
(a) Pressing the skin spreads the beneficial microorganisms
(b) Pressing is suggested before scratching
(c) Pressing the skin promotes breaks in the skin
(d) Pressing the skin stimulates nerve endings

**117. A patient arrives at the office of his physician complaining of a rash. The nurse assesses the patient and notes several palpable, elevated masses, each about 0.5 cm in diameter. What term would the nurse use to accurately describe these masses?**
(a) Erosions
(b) Macules
(c) Papules
(d) Vesicles

**118. A patient has thick, discolored nails with splintered hemorrhages, easily separated from the nail bed. There are also 'ice pick' pits and ridges. The nurse explains to the patient that these findings are most closely associated with:**
(a) Paronychia (b) Psoriasis
(c) Seborrhea (d) Scabies

**119. After the initial phase of a burn injury, the primary focus of a patient's cure is:**
(a) Enhancing self-esteem
(b) Promoting hygiene
(c) Reducing anxiety
(d) Preventing infection

**120. Which patient is at greatest risk for impaired wound healing after surgery?**
(a) A 65-year-old patient with hypertension
(b) A 60-year-old patient who is slightly overweight
(c) A 78-year-old patient in general good health
(d) A 75-year-old patient with poorly controlled diabetes mellitus

**121. A 28-year-old woman is scheduled for a glucose tolerance test. She asks the nurse what results indicate diabetes mellitus. The nurse should respond that the minimum parameter for indication of diabetes mellitus is a 2 hour blood glucose level greater than:**
(a) 120 mg/dL
(b) 150 mg/dL
(c) 200 mg/dL
(d) 250 mg/dL

**122. A patient is diagnosed with hyperthyroidism. The nurse should expect clinical signs and symptoms similar to:**
(a) Hypovolemic shock
(b) Sympathetic nervous system stimulation
(c) Benzodiazepine overdose
(d) Addison's disease

**123. A patient with thyroid cancer undergoes a thyroidectomy. After surgery, the patient develops peripheral numbness and tingling and muscle twitching and spasms. The nurse should expect to administer:**
(a) A thyroid supplement
(b) An antispasmodic
(c) A barbiturate
(d) IV calcium gluconate

**124. A patient with intractable asthma develops Cushing's syndrome. Development of this complication can most likely be attributed to long-term or excessive use of:**
(a) Prednisone
(b) Theophylline
(c) Metaproterenol (Alupent)
(d) Cromolyn (Intal)

**125. Which nursing diagnosis is most likely for a patient with an acute episode of diabetes insipidus?**
(a) Imbalanced nutrition: More than body requirements
(b) Deficient fluid volume
(c) Impaired gas exchange
(d) Ineffective tissue perfusion: Cardiopulmonary

**126. A patient presents with diaphoresis, palpitations, jitters, and tachycardia approximately 1½ hours after taking his regular morning insulin. Which treatment option is appropriate for this patient?**
(a) Blood glucose level monitoring and carbohydrate administration
(b) Nitroglycerin administration and ECG
(c) Pulse oximetry monitoring and oxygen therapy
(d) Salt restriction, diuretic administration and paracentesis

**127. When teaching a newly diagnosed diabetic patient about diet and exercise, the nurse should teach the patient how to:**
(a) Use fiber laxatives and bulk-forming agents
(b) Manage fluids, proteins and electrolytes
(c) Reduce calorie intake before exercising
(d) Manage caloric goals, diet and physical activity

**128. A 52-year-old patient reports weight gain and fatigue. On assessment, her vital signs are a blood pressure of 120/74 mm Hg, a pulse rate of 52 beats/minute, a respiratory rate of 20 breaths/minute, and a temperature of 98°F (36.7°C). Laboratory results show low T4 and T3 levels. The nurse knows these signs and symptoms are associated with which condition?**
(a) Tetany
(b) Hypothyroidism
(c) Hyperthyroidism
(d) Hypokalemia

**129. A patient is admitted with a diagnosis of hyperparathyroidism. Which of the following signs would the nurse expect to find?**
(a) Bulging eyes
(b) Renal calculi
(c) Weight gain
(d) Weight loss

**130. A 37-year-old patient complains of muscle weakness, anorexia, and darkening of his skin. The nurse reviews his laboratory data and notes findings of low serum sodium and high serum potassium levels. The nurse recognizes that these signs and symptoms are associated with which condition?**
(a) Addison's disease (b) Cushing's syndrome
(c) Diabetes insipidus (d) Thyroid storm

**131. The nurse is providing post procedure care for a patient who underwent extracorporeal shock-wave lithotripsy for the treatment of renal calculi. The nurse should instruct the patient to:**
(a) Limit oral fluid intake for 1 to 2 weeks
(b) Report the presence of fine, sandlike particles in the urine
(c) Notify the practitioner about cloudy or foul-smelling urine
(d) Report bright pink urine within 24 hours after the procedure

**132. The nurse is planning a teaching session for a female patient who had a UTI. Which point should the nurse include?**
(a) Limit fluid intake to reduce the need to urinate.
(b) Take the prescribed antibiotic until symptoms subside.
(c) Notify the practitioner if urinary urgency, burning, frequency, or difficulty occurs.
(d) Wear only nylon underwear to reduce the chance of irritation.

**133. The nurse is caring for a patient with acute renal failure. The nurse should expect hypertonic glucose, insulin infusions, and sodium bicarbonate to be used to treat:**
(a) Hypernatremia
(b) Hypokalemia
(c) Hypercalcemia
(d) Hyperkalemia

**134. The nurse is teaching a patient with chronic renal failure which foods to avoid. It would be most accurate for the nurse to teach the patient to avoid foods high in:**
(a) Monosaccharides (b) Disaccharides
(c) Iron (d) Protein

**135. A patient with acute renal failure is being assessed to determine whether the cause is prerenal, renal, or postrenal. If the cause is prerenal, which condition most likely caused it?**
(a) Heart failure
(b) Glomerulonephritis
(c) Ureterolithiasis
(d) Aminoglycoside toxicity

**136. When teaching a patient how to prevent the recurrence of acute glomerulonephritis, which instruction should the nurse include?**
(a) 'Avoid physical activity'
(b) 'Strain all urine'
(c) 'Seek early treatment for respiratory infections'
(d) 'Monitor urine specific gravity daily'

**137. A patient diagnosed with chronic renal failure is told he must start hemodialysis. During patient teaching, the nurse should instruct the patient to:**
(a) Follow a high-potassium diet
(b) Strictly follow the hemodialysis schedule
(c) Recognize that the disorder will cause lifestyle changes
(d) Use alcohol to clean the skin because of integumentary changes

**138. A patient has an indwelling urinary catheter, and urine is leaking from a hole in the collection bag. Which nursing intervention would be most appropriate?**
(a) Cover the hole with tape
(b) Remove the catheter and collection bag, replace the bag and insert a new catheter, using sterile technique
(c) Disconnect the drainage bag from the catheter and replace it with a new bag
(d) Place a towel under the bag to prevent spillage of urine on the floor, which could cause the patient to slip and fall

**139. During a health history, which statement by a patient indicates a risk of renal calculi?**
(a) 'I have been drinking a lot of cola and soft drinks lately'
(b) 'I have been jogging more than usual'
(c) 'I have had more stress since we adopted a child last year'
(d) 'I am a vegetarian and eat cheese two or three times each day'

**140. Diuretics are ordered for a patient. What would be the best time of day for the nurse to schedule this medication?**
(a) Anytime
(b) Night time
(c) Morning
(d) Noon

**141. Which patient has the highest risk of ovarian cancer?**
(a) A 30-year-old woman taking an oral contraceptive
(b) A 45-year-old woman who has never been pregnant
(c) A 40-year-old woman with three children
(d) A 36-year-old woman who had her first child at age 22

**142. A patient with a small, well-defined breast nodule asks the nurse about her treatment options. Which treatments would be considered for this patient?**
(a) Lumpectomy and radiation
(b) Partial mastectomy and radiation
(c) Partial mastectomy and chemotherapy
(d) Total mastectomy and chemotherapy

**143. The nurse is assessing a male patient with gonorrhea. Which symptom most likely prompted him to seek medical attention?**
(a) Rashes on the palms of the hands and soles of the feet
(b) Cauliflower-like warts on the penis
(c) Painful red papules on the shaft of the penis
(d) Foul-smelling discharge from the penis

**144. The nurse is speaking to a group of women about early detection of breast cancer. The average age of the women in the group is 47. Following the American Cancer Society guidelines, the nurse should recommend that the women:**
(a) Perform BSE annually
(b) Have a mammogram annually
(c) Have a hormonal receptor assay annually
(d) Have a practitioner conduct a clinical examination every 2 years

**145. The nurse is teaching a male patient to perform monthly testicular self-examinations. What is the appropriate point to make?**
(a) Testicular cancer is highly curable
(b) Testicular cancer is difficult to diagnose
(c) Testicular cancer is the number one cause of cancer deaths in men
(d) Testicular cancer is more common in older men

**146. On a follow-up visit after having a vaginal hysterectomy, a 32-year-old patient has an elevated temperature and decreased hematocrit. Which complication does this suggest?**
(a) Hematoma (b) Hypovolemia
(c) Infection (d) Thromboembolism

**147. An annual Pap test is most important in patients:**
(a) With a history of recurrent candidiasis
(b) Who became pregnant before age 20
(c) Infected with HPV
(d) Who have used oral contraceptives for a short time

**148. When planning to teach an adolescent female patient about PID, which of the following statements should the nurse include?**
(a) 'Good hygiene practices prevent the development of PID'
(b) 'The use of hormonal contraceptives decreases the risk of PID'
(c) 'PID can lead to long-term complications of the reproductive trac'
(d) 'Infants born to adolescents with PID are at risk for birth defects'

**149. Perineal pain in the absence of any observable cause suggests which condition?**
(a) Endometriosis (b) Internal hemorrhoids
(c) Prostatitis (d) Renal calculi

**150. Which statement should the nurse include when teaching a patient newly diagnosed with testicular cancer?**
(a) 'Testicular cancer is not responsive to chemotherapy, but it is highly curative with surgery'
(b) 'Radiation therapy is never used so that the unaffected testicle can remain healthy'
(c) 'Testicular self-examination is still important because having testicular cancer increases the risk of developing a second tumor'
(d) 'Taking testosterone after orchiectomy prevents changes in appearance and sexual function'

**151. The nurse is preparing a female patient with SLE for discharge. Which instructions should the nurse include in the teaching plan?**
(a) Exposure to sunlight will help control skin rashes
(b) No activity limitations are necessary between flare-ups
(c) Monitor body temperature
(d) Corticosteroids may be stopped when symptoms are relieved

**152. A patient with rheumatoid arthritis has a history of long-term NSAID use and, consequently, has developed peptic ulcer disease. To treat this condition, the nurse should expect to administer:**
(a) Cyanocobalamin (vitamin B12)
(b) Ticlopidine
(c) Prednisone
(d) Misoprostol

**153. The nurse is providing care for a patient with AIDS and *Pneumocystis jiroveci* pneumonia. The patient is receiving aerosolized pentamidine isethionate (Nebu-Pent). What's the best evidence that the therapy is working?**
(a) A sudden gain in lost body weight
(b) Whitening of lung fields on the chest X-ray
(c) Improved patient vitality and activity tolerance
(d) A febrile body temperature and development of leukocytosis

**154. A patient with SLE who receives immunosuppressants develops a fever. The nurse should:**
(a) Administer prescribed antipyretics.
(b) Place the patient in isolation.
(c) Apply cooling measures immediately.
(d) Help identify the cause.

**155. Which finding distinguishes rheumatoid arthritis from osteoarthritis and gouty arthritis?**
(a) Crepitus with ROM
(b) Symmetry of joint involvement
(c) Elevated serum uric acid levels
(d) Dominance in weight-bearing joints

**156. A patient is admitted with acute bronchitis. During the admission interview, he tells the nurse he is allergic to bananas. Based on this statement, he may also have an allergy to which drug or substance?**
(a) Iodine-containing drugs
(b) Cephalosporins
(c) Penicillins
(d) Latex

**157. A patient with AIDS is prescribed zidovudine (Retrovir), 200 mg by mouth every 4 hours. When teaching the patient about this drug, the nurse should provide which instruction?**
(a) 'Take zidovudine with meals'
(b) 'Take zidovudine on an empty stomach'
(c) 'Take zidovudine every 4 hours around the clock'
(d) 'Take OTC drugs to treat minor adverse reactions'

**158. In a patient who has HIV infection, the CD4+ level is measured to determine the:**
(a) Presence of opportunistic infections
(b) Level of the viral load
(c) Extent of immune system damage
(d) Resistance to antigens

**159. A 36-year-old patient complains of fatigue, weight loss, and a low-grade fever. He also has pain in his fingers, elbows, and ankles. Which condition is suspected?**
(a) Anemia (b) Leukemia
(c) Rheumatic arthritis (d) SLE

**160. Which WBCs are involved in releasing histamine during an allergic reaction?**
(a) Basophils
(b) Eosinophils
(c) Monocytes
(d) Neutrophils

**161. The nurse is caring for a patient who underwent stapedectomy. To prevent postoperative complications, the nurse should instruct the patient to:**
(a) Sneeze with her mouth open
(b) Frequently blow her nose
(c) Clean her operated ear with a cotton-tipped applicator twice a day
(d) Resume bending and straining when she is no longer experiencing ear pain

**162. The nurse is assessing a 32-year-old patient with otosclerosis. The nurse should be aware that the patient's hearing loss:**
(a) Will resolve in 4 to 6 weeks without intervention
(b) Typically affects both ears
(c) Occurred suddenly
(d) Is associated with ear pain

**163. The nurse is teaching a patient with a detached retina who underwent scleral buckling on the left eye. The procedure included gas injection into the vitreous. Which of the following statements indicates that the patient understands the nurse's instructions?**
(a) 'I should lie on my abdomen with my head turned to the right'
(b) 'I will lie face down with my head turned to the left'
(c) 'I will lie face up with my head turned to the right'
(d) 'I should lie on my back with my head turned to the left'

**164. The nurse is providing care for a patient following right cataract removal surgery. In which position should the nurse place the patient?**
(a) Right-side lying
(b) Prone
(c) Supine
(d) Trendelenburg's

**165. Which position would be the most appropriate for a patient who has undergone stapedectomy?**
(a) On the affected side
(b) On the unaffected side
(c) Prone
(d) Sims'

**166. Which symptom would occur in a patient with a detached retina?**
(a) Flashing lights and floaters
(b) Homonymous hemianopia
(c) Loss of central vision
(d) Ptosis

**167. A 72-year-old patient is being discharged from same-day surgery after having a cataract removed from his right eye. Which discharge instruction should the nurse give the patient?**
(a) 'Sleep on the operative side'
(b) 'Resume all activities as before'
(c) 'Do not rub or place pressure on the eyes'
(d) 'Wear an eye shield all day and remove it at night'

**168. Which of the following increases a 40-year-old patient's risk of developing cataracts?**
(a) A history of frequent streptococcal throat infections
(b) Maternal exposure to rubella during pregnancy
(c) Increased IOP
(d) Prolonged use of steroidal anti-inflammatory agents

**169. In caring for a patient after cataract surgery, the nurse should tell the patient to notify his physician of which of the following conditions?**
(a) Blurred vision (b) Eye pain
(c) Glare (d) Itching

**170. When assessing a patient with glaucoma, the nurse would expect which of the following findings?**
(a) Complaints of double vision
(b) Complaints of halos around lights
(c) An IOP of 15 mm Hg
(d) A soft globe on palpation

**171. A patient undergoes a surgical procedure that requires the use of general anesthesia. Following general anesthesia, the patient is most at risk for:**
(a) Atelectasis (b) Anemia
(c) Dehydration (d) Peripheral edema

**172. The nurse is administering preoperative medication to a patient going to the operating room for an ortobifemoral bypass. After administering preoperative medication to the patient, the nurse should:**
(a) Allow him to walk to the bathroom unassisted
(b) Place the bed in low position with the side rails up
(c) Tell him that he will be asleep before he leaves for surgery
(d) Take his vital signs

**173. The nurse is caring for a patient who was given pain medication before leaving the PACU. Upon returning to her room, the patient states that she is experiencing pain and requests more pain medication. Which is the best action for the nurse to take?**
(a) Tell the patient that she must wait 4 hours for more pain medication
(b) Give one-half of the ordered as-needed dose
(c) Document the patient's pain
(d) Notify the practitioner that the patient is continuing to experience pain

**174. The nurse is evaluating a patient postoperatively for infection. Which of the following would be most indicative of infection?**
(a) The presence of an indwelling urinary catheter
(b) A rectal temperature of 100°F (37.8°C)
(c) Redness, warmth, and tenderness in the incision area
(d) A white blood cell (WBC) count of 8,000/mL

**175. The nurse is caring for a patient with a postoperative wound evisceration. Which action should the nurse perform first?**
(a) Explain to the patient what is happening, and provide support
(b) Cover the protruding organs with sterile gauze moistened with sterile saline solution
(c) Push the protruding organs back into the abdominal cavity
(d) Ask the patient to drink as much fluid as possible

**176. A patient in the postoperative phase of abdominal surgery is to advance his diet as tolerated. The patient has tolerated ice chips and a clear liquid diet. As the next step, the nurse would expect the patient to advance to:**
(a) Fluid restriction
(b) A full-liquid diet
(c) A general diet
(d) A soft diet

**177. The patient's intake and output record contains the following information: milk, 180 mL; orange juice, 60 mL; one serving scrambled eggs; one slice toast; one can ensure oral nutritional supplement, 240 mL; IV dextrose 5% in water at 100 mL/hour; 50 mL water after twice daily medications. Medications are given at 9:00 am and 9:00 pm. What is the patient's total intake for the 7 am to 3 pm shift?**
(a) 1,000 mL
(b) 1,250 mL
(c) 1,330 mL
(d) 1,380 mL

**178. Which action is included in the principles of asepsis?**
(a) Maintaining a sterile environment
(b) Keeping the environment as clean as possible
(c) Testing for microorganisms in the environment
(d) Cleaning an environment until it is free from germs

**179. On the first day after thoracotomy, the nurse's assessment of the patient reveals a temperature of 100°F (37.8°C), a heart rate of 96 beats/minute, blood pressure of 136/86 mm Hg, and shallow respirations of 24 breaths/minute, with rhonchi heard at the lung bases. The patient complains of incisional pain. Which nursing action takes priority?**
(a) Medicating the patient for pain
(b) Helping the patient out of bed
(c) Administering ibuprofen (Motrin) as ordered to reduce fever
(d) Encouraging the patient to cough and deep-breathe

**180. Which intervention is most important to include in a nursing care plan for a patient with atelectasis?**
(a) Give oxygen continuously at 3 L/minute
(b) Have the patient cough and deep-breathe every 4 hours
(c) Have the patient use an incentive spirometer every hour
(d) Get the patient out of bed to a chair every day

**181. Excessive accumulation of endolymph in the membranous labyrinth results in:**
(a) Osteosclerosis (b) Otitis
(c) Menier's disease (d) Acousticneuroma

**182. Type of ulcer common in patient with extensive burn injury:**
(a) Cushing's ulcer (b) Curling's ulcer
(c) Both (a) and (b) (d) None of the above

**183. Group of disorders characterized by increased IOP, optic nerve atrophy and peripheral visual field loss:**
(a) Hordeolum (b) Glaucoma
(c) Keratoconus (d) Strabismus

**184. Shortening of scar tissue in the flexor tissue of the joint result in:**
(a) Contracture (b) Eschar
(c) Blister (d) None of the above

**185. Most common cause of cerebrovascular disease:**
(a) Atherosclerosis (b) Stress
(c) Heart failure (d) None of the above

**186. Disease characterized by slowness in the initiation and execution of movement, tremor at rest and impaired postural reflexes:**
(a) Parkinson's disease (b) Multiple sclerosis
(c) Alzheimer's disease (d) GB syndrome

**187. Farsightedness is also known as:**
(a) Presbyopia (b) Myopia
(c) Hyperopia (d) Astigmastin

**188. Confining to the room, crying and talking to one's long dead husband is a type of griving and is known as:**
(a) Dysfunctional (b) Adaptive
(c) Disruptive (d) Anticipatory

**189. The vibration of tactile fermitus is best assessed by using the nurse's:**
(a) Index finger (b) Finger tip
(c) Palm (d) Stethoscope

**190. The client on chemotherapy is placed in barrier nursing. The purpose is to:**
(a) Protect the client from infection
(b) Protect the nurse from infection
(c) Provide privacy
(d) Facilitate recovery

**191. Excessive accumulation of endolymph in the membrane labyrinth result in Meniere's disease. A client with Meniere's disease should:**
(a) Increase in sodium diet
(b) Decrease in sodium diet
(c) Increase in potassium diet
(d) Decrease in potassium diet

**192. A nursing measure to reduce increased Intra Cranial Pressure in a patient after head injury is to:**
(a) Administer codien to relieve neck spasm
(b) Control fever
(c) Minimize environmental stimulation
(d) Raise the head end of bed to 300

**193. Cataract is described as:**
(a) Inflammation of retina
(b) Opacity of lens
(c) Infection of cornea
(d) Obstruction of aqueous humor

**194. Following the head trauma the patient complains of hearing, ringing noise, this suggest injury to:**
(a) Frontal lobe
(b) Occipital lobe
(c) Abducent nerve
(d) Vestibular and cochlear nerve

**195. The inner most and smallest ossicle is:**
(a) Stapes (b) Mallens
(c) Incus (d) Labyrinth

**196. The position used for patient who is having epitaxis is:**
(a) Sitting up victim with head tilt forward
(b) Sitting up victim with head tilt backward
(c) Lying on the back with head turned to one side
(d) Lying straight with head elevated

**197. Primary responsibility of a nurse during a client with generalized seizure is:**
(a) Determine if an aura was experienced
(b) Inserting the plastic airway between teeth
(c) Cleaning the immediate environment for safety
(d) Administering PRN anticonvulsant

**198. Romberg's test is used to assess:**
(a) Visual acuty (b) Hearing
(c) Balance (d) Infertility

**199. Normal range of potassium 'K' in serum:**
(a) 136–146 m. eq/L (b) 3.5–4.5 m. eq/L
(c) 60–100 mg/C (d) 35 to 45%

**200. Digitalis is considered as:**
(a) Heart tonic (b) Coagulant
(c) Thrombolytic (d) Vasodilator

**201. Dexamethasom is administered to patient after stroke to:**
(a) To improve renal blood flow
(b) Maintain circulatory volume
(c) To reduce intracranial pressure
(d) To prevent development of thrombus

**202. Loss of accommodation associated with age is:**
(a) Presbyopia (b) Hyperopia
(c) Myopia (d) Astigmatin

**203. An example of distraction to provide pain relief is:**
(a) Tens (b) Music
(c) Exercise (d) Bio feedback

**204. Meniere's diseaseis characterized by:**
(a) Vertigo (b) Tinnitus
(c) Aural fullness (d) Pain

**205. Inflammation of the sebaceous gland in the eye lid is called:**
(a) Blepharitis (b) Conjunctivitis
(c) Chalazion (d) Keratitis

**206. While assessing partial thickness burn nurse should expect to find:**
(a) Exposed fascia
(b) Dry waxy appearance
(c) Red, shiny appearance
(d) Absence of blanching with pressure

**207. In which area should the nurse assess a patient who is on bed rest for the presence of edema:**
(a) Arms (b) Ankles
(c) Sternum (d) Sacrum

**208. Kidneys regulates blood pressure by the release of:**
(a) Epinephrine (b) Cytokines
(c) Aldosteron (d) Rennin

**209. The normal value of $PO_2$ in arterial blood gas (ABG) analysis is:**
(a) 80–100 mm of Hg (b) 73–100 mm of Hg
(c) 35–45 mm of Hg (d) 100–200 mm of Hg

**210. The most common factor for developing oral cancer is:**
(a) Family history (b) Lifestyle changes
(c) Infection (d) Age

**211. Hemorrhage into the inner ear occurs in which of the following:**
(a) Diabetes mellitus (b) Polycythemia
(c) Leukemia (d) Iron deficiency anemia

**212. The first step in cardio-pulmonary resuscitation (CPR) is to obtain:**
(a) Circulation (b) Pulse activity
(c) Breathing (d) Open airway

**213. Complication associated with tracheostomy tube includes:**
(a) Decreased cardiac output
(b) Damage to laryngeal nerve
(c) Pneumothorax
(d) Acute respiratory distress syndrome

**214. A pigskin graft used in skin grafting for burn patient is known as:**
(a) An isograft (b) An allograft
(c) Axenograft (d) A homograft

**215. The most common cancer in women is that of:**
(a) Cervix (b) Ovary
(c) Fallopian tube (d) Urinary bladder

**216. When a clients pupil is dilated which cranial nerve is involved:**
(a) 2nd cranial nerve (b) 4th cranial nerve
(c) 7th cranial nerve (d) 3rd cranial nerve

**217. Which muscle become weak and atrophied after just a few days of mechanical ventilation:**
(a) Cardiac muscle
(b) Respiratory muscle
(c) Abdominal muscle
(d) Facial muscle

**218. An indicator for fluid replacement therapy in a client during first 24 hours following burn is:**
(a) Falling CVP
(b) Slowing of previously rapid pulse
(c) Hematocrit levels rising from 50 to 55
(d) Changes in ECG pattern

**219. Treatment of choice for stage I cancer of larynx is:**
(a) Radical surgery
(b) Radiotherapy
(c) Chemotherapy
(d) Surgery followed by radiotherapy

**220. Which of the following nursing intervention to be followed after Lumbar laminectomy?**
(a) Encourage the client to cough frequently
(b) Log roll the client using the draw sheet
(c) Assess the client for indication of peritonitis
(d) Instruct the client to bend the knees

**221. The hemlich maneuver recommended for relieving the foreign body airway obstruction is a:**
(a) Subdiaphragmatic abdominal thrust
(b) Abdominal thrust
(c) Trachea thrust
(d) Diaphragmatic thrust

**222. In a client with heat stroke the temperature is recorded as:**
(a) 105°F (b) 100–102°F
(c) Greater than 105°F (d) Less then 100°F

**223. One of the earlier problems encountered in a client with paraplegia after spinal cord injury is:**
(a) Bladder control
(b) Nutritional intake
(c) Quadriceps setting
(d) Use of aids for ambulation

**224. Normal range of intraocular pressure:**
(a) 10–12 mm of Hg (b) 10–22 mm of Hg
(c) 10–20 mm of Hg (d) 10–30 mm of Hg

**225. While assessing a client with Parkinson's disease the nurse identifies bradykinesia when the client exhibit:**
(a) Muscle flassidity
(b) Tremors
(c) Paralysis of limbs
(d) Abnormal slow movements

**226. A client with open angle glaucoma is most likely to exhibit:**
(a) Constant blurring of vision
(b) Sudden stack of acute pain
(c) Impairment of peripheral vision
(d) A sudden loss of complete vision

**227. The protrusion of uterus beyond the introitus is called:**
(a) Prolapse (b) Procedentia
(c) Displaced uterus (d) Inverted uterus

**228. Iatrogenic traumatic facial nerve palsy is most commonly caused during:**
(a) Myringoplasty (b) Stapedectomy
(c) Mastoidectomy (d) Ossiculoplasty

**229. One of the following gastrointestinal complication resulting from burn trauma:**
(a) Paralytic ileus (b) Dumping syndrome
(c) Ascitis (d) Colitis

**230. A method for minimizing absorption of toxic substances in a client with ingested poisioning:**
(a) Activated charcoal (b) Syrup of ipecac
(c) Vinegar (d) Salt water

**231. Pulmonary fibrosis is an side effect of the following antineoplastic drug:**
(a) Bleomycin (b) 5- fluorouracil
(c) Cisplastin (d) Vincristine

**232. Neostigmine is prescribed for a client with myasthenia gravis. The drug act by:**
(a) Stimulating cerebral cortex
(b) Blocking the action of cholinesterase
(c) Replacing deficient neurotransmitter
(d) Accelerating transmission along neural sheet

**233. The primary purpose of estrogen replacement therapy following panhysterectomy is to prevent:**
(a) Arthritis (b) Pregnancy
(c) Breast cancer (d) Vasomotor instability

**234. When earring for client with head injury the nurse should assess for:**
(a) Decreased carotid pulse
(b) Bleeding from oral cavity
(c) Altered level of consciousness
(d) Absence of deep tendon reflexes

**235. Common symptoms in a client with cataract would be:**
(a) Halos and rainbow ground light
(b) Eye pain and irritation that worsen at night
(c) Blurred and hazy vision
(d) Eye strain and head ache

**236. Location of cardiac center in nervous center is found in:**
(a) Cerebrum (b) Hypothalamus
(c) Spinal cord (d) Medulla

**237. A patient is scheduled for vascular surgery. The patient is taking many drugs. Which medication should be stopped by the physician several days before the surgery:**
(a) Digoxin (b) Furosemide
(c) Warfarin (d) Famotidine

**238. After laryngectomy, which of the following assessment takes priority:**
(a) Airway patency (b) Nutritional status
(c) Lung sound (d) Peripheral pulse

**239. Foot/diet likely to contribute to development of certain type of cancer includes all of the following EXCEPT:**
(a) High fat diet
(b) Low fiber diet
(c) Smoked food
(d) Diet containing antioxidant

**240. The most important risk factor for lung cancer:**
(a) Smoking (b) Air pollution
(c) Alcohol (d) Genetic link

**241. Mydriatics are ocular medications that:**
(a) Dilate the pupil
(b) Constrict the pupil
(c) Increased the aqueous humor production
(d) Decrease the aqueous humor production

**242. Which of the following are least effective for contraception?**
(a) Condom with spermicide
(b) Douching
(c) Diaphragm with spermicide
(d) Oral contraceptive pills

**243. How soon after symptoms onset must the stroke victim receive thrombolytic treatment:**
(a) 1 hour (b) 2 hour
(c) 3 hour (d) 4 hour

**244. Which of the following are the modifiable risk factor for stroke:**
(a) Heredity (b) Age
(c) Sex (d) Obesity

**245. __________ is used to assess both air bone conduction:**
(a) Weber test (b) Rinne test
(c) Wisper test (d) Caloric test

**246. The technique for measuring intraocular pressure:**
(a) Tonometry
(b) Tomography
(c) Opthalmoscopy
(d) Fundoscopy

**247. Extent of electrical burn can be difficult to assess because:**
(a) Victims are in shock
(b) The entry and exit wound are deep
(c) Internal damage is not readily apparent
(d) Electrical injury is normally smaller then thermal

**248. The cherry red appeaence of skin color indicates:**
(a) Food poisoning
(b) Carbon monoxide poisoning
(c) Snake bite
(d) Chemical burn

**249. Interventions to prevent falls in older people include:**
(a) Good lightening
(b) Attention to postural hypotension
(c) Balance and gait training
(d) All of the above

**250. Acute toxicity of radiation occurs largely in:**
(a) Slow proliferating tissue
(b) Glands
(c) Rapid renewing tissue
(d) Normal tissue

**251. A massive uncompensated cardiovascular reaction mediated by the sympathetic nervous system in spinal cord injury is:**
(a) Sensory perception alteration
(b) Autonomic dysreflexia
(c) Spastic reflexes
(d) Arfelexia

**252. The weaning mode for ventilator is:**
(a) SIMV (b) CPAP
(c) PEEP (d) $FiO_2$

**253. Lack of coordination in articulating speech is called:**
(a) Dysphasia (b) Dysarthria
(c) Hyporeflexia (d) Akinesia

**254. When a nurse detects the ventricular fibrillation the first thing the nurse should administer:**
(a) Oxygenation
(b) Initiate CPR
(c) Defibrillate the patient
(d) Potassium chloride

**255. Visual acuty can be tested with the help of:**
(a) Speculum
(b) Spirit lamp and tuning fork
(c) Snellen's chart
(d) Tonometer

**256. The malignant tumor which originate from bone is known as:**
(a) Adenoma (b) Leiomyoma
(c) Sarcoma (d) Carcinoma

**257. A client with radium implanted for cancer cervix, prepare discharge plan that the nurse should explain the importance of:**
(a) Limiting fluid intake
(b) Regularly returning for medical follow up
(c) Continue with liquid diet
(d) Vitamin 'D' should be gained from the sunlight

**258. The most frequently occurring brain tumor is:**
(a) Glioma (b) Meningoma
(c) Neurofibroma (d) Pituitary adenoma

**259. First top priority nursing care, for the post operative patient laryngectomy patient is:**
(a) Ensure communication
(b) Alley anxiety
(c) Maintain patent airway
(d) Train for speech therapy

**260. Other name for inner ear is:**
(a) Eustachian tube (b) Tymphanic membrane
(c) Cochlea (d) Labyrinth

**261. A 37 years old AIDS patient who is homosexual has increased susceptibility to disease because of:**
(a) Immune suppression
(b) Young age
(c) Side effect of medicine
(d) Malnutrition

**262. Pilocarpine is drug used to treat glaucoma, it act as:**
(a) Papillary dilator
(b) Papillary constrictor
(c) Reduces production of aqueous humour
(d) Increases optic nerve stimulation

**263. Aphakia is corrected by:**
(a) Audiometer test
(b) Tonometric test
(c) Spectrotherapy
(d) Eye glasses

**264. The appropriate duration of tracheosomy suctioning at a time is NOT more then:**
(a) 5 to 10 sec (b) 15 to 20 sec
(c) 21 to 25 sec (d) 20 to 30 sec

**265. A Swan Ganz Catheter (pulmonary artery catheter) inserted to provide information of:**
(a) Stroke volume (b) Cardiac output
(c) Venous pressure (d) Left ventricular functioning

**266. A client has a chest tube attached to a water seal drainage system and the nurse detect that the fluid in the chest tube and in the water seal column was stopped fluctuating, this means:**
(a) The lung has fully expanded
(b) The lung has collapsed
(c) Chest tube is in plural space
(d) The meditational space has decreased

**267. In a leukemia patient the platlet count is very low. The nurse should monitor client's urine for the presence of:**
(a) Casts (b) Erythrocytes
(c) Leukocytes (d) Bacteria

**268. While performing cardiac compression it is essential to exert ventricular downward pressure which compresses the lower sternum at least:**
(a) 1.5 to 2 cm (1/2 to ¼ inch)
(b) 2–2.5 cm (3/4 inch)
(c) 2.5 to 4 cm (1–1 ½ inch)
(d) 4–5 cm (1 ½ to 2 inch)

**269. The primary responsibility of a nurse while caring for HIV positive client is to explain him the process to prevent:**
(a) AIDS (b) Social isolation
(c) Other infection (d) Kaposis sarcoma

**270. An intensive care nurse observes the multipara monitor for a patient with hypokalemia for:**
(a) Lowering of 'T' wave
(b) Elevation of 'ST' segment
(c) Shortening of PR interval
(d) Increased deflection of 'Q' wave

**271. Cardiogenic shock is:**
(a) An irreversible phenomena
(b) Failure of peripheral circulation
(c) Occurs as an reaction of pain
(d) Caused by cardiac overload

**272. The potential of injury during attack of Meniere's disease is great. The nurse should instruct the patient that when vertigo is experienced immediately:**
(a) Place your head between knees
(b) Concentrate on rhythmic deep breathing
(c) Close your eyes tightly
(d) Assume recline or flat position

**273. The most lethal effect of chemotherapy:**
(a) Alopecia
(b) Myelosuppression
(c) Nausea and vomiting
(d) Stomatitis

**274. Which of the following is not the cardiovascular changes related to ageing:**
(a) Increase in collagen in cardiac structure
(b) Decrease in heart rate
(c) Calcification of cardiac valves
(d) Decrease in number of pacemaker cell

**275. Following are the example of benign tumor:**
(a) Melanoma (b) Adenosarcoma
(c) Fibrosarcoma (d) Adenoma

**276. The drug of choice in endometriosis is:**
(a) Antibiotics (b) Corticosteroids
(c) Vaginal pessaries (d) Hormonal therapy

**277. The organism most common responsible for nosocomial infection in burn patient is:**
(a) Streptococci (b) Staphylococci
(c) E Coli (d) Salmonella

**278. The drug of choice to treat anaphylactic shock is:**
(a) Epinephrine (b) Dopamine
(c) Hydrocortisone (d) Nitroglycerine

**279. Patchy blindness (scotoma) is a clinical manifestation of:**
(a) Myasthenia gravis (b) Retinal detachment
(c) Glaucoma (d) Multiple sclerosis

**280. Following tonsillectomy operation, when ready, a child can be given:**
(a) Lime juice (b) Hot tea
(c) Ice-cream (d) Hot soups

**281. A patient was managed in casualty for epitaxis by placing anterior nasal packing. During discharge nurse should instruct the patient to:**
(a) Avoid vigorous nose blowing and strenuous activity
(b) Use aspirin to pain relief
(c) Remove the pack later that day
(d) Skip the next dose of anti hypertensive

**282. Syngeneic transplantation involves:**
(a) Receiving own bone marrow
(b) Obtaining stem cells from one identical twins and infusing them into other
(c) Infusing bone marrow from HLA matched donor to the recipient.
(d) Infusing bone marrow collected from other species

**283. An apparatus which applies cervical traction by means of a jacket like arrangement that allows greater mobility and wheel chair activities:**
(a) Philadelphia collar (b) Halo vest
(c) Body jacket (d) Gardner wells tongs

**284. Loss of skilled voluntary movement is known as:**
(a) Dysarthria (b) Hyporeflexia
(c) Akinesia (d) Dysphagia

**285. A failure of more then one organ system in an acutely ill patient in which homeostasis cannot be maintained without intervention:**
(a) ARDS (b) SIRS
(c) MODS (d) SIADM

**286. Which of the following is known as true tissue freezing:**
(a) Profound hypothermia
(b) Hypothermia
(c) Frost bite
(d) Moderate hypothermia

**287. If the cervix is at vaginal opening, the uterine prolapse is of:**
(a) 1st degree (b) 2nd degree
(c) 3rd degree (d) 4th degree

**288. The nursing measure to reduce ICP in a patient is:**
(a) Administer medicine for pain relief
(b) Control fever
(c) Minimize environmental stimulation
(d) Raise head end of the bed to 300

**289. The purpose of adding PEEP to positive pressure ventilation is:**
(a) Increase functional residual capacity
(b) Increase $FiO_2$ so as to wean the patient
(c) Avoid risk of pneumomediastinum
(d) Determine if patient is in synchrony with ventilator

**290. Stomatitis a common side effect of chemotherapeutic agent occurs because:**
(a) Site of malignancy is near oral cavity
(b) General health of a cancer patient is poor
(c) External local and irritating effect of chemotherapy
(d) Rapidly dividing cells of mucous membrane of mouth are being destroyed

**291. By rule of nine, calculate the percentage of burn in a person with a burn of anterior trunk, leg and perineum:**
(a) 37% (b) 32%
(c) 28% (d) 24%

**292. The use of various monitoring device which help patient to control their own physiological responses such as heart rate is called:**
(a) Psychotherapy (b) Imagery
(c) Reiki therapy (d) Bio feedback

**293. Following are the high risk factor for development of glaucoma:**
(a) Diabetes mellitus
(b) Migraine
(c) Prolonged used of corticosteroid
(d) Use of diuretics

**294. In which degree of burn the burn wound blanches with pressure:**
(a) Ist (b) IInd
(c) IIIrd (d) IVth

**295. Asom is:**
(a) An infection to inner ear
(b) An infection to mastoid
(c) An infection to middle ear
(d) Conduction disorder

**296. Which of the following virus is been associated with cancer of cervix:**
(a) Epstein Barr Virus
(b) Human Papilloma Virus
(c) HIV
(d) Hepatitis B

**297. BSE involves palpation of breast and:**
(a) A physical examination
(b) Inspection of both breast for skin changes
(c) Mammographic evaluation of the breast tissue
(d) A fine needle aspiration biopsy

**298. A patient who has sustain burns of his upper body part. A nurse assessing his potential problem of respiratory obstruction. Which of the following indicates potential problem of respiratory obstruction:**
(a) Deep breathing
(b) Pink frothy sputum
(c) Rapid abdominal breathing
(d) Hoarseness of voice

**299. Petrygium is:**
(a) Type of cataract
(b) Ptosis
(c) Glaucoma
(d) Sclera thickening in form of bad

**300. The concept of hospice care is:**
(a) Care of patient in his terminal illness phase
(b) Care of patient in the end stage of illness
(c) Place to provide care for older adult
(d) Place to keep cancer patient

**301. A patient with a tricuspid valve disorder will have impaired blood flow between the:**
(a) Vena cava and right atrium
(b) Left atrium and left ventical
(c) Right atrium and right ventrical
(d) Right ventrical and pulmonary artey

**302. A patient with an MI of the anterior wall of the left ventricle most likely has an occlusion of:**
(a) Left marginal artery
(b) Right marginal artery
(c) Right descending artery
(d) Left anterior descending artery

**303. If the purkinje system is damaged conduction of electrical impulses is impaired through the:**
(a) Atria (b) AV node
(c) Ventricle (d) Bundle of his

**304. The portion of the vascular system responsible for hemostasis is the:**
(a) Thin capillary vessel
(b) Endothelial layer of arteries
(c) Elastic middle layer of the veins
(d) Smooth muscle of the arterial wall

**305. A 'P' wave in ECG represents an impulse:**
(a) Arising from SA node and repolarisation of atria
(b) Arising from SA node and depolarisation of atria
(c) Arising from AV node and repolarisation of atria
(d) Arising from AV node and depolarisation of atria

**306. When checking the capillary filling time of the patient, the color return in 5 seconds the nurses recognizes this finding as indicative of:**
(a) A normal response
(b) Thrombus formation in vein
(c) Lymphatic obstruction of venious returns
(d) Impaired arterial flow to the extrimities

## ANSWERS

| 1. | (a) | 41. | (c) | 81. | (a) | 121. | (c) | 161. | (a) | 201. | (c) | 241. | (a) | 281. | (a) |
|---|---|---|---|---|---|---|---|---|---|---|---|---|---|---|---|
| 2. | (b) | 42. | (d) | 82. | (b) | 122. | (b) | 162. | (b) | 202. | (a) | 242. | (d) | 282. | (b) |
| 3. | (c) | 43. | (d) | 83. | (b) | 123. | (d) | 163. | (b) | 203. | (b) | 243. | (a) | 283. | (b) |
| 4. | (a) | 44. | (d) | 84. | (a) | 124. | (a) | 164. | (c) | 204. | (a) | 244. | (d) | 284. | (c) |
| 5. | (a) | 45. | (c) | 85. | (d) | 125. | (b) | 165. | (b) | 205. | (a) | 245. | (b) | 285. | (c) |
| 6. | (b) | 46. | (a) | 86. | (c) | 126. | (a) | 166. | (a) | 206. | (d) | 246. | (a) | 286. | (c) |
| 7. | (b) | 47. | (b) | 87. | (a) | 127. | (d) | 167. | (c) | 207. | (b) | 247. | (c) | 287. | (b) |
| 8. | (c) | 48. | (a) | 88. | (b) | 128. | (b) | 168. | (d) | 208. | (d) | 248. | (d) | 288. | (d) |
| 9. | (a) | 49. | (b) | 89. | (c) | 129. | (b) | 169. | (b) | 209. | (a) | 249. | (d) | 289. | (a) |
| 10. | (a) | 50. | (d) | 90. | (c) | 130. | (a) | 170. | (b) | 210. | (b) | 250. | (a) | 290. | (d) |
| 11. | (d) | 51. | (b) | 91. | (d) | 131. | (c) | 171. | (a) | 211. | (b) | 251. | (b) | 291. | (c) |
| 12. | (b) | 52. | (c) | 92. | (a) | 132. | (c) | 172. | (b) | 212. | (a) | 252. | (b) | 292. | (d) |
| 13. | (a) | 53. | (b) | 93. | (b) | 133. | (d) | 173. | (d) | 213. | (c) | 253. | (b) | 293. | (c) |
| 14. | (c) | 54. | (b) | 94. | (a) | 134. | (d) | 174. | (c) | 214. | (c) | 254. | (c) | 294. | (b) |
| 15. | (d) | 55. | (c) | 95. | (a) | 135. | (a) | 175. | (b) | 215 | (a) | 255. | (c) | 295. | (c) |
| 16. | (d) | 56. | (d) | 96. | (c) | 136. | (c) | 176. | (b) | 216. | (a) | 256. | (c) | 296. | (b) |
| 17. | (a) | 57. | (d) | 97. | (b) | 137. | (b) | 177. | (c) | 217. | (b) | 257. | (b) | 297. | (b) |
| 18. | (b) | 58. | (c) | 98. | (d) | 138. | (b) | 178. | (b) | 218. | (c) | 258. | (a) | 298. | (d) |
| 19. | (a) | 59. | (b) | 99. | (c) | 139. | (d) | 179. | (a) | 219. | (a) | 259. | (c) | 299. | (d) |
| 20. | (c) | 60. | (c) | 100. | (b) | 140. | (c) | 180. | (c) | 220. | (b) | 260. | (d) | 300. | (a) |
| 21. | (a) | 61. | (a) | 101. | (c) | 141. | (b) | 181. | (c) | 221. | (a) | 261. | (a) | 301. | (b) |
| 22. | (b) | 62. | (b) | 102. | (c) | 142. | (a) | 182. | (b) | 222. | (c) | 262. | (b) | 302. | (d) |
| 23. | (c) | 63. | (d) | 103. | (d) | 143. | (d) | 183. | (b) | 223. | (a) | 263. | (d) | 303. | (d) |
| 24. | (a) | 64. | (b) | 104. | (a) | 144. | (b) | 184. | (a) | 224. | (b) | 264. | (a) | 304. | (b) |
| 25. | (a) | 65. | (c) | 105. | (d) | 145. | (a) | 185. | (a) | 225. | (d) | 265. | (c) | 305. | (a) |
| 26. | (d) | 66. | (b) | 106. | (d) | 146. | (a) | 186. | (a) | 226. | (a) | 266. | (d) | 306. | (a) |
| 27. | (d) | 67. | (c) | 107. | (d) | 147. | (c) | 187. | (c) | 227. | (a) | 267. | (b) | | |
| 28. | (a) | 68. | (d) | 108. | (d) | 148. | (c) | 188. | (d) | 228. | (c) | 268. | (d) | | |
| 29. | (b) | 69. | (c) | 109. | (a) | 149. | (c) | 189. | (c) | 229. | (a) | 269. | (c) | | |
| 30. | (c) | 70. | (b) | 110. | (d) | 150. | (c) | 190. | (a) | 230. | (a) | 270. | (a) | | |
| 31. | (c) | 71. | (c) | 111. | (c) | 151. | (c) | 191. | (b) | 231. | (a) | 271. | (b) | | |
| 32. | (b) | 72. | (a) | 112. | (c) | 152. | (d) | 192. | (d) | 232. | (b) | 272. | (d) | | |
| 33. | (c) | 73. | (c) | 113. | (a) | 153. | (c) | 193. | (b) | 233. | (d) | 273. | (b) | | |
| 34. | (d) | 74. | (d) | 114. | (c) | 154. | (d) | 194. | (d) | 234. | (c) | 274. | (c) | | |
| 35. | (d) | 75. | (a) | 115. | (d) | 155. | (b) | 195. | (a) | 235. | (c) | 275. | (d) | | |
| 36. | (c) | 76. | (b) | 116. | (d) | 156. | (d) | 196. | (a) | 236. | (d) | 276. | (d) | | |
| 37. | (d) | 77. | (d) | 117. | (c) | 157. | (c) | 197. | (c) | 237. | (c) | 277. | (b) | | |
| 38. | (b) | 78. | (a) | 118. | (b) | 158. | (c) | 198. | (c) | 238. | (a) | 278. | (a) | | |
| 39. | (a) | 79. | (a) | 119. | (d) | 159. | (c) | 199. | (b) | 239. | (a) | 279. | (c) | | |
| 40. | (c) | 80. | (b) | 120. | (d) | 160. | (a) | 200. | (a) | 240. | (a) | 280. | (c) | | |

# QUICK REVIEW

## Child Health Nursing Review and Multiple Choice Questions

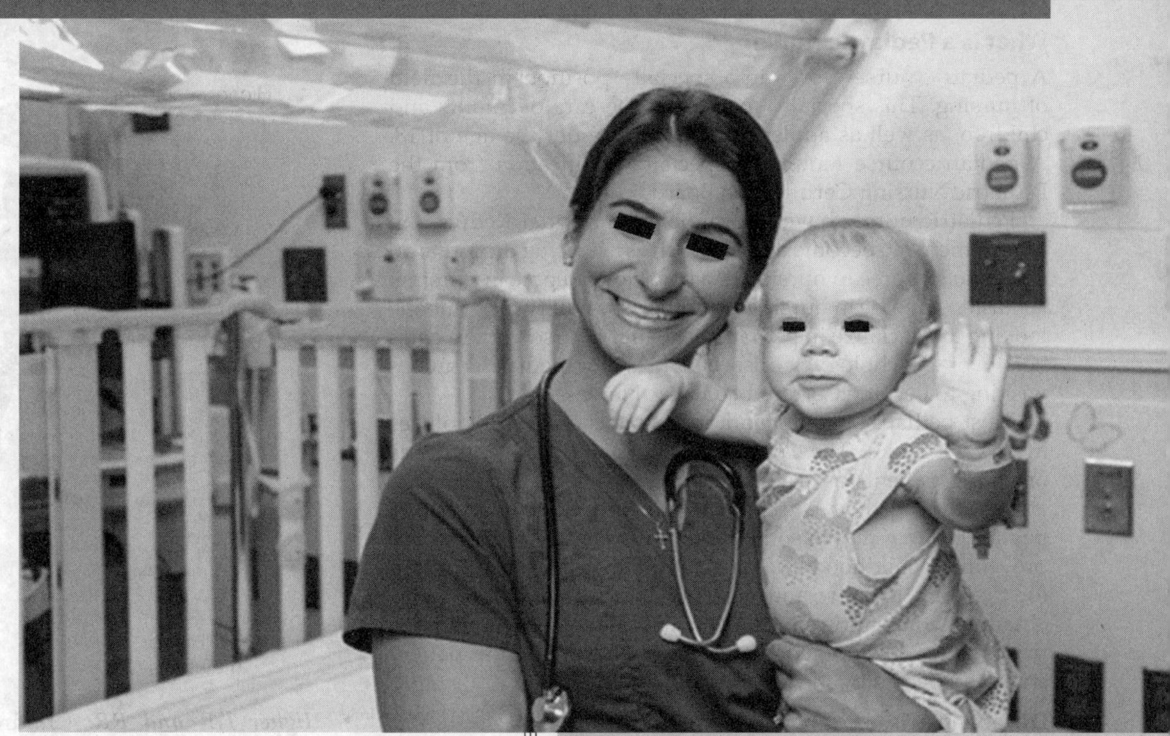

### HIGHLIGHTS

- Why is Specialist Pediatric Training Important?
- Concept of Growth and Development
- Freud's Theory of Psychosexual Development
- Erikson's Theory of Psychosocial Development
- Milestones of Growth and Development
- Severe Acute Malnutrition
- Pediatric Genitourinary Disorders
- Congenital Anomalies
- Infant Care
- Under 5 Clinic
- Multiple Choice Questions

# Child Health Nursing/Pediatric

## INTRODUCTION

### What is a Pediatric Nurse?

A pediatric nurse works in a specialty position in the field of nursing. This specialty focuses on the care of infants and children, as well as adolescents that are under the age of 18. A pediatric nurse requires a specialty certification from the Pediatric Nursing Certification Board.

Pediatric nurses have to complete the standard education requirements to become a nurse, such as a nursing diploma, an associate's degree in nursing or a bachelor's degree in nursing. A master's degree in nursing is another possibility for someone looking to specialize in pediatric nursing. Coursework in child health or psychology is also beneficial for pediatric nurses wishing to become Certified Pediatric Nurses.

Most pediatric nurses work in hospitals or doctor's offices in private clinics. They need an understanding of the needs of young patients as well as techniques for putting children at ease during their course of treatment or doctor's visit. A pediatric nurse may also be required to discuss methods for preventing childhood diseases and the necessary nutrition for the child to grow and develop. This role may also cover obtaining vital information from the child or their parents, performing developmental screenings and giving the patient shots as directed by the physician.

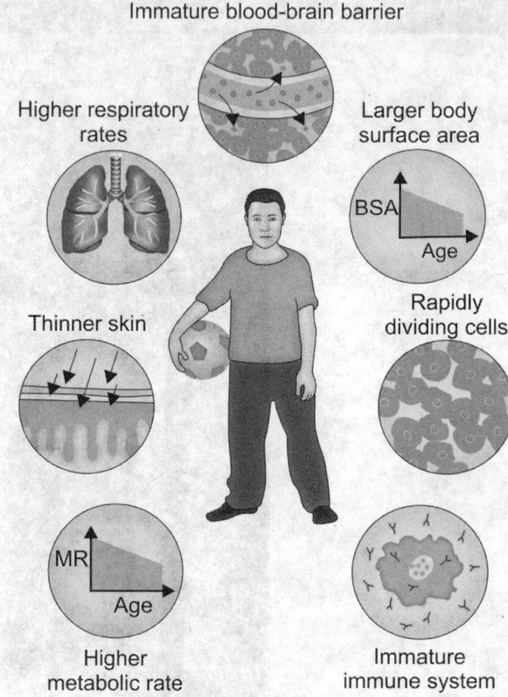


### Differences Between Children and Adults

There are many differences between children, adolescents and adults physiological, anatomical, cognitive, social and emotional of which all impact on the way illness and disease present in children and young people, as well as the way health care is provided.

### Overview of Differences

#### *Anatomical/Physiological*

- *Larger BSA:* Children have a proportionately larger body surface area (BSA) than adults do. The smaller the patient, the greater the ratio of surface area (skin) to size. As a result, children are at greater risk of excessive loss of heat and fluids; children are affected by more quickly and easily toxins that are absorbed through the skin.
- *Thinner skin:* Children have thinner skin than adults. Their epidermis is thinner and under-keratinized, compared with adults. As a result, children are at risk for on increased absorption of agents that can be absorbed through the skin.
- *Rapidly dividing cells:* Children cells divide into more rapidly than adults to assist in their rapid rate of growth. As a result, children are more susceptible to the effects of radiation than adults.
- *Higher HR and RR:* Children have higher respiratory rates than adults. Higher respiratory rates lead to proportionately higher minute volumes. As a result, children may be more susceptible to agents absorbed through the pulmonary route than adults with the same exposure. Children may also respond more rapidly to such agents. Signs and symptoms in children may be an 'early warning' of a chemical, biological, or radiological incident.
- *Immature blood/brain barrier:* Children have immature blood/brain barriers and enhanced central nervous system (CNS) receptivity.

  As a result, children may exhibit as a prevalence of neurological symptoms. Nerve agents may produce more symptoms in pediatric patients, requiring levels of treatment for children that are not indicated for adults with the same level of exposure.
- *Higher metabolic rate:* More susceptible to contaminants in food or water; greater risk for increased loss of water and when ill or stressed. Medication doses must be carefully calculated based on the child's weight and body size.
- *Immature immune systems:* Greater risk of infection; less hard immunity from some infections.

### Psychosocial Differences

Although adults continue to develop psychosocial, their values/behavior/social circles are generally far more defined and stable, whereas children and adolescents are rapidly developing and using the world around them and picking up cues from their environment to aid in that development. It is essential to be mindful of the way that clinicians interact and communicate with children, adolescents and their families play a role in this development, and to be well aware of the broader context of a child or adolescent's life, as this has much more significant impact on the way they experience and recover from illness or injury.

### Social

Unlike adult, children and adolescents are still in a period of social development which involves learning the values, knowledge and skills that enable them to relate to others. The goal is for children and adolescents to build a positive sense of their own identity and their role in relationships with people around them. These social skills and lessons can be learnt from those who care for them, as well as indirectly through negotiating social relationships with family or with friends, and through participation in the world around them e.g. coming to hospital.

Not of these relationships and experiences are positive, and the impact of negative influences also shapes of social behaviors. Hospitals and their staff can be part of a child/families social environment and therefore, it is important for clinicians to be mindful of how they conduct themselves in their social or professional relationships with a child's family and toward the child and adolescent themselves, as this has an impact on learning and development of their own social identity. It is also important to be mindful of different circumstances which shape social skills during the developmental process and influence behaviors and interactions with other people.

Children, and to a lesser extent adolescents, typically present more explicitly with their immediate social circle shown to the clinician- with the presentation of parents, grandparents, aunts and uncles etc at appointments.

### Emotional

Children and adolescents are still developing their ability to recognize and manage their emotions or feelings, and this can be influenced by many social and environmental factors. For infants and young children, their emotional bond of affection or 'attachment' to their caregivers is crucial to their emotional development.

### Effects of Secure Attachment

More resilient, competent toddlers with high self esteem. In pre-school display more persistence, curiosity, self-reliance, leadership and have better peer relations.

After age 11—better social skills, close friends, clinicians in a pediatric setting should be mindful of the disruption to this bond that may result in separation of anxiety which is emotional distress seen in many infants. When they are separated from people with whom they have formed an attachment, they should also be mindful that not all children and adolescents will come from an environment where they will have the consistency and stability in their everyday lives but also to allow them to form secure attachments, and this may be reflected in their coping and behavior.

### Cognitive

The growth of thought in children more so that in an adult environment, a clinician must be mindful of how they communicate with a patient, taking into account a child or adolescent's level of cognitive development.

### Examples

*Example for a Younger Child*

Four year old Susan was asked where she got her name.

- She answered, 'my mummy named me',
- 'What if your mother called you Jack?'
- 'Then I would be a boy'

*Example for an Older Child*

- ***Concrete:*** 'You said I should get it, if I missed my asthma inhalers, but I forgot them twice and I stayed fine so I do not need them anymore'
- ***Abstract:*** 'I missed my inhalers a couple of times but I think I got away with it because I wasn't doing much exercise. I think I will still need them in the future, if I am doing lots of exercise in cold weather'.

### Adolescence

It is important to not only acknowledge the differences in a child vs. adult population but also adolescence and the specific developmental challenges that it presents. Adolescents are generally more able to participate in decision-making about their own care, and have opinions and views which can challenge those of their families and/or health care providers so it is necessary to find the most appropriate way to work with each adolescent on an individual basis. This is the case in a pediatric or adult setting, as adolescents can often be seen in adult environments and can feel overwhelmed or insignificant without the opportunity to participate in their own health care decisions.

Adolescents can be more inclined to be experimental and can take part in high-risk behaviors which on impact of their health and their response to intervention. Adolescents and children are also more vulnerable as a result of their reliance on others to meet their different needs, and they can be more susceptible to the negative impacts of complex social situations and exploitation as they are not yet fully developed or independent. These factors can have a major impact on their presentation and behaviors, and are also a major factor in planning for discharge/future health care and wellness.

Adolescents will eventually occur transition to adult health-care environments, which can be a vastly different environment with new challenges and staff. It is important to help adolescents prepare for this transition by taking more responsibility for their own health care and enable them to negotiate their way through this new environment.

## WHY IS SPECIALIST PEDIATRIC TRAINING IMPORTANT?

### Children, Adolescents and Adults

Present with illness differently, so people working with children need the skills and knowledge to identify and diagnose illness in a child or adolescent, and be aware of illnesses specific to different age groups.

Often require different treatment or approaches to treatment, and also require specific age, appropriate treatment, approaches and environments (wherever it is possible).

### Have Different Contexts

Children and adolescents come with family, who generally has a greater role in their well-being, so health professionals need to work with family as well as the patient.

Activities are different for different ages- play becomes less important with age, but the need for stimulation and employment in other activities remains important. School in older children and adolescents moving towards work for older adolescents and adults.

Children and adolescents are still developing, so their responses to similar situations will be different and experiences they will have impact on their future development.

### *Summary*

As well as the more obvious physiological and cognitive differences between children and adults, working with children and adolescents requires the consideration for future development—physical, social, emotional cognitive as of primary importance. The need to be aware of the context in which a child or adolescent lives and functions is crucial for both the provision of appropriate management as well as planning for future health care.

## CONCEPT OF GROWTH AND DEVELOPMENT

Children develop as they interact with their surroundings. They learn skills at different ages, but the order in which they learn them is universal. Development is affected by factors such as nutrition and cultural practices, as well as the social situation in the country or neighborhood.

In this chapter, you will learn general principles of growth and development and will explore several theories related to childhood development, as well as their nursing applications.

## PRINCIPLES OF GROWTH AND DEVELOPMENT

It is essential to understand the concepts of growth and development when learning to care for children.

Nurses who work with children must not only understand the pathophysiology of disease practices, and the health promotion and health maintenance needs, but also must integrate knowledge of development into each encounter with a child. The pathophysiologic process, metabolism of medications, and healing process are influenced by the child's age and organ maturity. Health promotion needs regarding topics such as safety measures and immunizations are determined by age and developmental stage of the child, and these factors must also be considered for therapeutic communication to occur.

Growth refers to an increase in physical size. Growth represents quantitative changes such as height,weight, blood pressure, and number of words in the child's vocabulary. Development refers to an increase in capability or function. Developmental skills unfold in a complex manner as a relationship between the child's innate, unfolding capabilities with the stimuli and support provided in the environment. Examples include the ability to sit without support or to throw a ball overhand. Growth and development or quantitative and qualitative changes in body organ functioning, ability to communicate, and performance of motor skills unfold over time and are key components in the process of planning pediatric health care.

Each child displays a unique maturational pattern during the process of development. Although the exact age at which skills emerge differs, the sequence or order of skill performance is uniform among children. Skill development proceeds according to two processes: from the head down and from the center of the body out to the extremities. Development that proceeds from the head downward through the body and toward the feet is called cephalocaudal development. For example, at birth, an infant's head is much larger proportionately than the trunk or extremities. Similarly, infants learn to hold up their heads before sitting, and to sit before standing. Skills such as walking that involve the legs and feet develop last in infancy.

Development that proceeds from the center of the body outward to the extremities is called proximodistal development. For example, infants are first able to control the trunk, then the arms; only later are fine motor movements of the fingers possible. Pediatric nurses use these concepts of predictable and sequential developmental direction to analyze the infant's or child's present state and to partner with families to plan ways to encourage and support emerging developmental abilities.

## MAJOR THEORIES OF DEVELOPMENT

Child development is a complex process. Many theorists have attempted to organize their observations of behavior into a description of principles or a set of stages. Each theory focuses on a particular facet of development. No one theory provides all necessary information and stages are not absolute, i.e. there are differences in rates of progression among children and overlapping of stages within an specific child. Most developmental theorists separate children into age groups by common characteristics.

Some of the age groups and developmental characteristics commonly used to group children include:

- ***Prenatal period:*** Includes the time from conception to birth; influenced by the genetics of the baby and the health of parents, particularly the mother.
- ***Newborn:*** From birth to 1 month of life. Although part of infancy, the first month is marked by the need for adaptation to extrauterine life and requires special support and care.
- ***Infancy:*** From 1 to 12 months. Includes infants or babies upto 1 year of age who require a high level of care in daily activities.

- *Toddlerhood:* From 1 to 3 years. Characterized by increased motor ability and independent behavior.
- *Preschool:* From 3 to 6 years. The preschooler refines gross and fine motor ability and language skills and often participates in a preschool learning program.
- *School age:* From 6 to 12 years. Begins with entry into a school system and is characterized by growing intellectual skills, physical ability, and independence.
- *Adolescence:* From 12 to 18 years. Begins with entry into the teen years. Mature cognitive thought, formation of identity, and influence of peers are important characteristics.

## FREUD'S THEORY OF PSYCHOSEXUAL DEVELOPMENT

### Theoretical Framework

The psychoanalytic techniques used by Sigmund Freud led him to believe that early childhood experiences form the unconscious motivation for actions in later stages. He developed a theory that sexual energy is centered in specific parts of the body at certain ages. Unresolved conflict and unmet needs at a certain stage lead to a fixation of development at that stage (Lerner, 2002).

Freud viewed the personality as a structure with three parts: the id, the basic sexual energy that is present at birth and drives the individual to seek pleasure; the ego, the realistic part of the person, which develops during infancy and searches for acceptable methods of meeting impulses; and the superego, the moral and ethical system, which develops in childhood and contains a set of values and conscience (Craig and Baucum, 2001). He viewed all of these forces as largely out of conscious awareness.

Development and behaviors then unfold as the ego balances, the tension between the two, i.e. opposing forces of id and superego.

The ego diverts impulses of the id and protects itself from excess anxiety created by the superego by use of defense mechanisms.

These unconscious techniques distort reality to guide actions and prevent painful challenges to the personality.

### *Stages*

- *Oral (birth to 1 year):* The infant derives pleasure largely from the mouth,with sucking, eating, chewing, and mouthing objects as primary desires. These oral behaviors also release tension for the infant and play an important part in formation of the ego.
- *Anal (1 to 3 years):* The young child's pleasure is centered in the anal area, with control over body secretions as a prime force in behavior.
- *Phallic (3 to 6 years):* Sexual energy becomes centered in the genitalia and children explore touching their sexual organs.
  - Freud also viewed this period as the time that the child works out relationships with parents of the same and opposite sexes.
  - He believed that children love the parent of the opposite sex and want to take the place of the parent of their same sex. The child needs to accept the presence of both parents and begin to identify with the parent of the same sex.
- *Latency (6 to 12 years):* Sexual energy is at rest in the passage between earlier stages and adolescence. During this stage Freud believed that the child focused on other activities related to social and cognitive growth.
- *Genital (12 years to adulthood):* Mature sexuality is achieved as physical growth is completed, sexual pleasure reemerges, and relationships develop with others outside the family.

## ERIKSON'S THEORY OF PSYCHOSOCIAL DEVELOPMENT

### Theoretical Framework

Erikson's theory establishes psychosocial stages during eight periods of human life. For each stage, Erikson identifies a crisis, i.e. a particular challenge that exists for healthy personality development to occur (Erikson, 1963, 1968). The word ***crisis*** in this context refers to normal maturational social needs rather than to a single critical event. Each developmental crisis has two possible outcomes: when needs are met, the consequences is healthy and the individual moves on to future stages with particular strengths. When needs are not met, an unhealthy outcome occurs that will influence future social relationships.

### *Stages*

- *Trust Versus Mistrust (Birth to 1 Year):* The task of the first year of life is to establish trust in the people providing care. Trust is fostered by provision of food, clean clothing, touch, and comfort. If basic needs are not met, the infant will eventually learn to mistrust others. Developing a sense of trust leads to the child and eventually the adult to have confidence that the world is a good place and to approach life with a general sense of optimism.
- *Autonomy Versus Shame and Doubt (1 to 3 Years):* The toddler's sense of autonomy or independence is shown by controlling body excretions, saying no when asked to do something, and directing motor activity. Children who are consistently criticized for expressions of autonomy or for lack of control, e.g. during toilet training—will develop a sense of shame about themselves and doubt in their abilities.
  - Developing a healthy sense of autonomy results in a person who can function with independence and self-direction. It is also important for the toddler to recognize feelings and needs of others; excessive autonomy could lead to disregard and inability to work with others.
- *Initiative Versus Guilt (3 to 6 Years):* The young child is exposed to more people outside of the family and therefore initiates new activities and considers new ideas. This interest in exploring the world creates a child who is involved and busy. The child learns to assume new responsibilities and becomes aware of guiding principles for actions. Constant criticism for the child's activities, on the other hand, leads to feelings of guilt and a lack of purpose. Preschoolers' sense of initiative leads to the ability to start projects but they may not always see the value in completing them, a potentially frustrating situation for parents.
- *Industry Versus Inferiority (6 to 12 Years):* The middle years of childhood are characterized by development of new interests and by a focus on intellectual or cognitive

pursuits. The child takes pride in accomplishments in sports, school, home, and community. Developing a sense of industry provides the child with purpose and confidence in his or her ability to be successful. If the child cannot accomplish what is expected, however, the result will be a sense of inferiority. The child's sense of industry must be balanced by a realistic perspective gained over time, that there is always more to learn and that one cannot be the 'best' at every activity.

- *Identity Versus Role Confusion (12 to 18 Years):* In adolescence, as the body matures and thought processes become more complex, a new sense of identity or self is established. The adolescent tries out roles and examines what fits best for the self and family/society expectations. The self, family, peer group, and community are all examined and redefined. Identifying with values and roles provides guidance as the adolescent enters adulthood. The adolescent who is unable to establish a meaningful definition of self will experience confusion in one or more roles of life. On the other hand, a certain amount of role confusion is desirable as it is the impetus for self-examination and provides the basis for establishment of identity.

Although not discussed here, Erikson describes adulthood through three additional stages of development. They include intimacy versus isolation, generativity versus stagnation, and integrity versus despair.

## MILESTONES OF GROWTH AND DEVELOPMENT

### GROWTH AND DEVELOPMENT IN INFANT (0 TO 12 MONTHS)

| Age Group | Physical Growth | Fine Motor Abilities | Gross Motor Abilities | Sensory Abilities |
|---|---|---|---|---|
| Birth to 1 month | Gains 5–7 oz (140–200 g)/week<br>Grows 1.5 cm (1/2 inches ) in first month<br>Head circumference increases 1.5 cm (1/2 inches )/month | Holds hand in fist<br>Draws arms and legs to body when crying | Inborn reflexes such as startle and rooting are predominant activity<br>May lift head briefly if prone<br>Alerts to high-pitched voices | Prefers to look at faces and black and- white geometric designs<br>Follows objects in line of vision |
| 2–4 months | Gains 5–7 oz (140–200 g)/week<br>Grows 1.5 cm (1/2inches )/month<br>Head circumference increases 1.5 cm (1/2inches )/month<br>Posterior fontanel closes<br>Eats 120 mL/kg/24 hr (2 oz/lb/24 hr) | Holds rattle when placed in hand<br>Looks at and plays with own fingers<br>Readily brings objects from hand to mouth | Moro reflex fading in strength<br>Can turn from side to back and then return<br>Decrease in head lag when pulled to sitting; sits with head held in midline with some bobbing<br>When prone, holds head and supports weight on forearms | Follows objects 180 degrees<br>Turns head to look for voices and sounds |
| 4–6 months | Gains 5–7 oz (140–200 g)/week<br>Doubles birth weight 5–6 months<br>Grows 1.5 cm (1/2 inches )/month<br>Head circumference increases 1.5 cm (1/2 inches )/month<br>Teeth may begin erupting by 6 months<br>Eats 100 mL/kg/24 hr (1 1/2 oz/lb/24 hr) | Grasps rattles and other objects at will, drops them to pick up another offered object<br>Mouths objects<br>Holds feet and pulls to mouth<br>Holds bottle<br>Grasps with whole hand (palmar grasp)<br>Manipulates objects | Head held steady when sitting<br>No head lag when pulled to sitting<br>Turns from abdomen to back by 4 months and then back to abdomen by 6 months<br>When held standing supports much of own weight | Examines complex visual images<br>Watches the course of a falling object<br>Responds readily to sounds |
| 6–8 months | Gains 3–5 oz (85–140 g)/week<br>Grows 1 cm (3/8 inches )/month<br>Growth rate slower than first 6 months | Bangs objects held in hands<br>Transfers objects from one hand to the other<br>Beginning pincer grasp at times | Most inborn reflexes extinguished<br>Sits alone steadily without support by 8 months<br>Likes to bounce on legs when held in standing position | Recognizes own name and responds by looking and smiling<br>Enjoys small and complex objects at play |
| 8–10 months | Gains 3–5 oz (85–140 g)/week<br>Grows 1 cm (3/8 inches )/month | Picks up small objects<br>Uses pincer grasp well | Crawls or pulls whole body along floor by arms<br>Creeps by using hands and knees to keep trunk off floor<br>Pulls self to standing and sitting by 10 months<br>Recovers balance when sitting | Understands words such as 'no' and 'cracker'<br>May say one word in addition to 'mama' and 'dada'<br>Recognizes sound without difficulty |
| 10–12 months | Gains 3–5 oz (85–140 g)/week<br>Grows 1 cm (3/8 in.)/month<br>Head circumference equals chest circumference<br>Triples birth weight by 1 year | May hold crayon or pencil and make mark on paper<br>Places objects into containers through holes | Stands alone<br>Walks holding onto furniture<br>Sits down from standing | Plays peek-a-boo and patty cake |

## PSYCHOSOCIAL DEVELOPMENT IN INFANT

| Age | Play and toys | Communication |
|---|---|---|
| Birth–3 months | Prefers visual stimuli of mobiles, black-and-white patterns, mirrors<br>Auditory stimuli are music boxes, tape players, soft voices<br>Responds to rocking and cuddling<br>Moves legs and arms while adult sings and talks<br>Likes varying stimuli—different rooms, sounds, visual images | Coos<br>Babbles<br>Cries |
| 3–6 months | Prefers noise-making objects that are easily grasped like rattles<br>Enjoys stuffed animals and soft toys with contrasting colors | Vocalizes during play and with familiar people<br>Laughs<br>Cries less<br>Squeals and makes pleasure sounds<br>Babbles multisyllabically (mamamamama) |
| 6–9 months | Likes teething toys<br>Increasingly desires social interaction with adults and other children<br>Soft toys that can be manipulated and mouthed are favorites | Increases vowel and consonant sounds<br>Links syllables together<br>Uses speech like rhythm when vocalizing with others |
| 9–12 months | Enjoys large blocks, toys that pop apart and go back together, nesting cups and other objects<br>Laughs at surprise toys like jack-in-the-box<br>Plays interactive games like peek-a-boo<br>Uses push-and-pull toys | Understands 'no' and other simple commands<br>Says 'dada' and 'mama' to identify parents<br>Learns one or two other words<br>Receptive speech surpasses expressive speech |

## GROWTH AND DEVEOLOPMENT IN TODDLERS (1 YEAR TO 3 YEARS)

| Age Group | Physical Growth | Fine Motor Abilities | Gross Motor Abilities | Sensory Abilities |
|---|---|---|---|---|
| 1–2 years | Gains 8 oz (227 g) or more per month<br>Grows 3.5–5 inches (9–12 cm) during this year<br>Anterior fontanel closes | By end of 2nd year, builds a tower of four blocks (1)<br>Scribbles on paper (2)<br>Can undress self (3)<br>Throws a ball | Runs<br>Walks up and down stairs (5)<br>Likes push and pull toys | Visual activity 20/50 |
| 2–3 years | Gains 1.4–2.3 kg (3–5 lb)/year<br>Grows 5–6.5 cm (2–2.5 inches )/year | Draws a circle and other rudimentary forms<br>Learns to pour<br>Learning to dress self (4) | Jumps<br>Kicks ball (6)<br>Throws ball overhand | |

## PSYCHOSOCIAL DEVELOPMENT IN TODDLERS

| Age | Play and Toys | Communication |
|---|---|---|
| 1–3 years | Refines fine motor skills by use of cloth, books, large pencil and paper, wooden puzzles<br>Facilitates imitative behavior by playing kitchen, grocery shopping, toy telephone<br>Learns gross motor activities by riding Big Wheel tricycle, playing with soft ball and bat, molding water sand, tossing ball or bean bag<br>Cognitive skills develop by educational television shows, music, stories and books | Increasingly enjoys talking<br>Exponential growth of vocabulary especially when spoken and read to needs to release stress by pounding board, frequent gross motor activities, and occasional temper tantrums<br>Likes contact with other children and learns interpersonal skills |

## GROWTH AND DEVELOPMENT IN PRE SCHOOL CHILDREN

| Physical Growth | Fine Motor Abilities | Gross Motor Abilities | Sensory Abilities |
|---|---|---|---|
| Gains 1.5–2/5 kg (3–5 lb)/year<br>Grows 4–6 cm<br>(1 1/2–2 1/2 inches)/year | Uses scissors<br>Draws circle, square, cross<br>Draws at least a six-part person<br>Enjoys art projects such as pasting, stringing beads, using clay<br>Learns to tie shoes at end of preschool years<br>Buttons<br>Brushes teeth | Throws a ball overhand<br>Climbs well<br>Rides tricycle | Visual acuity continues to improve<br>Can focus on and learn letters and numbers |

## PSYCHOLOGICAL DEVELOPMENT IN PRE SCHOOL CHILDRENS

| Age | Play And Toys | Communication |
|---|---|---|
| 3–6 years | Associative play is facilitated by simple games, puzzles, nursery rhymes, songs<br>Dramatic play is fostered by dolls and doll clothes, play houses and hospitals, dress-up clothes, puppets<br>Stress is relieved by pens, paper, glue, scissors<br>Cognitive growth is fostered by educational television shows, music, stories and books | All parts of speech are developed and used, occasionally incorrectly<br>Communicates with a widening array of people<br>Play with other children is a favorite activity<br>Health professionals can<br>• Verbalize and explain procedures to children<br>• Use drawings and stories to explain care<br>• Use accurate names for bodily functions<br>• Allow the child to talk, ask questions, and make choices |

## GROWTH AND DEVELOPMENT IN SCHOOL AGE CHILDREN

| Physical Growth | Fine Motor Abilities | Gross Motor Abilities | Sensory Abilities |
|---|---|---|---|
| Gains 1.4–2.2 kg (3–5 lb)/year<br>Grows 4–6 cm (1 1/2–2 1/2 in.)/year | Enjoys craft projects<br>Plays card and board games | Rides two-wheeler<br>Jumps rope<br>Roller skates or ice skates | Can read<br>Able to concentrate for longer periods on activities by filtering out surrounding sounds |

## PSYCHOLOGICAL DEVELOPMENT IN SCHOOL AGE CHILDREN

| Age | Play and Toys | Communication |
|---|---|---|
| 6–12 years | Gross motor development is fostered by ball sports, skating, dance lessons, water and snow skiing/boarding, biking<br>A sense of industry is fostered by playing a musical instrument, gathering collections, starting hobbies, playing board and video games<br>Cognitive growth is facilitated by reading, crafts, word puzzles, school work | Mature use of language<br>Ability to converse and discuss topics for increasing lengths of time<br>Spends many hours at school and with friends in sports or other activities<br>Health professionals can:<br>• Assess child's knowledge before teaching<br>• Allow the child to select rewards following procedures<br>• Teach techniques such as counting or visualization to manage difficult situations<br>• Include both parent and child in health care decisions |

## GROWTH AND DEVELOPMENT IN ADOLESCENCE

| Physical Growth | Fine Motor Abilities | Gross Motor Abilities | Sensory Abilities |
|---|---|---|---|
| Variation in age of growth spurt. During growth spurt, girls gain 7–25 kg (15–55 lb) and grow 2.5–20 cm (2–8 in.); boys gain approximately 7–29.5 kg (15–65 lb) and grow 11–30 cm (41/2–12 in.) | Skills are well developed | New sports activities ttempted and muscle development continues<br>Some lack of coordination common during growth spurt | Fully developed |

## PSYCHOLOGICAL DEVELOPMENT IN ADOLESCENCE

| Age | Play and Toys | Communication |
|---|---|---|
| 12–18 years | Sports—ball games, gymnastics, water and snow skiing/boarding, swimming, school sports<br>School activities—drama, yearbook, class, office, club participation<br>Quiet activities—Reading, school work, television, computer, video games, music | Increasing communication and time with peer group—movies, dances, driving, eating out, attending sports events.<br>Applying abstract thought and analysis in conversations at home and school |

## Neonatal Resuscitation: Steps and Process

There is no need to slap the infant; rubbing the back two or three times in addition to thorough drying is enough for stimulation.

### *Airway*

- Keep the infant's head in a slightly extended position to open the airway.
- Do not suction routinely. Suction the airway if there is meconium-stained fluid and the infant is not crying and moving limbs. When the amniotic fluid is clear, suction only if the nose or mouth is full of secretions.
- Suck the mouth, nose and oropharynx by direct vision; do not suck right down the throat, as this can cause apnea or bradycardia.

### *Breathing*

- Choose a mask size that fits over the nose and mouth: size 1 for normal-weight infant, size 0 for small (< 2.5 kg) infants
- Ventilate with bag and mask at 40–60 breaths/min.
- Make sure the chest moves up with each press on the bag; in a very small infant, make sure the chest does not move too much (danger of causing pneumothorax).

### *Circulation*

- Give chest compressions, if the heart rate is < 60/min after 30–60s of ventilation with adequate chest movements: 90 compressions coordinated with 30 breaths/min (three compressions: one breath every 2 seconds).
- Place thumbs just below the line connecting the nipples on the sternum.
- Compress one third the anterior–posterior diameter of the chest.

This chapter provides guidance on essential newborn care and the management of problems in neonates and young infants, from birth to 2 months of age. It includes neonatal resuscitation, the recognition and management of neonatal sepsis and other bacterial infections, and the management of preterm and low-birth-weight infants.

## Essential Newborn Care at Delivery

Most newborns require only simple supportive care at and after delivery.

- Dry the infant with a clean towel.
- Observe the infant while drying.
- Maintain the infant in skin-to-skin contact position with the mother.
- Cover the infant to prevent heat loss.
- Clamp and cut the cord at least 1 min after birth.
- Encourage the mother to initiate breastfeeding within the first hour.

Skin-to-skin contact and early breastfeeding are the best ways to keep an infant warm and prevent hypoglycemia. Term and low-birth-weight neonates weighing > 1200 g who do not have complications and are clinically stable should be put in skin-to-skin contact with the mother soon after birth after they have been dried thoroughly to prevent hypothermia.

## Neonatal Resuscitation

Resuscitation may be required for some infants, such as those born to mothers with chronic illness, to mothers who had a previous fetal or neonatal death, to mothers with pre-eclampsia, in multiple pregnancies, in preterm delivery, in abnormal presentation of the fetus, infants with a prolapsed cord, or after prolonged labor, rupture of membranes or meconium-stained liquor.

For many infants, resuscitation cannot be anticipated before delivery.

Therefore be prepared for resuscitation at every delivery, follow the assessment steps.

## Post Resuscitation Care

Infants who require resuscitation are at risk for deterioration after their vital signs have returned to normal. Once adequate ventilation and circulation has been established:

- Stop ventilation.
- Return to mother for skin-to-skin contact as soon as possible.
- Closely monitor breathing difficulties, signs of asphyxia and anticipate need for further care.

## Cessation of Resuscitation

It is appropriate to consider discontinuing after effective resuscitation efforts if:

- Infant is not breathing and heartbeat is not detectable beyond 10 minutes, stop resuscitation.
- If no spontaneous breathing and heart rate remains below 60/min after 20 minutes of effective resuscitation, discontinue active resuscitation.

Record the event and explain to the mother or parents that the infant has died.

Give them the infant to hold if they wish so.

## Routine Care for all Newborns After Delivery

The routine care described below applies to all newborns, either born in hospital or born outside and brought to the hospital.

- Keep the baby in skin-to-skin contact on the mother's chest or at her side, in a warm, draft-free room.
- Start breastfeeding within the first hour as soon as the baby shows signs of readiness to feed.
- Let the infant breastfed on demand if able to suck.
- Give IM vitamin K (phytomethadione) to all newborns.
- 1 ampoule (1 mg/0.5 mL or 1 mg/mL) once. (Do not use 10 mg/mL ampoule).
- For preterm neonates, give 0.4 mg/kg IM (maximum dose, 1 mg).
- Keep umbilical cord clean and dry.
- Apply antiseptic eye drops or ointment (e.g. tetracycline ointment) to both eyes once, according to national guidelines.
- Give oral polio, hepatitis B and bacille Calmette-Guérin (BCG) vaccines, depending on national guidelines.

Neonatal Resuscitation Chart

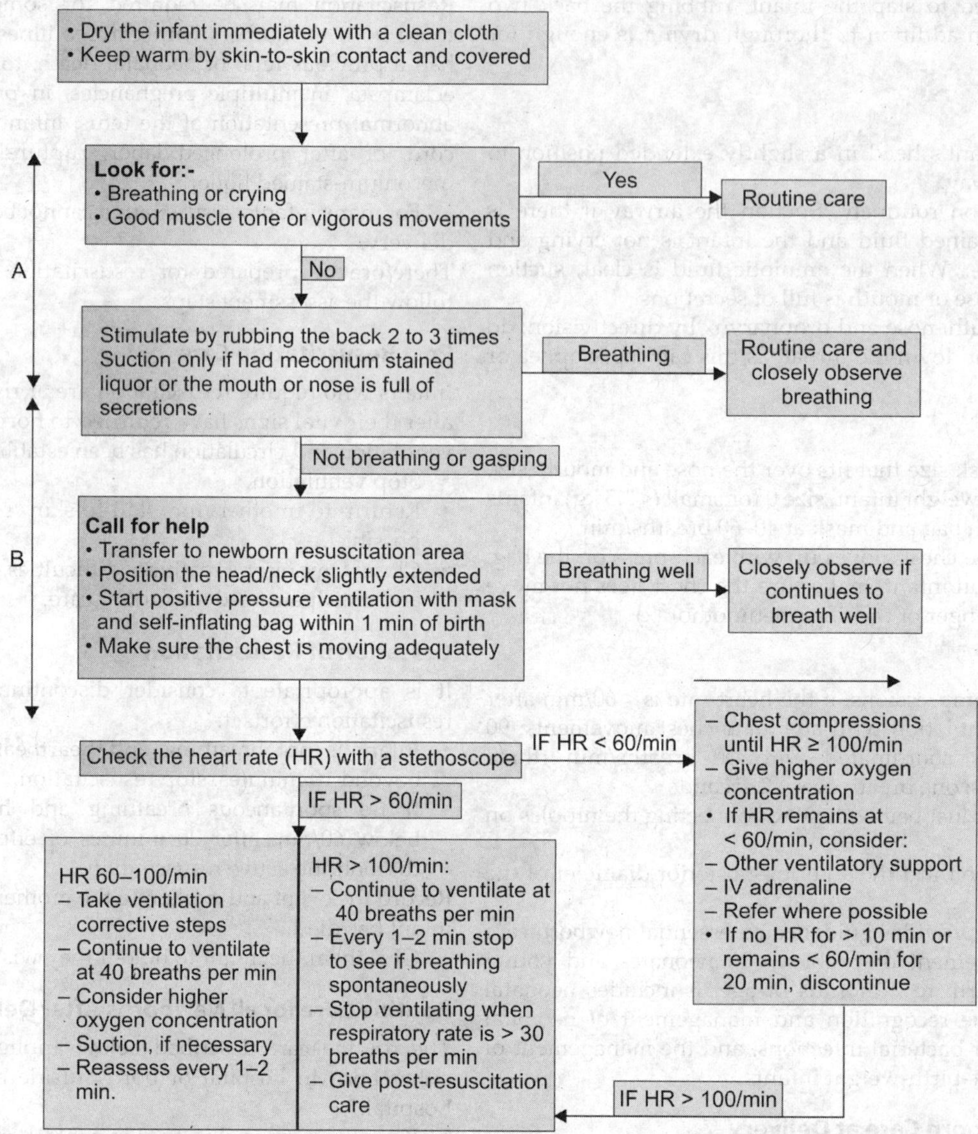


## Prevention of Neonatal Infections

Many early neonatal infections can be prevented by:

- Avoiding unnecessary separation of the newborn from the mother e.g. baby unit
- Handwashing before delivering and handling the infant
- Good basic hygiene and cleanliness during delivery (e.g. chlorhexidine cream for all maternal vaginal examinations).
- Appropriate umbilical cord care
- Appropriate eye care

Give prophylactic antibiotics only to neonates with documented risk factors for infection:

- Membranes ruptured > 18 h before delivery.
- Mother had fever > 38°C before delivery or during labor.
- Amniotic fluid was foul-smelling or purulent.
- Give IM or IV ampicillin and gentamicin for at least 2 days and reassess; continue treatment only if there are signs of sepsis (or a positive blood culture).

Many late neonatal infections are acquired in hospitals. These can be prevented by:

- Exclusive breastfeeding
- Strict procedures for handwashing or alcohol hand rubs for all staff and for families before and after handling infants
- Using Kangaroo mother care and avoiding use of incubators for preterm infants. If an incubator is used, do not use water for humidification (where Pseudomonas will easily colonize) and ensure that it was thoroughly cleaned with an antiseptic.
- Strict sterility for all procedures

- Clean injection practices
- Removing intravenous drips when they are no longer necessary.

## Danger Signs in Newborns and Young Infants

Neonates and young infants often present with non-specific symptoms and signs that indicate severe illness. These signs might be present at or after delivery or in a newborn presenting to hospital or develop during hospital stay. The aim of initial management of a neonate presenting with these signs is stabilization and preventing deterioration. The signs include:

- not feeding well
- convulsions
- drowsy or unconscious
- movement only when stimulated or no movement at all
- fast breathing (60 breaths per min)
- grunting
- severe chest indrawing
- raised temperature, > 38°C
- hypothermia, < 35.5°C
- central cyanosis.

## Emergency Management of Danger Signs

- Open and maintain airway. Give oxygen by nasal prongs if the young infant is cyanosed or in severe respiratory distress or hypoxemic (oxygen saturation ≤ 90%).
- Give bag and mask ventilation with oxygen (or room air if oxygen is not available) if there is apnea, gasping or respiratory rate too slow (< 20).
- Insert venous cannula.
- Give ampicillin (or penicillin) and gentamicin. If drowsy, unconscious or convulsing, check blood glucose. If glucose < 2.2 mmol/L (< 40 mg/100 mL), give 10% glucose at 2 mL/kg IV. Then give a sustained IV infusion of 5 mL/kg per h of 10% glucose for the next few days while oral feds are built up.

  If you cannot check blood glucose quickly, assume hypoglycemia and give glucose IV. If you cannot insert an IV drip, give expressed breast milk or glucose through a nasogastric tube.
- Give phenobarbital if convulsing.
- Admit.
- Give vitamin K (if not given before).
- Monitor the infant frequently (see below).

## Supportive Care for Sick Neonates

### *Thermal Environment*

- Keep the young infant dry and well wrapped.
- A hat can reduce heat loss. Keep the room warm (at least 25°C). Keeping a young infant in close skin-to-skin contact with the mother (Kangaroo mother care) for 24 h/day is an effective way of keeping the infant warm. An external heating device may be needed when the mother is asleep or too ill.
- Pay special attention to avoid chilling the infant during an examination or investigation.
- Check regularly that the infant's temperature is maintained in the range 36.5–37.5°C (97.7–99.5 °F) rectal or 36.0–37.0°C (96.8–98.6 °F) axillary.

  Use a low-reading thermometer to ensure detection of hypothermia.

### *Fluid Management*

Encourage the mother to breastfed frequently to prevent hypoglycemia. If the infant is unable to feed, give expressed breast milk by nasogastric tube.

- Withhold oral feeding if there is bowel obstruction, necrotizing enterocolitis, or the feds are not tolerated, indicated, e.g. by increasing abdominal distension or vomiting everything.
- Withhold oral feeding in the acute phase in infants who are lethargic, unconscious or having frequent convulsions.

If IV fluids are given, reduce the rate as the volume of oral or gastric milk feeds increases. IV fluids should ideally be given with an in-line burette to ensure the exact doses of fluids prescribed.

Increase the amount of fluid given over the first 3–5 days (total amount, oral plus IV).

- Day 1 60 mL/kg per day
- Day 2 90 mL/kg per day
- Day 3 120 mL/kg per day
- Day 4 and 5 150 mL/kg per day

When the infant tolerates oral feds well, the amount of fluid might be increased to 180 mL/kg per day after some days. Be careful in giving parenteral IV fluids, which can quickly overhydrate a child. Do not exceed 100 mL/kg per day of IV fluids, unless the infant is dehydrated or under phototherapy or a radiant heater.

This amount is the total fluid intake an infant needs, and oral intake must be taken into account when calculating IV rates.

- Give more fluid if the infant is under a radiant heater (1.2–1.5 times).
- During the first 2 days of life give 10% glucose infusion IV. Do not use IV glucose without sodium after the first 2 days of life. Suitable alternative IV fluids after the first 2 days are half normal saline and 5% dextrose.

Monitor the IV infusion very carefully (ideally through an in-line burette).

- Use a monitoring sheet.
- Calculate the drip rate.
- Check the drip rate and volume infused every hour.
- Weigh the infant daily.
- Watch for facial swelling: if this occurs, reduce the IV fluid to a minimum or take out the IV line. Introduce breastfeeding or milk feeding by orogastric or nasogastric tube as soon as it is safe to do so.

### *Oxygen Therapy*

- Give oxygen to neonates or young infants with any of the following:
- Central cyanosis or gasping
- Grunting with every breath

- Difficulty in feeding due to respiratory distress
- Severe lower chest wall indrawing
- Head nodding (i.e. a nodding movement of the head, synchronous with the respiration and indicating severe respiratory distress)

Use a pulse oximeter to guide oxygen therapy. Oxygen should be given if the oxygen saturation is ≤ 90%, and the oxygen flow should be regulated to maintain saturation of > 90%. Oxygen can be discontinued once the infant can maintain saturation > 90% in room air.

Nasal prongs are the preferred method for delivering oxygen to this age group, with a flow rate of 0.5–1 liter/min, increased to 2 liters/min in severe respiratory distress to achieve oxygen saturation > 90%. Thick secretions should be cleared from the throat by intermittent suction under direct observation, if they are obstructing the airway and the infant is too weak to clear them. Oxygen should be stopped when the infant's general condition improves and the above signs are no longer present.

### *High Fever*

Do not use antipyretic agents such as paracetamol to control fever in young infants; control the environment. If necessary, undress the child.

### Preterm and low-birth-weight infants Infants with a birth weight of 2.0–2.5 kg (35–36 weeks' gestation)

These infants are usually strong enough to breastfed and maintain their body temperature. Start feds within 1 h of delivery. Their mothers usually need additional support for exclusive breastfeeding. They should be kept warm at all times. All low-birth-weight infants are at risk of infection and should be closely observed for infection control.

### Infants with a birth weight < 2.0 kg (< 35 weeks' gestation)

All infants with a gestation < 35 weeks or a birth weight < 2.0 kg should be admitted to a special care unit. These infants are at risk of hypothermia, feeding problems, apnea, respiratory distress syndrome and necrotizing enterocolitis.

The smaller the infant, the higher the risk. The risks associated with keeping the child in hospital (e.g. hospital-acquired infections) should be balanced against the potential benefit of better care. See the infants at least twice a day to assess feeding ability, fluid intake or the presence of any **danger signs** or signs of serious bacterial infection.

If any of these signs is present, it should be closely monitored. Management of common problems is discussed below.

### Preventing Hypothermia

Low-birth-weight neonates (weighing < 2000 g) who are clinically stable should be given Kangaroo mother care starting soon after birth and ensured at all times, day and night. To provide Kangaroo mother care:

- Dress the infant only in a nappy, hat and socks.
- Place the infant skin-to-skin on the mother's chest between her breasts, with the infant's head turned to one side.
- Tie the infant to the mother with a cloth.
- Cover the mother and infant with the mother's clothes.
- Encourage the mother to breastfed the infant frequently.

Aim for a core body temperature of 36–37°C, with the feet warm and pink.

If the mother is unable to provide Kangaroo mother care, a clean incubator can be used. Incubators should be washed with disinfectant between infants and should be of a basic design that can be used appropriately by the staff available.

### Feeding

Many low-birth-weight infants will be able to suckle at the breast. Infants who can suckle should be breastfed. Those who cannot breastfed should be given expressed breast milk with a cup and spoon. When the infant is sucking well at the breast and gaining weight, reduce the cup feds. Infants unable to fed from a cup and spoon should be given intermittent bolus feds through a gastric tube.

Fed the infant only the mother's own milk. In exceptional situations, when this is not possible, donor human milk should be given, if safe milk-banking facilities are available. Formula should be given only if neither of the above is possible.

### Special Feeding Considerations for Infants Weighing < 1.5 kg at Birth

These infants are at the highest risk of feeding problems and necrotizing enterocolitis. The smaller the infant, the higher the risk.

- Starting on the first day, give 10 mL/kg per day of enteral feds, preferably expressed breast milk, with the remaining fluid requirement at 50 mL/kg per day met by IV fluids. If the infant is well and active and not receiving IV fluids, give 2–4 mL of expressed breast milk every 2 h through a nasogastric tube, depending on the weight of the infant.
- If the infant cannot tolerate enteral feds, give IV fluids at 60 mL/kg per day for the first day of life. It is best to use a pediatric (100 mL) intravenous burette; 60 drops = 1 mL, therefore one drop per minute = 1 mL/hour.
- Check blood sugar every 6 h until enteral feds are established, especially if the infant is apnoeic, lethargic or convulsing. Very low-birth-weight infants may need a 10% glucose solution. Add 10 mL of 50% glucose to every 90 mL of 4.3% glucose + 0.18% normal saline, or use 10% glucose in water solution.
- Start enteral feeding when the condition of the infant is stable and there is no abdominal distension or tenderness, bowel sounds are present, meconium passed and no apnea.
- Calculate exact amounts for feeding and the timing of feds.
- Use a prescription chart.
- Increase daily if well-tolerated.
- When commencing milk feds, start with 2–4 mL every 1–2 h by orogastric or nasogastric tube. Some active very-low-birth-weight infants can be fed with a cup and spoon or an eyedropper, which must be sterilized before each fed. Use only expressed breast milk if possible. If a 2–4 mL volume is tolerated with no vomiting, abdominal distension or gastric aspirates of more than half the fed, the volume

can be increased by 1–2 mL per fed each day. Reduce or withhold feds if there are signs of poor tolerance.

Aim to establish feeding within the first 5–7 days so that the IV drip can be removed, to avoid infection.

- The feds may be increased during the first 2 weeks of life to 150–180 mL/kg per day (3-hourly feeds of 19–23 mL for a 1 kg infant and 28–34 mL for a 1.5 kg infant). As the infant grows, recalculate the fed volume on the basis of the higher weight.
- Give daily supplements when the infant is accepting full enteral feds:
  - vitamin D at 400 IU
  - calcium at 120–140 mg/kg
  - phosphorus at 60–90 mg/kg.
- Start iron supplements at 2 weeks of age at a dosage of 2–4 mg/kg per day until 6 months of age.

### Preventing Apnea

- Give caffeine citrate and aminophylline to prevent apnea in premature infants. Caffeine is preferred if it is available.
  - The loading dose of caffeine citrate is 20 mg/kg orally or IV (given slowly over 30 min). A maintenance dose of 5 mg/kg per day should be prescribed 24 h later and can be increased by 5 mg/kg every 24 h to a maximum of 20 mg/kg per day, unless side-effects develop. Continue 4–5 days after cessation of apnea.
  - If caffeine is not available, give a loading dose of aminophylline at 6 mg/kg IV over 20 min, followed by a maintenance dose of 2.5 mg/kg every 12 h.
- If an apnea monitor is available, this should be used.
- If an apnea monitor is not available, a pulse oximeter with the alarm turned on for hypoxemia may help to detect apnea if the neonate is breathing room air.

### Common Problems of Low-birth-weight Infants

### Respiratory Distress Syndrome

Preterm infants are at risk for respiratory distress syndrome due to surfactant deficiency. This can be reduced if pregnant mothers at risk for premature delivery (e.g. premature contractions or premature rupture of membranes) are given dexamethasone at two doses of 12 mg 24 h apart. Respiratory distress usually occurs in a preterm infant during the first 3 days of life. It is a self- limiting condition, because birth triggers an increase in surfactant production.

The challenge is to support the infant for the first few days of life until such time as the deficiency resolves.

The key clinical features usually become obvious within 4 h of birth and include:

- Tachypnea
- An expiratory 'grunt'
- Intercostal and/or subcostal recession and
- Cyanosis.

### Treatment

The principles of treatment are:

- Minimal handling of the infant
- Supplementary oxygen if needed to keep the oxygen saturation > 90% but < 95% to avoid eye damage
- Initially no oral feeding
- IV fluids
- Maintenance of a normal temperature range
- IV antibiotics for neonatal sepsis, as it is difficult to exclude pneumonia as a cause of respiratory distress

Continuous positive airway pressure is used, even in expiration, to prevent airway collapse, improve oxygenation and reduce breathing fatigue.

If there is persistent respiratory distress or hypoxemia, do chest X-ray to check for pneumothorax.

### Discharge and follow-up of Low-birth-weight Infants

Low-birth-weight infants can be discharged when:

- They have no **danger** signs or signs of serious infection
- They are gaining weight on breastfeeding alone
- They can maintain their temperature in the normal range (36–37°C) in an open cot
- The mother is confident and able to care for the infant.

Low-birth-weight infants should be given all the scheduled vaccines at the time of birth and any second doses that are due by the time of discharge.

### Counseling on Discharge

Counsel parents before discharge on

- Exclusive breastfeeding
- Keeping the infant warm
- Danger signs for seeking care

Low-birth-weight infants should be followed up weekly for weighing and assessment of feeding and general health, until they have reached 3 kg.

### Other Common Neonatal Problems

#### *Jaundice*

More than 50% of normal newborns and 80% of preterm infants have some jaundice. Jaundice may be normal or abnormal:

#### *Normal (Physiological)*

Skin and eyes yellow but none of the signs of abnormal jaundice below.

#### *Abnormal (Non-physiological)*

- Starting on the first day of life
- Lasting > 14 days in term and > 21 days in preterm infants
- With fever
- Deep jaundice: Palms and soles of the infant deep yellow

Abnormal jaundice may be due to:

- Serious bacterial infection
- Hemolytic disease due to blood group incompatibility or glucose 6-phosphate dehydrogenase deficiency
- Congenital syphilis or other intrauterine infection
- Liver disease such as hepatitis or biliary atresia (stools pale and urine dark)
- Hypothyroidism

#### *Investigations for Abnormal Jaundice*

All newborns should be monitored for the development of jaundice, which should be confirmed by a bilirubin measurement, when possible, in all:

- Infants if jaundice appears on day 1
- Preterm infants (< 35 weeks) if jaundice appears on day 2
- Infants if palms and soles are yellow at any age.

The investigations depend on the probable diagnosis and what tests are available but may include:

- Hb or packed cell volume
- Full blood count to identify signs of serious bacterial infection (high or low neutrophil count with > 20% band forms) and signs of hemolysis
- Blood type of infant and mother and Coombs test
- Syphilis serology, such as venereal disease research laboratory tests
- Glucose 6-phosphate dehydrogenase screening, thyroid function tests, liver ultrasound

### Treatment

- Phototherapy if
- Jaundice on day 1
- Deep jaundice involving palms and soles of the feet
- Prematurity and jaundice
- Jaundice due to hemolysis

Continue phototherapy until the serum bilirubin level is lower than the threshold range or until the infant is well and there is no jaundice of palms and soles.

If the bilirubin level is very high and you can safely do exchange transfusion, consider doing so.

#### *Antibiotics*

If infection or syphilis is suspected, treat for serious bacterial infection.

#### *Antimalarials*

- If fever is present and the infant is from a malarious area, check blood films for malaria parasites, and give antimalarials if positive.
- Encourage breastfeeding.

## Cough or Difficulty in Breathing

Cough and difficulty in breathing are common problems in young children. The causes range from a mild, self-limited illness to severe, life-threatening disease.

This chapter provides guidelines for managing the most important conditions that cause cough, difficulty in breathing or both in children aged 2 months to 5 years.

### Child Presenting with Cough

### History

Pay particular attention to:

- Cough
  - Duration in days
  - Paroxysms with whoops or vomiting or central cyanosis
- Exposure to someone with TB (or chronic cough) in the family
- History of choking or sudden onset of symptoms
- Known or possible HIV infection
- Vaccination history: BCG; diphtheria, pertussis, tetanus (DPT); measles; Hemophilus infl uenzae type b and pneumococcus
- Personal or family history of asthma.

### Examination

The symptoms and signs listed below are a guide for the clinician to reach a diagnosis. Not all children will show every symptom or sign.

#### *General*

- Central cyanosis
- Apnea, gasping, grunting, nasal flaring, audible wheeze, stridor
- Head nodding (a movement of the head synchronous with inspiration indicating severe respiratory distress)
- Tachycardia
- Severe palmar pallor.

#### *Chest*

- Respiratory rate (count during 1 min when the child is calm)
- Fast breathing:
  - < 2 months, ≥ 60 breaths
  - 2–11 months, ≥ 50 breaths
  - 1–5 years, ≥ 40 breaths
- Lower chest wall indrawing
- Hyperinflated chest
- Apex beat displaced or trachea shifted from midline
- Raised jugular venous pressure
- On auscultation, coarse crackles, no air entry or bronchial breath sounds or wheeze
- Abnormal heart rhythm on auscultation
- Percussion signs of pleural effusion (stony dullness) or Pneumothorax (hyper-resonance)

***Note:*** *Lower chest wall indrawing is when the lower chest wall goes in when the child breathes in; if only the soft tissue between the ribs or above the clavicle goes in when the child breathes, this is not lower chest wall indrawing.*

#### *Abdomen*

- Abdominal masses (e.g. lymphadenopathy)
- Enlarged liver and spleen

### Investigations

- Pulse oximetry to detect hypoxia and as a guide to when to start or stop oxygen therapy
- Full blood count
- Chest X-ray only for children with severe pneumonia or pneumonia that does not respond to treatment or complications or unclear diagnosis or associated with HIV.

### Pneumonia

Pneumonia is caused by viruses or bacteria. It is usually not possible to determine the specific cause of pneumonia by clinical features or chest X-ray appearance. Pneumonia is classified as severe or non-severe on the basis of clinical features, the management being based on the classification. Antibiotic therapy should be given in most cases of pneumonia and severe pneumonia.

Severe pneumonia may require additional supportive care, such as oxygen, to be given in hospital.

## Severe Pneumonia

### Diagnosis

Cough or difficulty in breathing, plus at least one of the following:

- Central cyanosis or oxygen saturation < 90% on pulse oximetry
- Severe respiratory distress (e.g. Grunting, very severe chest indrawing)
- Signs of pneumonia with a general danger sign:
  - Inability to breastfed or drink,
  - Lethargy or unconscious,
  - Convulsions.
- In addition, some or all of the other signs of pneumonia may be present, such as:
  - Signs of pneumonia
- Fast breathing:
  - Age 2–11 months, ≥ 50/min
  - Age 1–5 years, ≥ 40/min
- Chest indrawing: lower chest wall indrawing (i.e. Lower chest wall goes in when the child breathes in)
  - Chest auscultation signs:
- Decreased breath sounds
- Bronchial breath sounds
- Crackles
- Abnormal vocal resonance (decreased over a pleural effusion or empyema, increased over lobar consolidation)
- Pleural rub

| Sign or symptom | Classification | Treatment |
|---|---|---|
| Cough or difficulty in breathing with:<br>• Oxygen saturation < 90% or central cyanosis<br>• Severe respiratory distress (e.g. grunting, very severe chest indrawing)<br>• Signs of pneumonia with a general danger sign (inability to breastfed or drink, lethargy or reduced level of consciousness, convulsions) | **Severe pneumonia** | • Admit to hospital<br>• Give oxygen if saturation < 90%<br>• Manage airway as appropriate<br>• Give recommended antibiotic<br>• Treat high fever if present |
| • Fast breathing:<br>– ≥ 50 breaths/min in a child aged 2–11 months<br>– ≥ 40 breaths/min in a child aged 1–5 years<br>• Chest indrawing | **Pneumonia** | • Home care<br>• Give appropriate antibiotic<br>• Advise the mother when to return immediately if symptoms of severe<br>• Pneumonia<br>• Followup after 3 days. |
| • No signs of pneumonia or severe pneumonia | **No pneumonia: Cough or cold** | • Home care<br>• Soothe the throat and relieve cough with safe remedy.<br>• Advise the mother when to return<br>• Follow up after 5 days if not improving<br>• If coughing for more than 14 days, refer to chronic cough |

### Investigations

- Measure oxygen saturation with pulse oximetry in all children suspected of having pneumonia.
- If possible, obtain a chest X-ray to identify pleural effusion, empyema, pneumothorax, pneumatocoele, interstitial pneumonia or pericardial effusion.

### Treatment

Admit the child to hospital.

#### *Oxygen Therapy*

Ensure continuous oxygen supply, either as cylinders or oxygen concentrator, at all times.

- Give oxygen to all children with oxygen saturation < 90%.
- Use nasal prongs as the preferred method of oxygen delivery to young infants; if not available, a nasal or nasopharyngeal catheter may be used.
- Use a pulse oximetry to guide oxygen therapy (to keep oxygen saturation > 90%). If a pulse oximeter is not available, continue oxygen until the signs of hypoxia (such as inability to breastfed or breathing rate ≥ 70/min) are no longer present.
- Remove oxygen for a trial period each day for stable children while continuing to use a pulse oximeter to determine oxygen saturation. Discontinue oxygen if the saturation remains stable at > 90% (at least 15 min on room air).

Nurses should check every 3 h that the nasal prongs are not blocked with mucus and are in the correct place and that all connections are secure.

#### *Antibiotic Therapy*

- Give intravenous ampicillin (or benzylpenicillin) and gentamicin.
  - Ampicillin 50 mg/kg or benzylpenicillin 50000 U/kg IM or IV every 6 h for at least 5 days
  - Gentamicin 7.5 mg/kg IM or IV once a day for at least 5 days.
- If the child does not show signs of improvement within 48 h and staphylococcal pneumonia is suspected, switch to gentamicin 7.5 mg/kg IM or IV once a day and cloxacillin 50 mg/kg IM or IV every 6 hour.
- Use ceftriaxone (80 mg/kg IM or IV once daily) in cases of failure of firstline treatment.

### Supportive Care

- Remove by gentle suction any thick secretions at the entrance to the nasal passages or throat, which the child cannot clear.
- If the child has fever (≥ 39°C or e 102.2 °F) which appears to be causing distress, give paracetamol.
- If wheeze is present, give a rapid-acting bronchodilator, and start steroids when appropriate.
- Ensure that the child receives daily maintenance fluids appropriate for his or her age, but avoid over-hydration.
- Encourage breastfeeding and oral fluids.
- If the child cannot drink, insert a nasogastric tube and give maintenance fluids in frequent small amounts. If the child

is taking fluids adequately by mouth, do not use a nasogastric tube as it increases the risk for aspiration pneumonia and obstructs part of the nasal airway. If oxygen is given by nasal catheter at the same time as nasogastric fluids, pass both tubes through the same nostril.

- Encourage the child to eat as soon as food can be taken.

### Monitoring

The child should be checked by a nurse at least every 3 h and by a doctor at least twice a day. In the absence of complications, within 2 days there should be signs of improvement (breathing slower, less in drawing of the lower chest wall, less fever, improved ability to eat and drink, better oxygen saturation).

### Other Alternative Diagnosis and Treatment

- If the child has not improved after 2 days or if the child's condition has worsened, look for complications or alternative diagnoses. If possible, obtain a chest X-ray. The commonest other possible diagnoses are:

*Staphylococcal pneumonia.* This is suggested if there is rapid clinical deterioration despite treatment, by a pneumatocoele or pneumothorax with effusion on chest X-ray, numerous Gram-positive cocci in a smear of sputum or heavy growth of *S. aureus* in cultured sputum or empyema fluid. The presence of septic skin pustules supports the diagnosis.

- Treat with cloxacillin (50 mg/kg IM or IV every 6 h) and gentamicin (7.5 mg/kg IM or IV once a day). When the child improves (after at least 7 days of IV or IM antibiotics), continue cloxacillin orally four times a day for a total course of 3 weeks. Note that cloxacillin can be replaced by another antistaphylococcal antibiotic, such as oxacillin, flucloxacillin or dicloxacillin.

***Tuberculosis:*** A child with persistent cough and fever for more than 2 weeks and signs of pneumonia after adequate antibiotic treatment should be evaluated for TB. If another cause of the fever cannot be found, TB should be considered, particularly in malnourished children. Further investigations and treatment for TB, following national guidelines, may be initiated and response to anti-TB treatment evaluated. The HIV status of all children suspected of having TB should be confirmed if not known.

***HIV infection or exposure to HIV:*** Some aspects of antibiotic treatment are different for children who are HIV positive or in whom HIV infection is suspected.

Although pneumonia in many of these children has the same etiology as that in children without HIV, *Pneumocystis* pneumonia (PCP), often at the age of 4–6 months is an important cause to be suspected and treated.

- Treat as for severe pneumonia above; give ampicillin plus gentamicin IM or IV for 10 days.
- If the child does not improve within 48 h, switch to ceftriaxone at 80 mg/kg IV once daily over 30 min. If ceftriaxone is not available, give gentamicin plus cloxacillin, as above.
- For children < 12 months, also give high-dose co-trimoxazole (8 mg/kg trimethoprim and 40 mg/kg sulfamethoxazole IV every 8 h or orally three times a day) for 3 weeks. For a child aged 12–59 months, give this treatment only if there are clinical signs of PCP (such as chest X-ray findings of interstitial pneumonia).
- For further management of the child, including PCP prophylaxis.

### Discharge

Children with severe pneumonia can be discharged when:

- Respiratory distress has resolved.
- There is no hypoxemia (oxygen saturation, > 90%).
- They are feeding well.
- They are able to take oral medication or have completed a course of parenteral antibiotics.
- The parents understand the signs of pneumonia, risk factors and when to return.

### Follow-up

Children with severe pneumonia may cough for several weeks. As they have been very sick, their nutrition is often poor. Give the vaccinations that are due, and arrange follow-up 2 weeks after discharge, if possible, to check the child's nutrition. Also address risk factors such as malnutrition, indoor air pollution and parental smoking.

## Pneumonia

#### *Diagnosis*

Cough or difficult breathing plus at least one of the following signs:

- Fast breathing: age 2–11 months, ≥ 50/min age 1–5 years, ≥ 40/min
- Lower chest wall indrawing

In addition, either crackles or pleural rub may be present on chest auscultation.

Check that there are no signs of severe pneumonia, such as:

- Oxygen saturation < 90% on pulse oximetry or central cyanosis
- Severe respiratory distress (e.g. grunting, very severe chest indrawing)
- Inability to breastfed or drink or vomiting everything
- Convulsions, lethargy or reduced level of consciousness
- Auscultatory findings of decreased or bronchial breath sounds or signs of pleural effusion or empyema.

### Treatment

- Treat child as outpatient.
- Advise carers to give normal fluid requirements plus extra breast milk or fluids if there is a fever. Small frequent drinks are more likely to be taken and less likely to be vomited.

#### *Antibiotic Therapy*

- Give the first dose at the clinic and teach the mother how to give the other doses at home.
- Give oral amoxicillin:
  - In settings with high HIV infection rate, give oral amoxicillin at least 40 mg/kg per dose twice a day for 5 days.
  - In areas with low HIV prevalence, give amoxicillin at least 40 mg/kg per dose twice a day for 3 days.

- Avoid unnecessary harmful medications such as remedies containing atropine, codeine derivatives or alcohol.

### Follow-up

Encourage the mother to fed the child. Advise her to bring the child back after 3 days, or earlier if the child becomes sicker or is unable to drink or breastfed.

When the child returns, check:

- Whether the breathing has improved (slower), there is no chest indrawing, less fever, and the child is eating better; complete the antibiotic treatment.
- If the breathing rate and/or chest indrawing or fever and/ or eating have not improved, exclude a wheeze. If no wheeze, admit to hospital for investigations to exclude complications or alternative diagnosis.
- If signs of severe pneumonia are present, admit the child to hospital and treat as above.
- Address risk factors such as malnutrition, indoor air pollution and parental smoking.

### *Pneumonia in Children with HIV Infection*

Admit to hospital and manage as severe pneumonia. For further management of these children, including PCP prophylaxis

### Complications of Pneumonia

Septicemia is the most common pneumonia complication and occurs when the bacteria causing pneumonia spreads into the bloodstream. The spread of bacteria can lead to septic shock or metastatic secondary infections like meningitis especially in infants, peritonitis, and endocarditis especially in patients with vulvar heart disease or septic arthritis. Other common complication include pleural effusion, empyema and lung abscess.

### Lung Abscess

A lung abscess is a circumscribed, thick-walled cavity in the lung that contains purulent material resulting from suppuration and necrosis of the involved lung parenchyma. It frequently develops in an unresolved area of pneumonia. This could be a result of pulmonary aspiration, diminished clearance mechanisms, embolic phenomena, or hematogenous spread.

### Diagnosis

Common signs and symptoms:

- Fever
- Pleuritic chest pain
- Sputum production or hemoptysis
- Weight loss
- *On examination:* Reduced chest movement, decreased breath sounds, dullness to percussion, crackles, and bronchial breathing.
- *Chest X-ray:* Solitary, thick-walled cavity in the lung with or without air fluid level.
- Ultrasonography and CT scan: To localize the lesion and guide drainage or needle aspiration.

### Treatment

The choice of antibiotic is usually empirical and is based on the underlying condition of the patient and the presumed etiological agent.

- Give ampicillin or cloxacillin or flucloxacillin (50 mg/kg IM or IV every 6 h) and gentamicin (7.5 mg/kg IM or IV once a day). Continue treatment as in empyema for up to 3 weeks.
- Surgical management is considered in cases of large lung abscess especially when associated with hemoptysis or clinical deterioration despite appropriate antibiotic therapy. Drainage is usually through percutaneous tube drainage or ultrasound guided needle aspiration.

### Pneumothorax

Pneumothorax is usually secondary to an accumulation of air in the pleural spaces from alveolar rupture or from infection with gas-producing microorganisms.

### Diagnosis

- Signs and symptoms may vary according to the extent of lung collapse, degree of intrapleural pressure, and rapidity of onset.
- *On examination:* chest bulging on the affected side if one side is involved, shift of cardiac impulse away from the site of the pneumothorax, decreased breath sounds on the affected side, grunting, severe respiratory distress and cyanosis may occur late in the progression of the complication.
- Differential diagnosis include lung cyst, lobar emphysema, bullae, diaphragmatic hernia
- Chest X-ray is crucial in the confirmation of diagnosis.

### Treatment

Insert needle for urgent decompression, before insertion of an intercostals chest drain.

### Cough or Cold

These are common, self-limited viral infections that require only supportive care. Antibiotics should not be given. Wheeze or stridor may occur in some children, especially infants. Most episodes end within 14 days. Cough lasting 14 days or more may be caused by TB, asthma, pertussis or symptomatic HIV infection.

### Diagnosis

Common features:

- Cough
- Nasal discharge
- Mouth breathing
- Fever

The following are absent:

- General danger signs.
- Signs of severe pneumonia or pneumonia
- Stridor when the child is calm

Wheezing may occur in young children (*See* below).

### Treatment

- Treat the child as an outpatient.
- Soothe the throat and relieve the cough with a safe remedy, such as a warm, sweet drink.

- Relieve high fever (≥ 39°Core 102.2 °F) with paracetamol if the fever is causing distress to the child.
- Clear secretions from the child's nose before feds with a cloth soaked in water that has been twisted to form a pointed wick.

Give normal fluid requirements plus extra breast milk or fluids if there is fever.

Small frequent drinks are more likely to be taken and less likely to be vomited.

- Do not give any of the following:
  - An antibiotic (they are not effective and do not prevent pneumonia)
  - Remedies containing atropine, codeine or codeine derivatives, or alcohol (these may be harmful) or mucolytics
  - Medicated nose drops.

## Follow-up

Advise the mother to:

- Fed the child
- Watch for fast or difficult breathing and return if either develops
- Return if the child becomes sicker or is unable to drink or breastfed.

## Bronchiolitis

Bronchiolitis is a lower respiratory viral infection, which is typically most severe in young infants, occurs in annual epidemics and is characterized by airways obstruction and wheezing. It is most commonly caused by respiratory syncytial virus. Secondary bacterial infection may occur. The management of bronchiolitis associated with fast breathing or other sign of respiratory distress is therefore similar to that of pneumonia. Episodes of wheeze may occur for months after an attack of bronchiolitis, but will eventually stop.

## Diagnosis

Typical features of bronchiolitis, on examination, include:

- Wheezing that is not relieved by up to three doses of a rapid-acting bronchodilator
- Hyperinflation of the chest, with increased resonance to percussion
- Lower chest wall indrawing
- Fine crackles and wheeze on auscultation of the chest
- Difficulty in feeding, breastfeeding or drinking owing to respiratory distress
- Nasal discharge, which can cause severe nasal obstruction.

## Treatment

Most children can be treated at home, but those with the following signs of severe pneumonia should be treated in hospital:

- Oxygen saturation < 90% or central cyanosis.
- Apnea or history of apnea
- Inability to breastfed or drink, or vomiting everything
- Convulsions, lethargy or unconsciousness
- Gasping and grunting (especially in young infants).

### *Oxygen*

- Give oxygen to all children with severe respiratory distress or oxygen saturation ≤ 90%. The recommended method for delivering oxygen is by nasal prongs or a nasal catheter.
- The nurse should check, every 3 hour, that the prongs are in the correct position and not blocked with mucus, and that all connections are secure.

### *Antibiotic Treatment*

- If the infant is treated at home, give amoxicillin (40 mg/kg twice a day) orally for 5 days only if the child has signs of pneumonia (fast breathing and lower chest wall indrawing).
- If there are signs of severe pneumonia, give ampicillin at 50 mg/kg or benzylpenicillin at 50,000 U/kg IM or IV every 6 h for at least 5 days and gentamicin 7.5 mg/kg IM or IV once a day for at least 5 days.

## Supportive Care

- If the child has fever (≥ 39°C or e 102.2 °F) that appears to be causing distress, give paracetamol.
- Ensure that the hospitalized child receives daily maintenance fluids appropriate for age, but avoid overhydration. Encourage breastfeding and oral fluids.
- Encourage the child to eat as soon as food can be taken. Nasogastric feeding should be considered in any patient who is unable to maintain oral intake or hydration (expressed breast milk is the best).
- Gentle nasal suction should be used to clear secretions in infants where nasal blockage appears to be causing respiratory distress.

## Monitoring

A hospitalized child should be assessed by a nurse every 6 hour (or every 3 hour if there are signs of very severe illness) and by a doctor at least once a day.

Watch for signs of respiratory failure, i.e. increasing hypoxia and respiratory distress leading to exhaustion.

## Complications

If the child fails to respond to oxygen therapy or the child's condition worsens suddenly, obtain a chest X-ray to look for evidence of pneumothorax. Tension pneumothorax associated with severe respiratory distress and shift of the heart requires immediate relief by placing a needle to allow the air that is under pressure to escape (needle thoracocentesis). Following this, a continuous air exit should be assured by inserting a chest tube with an underwater seal until the air leak closes spontaneously and the lung expands.

If respiratory failure develops, continuous positive airway pressure may be helpful.

## Infection Control

It is very infectious and dangerous to other young children in hospital with other conditions. The following strategies may reduce cross-infection:

- Handwashing by personnel between patients
- Ideally isolate the child, but maintain close observation

- During epidemics, restrict visits to children by parents and siblings with symptoms of upper respiratory tract infection.

### Discharge

An infant with bronchiolitis can be discharged when respiratory distress and hypoxemia have resolved, when there is no apnea and the infant is feeding well.

Infants are at risk for recurrent bronchiolitis if they live in families where adults smoke or if they are not breastfed. So, advise the parents against smoking.

### Follow-up

Infants with bronchiolitis may have cough and wheeze for upto 3 weeks. As long as they are well with no respiratory distress, fever or apnea and are feeding well they do not need antibiotics.

## Asthma

Asthma is a chronic inflammatory condition with reversible airways obstruction. It is characterized by recurrent episodes of wheezing, often with cough, which respond to treatment with bronchodilators and anti-inflammatory drugs.

Antibiotics should be given only when there are signs of pneumonia.

### Diagnosis

History of recurrent episodes of wheezing, often with cough, difficulty in breathing and tightness in the chest, particularly if these are frequent and recurrent or are worse at night and in the early morning. Findings on examination may include:

- Rapid or increasing respiratory rate
- Hyperinflation of the chest
- Hypoxia (oxygen saturation ≤ 90%)
- Lower chest wall indrawing
- Use of accessory muscles for respiration (best noted by feeling the neck muscles)
- Prolonged expiration with audible wheeze
- Reduced or no air intake when obstruction is life-threatening
- Absence of fever
- Good response to treatment with a bronchodilator.

If the diagnosis is uncertain, give a dose of a rapid-acting bronchodilator. A child with asthma will often improve rapidly with such treatment, showing signs such as slower respiratory rate, less chest wall indrawing and less respiratory distress. A child with severe asthma may require several doses in quick succession before a response is seen.

### Treatment

- A child with a **first episode of wheezing and no respiratory distress** can usually be managed at home with supportive care. A bronchodilator is not necessary.
- If the child is in **respiratory distress (acute severe asthma) or has recurrent wheezing**, give salbutamol by metered-dose inhaler and spacer device or, if not available, by nebulizer. If salbutamol is not available, give subcutaneous adrenaline.
- Reassess the child after 15 min to determine subsequent treatment:
- If respiratory distress has resolved, and the child does not have fast breathing, advise the mother on home care with inhaled salbutamol from a metered dose inhaler and spacer device (which can be made locally from plastic bottles).
- If respiratory distress persists, admit to hospital and treat with oxygen, rapid-acting bronchodilators and other drugs.

#### *Severe Life-threatening Asthma*

- If the child has life-threatening acute asthma, is in severe respiratory distress with central cyanosis or reduced oxygen saturation ≤ 90%, has poor air entry (silent chest), is unable to drink or speak or is exhausted and confused, admit to hospital and treat with oxygen, rapid-acting bronchodilators and other drugs, as described below.
- In children admitted to hospital, promptly give oxygen, a rapid-acting bronchodilator and a first dose of steroids.

#### *Oxygen*

- Give oxygen to keep oxygen saturation > 95% in all children with asthma who are cyanosed (oxygen saturation ≤ 90%) or whose difficulty in breathing interferes with talking, eating or breastfeeding.

#### *Rapid-acting Bronchodilators*

- Give the child a rapid-acting bronchodilator, such as nebulized salbutamol or salbutamol by metered-dose inhaler with a spacer device. If salbutamol is not available, give subcutaneous adrenaline.

#### *Nebulized Salbutamol*

The driving source for the nebulizer must deliver at least 6–9 liters/min. Recommended methods are an air compressor, ultrasonic nebulizer or oxygen cylinder, but in severe or life-threatening asthma oxygen must be used. If these are not available, use an inhaler and spacer. An easy-to-operate foot pump may be used but is less effective.

- Put the dose of the bronchodilator solution in the nebulizer compartment, add 2–4 mL of sterile saline and nebulize the child until the liquid is almost all used up. The dose of salbutamol is 2.5 mg (i.e. 0.5 mL of the 5 mg/mL nebulizer solution).
- If the response to treatment is poor, give salbutamol more frequently.
- In severe or life-threatening asthma, when a child cannot speak, is hypoxic or tiring with lowered consciousness, give continuous back-to-back nebulizers until the child improves, while setting up an IV cannula. As asthma improves, a nebulizer can be given every 4 hour and then every 6–8 hour.

#### *Giving Salbutamol by Metered-dose Inhaler with a Spacer Device*

Spacer devices with a volume of 750 mL are commercially available.

- Introduce two puffs (200 μg) into the spacer chamber. Then, place the child's mouth over the opening in the spacer and allow normal breathing for three to five breaths. This can be repeated in rapid succession until six puffs of the drug have been given to a child < 5 years, 12 puffs for > 5 years of age. After 6 or 12 puffs, depending on age, assess the response and repeat regularly until the child's condition improves. In severe cases, 6 or 12 puffs can be given several times an hour for a short period.

- Some infants and young children cooperate better when a face mask is attached to the spacer instead of the mouthpiece. If commercial devices are not available, a spacer device can be made from a plastic cup or a 1-liter plastic bottle. These deliver three to four puffs of salbutamol, and the child should breathe from the device for upto 30 second.

### *Subcutaneous Adrenaline*

If the above two methods of delivering salbutamol are not available, give a subcutaneous injection of adrenaline at 0.01 mL/kg of 1:1000 solution (up to a maximum of 0.3 mL), measured accurately with a 1 mL syringe. If there is no improvement after 15 min, repeat the dose once.

### *Steroids*

- If a child has a severe or life-threatening acute attack of wheezing (asthma), give oral prednisolone, 1 mg/kg, for 3–5 days (maximum, 60 mg) or 20 mg for children aged 2–5 years. If the child remains very sick, continue the treatment until improvement is seen.

Repeat the dose of prednisolone for children who vomit, and consider IV steroids if the child is unable to retain orally ingested medication. Treatment for up to 3 days is usually sufficient, but the duration should be tailored to bring about recovery. Tapering of short courses (7–14 days) of steroids is not necessary.

IV hydrocortisone (4 mg/kg repeated every 4 hour) provides no benefit and should be considered only for children who are unable to retain oral medication.

### *Magnesium Sulfate*

Intravenous magnesium sulfate may provide additional benefit in children with severe asthma treated with bronchodilators and corticosteroids. Magnesium sulfate has a better safety profile in the management of acute severe asthma than aminophylline. As it is more widely available, it can be used in children who are not responsive to the medications.

- Give 50% magnesium sulfate as a bolus of 0.1 mL/kg (50 mg/kg) IV over 20 min.

### *Aminophylline*

Aminophylline is not recommended in children with mild-to-moderate acute asthma. It is reserved for children who do not improve after several doses of a rapid-acting bronchodilator given at short intervals plus oral prednisolone. If indicated in these circumstances:

- Admit the child ideally to a high-care or intensive-care unit, if available, for continuous monitoring.
- Weigh the child carefully and then give IV aminophylline at an initial loading dose of 5–6 mg/kg (up to a maximum of 300 mg) over at least 20 min but preferably over 1 hour, followed by a maintenance dose of 5 mg/kg every 6 hour. IV aminophylline can be dangerous at an overdose or when given too rapidly.
- Omit the initial dose if the child has already received any form of aminophylline or caffeine in the previous 24 hour.
- Stop giving it immediately if the child starts to vomit, has a pulse rate > 180/min, develops a headache or has a convulsion.

## Oral Bronchodilators

Use of oral salbutamol (in syrup or tablets) is **not** recommended in the treatment of severe or persistent wheeze. It should be used only when inhaled salbutamol is not available for a child who has improved sufficiently to be discharged home.

### *Dosage*

- *Age 1 month to 2 years:* 100 μg/kg (maximum, 2 mg) upto four times daily
- *Age 2–6 years:* 1–2 mg upto four times daily.

### *Antibiotics*

Antibiotics should not be given routinely for asthma or to a child with asthma who has fast breathing without fever. Antimicrobial treatment is indicated, however, when there is persistent fever and other signs of pneumonia.

## Supportive Care

Ensure that the child receives daily maintenance fluids appropriate for his or her age. Encourage breastfeeding and oral fluids. Encourage adequate complementary feeding for the young child, as soon as food can be taken.

## Monitoring

A hospitalized child should be assessed by a nurse every 3 hour or every 6 hour as the child shows improvement (i.e. slower breathing rate, less lower chest wall indrawing and less respiratory distress) and by a doctor at least once a day. Record the respiratory rate, and watch especially for signs of respiratory failure—increasing hypoxia and respiratory distress leading to exhaustion.

## Complications

If the child fails to respond to the above therapy, or the child's condition worsens suddenly, obtain a chest X-ray to look for evidence of pneumothorax.

Be very careful in making this diagnosis as per the hyperinflation in asthma can mimic a pneumothorax on a chest X-ray.

## Follow-up Care

Asthma is a chronic and recurrent condition.

- Once the child has improved sufficiently to be discharged home, inhaled salbutamol through a metered dose inhaler should be prescribed with a suitable (not necessarily commercial) spacer and the mother instructed on how to use it.

- A long-term treatment plan should be made on the basis of the frequency and severity of symptoms. This may include intermittent or regular treatment with bronchodilators, regular treatment with inhaled steroids or intermittent courses of oral steroids. Up-to-date international or specialized national guidelines should be consulted for more information.

### Tuberculosis

Most children infected with *M. tuberculosis* do not develop TB. The only evidence of infection may be a positive skin test. The development of TB depends on the competence of the immune system to resist multiplication of the *M. tuberculosis* infection. This competence varies with age, being least in the very young. HIV infection and malnutrition lower the body's defenses, and measles and whooping cough temporarily impair the strength of the immune system. In the presence of any of these conditions, TB can develop more easily. TB is most often severe when it is located in the lungs, meninges or kidney.

Cervical lymph nodes, bones, joints, abdomen, ears, eyes and skin may also be affected. Many children present only with failure to grow normally, weight loss or prolonged fever. Cough for > 14 days can also be a presenting sign; in children, however, sputum-positive pulmonary TB is rarely diagnosed.

### Diagnosis

The risk for TB is increased when there is an active case (infectious, smear-positive pulmonary TB) in the same house or when the child is malnourished, has HIV/AIDS or had measles in the past few months. Consider TB in any child with:

#### *A History of*

- Unexplained weight loss or failure to grow normally
- Unexplained fever, especially when it continues for longer than 2 weeks
- Chronic cough (i.e. cough for > 14 days, with or without a wheeze)
- Exposure to an adult with probable or definite infectious pulmonary TB.

#### *On Examination*

- Fluid on one side of the chest (reduced air entry, stony dullness to percussion)
- Enlarged non-tender lymph nodes or a lymph node abscess, especially in the neck
- Signs of meningitis, especially when these develop over several days and the spinal fluid contains mostly lymphocytes and elevated protein
- Abdominal swelling, with or without palpable lumps
- Progressive swelling or deformity in the bone or a joint, including the spine.

### Investigations

- Try to obtain specimens for microscopic examination of acid-fast bacilli (Ziehl-Neelsen stain) and for culture of tubercle bacilli. Possible specimens include three consecutive early-morning, fasting gastric aspirates, CSF (if clinically indicated) and pleural fluid and ascites fluid (if present). As the detection rates with these methods are low, a positive result confirms TB, but a negative result does not exclude the disease.
- New rapid diagnostic tests are more accurate and may be more widely available in future.
- Obtain a chest X-ray. A diagnosis of TB is supported when a chest X-ray shows a miliary pattern of infiltrates or a persistent area of infiltrate or consolidation, often with pleural effusion, or a primary complex.
- Perform a purified protein derivative skin test *(PPD or mantoux test)*. The test is usually positive in children with pulmonary TB (reactions of > 10 mm suggest TB; < 10 mm in a child previously vaccinated with BCG is equivocal). The purified protein derivative test may be negative in children with TB who have HIV/AIDS, miliary disease, severe malnutrition or recent measles.
- Xpert MTB/RIF should be used as the initial diagnostic test in children suspected of having multidrug-resistant TB (MDR-TB) or HIV-associated TB.
- Routine HIV testing should be offered to all children suspected of TB.

### Treatment

- Give a full course of treatment to all confirmed or strongly suspected cases.
- When in doubt, e.g. in a child with strongly suspected TB or who fails to respond to treatment for other probable diagnoses, give treatment for TB.

Treatment failures for other diagnoses include antibiotic treatment for apparent bacterial pneumonia (when the child has pulmonary symptoms), for possible meningitis (when the child has neurological symptoms) or for intestinal worms or giardiasis (when the child fails to thrive or has diarrhea or abdominal symptoms).

- Suspected or confirmed childhood TB should be treated with a combination of anti-TB drugs, depending on the severity of disease, HIV status and level of isoniazid resistance.
- Follow the national TB programme guidelines for recommended treatment.
- To reduce the risk for drug-induced hepatotoxicity in children, follow the recommended dosages:
  - Isoniazid (H): 10 mg/kg (range, 10–15 mg/kg), maximum dose, 300 mg/day
  - Rifampicin (R): 15 mg/kg (range, 10–20 mg/kg), maximum dose, 600 mg/ kg per day
  - Pyrazinamide (Z): 35 mg/kg (range, 30–40 mg/kg)
  - Ethambutol (E): 20 mg/kg (range, 15–25 mg/kg).

#### *Treatment Regimens*

If national recommendations are not available, follow the WHO guidelines according to the regimens given below:

- ***Four-drug regimen:*** HRZE for 2 months, followed by a two-drug (HR) regimen for 4 months for all children with suspected or confirmed pulmonary TB or peripheral

lymphadenitis living in an area of high HIV prevalence or where resistance to H is high or children with extensive pulmonary disease living in areas of low HIV prevalence or low H resistance;
- *Three-drug regimen:* HRZ for 2 months, followed by a two-drug (HR) regimen for 4 months for children with suspected or confirmed pulmonary TB or tuberculous peripheral lymphadenitis living in areas of low HIV prevalence or low H resistance or HIV-negative;
- In cases of suspected or confirmed tuberculous meningitis, spinal TB with neurological signs or osteo-articular TB, treat for 12 months with a fourdrug regimen (HRZE) for 2 months, followed by a two-drug (HR) regimen for 10 months;
- In infants (aged 0–3 months) with suspected or confirmed pulmonary TB or tuberculous peripheral lymphadenitis, treat promptly with the standard regimens described above, with adjustment of doses to reconcile the effect of age and possible toxicity in young infants.

*Intermittent regimens:* In areas with well-established directly observed therapy, thrice-weekly regimens can be considered for children known to be HIV-negative.

They should not be used in areas with a high HIV prevalence, because there is a high risk of treatment failure and development of multidrug-resistant TB.

***Precautions:*** Streptomycin should not be used as part of first-line treatment regimens for children with pulmonary TB or tuberculous peripheral lymphadenitis.

It should be reserved for the treatment of multidrug-resistant TB in children with known susceptibility to this medicine.

## Multidrug-resistant TB

In cases of MDR TB, treat children with proven or suspected pulmonary TB or tuberculous meningitis with a fluoroquinolone or other second-line TB drug. An appropriate MDR TB treatment regimen in the context of a well-functioning MDR TB control programme should be used. The decision to treat should be taken by a clinician experienced in managing pediatric TB.

## Monitoring

Confirm that the medication is being taken as instructed, by direct observation of each dose. Monitor the child's weight gain daily and temperature twice a day in order to check for resolution of fever. These are signs of response to therapy. When treatment is given for suspected TB, improvement should be seen within 1 month. If this does not occur, review the patient, check compliance, reinvestigate and reconsider the diagnosis.

## Public Health Measures

- Notify the case to the responsible district health authorities. Ensure that treatment is monitored as recommended by the national TB program
  Check all household members of the child (and, if necessary, school contacts) for undetected cases of TB, and arrange treatment for any that are found.
- Children < 5 years of age who are household or close contacts of people with TB and who, after an appropriate clinical evaluation, are found not to have active TB should be given 6 months of isoniazid preventive therapy (10 mg/kg/day, range 7–15 mg/kg, maximum dose 300 mg/day).

## Follow-up

A program of 'active' follow-up, in which a health worker visits the child and his or her family at home, can reduce default from TB treatment. During follow-up at home or in hospital, health workers can:
- Check whether medications for TB are being taken regularly.
- Remind the family and the treatment supporter about the importance of taking medications regularly, even if the child is well, for the full duration of treatment.
- Screen family contacts, including other children in the family, by inquiring about cough, and start these children on isoniazid preventive therapy.
- Suggest how the family's home environment might be made healthier for children, such as eliminating smoking inside the house, good ventilation and handwashing.
- Discuss with the parents the importance of nutrition in recovery from TB and any problems in providing good nutrition for their children.
- Check the child for growth, nutritional state and signs of TB and other treatable conditions. If problems are found, the health worker should recommend how these can be treated or refer the family to a pediatrician.
- Check the child's health record, and tell the parents when and where they should bring the child for doses of vaccine.
- Ask the parents if they have any questions or concerns, and answer or discuss these, or refer the family to a pediatrician.
- Record their observations on the TB treatment card.

## Foreign Body Inhalation

Nuts, seeds or other small objects may be inhaled, most often by children < 4 years of age. The foreign body usually lodges in a bronchus (more often in the right) and can cause collapse or consolidation of the portion of lung distal to the site of blockage. Choking is a frequent initial symptom. This may be followed by a symptom-free interval of days or weeks before the child presents with persistent wheeze, chronic cough or pneumonia, which fails to respond to treatment. Small sharp objects can lodge in the larynx, causing stridor or wheeze. Rarely, a large object lodged in the larynx can cause sudden death from asphyxia, unless it can be dislodged or an emergency tracheostomy be done.

## Diagnosis

Inhalation of a foreign body should be considered in a child with the following signs.
- Sudden onset of choking, coughing or wheezing; or
- Segmental or lobar pneumonia that fails to respond to antibiotic therapy.

Examine the child for:
- Unilateral wheeze

• An area of decreased breath sounds that is either dull or hyper-resonant on percussion
• Deviation of the trachea or apex beat.

Obtain a chest X-ray at full expiration to detect an area of hyperinflation or collapse, mediastinal shift (away from the affected side) or a foreign body if it is radio-opaque.

### Treatment

*Emergency first aid for the choking child*: Attempt to dislodge and expel the foreign body. The management depends on the age of the child.

#### *For infants:*

• Lay the infant in a head-down position on one of your arms or on your thigh.
• Strike the middle of the infant's back five times with the heel of your hand.
• If the obstruction persists, turn the infant over and give five firm chest thrusts with two fingers on the lower half of the sternum.
• If the obstruction persists, check the infant's mouth for any obstruction that can be removed.
• If necessary, repeat this sequence with back slaps.

#### *For Older Children:*

• While the child is sitting, kneeling or lying, strike the child's back five times with the heel of the hand.
• If the obstruction persists, go behind the child and pass your arms around the child's body, form a first with one hand immediately below the sternum, place the other hand over the fist and thrust sharply upwards into the abdomen.

Repeat this up to five times.

• Then check the child's mouth for any obstruction that can be removed.
• If necessary, repeat the sequence with back slaps.

Once this has been done, it is important to check the patency of the airway by:

• Looking for chest movements
• Listening for breath sounds and
• Feeling for breath.
• Later treatment of suspected foreign body aspiration. If a foreign body is suspected, refer the child to a hospital where diagnosis is possible and the object can be removed after bronchoscopy. If there is evidence of pneumonia, begin treatment with ampicillin (or benzylpenicillin) and gentamicin, as for severe pneumonia, before attempting to remove the foreign body.

### Heart Failure

Heart failure causes fast breathing and respiratory distress. The underlying causes include congenital heart disease (usually in the first months of life), acute rheumatic fever, cardiac arrhythmia, myocarditis, suppurative pericarditis with constriction, infective endocarditis, acute glomerulonephritis, severe anemia, severe pneumonia and severe malnutrition. Heart failure can be precipitated or worsened by fluid overload, especially when large volumes of IV fluids are given.

### Diagnosis

The commonest signs of heart failure, on examination, are:

• Tachycardia (heart rate > 160/min in a child < 12 months; > 120/min in a child aged 12 months to 5 years)
• Gallop rhythm with basal crackles on auscultation
• Enlarged, tender liver
• In infants, fast breathing (or sweating), especially when feeding; in older children, oedema of the feet, hands or face or distended neck veins (raised jugular venous pressure) Severe palmar pallor may be present if severe anemia is the cause of the heart failure.

Heart murmur may be present in rheumatic heart disease, congenital heart disease or endocarditis.

If the diagnosis is in doubt, a chest X-ray can be taken and may show an enlarged heart or abnormal shape.

Measure blood pressure if possible. If it is raised, consider acute glomerulonephritis.

### Treatment

Treatment depends on the underlying heart disease (Consult international or national pediatric guidelines). The main measures for treating heart failure in children who are not severely malnourished are:

• Oxygen. Give oxygen if the child has a respiratory rate of ≥ 70/min, shows signs of respiratory distress, or has central cyanosis or low oxygen saturation.

Aim to keep oxygen saturation > 90%.

• Diuretics. Give furosemide: A dose of 1 mg/kg should increase urine flow within 2 h. For faster action, give the drug IV. If the initial dose is not effective, give 2 mg/kg and repeat in 12 hour, if necessary. Thereafter, a single daily dose of 1–2 mg/kg orally is usually sufficient.
• Digoxin. Consider giving digoxin.
• Supplemental potassium. Supplemental potassium is not required when furosemide is given alone for treatment lasting only a few days. When digoxin and furosemide are given, or if furosemide is given for more than 5 days,give oral potassium at 3–5 mmol/kg per day.

### Supportive Care

• Avoid giving IV fluids, if possible.
• Support the child in a semi-seated position with head and shoulders elevated and lower limbs dependent.
• Relieve any fever with paracetamol to reduce the cardiac workload.
• Consider transfusion if severe anemia is present.

### Monitoring

The child should be checked by a nurse every 6 hour (every 3 hour while on oxygen therapy) and by a doctor once a day. Monitor both respiratory and pulse rates, liver size and body weight to assess the response to treatment. Continue treatment until the respiratory and pulse rates are normal and the liver is no longer enlarged.

### Rheumatic Heart Disease

Chronic rheumatic heart disease is a complication of acute rheumatic fever, which leaves permanent damage to the heart valves. In some children, antibodies produced in response to group A â-hemolytic streptococci lead to varying degrees of pancarditis, with associated valve insufficiency in the acute phase.

The risk for rheumatic heart disease is higher with repeated episodes of acute rheumatic fever. It leads to valve stenosis, with varying degrees of regurgitation, atrial dilatation, arrhythmia and ventricular dysfunction. Chronic rheumatic heart disease is a major cause of mitral valve stenosis in children.

### Diagnosis

Rheumatic heart disease should be suspected in any child with a previous history of rheumatic fever who presents with heart failure or is found to have a heart murmur. Diagnosis is important because penicillin prophylaxis can prevent further episodes of rheumatic fever and avoid worse damage to the heart valves.

The presentation depends on the severity. Mild disease may cause few symptoms except for a heart murmur in an otherwise well child and is rarely diagnosed. Severe disease may present with symptoms that depend on the extent of heart damage or the presence of infective endocarditis.

### History

- Chest pain
- Heart palpitations
- Symptoms of heart failure (including orthopnea, paroxysmal nocturnal dyspnea and edema)
- Fever or stroke usually associated with infection of damaged heart valves breathlessness on exertion or exercise
- Fainting (syncope).

### Examination

- Signs of heart failure
- Cardiomegaly with a heart murmur
- Signs of infective endocarditis (e.g. conjunctival or retinal hemorrhages, hemiparesis, Osler nodes, Roth spots and splenomegaly)

### Investigations

- Chest x-ray: Cardiomegaly with congested lungs
- An echocardiogram, if available, is useful for confirming rheumatic heart disease, the extent of valve damage and evidence of infective endocarditis.
- Full blood count
- Blood culture.

### Management

- Admit the child if in heart failure or has suspected bacterial endocarditis.
- Treatment depends on the type and extent of valvular damage.
- Manage heart failure if present.
- Give diuretics to relieve symptoms of pulmonary congestion and vasodilators when necessary.
- Give penicillin or ampicillin or ceftriaxone plus gentamicin IV or IM for 4–6 weeks for infective endocarditis.
- Refer for echocardiographic evaluation and decision on long-term management.

May require surgical management in severe valvular stenosis or regurgitation.

### Follow-up Care

- All children with rheumatic heart disease should receive routine antibiotic prophylaxis.
- Give benzathine benzylpenicillin at 600,000 U IM every 3–4 weeks
- Ensure antibiotic prophylaxis for endocarditis before dental and invasive surgical procedures.
- Ensure that vaccinations are up to date.
- Review every 3–6 months, depending on severity of valvular damage.

### Complications

Infective endocarditis is more common. It presents with fever and heart murmur in a very unwell child. Treat with ampicillin and gentamicin for 6 weeks.

Atrial fibrillation or thromboembolism may occur, especially in the presence of mitral stenosis.

## Diarrhea

This chapter gives treatment guidelines on the management of acute diarrhea (with severe, some or no dehydration), persistent diarrhea and dysentery in children aged 1 week to 5 years.

The three essential elements in the management of all children with diarrhea are rehydration therapy, zinc supplementation and counseling for continued feeding and prevention.

In diarrhea, there is excess loss of water, electrolytes (sodium, potassium, and bicarbonate) and zinc in liquid stools. Dehydration occurs when these losses are not adequately replaced and there are deficits of water and electrolytes.

The degree of dehydration is graded according to symptoms and signs that reflect the amount of fluid lost The rehydration regimen is selected according to the degree of dehydration. All children with diarrhea should receive zinc supplements.

During diarrhea, decreased food intake and nutrient absorption and increased nutrient requirements often combine to cause weight loss and failure to grow.

Malnutrition can make diarrhea more severe, more prolonged and more frequent than in well-nourished children. This vicious circle can be broken by giving nutrient-rich foods during and continuing after the diarrhea episode, when the child is well.

Antibiotics should not be used except for children with bloody diarrhea (probable shigellosis), suspected cholera with severe dehydration and other serious non-intestinal infections such as pneumonia and urinary tract infection.

Antiprotozoal drugs are rarely indicated. 'Antidiarrheal' drugs and anti-emetics should not be given to young children with acute or persistent diarrhea or dysentery: they do not prevent dehydration or improve nutritional status, and some have dangerous, sometimes fatal, sideeffects.

## Child Presenting with Diarrhea

### *History*

A careful feeding history is essential in the management of a child with diarrhea. Inquiries should also be made about:
- Frequency of stools
- Number of days of diarrhea
- Blood in stools
- Report of a cholera outbreak in the area
- Recent antibiotic or other drug treatment
- Attacks of crying with pallor in an infant.

### *Examination*

Look for:
- Signs of some dehydration or severe dehydration:
  - Restlessness or irritability
  - Lethargy or reduced level of consciousness
  - Sunken eyes
  - Skin pinch returns slowly or very slowly
  - Thirsty or drinks eagerly, or drinking poorly or not able to drink
- Blood in stools
- Signs of severe malnutrition
- Abdominal mass
- Abdominal distension.

There is no need for routine stool microscopy or culture in children with nonbloody diarrhea.

### *Differential Diagnosis in a Child Presenting with Diarrhea*

*Acute (Watery) Diarrhea*
- More than three loose stools per day
- No blood in stools

*Cholera*
- Profuse watery diarrhea with severe dehydration during cholera outbreak
- Positive stool culture for *Vibrio cholerae*

*Dysentery*

Blood mixed with the stools (seen or reported).

*Persistent Diarrhea*

Diarrhea lasting ≥ 14 days.

*Diarrhea with Severe Malnutrition*

Any diarrhea with signs of severe acute malnutrition.

*Diarrhea Associated with Recent Antibiotic Use*

Recent course of broad-spectrum oral antibiotics.

## Intussusception

- Blood and mucus in stools
- Abdominal mass
- Attacks of crying with pallor in infant or young child.

## Acute Diarrhea Assessing Dehydration

For all children with diarrhea, their hydration status should be classified as ***severe dehydration, some dehydration*** or ***no dehydration*** and appropriate treatment given. In a child with diarrhea, assess the general condition, look for sunken eyes, make a skin pinch, and offer the child fluid to see if he or she is thirsty or drinking poorly.

| Classification | Signs or symptoms | Treatment |
|---|---|---|
| **Severe dehydration** | Two or more of the following signs:<br>• Lethargy or unconsciousness<br>• Sunken eyes<br>• Unable to drink or drinks poorly<br>• Skin pinch goes back very slowly (≥ 2 s) | • Give fluids for severe dehydration |
| **Some dehydration** | Two or more of the following signs:<br>• Restlessness, irritability<br>• Sunken eyes<br>• Drinks eagerly, thirsty<br>• Skin pinch goes back slowly | • Give fluid and food for some dehydration<br>• After rehydration, advise mother on home treatment and when to return immediately<br>• Follow-up in 5 days if not improving. |
| **No dehydration** | Not enough signs to classify as some or severe dehydration | • Give fluid and food to treat diarrhea at home<br>• Advise mother on when to return immediately<br>• Followup in 5 days if not improving. |

## Severe Dehydration

Children with severe dehydration require rapid IV rehydration with close monitoring, followed by oral rehydration and zinc once the child starts to improve sufficiently. In areas where there is a cholera outbreak, give an antibiotic effective against cholera.

## Diagnosis

Severe dehydration should be diagnosed if any two signs or symptoms of severe dehydration are present in a child with diarrhea.

## Treatment

Children with severe dehydration should be given rapid IV rehydration followed by oral rehydration therapy.
- Start IV fluids immediately. While the drip is being set up, give ORS solution if the child can drink.

***Note:*** *The best IV fluid solutions for rehydration are isotonic solutions: Ringer's lactate solution (called Hartmann's solution for Injection) and normal saline solution (0.9% NaCl). Do not use 5% glucose (dextrose) solution or 0.18% saline with 5% dextrose solution, as they increase the risk for hyponatremia, which can cause cerebral edema.*

- Give 100 mL/kg of the chosen solution, divided as shown in Table.

*Administration of Intravenous Fluids to a Severely Dehydrated Child*

| Age (months) | First, give 30 mL/kg in: | Then, give 70 mL/kg in: |
|---|---|---|
| < 12 | 1 h | 5 h |
| ≥ 12 | 30 min | 2.5 h |

### *Cholera*

- Suspect cholera in children > 2-years-old who have acute watery diarrhea and signs of severe dehydration or shock, if cholera is present in the area.
- Assess and treat dehydration as for other acute diarrhea.
- Give an oral antibiotic to which strains of V cholerae in the area are known to be sensitive. Possible choices are: erythromycin, ciprofloxacin and cotrimoxazole.
- Prescribe zinc supplementation as soon as vomiting stops.

### Monitoring

Reassess the child every 15–30 min until a strong radial pulse is present. Thereafter, reassess the child by checking skin pinch, level of consciousness and ability to drink at least every hour, in order to confirm that hydration is improving. Sunken eyes recover more slowly than other signs and are less useful for monitoring. When the full amount of IV fluid has been given, reassess the child's hydration status fully using chart.

- *If signs of severe dehydration are still present*, repeat the IV fluid infusion outlined earlier. Persistent severe dehydration after IV rehydration is unusual; it usually occurs only in children who pass large watery stools frequently during the rehydration period.
- *If the child is improving but still shows signs of some dehydration*, discontinue IV treatment and give ORS solution for 4 hour. If the child is usually breastfed, encourage the mother to continue breastfeeding frequently.
- *If there are no signs of dehydration*, follow the guidelines in section and treatment plan A. When appropriate, encourage the mother to continue breastfeeding frequently. Observe the child for at least 6 hour before discharge, to confirm that the mother is able to maintain the child's hydration by giving ORS solution.

All children should start to receive some ORS solution (about 5 mL/kg per hour) by cup when they can drink without difficulty (usually within 3–4 hour for infants and 1–2 hour for older children). ORS provides additional base and potassium, which may not be adequately supplied by IV fluid.

When severe dehydration is corrected, prescribe zinc.

### Some Dehydration

In general, children with some dehydration should be given ORS solution for the first 4 hour at a clinic, while the child is monitored and the mother is taught how to prepare and give ORS solution.

### Diagnosis

If the child has two or more of the following signs, he or she has some dehydration:

- Restlessness or irritability
- Thirsty and drinks eagerly
- Sunken eyes
- Skin pinch goes back slowly.

Note that if a child has only one of the above signs and one of the signs of severe dehydration (e.g. restlessness or irritable and drinking poorly), then the child also has some dehydration.

### Treatment

- In the first 4 hour, give the child ORS solution according to the child's weight or age if the weight is not known. If the child wants more to drink, give more.
- Show the mother how to give the child ORS solution: a teaspoonful every 1–2 min if the child is < 2 years, frequent sips from a cup for an older child.
- Check regularly to see whether there are problems.
- If the child vomits, wait 10 min; then, resume ORS solution more slowly (e.g. a spoonful every 2–3 min).
- If the child's eyelids become puffy, stop ORS solution, reduce the fluid intake and continue with breast milk. Weigh the child, and monitor urine output.
- Advise breastfeeding mothers to continue to breastfeed whenever the child wants.
- Check blood glucose or electrolytes if possible in a child who is restless or irritable and convulsing, in case hypoglycemia or hypernatremia is present. Manage the child accordingly; if blood glucose measurement is not possible, give IV glucose or oral sugar.
- If the mother cannot stay for 4 hour, show her how to prepare ORS solution and give her enough ORS packets to complete rehydration at home plus enough for 2 more days.
- Reassess the child after 4 hour, checking for signs of dehydration listed earlier.

***Note:*** *Reassess the child before 4 hour if he or she is not taking the ORS solution or seems to be getting worse.*

If there is no dehydration, teach the mother the four rules of home treatment:

1. Give extra fluid.
2. Give zinc supplements for 10–14 days.
3. Continue feeding.
4. Return if the child develops any of the following signs:
   - Drinking poorly or unable to drink or breastfed
   - Develops a general danger sign
   - Becomes sicker
   - Develops a fever
   - Has blood mixed with the stools or more than a few drops on the outside of the stool.

- If the child still has some dehydration, repeat treatment with ORS solution for another 4 hour, as above, and start to offer food, milk or juice and breastfed frequently.

### *Give Zinc Supplements*

Zinc is an important micronutrient for a child's overall health and development but is lost in greater quantities during diarrhea. Replacement helps the child's recovery, reduces the duration and severity of the episode, and lowers the incidence of diarrhea in the following 2–3 months.

- Give zinc and advise the mother how much to give:
  - ≤ 6 months: Half tablet (10 mg) per day for 10–14 days
  - ≥ 6 months: One tablet (20 mg) per day for 10–14 days.

### Feeding

Continuation of nutritious feeding is an important element in the management of diarrhea. In the initial 4-h rehydration period, do not give any food except breast milk. Breastfed children should continue to breastfed frequently throughout the episode of diarrhea. If they cannot suck from the breast, consider giving expressed breast milk either orally from a cup or by nasogastric tube.

- After 4 h, if the child still has some dehydration and ORS continues to be given, give food every 3–4 h.
- All children > 6 months should be given some food before being sent home. If the child is not normally breastfed, explore the feasibility of relactation or give the usual breast milk substitute. If the child is ≥ 6 months or already taking solid food, give freshly prepared foods– cooked, mashed or ground. The following are recommended:
- Cereal or another starchy food mixed with pulses, vegetables and meat or fish, if possible, with 1–2 teaspoons of vegetable oil added to each serving
- Local complementary foods recommended by the imci in that area
- Fresh fruit juice or mashed banana to provide potassium.
- Encourage the child to eat by offering food at least six times a day. Give the same foods after the diarrhea stops, and give an extra meal a day for 2 weeks.

## No Dehydration

Children with diarrhea but no dehydration should receive extra fluids at home to prevent dehydration. They should continue to receive an appropriate diet for their age, including continued breastfeeding.

## Diagnosis

*Diarrhea with no dehydration* should be diagnosed if the child does not have two or more signs that characterize some or severe dehydration, as described above.

## Treatment

- Treat the child as an outpatient.
- Counsel the mother on the four rules of home treatment:
- Give extra fluid.
- Give zinc supplements.
- Continue feeding.
- Know when to return to the clinic.
- Give extra fluid, as follows:
- If the child is being breastfed, advise the mother to breastfed frequently and for longer at each fed. If the child is exclusively breastfed, give ORS solution or clean water in addition to breast milk. After the diarrhea stops, exclusive breastfeeding should be resumed, if appropriate to the child's age.
- In non-exclusively breastfed children, give one or more of the following:
- ORS solution
- food-based fluids (such as soup, rice water and yoghurt drinks)
- clean water.

To prevent dehydration, advise the mother to give as much extra-fluids as the child will take:

- for children < 2 years, about 50–100 mL after each loose stool
- for children ≥ 2 years, about 100–200 mL after each loose stool.

Tell the mother to give small sips from a cup. If the child vomits, wait 10 min, and then give more slowly. She should continue giving extra fluid until the diarrhea stops.

Teach the mother how to mix and give ORS solution, and give her two packets of ORS to take home.

- Give zinc supplements
- Tell the mother how much zinc to give:
- ≤ 6 months: half tablet (10 mg) per day
- ≥ 6 months: one tablet (20 mg) per day for 10–14 days
- Show the mother how to give the zinc supplement:
  - For infants, dissolve the tablet in a small amount of clean water, expressed milk or ORS.
  - Older children can chew the tablet or drink it dissolved.
- Remind the mother to give the zinc supplement for the full 10–14 days.
- Continue feeding
- Advise the mother on when to return.

## Follow-up

- Advise the mother to return immediately to the clinic if the child becomes sicker, is unable to drink or breastfed, drinks poorly, develops a fever or has blood in the stool. If the child shows none of these signs but is still not improving, advise the mother to return for follow-up after 5 days.

Also explain that the same treatment should be given in the future as soon as diarrhea develops.

## Persistent Diarrhea

Persistent diarrhea is the diarrhea, with or without blood, that begins acutely and lasts for ≥ 14 days. When there is some or severe dehydration, persistent diarrhea is classified as 'severe'.

The following guidelines are for children with persistent diarrhea who are not severely malnourished. Severely malnourished children with severe persistent diarrhea require hospitalization and specific treatment. *In areas where HIV infection is highly prevalent*, suspect HIV infection if there are other suggestive clinical signs, and assess the child for HIV infection and do an appropriate HIV test. Perform stool microscopy for parasites such as *Isospora* and *Cryptosporidium*.

## Severe Persistent Diarrhea Diagnosis

- Infants or children with diarrhea lasting ≥ 14 days with signs of dehydration have severe persistent diarrhea and require hospital treatment.
- Assess the child for signs of dehydration.

## Treatment

*Give fluids according to treatment plan B or C, as appropriate*

ORS solution is effective for most children with persistent diarrhea. A few children, however, may have impaired glucose absorption, and ORS solution may not be as effective. When these children are given ORS, their stool volume increases markedly, thirst increases, signs of dehydration develop or worsen, and the stools contain a large amount of unabsorbed glucose. These children require IV rehydration until ORS solution can be taken without causing the diarrhea to worsen.

Routine treatment of persistent diarrhea with antibiotics is not effective and should not be done. Some children, however, have non-intestinal or intestinal infections that require specific antibiotic therapy.

- Examine every child with persistent diarrhea for non-intestinal infections such as pneumonia, sepsis, urinary tract infection, oral thrush and otitis media, and treat appropriately.
- Give micronutrients and vitamins
- Treat persistent diarrhea with blood in the stools with an oral antibiotic effective for Shigella,

Give oral metronidazole at 10 mg/kg three times a day for 5 days only if:

- Microscopic examination of fresh faeces reveals trophozoites of *Entamoeba histolytica* within red blood cells; **or** – trophozoites or cysts of giardia are seen in the feces, **or** – two different antibiotics that are usually effective for *Shigella* locally have been given without clinical improvement.
- if stool examination is not possible, when diarrhea persists for > 1 month.

## Feeding

Careful attention to feeding is essential for all children with persistent diarrhea.

Breastfeeding should be continued for as often and as long as the child wants.

Other food should be withheld for 4–6 h only for children with dehydration

### Hospital Diet

Children treated in hospital require special diets until their diarrhea lessens and they are gaining weight. The goal is to give a daily intake of at least 110 calories/kg.

*Infants Aged < 6 Months*

- Encourage exclusive breastfeeding. Help mothers who are not breastfeeding exclusively to do so.
- If the child is not breastfeeding, give a breast milk substitute that is low in lactose, such as yoghurt, or is lactose-free. Use a spoon or cup; do not use a feeding bottle. Once the child improves, help the mother to re-establish lactation.
- If the mother is not breastfeeding because she is HIV-positive, she should receive appropriate counselling about the correct use of breast milk substitutes.

*Children Aged ≥ 6 Months*

Feeding should be restarted as soon as the child can eat. Food should be given six times a day to achieve a total intake of at least 110 calories/kg per day.

Many children will eat poorly, however, until any serious infection has been treated for 24–48 h. These children may require nasogastric feeding initially.

### Two Recommended Diets

Tables A and B show two diets recommended for children and infants aged > 6 months with severe persistent diarrhea. If there are signs of dietary failure or if the child is not improving after 7 days of treatment, the first diet should be stopped and the second diet given for 7 days.

***First diet for persistent diarrhea: A starch-based, reduced-milk (low-lactose) diet***

The diet should contain at least 70 calories/100 g, provide milk or yoghurt as a source of animal protein, but no more than 3.7 g lactose/kg per day and should provide at least 10% of calories as protein. The following example provides 83 calories/100 g, 3.7 g lactose/kg per day and 11% of calories as protein:

| | |
|---|---|
| • full-fat dried milk (or whole liquid milk: 85 mL) | 11 g |
| • rice | 15 g |
| • vegetable oil | 3.5 g |
| • cane sugar | 3.0 g |
| • water to make up | 200 mL |

***Second diet for persistent diarrhea: A reduced-starch (cereal) no-milk (lactose-free) diet***

The diet should contain at least 70 calories/100 g and provide at least 10% of calories as protein (egg or chicken). The following example provides 75 calories/100 g:

| | |
|---|---|
| • whole egg | 64 g |
| • rice | 3 g |
| • vegetable oil | 4 g |
| • glucose | 3 g |
| • water to make up | 200 mL |

Finely ground, cooked chicken (12 g) can be used in place of egg to give a diet providing 70 calories/100 g

*Successful treatment* with either diet is characterized by:

- Adequate food intake
- Weight gain
- Fewer diarrheal stools
- Absence of fever.

The most important criterion is weight gain. Weight should increase for at least three successive days before weight gain can be assumed.

Give additional fresh fruit and well-cooked vegetables to children who are responding well. After 7 days of treatment with the effective diet, they should resume an appropriate diet for their age, including milk, which provides at least 110 calories/kg per day. Children may then return home but must be followed up regularly to ensure continued weight gain and compliance with feeding advice.

*Dietary failure is indicated by:*

- an increase in stool frequency (usually to > 10 watery stools a day), often with a return of signs of dehydration (usually shortly after a new diet is begun)
- failure to establish daily weight gain within 7 days.

***Supplementary multivitamins and minerals***

Give all children with persistent diarrhea daily supplementary multivitamins and minerals for 2 weeks. These should provide as broad a range of vitamins and minerals as possible, including at least two recommended daily allowances of folate, vitamin A, zinc, magnesium and copper.

As a guide, one recommended daily allowance for a child aged 1 year is:

| | |
|---|---|
| • folate | 50 μg |
| • zinc | 10 mg |
| • vitamin A | 400 μg |
| • iron | 10 mg |
| • copper | 1 mg |
| • magnesium | 80 mg |

### Persistent Diarrhea (Non-severe)

Children with non-severe persistent diarrhea do not require hospital treatment but need special feeding and extra fluids at home.

### Diagnosis

Children with diarrhea lasting ≥ 14 days but with no signs of dehydration or severe malnutrition.

### Treatment

- Treat the child as an outpatient.
- Give supplementary multivitamins and minerals as shown in the box above.

#### *Prevent Dehydration*

Give fluids according to treatment plan A. ORS solution is effective for most children with persistent diarrhea. In a few, however, glucose absorption is impaired, and when they are given ORS solution their stool volume increases markedly, thirst increases, signs of dehydration develop or worsen, and the stools contain a large amount of unabsorbed glucose.

These children require admission to hospital for IV rehydration until ORS solution can be taken without aggravating the diarrhea.

#### *Identify and Treat Specific Infections*

- Do not routinely treat with antibiotics, as they are not effective; however, give antibiotic treatment to children with specific non-intestinal or intestinal infections. Until these infections are treated correctly, persistent diarrhea will not improve.
- Non-intestinal infections. Examine every child with persistent diarrhea for non-intestinal infections, such as pneumonia, sepsis, urinary tract infection, oral thrush and otitis media. Treat each specific disease.
- Intestinal infections. Treat persistent diarrhea with blood in the stools with an oral antibiotic that is effective for Shigella,

### Feeding

Careful attention to feeding is essential for all children with persistent diarrhea.

These children may have difficulty in digesting animal milk other than breast milk.

- Advise the mother to reduce the amount of animal milk in the child's diet temporarily.
- Continue breastfeeding and give appropriate complementary foods:
  - If still breastfeeding, give more frequent, longer breastfeds, day and night.
  - If taking other animal milk, explore the feasibility of replacing animal milk with fermented milk products (e.g. yoghurt), which contain less lactose and are better tolerated.
  - If replacement of animal milk is not possible, limit animal milk to 50 mL/kg per day. Mix the milk with the child's cereal, but do not dilute it.
  - Give other foods appropriate for the child's age to ensure an adequate caloric intake. Infants aged > 4 months whose only food has been animal milk should begin to take solid foods.
  - Give frequent small meals, at least six times a day.

*Supplementary micronutrients, including zinc.*

### Follow-up

- Ask the mother to bring the child back for reassessment after 5 days, or earlier if the diarrhea worsens or other problems develop.
- Fully reassess children who have not gained weight or whose diarrhea has not improved in order to identify the cause, such as dehydration or infection, which requires immediate attention or admitted to hospital.

Those who have gained weight and who have three or fewer loose stools per day may resume a normal diet for their age.

### Dysentery

Dysentery is diarrhea presenting with frequent loose stools mixed with blood (not just a few smears on the surface). Most episodes are due to *Shigella*, and nearly all require antibiotic treatment. Shigellosis can lead to life-threatening complications, including intestinal perforation, toxic megacolon and hemolytic uremic syndrome.

### Diagnosis

The diagnostic signs of dysentery are frequent loose stools mixed with visible red blood. Other findings on examination may include:

- Abdominal pain
- Fever
- Convulsions
- Lethargy
- Dehydration
- Rectal prolapse

### Treatment

Most children can be treated at home.

- Admit to hospital:
  - Young infants (< 2 months old)
  - Severely ill children, who look lethargic, have abdominal distension and tenderness or convulsions
  - Children with any another condition requiring hospital treatment.
  - Give an oral antibiotic (for 5 days) to which most local strains of *Shigella* are sensitive.
  - Give ciprofloxacin at 15 mg/kg twice a day for 3 days if antibiotic sensitivity is unknown. If local antimicrobial sensitivity is known, follow local guidelines.
  - Give ceftriaxone IV or IM at 50–80 mg/kg per day for 3 days to severely ill children or as second-line treatment.
  - Give zinc supplements as for children with watery diarrhea.

***Note:*** *There is widespread Shigella resistance to ampicillin, co-trimoxazole, chloramphenicol, nalidixic acid, tetracycline, gentamicin and first- and secondgeneration cephalosporin, which are no longer effective. There is also already reported resistance to ciprofloxacin in some countries.*

### Follow-up

Follow up children after 2 days, and look for signs of improvement, such as no fever, fewer stools with less blood, improved appetite.

- If there is no improvement after 2 full days of treatment:
  - Check for other conditions
  - Stop the first antibiotic, and give a second-line antibiotic or a known effective against Shigella in the area.
- If the two antibiotics that are usually effective against Shigella in the area have each been given for 2 days, with no sign of clinical improvement, check for other conditions.
  - If amebiasis is possible, give metronidazole at 10 mg/kg three times a day for 5 days.
- Admit the child if there is an indication requiring hospital treatment.

### *Infants and Young Children*

Consider surgical causes of blood in the stools and refer to a surgeon, if appropriate. Dysentery is unusual in neonates and young infants; therefore, consider life-threatening bacterial sepsis.

- For suspected sepsis give IM or IV ceftriaxone at 100 mg/kg once daily for 5 days.

### *Severely Malnourished Children*

- Treat for *Shigella* first and then for amebiasis on clinical grounds if laboratory examination is not possible.
- If microscopic examination of fresh stools in a reliable laboratory is possible, check for trophozoites of *Entamoeba histolytica* in red blood cells and treat for amebiasis, if present. Also examine stools for trophozoites of *Giardia lamblia* and treat if present.

### Supportive Care

Supportive care includes the prevention or correction of dehydration and continued feeding.

Never give drugs for symptomatic relief of abdominal or rectal pain or to reduce the frequency of stools, as these drugs can increase the severity of the illness.

### *Treatment of Dehydration*

Assess the child for signs of dehydration and give fluids as appropriate.

### *Nutritional Management*

Ensuring a good diet is important, as dysentery has a marked adverse effect on nutritional status. Feeding is often difficult because of lack of appetite; return of appetite is an important sign of improvement.

- Breastfeeding should be continued throughout the course of the illness, more frequently than normal, if possible, because the infant may not take the usual amount per fed.
- Children aged 6 months or more should receive their normal foods. Encourage the child to eat, and allow the child to select preferred foods.

### Complications

- *Dehydration:* Dehydration is the commonest complication of dysentery, and children should be assessed and managed for dehydration irrespective of any other complication. Give fluids as appropriate.
- *Potassium depletion:* Potassium depletion can be prevented by giving ORS solution (when indicated) or potassium-rich foods such as bananas, coconut water or dark-green leafy vegetables.
- *High fever:* If the child has high fever (≥ 39°C or e 102.2°F) that appears to be causing distress, give paracetamol and consider severe bacterial infection.
- *Rectal prolapse:* Gently push back the rectal prolapse using a surgical glove or a wet cloth. Alternatively, prepare a warm solution of saturated magnesium sulfate, and apply compresses with this solution to reduce the prolapse by decreasing edema.
- *Convulsions:* A single convulsion is the commonest finding. If they are prolonged or repeated, give diazepam. Avoid giving rectal diazepam. Always check for hypoglycemia.
- *Hemolytic uremic syndrome:* Where laboratory tests are not possible, suspect hemolytic uremic syndrome in patients with easy bruising, pallor, altered consciousness and low or no urine output.
- *Toxic megacolon:* Toxic megacolon usually presents with fever, abdominal distension, pain and tenderness with loss of bowel sounds, tachycardia and dehydration. Give IV fluids for dehydration, pass a nasogastric tube, and start antibiotics.

## SEVERE ACUTE MALNUTRITION

Severe acute malnutrition is defined in these guidelines as the presence of edema of both feet or severe wasting (weight-for-height/length <-3SD or mid-upper arm circumference < 115 mm). No distinction is made between the clinical conditions of kwashiorkor or severe wasting because their treatment is similar.

Children who are <-3SD weight-for-age may be stunted (short stature) but not severely wasted. Stunted children who are not severely wasted do not require hospital admission unless they have a serious illness.

### Diagnosis

The main diagnostic features are:

- weight-for-length/height < -3SD (wasted) or
- mid-upper arm circumference < 115 mm or
- oedema of both feet (kwashiorkor with or without severe wasting).

Children with severe acute malnutrition should first be assessed with a full clinical examination to confirm whether they have any general danger sign, medical complications and an appetite.

Children with severe acute malnutrition with loss of appetite or any medical complication have ***complicated severe acute malnutrition*** and should be admitted for inpatient care. Children who have a good appetite and no medical complications can be managed as outpatients.

### Initial Assessment

Assess for general danger signs or emergency signs and take a history concerning:

- Recent intake of food and fluids
- Usual diet before the current illness
- Breastfeeding
- Duration and frequency of diarrhea and vomiting
- Type of diarrhea (watery/bloody)
- Loss of appetite
- Family circumstances
- Cough > 2 weeks
- Contact with tb
- Recent contact with measles
- Known or suspected HIV infection/exposure.

*On examination, Look for:*

- ***Shock:*** lethargic or unconscious; with cold hands, slow capillary refi ll (> 3 s), or weak (low volume), rapid pulse and low blood pressure
- Signs of dehydration
- Severe palmar pallor
- Bilateral pitting edema
- Eye signs of vitamin a deficiency:
  - Dry conjunctiva or cornea, bitot spots
  - Corneal ulceration
  - Keratomalacia

Children with vitamin A deficiency are likely to be photophobic and will keep their eyes closed. It is important to examine the eyes very gently to prevent corneal rupture.

- Localizing signs of infection, including ear and throat infections, skin infection or pneumonia
- Signs of hiv infection
- Fever (temperature ≥ 37.5°C or ≥ 99.5°F) or hypothermia (rectal temperature < 35.5°C or < 95.9°F)
- Mouth ulcers
- Skin changes of kwashiorkor:
  - Hypo- or hyperpigmentation
  - Desquamation
  - Ulceration (spreading over limbs, thighs, genitalia, groin and behind the ears)
  - Exudative lesions (resembling severe burns) often with secondary infection (including *Candida*).
- Conduct an appetite test:
  - Check if the child has appetite by providing ready-to-use therapeutic food.

Laboratory investigations should be conducted for HB or EVF, especially if there is severe palmar pallor.

### General Management

#### *Plan for Inpatient Care*

When there is corneal ulceration, give vitamin A, instil chloramphenicol or tetracycline and atropine drops into the eye, cover with a saline-soaked eye pad, and bandage. Severe anemia, if present, will require urgent treatment.

General treatment involves 10 steps in two phases: initial stabilization and rehabilitation

1. Hypoglycemia
2. Hypothermia
3. Dehydration
4. Electrolytes
5. Infection
6. Micronutrients
7. Initiate feeding
8. Catch-up feeding
9. Sensory stimulation
10. Prepare for follow-up

### Hypoglycemia

All severely malnourished children are at risk of hypoglycemia and, immediately on admission, should be given a feed or 10% glucose or sucrose (see below). Frequent 2 h feeding is important.

### Diagnosis

If there is any suspicion of hypoglycemia and when blood glucose can be measured quickly (e.g. with Dextrostix®), this should be done immediately.

Hypoglycemia is present when the blood glucose is < 3 mmol/liter (< 54 mg/dl). If blood glucose cannot be measured, it should be assumed that all children with severe acute malnutrition are hypoglycemic and given treatment.

### Treatment

- Give 50 mL of 10% glucose or sucrose solution (one rounded teaspoon of sugar in three tablespoons of water) orally or by nasogastric tube, followed by the first fed as soon as possible
- Give the first fed of F-75 therapeutic milk, if it is quickly available, and then continue with feds every 2 h for 24 h; then continue feds every 2 or 3 h, day and night.
- If the child is unconscious, treat with IV 10% glucose at 5 mL/kg or, if IV access cannot be quickly established, then give 10% glucose or sucrose solution by nasogastric tube. If IV glucose is not available, give one teaspoon of sugar moistened with one or two drops of water sublingually, and repeat every 20 min to prevent relapse. Children should be monitored for early swallowing, which leads to delayed absorption; in this case another dose of sugar should be given. Continue with 2 h oral or nasogastric feds to prevent recurrence.
- Start on appropriate IV or IM antibiotics.

### Monitoring

If the initial blood glucose was low, repeat the measurement (using finger or heel prick blood and measure with the dextrostix, when available) after 30 min.

- If blood glucose falls to < 3 mmol/liter (< 54 mg/dl), repeat the 10% glucose or oral sugar solution.
- If the rectal temperature falls to < 35.5°C, or if the level of consciousness deteriorates, repeat the Dextrostix measurement and treat accordingly.

### Prevention

- Fed every 2 h, starting immediately or, when dehydrated, rehydrate first. Continue feeding throughout the night.

- Encourage mothers to watch for any deterioration, help fed and keep the child warm.
- Check on abdominal distension.

## Hypothermia

Hypothermia is very common in malnourished children and often indicates coexisting hypoglycemia or serious infection.

### Diagnosis

If the axillary temperature is < 35°C (< 95°F) or does not register on a normal thermometer, assume hypothermia. When a low-reading thermometer is available, take the rectal temperature (< 35.5°C or < 95.9°F) to confirm hypothermia.

### Treatment

All children with hypothermia should be treated routinely for hypoglycemia and infection.

- Feed the child immediately and then every 2 h unless they have abdominal distension; if dehydrated, rehydrate first.
- *Re-warm the child:* Make sure the child is clothed (especially the head); cover with a warmed blanket and place a heater (not pointing directly at the child) or lamp nearby, or put the child on the mother's bare chest or abdomen (skin-to-skin) and cover them with a warmed blanket and/or warm clothing.
- Keep the child away from draughts.
- Give appropriate IV or IM antibiotics.

### Monitoring

- Take the child's rectal temperature every 2 h until it rises to > 36.5°C. Take it every 30 min if a heater is being used.
- Ensure that the child is covered at all times, especially at night. Keep the head covered, preferably with a warm bonnet, to reduce heat loss.
- Check for hypoglycemia whenever hypothermia is found.

### Prevention

- Fed immediately and then every 2–3 h, day and night.
- Place the bed in a warm, draught-free part of the ward, and keep the child covered.
- Use the Kangaroo technique for infants, cover with a blanket and let the mother sleep with child to keep the child warm.
- Avoid exposing the child to cold (e.g. after bathing or during medical examinations).
- Change wet nappies, clothes and bedding to keep the child and the bed dry.
  Dry carefully after bathing, but do not bathe if very ill.
- Use a heater or incandescent lamp with caution.
- Do not use a hot water bottle or fluorescent lamp.

## Dehydration

### *Diagnosis*

Dehydration tends to be overdiagnosed and its severity overestimated in children with severe acute malnutrition because it is difficult to determine dehydration accurately from clinical signs alone. Assume that all children with watery diarrhea or reduced urine output have some dehydration. It is important to note that poor circulatory volume or perfusion can co-exist with edema.

### *Treatment*

Do not use the IV route for rehydration, except in cases of shock.

Rehydrate slowly, either orally or by nasogastric tube, using oral rehydration solution for malnourished children (5–10mL/kg per h up to a maximum of 12 hours). The standard WHO ORS solution for general use has a high sodium and low potassium content, which is not suitable for severely malnourished children. Instead, give special rehydration solution for malnutrition, ReSoMal.

- Give the ***ReSoMal rehydration fluid orally*** or by nasogastric tube, more slowly than you would rehydrating a well-nourished child.
  - Give 5 mL/kg every 30 min for the first 2 h.
  - Then give 5–10 mL/kg per h for the next 4–10 h on alternate hours, with F-75 formula. The exact amount depends on how much the child wants, the volume of stool loss and whether the child is vomiting.
- If not available then give ***half strength*** standard WHO oral rehydration solution with added potassium and glucose as per the ReSoMal recipe below, unless the child has cholera or profuse watery diarrhea.
- If rehydration is still required at 10 h, give starter F-75 instead of ReSoMal, at the same times. Use the same volume of starter F-75 as of ReSoMal.
- If in shock or severe dehydration but cannot be rehydrated orally or by nasogastric tube, give IV fluids, either Ringer's lactate solution with 5% dextrose or half-strength Darrow's solution with 5% dextrose. If neither is available, 0.45% saline with 5% dextrose should be used.

**Recipe for ReSoMal using standard WHO ORS**

| Ingredient | Amount |
|---|---|
| Water | 2 liters |
| WHO ORS | One 1-liter packet |
| Sucrose | 50 g |
| Electrolyte/mineral solution | 40 mL |

a. 2.6 g sodium chloride, 2.9 g trisodium citrate dihydrate, 1.5 g potassium chloride, 13.5 g glucose
b. If you use a commercially prepared electrolyte and mineral powder, follow the manufacturer's instructions. If these cannot be made up, use 45 mL of potassium chloride solution (100 g potassium chloride in 1 liter of water) instead.

ReSoMal contains approximately 45 mmol sodium, 40 mmol potassium and 3 mmol magnesium per liter.

### Monitoring

During rehydration, respiration and pulse rate should fall and urine start to be passed. The return of tears, a moist mouth, less sunken eyes and fontanelle, and improved skin turgor are also signs that rehydration is proceeding, but many severely malnourished children will not show these changes even when fully rehydrated. Monitor weight gain.

Monitor the progress of rehydration every 30 min for 2 h, then every hour for the next 4–10 h. Be alert for signs of overhydration, which is very dangerous and may lead to heart failure. Check for:
- weight gain to ensure that it is not quick and excessive.
- increase in respiratory rate
- increase in pulse rate
- urine frequency (Has the child urinated since last checked?)
- enlarging liver size on palpation
- frequency of stools and vomit.

If you find signs of overhydration (early signs are respiratory rate increasing by 5/min and pulse rate by 25/min), stop ReSoMal immediately and reassess after 1 h.

## Prevention

Measures to prevent dehydration due to continuing watery diarrhea are similar to those for well-nourished children, except that ReSoMal fluid is used instead of standard ORS.
- If the child is breastfed, continue breastfeeding.
- Initiate re-feeding with starter F-75.
- Give ReSoMal between feeds to replace stool losses. As a guide, give 50–100 mL after each watery stool.

## Electrolyte Imbalance

All severely malnourished children have deficiencies of potassium and magnesium, which may take about 2 weeks to correct. Edema is partly a result of potassium deficiency and sodium retention. Do not treat edema with a diuretic. Excess body sodium exists even though the plasma sodium may be low. Giving high sodium loads could kill the child.

## Treatment

- Give extra potassium (3–4 mmol/kg per day).
- Give extra magnesium (0.4–0.6 mmol/kg per day).

The extra potassium and magnesium should be added to the fed during its preparation if not pre-mixed. Add 20 mL of this solution to 1 liter of feed to supply the extra potassium and magnesium required. Alternatively, use commercially available pre-mixed sachets (specially formulated for malnourished children).
- When rehydrating, give low sodium rehydration fluid (ReSoMal).
- Prepare food without added salt.

## Infection

In severe acute malnutrition, the usual signs of bacterial infection, such as fever, are often absent, yet multiple infections are common. Therefore, assume that all children with severe acute malnutrition have an infection on their arrival in hospital, and treat with antibiotics immediately. Hypoglycemia and hypothermia are often signs of severe infection.

## Treatment

Give all severely malnourished children:
- a broad-spectrum antibiotic
- measles vaccine if the child is ≥ 6 months and not vaccinated or was vaccinated before 9 months age. Delay vaccination if the child is in shock.

### *Choice of Broad-spectrum Antibiotics*

- If the child has uncomplicated severe acute malnutrition, give oral amoxicillin for 5 days.
- If there are complications (hypoglycemia, hypothermia or the child looks lethargic or sickly) or any other medical complication, give parenteral antibiotics:
  - benzylpenicillin (50000 U/kg IM or IV every 6 h) or ampicillin (50 mg/kg IM or IV every 6 h) for 2 days, then oral amoxicillin (25–40 mg/kg every 8 h for 5 days) plus
  - gentamicin (7.5 mg/kg IM or IV) once a day for 7 days.

These regimens should be adapted to local resistance patterns.

***Note:*** *Metronidazole 7.5 mg/kg every 8 h for 7 days may be given in addition to broad-spectrum antibiotics; however, the efficacy of this treatment has not been established in clinical trials.*
- Treat other infections as appropriate:
  - If meningitis is suspected, do a lumbar puncture for confirmation, where possible, and treat with the antibiotic regime.
  - If you identify other specific infections (such as pneumonia, dysentery, skin or soft-tissue infections), give antibiotics as appropriate.
  - Add antimalarial treatment if the child has a positive blood film for malaria parasites or a positive malaria rapid diagnostic test.
  - TB is common, but anti-TB treatment should be given only if TB is diagnosed or strongly suspected.

### *Treatment for Parasitic Worms*

If there is evidence of worm infestation, treatment should be delayed until the rehabilitation phase. Give albendazole as a single dose or mebendazole 100 mg orally twice a day for 3 days. In countries where infestation is prevalent, also give mebendazole to children with no evidence of infestation 7 days after admission.

### *HIV Infection*

Where HIV infection is common, children with severe acute malnutrition should be tested for HIV to determine their need for antiretroviral therapy (ART). If the child is infected with HIV, start ART as soon as possible after stabilization of metabolic complications and sepsis. They should be monitored closely (inpatient and outpatient) in the first 6–8 weeks following initiation of ART to identify early metabolic complications and opportunistic infections.

## Monitoring

If the child is still anorexic after 7 days of antibiotic treatment, continue for a full 10-day course. If anorexia persists, reassess the child fully.

## Micronutrient Deficiencies

All severely malnourished children have vitamin and mineral deficiencies.

Although anemia is common, do not give iron initially, but wait until the child has a good appetite and starts gaining weight (usually in the second week), because iron can make infections worse.

Multvitamins including vitamin A and folic acid, zinc and copper are already present in F-75, F-100 and ready-to-use therapeutic food packets. When premixed packets are used, there is no need for additional doses.

In addition, if there are no eye signs or history of measles, then do not give a high dose of vitamin A because the amounts already present in therapeutic foods are enough.

## Treatment

- Give vitamin A on day 1 and repeat on days 2 and 14 only if child has any signs of vitamin A deficiency like corneal ulceration or a history of measles – < 6 months, 50 000 U – 6–12 months, 100 000 U – > 12 months, 200 000 U
- Start iron at 3 mg/kg per day after 2 days on F-100 catch-up formula. Do not give iron in the stabilization phase, and do not give iron if the child is receiving ***ready-to-use therapeutic food (RUTF)***.

  If child is **not** on any of the pre-mixed therapeutic foods, give the following micronutrients daily for at least 2 weeks:
- folic acid at 5 mg on day 1; then 1 mg daily
- multivitamin syrup at 5 mL
- zinc at 2 mg/kg per day
- copper at 0.3 mg/kg per day.

## Initial Re-feeding

In the initial phase, re-feeding should be gradual.

## Treatment

The essential features of initial feeding are:

- frequent (every 2–3 h) oral small feeds of low osmolality and low lactose
- nasogastric feeding if the child is eating ≤ 80% of the amount offered at two consecutive feeds
- calories at 100 kcal/kg per day
- protein at 1–1.5 g/kg per day
- liquid at 130 mL/kg per day or 100 mL/kg per day if the child has severe oedema
- in addition, if the child is breastfed, encourage continued breastfeeding, but make sure the prescribed amounts of starter formula are given:

| Days | Frequency | Volume/kg fed | Volume/kg per day |
|---|---|---|---|
| 1–2 | 2 h | 11 mL | 130 mL |
| 3–5 | 3 h | 16 mL | 130 mL |
| > 6 | 4 h | 22 mL | 130 mL |

## Monitoring

Monitor and record:

- amounts of fed offered and left over
- vomiting
- stool frequency and consistency
- daily body weight.

## Catch-up Growth Feeding

Children in the catch-up phase should in most cases be managed as outpatients.

Signs that a child has reached rehabilitation phase for catch-up growth are:

- Return of appetite
- No episodes of hypoglycemia (metabolically stable)
- Reduced or disappearance of all edema.

## Monitoring

***Avoid causing heart failure***. Monitor for early signs of congestive heart failure (rapid pulse, fast breathing, basal lung crepitations, enlarging liver, gallop heart rhythm, raised jugular venous pressure). If both pulse and breathing rates increase (breathing by 5 breaths/min and pulse by 25 beats/min), and the increase is sustained for two successive 4-hourly readings, then:

- Reduce the volume fed to 100 mL/kg per day for 24 h.
- Then, gradually increase as follows:
  - 115 mL/kg per day for next 24 h
  - 130 mL/kg per day for the following 48 h
- Thereafter, increase each feed by 10 mL as described earlier.

***Assess progress***. After the transition, monitor progress by the rate of weight gain:

- Weigh the child every morning before feeding, and plot the weight.
- Calculate and record the weight gain every 3 days as g/kg per day If the weight gain is:
  - Poor (< 5 g/kg per day), the child requires a full re-assessment
  - Moderate (5–10 g/kg per day), check whether the intake targets are being met or if infection has been overlooked
- Good (> 10 g/kg per day).

## Sensory Stimulation

Provide:

- Tender loving care
- A cheerful, stimulating environment
- Structured play therapy for 15–30 min/day
- Physical activity as soon as the child is well enough
- Support for as much maternal involvement as possible (e.g. comforting, feeding, bathing, playing).

  Provide suitable toys and play activities for the child.

## Discharge from Nutritional Treatment

Children with severe acute malnutrition should be discharged from the nutritional treatment program only when their:

- Weight-for-height/length is at least ≥ -2 z score and they have had no edema for at least 2 weeks, or
- Mid-upper-arm circumference is ≥ 125 mm and they have had no edema for at least 2 weeks.

The decision should be based on the same anthropometric indicator that was used on admission. Thus, if mid-upper arm circumference was used, then it should be used to assess and confirm nutritional recovery, and similarly for weight for length/height. Children admitted with only bilateral pitting edema, should be discharged on the basis of either mid-upper arm circumference or weight for height/length depending on the indicator used routinely in the national nutrition program. Percentage weight gain should not be used as a discharge criterion.

The child should be fed at least five times a day with foods that contain approximately 100 kcal and 2–3 g protein per 100 g of food. It is essential to give frequent meals with a high energy and protein content. The mother should be counseled on appropriate feeding to:

- give appropriate meals (and the correct quantity of food) at least five times daily.
- give high-energy snacks between meals (e.g. milk, banana, bread, biscuits).
- assist and encourage the child to complete each meal.
- give food separately to the child so that the child's intake can be checked.
- breastfed as often as the child wants.

### Follow-up

When a child is discharged to outpatient, make a plan for following up of the child until full recovery, and contact the outpatient department, nutrition rehabilitation centre, local health clinic or health worker who will take responsibility for continuing supervision of the child. In general, the child should be weighed weekly after discharge.

If he or she fails to gain weight over a 2-week period or loses weight between two measurements or develops loss of appetite or edema, the child should be referred back to hospital for further assessment. Once discharged from the nutritional treatment, he or she should be periodically monitored to avoid relapse.

## PEDIATRIC GENITOURINARY DISORDERS

### Enuresis

Repeated involuntary voiding or incontinence by a child past the age of toilet training about 5-6 years of age.

Multi-treatment Approach:

- Fluid Restriction
- Bladder exercises
- Timed voiding
- Enuresis alarms
- Reward system
- Medications

### Urinary Tract Infection

- Etiology and Pathophysiology
  - Tend to occur more in girls than in boys because the urethra is shorter in girls and is located close to the vagina and anus.
  - Pathogens enter as an ascending infection
  - Most common causative organism is *Escherichia coli*
- Typical symptoms of older children and adults—dysuria, frequency, urgency, burning,hematuria – may not be present.
- Symptoms not always clear
  - Fever
  - Mild abdominal pain
  - Bedwetting (enuresis)
  - If gets worse–high fever, flank pain, vomiting, malaise
- Urine for culture and sensitivity
  - Clean catch
  - Suprapubic aspiration
  - Catheterization
- A Positive Test
  - Bacteria colony count is more than 100.000/mL.
  - Proteinuria may also be present indicating presence of bacteria.
- Drug Therapy
  - Antibiotics–specific to causative organism
  - Analgesics–Tylenol
- Nursing Care
  - Force fluids – childs choice
  - Dysuria – sit in warm water in bathtub and void into the water
- Parent Teaching
  - Change diaper frequently
  - Teach girls to wipe front to back
  - Discourage bubble baths
  - Encourage children to drink periodically during the day
  - Bathe daily
  - Adolescent start menstruating – encourage change of pad every 4 hours
  - When girls become sexually active – teach to urinate immediately after intercourse
- Follow up
  - Return for repeat urinalysis – usually after 72 hours of treatment to be sure treatment is working
  - Girls who have more than three UTI's, and boys with first UTI should be referred to urologist for further evaluation.

### Vesicoureteral Reflux

Common Sites for Obstruction

- Stenosis of ureteropelvic valve
- Stenosis of ureterovescicular junction
- Stenosis of the posterior urethral valve
- Reflux occurs because the valve that guards the entrance from the bladder to the ureter is defective from:
  - Primary reflux—congenital abnormal insertion of ureters into the bladder
  - Secondary reflux—repeated UTI's cause scarring of valve
  - Bladder pressure that is stronger than usual, neurogenic bladder
- Backflow happens at voiding when bladder contracts, urine is swept up the ureters
- Results in stasis of urine in ureters or kidneys which in turn leads to infection or **hydronephrosis**.

#### *Clinical Manifestations*

- Fever
- Vomiting
- Chills
- Straining or crying on urination, poor urine stream,
- Enuresis (bedwetting), incontinence in a toilet trained child, frequent urination.
- Strong smelling urine
- Abdominal or back/flank pain.

#### *Diagnostic Tests*

- Urine culture—done every 2–3 months
- Cystourethrogram

- Renal ultrasound—a non-invasive test in which a transducer is passed over the kidney producing sound waves which bounce off the kidney, transmitting a picture of the organ on a video screen. The test is used to determine the size and shape of the kidney, and to detect a mass, kidney stone, cyst, or other obstruction or abnormalities.

### *Drug Therapy*

1. Antibiotics
   - Penicillin
   - Cephalosporins
2. Urinary Antiseptics
   - Nitrofurantoin
   - Surgery
3. Repair of significant anatomical anomalies, uretheral implantation

- Keep accurate record of intake and output. Keep records from stents and catheter separate. Decreased output from stent could indicate obstruction.
- Secure stents and catheter to prevent displacement.
- Assess vital signs for signs of infection.
- Assess pain. Handle child gently
- Administer pain medications
- Patient Teaching
  - regarding prevention of UTI,
  - importance of taking all antibiotics, continue taking antiseptics even when have no symptoms.
- Follow-up
  - Go in for a VCUG (voiding cystourethrogram) after a few months

### Structural Defects

- **Cryptorchidism**
- **Hypospadius/Epispadius**

### Cryptorchisism

Failure of one or both of the testes to descend from abdominal cavity to the scrotum

- Testes usually descend into the scrotal sac during the 7–9 month gestation
- They may descend anytime up to 6 weeks after birth. Rarely descend after that time.
- Cause unknown
- Theories
  - Inadequate length of spermatic vessels
  - Lowered testosterone levels
- Why is it important that the testes are in the scrotal sac?
  - The higher temperatures in the abdomen than in the scrotum results in morphologic changes to the testis – mainly concerned with lower sperm counts at sexual maturity.
- Diagnosed on Newborn Physical Exam
  - Palpate the testes separately between thumb and forefinger, with thumb and forefinger of other hand over the inguinal canal.
- Surgery
- Orchiopexy done via laproscopy
- Done around 1 year of age
- Nursing Care—Post-operative
- Minimal activity for few day to ensure that the internal sutures remain intact
- Allow opportunity to express fears about mutilation or castration by playing with puppets or dolls.

### Hypospadias/Epispadias

- **Hypospadias**
  - Congenital urethral defect in which the uretheral opening is on the lower aspect of the penis and not on the tip.
- **Epispadias**
  - Congenital urethral defect in which the uretheral opening is on the upper aspect of the penis and not on the end

### Etiology and Pathophysiology

- **Etiology**–rare and often associated with extrophy of bladder.
- **Pathophysiology**
  - Occurs from incomplete development of urethra in utero.
  - Occurs in 1 of 100 male children. Increased risk if father or siblings have defect.
  - Defect ranges from mild (meatus is just below tip); to meatus on the perineum between scrotum, ventral foreskin lacking
  - May have accompanying chordee (a fibrous band that causes the penis to curve downward),
  - Undescended testes – found in conjunction with hypospadias
  - Might interfere with fertility in the mature male if not corrected.

### Assessment

Usually discovered during Newborn Physical Assessment

- Why would the nurse question an order to prepare the infant for a circumcision?

The nurse would question the order for a circumcision because the foreskin is used in reconstruction and repair of the defect.

What is the relation of epispadius or hypospadius to *infertility?*

- If the urethral opening is not at the end of the penis, then the male will not be able to deposit his sperm at the opening of the os of the cervix.
- Medical Treatment:
  - Surgery
    - ➢ Reconstructive–repositions uretheral opening at tip of penis
    - ➢ Stent placed in urethra to maintain patency
    - ➢ Chordee–released and urethra lengthened.
- The reason for surgery at about 1 year of age is because:
  - children will experience less pain
  - chordee may be reabsorbed
  - the child has not developed body image and castration anxiety
  - the repair is easier before toilet training
- Post-operative Nursing Care
  - Assess bleeding—Bleeding is controlled post-operatively by the use of pressure dressings. However, a small

amount of bleeding for the first several days post-operatively is normal. A few drops of blood or a spot no larger than a quarter on the diaper is acceptable.
- Maintain urinary drainage—care for catheter–foley/ suprapubic, or urethral stent. Use double diapering.
- Control Bladder Spasms—usually due to the presence of the in-dwelling catheters are common post-operatively and are controlled by medications that relax the bladder (ie. Antispasmotics- Pro-Banthine and Ditropan)
- Control Pain – may be given Tylenol
- Increase fluids intake–assists in maintaining hydration and free flow of urine.
- Do not allow to play on any straddle toys.
- Prevent infection – no bathing or swimming until
- stents removed.
- Call Dr if:
  - ➢ Temp is over 101
  - ➢ Loss of appetite
  - ➢ Pus or increased bleeding from stent
  - ➢ Cloudy or foul smelling urine.

## Acute Postinfectious Glomerulonephritis

Immune-complex disease which causes inflammation of the glomeruli of the kidney as a result of an infection elsewhere in the body.

## Etiology and Pathophysiology

- Usual organism is Group A beta-hemolytic streptococcus
- Organism not found in kidney, but the antigen-antibody complexes become trapped in the membrane of the glomeruli causing inflammation, obstruction and edema in kidney
- The glomeruli become inflamed and scarred, and slowly lose their ability to remove wastes and excess water from the blood to make urine.
- Decreased glomerular filtration leads to accumulation of sodium and water in bloodstream causing increased intravascular and interstitial fluid volume, or edema
- Protein molecules filter through the damaged glomeruli – proteinuria
- Damage to glomeruli leads to hematuria.
- High B/P, Heart failure may result
- Common in boy 5–10 years old. Occurs 1–2 weeks after a Strep respiratory infection or after impetigo.
- Has 2 phases
- Edematous phase—4-10 days
- Diuresis phase.

## Assessment

- Renal:
  - Moderate Proteinuria
  - Sudden onset of hematuria (tea-colored, reddish-brown, or smoky) and next develops oliguria
  - Excessive foaming of urine
- Cardiovascular:
  - Edema-usually eyes, hands, feet, not generalized
  - Hypertension from hypervolemia which can lead to
  - Cardiac involvement CHF- orthopnea/ dyspnea, cardiac enlargement, pulmonary edema
- Neuro:
  - Encephalopathy (headache, irritability, convulsions, coma-from cerebral edema)

## Diagnostic Tests

Urinalysis- protein (moderate), RBC's, WBC's, Specific Gravity elevated.

All children should have a urinalysis 2 weeks after strep infection.

*Blood*

- ASO titer (anti-streptolysin O) (antibody formation against Streptococcus) is elevated, indicating a recent hemolytic streptococcal infection Normal titer is 170-330 Todd units; IgG antibodies against Streptococcus may be found
- ESR (erythrocyte sedimentation rate) elevated showing inflammatory process
- BUN (urea nitrogen) and creatinine elevated indicating glomeruli damage

Therapeutic Interventions

- Depends on the severity of the disease. No specific treatment. Bedrest encouraged. Disease is self-limiting.
- Treat at home if normal BP and adequate output.
- Must be hospitalized if:
  - BP increases
  - Gross hematuria
  - Oliguria present.
- This way the child can be monitored closely and prevent complications. Rarely develops into acute renal failure

*Main Goals*

Relieve Hypertension

Reestablish fluid and electrolyte balance by:

- Keep accurate record of I and O. Be sure that child does not exceed maximum intake ordered.
- Record characteristics of urine output including presence of proteinuria and hematuria.
- Check and record specific gravity with each voiding
- Monitor vital signs and neuro vital signs
- Monitor and record amount of edema at least once a shift.
- Daily weights
- Bedrest for 4–10 days during acute phase. Semi-Fowler's position to assist with breathing. Quiet play.
- Oxygen therpay
- Diet therapy
- Limit salt intake with hypertension or edema
- Limit protein if BUN elevated
- Decrease intake of potassium if output decreased
- Drug therapy
- Antibiotics
- Digitalization
- Antihypertensives- vasodilators

*Nephrotic Syndrome*

Chronic renal disorder in which the basement membrane surfaces of the glomeruli are affected, causing loss of protein in the urine.

The glomeruli membrane has increased permeability permitting albumin and protein to pass through the membrane and excreted in the urine.

*Clinical Manifestations*

Four most common characteristics:

- *Edema*—May have periorbital edema upon rising in morning and shifts during the day.
- Massive *proteinuria* and *hypoproteinemia*
- *Hypoalbuminemia*
- *Hyperlipidemia*

*Other Signs and Symptoms*

- Fatigue
- Anorexia
- Weight gain
- Abdominal pain – from large amount of fluid in abdominal

*Diagnostic Tests*

- Urinalysis–protein-to-creatitine (PR/CR) ratio of first morning void to assess for proteinuria. Urine appears dark and frothy.
- Blood tests–hypoalbuminemia, elevated cholesterol and triglycerides, elevated hgb, hct, platelets

*Complications*

- Children with Nephrotic Syndrome are prone to infection related to:
- Loss of immunoglobins in the urine
- Corticosteroid Therapy

*Therapeutic Interventions*

- Administer medications–assess for side effects
  - Prednisone, Albumin, Diuretics
- Prevention of infection – avoid people with infections.
  - May be placed on protective isolation.
- Keep accurate record of I and O. Measure abdominal girth, weigh daily.
- Test urine for protein and specific gravity to see if treatment is effective
- Diet:
  - Normal diet for child's age
  - A 'no added salt' diet is recommended during steroid treatment.
- Promote rest
- Discharge teaching

## CONGENITAL ANOMALIES

### Key Facts

- An estimated 303000 newborns die within 4 weeks of birth every year, worldwide, due to congenital anomalies.
- Congenital anomalies can contribute to long-term disability, which may have significant impacts on individuals, families, health-care systems, and societies.
- The most common, severe congenital anomalies are heart defects, neural tube defects and Down syndrome.
- Although congenital anomalies may be the result of one or more genetic, infectious, nutritional or environmental factors, it is often difficult to identify the exact causes.
- Some congenital anomalies can be prevented. Vaccination, adequate intake of folic acid or iodine through fortification of staple foods or supplementation, and adequate antenatal care are just 3 examples of prevention methods.

Congenital anomalies are important causes of infant and childhood deaths, chronic illness and disability.

### Definition

Congenital anomalies are also known as birth defects, congenital disorders or congenital malformations. Congenital anomalies can be defined as structural or functional anomalies (for example, metabolic disorders) that occur during intrauterine life and can be identified prenatally, at birth, or sometimes may only be detected later in infancy, such as hearing defects.

In simple terms, congenital refers to the existence at or before birth.

### Causes and Risk Factors

Although approximately 50% of all congenital anomalies cannot be linked to a specific cause, there are some known genetic, environmental and other causes or risk factors.

#### *Genetic Factors*

Genes play an important role in many congenital anomalies. This might be through inherited genes that code for an anomaly, or resulting from sudden changes in genes known as mutations.

Consanguinity (when parents are related by blood) also increases the prevalence of rare genetic congenital anomalies and nearly doubles the risk for neonatal and childhood death, intellectual disability and other anomalies.

Some ethnic communities (such as Ashkenazi Jews or Finns) have a comparatively high prevalence of rare genetic mutations such as Cystic Fibrosis and Hemophilia C.

#### *Socioeconomic and Demographic Factors*

Low-income may be an indirect determinant of congenital anomalies, with a higher frequency among resource-constrained families and countries. It is estimated that about 94% of severe congenital anomalies occur in low- and middle-income countries. An indirect determinant, this higher risk relates to a possible lack of access to sufficient, nutritious foods by pregnant women, an increased exposure to agents or factors such as infection and alcohol, or poorer access to health care and screening. Factors often associated with lower-income may induce or increase the incidence of abnormal prenatal development.

Maternal age is also a risk factor for abnormal intrauterine fetal development. Advanced maternal age increases the risk of chromosomal abnormalities, including Down syndrome.

#### *Environmental Factors*

Maternal exposure to certain pesticides and other chemicals, as well as certain medications, alcohol, tobacco and radiation during pregnancy, may increase the risk of having a fetus or neonate affected by congenital anomalies. Working or living near, or in, waste sites, smelters or mines may also be a risk factor, particularly if the mother is exposed to other environmental risk factors or nutritional deficiencies.

### *Infections*

Maternal infections such as syphilis and rubella are a significant cause of congenital anomalies in low- and middle-income countries.

More recently, the effect of in utero exposure to Zika virus on the developing fetus has been reported. In 2015, Brazil detected cases of Zika virus and a spatio-temporally associated increase in microcephaly. By 2016, Brazil reported that of 4180 suspected cases of microcephaly, 270 were confirmed, 462 were discarded and 3448 are still under investigation. This is compared to an average of 163 microcephaly cases recorded nationwide per year. With 6 of the 270 confirmed cases of microcephaly showing evidence of Zika infection, health authorities and agencies are investigating and conducting comprehensive research to confirm a causal link. Following the Zika outbreak in French Polynesia, health authorities reported an unusual increase in the number of congenital malformations in babies born between March 2014 and May 2015.

### Maternal Nutritional Status

Maternal folate insufficiency increases the risk of having a baby with a neural tube defect while excessive vitamin A intake may affect the normal development of an embryo or fetus.

### Prevention

Preventive public health measures work to decrease the frequency of certain congenital anomalies through the removal of risk factors or the reinforcement of protective factors. Important interventions and efforts include:

- Ensuring adolescent girls and mothers have a healthy diet including a wide variety of vegetables and fruit, and maintain a healthy weight;
- Ensuring an adequate dietary intake of vitamins and minerals, and particularly folic acid in adolescent girls and mothers;
- Ensuring mothers avoid harmful substances, particularly alcohol and tobacco;
- Avoidance of travel by pregnant women (and sometimes women of child-bearing age) to regions experiencing outbreaks of infections known to be associated with congenital anomalies;
- Reducing or eliminating environmental exposure to hazardous substances (such as heavy metals or pesticides) during pregnancy;
- Controlling diabetes prior to and during pregnancy through counseling, weight management, diet and administration of insulin when required;
- Ensuring that any exposure of pregnant women to medications or medical radiation (such as imaging rays) is justified and based on careful health risk–benefit analysis;
- Vaccination, especially against the rubella virus, for children and women;
- Increasing and strengthening education of health staff and others involved in promoting prevention of congenital anomalies;
- Screening for infections, especially rubella, varicella, and syphilis, and consideration of treatment.

### List of Congenital Anomalies Head to Toe

- Nervous system
  - Anencephalus
  - Spina bifida
  - Hydrocephalus
  - Microcephalus
- Eye
  - Anophthalmos
  - Cystic eyeball
  - Cryptophthalmos
  - Microphthalmos
  - Buphthalmos
  - Congenital cataract
  - Coloboma
  - Aniridia
- Ear
  - Accessory auricle
  - Macrotia
  - Microtia
  - Preauricular sinus
- Face
  - Macrocheilia
  - Microcheilia
  - Macrostomia
  - Microstomia
- Neck
  - Webbing of neck
- Circulation and Heart:
  - Common truncus
  - Transposition of great vessels
  - Tetralogy of fallot
  - Common ventricle
  - Ventricular septal defect
  - Atrial septal defect
  - Tricuspid atresia and stenosis congenital
  - Ebstein's anomaly
  - Congenital stenosis of aortic valve
  - Congenital insufficiency of aortic valve
  - Congenital mitral stenosis
  - Congenital mitral insufficiency
  - Hypoplastic left heart syndrome
  - Congenital heart block
  - Malposition of heart and cardiac apex [dextrocardia]
  - Brugada syndrome
  - Coarctation of aorta
- Respiratory System
  - ARDS
  - Choanal atresia
  - Tracheoesophageal fistulas
  - Ectopic lung lobes
  - Congenital cysts of the lung

- Digestive System
  - Cleft palate
  - Cleft lip
  - Tongue tie
  - Microglossia
  - Macroglossia
  - Esophageal fistula
  - Congenital hypertrophic pyloric stenosis
  - Congenital hiatus hernia
  - Meckel's diverticulum
  - Congenital atresia and stenosis of small intestine
  - Imperforate anus
  - Hirschsprung's disease
- Urinary System
  - Renal dysplasias
  - Renal agenesis
  - Polycystic kidney
  - Hoarseshoe kidney
  - Floating kidney
  - Duplication of the ureter
  - Pelvic kidney
  - Accessory renal arteries
  - Urachal fistula
  - Urachal cyst
  - Urachal sinus
  - Exstrophy of the bladder
- Genital System
  - Duplications of the uterus
  - Uterus bicornis
  - Uterus arcuatus
  - Hypospadias
  - Epispadias
  - Micropenis
  - Bifid penis or double penis
  - Gonadal dysgenesis
  - Congenital inguinal hernia and hydroceles
  - Cryptorchidism
- Limbs
  - Meromelia
  - Amelia
  - Phocomelia
  - Micromelia
  - Brachydactyly
  - Syndactyly
  - Polydactyly
  - Ectrodactyly
  - Cleft hand and foot (lobster claw deformity)
  - Osteogenesis imperfect
  - Clubfoot
  - Craniosynostosis-radial aplasia syndrome

## Approach to Patients with Congenital Heart Disease

### *Congenital Heart Disease*

- Congenital cardiac malformations resulting from defective embryonic development without obvious cause.
- Between 3-8 weeks 'gestation' all the fetal heart structures are formed 'organogenesis'

### Incidence

- Incidence is more in:
  - Premature
  - Abortions
  - Still births
- Incidence increased for siblings.
  - 2–6%, 10–12%, 25%

### Etiology

Multifactorial inheritance pattern 'mostly'

- Chromosomal abnormality (5-10%).
  - Trisomy 21 (50%) > A-V canal, VSD, ASD, others.
  - Trisomy 18 (80%)> VSD, ASD, others.
  - Trisomy 13 (40%)> VSD, ASD, PDA, others.
  - Turner syndrome (xo)> Bicuspid aortic valve and co-ao
  - others.

*Adverse Maternal Conditions (Enviromential)*

- Maternal infections > Rubella: PDA, PS
- Maternal diseases > PKU-VSD, ASD
- DM: Left septal hypertrophy
- Drugs > fetal hydntoin syndrome- VSD
- Valproate effect-co ao left heart hypoplasia
- Fetal alcohol syndrome > VSD, ASD, CO-AO.
- Advance maternal age.

*Syndrome Complexes*

- VACTREL syndrome
  Vertebral, Anorectal, Cardiac (VSD, TOF and others), tracheal, Renal, Esophageal and Limb abnormalities.
- CHARGE syndrome
  'Coloboma, Heart (VSD, TOF, A-V canal), Atresia choanal, Retardation, Gential, Ear abnormalties.
- Kartagener syndrome Dextrocardia
- TAR syndrome
  Majority of cases of the congenital heart diseases are unknown cause

### Classification

- CHD with little or no cyanosis 'acyanotic'
  a-With Lt. ventricular enlargement
  ex. PDA=8% ,CO-Ao= 5%
  - aortic stenosis =7%
  b-With Rt. Ventricular enlargement
  ex. ASD=10% ,PS=6%,MS
  c-With both ventricular enlargement
  ex. VSD= 25%

*Common Acyanotic Lesions*

- Ventricular septal defects
- Atrial septal defects
- Atrio-ventricular septal defects
- Patent ductus arteriosus
- Truncus arteriosus
- Aortic stenosis
- Mitral stenosis/incompetence
- Coarctation of aorta
- Tricuspid regurgitation

- CHD with cyanosis 'mainly Rt. Lt. shunt'
  A -With decrease pulmonary vascularity
  ex.-TOF=5% , Tricuspid Artesia=1-3%
  - PS with or without VSD=5%
  B -With increase pulmonary vascularity
  ex.-TGA =5% ,Truncus arteriosus=2%
  -TAPVR=1%

*Common Cyanotic Lesions*

Decreased flow

- Tetralogy of Fallot
- Tricuspid Atresia
- Severe Pulmonic Stenosis
- Ebstein's anamoly

Increased flow

- Transposition of great vessles
- VSD with pulmonary atresia
- Truncus Arteriosus
- Hypoplastic left heart
- Single ventricle
- TAPVR with infradiaphragmatic obstruction
  - Cyanotic: 22%
  - Acyanotic: 68%
    - ➢ VSD 25%
    - ➢ ASD 6%
    - ➢ PDA 6%
    - ➢ TOF 5%
    - ➢ PS 5%
    - ➢ AS 5%

## Diagnosis

- Early diagnosis of CHD mean better results.
- 40% of CHD are diagnosed at 1st week of life.
- 50–60% diagnosed at 1st two months .
- Others are usually later during routine medical examination.
- Diagnosis depend on good clinical history + good medical examination and investigations.

## Physical Examination

Inspection look for:

- Cyanosis
- Digital clubbing
- Tachypnea
- Prominence of the precordium (cardiomegaly, Rt. heart enlargement)
- Jugular veins engorgement 'older children'
- Any associated defects or findings (down syndrome, Digorge syndrome…etc.)
- Focal neurological lesion.

## Palpation

- Pulses (rate, rythem, volume, peripheral pulses, brachio-femoral delay)
- Cardiac impulses
- Thrill
- Hyper dynamic precordium.
- Hepato-splenomegaly
- Sacral edema(neonate, and infancy), Lower limb edema in older children

## Auscultation

a. First heart sound (A-V valves closure)
   'Best heard at the Lt. lower sternal border or apex'
b. Second heart sound (semilunar valve closure)
   'Best heard on the 1st and 2nd ICS, normally there is normal splitting of the 2nd heart sound,
   - Single ⟶ Aortic atresia, Pulmonary Artesia
   - Fixed splitting ⟶ ASD, PS, Rt. BBB
c. Murmurs ⟶ Systolic

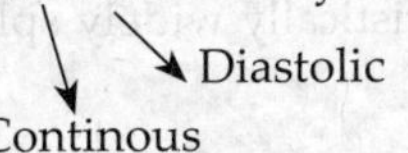


## Blood Pressure

- Methods sphingnonaometer (different cuffs)
  - Flush method
  - Palpation method
  - Doppler method
- Wide pulse pressure
  - Aortic insufficiency
  - A-V communication
  - PDA
- Low blood pressure (HF, pericardial tamponade, cardiomyopathy).
- Difference in BP between upper and lower extremities Co-ao.

**If we suspect CHD**

**Investigation**

- CBC—polycythemia, anemia….etc.
- CXR—heart size and shape
- ECG—HR, axis rythm LVH, RVH, BVH, BBB.
- Echocardiography
- MRI
- Cardiac catheterization

Cyanosis: is it a cardiac cause or lung cause

- Hyperoxia test
  - Neonates with cyanotic congenital heart disease usually do not have significantly raised arterial $PaO_2$ during administration of 100% oxygen.

### *Ventricular Defect*

- Small VSD
  - Asymptomatic
  - A loud, harsh, or blowing holosystolic murmur.
- Large VSD
  - dyspnea, feeding difficulties, poor growth, profuse perspiration, recurrent pulmonary infections, and cardiac failure in early infancy.

### *Ventricular Septal Defects*

- 30–50% of small defects close spontaneously, most frequently during the first two years of life.
- Small muscular VSDs are more likely to close (up to 80%) than membranous VSDs are (up to 35%).
- Infants with large defects have repeated episodes of respiratory infection and heart failure despite optimal medical management.

- Surgical repair prior to development of an irreversible increase in pulmonary vascular resistance (usually prior to the patient's second birthday).

### Atrial Septal Defects: Secundum

- Most common form of ASD (fossa ovalis)
- In large defects, a considerable shunt of oxygenated blood flows from the left to the right atrium.
- Mostly asymptomatic
- The 2nd heart sound is characteristically widely split and fixed.

### Atrial Septal Defects: Primum

- Situated in the lower portion of the atrial septum and overlies the mitral and tricuspid valves. In most instances, a cleft in the anterior leaflet of the mitral valve is also noted.
- Combination of a left-to-right shunt across the atrial defect and mitral insufficiency
- C/F similar to that of an ostium secundum ASD

### Atrial Septal Defect

- ciprofloxacin Enlargement of the right ventricle
- ciprofloxacin Enlargement of atrium
- ciprofloxacin Large pulmonary artery
- ciprofloxacin increased pulmonary vascularity is.
- Atrial Septal Defects
- ciprofloxacin Secundum ASDs are well tolerated during childhood.
- ciprofloxacin Antibiotic prophylaxis for isolated secundum ASDs is not recommended.
- ciprofloxacin Surgery or transcatheter device closure is advised for all symptomatic patients and also for asymptomatic patients with a Qp:Qs ratio of at least 2:1.
- ciprofloxacin Ostium primum defects are approached surgically

### Patent Ductus Arteriosus

- Small defect no symptoms.
- Large defect:
  - Wide pulse pressure
  - Enlarged heart
  - Thrill in L second IS
  - Continuous murmur
  - *X-ray:* prominent pulmonary artery with increased vascular markings.

### Primary Pulmonary Hypertension

- Prominent pulmonary artery.
- Prominent right ventricle
- Prominent vascularity in the hilar areas
- Decreased vascualr marking in the periphery.
- No treatment

### Cardiac Disease with Normal/Decreased Vasculature

- Tetralogy of Fallot
- Pulmonary atresia
- Tricuspid atresia
- Endocardial fibroelastosis
- Aberrant left coronary artery
- Cystic medial necrosis
- IODM 'septal hypertrophy'

### Tetralogy of Fallot

- Ventricular septal defect
- Pulmonic stenosis
- Overriding aorta
- Right ventricular hypertrophy

### Cardiac Disease with Increased Vasculature

- Atrioventricular septal defects
- Congestive cardiac failure
- Transposition of great arteries with VSD
- Total anomalous pulmonary venous drainage
- Truncus arteriosus
- Single ventricle without pulmonary stenosis
- Hypoplastic left heart syndrome

### Treatment of CHD

- This is depend on the type of the C.H.D.
- No treatment (observation + reassurance)
- Medical treatment (antifailure, antiarrythmic.etc.).
- Surgical treatment (palliative or curative).
- Cardiac transplant or lung heart transplant.

### General Measures

- Special positions. (semisiting, knee chest position)
- O2 (most patients need O2 and other need little O2).
- IVF (again depend on type of CHD, some need IVF as PDA and PS, OTHERS need IVF when ever there are pulmonary congestion or volume overload).
- Salt restriction.
- Exercise restriction.
- Rx of anemia.
- Rx of polycythemia. PCV > 65
- Avoidances of dehydration mainly polycythemic patients.
- Avoidances of high altitude.
- Avoidance of contraceptive 'thrombosis + hypertension'.
- Correction of acidosis.
- Correction of electrolyte disturbances.
- Careful monitoring during surgery.

### Rx of Congestive Heart Failure

- Digoxin, Digitalization '0.04 mg/kg'
- Maintenance '0.01mg/kg'
- Loop diuretics 'frusemide 1-2 mg/kg/day'.
- Potassium sparing diuretics 'spironlactone'
- After load reducing agents
  e.g. Captopril 0.5-6 mg /kg/24 hours.
- Positive intropic agents. 'dopamine and dobutamine'

### Rx of Cardiac Arrhythmias

- Digoxin (be aware of toxicity– nausia, vomiting, AV block, K, ca).
- Quinidine (hemolytic anemia. SLE, perodic paralysis)

- Procainamide (agranulocytosis, +ve coombs hemolytic anemia)
- Lidocaine (confusion, convulsion ,respiratory failure, AV block).
- Propranolol (bradycardia, bronchspasm, hypotension etc).
- Verapamil (bradycardia, PR interval prolongation, CHF).
- Adenosine (chest pain, flushing, bronchospasm, bradycardia)

### *Rx of the Cyanotic Spells*

- Try to calm the patient .
- Knee chest position,
- $O_2$
- Propranolol IV.
- Morphine s.c
- $NaHCO_3$ IV
- Increase IV fluid.

### *Prophylaxis Against Infective Endocarditis*

- By oral or parental antibiotics.
- Given in case of dental procedures, urinary and GIT.
- Instrumental 'proctoscopy, cystescopy'.
- Now a days lot of controversy about who should take the prophylactic antibiotics.

*New Guidelines Regarding Antibiotics to Prevent Infective Endocarditis*

The American Heart Association recently updated its guidelines regarding which patients should take a precautionary antibiotic to prevent infective endocarditis (IE) before a trip to the dentist.

The guidelines, published in *Circulation: Journal of the American Heart Association,* are based on a growing body of scientific evidence that shows that, for most people, the risks of taking prophylaxis antibiotics for certain procedures outweigh the benefits. These guidelines represent a major change in philosophy.

The new guidelines show taking preventive antibiotics is not necessary for most people and, in fact, might create more harm than good. Unnecessary use of antibiotics could cause allergic reactions and dangerous antibiotic resistance.

Only the people at greatest risk of bad outcomes from infective endocarditis—an infection of the hearts inner lining or the heart valves—should receive short-term preventive antibiotics before common, routine dental and medical procedures.

Patients at the greatest danger of bad outcomes from IE and for whom preventive antibiotics are worth the risks include those with:

- Artificial heart valves
- A history of having had IE
- Certain specific, serious congenital (present from birth) heart conditions, including:
  - unrepaired or incompletely repaired cyanotic congenital heart disease, including those with palliative shunts and conduits
  - a completely repaired congenital heart defect with prosthetic material or device, whether placed by surgery or by catheter interventions, during the first six months after the procedure
  - Any repaired congenital heart defect with residual defect at the site or adjacent to the site of a prosthetic patch or prosthetic device
- A cardiac transplant which develops a problem in a heart valve

Do not forget prostglandin PGE2, AND indomethacine for selective cases of CHD.

## Congenital Malformations of the Gastrointestinal Tract

Sometimes babies are born with malformations somewhere along the gastrointestinal (GI) tract. These malformations are not caused by prematurity and are rare. They range from minor to serious and can occur anywhere from the esophagus to the anus. Many of these conditions can be surgically treated, with an excellent chance at normal development and function later on as the baby grows into childhood and beyond. Other malformations have outcomes that are not as good. Some of the more common malformations are.

## Esophageal Atresia and Fistula

Esophageal atresia and fistula are malformations in which the natural breathing tube, known as the trachea, and the feeding tube, called the esophagus, are improperly formed. Most often the upper esophagus lacks a connection to the stomach while the lower esophagus connects to the trachea through an abnormal passage called a fistula. Babies with these types of malformations are fed with total parenteral nutrition (TPN) or with a feeding tube directly into the stomach. During this time, the baby gains strength and the esophagus will continue to grow. After several weeks, the malformation is repaired with surgery. About 20% of babies with these types of malformations will also have other complications, such as heart disease.

### *Tracheoesophageal Fistula and Esophageal Atresia*

Tracheoesophageal fistula is a small opening between the windpipe and the esophagus. It often occurs in combination with esophageal atresia, a condition in which the esophagus is not properly connected to the stomach.

Babies born with these conditions are fed with a feeding tube directly into the stomach. After several weeks, the malformations are repaired with surgery.

## Intestinal Atresias

Intestinal atresias are malformations of the intestines in which a segment of bowel is very narrow or is disconnected from the rest of the GI tract. Most commonly, these occur in or near the duodenum, just below the stomach. Although atresias are rare, babies born with this condition are often small for their gestational age and some may also have Down syndrome. Depending on exactly where the malformation is, bile may be released into the GI tract with nowhere to go but up, appearing in the esophagus. As with esophageal atresia, the malformation is repaired with surgery, though the exact nature of the malformation may mean surgery will be performed sooner rather than later.

**Intestinal Atresia**

Intestinal atresia is a malformation where part of the intestine is very narrow or disconnected from the rest of the gastrointestinal tract. Most often, this occurs at a spot just below the stomach called the duodenum. Intestinal atresia can be repaired with surgery.

## Malrotation with Volvulus

Until about the 10th week of pregnancy, a fetus's GI tract develops, in part, in the umbilical cord. At this point, it returns to the abdomen and rotates 90 degrees to the right. The individual components of the GI tract, including the duodenum, which connects the stomach and the intestines, and the intestines themselves, rearrange themselves and begin to settle into a position that will then remain unchanged for the rest of a person's life. At the end of this process, the GI tract is normally fixed; that is, it is contained and supported, and does not move.

Occasionally, this series of maneuvers and migrations is not performed properly and part of the GI tract, though still connected, ends up in the wrong place. This malrotation, as it is called, can also leave the GI tract unfixed. In some cases, this is not a problem; some people end up leading a normal life with an unfixed and rotated bowel. However, many babies have severe symptoms. Occasionally, as the GI tract settles itself into place, it loops around itself, reducing its blood supply or causing an obstruction. This is called volvulus. Malrotation with volvulus requires emergency surgery to correct the problem.

**Malrotation with Volvulus**

If the gastrointestinal tract does not develop properly, parts of it can end up in the wrong place. This is called malrotation. Sometimes the gastrointestinal tract ends up looping around itself to the extent that a blockage forms that could reduce the blood supply, and this is called volvulus. Malrotation with volvulus requires emergency surgery.

## Hirschsprung's Disease

Hirschsprung's disease is a condition in which nerve cells called ganglia have not formed on the inner wall of the bowel. This causes the bowel to contract and not relax, obstructing the lower intestine. Boys are about 10 times more likely to have the disease than girls. Again, surgery is used to correct the malformation. Surgeons will identify the bowel section without ganglia, cut it out, and reattach the two ends of healthy bowel. Sometimes a colostomy, or the surgical removal of some of the bowels, is necessary, and the surgeons will do the final repair at six to 12 months of age. Many babies who have undergone this procedure will develop and lead normal lives, since enough functioning bowel remains for digestion. However, a small number of babies with Hirschsprung's disease also have an inflammation of the large intestine called colitis, which may complicate surgery and can be life-threatening.

## Anorectal Malformations

Some babies are born with malformations of the anus, rectum, or both. There are several general types. They have varying degrees of severity and are treated with surgery. These malformations are often specific to boys and girls. The malformation can come in the form of an absence of an opening where the anus should be; a fistula, or small opening from the rectum to the urinary tract or to the vagina; and many variations from these general categories. Depending on the exact nature and severity of the malformation, babies may be left completely continent, with full control over their bowel movements; partially continent; or incontinent. In general, surgeons will close the fistula and, in the case of a missing anus, create an opening and gently pull though the bottom of the bowel, creating a new anus.

## Abdominal wall Defects

A defect in the abdominal wall may allow some of the digestive system to develop outside the baby's body in the amniotic fluid of the womb. These rare abnormalities are usually very small and only a small portion of the intestines are exposed. Gastroschisis occurs on the abdominal wall. Omphalocele occurs on the umbilicus, or belly button. Each of these defects allows some of the digestive system to develop outside the body. They can be small or large, and involve one organ or several.

Sometimes, these conditions can be diagnosed before birth. Exposure to the amniotic fluid can cause damage to the intestines. For this reason, some hospitals may suggest a planned early caesarean section to limit the extent of intestinal exposure to amniotic fluid. There is still debate about whether this is the best course of action. The treatment is surgical reinsertion of the intestines into the body. Depending on the size and extent of the condition, there may be more than one surgery needed to accomplish this goal.

Though in general they are very rare, there are many other types of malformations not mentioned on this page.

## Diagnosis of Congenital Malformations of the Gastrointestinal Tract

Abnormalities, also called lesions, of the upper GI tract will have symptoms such as feeding intolerance and vomiting, possibly of both food and bile from the stomach. A distension or abnormal enlargement of the abdomen may also be apparent. At times, the stomach may continue to fill up but may not pass its contents further down the GI tract, enlarging the stomach to a surprisingly large extent. Meconium, a baby's black and tarry first stool, may have passed or may continue to pass.

Intermediate lesions, found in the duodenum, will have similar symptoms as upper GI tract malformations. If there is distension of the abdomen, it may be even larger than the distension normally seen as a result of lesions of the upper GI tract.

In general, lesions of the lower GI tract have some or all the following symptoms: a delayed passage of meconium, poor passage of stool, and abdominal distension. If vomiting occurs, it usually does not occur immediately and it may contain feces.

Abdominal X-rays may reveal the malformation. It is also common to use both upper and lower GI tract tests called 'series' when trying to diagnose a malformation. In these tests, a substance such as barium is given. The baby's GI system is monitored with an X-ray machine called a fluoroscope as the barium makes its way through. This can reveal important details that will not be seen with X-ray. Even with fluoroscopy, diagnosis can remain unclear.

The usual blood tests will also be conducted to look for evidence of infection, electrolyte imbalances, hypoglycemia, or metabolic acidosis, among others.

### Esophageal Atresia X-ray

Normally, a very thin tube called a nasogastric tube can be passed down the esophagus and into the stomach. With an esophageal atresia, there is not a proper connection from the esophagus to the stomach. The nasogastric tube can only be passed as far down as the upper esophagus. There is usually a fistula, or small passageway, between the esophagus and trachea.

### Bowel Obstruction X-ray

The bowel pattern on the right is abnormal and is highly suggestive of an obstruction somewhere in the GI tract. The cause of the obstruction could be intestinal atresia, malrotation with volvulus, or Hirschprung's disease.

### Treatment of Congenital Malformations of the Gastrointestinal Tract

Congenital malformations of the gastrointestinal (GI) tract are extremely rare. There are many different types of malformations that can occur. In all but a few cases, these malformations require surgical intervention. Surgery may happen immediately or may have to wait until a baby is older and stronger. Additionally, some malformations require more than one surgery to repair. Before surgery and for a time afterwards, it is likely the baby will be fed intravenously, giving the bowel time to heal.

Congenital anomalies of urinary system

*Renal Problems*

- Hypertension
- Renal Masses
  - Renal
  - Juxtarenal
- Renal Failure

*Genitourinary Problems*

- Obstructive uropathies (PUV,UPJ,UVJ)
- Vesicourethral reflux
- Bladder exstrophy
- Cloacal exstrophy
- Prune Belly Syndrome
- Ambiguous genitalia
- Hypo/Epispadias

*Neonatal Hypertension*

- Healthy newborns – 0.2%
- Babies after NICU care – 2.6%
- Infants with CLD – up to 40%
- Worry about end organ damage
  - Cardiac – Heart failure
  - Retinal – Retinopathy
  - CNS – Encephalopathy
  - Renal

*Getting the Correct BP*

- First reading frequently higher than third
- Nwanko et. al. recommends following protocol:
  - Check BP 1.5 hours after the last feeding or intervention
  - Apply appropriately sized cuff
- 2/3 the length of the limb segment
- Defined size markers on cuffs
  - Wait 15 minutes/until patient still
  - obtaining three successive readings at 2-minute intervals.

*Definition of HTN*

- AAP 2nd task force (70,000 American/British Children)
  - BP > 95% for age on three separate occasions
  - In newborn, only systolic values used
- Term 95th Percentile
  - DOL #1 96 mmHg
  - DOL #8–30 104 mmHg
- Term 99th Percentile
  - DOL #7–10 110–115 mmHg

*Causes of Hypertension*

**Table:** Common causes of hypertension in neonates

| |
|---|
| **Renovascular*** |
| • Thromboembolism<br>• Renal artery stenosis<br>• Renal venous thrombosis<br>• Compression of renal artery |
| **Cardiac*** |
| • Coarctation of aorta |
| **Pulmonary*** |
| • Bronchopulmonary dysplasia |
| **Renal disease*** |
| • Congenital<br>– Polycystic kidney disease<br>– Multicystic-dysplastic kidney disease<br>– Ureteropelvic junction obstruction<br>• Acquired<br>– Acute tubular necrosis<br>– Hemolytic-uremic syndrome<br>– Obstruction by tumor |
| **Endocrine** |
| • Congenital adrenal hyperplasia<br>• Pseudohypoaldosteronism type II |
| **Medications/Intoxications** |
| • Maternal<br>– Opioids (cocaine, heroin)<br>• Infant<br>– Dexamethasone<br>– Theophylline<br>– Caffeine<br>– Pancuronium<br>– Phenylephrine |

*Contd...*

*Contd...*

| |
|---|
| **Neoplasms**<br>• Wilms tumor<br>• Mesoblastic nephroma<br>• Neuroblastoma |
| **Neurologic**<br>• Pain<br>• Intracranial hypertension<br>• Seizures |
| **Miscellaneous**<br>• Closure of abdominal wall defect<br>• Adrenal hemorhage<br>• Hypercalcemia<br>• Extracorporeal membrane oxygenation<br>• Birth asphyxia |

*These categories account for the majority of cases.

*Treatment of HTN*

- Treat at SBP >99% or >95% with end-organ involvement
- Medications:
  - Emergent – use drips or IV medications
    - Nicardipine or nitroprusside/labetalol or hydralazine
  - Non-emergent
    - β-blocker – Propranolol – most extensively used
    - Diuretic – limited use in neonates for HTN
    - Calcium channel blocker – Amlodipine, Nifedipine
    - ACE inhibitor – Captopril

*Differential of Abdominal Mass–Renal*

- Hydronephrosis
- Cystic diseases of kidney
  - PCKD
  - MCDK
- Renal vein thrombosis
- Solid tumors of kidneys
  - Mesoblastic Nephroma
  - Wilm's Tumor
- Horseshoe or ectopic kidneys

*Differential of Abdominal Mass – Juxtarenal*

- Neuroblastoma
- Adrenal Hemorrhage
- Pheochromocytoma
- Teratoma
- Sarcoma
- Meconium Cyst

*Lab Evaluation:*

- Basic Metabolic Profile
- Urinalysis
- Urinary Electrolytes – Renal Failure
- Urine HVA/VMA – Neuroblastoma
- Teratoma - B-HCG and AFP
- Renin – Renal Artery Stenosis
- Urinary Catecholamines – Pheochromocytoma

*Imaging Evaluation*

- Imaging
- Start with plain film
- Abdominal/Renal U/S
- MRI
- CT +/- contrast

*Differential of Abdominal Mass - Renal Hydronephrosis*

- Most common congenital condition on prenatal ultrasound (1:500 to 1:700 deliveries)
- Causes are varied
  - Physiologic (usually mild, up to 15%)
  - UPJ or UVJ obstruction
  - Vesicoureteral reflux
  - Eagle-Barrett syndrome
  - Posterior urethral valves

*Pyelectasis*

- Also known as renal pelvis dilation
- Typically defined when renal pelvic dilation is more than 4 mm but less than 10 mm
- 90% of cases improves on its own
- Diagnosis is done by ultrasound

*Cystic Diseases of Kidneys*

- Multicystic Dysplastic Kidney (MCDK)
- Polycystic Kidney Disease
  - Autosomal Recessive
  - Autosomal Dominant

*Multicystic Dyplastic Kidney MCDK*

- Most severe form of renal dysplasia
- Multiple large cysts/ureteral atresia
- Unilateral
- Sporadic (+/- VACTERL)
- Involutes over time
- Follow with serial U/S and remove if doesn't involute
- Urological testing on healthy kidney

*Polycystic Kidney Disease*

- Genetic, with variable expression
- Most commonly inherited kidney disease
- Bilateral involvement
- Cysts may also be in liver
- Results in hypertension

| | Autosomal Recessive 'Infantile' PKD | Autosomal Dominant Adult PKD |
|---|---|---|
| Frequency | 1/40,000 | 1/10,000 |
| Chromosome | 6p21 | 16 (Codes for polycystin) |
| Diagnosis | Fetal U/S: large echogenic kidneys, oligohydramnios | Rarely findings at birth |
| Cysts | Kidneys and liver, as older Large > 2 cms | Kidney, liver, pancreas, spleen. Variable size |
| Problems | Severe HTN, hepatic fibrosis, biliary dysgenesis, Potter's Sequence | HTN, renal insufficiency. Worse as older |

Renal vein thrombosis

## Flank Mass, Hematuria and Renal Failure

- Usually with in first 3 DOL, dx RUS watch for doppler
- Risk factors: Maternal diabetes, dehydration, sepsis, hypovolemia, DIC, polycythemia, hypercoagulable state.
- Conservative, non-operative management
- Thrombocytopenia (consumptive)
- Most frequent vascular condition

*Tumors of Neonate*

- **Renal:**
  - Mesoblastic Nephroma
  - Less common:
- Wilms (aka nephroblastoma)
- Clear cell
- Rhabdoid Tumor
- **Adrenal:**
  - Pheochromocytoma (medulla of adrenals)
  - Neuroblastoma

*Mesoblastic Nephroma*

- Can be seen with polyhydramnios (from excessive fetal urine production)
- Peak age at presentation: 3 months
  - Usually watch for large, palpable abdominal mass
- Males = females

*Wilm's Tumor*

- Common tumor, but rarely diagnosed in the first month of life
  - 80% diagnosed between 1 and 5 years of age
- 15% associated with other syndromes
  - WAGR
  - Hemihypertrophy
  - Beckwith-Wiedemann
- Most have good prognosis and are cured with primary nephrectomy

*Ectopic Kidney*

- Kidney not located in usual position
- 1 in 1,000 births, but only about one in 10 of these are ever diagnosed; up to 10% bilateral

*Most Common*

Horseshoe Kidney
Unilateral renal agenesis
Pelvic kidney
(Left kidney more likely to be abnormal)

*Ectopic Kidney*

- Function is generally normal initially, but…
- Abnormal position leads to obstruction in 50% of ectopic kidneys
- Increased risk UTI, kidney stones, VUR
- Frequently associated with abnormalities of other organ systems (uterine, cardiac, skeletal)

*Horseshoe Kidney*

- Most common renal fusion anomaly (1:400)
- As kidneys rise from pelvic area they fuse at lower pole (90%)
- 33% without symptoms, although associated with Turner Syndrome, Trisomy 18
- Commonly present with UTI
- Diagnosis: Renal Ultrasound, VCUG
- Supportive Management, prophylactic antibiotics, surgical intervention (stones)

*Patient Course*

- Patient underwent exploratory laparotomy and resection of mass
- Findings: Pararenal immature teratoma with no malignancy identified

*Differential of Acute Renal Failure*

- Prerenal
- Intrinsic
- Obstructive

**Prerenal**

- Decreased true intravascular volume
  - Perinatal hemorrhage
  - Dehydration
  - Third space losses (sepsis, traumatized tissue, nectotizing enterocolitis)
  - Gastointestinal losses
  - Hypoalbuminemia
- Decreased effective intravascular volume
  - Congestive heart failure
  - Pericarditis, cardiac tamponade

**Intrinsic Renal**

- Acute tubular necrosis
  - Perinatal asphyxia
  - Ischemic/hypoxic insults
  - Drug-induced
    - Aminoglycosides
    - Intravenous contrast media
    - Non-steroidal anti-inflammatory drugs (indomethacin)
    - Angiotensin-converting enzyme inhibitors (captopril, enalapril)
    - Amphotericin B
- Interstitial nephritis
- Vascular lesions
  - Renal artery thrombosis
  - Renal vein thrombosis
  - Cortical necrosis
- Infectious causes
  - Sepsis
  - Pyelonephritis
  - Symphilis
  - Toxoplasmosis
  - Candidiasis

**Postrenal/Obstructive**

- Obstruction in a solitary kidney
- Bilateral ureteral obstruction
  - Bilateral fungal bezoar
- Urethral obstruction
  - Posterior urethral valves
- Neurogenic bladder due to myelomeningocele

*Dialysis – Indications*

- Fluid Overload
- Hyperkalemia/Electrolyte Disturbances
- Severe metabolic acidosis
- Catabolism/Malnutrition

- Symptomatic uremia
- Drug toxicity (renally excreted)

*Genitourinary Problems*

- Obstructive uropathies (PUV, UPJ, UVJ)
- Vesicourethral reflux
- Bladder exstrophy
- Cloacal exstrophy
- Ambiguous genitalia
- Hypo/Epispadias
- Urachal Anomalies

*Obstructive Uropathies*

- Posterior Urethral Valves (PUV)
- Ureteropelvic Junction Obstruction (UPJ)
- Ureterovesical Junction Obstruction (UVJ)
  - Ureterocele

*Posterior Urethral Valves*

- Most common cause of obstructive uropathy in males
  - Does not affect females
- Incidence: 1/5000-1/8000
- Cause: Congenital membrane which (partially) obstructs urethra
- Clinical presentation:
  - bilateral flank masses (hydronephrosis)
  - distended bladder
  - poor urinary stream (+/- dribbling)
- Diagnostic test: VCUG
- Therapeutic Goal: Preserve renal function, avoid renal failure
  - 30% at risk for progressive renal insufficiency
- Immediate: Place Foley, Decompress Bladder
- Surgical therapy: Ablation of valves, urinary diversion
  - Fetal therapy with vesicoamniotic shunt
- Severe cases can present with Potter's Sequence
  - Oligohydramnios, pulmonary hypoplasia, uterine molding

*UPJ Obstruction*

- Most common cause of congenital hydronephrosis
- Cause: Abnormal muscle development at UPJ
- Males > Females
- Can be associated with other congenital abnormalities (e.g. VATER)
- Clinical/Prenatal Presentation:
- Prenatal: Hydronephrosis (unilateral)
- Post-natal: Renal mass (hydronephrosis) or work-up after urinary tract infection
- Diagnosis: Obstructive pattern on diuretic enhanced radionucleotide scan

*UPJ Obstruction: Surgical Repair*

- Pyeloplasty: involves removing the blockage, and reconnecting the ureter to the renal pelvis.
  - Stent may be left across the pyeloplasty or a nephrostomy may be left above the repair to decompress the kidney

*UVJ Obstruction*

- Second most common cause of hydronephrosis
- Cause: Deficient development of uereter or a ureterocele
- Do not have dilated ureter in UPJ obstruction:
- Clinical/Prenatal Presentation:
- Prenatal: Hydronephrosis (+/- Hydroureter)
- Post-natal: Renal mass (hydronephrosis) or workup after urinary tract infection
- Diagnosis: Renal Ultrasound, Radionucleotide Scan, VCUG
- Treatment:
- Surgical resection of obstruction
- May require stent placement, ~10% recurrence

*Vesicoureteral Reflux (VUR)*

- Accounts for 25–30% of antenatal hydronephrosis and 1% of newborns
- Most (75%) children outgrow this during childhood
- Presentation: UTI, hydronephrosis
  - Up to 30% with other GU anomalies
  - Males present earlier due to shorter ureters but girls 2x more likely to have reflux
  - 3x greater in whites > blacks
- Concern: increased risk of UTI, renal scarring in 30–60% of Grade IV and V Reflux
- Medical Treatment:
  - Antibiotic prophylaxis (controversial)
- Amoxicillin for < 2mo
- TMP-SMX or Nitrofurantoin QHS
  - Surveillance ultrasounds
  - VCUG
- Surgical Treatment
  - open vs endoscopic - DEFLUX

*VUR – Monitoring*

- Ismaili et al., prospective study of 43 patients
- At 2 years:
  - Mild VUR spontaneously resolved in 91 percent with low-grade reflux (grades I to III).
  - In patients with high-grade reflux (grades IV and V), VUR resolved in only 2 of 11 patients.

*Genitourinary Malformations*

- Bladder exstrophy
- Cloacal exstrophy
- Ambiguous genitalia
- Hypo/Epispadias
- Urachal Anomalies

*Bladder Exstrophy*

- Spectrum of severity
- Small defect can result in epispadias
- large defect can result in exposure of posterior bladder wall
- Occurs 1 in 30,000 births
- Exposed bladder mucosa is edematous and friable
- Moist, fine-mesh gauze or vaseline gauze to cover exposed bladder
- Antibiotics
- Renal ultrasound
- Transfer infant to surgical center
- Want surgical correction by 48–72 hours of life
- Sacroiliac joints are still pliable and the pelvis can be 'molded' to allow better approximation of the pubic rami

- IVP of limited utility b/c of poor concentrating ability of neonatal kidney

*Surgery*
- Turn-in of the bladder to preserve bladder function
- Symphysis pubis is approximated
- Iliac osteotomies are not necessary if repair is within 48 HOL (bones are still pliable from circulating maternal estrogens)
- Epispadiac urethra is reconstructed later

*Cloacal Exstrophy*
- Very rare: 1 in 200,000 births
- Sporadic occurrence
- Complex of GI and GU anomalies:
  - Imperforate anus
  - Exstrophy of the bladder
  - Omphalocele
  - Vesicointestinal fistula
  - Frequently with prolapse of bowel through the fistula on bladder mucosa

*Preoperative*
- Cover exposed mucosa (vaseline/saline gauze) and/or plastic wrap to minimize heat loss
- Gender assignment/diagnosis
  - Karyotype / FISH
  - Controversial regarding assignment
- NG suction to relieve partial intestinal obstruction.
  - Stool frequently excreted through a vesico-intestinal fistula that is often partially obstructed

*Operative*
- Survival 80%: mortality due to sepsis and bowel obstruction
- Prompt surgery to separate fecal and urinary streams
- Bladder can be closed during initial procedure if baby stable
- Subsequent procedures to reduce the number of stomas and create genitalia

*Cloacal Exstrophy*
- Multiple Long term problems:
- Psychosocial/Gender Identification
- Recurrent UTIs
- Bowel/Bladder Incontinence
- Sexual function in later life

*Ambiguous Genitalia – CAH*
- CAH is the most common diagnosis in virilized XX infants
- Presentation
  - Hypoglycemia, vomiting, diarrhea, hypovolemia, hyponatremia with hyperkalemia, and shock
- Management
  - Monitor electrolytes, glucose
  - 17-OHP high (Newborn screen/Lab Studies)
- Treatment: glucocorticoids (hydrocortisone)
- May require mineralocorticoids in salt-wasters

*Hypospadias*
- Incidence: up to 1:250 births
- Associations: undescended testicles (DSD), inguinal hernias
- Management: recognition, avoidance of circumcision
- Surgery: usually by 2 years of life

*Epispadias*
- Incidence: 1:10,000 to 1:20,000
- Associations: Bladder exstrophy, VUR (40%)
- Management: recognition, avoidance of circumcision
- Surgery: multistaged reconstruction

*Urachal abnormalities*
- Patent urachus:
  - Connection remains between allantois and fetal bladder
  - Drainage/urine leakage through umbilicus
  - Surgically remove mole
- Urachal sinus:
  - Drains to umbilicus
  - Intermittent drainage from umbilicus (may be serous or serosanguinous
- Urachal cyst:
  - Fluid-filled structure occurring in between the two obliterated ends of the urachus (distal end)

## Central Nervous System Birth Defects

Birth defects of the central nervous system are called neural tube defects (NTDs). NTDs include conditions called *spina bifida, anencephaly* and *encephalocele*. They are all present at birth and are due to a problem with the development of the brain and/or spinal cord in the developing baby (fetus).

The brain and spinal cord of a growing fetus develop from a simple structure called the *neural tube*. The neural tube 'zips up' along its length to close and protect the brain and spinal cord. If the neural tube does not close at any part along its length, the baby will have a neural tube defect. The types of neural tube defects (*spina bifida, anencephaly* and *encephalocele*) are due to the place along the neural tube that has not closed, leaving parts of the brain and/or spinal cord exposed.

A range of genetic and environmental factors are thought to be responsible for NTDs, including the mother having not enough of the vitamin folate and some epilepsy medications. Taking folate (folic acid) before and during early pregnancy can significantly reduce the chance that a mother will have a baby with this kind of birth defect.

## The Central Nervous System (CNS)

The central nervous system consists of the brain and spinal cord. Both are wrapped in a thin lining called *meninges* and are surrounded by a fluid called *cerebrospinal fluid*. The brain is attached to the spinal cord by the brain stem, located at the base of the brain. The spinal cord runs the length of the backbone and is protected by the bones (vertebrae) of the spine. Nerves branch off from the spinal cord into the parts of the body.

## Development of the Fetal CNS

The central nervous system of a growing fetus starts with a simple structure called the 'neural groove' that folds in to form the 'neural tube'. This then develops into the spinal cord and brain. By day 28 after conception, the neural tube should be closed and fused. If it does not close, the result is a neural tube defect.

In many cases, these defects can be diagnosed during pregnancy with ultrasound scans and, rarely, with other tests such as amniocentesis (analysing a sample of amniotic fluid).

## Risk Factors and Prevention of CNS Birth Defects

Neural tube defects are thought to be caused by a range of genetic and environmental factors working in combination. Some of these factors include:

- *The mother has a folate deficiency:* if the mother is lacking some nutrients, especially the B-group vitamin called folate (folic acid), the chance of having a baby with a NTD is increased. If folate is taken before conception and at least for the first four weeks of pregnancy, around seven out of 10 cases of NTDs can be prevented. You should talk to your doctor about how much folate you should take if you are thinking of becoming pregnant.
- *Genetics:* the exact genetic association is unclear, but a woman is at increased risk of having a baby with a neural tube defect if she has a close relative who has had a baby with the condition (a family history). A woman who has already given birth to a child with a neural tube defect is also at increased risk of having subsequent babies with a similar condition.
- Having a personal or family history of a NTD can influence the amount of folate needed to reduce the chance of having a baby with a neural tube defect. You should talk to your doctor about how much folate you should take if you are thinking of becoming pregnant.
- In some cases, however, there is evidence to suggest that some forms of neural tube defects are caused by specific genetic changes (mutations) that are not related to folate. In these cases, the neural tube defect is caused by the baby inheriting faulty gene copies from both parents. These faulty genes prevent the baby from making use of folate, i.e. necessary to grow and develop in pregnancy (even if the folate is present in the right amount). In these cases, taking folate before and during pregnancy will not prevent the condition.
- *Medication:* particular medications used to treat and control epilepsy are thought to contribute to the risk of neural tube defect.

## Spina Bifida

In a baby with *spina bifida,* the bones (vertebrae) of the spine fail to fuse. The spinal cord and nerves protrude (or 'pop out') through the gap that has been created due to a failure of closure of the neural tube. This can affect the nerves that spread from this area into the abdomen and legs. *Spina bifida* can occur anywhere along the length of the spine, but more commonly appears in the lower back.

Nine out of 10 affected babies also have a build-up of cerebrospinal fluid inside the brain. This condition is called hydrocephalus and is sometimes referred to as 'water on the brain'. The incidence of spina bifida in Victoria is around one in every 1,235 births.

Spina bifida can be mild, moderate or severe and is graded according to the degree of the defect into:

- *Occulta:* the bones (vertebrae) have not closed completely, but the spinal cord is unharmed. The characteristic soft lump may be missing, which is why this form of spina bifida is sometimes diagnosed later in life.
- *Meningocele:* the membrane (meninges) covering the spinal cord protrudes or bulges out through the gap in the spine.
- *Myelomeningocele:* the meninges, spinal cord and blood vessels protrude through the gap.

  *Spina bifida* is incurable. The main form of treatment is surgery to seal the gap. If the baby has *hydrocephalus,* a shunt is inserted into the brain to drain the excess cerebrospinal fluid.

## Treatment

There is no known cure for nerve damage caused by spina bifida. Standard treatment is surgery after delivery. This surgery aims to prevent further damage of the nervous tissue and to prevent infection, pediatric neurosurgeons operate to close the opening on the back. The spinal cord and its nerve roots are put back inside the spine and covered with meninges. In addition, a shunt may be surgically installed to provide a continuous drain for the excess cerebrospinal fluid produced in the brain, as happens with hydrocephalus. Shunts most commonly drain into the abdomen or chest wall.

## Pregnancy

Standard treatment is after delivery. There is tentative evidence about treatment before delivery while the baby is inside the womb for severe disease. As of 2014 the evidence; however, remains insufficient to determine benefits and harms.

Treatment of spina bifida during pregnancy is not without risk. To the mother, this includes scarring of the uterus. To the baby, there is the risk of preterm birth.

Broadly, there are two forms of prenatal treatment. The first is open fetal surgery, where the uterus is opened and the spina bifida repair performed. The second is via fetoscopy. These techniques may be an option to standard therapy.

## Childhood

Most individuals with myelomeningocele will need periodic evaluations by a variety of specialists:

- *Physiatrists* coordinate the rehabilitation efforts of different therapists and prescribe specific therapies, adaptive equipment, or medications to encourage as high of a functional performance within the community as possible.
- *Orthopedists* monitor growth and development of bones, muscles, and joints.
- *Neurosurgeons* perform surgeries at birth and manage complications associated with tethered cord and hydrocephalus.
- *Neurologists* treat and evaluate nervous system issues, such as seizure disorders
- *Urologists* to address kidney, bladder, and bowel dysfunction - many will need to manage their urinary systems with a program of catheterization. Bowel management programs aimed at improving elimination are also designed.
- *Ophthalmologists* evaluate and treat complications of the eyes.

- *Orthotists* design and customize various types of assistive technology, including braces, crutches, walkers, and wheelchairs to aid in mobility. As a general rule, the higher the level of the spina bifida defect, the more severe the paralysis, but paralysis does not always occur. Thus, those with low levels may need only short leg braces, whereas those with higher levels do best with a wheelchair, and some may be able to walk unaided.
- *Physical therapists, occupational therapists, psychologists*, and *speech/language pathologists* aid in rehabilitative therapies and increase independent living skills.

## Transition to Adulthood

Although many children's hospitals feature integrated multidisciplinary teams to coordinate health care of youth with spina bifida, the transition to adult health care can be difficult because the above health care professionals operate independently of each other, requiring separate appointments and communicate among each other much less frequently. Healthcare professionals working with adults may also be less knowledgeable about spina bifida because it is considered a childhood chronic health condition. Due to the potential difficulties of the transition, adolescents with spina bifida and their families are encouraged to begin to prepare for the transition around ages 14–16, although this may vary depending on the adolescent's cognitive and physical abilities and available family support. The transition itself should be gradual and flexible. The adolescent's multidisciplinary treatment team may aid in the process by preparing comprehensive, up-to-date documents detailing the adolescent's medical care, including information about medications, surgery, therapies, and recommendations. A transition plan and aid in identifying adult health care professionals are also helpful to include in the transition process.

Further complicating the transition process is the tendency for youths with spina bifida to be delayed in the development of autonomy, with boys particularly at risk for slower development of independence. An increased dependence on others (in particular family members) may interfere with the adolescent's self-management of health-related tasks, such as catheterization, bowel management, and taking medications. As part of the transition process, it is beneficial to begin discussions at an early age about educational and vocational goals, independent living, and community involvement.

## Anencephaly

When the neural tube does not close at the head, this may cause the uppermost brain tissue, the meninges, top of the skull (calvarium) and the scalp to be partially or completely missing. For reasons unknown, *anencephaly* occurs twice as often in females as males. Around one in 10 affected babies is one of a pair of twins. In some cases, the baby has other problems such as congenital heart disease and cleft palate. The incidence of *anencephaly* in Victoria is around one in every 1,370 births.

A baby with *anencephaly* is not able to live. Most are stillborn or die within a few days of birth.

### Prognosis

There is no cure or standard treatment for anencephaly and the prognosis for patients is death. Most anencephalic fetuses do not survive birth, accounting for 55% of non-aborted cases. Infants that are not *stillborn* will usually die within a few hours or days after birth from *cardiorespiratory arrest*.

Four recorded cases of anencephalic children surviving for longer periods of time are *Stephanie Keene* of *Falls Church, Virginia*, USA, who lived for 2 years 174 days; Vitoria de Cristo, born in Brazil in January 2010 and surviving until July 17, 2012; Nickolas Coke of *Pueblo, Colorado*, USA, who lived for 3 years and 11 months, and died October 31, 2012; and Angela Morales, from Providence, Rhode Island.

In almost all cases, anencephalic infants are not aggressively *resuscitated* because there is no chance of the infant's ever achieving a conscious existence. Instead, the usual clinical practice is to offer *hydration, nutrition*, and *comfort measures* and to 'let nature take its course'. Artificial ventilation, surgery (to fix any co-existing congenital defects), and drug therapy (such as antibiotics) are usually regarded as futile efforts. Some clinicians and medical ethicists view even the provision of nutrition and hydration as medically futile.

## Encephalocele

In this rare form of neural tube defect, the meninges and brain tissue bulge out through a gap in the skull. In severe cases, the brain is pushed out to such an extent that the bundle of brain tissue covered by the meninges (membranes) may be larger than the baby's head. Infection can occur if the membrane breaks and exposes the brain tissue. Other problems associated with *encephalocele* can include cleft lip or palate, additional fingers (polydacty) and abnormalities of the sex organs. The incidence of *encephalocele* in Victoria is around one in every 6,667 births.

If there is a significant amount of brain tissue that has been pushed out, surgery may not be possible. Treatment options include the use of a shunt to remove the fluid build-up (treat the hydrocephalus), if necessary. The baby will experience a range of difficulties that can include intellectual impairment, difficulty in controlling muscles (spasticity) and fits (convulsions). Physiotherapy and anticonvulsant medication may help.

### Treatment

Currently, the only effective treatment for encephaloceles is reparative surgery, generally performed during *infancy*. The extent to which it can be corrected depends on the location and size of the encephaloceles; however, large protrusions can be removed without causing major disability. Surgery repositions the bulging area back into the skull, removes the protrusions, and corrects the deformities, typically relieving pressure that can delay normal brain development. Occasionally, *shunts* are placed to drain excess cerebrospinal fluid from the brain.

*The Goals of Treatment Include*

- Closure of open skin defects to prevent infection and desiccation of brain tissue

- Removal of nonfunctional extracranial cerebral tissue with water-tight closure of the dura
- Total craniofacial reconstruction with particular emphasis on avoiding the long-nose deformity (nasal elongation that results from depression of the cribiform plate and nasal placode). Without proper management, the long-nose deformity can be more obvious after repair.

## INFANT CARE

- The health services given to a baby during the first year of life.
- It is a function of the MCH centers (in PHCC, and in some hospitals)
- It is done through the 'well baby clinics' = the clinics that are concerned with health care for all children under the age of 5 years.

### Well Baby Clinic

- Frequency of visits: (15)
  - seven visits in first year (including visits at time of vaccination)
  - Two visits each year from 2–5 years
  - Wt, and Ht For each prn visit
- ***Every infant has a health card kept in the PHCC containing the following information:***
  - Name of parents
  - Date of birth
  - Place of delivery
  - Attendance at labor
  - Type of delivery (NSVD, forceps, CS,…)
  - Health condition at birth (weight, length, and any congenital anomalies)
  - Social data of the family
  - PMH, PSH
  - Immunizations
  - Measurements of wt, length, HC and comparison with the normal

### Equipments of WBC

- Newborn baby weighing scales
- Weighing scales for older children
- Height scale fixed on the wall
- Measuring tape
- Infantometer
- Stethoscope and sphygmomanometer with small cuff (pediatric)
- Torch
- Examination table (couch)
- ENT and eye diagnostic sets
- Some attractive toys for babies
- Well baby register records and growth charts
- Posters denoting child growth and development at different ages should be provided
- Health education materials and facilities should be readily available.

### Process

- General examination: appearance, clothing
- Examine vision: ask the parents and observe the child (measure visual acuity at school entry and color testing at 9–13 years)
- Examine hearing:
  - Examine hearing abilities for those under 5 years.
  - Test child's attention to noise/voice at 8–12 months of age
  - Take parent's notes on hearing
  - Arrange for audiometry for children before school age
  - Growth measurements plotted on the charts.
  - Children outside the averages are re-examined, investigated, and treated or referred
  - Developmental milestones are checked
  - Detection and treatment of malnourished
  - Health education to the mothers
  - For ill children: vital signs, preparation and teaching of ORS, nurse-doctor referral, and giving injections when needed

*Growth Indices–Weight*

- At birth: 3–3.5 kg
- 1st 4 months: 3/4 kg per month
- 2nd 4 months :1/2 kg per month
- 3rd 4 months: 1/4 kg per month
- At the end of 4th month: 6 kg
- At the end of 1st year: 9 kg
- After 1st year: 2 kg per year

*Abnormal Weight*

- Above 90th percentile
- Below 5th percentile
- No increase over 3 subsequent months
- Curve down in 2 subsequent visits

*Growth Indices – HC*

- Between 97th and 3rd percentile
- At birth: 35 cm
- At 6 months: 43.8 cm
- At 1 year: 46.8 cm
- At 2 year: 49.1 year
- At 3 years: 50.2 cm
- At 4 years: 50.8 cm
- At 5 years: 51.3 cm

*Growth Indices-Height*

- At birth: 50 cm
- At the end of 1st year: 75 cm
- Thereafter: 5 cm per year
- Between 90th and 5th percentile

*Home Visits*

- Should be done by the nurse of the WBC for the following children:
  - Delayed mile stones or delayed growth
  - Diarrhea: chronic or recurrent acute
  - Social or psychiatric problems
  - Defaulters

*At Risk Children*

I. Group A:
- Babies of working mothers
- Babies of poor family (low income)
- Loss of a parents, or divorce
- History of mental or psychiatric disturbance of a parent
- More than 7 children in the family
- Non–breast feeders
- Early weaning
- Twins

Management
- Registration in risk records
- Regular follow up
- Call for defaulters
- Comprehensive health education
- Take out of registry if no problems by 6 months of follow-up

II. Group B:
- Birth weight < 2500 gm.
- Failure to gain weight in 3 successive visits.
- Loss of weight in 2 successive visits
- Weight below 80% of expected weight for his age

III. Group C:
- Congenital abnormalities
- Bronchial asthma
- Diabetes mellitus
- Handicapped (mental or physical)

### Health Education Contents

- Care of newborn
- Dealing with infantile common problems
- Nutritional education (especially breast feeding, weaning, and hygienic preparation of bottle feeding )
- Family planning
- Growth curve and its importance

## UNDER 5 CLINIC

### Aims and Objectives

1. *Care in illness:* it is mothers felt need.
   - 70%–80% of illnesses can be treated with trained nurses.
   a. Diagnosis and treatment of acute illness, chronic illnesses and disorders of growth and development.
   b. X-ray and laboratory services
   c. Referral services
2. Preventive care:
   a. Immunization
   b. Nutritional surveillance
      - sub-clinical nutrition
      - Food supplementation
   c. Health check ups – every 3-6 months. The child health card is maintained.
   d. Oral rehydration solution for diarrhea. The child gets 2–6 attacks in a year.
   e. Family planning
   f. Health education
3. Growth monitoring – on growth chart also called as *Road to health card.*
   a. Every month – up to 1 year
   b. 2 monthly – up to 2 years
   c. 3 monthly – up to 5 years
   d. The weight is plotted according to the age of child.

### Growth Chart Used In India

- It has four reference curves.
- Top most curve—80% of the median (50th percentile) of the WHO reference standard.
  Lower lines represent 70%, 60% and 50% of the standard.
- 80% median weight is approximately equal to 2 SD below the median which is the conventional lower limit of 'normal range'.
- Purpose of reference curve—It indicates degree of malnutrition.

II. IAP recommended vaccines for High-risk* children (Vaccines under special circumstances):
- Influenza Vaccine
- Meningococcal Vaccine
- Japanese Encephalitis Vaccine
- Cholera Vaccine
- Rabies Vaccine
- Yellow Fever Vaccine
- Pneumococcal Polysaccharide vaccine (PPSV 23)
- *High-risk category of children:
- Congenital or acquired immunodeficiency (including HIV infection),
- Chronic cardiac, pulmonary (including asthma if treated with prolonged high-dose oral corticosteroids), hematologic, renal (including nephrotic syndrome), liver disease and diabetes mellitus
- Children on long term steroids, salicylates, immunosuppressive or radiation therapy
- Diabetes mellitus, Cerebrospinal fluid leak, Cochlear implant, Malignancies,
- Children with functional/anatomic asplenia/ hyposplenia
- During disease outbreaks
- Laboratory personnel and health care workers
- Travelers
- Children having pets in home
- Children perceived with higher threat of being bitten by dogs such as hostellers, risk of stray dog menace while going outdoor.

### Pentavalent Vaccine

A pentavalent vaccine is a combined vaccine with five individual vaccines conjugated into one, intended to actively protect people from 5 potentially deadly diseases. The main example is a vaccine that protects against Haemophilus Influenza type B (a bacterium that causes meningitis, pneumonia and otitis), whooping cough, tetanus, hepatitis B and diphtheria.

During studies and tests, the conjugated liquid DTwP-HepB-Hib vaccine was found to have positive safety when administered as a booster to young children who have been given a vaccination course with another pentavalent booster that requires a change in constitution and was also found to be adequately immunogenic.

## IAP Immunization Schedule 2016

| Age (completed weeks/ months/years) | Vaccines | Comments |
|---|---|---|
| Birth | BCG<br>OPV 0<br>Hep-B 1 | Administer these vaccines to all newborns before hospital discharge |
| 6 weeks | DTwP 1<br>IPV 1<br>Hep-B 2<br>Hib 1<br>Rotavirus 1<br>PCV 1 | *DTP:*<br>• DTaP/DTwP vaccine/combinations should preferably be avoided for the primary series<br>• DTaP/DTwP vaccine/combinations should be preferred in certain specific circumstances/conditions only<br>• No need of repeating/giving additional doses of whole-cell pertussis (wP) vaccine to a child who has earlier completed their primary schedule with acellular pertussis (aP) vaccine-containing products<br>*Polio:*<br>• All doses of IPV may be replaced with OPV if administration of the former is unfeasible<br>• Additional doses of OPV on all supplementary immunization activities (SIAs)<br>• Two doses of IPV instead of 3 for primary series if started at 8 weeks, and 8 weeks interval between the doses<br>• No child should leave the facility without polio immunization (IPV or OPV), if indicated by the schedule<br>• See footnotes under figure titled IAP recommended immunization schedule (with range) for recommendations on intradermal IPV<br>*Rotavirus:*<br>• 2 doses of RV1 and 3 doses of RV5 and RV 116E<br>• RV1 should be employed in 10 and 14 week schedule, 10 and 14 week schedule of RV1 is found to be more immunogenic than 6 and 10 week schedule |
| 10 weeks | DTwP 2<br>IPV 2<br>Hib 2<br>Rotavirus 2<br>PCV 2 | Rotavirus:<br>If RV1 is chosen, the first dose should be given at 10 weeks |
| 14 weeks | DTwP 3<br>IPV 3<br>Hib 3<br>Rotavirus 3<br>PCV 3 | *Rotavirus:*<br>• Only 2 doses of RV1 are recommended.<br>• If RV1 is chosen, the 2nd dose should be given at 14 weeks |
| 6 months | OPV 1<br>Hep-B 3 | *Hepatitis-B:*<br>• The final (3rd or 4th) dose in theHepB vaccine series should be administered no earlier than age 24 weeks and at least 16 weeks after the first dose. |
| 9 months | OPV 2<br>MMR-1 | *Hepatitis-B:*<br>• Measles-containing vaccine ideally should not be administered before completing 270 days or 9 months of life;<br>• The 2nd dose must follow in 2nd year of life;<br>• No need to give stand-alone measles vaccine |
| 9 to 12 months | Typhoid Conjugate Vaccine | • Currently, two typhoid conjugate vaccines, Typbar-TCV® and PedaTyph® available in Indian market;either can be used<br>• An interval of at least 4 weeks with the MMR vaccine should be maintained while administering this vaccine |
| 12 months | Hep-A 1 | *Hepatitis-A:*<br>• Single dose for live attenuated H2-strain Hep-A vaccine<br>• Two doses for all inactivated Hep-A vaccines are recommended |
| 15 months | MMR 2<br>Varicella 1<br>PCV booster | *MMR:*<br>• The 2nd dose must follow in 2nd year of life<br>• However, it can be given at anytime 4-8 weeks after the 1st dose<br>*Varicella:* The risk of breakthrough varicella is lower if given 15 months onwards |

*Contd...*

*Contd...*

| Age (completed weeks/ months/years) | Vaccines | Comments |
|---|---|---|
| 16 to 18 months | DTwP B1/<br>DTaP B1<br>IPV B1<br>Hib B1 | The first booster (4th dose) may be administered as early as age 12 months, provided at least 6 months have elapsed since the third dose<br>*DTP:*<br>• First and second boosters should preferably be of DTwP<br>• Considering a higher reactogenicity of DTwP/DTaP can be considered for the boosters |
| 18 months | Hep-A 2 | *Hepatitis A:*<br>2nd dose for inactivated vaccines only |
| 2 years | Booster of Typhoid Conjugate Vaccine | • A booster dose of Typhoid conjugate vaccine (TCV), if primary dose is given at 9–12 months<br>• A dose of Typhoid Vi-polysaccharide(Vi-PS) vaccine can be given if conjugate vaccine is not available or feasible;<br>• Revaccination every 3 years with Vi-polysaccharide vaccine<br>• Typhoid conjugate vaccine should be preferred over Vi-PS vaccine |
| 4 to 6 years | DTwP B2/<br>DTaP B2<br>OPV 3<br>Varicella 2<br>MMR 3 | *Varicella:*<br>The 2nd dose can be given at anytime 3 months after the 1st dose.<br>*MMR:*<br>The 3rd dose is recommended at 4–6 years of age. |
| 10 to 12 years | Tdap/Td<br>HPV | *Tdap:*<br>is preferred to Td followed by Td every 10 years<br>*HPV:*<br>• Only 2 doses of either of the two HPV vaccines for adolescent/preadolescent girls aged 9-14 years;<br>• For girls 15 years and older, and immunocompromised individuals 3 doses are recommended<br>• For two-dose schedule, the minimum interval between doses should be 6 months.<br>• For 3 dose schedule, the doses can be administered at 0, 1-2 (depending on brand) and 6 months |

A typical wholesale cost of a DTwP-HepB-Hib pentavalent vaccine was about 15.40 USD in 2014.

## Types

Common versions of pentavalent vaccines include ComBE Five, Pentavac PFS, Easyfive, Pentaxim (DTaP), shan-5, and Quinvaxem (DTwP).

## Pentavac PFS

Pentavac PFS is a pentavalent vaccine manufactured in India by Pune-based pharmaceutical company Serum Institute of India and was the lowest cost pentavalent vaccine in India.

## Easyfive TT

Produced by Panacea Biotec, Easyfive was removed from the WHO's list of pre-approved and prequalified vaccines in mid-2011. Thereafter, in September 2013, WHO re-approved Easyfive after a positive result in the re-evaluation of the vaccine.

## Shan-5

Shan-5 is an efficient vaccine against Diphtheria, Tetanus, Pertusis, Hepatitis-b and HIB; produced by Shantha Biotech (A Sanofi Company). Shan-5 is WHO Prequalified vaccine and got WHO approval in the year 2014.

## ComBE Five

ComBE Five is the pentavalent vaccine manufactured in India by Hyderabad-based Pharmaceutical and Biologics company Biological E and was one of the lowest cost pentavalent vaccine in India with WHO approval.

## Quinvaxem

In March 2006, the Korea Food and Drug Administration (KFDA) awarded Quinvaxem the rights to distribution and sale. The vaccine was being developed and manufactured by Crucell in Korea and was co-produced by Chiron Corporation (that was eventually purchased by Novartis International AG on April 20, 2006), which provides four out of the five vaccine elements in bulk.

## Side Effects

- Gastrointestinal disorders: Common: diarrhea, vomng.
- General disorders and administration site conditions: Very common: Injection site pain and swelling accompanied by fever.
- Common: Injection site redness.
- Metabolism and nutrition disorders: Very common: feeding disorders.
- Nervous system disorders: Very common: sleepiness.
- Psychiatric disorders: Very common: irritability. Common: crying.

**Controversy**

***India***

Late 2013, it was found that the Pentavalent vaccine manufacturer—The Serum Institute in India was distributing 2 sets of Pentavac PFS vaccines for administration. One set with manufacturing and expiry dates was being provided to private hospitals, while the other set without manufacturing and expiry dates was being distributed to government hospitals. It was later clarified that the dates not appearing on one set of vaccines did not contravene any regulations as they were supplied by UNICEF and was legal under Rule 94 applicable to exports under Indian Law.

## MULTIPLE CHOICE QUESTIONS

1. **Temperature of the nursery must be maintained at:**
   (a) 26 +/- 2 degree centigrade
   (b) 30 +/- 2 degree centigrade
   (c) 28 +/- 2 degree centigrade
   (d) 36 +/- 2 degree centigrade
2. **Ballard scoring is used to assess neonates:**
   (a) Gestational age (b) Serum bilirubin level
   (c) Nutritional status (d) Asphyxia
3. **Confirmatory diagnostic tool for congenital aganglionic megacolon is:**
   (a) Barium swallow (b) Rectal biopsy
   (c) Barium enema (d) Rectosegmoidoscopy
4. **Anterior fontanel closes by:**
   (a) 1½ month (b) 12 month
   (c) 6 month (d) 18 month
5. **Febrile convulsion generally occurs between age of:**
   (a) 6 month–5 yrs (b) 1–5 yrs
   (c) 0–1 yr (d) Birth–5 yrs
6. **Vaccine given at the birth are:**
   (a) OPV + DPT (b) OPV + BCG
   (c) BCG + DPT (d) BCG + Measles
7. **As per 2004 census infant mortality rate is:**
   (a) 85/1000 live birth (b) 51/1000 live birth
   (c) 58/1000 live birth (d) 60/1000 live birth
8. **The ratio of chest compression to ventilation in new born ventilation is:**
   (a) 2:1 (b) 3 :1
   (c) 5 :2 (d) 3 :2
9. **The volume of blood required to be transfused in double volume exchange transfusion is:**
   (a) 80 mL/hr (b) 120 mL/hr
   (c) 160 mL/hr (d) 240 mL/hr
10. **Psychological development for adolescent is:**
    (a) Identity vs role confusion
    (b) Initiative vs guilt
    (c) Trust vs mistrust
    (d) Industry vs Inferiority
11. **A child with single transverse palmar crease, short neck with excessive skin at neck, a depressed nasal bridge and cardiac defect is most likely to have:**
    (a) Trisomy 21 (b) Trisomy 18
    (c) Trisomy 14 (d) Trisomy 13
12. **World breastfeeding week is celebrated from:**
    (a) 1st–7th August (b) 8th–14th August
    (c) 1st–7th September (d) 8th–14th September
13. **Components of integrated child development scheme are all EXCEPT:**
    (a) Supplementary nutrition
    (b) Immunization
    (c) Care in illness
    (d) Health check up
14. **Child achieves gratification by sucking at the breast of mouth and nipple of the bottle. The child is in:**
    (a) Anal stage (b) Phallic stage
    (c) Latency stage (d) Oral stage
15. **At well baby clinic, hydrocephalus may be suspected in an infant if on assessment nurse find:**
    (a) Overlapping of suture
    (b) Rapid increase in head circumference
    (c) Sunken fontales
    (d) Rapid increase in weight
16. **Visible peristaltic wave across the epigastrium region is indicative of:**
    (a) Infantile hypertropic pyloric stenosis
    (b) Imperforated anus
    (c) Intussusception
    (d) Short gut syndrome
17. **Desferal infusion is given to prevent toxicity caused by:**
    (a) Zinc (b) Calcium
    (c) Iron (d) Potassium
18. **Protein contain of 100mL breast milk is:**
    (a) 1.1 mg (b) 1.5 mg
    (c) 2.2 mg (d) 2.5 mg
19. **Nephritic syndrome is characterized by:**
    (a) Proteinuria (b) Hematuria
    (c) Hypertension (d) Weight loss
20. **Neural tube defect can be prevented by ingestion of:**
    (a) Riboflavin (b) Niacin
    (c) Iron (d) Folic acid
21. **Wasing and undernutrition is indicated if midarm circumference is:**
    (a) <13.5 (b) <12.5
    (c) <13 (d) <12
22. **Infant should be exclusively breast fed:**
    (a) Till 3 months of age (b) Till 5 months of age
    (c) Till 6 months of age (d) Till 9 months of age

**23. Subpriostal collection of blood secondary to injury during vaginal delivery:**
(a) Cephal hematoma
(b) Caput succedanum
(c) Toxic erythma
(d) Sub conjuctival hemorrhage

**24. In moderate dehydration the child is treated with:**
(a) Home made fluid (b) ORS
(c) IV fluid (d) Nil orally

**25. Septic meningitis is also called:**
(a) Fungal meningitis
(b) Bacterial meningitis
(c) Viral meningitis
(d) Tubercular meningitis

**26. Commonest malignancy is also called:**
(a) Acute lymphocytic leukemia
(b) Astrocytoma
(c) Wilms tumor
(d) Lymphoma

**27. Iron deficiency anemia can be differentiated by thalesemia by:**
(a) PBS (b) Hb F estimation
(c) Good history (d) Hb estimation

**28. The commonest preventable cause of mental retardation is:**
(a) Congenital hypothyroidism
(b) Down syndrome
(c) Birth asphyxia
(d) Congenital infection

**29. Drug used in patent ductus arteriosis is:**
(a) Prostaglandins (b) Indomethacin
(c) Sodium bicarbonate (d) Sidenafil

**30. Birth injury to spinal root of brachial plexus result in:**
(a) Apnea (b) Paralysis of arm
(c) Paralysis of leg (d) Shock

**31. Meatal opening located on the dorsal surface of penis is called:**
(a) Epispadiais (b) Hypospadias
(c) Chordee (d) Phimosis

**32. Common gastrointestinal sign for digoxin toxicity in children is:**
(a) Nausea/vomiting (b) Diarrhea
(c) Acidity (d) Colic pain

**33. Protrusion of abdominal organ through an opening in diaphragm is which type of hernia:**
(a) Hiatal (b) Diaphragmatic
(c) Abdominal (d) Inguinal

**34. Cervical esophagostomy is done in esophageal atresia to allow the passage of:**
(a) Mucus (b) Water
(c) Saliva (d) Pus

**35. Histamine (H2) receptors antagonist act to suppress the production of:**
(a) Acetic acid (b) Gastric acid
(c) Nitric acid (d) Sulphuric acid

**36. When photographic scale is used for rating pain in schooler, the number 5 or 10 means:**
(a) No hurt (b) Hurt little bit
(c) Hurts worst (d) Hurts even more

**37. Postural drainage helps to removethe excessive fluid or mucus in bronchi by:**
(a) Gravity (b) Siphon method
(c) Height (d) Weight

**38. Average weight gain during first 3 months of life is:**
(a) 30 gm/day (b) 10 gm/day
(c) 15 gm/day (d) 20 gm/ay

**39. The characteristic play during infancy is:**
(a) Parallel play (b) Associative play
(c) Solitary play (d) Cooperative play

**40. The psychological development attained by a school aged child is:**
(a) Autonomy vs shame or doubt
(b) Turst vs mistrust
(c) Initiative vs guilt
(d) Industry vs inferiority

**41. At the age of 5 years the head circumference will be:**
(a) 45 cm (b) 50 cm
(c) 48 cm (d) 53 cm

**42. A newborn weighing 2000 gms would be expected to have a head circumference of:**
(a) 25–26 cm (b) 27–28 cm
(c) 31–32 cm (d) 34–35 cm

**43. The caloric requirement of newborn in the second week of life is:**
(a) 80 cal/kg (b) 100 cal/kg
(c) 150 cal/kg (d) 120 cal/kg

**44. Prehension appear at the age of:**
(a) 6 months (b) 7 months
(c) 9 months (d) 12 months

**45. Which of the following finding confirm esophageal atresia:**
(a) Radiographs showing air in stomach and intestine
(b) Abdomen flat and scaphoid
(c) Repeated history of pneumonia
(d) Inbility to pass radio opaque catheter

**46. An increase in stool frequency and increase in water content with duration more than 14 days is which type of diarrhea:**
(a) Acute (b) Chronic
(c) Intractable (d) Chronic non specific

**47. Eating disorder characterized by repeated episode of consumption of large amount of caloric food is called:**
(a) Bulimia (b) Anorexia nervosa
(c) Over eating (d) Under eating

**48. Nacater amerianus (hook worm) in children causes:**
(a) Severe anemia (b) Fever
(c) Enlarged abdomen (d) Anorexia

**49. The developmental task of acquiring sense of autonomy while overcoming a sense of doubt and shame is in:**
(a) Infant (b) Toddler
(c) Preschool (d) Schooler

**50. An infant born between beginning of 38 weeks and completion of 42 week of gestation, regardless of birth weight is:**
(a) Pre-mature infant (b) Full term baby
(c) Post mature infant (d) Small infant

**51. To prevent the cremastic reflex, the child is made to sit in which position:**
(a) Fowler's position (b) Supine
(c) Tailor (d) Prone

**52. The site of injection to administer Inj. Vitamin K in neonate is:**
(a) Deltoid (b) Vastus lateralis
(c) Supra pubic (d) Abdominal muscle

**53. Rupture of blood vessel during delivery to produce bleeding between cranium bone and its perostenum is called:**
(a) Cephal edama (b) Cephal hematoma
(c) Caput succedaneum (d) Caput marginata

**54. The side effect of phototherapy in neonate are all from the following EXCEPT:**
(a) Greenish stool (b) Skin rashes
(c) Hypothermia (d) Hyperthermia

**55. The blood pressure should be measured with the cubital fossa at what level:**
(a) Eye level (b) Heart level
(c) Ear level (d) Nose level

**56. Bilateral or unilateral enlargement of breast in young boys during puberty is called:**
(a) Gynecomastia (b) Mastitis
(c) Breast engorgement (d) Enlarged breast

**57. Reducing the excretion of urinary protein and fluid retention in tissue is the therapeutic objective of:**
(a) Urinary infection (b) Cystitis
(c) Nephritic syndrome (d) Cellulitis

**58. The dilation of the renal pelvis from distention caused by collected urine above the obstruction is:**
(a) Hydronephrosis
(b) Glomerulonephrosis
(c) Pyelonephritis
(d) Caliculi

**59. The clinical manifestation of idiopathic thrombocytopenic purpura is:**
(a) Swelling (b) Petechiae
(c) Rash (d) Sneezing

**60. The eyes rolled upward, and immediate loss of consciousness is which type of seizure?**
(a) Partial (b) Generalized
(c) Complex (d) Atomic

**61. To prevent hypoxia, tracheal suctioning in children should be for:**
(a) 10 to 25 seconds (b) 30 to 55 seconds
(c) 60 to 75 seconds (d) 80 to 90 seconds

**62. In infant chest compression is done using two finger compression, compressing sternum to the depth of:**
(a) ½ to 1 inch (b) 2½ to 3 inch
(c) 4½ to 5 inch (d) 6½ to 7 inch

**63. Ototscopy is examination of which part of the body?**
(a) Lungs (b) Ears
(c) Eyes (d) Noses

**64. A type of skin traction with the lungs in an extended position is:**
(a) Russel traction (b) Buck traction
(c) Balance traction (d) Dunlop traction

**65. Fredet Ramstedt operation is done for:**
(a) Achalasia
(b) Gastroesophageal reflux disorder
(c) Congenital pyloric stenosis
(d) Hirchsprung disease

**66. 'Appropriate for gestational age' (AGA) is an infant whose weight falls between:**
(a) 10th and 90th percentile
(b) 20th and 90th percentile
(c) 30th and 90th percentile
(d) 40th and 90th percentile

**67. Which glands are enlarged when a child is suffering from mumps?**
(a) Pituitary (b) Salivary
(c) Parotid (d) Sweat

**68. 'Ego mastery' through play and environment is achieved by which age group children?**
(a) Infant (b) Toddler
(c) Pre- schooler (d) School –age

**69. Which of the following is NOT a cyanotic heart disease?**
(a) Trunchus arteriosus
(b) Tricuspid atresia
(c) Coarctation of aorta
(d) Tetralogy of fallot

**70. Bronchiolitis is caused by:**
(a) Pneumococcus
(b) Staphylococcus
(c) Respiratory syncytial virus
(d) Streptococcus

**71. Nephritic syndrome is charaterized by**
(a) Proteinuria, hypoalbuminemia and hypocholesterolemia
(b) Edema, albuniuria, hyperalbuminemia
(c) Proteinuria, hypoalbuminemia, hyperlipidemia and edema
(d) Hyperalbuminemia, edema and hematiria

**72. The following is not a major manifestation in Rh–fever according to modified jone's criteria:**
(a) Carditis
(b) Chorea
(c) Arthralgia
(d) Erythema marginatum

**73. In tetralogy of fallot, breathlessness is relivd by squatting position due to:**
(a) Increased systemic vascular resistance and reducing right to let shunt
(b) Increased venous return
(c) Improved blood flow
(d) Improved arterial bold flow

**74. Which of the following is NOT a component of tetralogy of fallot?**
(a) Left ventricular hypertrophy
(b) VSD
(c) Pulmonary stenosis
(d) Overriding of aorta

**75. Febrile seizure generally occur in the age group of:**
(a) 0 to 6 month (b) 6 months to 5 years
(c) 3 years to 8 years (d) 6 years to 10 years

**76. Persistence of a seizure for more than 10 min. or recurrent seizures without gain of consciousness is:**
(a) Unconsciousness (b) Grandma seizure
(c) Petimal seizure (d) Status epilepticus

**77. Pea soup stool and rose red spot over the abdomen are seen in case of:**
(a) Dengue fever (b) Cholera
(c) Typhoid fever (d) Diphtheria

**78. A painless palpable abdominal mas in one of the flanks is the cardinal presenting symptom in a case of:**
(a) Hydronephrosis (b) Nephroblastoma
(c) Polyystic kidney (d) Neuroblastoma

**79. A difference in blood pressure recorded in the upper and lower extremity is seen in case of:**
(a) Pulmonary stenosis (b) Aortic stenosis
(c) Coarctation of aorta (d) Systemic hypertension

**80. The fine downy hair covering the skin of a newborn is:**
(a) Vernix caseosa (b) Aortic stenosis
(c) Milia (d) Erythema toxicum

**81. Incubation period of chickenpox is:**
(a) 14–21 days (b) 10–12 days
(c) 8–12 days (d) 7–14 days

**82. The premature teeth that would erupt first are:**
(a) Incisors (b) Molar
(c) Pre-molar (d) Canines

**83. While lanning the care for a child with tetanus, the primary consideration should be to:**
(a) Reduce tactile and auditory stimuli
(b) Fed the child
(c) Give emotional support
(d) Administer oxygen

**84. Congenital hypoplasia of the lung on the affected side is seen incase of:**
(a) Omphalogocele (b) Hiatus hernia
(c) Inguinal hernia (d) Meningomyelocele

**85. Caput succedaneum disappears by the:**
(a) 3rd day (b) First week
(c) 10th days (d) Second week

**86. One ounce of milk gives approximately:**
(a) 10 calories (b) 20 calories
(c) 25 calories (d) 30 calories

**87. Following are the manifestations of increased intracranial pressure EXCEPT:**
(a) Rising BP (b) Rising pulse
(c) Vomiting (d) Headache

**88. Depostition of irón in various tissue of the body is known as:**
(a) Hemopoiesis (b) Hemolysis
(c) Hemosiderosis (d) Thrombolysis

**89. A viral infection in achild charaterized by a blotchy rash and koplik's spot the month is a case of:**
(a) Mumps (b) Rubella
(c) Rubeola (d) Chickenpox

**90. In terms of preventive care teaching, the parents of a one year old child should be given advise regarding:**
(a) Accidents (b) Toilet training
(c) Bonding (d) Sexual development

**91. The nurse should encourage two to 6 years old boys in playroom to play with:**
(a) Clay (b) Checkers
(c) A board game (d) A building block

**92. The man known as father of Pediatrics:**
(a) Benjami Spock (b) Abrahim Jacobi
(c) Hippocrates (d) Samhita

**93. In INDIA, baby friendly hospital concept was launched in the year:**
(a) 1990 (b) 1994
(c) 1992 (d) 1996

**94. The chrateristic play seen toddler is:**
(a) Independent play (b) Parallel play
(c) Onlooker play (d) Co-oprative play

**95. Commonest cause of neonatal death in India:**
(a) Prematurity (b) Metabolic diseases
(c) Birth injury (d) Congenital diseases

**96. Neonatal period extends upto:**
(a) 21 days (b) 28 days
(c) 30 days (d) 31 days

**97. The fine downey hair devoid of medulla, covering fetus is:**
(a) Smegrna (b) Vernix cseosa
(c) Languo (d) Mucus

**98. One of the following is not normal features of neonate:**
(a) Vaginal bleeding
(b) Hypospadiasis
(c) Witch's milk
(d) Scortam apperars pigmented with rugae

**99. In phototherapy distance between baby and the source of light in inches is:**
(a) 18 (b) 40
(c) 45 (d) 60

**100. The shape of posterior fontanel is..........:**
(a) Diamond (b) Square
(c) Circular (d) Triangular

**101. Umbilical cord has:**
(a) 2 veins and 2 arteries (b) 1 vein and 2 arteries
(c) 2 vein and 1 arteries (d) 1 vein and 1 artery

**102. Commonest cause of pathological hyerbilirubinemia in INDIA is:**
(a) ABO incompatibility (b) Rh incompatibility
(c) Infection (d) G6PD deficiency

**103. Fetal Hb is eplaced by adult Hb completely at:**
(a) At birth (b) 2 Months
(c) 4 Months (d) 6 Months

**104. Diagnosis for rheumatic fever is well confirmed by:**
(a) Throat swab culture (b) ASLO Titer
(c) Raised ESR (d) ECG changes

**105. In nephritic syndrome the essential feature is:**
(a) Proteinuria (b) Hypoalbuminemia
(c) Hyperlipemia (d) Edema

**106. The drug of choice for status epilectic in children is:**
(a) Hydantoin (b) Phenobarbiturate
(c) Diazepam (d) Carbamezapine

**107. Most common presentation in neonatal meningitis is:**
(a) Bulging fontanels (b) Poor feeding
(c) Nuchal rigidity (d) Convulsion

**108. Normal pressure hydrocephalus is characterized by:**
(a) Aphesia (b) Dementia
(c) Ataxia (d) Urinary disturbance

**109. Which is the syndrome of over worked myocardium:**
(a) Congestive cardiac failure
(b) Acute respiratory failure
(c) Cardiac arrest
(d) Cancer

**110. Among which of the following in not a live vaccine?**
(a) Polio (b) Typhoid
(c) Plague (d) Hepatitis B

**111. Psychosexual theory of growth and development is given by:**
(a) Jean piaget (b) Erikson
(c) Kholberg (d) Freuid

**112. First permanent tooth which erupt is:**
(a) 1st molar (b) 1st premolar
(c) 1st incisor (d) 2nd premolar

**113. The period of ovum is:**
(a) 0 to 14 days (b) 14 days to 9 weeks
(c) 280 days (d) 9 weeks to birth

**114. Visual acuity reaches the adult acuity by the age of:**
(a) 7 (c) 5
(b) 9 (d) 3

**115. In a child cessation of breath for 20 sec. with bradycardia is:**
(a) Apnea (b) Dyspnea
(c) Arrhythmia (d) Seizures

**116. The earlier indicator of PEM is:**
(a) Hair changes (b) Edema
(c) Under weight for age (d) Restlessness

**117. Organism responsible for bronchiolitis is:**
(a) Adenovirus (b) Influenza virus
(c) Rhino virus (d) RSV

**118. Which of the following is not seen in nephritic syndrome:**
(a) Proteinurea
(b) Hyperalbuminemia
(c) Hyperlipedemia
(d) Edema

**119. Obstruction of outflow of CSF with in the ventricular system is:**
(a) Communicating hydrocephalus
(b) Non communicating hydrocephalus
(c) Meningocele
(d) Myelomeninggocele

**120. Regression is common in:**
(a) Toddler (b) Infant
(c) Pre-school (d) Schooler

**121. Telescoping of bowel into an adjacent section is called:**
(a) Obstruction (b) Strangulation
(c) Volvulus (d) Intussuception

**122. Swensens technique of surgical management is used in:**
(a) Pyloric stenosis (b) Esophageal atresia
(c) Imperforated anus (d) Megacolon

**123. Congenital absence of an opening or canal is called:**
(a) Agenesis (b) Atresia
(c) Fistula (d) None of the above

**124. Tricyclic antidepressant is the drug of choice in:**
(a) Enurasis (b) Failure of thrive
(c) Undescended testis (d) Hypospediasis

**125. Color of diptheric membrane is:**
(a) Yellow (c) Cream
(b) Grey (d) White

**126. Chicken pox is caused by:**
(a) Vericella zoster (b) RSV
(c) Myxovirus (d) H influenza

**127. Finger sucking can cause:**
(a) Malocclusion (b) Facial distortion
(c) Speech difficulty (d) All the above

**128. Eating of non-edible items is known as:**
(a) Pica (b) Enuresis
(c) Encopresis (d) Somnambulism

**129. A child develops leg pain, headache, abdominal pain fever and refusal to school is suspected for:**
(a) Conversion neurosis (b) Stealing
(c) School phobia (d) Lying

**130. Denver developmental screening test is used for:**
(a) Mental retardation (b) Cerebral palsy
(c) Visual palsy (d) Healing impairment

**131. Passes of stool at inappropriate places is known as:**
(a) Enurasis (b) Somnambulism
(c) Encopresis (d) Tics

**132. Squint or cross eye is known as:**
(a) Opacity of lens (b) Glaucoma
(c) Cataract (d) Strabismus

**133. Herniation of abdominal organ into umbilical cordis known as:**
(a) Fistula (b) Fissure
(c) Intussusceptions (d) Omphalocele

**134. Vitamin B1 is also known as:**
(a) Thiamine (b) Riboflavin
(c) Niacin (d) Cobalamin

135. **Mostely death in PEM is due to all EXCEPT:**
(a) Hypothermia (b) CCF
(c) Worm infestation (d) Electrolytic imbalance

136. **Indecation of fetal distress:**
(a) Decrease in fetal scalp blood
(b) Meconium staining
(c) Late declaration of heart rate
(d) All the above

137. **In kernicture which is increased:**
(a) Conjugated bilirubin
(b) Unconjugated bilirubin
(c) Both
(d) None

138. **The shape of anterior fontanel is:**
(a) Circular (b) Square
(c) Diamond (d) Triangle

139. **Tetrology of fallot includes all except:**
(a) Atrial septal defect
(b) Pulmonary stenosis
(c) Overriding of aorta
(d) Right ventricular hypertrophy

140. **The most common type of esophageal atresia with trachio-esophageal fistula is:**
(a) Esophageal atresia
(b) Esophageal atresia with proximal TEF
(c) Esophageal atresia with distal TEF
(d) Trachio- esophageal fistula

141. **Convulsion is a side effect of:**
(a) OPV (c) BCG
(b) DPT (d) Measles.

142. **The term development refers to:**
(a) Functional maturity
(b) Increase in cell size and function
(c) Increase in cell size
(d) Increase in intracellular substances

143. **The most important factor affecting growth and development is:**
(a) Teratogens
(b) Diseases
(c) Genetics and environment
(d) Genetics and nutrition

144. **Shakirs tape is used for:**
(a) Measurement of height
(b) Measurement of length
(c) Measurement of mid-arm circumference
(d) Measurement of skin pad thickness

145. **The papules on the face of new born are:**
(a) Milia (b) Urticaria
(c) Exanthema (d) Sebaceous glands

146. **One of the major intervention to bring down the infant mortality rate is:**
(a) Integrated management of neonatal and childhood illness
(b) Panchayati Raj
(c) Primary Health Center
(d) Sub-center

147. **Z plasty is a surgical procedure done for the repair of:**
(a) Cleft lip (b) Cleft palate
(c) Both (a) and (b) (d) None of the above

148. **Characteristic feature in the pre-eruptive phase of measles is:**
(a) Vesicles (b) Sore throat
(c) Koplik spots (d) Boils

149. **The most common acyanotic congenital heart disease with left to right shuntis:**
(a) Atrial septal defect
(b) Ventricular septal defect
(c) Patent ductus arteriosis
(d) Etrology fallot

150. **The condition which is characterized anemia, thrombocytopenia and neutropenia specially granulocytopenia is:**
(a) Leukemia
(b) Thalesemia
(c) Hemophilia
(d) Thrombocytopenia purpura

151. **Bag and mask ventilation is contraindicated in:**
(a) Cleft lip
(b) Trachea- esophageal fistula
(c) Meningo-myelocoele
(d) Diaphragmatic hernia

152. **The clinical parameters normally affected in Protein – Energy malnutrition is:**
(a) Height
(b) Weight
(c) Mid arm circumference
(d) Head circumference

153. **The ideal method of administration of oxygen to children is by:**
(a) Hood (b) Nasel catheter
(c) Mask (d) Ventilator

154. **In Thalesemia major blood is transfused to maintain hemoglobin level above:**
(a) 8–10 gm/dl (b) 10–12 gm/dl
(c) 12–14 gm/dl (d) 14–16 gm/dl

155. **The failure of one or both testes to descent from abdominal cavity to the scrotum is known as:**
(a) Hydrocoele (b) Hernia
(c) Phimosis (d) Crypto- orchidism

156. **In NALS protocol heart rate is counted for:**
(a) 5 sec (b) 6 sec
(c) 15 sec (d) 60 sec

157. **Moro's reflex completes at gestation of:**
(a) 40 weeks (b) 36 weeks
(c) 32 weeks (d) 24 weeks

158. **Child presenting with painless abdominal mass, fever, abdominal pain and hematuria is suspected for:**
(a) Neuroblastoma
(b) Retinoblastoma
(c) Chronic lymphoid leukemia
(d) Wims tumor

**159. The organism isolated by Shick test is:**
(a) Cornybacterium diphtheria
(b) N gonorrhea
(c) Meningococci
(d) Pnemococci

**160. The curative treatment for congenital syphilis includes:**
(a) Prenidolone
(b) Streptomycin
(c) 1.2 Mega unit of Benzathine penicillin
(d) Tetracycline

**161. In IMNCI guidelines the pin color refers to:**
(a) Suggestion for referral
(b) Treatment in health facilities
(c) Management at home
(d) None of the above

**162. Carneotabes in infant below six months of age is an early signs of:**
(a) Rickets
(b) Hydrocephalus
(c) Scurvy
(d) Beriberi

## ANSWERS

| | | | | | | | | | | | |
|---|---|---|---|---|---|---|---|---|---|---|---|
| **1.** | (d) | **31.** | (b) | **61.** | (a) | **91.** | (c) | **121.** | (a) | **151.** | (d) |
| **2.** | (a) | **32.** | (a) | **62.** | (a) | **92.** | (b) | **122.** | (c) | **152.** | (b) |
| **3.** | (c) | **33.** | (b) | **63.** | (b) | **93.** | (c) | **123.** | (b) | **153.** | (a) |
| **4.** | (d) | **34.** | (b) | **64.** | (d) | **94.** | (a) | **124.** | (a) | **154.** | (b) |
| **5.** | (d) | **35.** | (b) | **65.** | (c) | **9.5.** | (c) | **125.** | (c) | **155** | (d) |
| **6.** | (b) | **36.** | (b) | **66.** | (a) | **96.** | (b) | **126.** | (a) | **156.** | (c) |
| **7.** | (c) | **37.** | (a) | **67.** | (b) | **97.** | (c) | **127.** | (c) | **157.** | (b) |
| **8.** | (b) | **38.** | (d) | **68.** | (c) | **98.** | (a) | **128.** | (a) | **158.** | (d) |
| **9.** | (c) | **39.** | (b) | **69.** | (c) | **99.** | (c) | **129.** | (c) | **159.** | (a) |
| **10.** | (a) | **40.** | (d) | **70.** | (c) | **100.** | (d) | **130.** | (a) | **160.** | (c) |
| **11.** | (a) | **41.** | (b) | **71.** | (c) | **101.** | (b) | **131.** | (c) | **161.** | (a) |
| **12.** | (a) | **42.** | (d) | **72.** | (c) | **102.** | (b) | **132.** | (d) | **162.** | (b) |
| **13.** | (c) | **43.** | (b) | **73.** | (b) | **103.** | (d) | **133.** | (d) | | |
| **14.** | (d) | **44.** | (a) | **74.** | (a) | **104.** | (b) | **134.** | (a) | | |
| **15.** | (b) | **45.** | (d) | **75.** | (b) | **105.** | (a) | **135.** | (b) | | |
| **16.** | (a) | **46.** | (b) | **76.** | (d) | **106.** | (c) | **136.** | (d) | | |
| **17.** | (c) | **47.** | (a) | **77.** | (c) | **107.** | (d) | **137.** | (b) | | |
| **18.** | (a) | **48.** | (a) | **78.** | (b) | **108.** | (b) | **138.** | (c) | | |
| **19.** | (a) | **49.** | (b) | **79.** | (c) | **109.** | (a) | **139.** | (d) | | |
| **20.** | (d) | **50.** | (b) | **80.** | (a) | **110.** | (a) | **140.** | (c) | | |
| **21.** | (d) | **51.** | (c) | **81.** | (a) | **111.** | (b) | **141.** | (b) | | |
| **22.** | (c) | **52.** | (b) | **82.** | (a) | **112.** | (c) | **142.** | (a) | | |
| **23.** | (a) | **53.** | (b) | **83.** | (a) | **113.** | (a) | **143.** | (d) | | |
| **24.** | (b) | **54.** | (d) | **84.** | (b) | **114.** | (c) | **144.** | (c) | | |
| **25.** | (b) | **55.** | (b) | **85.** | (a) | **115.** | (a) | **145.** | (a) | | |
| **26.** | (c) | **56.** | (a) | **86.** | (b) | **116.** | (c) | **146.** | (a) | | |
| **27.** | (d) | **57.** | (c) | **87.** | (b) | **117.** | (d) | **147.** | (b) | | |
| **28.** | (a) | **58.** | (a) | **88.** | (c) | **118.** | (b) | **148.** | (c) | | |
| **29.** | (b) | **59.** | (b) | **89.** | (b) | **119.** | (b) | **149.** | (a) | | |
| **30.** | (b) | **60.** | (b) | **90.** | (a) | **120.** | (a) | **150.** | (a) | | |

# QUICK REVIEW

## Mental Health Nursing Review and Multiple Choice Questions

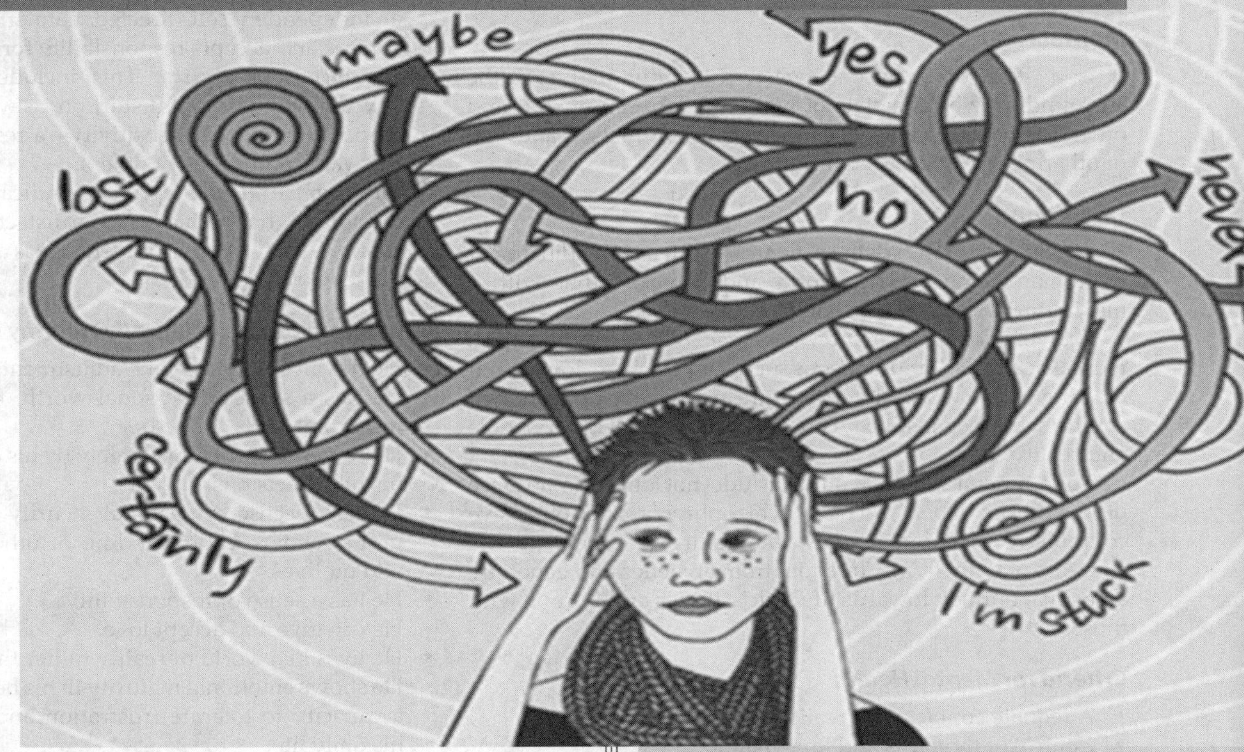


### HIGHLIGHTS

- Mental Health and Mental Illness
- Principles and Concepts of Mental Health Nursing
- Concepts of Personality Development
- The Therapeutic Nurse-Patient Relationship
- The Individual with Functional Psychiatric Disorder
- Classification of Organic Mental Disorders
- Organic Amnestic Syndrome
- Childhood Psychiatric Disorders
- Therapeutic Modalities in Psychiatry
- Legal Aspects of Mental Health Nursing
- Multiple Choice Questions

# Mental Health Nursing or Psychiatric Nursing

## MENTAL HEALTH AND MENTAL ILLNESS

### Mental Health

It is a state of balance between the individual and the surrounding world, a state of harmony between oneself and others, a coexistence between the realities of the self and that of other people and the environment.

#### *Definitions*

*Karl Menninger* (1947) defines mental health as 'An adjustment of human beings to the world and to each other with a maximum of effectiveness and happiness.'

*The American Psychiatric Association* (APA, 1980) defines mental health as: 'Simultaneous success at working, loving and creating with the capacity for mature and flexible resolution of conflicts between instincts, conscience, important other people and reality'.

Thus mental health would include not only the absence of diagnostic labels such as schizophrenia and obsessive compulsive disorder, but also the ability to cope with the stressors of daily living, freedom from anxieties and generally a positive outlook towards life's vicissitudes and to cope with those.

#### *Criteria for Mental Health*

- Adequate contact with reality
- Control of thoughts and imagination
- Efficiency in work and play
- Social acceptance
- Positive self-concept
- A healthy emotional life

#### *Indicators of Mental Health*

Jahoda (1958) has identified six indicators of mental health which include:

1. ***A positive attitude towards self:*** This includes an objective view of self, including knowledge and acceptance of strengths and limitations. The individual feels a strong sense of personal identity and security within the environment.
2. ***Growth, development and the ability for self-actualization:*** This indicator correlates with whether the individual successfully achieves the tasks associated with each level of development.
3. ***Integration:*** Integration includes the ability to adaptively respond to the environment and the development of a philosophy of life, both of which help the individual maintain anxiety at a manageable level in response to stressful situations.
4. ***Autonomy:*** It refers to the individual's ability to perform, in an independent self-directed manner; the individual makes choices and accepts responsibility for the outcomes.
5. ***Perception of reality:*** This includes perception of the environment without distortion, as well as the capacity for empathy and social sensitivity—a respect and concern for the wants and needs of others.
6. ***Environmental mastery:*** This indicator suggests that the individual has achieved a satisfactory role within the group, society or environment. He is able to love and accept the love of others.

#### *Characteristics of a Mentally Healthy Person*

- He has an ability to make adjustments.
- He has a sense of personal worth, feels worthwhile and important.
- He solves his problems largely by his own effort and makes his own decisions.
- He has a sense of personal security and feels secure in a group, shows understanding of other people's problems and motives.
- He has a sense of responsibility.
- He can give and accept love.
- He lives in a world of reality rather than fantasy.
- He shows emotional maturity in his behavior, and develops a capacity to tolerate frustration and disappointments in his daily life.
- He has developed a philosophy of life that gives meaning and purpose to his daily activities.
- He has a variety of interests and generally lives a well-balanced life of work, rest and recreation.

### Mental Illness

Mental illness is maladjustment in living. It produces a disharmony in the person's ability to meet human needs comfortably or effectively and function within a culture.

A mentally ill person loses his ability to respond according to the expectations he has for himself and the demands that society has for him. In general an individual may be considered to be mentally ill if:

- The person's behavior is causing distress and suffering to self and/or others.
- The person's behavior is causing disturbance in his day-to-day activities, job and interpersonal relationships.

#### *Definition*

Mental and behavioral disorders are understood as clinically significant conditions characterized by alterations in thinking, mood (emotions) or behavior associated with personal distress and/ or impaired functioning. *(WHO, 2001)*

### Characteristics of Mental Illness

- Changes in one's thinking, memory, perception, feeling and judgment resulting in changes in talk and behavior which appear to be deviant from previous personality or from the norms of community.
- These changes in behavior cause distress and suffering to the individual or others or both.
- Changes and the consequent distress cause disturbance in day-to-day activities, work and relationship with important others (social and vocational dysfunction).

### Features of Mental Illness

The features of mental illness are classified under four headings. These are:

1. Disturbances in bodily functions
2. Disturbances in mental functions
3. Changes in individual and social activities
4. Somatic complaints.

### Common Signs and Symptoms of Mental Illness

- *Disturbances in motor behavior*
  - Motor retardation, stupor, stereotypes, negativism, ambitendence, waxy flexibility, echopraxia, restlessness, agitation and excitement.
- *Disorders of thought, language and communication*
  - Pressure of speech, poverty of speech, dysarthria, flight of ideas, circumstantiality, loosening of association, tangentiality, incoherence, perseveration, neologism, clang association, thought block, thought insertion, thought broadcasting, echolalia, delusions, obsessions and phobias.
- *Disorders of perception*
  - Illusions, hallucinations, depersonalization, derealization.
- *Disorders of emotion*
  - Blunt affect, labile affect, elated mood, euphoria, ecstasy, dysphoric mood, depression, anhedonia.
- *Disturbances of consciousness*
  - Clouding of consciousness, delirium and coma.
- *Disturbances in attention*
  - Distractibility, selective inattention.
- *Disturbances in orientation*
  - Disorientation of time, place or person.
- *Disturbances of memory*
  - Amnesia, confabulation.
- *Impaired judgment*
- *Disturbances in biological function*
  - Persistent deviations in temperature, pulse and respiration, nausea, vomiting, headache, loss of appetite, increased appetite, loss of weight, pain, fatigue, weight gain, insomnia, hypersomnia and sexual dysfunction.

## ETIOLOGY OF MENTAL ILLNESS

Many factors are responsible for the causation of mental illness. These factors may predispose an individual to mental illness, precipitate or perpetuate the mental illness.

### Predisposing Factors

These factors determine an individual's susceptibility to mental illness. They interact with precipitating factors resulting in mental illness. These are:

- Genetic make up
- Physical damage to the central nervous system
- Adverse psychosocial influence.

### Precipitating Factors

These are events that occur shortly before the onset of a disorder and appear to have induced it. These are:

- Physical stress
- Psychosocial stress.

### Perpetuating Factors

These factors are responsible for aggravating or prolonging the diseases already existing in an individual. Psychosocial stress is an example. Thus etiological factors of mental illness can be:

- Biological factors
- Physiological changes
- Psychological factors
- Social factors.

### Biological Factors

*Heredity*

What one inherits is not the illness or its symptoms, but a predisposition to the illness, which is determined by genes that we inherit directly. Studies have shown that three-fourths of mental defectives and one-third of psychotic individuals owe their condition mainly to unfavorable heredity.

*Biochemical Factors*

Biochemical abnormalities in the brain are considered to be the cause of some psychological disorders. Disturbance in neurotransmitters in the brain is found to play an important role in the etiology of certain psychiatric disorders.

*Brain Damage*

Any damage to the structure and functioning of the brain can give rise to mental illness. Damage to the structure of the brain may be due to one of the following causes:

- Infection: For example, neurosyphilis, encephalitis, HIV infection, etc.
- Injury: Loss of brain tissue due to head injury.
- Intoxication: Damage to brain tissue due to toxins such as alcohol, barbiturates, lead, etc.
- Vascular: Poor blood supply, bleeding (intracranial hemorrhage, subarachnoid hemorrhage, subdural hemorrhage).
- Alteration in brain function: Changes in blood chemistry that interfere with brain functioning such as disturbance in blood glucose levels, hypoxia, anoxia, and fluid and electrolyte imbalance
- Tumors: Brain tumors
- Vitamin deficiency and malnutrition, in particular deficiency of vitamin B-complex.
- Degenerative diseases: Dementia

- Endocrine disturbances: Hypothyroidism, thyrotoxicosis, etc.
- Physical defects and physical illness: Acute physical illness as well as chronic illnesses with all their handicapping conditions may result in loss of mental capacities.

### Physiological Changes

It has been observed that mental disorders are more likely to occur at certain critical periods of life namely—puberty, menstruation, pregnancy, delivery, puerperium and climacteric. These periods are marked not only by physiological (endocrine) changes, but also by psychological issues that diminish the adaptive capacity of the individual. Thus the individual becomes more susceptible to mental illness during this period.

### Psychological Factors

- It is observed that some specific personality types are more prone to develop certain psychological disorders. For example, those who are unsocial and reserved (schizoid) are vulnerable to schizophrenia when they face adverse situations and psychosocial stresses.
- Psychological factors like strained interpersonal relationships at home, place of work, school or college, bereavement, loss of prestige, loss of job, etc.
- Childhood insecurities due to parents with pathological personalities, faulty attitude of parents (overstrictness, over leniency), abnormal parent-child relationship (over-protection, rejection, unhealthy comparisons), deprivation of child's essential psychological and social needs, etc.
- Social and recreational deprivations resulting in boredom, isolation and alienation.
- Marriage problems like forced bachelorhood, disharmony due to physical, emotional, social, educational or financial incompatibility, childlessness, too many children, etc.
- Sexual difficulties arising out of improper sex education, unhealthy attitudes towards sexual functions, guilt feelings about masturbation, pre and extramarital sex relations, worries about sexual perversions.
- Stress, frustration and seasonal variations are sometimes noted in the occurrence of mental diseases.

### Social Factors

- Poverty, unemployment, injustice, insecurity, migration, urbanization
- Gambling, alcoholism, prostitution, broken homes, divorce, very big family, religion, traditions, political upheavals and other social crises.

## MENTAL HEALTH TEAM OR MULTIDISCIPLINARY TEAM

Multidisciplinary approach refers to collaboration between members of different disciplines who provide specific services to the patient. The multidisciplinary team includes:

- *A psychiatrist* is a medical doctor with special training in psychiatry. He is accountable for the medical diagnosis and treatment of patient. Other important functions are:
  - Admitting patient into acute care setting
  - Prescribing and monitoring psychopharmacologic agents
  - Administering electroconvulsive therapy
  - Conducting individual and family therapy
  - Participating in interdisciplinary team meetings
  - Owing to their legal power to prescribe and to write orders, psychiatrists often function as leaders of the team.
- *A psychiatric nurse* is a registered nurse with specialized training in the care and treatment of psychiatric patients, she may have a Diploma, MSc, MPhil or PhD in psychiatric nursing. She is accountable for the biopsychosocial nursing care of patients and their milieu. Other functions include:
  - Administering and monitoring medications
  - Assisting in numerous psychiatric and physical treatments
  - Participate in interdisciplinary team meetings
  - Teach patients and families
  - Take responsibility for patient's records
  - Act as patient's advocate
  - Interact with patients' significant others.
- *A clinical psychologist* should have a Masters Degree in Psychology or PhD in clinical psychology with specialized training in mental health settings. He is accountable for psychological assessments, testing, and treatments. He offers direct services such as individual, family or marital therapies.
- *A psychiatric social worker* should have a Masters Degree in Social Work or PhD degree with specialized training in mental health settings. He is accountable for family case work and community placement of patients. He conducts group therapy sessions. He emphasizes intervention with the patient in social environment in which he will live.
- *An occupational therapist or an activity therapist* is accountable for recreational, occupational and activity programs. He assists the patients to gain skills that help them cope more effectively to gain or retain employment, to use leisure time.
- *A pharmacist and a dietitian*
- *A counselor* provides basic supportive counseling and assists in psycho educational and recreational activities.

## CLASSIFICATION OF MENTAL DISORDERS

### ICDIO (International Statistical Classification of Disease and Related Health Problems)—1992

This is WHO's classification for all diseases and related health problems. The chapter 'F' classifies psychiatric disorders as mental and behavioral disorders and codes them on an alphanumeric system from F00 to F99.

#### The Main Categories in ICDIO F00–F09 Organic, Including Symptomatic, Mental Disorders

| | |
|---|---|
| F00 | Dementia in Alzheimer's disease |
| F01 | Vascular dementia |
| F04 | Organic amnestic syndrome |
| F05 | Delirium |
| F06 | Other mental disorders due to brain damage and dysfunction and to physical disease |
| F07 | Personality and behavioral disorders due to brain disease, damage and dysfunction. |

***F10–F19 Mental and Behavioral Disorders Due to Psychoactive Substance Use***

F10 Mental and behavioral disorders due to use of alcohol
F11 Mental and behavioral disorders due to use of opioids
F12 Mental and behavioral disorders due to use of cannabinoids
F13 Mental and behavioral disorder due to sedative or hypnotic
F14 Mental or behavioral disorder due to cocaine
F16 Mental or behavioral disorder due to use of hallucinogens.

***F20–F29 Schizophrenia, Schizotypal and Delusional Disorder***

F20 Schizophrenia
F20.0 Paranoid schizophrenia
F20.1 Hebephrenic schizophrenia
F20. 2 Catatonic schizophrenia
F20. 3 Undifferentiated schizophrenia
F20.4 Postschizophrenic depression
F20.5 Residual schizophrenia
F20.6 Simple schizophrenia
F21 Schizotypal disorder
F22 Persistent delusional disorders
F23 Acute and transient psychotic disorders
F24 Induced delusional disorders
F25 Schizoaffective disorders.

***F30–F39 Mood (Affective) Disorders***

F30 Manic episode
F31 Bipolar affective disorder
F32 Depressive episode
F33 Recurrent depressive disorder
F34 Persistent mood disorder

***F40–F49 Neurotic, Stress-related and Somatoform Disorders***

F40 Phobic anxiety disorders
F41 Other anxiety disorders
F42 Obsessive compulsive disorder
F43 Reaction to severe stress, and adjustment disorders
F44 Dissociative (conversion) disorders
F45 Somatoform disorders.

***F50–F59 Behavioral Syndromes Associated with Physiological Disturbances and Physical Factors***

F50 Eating disorders
F51 Nonorganic sleep disorders
F52 Sexual dysfunction, not caused by organic disorder or disease

***F60–F69 Disorders of Adult Personality and Behavior***

F60 Specific personality disorders
F60.0 Paranoid personality disorder
F60.1 Schizoid personality disorder
F60.2 Dissocial personality disorder
F60.3 Emotionally unstable personality disorder
F60.4 Histrionic personality disorder
F60.5 Anankastic personality disorder
F60.6 Anxious personality disorder
F60.7 Dependent personality disorder
F61 Mixed and other personality disorders
F62 Enduring personality changes, not Attributable to brain damage and disease
F63 Habit and impulse disorders
F64 Gender identity disorders
F65 Disorders of sexual preference.

***F70–F79 Mental Retardation***

F70 Mild mental retardation
F71 Moderate mental retardation
F72 Severe mental retardation
F73 Profound mental retardation

***F80–F89 Disorders of Psychological Development***

F80 Specific developmental disorders of speech and language
F81 Specific developmental disorders of scholastic skills
F82 Specific developmental disorder of motor function
F83 Mixed specific developmental disorders
F84 Pervasive developmental disorders

***F90–F98 Behavioral and Emotional Disorders with Onset Usually Occurring in Childhood and Adolescence***

F90 Hyperkinetic disorders
F91 Conduct disorders
F93 Emotional disorders with onset specific to childhood
F94 Disorders of social functioning with onset specific to childhood and adolescence
F95 Tic disorders
F98 Other behavioral and emotional disorders with onset usually occurring in childhood and adolescence.

***F99 Unspecified Mental Disorder***

## DSM IV (Diagnostic and Statistical Manual)–1994

This is the classification of mental disorders by the American Psychiatric Association (APA). The pattern adopted by DSM IV is of multiaxial systems. A multiaxial system that evaluates patients along several versatiles contains five axes. Axis I and II make up the entire classification which contains more than 300 specific disorders. The five axes of DSM IV are:

1. *AXIS I:* Clinical psychiatric diagnosis
2. *AXIS II:* Personality disorder and mental retardation
3. *AXIS III:* General medical conditions
4. *AXIS IV:* Psychosocial and environmental problems
5. *AXIS V:* Global assessment of functioning in current and past one year.

## Indian Classification

In India Neki (1963),Wig and Singer (1967), Vahia (1961) and Varma (1971) have attempted some modifications of ICD8 to suit Indian conditions. They are broadly grouped as follows:

### Psychosis

- Functional
  - Schizophrenia
  - Hebephrenic schizophrenia
  - Catatonic schizophrenia
  - Paranoid schizophrenia
- Affective
  - Mania
  - Depression
- Organic
  - Acute
  - Chronic.

### Neurosis

- Anxiety neurosis
- Depression neurosis
- Hysterical neurosis
- Obsessive compulsive neurosis
- Phobic neurosis.

### Special Disorder

- Childhood disorder
  - Conduct disorder
  - Emotional disorder
- Personality disorder
  - Sociopath
  - Psychopath
- Substance abuse
  - Alcohol abuse
  - Drug abuse
- Psychophysiological disorder
  - Asthma
  - Psoriasis
- Mental retardation
  - Mild
  - Moderate
  - Severe
  - Profound.

## PRINCIPLES AND CONCEPTS OF MENTAL HEALTH NURSING

### Psychiatry

It is a branch of medicine that deals with the diagnosis, treatment and prevention of mental illness.

### Psychiatric Nursing

It is a specialized area of nursing practice, employing theories of human behavior as it is a science, and the purposeful use of self as it is an art, in the diagnosis and treatment of human responses to actual or potential mental health problems. (American Nurses Association, 1994).

### Psychiatric Nursing Skills

Mental health nursing is the practice of promoting mental health as well as caring for people who have mental illness, potentiating their independency and restoring their dignity.

### Prerequisites for a Mental Health Nurse

*Personal Skills*

- ***Self-awareness:*** It is a key component of psychiatric nursing experience. It is an answer to the question, 'who am I'. The nurse must be able to examine personal feelings, actions and reactions as a provider of care. A firm understanding and acceptance by the nurse allows acknowledging a patient's differences and uniqueness.
- ***Adaptability:*** A mental health nurse needs to be adaptable to different settings and cultures. A mental health nurse also needs to cope with a variety of social and cultural settings. Social settings involve the class and status of the individuals while cultural settings involve race, ethnicity and gender. Therefore she may need to be familiar with the issues that arise in cross cultural mental health nursing.

*Care Values and Attitudes*

These include:

- Self-awareness and self-esteem
- Respecting the person's rights
- Listening
- Responding with care and respect
- Supporting with trust and confidence
- Reassuring with explanation and honesty
- Physically nursing the helpless with compassion
- Carrying out procedures skillfully
- Working within personal and ethical boundaries.

*Counseling Skills*

These include:

- Unconditional positive regard/nonjudgmental approach
- Empathy
- Warmth and genuineness
- Confidentiality
- Nonverbal sensitivity, nonverbal attending, nonverbal responding
- Other interpersonal skills required are paraphrasing, reflecting, clarifying, summarizing.

*Behavioral Skills*

These are based on Pavlovian principles and Skinner's principles. They include:

- To increase adaptive behavior:
  - Positive reinforcement
  - Negative reinforcement
  - Token economy.
- To decrease maladaptive behavior:
  - Extinction
  - Time out
  - Restraining
  - Over correction.
- To teach new behavior:
  - Modeling
  - Shaping
  - Chaining
  - Cueing.

*Supervisory Skills*

Supervision is an integral necessity for any worker in the caring profession, to ensure the best quality service for clients and best quality developmental opportunities for workers. A good supervisor requires interpersonal and professional skills, technical knowledge, leadership qualities and human skills.

*Crisis Skills*

Aggressive and assaultive behavior of violent patients, self-harm, acute alcohol intoxication are some of the cases a nurse is likely to encounter in the course of her practice. Such situations may cause the nurse to feel overwhelmed with feelings of helplessness, powerlessness and inadequacy. Exercise of self-control, calm, rational thinking and identifying ways of obtaining help from the other people are some of the skills to be cultivated by the psychiatric nurse when confronted with such crises situations.

*Teaching Skills*

This relates to the nurse's ability to explain, enabling full understanding on the part of the client. It also involves enhancing the client's environment in order to maximize his awareness of the things around him. It is necessary for the nurse to be enthusiastic about activities and choices of the clients and also give the client every opportunity to use his power of judgment in order to make decisions.

## STANDARDS OF MENTAL HEALTH NURSING

The standards presented here are a revision of the standards enunciated by the Division on Psychiatric and Mental Health Nursing Practice in 1973.

### Professional Practice Standards

#### *Standard I: Theory*

The nurse applies appropriate theory that is scientifically sound as a basis for decisions regarding nursing practice.

#### *Standard II: Data Collection*

The nurse continuously collects data that are comprehensive, accurate and systematic.

#### *Standard III: Diagnosis*

The nurse utilizes nursing diagnoses and/ or standard classification of mental disorders to express conclusions supported by recorded assessment data and current scientific premises.

#### *Standard IV: Planning*

The nurse develops a nursing care plan with specific goals and interventions delineating nursing actions unique to each client's needs. The nursing care plan is used to guide therapeutic intervention and effectively achieve the desired outcomes.

#### *Standard V: Intervention*

The nurse intervenes as guided by the nursing care plan to implement nursing actions that promote, maintain or restore physical and mental health, prevent illness and effect rehabilitation.

#### *Standard VI: Evaluation*

The nurse evaluates client responses to nursing actions in order to revise the database, nursing diagnoses and nursing care plan.

### Professional Performance Standards

#### *Standard VII: Peer Review*

The nurse participates in peer review and other means of evaluation to assure quality of nursing care provided for clients.

#### *Standard VIII: Continuing Education*

The nurse assumes responsibility for continuing education and professional development and contributes to the professional growth of others.

#### *Standard IX: Interdisciplinary Collaboration*

The nurse collaborates with other health care providers in assessing, planning, implementing and evaluating programs and other mental health activities.

#### *Standard X: Utilization of Community Health Systems*

The nurse participates with other members of the community in assessing, planning, implementing and evaluating mental health services and community systems that include the promotion of the broad continuum of primary, secondary and tertiary prevention of mental illness.

## GENERAL PRINCIPLES OF PSYCHIATRIC NURSING

The following principles are general in nature and form guidelines for emotional care of a patient.

### Patient is Accepted Exactly as he is

Accepting means being nonjudgmental. Acceptance conveys the feeling of being loved and cared. Acceptance is expressed in the following ways:

#### *Being Nonjudgmental and Nonpunitive*

The patient's behavior is not judged as right or wrong, good or bad. Patient is not punished for his undesirable behavior. All direct (chaining, restraining, putting him in a separate room) and indirect (ignoring his presence or withdrawing attention) methods of punishment must be avoided.

#### *Being Sincerely Interested in the Patient*

Being sincerely interested in another individual means considering the other individual's interest. This can be demonstrated by:

- Studying patient's behavior pattern.
- Allowing him to make his own choices and decisions as far as possible.
- Being aware of his likes and dislikes.
- Being honest with him.
- Taking time and energy to listen to what he is saying.
- Avoiding sensitive subjects and issues.

### *Recognizing and Reflecting on Feelings which Patient may Express*

When patient talks, it is not the content that is important to note, but the feeling behind the conversation, which has to be recognized and reflected.

### *Talking with a Purpose*

The nurse's conversation with a patient must revolve around his needs, wants and interests. Indirect approaches like reflection, open-ended questions, focusing on a point, presenting reality are more effective when the problems are not obvious.

### *Listening*

Listening is an active process. The nurse should take time and energy to listen to what the patient is saying. She must be a sympathetic listener and show genuine interest.

### *Permitting Patient to Express Strongly-held Feelings*

Strong emotions bottled up are potentially explosive and dangerous. It is better to permit the patient to express his strong feelings without disapproval or punishment. Expression of negative feelings (anxiety, fear, hostility and anger) may be encouraged in a verbal or symbolic manner.

### Use Self-understanding as a Therapeutic Tool

A psychiatric nurse should have a realistic self-concept and should be able to recognize one's own feelings, attitudes and responses. Her ability to be aware and to accept her own strengths and limitations should help her to see the strengths and limitations in other people too.

### Consistency is used to Contribute to Patient's Security

This means that there should be consistency in the attitude of the staff, ward routine and in defining the limitations placed on the patient.

### Reassurance should be given in a Subtle and Acceptable Manner

Reassurance is building patient's confidence. To give reassurance, the nurse needs to understand and analyze the situation as to how it appears to the patient. False reassurance can also reflect a lack of interest and understanding or unwillingness on the part of the nurse to empathize with the patient's life situation.

### Patient's Behavior is Changed through Emotional Experience and not by Rational Interpretation

Major focus in psychiatry is on feelings and not on the intellectual aspect. Advising or rationalizing with patients is not effective in changing behavior. Role-play and socio-drama are a few avenues of providing corrective emotional experiences to a patient and facilitating insight into his own behavior.

### Unnecessary Increase in Patient's Anxiety should be Avoided

The following approaches may increase the patient's anxiety and should, therefore, be avoided:
- Showing nurse's own anxiety.
- Showing attention to the patient's deficits.
- Making the patient to face repeated failures.
- Placing demands on patient which he obviously cannot meet.
- Direct contradiction of patient's psychotic ideas.
- Passing sharp comments and showing indifference.

### Objective Observation of Patient to Understand his Behavior

Objectivity is an ability to evaluate exactly what the patient wants to say and not mix up one's own feelings, opinion or judgment. To be objective, the nurse should indulge in introspection and make sure that her own emotional needs do not take a precedence over patient's needs.

### Maintain Realistic Nurse-Patient Relationship

Realistic or professional relationship focuses upon the personal and emotional needs of the patient and not on nurse's needs. To maintain professional relationship the nurse should have a realistic self-concept and should be able to empathize and understand the feelings of the patient and the meaning of behavior.

### Avoid Physical and Verbal Force as Much as Possible

All methods of punishment must be avoided. If the nurse is an expert in predicting patient behavior, she can mostly prevent an onset of undesirable behavior.

### Nursing Care is Centered on the Patient as a Person and not on the Control of Symptoms

Analysis and study of symptoms is necessary to reveal their meaning and their significance to the patient. Two patients showing the same symptoms may be expressing two different needs.

### All Explanations of Procedures and other Routines are Given According to the Patient's Level of Understanding

The extent of explanation that can be given to a patient depends on his span of attention, level of anxiety and level of ability to decide.

### Many Procedures are Modified but Basic Principles Remain Unaltered

In psychiatric nursing field, many methods are adapted to individual needs of the patients, but the underlying nursing scientific principles remain the same. Some nursing principles to be kept in mind are: safety, comfort, privacy, maintaining therapeutic effectiveness, economy of time, energy and material.

## FUNCTIONS OF A PSYCHIATRIC NURSE

- Assessing the client and planning nursing care.
- Providing safe nursing care, including medication administration and participation in various therapies, individual interactions, formal and informal group situations, role playing, advocating on behalf of the client, and so forth.
- Providing a safe environment, including protecting the client and others from injury.
- Accurately observing and documenting the client's behavior.
- Providing feedback to the client based on observations of his behavior.
- Teaching the client and significant others.
- Involving the client and the client's significant others in the nursing process.
- Providing opportunities for the client to make his own decisions and to assume responsibility for his emotions and life.
- Cooperating with other professionals in various aspects of the client's care; thereby, facilitating an interdisciplinary approach to care.
- Continuing nursing education and the exploration of new ideas, theories, and research.

## QUALITIES OF A PSYCHIATRIC NURSE

Certain attitudes are necessary for a psychiatric nurse to deal with psychiatric patients.

### Self-awareness

A psychiatric nurse should have a realistic self- concept and should be able to recognize her own feelings, fantasies and fears. She should analyze her own professional strengths and limitations.

### Self-acceptance

The nurse should not only be aware, but also accept her strengths as well as her limitations.

### Accepting the Patient

Accepting means, being nonjudgmental. Acceptance conveys the feeling of being loved and cared. The nurse should accept the patient as he is, as a sick person, regardless of caste, color, race or behavior.

### Being Sincerely Interested in Patient Care

Being sincerely interested in patient care means considering the patients interest. This can be demonstrated by:

- Studying patient's behavior pattern
- Allowing him to make his own choices and decisions as far as possible
- Being aware of his likes and dislikes
- Being honest with him
- Active listening.

### Being Available

Being available means nurse should be approachable all the time to the patient.

### Empathizing with the Patient

Empathy is an important tool in understanding others' feelings. Empathy is a process when a person gets into another person's situation and experiences what the other person feels and then is able to step back and analyze the situation.

### Reliability

The nurse must demonstrate honesty, truthfulness, resourcefulness and competence in her dealings with the patients and their families.

### Professionalism

Developing the professional skills of a psychiatric nurse is dependent upon learning as much as possible about the patient, his illness and the helping role of the nurse as it specifically applies to the patient.

### Accountability

Mental health nurses are accountable for the nature of the effort they make on behalf of patients and answerable to patients for the quality of their efforts.

### The Ability to Think Critically

The ability to think critically is crucial for mental health nurses. A critical thinker analyzes information before drawing conclusions about it. It is purposeful, reasonable, reflective thinking that drives problem solving and decision making and aims to make judgments based on evidence.

## CONCEPTS OF PERSONALITY DEVELOPMENT

### Definition of Personality

'Personality refers to deeply ingrained patterns of behavior, which include the way one relates to, perceives, and thinks about the environment and one self'.—American Psychiatric Association (APA) 1987.

The *Diagnostic and Statistical Manual of Mental Disorders, Fourth Edition, Text Revision* (*DSM-IV-TR*) (American Psychiatric Association [APA], 2000) defines *personality traits* as 'enduring patterns of perceiving, relating to, and thinking about the environment and oneself that are exhibited in a wide range of social and personal contexts'.

### Personality

The combination of character, behavioral, temperamental, emotional, and mental traits that is unique to each specific individual.

## PSYCHOANALYTIC THEORY

Sigmund Freud (1961), who has been called the father of psychiatry, is credited as the first to identify development by stages. He considered the first 5 years of a child's life to be the most important because he believed that an individual's basic character had been formed by the age of 5.

### Structure of the Personality

Freud organized the structure of the personality into three major components: i. The *id,* ii. *ego,* and iii. *superego.*

### *Id*

The *id* is the locus of instinctual drives—the 'pleasure principle.' Present at birth, it endows the infant with instinctual drives that seek to satisfy needs and achieve immediate gratification. Id-driven behaviors are impulsive and may be irrational.

### *Ego*

The *ego*, also called the *rational self* or the 'reality principle,' begins to develop between the ages of 4 and 6 months. The ego experiences the reality of the external world, adapts to it, and responds to it. A primary function of the ego is one of mediator, that is, to maintain harmony among the external world, the id, and the superego.

### *Superego*

If the id is identified as the pleasure principle, and the ego the reality principle, the *superego* might be referred to as the 'perfection principle.' The superego, which develops between ages 3 and 6 years, internalizes the values and morals set forth by primary caregivers. Derived from a system of rewards and punishments, the superego is composed of two major components: i. the *ego-ideal* and ii. the *conscience*. When a child is consistently rewarded for 'good' behavior, the self-esteem is enhanced, and the behavior becomes part of the ego-ideal; that is, it is internalized as part of his or her value system. The conscience is formed when the child is consistently punished for 'bad' behavior. The child learns what is considered morally right or wrong from feedback received from parental figures and from society or culture.

The superego is important in the socialization of the individual because it assists the ego in the control of id impulses. When the superego becomes rigid and punitive, however, problems with low self-confidence and low self-esteem arise.

### Structure of the Personality

| Id | Ego | Superego |
|---|---|---|
| 'I found this wallet; I will keep the money' | 'I already have money. This money does not belong to me. May be the person who owns this wallet does not have any money' | 'It is never right to take something that does not belong to you' |
| 'Mom and dad are gone. Let's party!' | 'Mom and dad said no friends over while they are away. Too risky' | 'Never disobey your parents' |
| 'I will have sex with whomever I please, whenever I please' | 'Promiscuity can be very dangerous.' | 'Sex outside of marriage is always wrong' |

## FREUD'S STAGES OF PERSONALITY DEVELOPMENT

Freud described formation of the personality through five stages of *psychosexual* development.

### Oral Stage: Birth to 18 Months

During the oral stage, behavior is directed by the id, and the goal is immediate gratification of needs. The focus of energy is the mouth, and behaviors include sucking, chewing, and biting. The infant feels a sense of attachment and is unable to differentiate the self from the person who is providing the mothering. With the beginning of development of the ego at age 4 to 6 months, the infant starts to view the self as separate from the mothering figure. A sense of security and the ability to trust others are derived out of gratification from fulfillment of basic needs during this stage.

### Anal Stage: 18 Months to 3 Years

The major task in the anal stage is gaining independence and control, with particular focus on the excretory function. Freud believed that the manner in which the parents and other primary caregivers approach the task of toilet training may have far-reaching effects on the child in terms of values and personality characteristics. When toilet training is strict and rigid, the child may choose to retain the feces, becoming constipated. Adult retentive personality traits influenced by this type of training include stubbornness, stinginess, and miserliness. An alternate reaction to strict toilet training is for the child to expel feces in an unacceptable manner or at inappropriate times. Far-reaching effects of this behavior pattern include malevolence, cruelty to others, destructiveness, disorganization, and untidiness. Toilet training that is more permissive and accepting attaches the feeling of importance and desirability to feces production. The child becomes extroverted, productive, and altruistic.

### Phallic Stage: 3 to 6 Years

In this stage, the focus of energy shifts to the genital area. Discovery of differences between genders results in a heightened interest in the sexuality of self and others. This interest may be manifested in sexual self-exploratory or group-exploratory play. Freud proposed that the development of the *Oedipus complex* (males) or *Electra complex* (females) occurred during this stage of development. He described this as the child's unconscious desire to eliminate the parent of the same gender and to possess the parent of the opposite gender for himself or herself.

### *Freud's Stages of Psychosexual Development*

| Age | Stage | Major developmental tasks |
|---|---|---|
| Birth to 18 months | Oral | Relief from anxiety through oral gratification of needs |
| 18 months to 3 years | Anal | Learning independence and control, with focus on the excretory function |
| 3–6 years | Phallic | Identification with parent of same gender, development of sexual identity focus on genital organs |
| 6–12 years | Latency | Sexuality repressed, focus on relationships with same gender peers |
| 13–20 years | Genital | Libido reawakened as genital organs mature, focus on relationships with members of the opposite gender |

### Latency Stage: 6 to 12 Years

During the elementary school years, the focus changes from egocentrism to one of more interest in group activities, learning, and socialization with peers. Sexuality is not absent during this period but remains obscure and imperceptible to others. Children of this age show a distinct preference for same-gender relationships, even rejecting members of the opposite gender.

### Genital Stage: 13 to 20 Years

In the genital stage, the maturing of the genital organs results in a reawakening of the libidinal drive. The focus is on relationships with members of the opposite gender and preparations for selecting a mate.

## INTERPERSONAL THEORY

Sullivan (1953) believed that individual behavior and personality development are the direct result of interpersonal relationships.

### Sullivan's Stages of Personality Development

Sullivan describes six stages of personality development. An outline of the stages of personality development according to Sullivan's interpersonal theory is presented in table.

| Age | Stage | Major developmental tasks |
|---|---|---|
| Birth to 18 months | Infancy | Relief from anxiety through oral gratification of need |
| 18 months to 6 years | Childhood | Learning to experience a delay in personal gratification without undue anxiety |
| 6–9 years | Juvenile | Learning to form satisfactory peer relationships |
| 9–12 years | Preadole-scence | Learning to form satisfactory relationships with persons of same gender initiating feeling of affection for another person |
| 12–14 years | Early adolescence | Learning to form satisfactory relationship with persons of the opposite gender, developing a sense of identity |
| 14–21 years | Late adolescence | Establishing self-identifty, experiencing satisfying relationships, working to develop a lasting intimate opposite gender relationship |

### Infancy: Birth to 18 Months

During this beginning stage, the major developmental task for the child is the gratification of needs. This is accomplished through activity associated with the mouth, such as crying, nursing, and thumb sucking.

### Childhood: 18 Months to 6 Years

At ages 18 months to 6 years, the child learns that interference with fulfillment of personal wishes and desires may result in delayedgratification. He or she learns to accept this and feel comfortable with it, recognizing that delayed gratification often results in parental approval, a more lasting type of reward. Tools of this stage include the mouth, the anus, language, experimentation, manipulation, and identification.

### Preadolescence: 9 to 12 Years

The tasks of the preadolescence stage focus on developing relationships with persons of the same gender. One's ability to collaborate with and show love and affection for another person begins at this stage.

### Early Adolescence: 12 to 14 Years

During early adolescence, the child is struggling with developing a sense of identity, separate and independent from the parents. The major task is formation of satisfactory relationships with members of the opposite gender. Sullivan saw the emergence of lust in response to biological changes as a major force occurring during this period.

### Late Adolescence: 14 to 21 Years

The late adolescent period is characterized by tasks associated with the attempt to achieve interdependence within the society and the formation of a lasting, intimate relationship with a selected member of the opposite gender. The genital organs are the major developmental focus of this stage.

## ERIKSON'S STAGES OF PERSONALITY DEVELOPMENT

### Trust Versus Mistrust: Birth to 18 Months

In this stage, the major task is to develop a basic trust in the mothering figure and be able to generalize it to others.

- Achievement of the task results in self-confidence, optimism, faith in the gratification of needs and desires, and hope for the future. The infant learns to trust when basic needs are met consistently.
- Nonachievement results in emotional dissatisfaction with the self and others, suspiciousness, and difficulty with interpersonal relationships.

### Autonomy Versus Shame and Doubt: 18 Months to 3 Years

The major task in this stage is to gain some self-control and independence within the environment.

- Achievement of the task results in a sense of self-control and the ability to delay gratification, and a feeling of self-confidence in one's ability to perform. Autonomy is achieved when parents encourage and provide opportunities for independent activities.
- Nonachievement results in a lack of self-confidence, a lack of pride in the ability to perform, a sense of being controlled by others, and a rage against the self. The task remains unresolved when primary caregivers restrict independent behaviors, both physically and verbally, or set the child up for failure with unrealistic expectations.

### Initiative Versus Guilt: 3 to 6 Years

During this stage the goal is to develop a sense of purpose and the ability to initiate and direct one's own activities.

- Achievement of the task results in the ability to exercise restraint and self-control of inappropriate social behaviors. Assertiveness and dependability increase, and the child enjoys learning and personal achievement.

- Nonachievement results in feelings of inadequacy and a sense of defeat. Guilt is experienced to an excessive degree, even to the point of accepting liability in situations for which one is not responsible.

| Age | Stage | Major developmental tasks |
|---|---|---|
| Infancy (Birth to 18 months) | Trust vs mistrust | To develop a basic trust in the mothering figure and be also able to generalize it to others |
| Early childhood (18 months to 3 years) | Autonomy vs shame and doubt | To gain some self-control and independence within the environment |
| Late childhood (3–6 years) | Initiative vs guilt | To develop a sense of purpose and the ability to initiate and direct own activities |
| School age (6–12 years) | Industry vs inferiority | To achieve a sense of self-confidence by learning, competing, performing successfully, and receiving recognition from significant other, peers and acquaintances |
| Adolescence (12–20 years) | Identity vs role confusion | To integrate the tasks mastered in the previous stages into a secure sense of self |
| Young adulthood (20–30 years) | Intimacy vs isolation | To form an intense, lasting relationship or a commitment to another person, cause, institution, or creative effort |
| Adulthood (30–65 years) | Generativity vs stagnation | To achieve the life goals established for oneself, while also considering the welfare to future generations |
| Old age (65 years to death) | Ego integrity vs despair | To review one's life and derive meaning from both positive and negative events, while achieving a positive sense of self-worth |

### Industry Versus Inferiority: 6 to 12 Years

The major task of this stage is to achieve a sense of self-confidence by learning, competing, performing successfully, and receiving recognition from significant others, peers, and acquaintances.

- Achievement of the task results in a sense of satisfaction and pleasure in the interaction and involvement with others. The individual masters reliable work habits and develops attitudes of trustworthiness.
- Nonachievement results in difficulty in interpersonal relationships because of feelings of personal inadequacy. The individual can neither cooperate and compromise with others in group activities nor problem solve or complete tasks successfully. He or she may become either passive and meek or overly aggressive to cover up feelings of inadequacy.

### Identity Versus Role Confusion: 12 to 20 Years

At this stage, the goal is to integrate the tasks mastered in the previous stages into a secure sense of self.

- Achievement of the task results in a sense of confidence, emotional stability, and a view of the self as a unique individual. Commitments are made to a value system, to the choice for a career, and to relationships with members of both genders.
- Nonachievement results in a sense of self- consciousness, doubt, and confusion about one's role in life. Personal values or goals for one's life are absent. Commitments to relationships with others are nonexistent or superficial and brief. A lack of self-confidence is often expressed by delinquent and rebellious behavior.

### Intimacy Versus Isolation: 20 to 30 Years

The objective during this stage is to form an intense, lasting relationship or a commitment to another person, a cause, an institution, or a creative effort.

- Achievement of the task results in the capacity for mutual love and respect between two people and the ability of an individual to pledge a total commitment to another. The intimacy goes far beyond the sexual contact between two people. It describes a commitment in which personal sacrifices are made for another, whether it be another person, or if one chooses, a career or other type of cause or endeavor to which an individual elects to devote his or her life.
- Nonachievement results in withdrawal, social isolation, and aloneness. The individual is unable to form lasting, intimate relationships, often seeking intimacy through numerous superficial sexual contacts. No career is established; he or she may have a history of occupational changes (or may fear change and thus remain in an undesirable job situation).

### Generativity Versus Stagnation or Self-absorption: 30 to 65 Years

The major task of this stage is to achieve the life goals established for oneself while also considering the welfare of future generations.

- Achievement of the task results in a sense of gratification from personal and professional achievements and from meaningful contributions to others. The individual is active in the service of and to society. Generativity is achieved when the individual expresses satisfaction with this stage in life and demonstrates responsibility for leaving the world a better place in which to live.
- Nonachievement results in lack of concern for the welfare of others and total preoccupation with the self. He or she becomes withdrawn, isolated, and highly self-indulgent, with no capacity for giving of the self to others.

## THE THERAPEUTIC NURSE-PATIENT RELATIONSHIP

A relationship is defined as a state of being related or a state of affinity between two individuals. The nurse and client interact with each other in the health care system with the goal of assisting the client to use personal resources to meet his or her unique needs. In a therapeutic relationship the nurse and client work together towards the goal of assisting the client to regain the inner resources to meet life challenges and facilitate growth. The interaction is purposefully established, maintained and carried out with the anticipated outcome of helping the client gain new coping and adaptation skills.

### Social Relationships

A social relationship can be defined as a relationship that is primarily initiated with the purpose of friendship, socialization, enjoyment or accomplishing a task. Mutual needs are met during social interaction.

### Intimate Relationships

An intimate relationship occurs between two individuals who have an emotional commitment to each other.

### Therapeutic Relationships

The therapeutic relationship between nurse and client differs from both a social and an intimate relationship in that the nurse maximizes inner communication skills, understanding of human behavior and personal strengths, in order to enhance the client's growth.

## GOALS OF THERAPEUTIC RELATIONSHIP

- Facilitating communication of distressing thoughts and feelings.
- Assisting the client with problem solving.
- Helping clients examine self-defeating behaviors and test alternatives.
- Promoting self-care and independence.

### Rapport

Rapport is a relationship or communication especially when useful and harmonious. It is the crux of a therapeutic relationship between the nurse and the patient is:
- A willingness to become involved with another person
- Growth towards mutual acceptance and understanding of individuality
- The end result of one's care and concern for another. The nurse establishes rapport through demonstration of understanding, warmth and nonjudgmental attitude.

### Empathy

Empathy is an ability to feel with the patient while retaining the ability to critically analyze the situation. It is the ability to put oneself in another person's circumstances and feelings. The nurse need not necessarily have to experience it, but has to be able to imagine the feelings associated with the experience.

### Warmth

Warmth is the ability to help the client feel cared for and comfortable. It shows acceptance of the client as a unique individual. It involves a non-possessive caring for the client as a person and a willingness to share the client's joys and sorrows.

### Genuineness

Genuineness involves being one's own self. This implies that the nurse is aware of her thoughts, feelings, values and their relevance in the immediate interaction with a client. The nurse's response to the client is sincere and reflects her internal response.

## PHASES OF THERAPEUTIC RELATIONSHIP

Four phases of relationship process have been identified.

### Preinteraction Phase

This phase begins when the nurse is assigned to initiate a therapeutic relationship and includes all that the nurse thinks, feels or does immediately prior to the first interaction with the patient.

#### *Nurse's Tasks in the Preinteraction Phase*

- Explore own feelings, fantasies and fears
- Analyze own professional strengths and limitations
- Gather data about patient whenever possible
- Plan for first meeting with patient.

### Introductory or Orientation Phase

It is during the introductory phase that the nurse and patient meet for the first time. One of the nurse's primary concerns is to find out why the patient sought help. Nurse's tasks in the orientation phase are:
- Establish rapport, trust and acceptance
- Establish communication; assist in the verbal expression of thoughts and feelings
- Gather data, including the client's feelings, strengths and weaknesses
- Define client's problems, set priorities for nursing intervention
- Mutually set goals.

### Working Phase

Most of the therapeutic work is carried out during the working phase. The nurse and the patient explore relevant stress and promote the development of insight in the patient. Nurse's tasks in the working phase:
- Gather further data, explore relevant stressors
- Promote patient's development of insight and use of constructive coping mechanisms
- Facilitate behavioral change; encourage him to evaluate the results of his behavior
- Provide him with opportunities for independent functioning
- Evaluate problems and goals and redefine as necessary.

### Termination Phase

This is the most difficult, but most important phase of the therapeutic nurse-patient relationship. The goal of this phase is to bring a therapeutic end to the relationship. Nurse's tasks in the termination phase:
- Establish reality of separation
- Mutually explore feelings of rejection, loss, sadness, anger and related behavior
- Review progress of therapy and attainment of goals
- Formulate plans for meeting future therapy needs.

## THERAPEUTIC COMMUNICATION TECHNIQUES

- ***Listening:*** It is an active process of receiving information.
- ***Broad openings***: Encouraging the patient to select topics for discussion.
- ***Restating***: Repeating the main thought expressed by the patient.
- ***Clarification***: Attempting to put vague ideas or unclear thoughts of the patient into words to enhance the nurse's understanding or asking the patient to explain what he means.

- ***Reflection***: Directing back the patient's ideas, feelings, questions and content.
- ***Humor***: The discharge of energy through comic enjoyment of the imperfect.
- ***Informing***: The skill of information giving.
- ***Focusing***: Questions or statements that help the patient expand on a topic of importance.
- ***Sharing perceptions***: Asking the patient to verify the nurse's understanding of what the patient is thinking or feeling.
- ***Theme identification***: This involving identification of underlying issues or problems experienced by the patient that emerge repeatedly during the course of the nurse-patient relationship.
- ***Silence***: Lack of verbal communication for a therapeutic reason.
- ***Suggesting***: Presentation of alternative ideas for the patient's consideration relative to problem-solving.

## THE INDIVIDUAL WITH FUNCTIONAL PSYCHIATRIC DISORDER

### Schizophrenia

The word 'schizophrenia' was coined in 1908 by the Swiss psychiatrist Eugen Bleuler. It is derived from the Greek words *skhizo* (split) and *phren* (mind). In ICDlO, schizophrenia is classified under code F2.

### *Definition*

Schizophrenia is a psychotic condition characterized by a disturbance in thinking, emotions, volitions and faculties in the presence of clear consciousness, which usually leads to social withdrawal.

### *Etiology*

The cause of schizophrenia is still uncertain. Some of the factors involved may be:

#### *Genetic Factors*

The disease is more common among people born of consanguineous marriages. The prevalence rate among family members of schizophrenics is as follows:

- Children with one schizophrenic parent: 12%
- Children with both schizophrenic parents: 40%
- Siblings of schizophrenic patient: 8%
- Second-degree relatives: 5–6%
- Dizygotic twins of schizophrenic patients: 12%
- Monozygotic twins of schizophrenic patients: 47%.

#### *Stress-Diathesis Model*

According to the stress-diathesis model for the integration of biological, psychosocial and environmental factors, a person may have a specific vulnerability (diathesis) that, when acted on by a stressful influence, allows the symptoms of schizophrenia to develop.

#### *Biochemical Factors*

- ***Dopamine hypotheses:*** This theory suggests that an excess of dopamine-dependent neuronal activity in the brain may cause schizophrenia.
- ***Other biochemical hypotheses:*** Various other biochemicals have been implicated in the predisposition to schizophrenia. These include abnormalities in the neurotransmitters norepinephrine, serotonin, acetylcholine and gamma-aminobutyric acid (GABA), and neuroregulators such as prostaglandins and endorphins.

#### *Psychological Factors*

Family relationships act as major influence in the development of illness:

- ***Mother-child relationship:*** Early theorists characterized the mothers of schizophrenics as cold, over-protective, and domineering, thus retarding the ego development of the child.
- ***Dysfunctional family system:*** Hostility between parents can lead to a schizophrenic daughter (marital skew and schism).
- ***Double-bind communication (Bateson et al. 1956):*** Parents convey two or more conflicting and incompatible messages at the same time.

#### *Social Factors*

Studies have shown that schizophrenia is more prevalent in areas of high social mobility and disorganization, especially among members of very low social classes.

### Clinical Features

The predominant clinical features in acute schizophrenia are *delusions, hallucinations* and *interference with thinking.* Features of this kind are often called positive symptoms or psychotic features while most of the patients recover from acute illness, some progress to the chronic phase, during which rime the main features are *affective flattening or blunting, avolition-apathy (lack of initiative), attentional impairment, anhedonia (inability to experience pleasure), asociality, alogia (lack of speech output).* These are called as negative symptoms.

Once the chronic syndrome is established, few patients recover completely. The signs and symptoms commonly encountered in schizophrenic patients may be grouped follows:

### *Thought and Speech Disorders*

- Autistic thinking (preoccupations totally removing a person from reality).
- Loosening of associations (a pattern of spontaneous speech in which the things said in juxtaposition lack a meaningful relationship with each other).
- Thought blocking (a sudden interruption in the thought process).
- Neologism (a word newly coined, or an everyday word used in a special way, not readily understood by others).
- Poverty of speech (decreased speech production).
- Poverty of ideation (speech amount is adequate but content conveys little information).
- Echolalia (repetition or echo by patient of the words or phrases of examiner).
- Perseveration (persistent repetition of words or themes beyond the point of relevance).
- Verbigeration (senseless repetition of some words or phrases over and over again).

- Delusions of various kinds, i.e. delusions of persecution (being persecuted against); delusions of grandeur (belief that one is especially very powerful, rich, born with a special mission in life); delusions of reference (being referred to by others); delusions of control (being controlled by an external force); somatic delusions.
- Other thought disorders are over inclusion (tending to include irrelevant items in speech), impaired abstraction, concreteness and ambivalence.

### *Disorders of Perception*

- Auditory hallucinations.
- Visual hallucinations may sometimes occur along with auditory hallucinations; tactile, gustatory and olfactory types are far less common.

### *Disorders of Affect*

These include apathy, emotional blunting, emotional shallowness, anhedonia and inappropriate emotional response. The incapacity of the patient to establish emotional contact leads to lack of rapport with the examiner.

### *Disorders of Motor Behavior*

There can be either an increase or a decrease in psychomotor activity. Mannerisms, grimacing, stereotypes, decreased self-care and poor grooming are common features.

### *Other Features*

- Decreased functioning in work, social relations and self-care, as compared to earlier life.
- Loss of ego boundaries.
- Loss of insight.
- Poor judgment.
- Suicide can occur due to the presence of associated depression, command hallucinations, impulsive behavior, or return of insight that causes the patient to comprehend the devastating nature of the illness and take his life.
- There is usually no disturbance of consciousness, orientation, attention, memory and intelligence.
- There is no underlying organic cause.

## Clinical Types

Schizophrenia can be classified into the following subtypes:

- Paranoid
- Hebephrenic (disorganized)
- Catatonic
- Residual
- Undifferentiated
- Simple
- Postschizophrenic depression

### *Paranoid Schizophrenia*

The word 'paranoid' means 'delusional.' Paranoid schizophrenia is at present the most common form of schizophrenia. It is characterized by the following features (in addition to the general features already described).

- Delusions of persecution
- Delusions of jealousy
- Delusions of grandiosity
- Hallucinatory voices that threaten or command the patient, or auditory hallucinations without verbal form. Paranoid schizophrenia has a good prognosis if treated early. Personality deterioration is minimal and most of these patients are productive and can lead a normal life.

### *Hebephrenic (Disorganized) Schizophrenia*

It has an early and insidious onset and is often associated with poor premorbid personality. The essential features include marked thought disorder, incoherence, severe loosening of associations and extreme social impairment. Delusions and hallucinations are fragmentary and changeable.

Other oddities of behavior include senseless giggling, mirror-gazing, grimacing, mannerisms and so on. The course is chronic and progressively downhill without significant remissions. Recovery classically never occurs and it has one of the worst prognoses among all the subtypes.

### *Catatonic Schizophrenia*

Catatonic (Cata-disturbed) schizophrenia is characterized by marked disturbance of motor behavior. This may take the form of catatonic stupor, catatonic excitement and catatonia alternating between excitement and stupor.

*Clinical Features of Excited Catatonia*

- Increase in psychomotor activity.
- Increase in speech production.
- Loosening of associations and frank incoherence. Sometimes excitement becomes very severe and is accompanied by rigidity, hyperthermia and dehydration and can result in death. It is then known as *acute lethal catatonia* or *pernicious catatonia. Clinical features of retarded catatonia (catatonic stupor):*
  - Mutism: Absence of speech.
  - Rigidity: Maintenance of rigid posture against efforts to be moved.
  - Negativism: A motiveless resistance to all commands and attempts to be moved, or doing just the opposite.
  - Posturing: Voluntary assumption of an inappropriate and often bizarre posture for long periods of time.
  - Stupor: Does not react to his surroundings and appears to be unaware of them.
  - Echolalia: Repetition or mimicking of phrases or words heard.
  - Echopraxia: Repetition or mimicking of actions observed.
  - Waxy flexibility: Parts of body can be placed in positions that will be maintained for long periods of time, even if very uncomfortable (flexible like wax).
  - Ambitendency: A conflict to do or not to do, e.g. on asking to put out tongue, it is slightly protruded but taken back again.
  - Automatic obedience: Obeys every command irrespective of their nature.

### *Residual Schizophrenia*

Symptoms of residual schizophrenia include emotional blunting, eccentric behavior, illogical thinking, social withdrawal and loosening of associations.

### Undifferentiated Schizophrenia

This category is diagnosed either when features of no subtype are fully present or features of more than one subtype are exhibited.

### Simple Schizophrenia

It is characterized by an early and insidious onset, progressive course, presence of characteristic negative symptoms, vague hypochondriacal features, wandering tendency, self-absorbed idleness and aimless activity. It differs from residual schizophrenia in that there never has been an episode with all the typical psychotic symptoms. The prognosis is very poor.

### Postschizophrenic Depression

Depression features develop in the presence of residual or active features of schizophrenia and are associated with an increased risk of suicide.

## Treatment

### Pharmacotherapy

An acute episode of schizophrenia typically responds to treatment with classic antipsychotic agents, which are most effective in its treatment.Some commonly used drugs include:

- Chlorpromazine: 300–1500 mg/day PO; 50–100 mg/day IM
- Fluphenazine decanoate: 25–50 mg IM every 1–3 weeks
- Haloperidol: 5–100 mg/day PO, 5–20 mg/day IM
- Trifluoperazine: 15–60 mg/day PO, 1–5 mg/day IM
- Clozapine: 25–450 mg/day PO
- Risperidone: 2–10 mg/day PO
- Olanzapine: 10–20 mg/day PO

### Electroconvulsive Therapy (ECT)

Indications for ECT in schizophrenia include:

- Catatonic stupor
- Uncontrolled catatonic excitement
- Severe side-effects with drugs
- Schizophrenia refractory to all other forms of treatment. Usually 8–12 ECTs are needed.

### Psychological Therapies

- *Group therapy:* The social interaction, sense of cohesiveness, identification, and reality testing achieved within the group setting have proven to be highly therapeutic for these individuals.
- *Behavior therapy:* Behavior therapy is useful in reducing the frequency of bizarre, disturbing and deviant behavior, and increasing appropriate behaviors.
- *Social skills training:* Social skills training addresses behaviors such as poor eye contact, odd facial expressions and lack of spontaneity in social situations through the use of videotapes, role playing and homework assignments.
- *Cognitive therapy:* Used to improve cognitive distortions like reducing distractibility and correcting judgment.
- *Family therapy:* Family therapy typically consists of a brief program of family education about schizophrenia. It has been found that relapse rates of schizophrenia are higher in families with high expressed emotions (EE), where significant others make *critical comments, express hostility* or show *emotional over-involvement*. The significant others are, therefore, taught to decrease expectations and family tensions, apart from being given social skills training to enhance communication and problem-solving.

### Psychosocial Rehabilitation

This includes activity therapy to develop the work habit, training in a new vocation or retraining in a previous skill, vocational guidance and independent job placement.

## Nursing Management

### Nursing Diagnosis I

Alteration in thought processes related to inability to trust, panic anxiety, evidenced by delusional thinking, inability to concentrate, impaired volition, extreme suspiciousness of others.

*Objective*

Patient will eliminate patterns of delusional thinking and demonstrate trust in others.

*Intervention*

- Convey acceptance of the patient's need for the false belief, but that you do not share the belief.
- Do not argue or deny the belief.
- Reinforce and focus on reality. Discourage long discussions about the irrational thinking. Instead talk about real events and real people.
- If the client is highly suspicious, the following interventions may help:
  - Use same staff as far as possible
  - Be honest and keep all promises
  - Avoid physical contact in the form of touching the patient, etc.
  - Avoid laughing, whispering or talking quietly where the client can see but cannot hear what is being said
  - Avoid competitive activities; use assertive, matter-of-fact yet friendly approach.

### Nursing Diagnosis II

Sensory-perceptual alteration: Auditory/visual, related to panic anxiety, withdrawal into self, evidenced by inappropriate responses, disordered thought process, poor concentration and disorientation.

*Objective*

Patient will be able to define and test reality, eliminating the occurrence of hallucinations.

*Intervention*

- Observe the client for signs of hallucinations (listening pose, laughing or talking to self, stopping in mid-sentence).
- Avoid touching the client without warning.
- An attitude of acceptance will encourage the patient to share the content of the hallucination with you.
- Do not reinforce the hallucinations. Use 'the voices' instead of words like 'they' that imply validation. Say 'even though I realize the voices are real to you, I do not hear any voices speaking.'

- Help the client understand the connection between anxiety and hallucinations.
- Try to distract the client away from the hallucinations and involve him in interpersonal activities and actual situations.

### Nursing Diagnosis III

Social isolation related to inability to trust, panic anxiety, delusional thinking, evidenced by withdrawal, sad, dull affect, preoccupation with own thoughts, expression of feelings of rejection of aloneness imposed by others.

*Objective*

Patient will voluntarily spend time with other patients and staff members in group activities on the unit.

*Intervention*

- Convey an accepting attitude by making brief, frequent contacts. Show unconditional positive regard.
- Offer to be with the client during group activities that he finds frightening or difficult. Involve the client gradually in different activities on the unit.
- Give recognition and positive reinforcement for the client's voluntary interaction with others.

### Nursing Diagnosis IV

Potential for violence, self-directed or directed at others, related to extreme suspiciousness, panic anxiety, catatonic excitement, rage reactions, command hallucinations, evidenced by physical violence, destruction of objects in the environment, self-destructive behavior or active aggressive suicidal acts.

*Objective*

Patient will not harm self or others.

*Intervention*

- Maintain low level of stimuli in the client's environment (low lighting, low noise, few people, simple decoration, etc.).
- Observe client's behavior frequently.
- Do this while carrying out routine activities.
- Remove all dangerous objects from the client's environment.
- Redirect violent behavior with physical outlets for the anxiety.
- Staff should maintain a calm attitude towards the client.
- Have sufficient staff available to indicate a show of strength to the client if it becomes necessary.
- Administer tranquilizers as prescribed. Use of mechanical restraints may become necessary in some cases.

### Nursing Diagnosis V

Impaired verbal communication related to panic anxiety, disordered, unrealistic thinking, evidenced by loosening of associations, echolalia, verbalizations that reflect concrete thinking, and poor eye contact.

*Objective*

Patient will be able to communicate appropriately and comprehensibly by the time of discharge.

*Intervention*

- Attempt to decode incomprehensible communication pattern. Seek validation and clarification by stating 'Is it what you mean..?'or 'I do not understand what you mean by that. Would you please clarify it for me?'
- Facilitate trust and understanding by maintaining staff assignments as consistently as possible.
  - The techniques of verbalizing: The implied is used with the client who is mute (either unable or unwilling to speak). For example, 'That must have been a very difficult time for you when your mother left. You must have felt all alone.'
- Anticipate and fulfill client's needs until functional communication pattern returns.

### Nursing Diagnosis VI

Self-care deficit related to withdrawal, panic anxiety, perceptual or cognitive impairment, evidenced by difficulty in carrying out tasks associated with hygiene, dressing, grooming, eating and toileting.

*Objective*

Patient will demonstrate ability to meet self-care needs independently.

*Intervention*

- Provide assistance with self-care needs as required. Some patients who are severely withdrawn may require total care.
- Encourage client to perform independently as many activities as possible. Provide positive reinforcement for independent accomplishments.
- Creative approaches may need to be used with the client who is not eating because he is suspicious of being poisoned (e.g. allow client to open own canned or packaged foods, etc.). If elimination needs are not being met, establish structured schedule to help the client fulfill these needs until he is able to do so independently.

### Nursing Diagnosis VII

Ineffective family coping related to highly ambivalent family relationships, impaired family communication, evidenced by neglectful care of the client, extreme denial or prolonged overconcern regarding his illness.

*Objective*

Family will identify more adaptive coping strategies for dealing with patient's illness and treatment regimen.

*Intervention*

- Identify role of the client in the family and how it is affected by his illness. Identify the level of family functioning. Assess communication patterns, interpersonal relationships between the members, problem solving skills and availability of support systems.
- Provide information to the family about the client's illness, the treatment regimen, long-term prognosis.
- Practice with family members, how to respond to bizarre behavior and communication patterns and when the client becomes violent.

## MOOD DISORDERS

Mood disorders are characterized by a disturbance of mood, accompanied by a full or partial manic or depressive syndrome, which is not due to any other physical or mental disorder.

## Classification of Mood Disorders

According to ICD-10 (F3) mood disorders are classified as follows:

- Manic episode
- Depressive episode
- Bipolarmood (affective)disorders
- Recurrent depressive disorder
- Persistent mood disorder (including cyclothymia and dysthymia)
- Other mood disorders.

## Etiology

The etiology of mood disorders is currently unknown. However, several theories have been propounded which include:

### Biological Theories

- *Genetic hypothesis:* Genetic factors are very important in predisposing an individual to mood disorders. The lifetime risk for the first-degree relatives of patients with bipolar mood disorder is 25% and of normal controls is 7%. The lifetime risk for the children of one parent with mood disorder is 27% and of both parents with mood disorder is 74%. The concordance rate for monozygotic twins is 65% and for dizygotic twins is 15%.
- *Biochemical theories:* A deficiency of norepinephrine and serotonin has been found in depressed patients and they are elevated in mania. Dopamine, GABA and acetylcholine are also presumably involved.

### Psychosocial Theories

- *Psychoanalytic theory:* According to Freud (1957) depression results due to loss of a 'loved object', and fixation in the oral sadistic phase of development. In this model, mania is viewed as a denial of depression.
- *Behavioral theory:* This theory of depression connects depressive phenomena to the experience of uncontrollable events. According to this model, depression is conditioned by repeated losses in the past.
- *Cognitive theory:* According to this theory depression is due to negative cognitions which includes:
  - Negative expectations of the environment
  - Negative expectations of the self
  - Negative expectations of the future
  - These cognitive distortions arise out of a defect in cognitive development and cause the individual to feel inadequate, worthless and rejected by others.
- *Sociological theory:* Stressful life events, e.g. death, marriage, financial loss before the onset of the disease or a relapse probably have a formative effect.

## MANIC EPISODE

Mania refers to a syndrome in which the central features are overactivity, mood change (which may be towards elation or irritability) and selt important ideas.

The lifetime risk of manic episode is about 0.8–1%. This disorder occurs in episodes lasting usually 3 to 4 months, followed by complete recovery.

## Classification of Mania (ICD10)

- Hypomania
- Mania without psychotic symptoms
- Mania with psychotic symptoms
- Manic episode unspecified.

## Clinical Features

An acute manic episode is characterized by the following features which should last for at least 1 week:

### Elevated, Expansive or Irritable Mood

Elevated mood in mania has four stages depending on the severity of manic episodes:

1. Euphoria (Stage I): Increased sense of psychological well-being and happiness not in keeping with ongoing events.
2. Elation (Stage II): Moderate elevation of mood with increased psychomotor activity.
3. Exaltation (Stage III): Intense elevation of mood with delusions of grandeur.
4. Ecstasy (Stage IV): Severe elevation of mood, intense sense of rapture or blissfulness seen in delirious or stuporous mania.

### Psychomotor Activity

There is an increased psychomotor activity ranging from overactiveness and restlessness to manic excitement.

### Speech and Thought

- Flight of ideas: Thoughts racing in mind, rapid shifts from one topic to another
- Pressure of speech: Speech is forceful, strong and difficult to interrupt. Uses playful language with punning, rhyming, joking and teasing and speaks loudly
- Delusions of grandeur
- Delusions of persecution
- Distractibility.

### Other Features

- Increased sociabilities
- Impulsive behavior
- Disinhibition
- Hypersexual and promiscuous behavior
- Poor judgment
- High-risk activities (buying sprees, reckless driving, foolish business investments, distributing money or articles to unknown persons)
- Dressed up in gaudy and flamboyant clothes although in severe mania there may be poor self care
- Decreased need for sleep (< 3 hr)
- Decreased food intake due to overactivity
- Decreased attention and concentration
- Poor judgment
- Absent insight.

### Symptoms of Hypomania

Hypomania is a lesser degree of mania. There is a persistent mild elevation of mood and increased sense of psychological well-being and happiness not in keeping with ongoing events. In some cases irritability, conceit, and boorish behavior may take the place of the more usual euphoric sociability. The features of hypomania may be specified as follows:

- A distinct period of persistently elevated, expansive, or irritable mood, lasting throughout 4 days, that is clearly different from the usual nondepressed mood.
- During the period of mood disturbance, three or more of the following symptoms are persistent (four, if the mood is only irritable) and present to a significant degree:
  - inflated self-esteem or grandiosity
  - decreased need for sleep (e.g. feels rested after only 3 hours of sleep)
  - more talkative than usual
  - flight of ideas or subjective experience that thoughts are racing
  - distractibility (i.e. attention too easily drawn to unimportant or irrelevant external stimuli)
  - increase in goal-directed activity (either socially, at work or school, or sexually) or psychomotor agitation
  - excessive involvement in pleasurable activities that have a high potential for painful consequences (e.g. the person engages in unrestrained buying sprees, foolish business investments or sexual indiscretions).
- The episode is associated with an unequivocal change in functioning that is uncharacteristic of the person when not symptomatic.
- The disturbance in mood and the change in functioning are observable by others.
- The episode is not severe enough to cause marked impairment in social or occupational functioning, or to necessitate hospitalization, and there are no psychotic features.

## Treatment

### *Pharmacotherapy*

- Lithium: 900–2100 mg/day
- Carbamazepine: 600–1800 mg/day
- Sodium valproate: 600–2600 mg/day
- Other drugs: Clonazepam, calcium channel blockers, etc.

### *Electroconvulsive Therapy (ECT)*

Electroconvulsive therapy (ECT) can also be used for acute manic excitement if not adequately responding to antipsychotics and lithium.

### *Psychosocial Treatment*

Family and marital therapy is used to decrease intrafamilial and interpersonal difficulties and to reduce or modify stressors. The main purpose is to ensure continuity of treatment and adequatedrug compliance.

## Nursing Management for Mania

### *Nursing Diagnosis I*

High-risk for injury related to extreme hyperactivity and impulsive behavior, evidenced by lack of control over purposeless and potentially injurious movements.

*Objective*

Patient will not injure self.

*Intervention*

- Keep environmental stimuli to a minimum; assign single room; limit interactions with others; keep lighting and noise level low. Keep his room and immediate environment minimally furnished.
- Remove hazardous objects and substances, caution the patient when there is possibility of an accident.
- Assist patient to engage in activities, such as writing, drawing and other physical exercise.
- Stay with patient as hyperactivity increases.
- Administer medication as prescribed by physician.

### *Nursing Diagnosis II*

High-risk for violence, self-directed or directed at others related to manic excitement, delusional thinking and hallucinations.

*Objective*

Patient will not harm self or others.

*Intervention*

- Maintain low level of stimuli in patient's environment, provide unchallenging environment.
- Observe patient's behavior at least every 15 minutes. Ensure that all sharp objects, glass or mirror items, belts, ties, matchboxes have been removed from patient's environment.
- Redirect violent behavior with physical outlet.
- Encourage verbal expression of feelings.
- Engage him in some physical exercises like aerobics.
- Maintain and convey a calm attitude to the patient. Respond matter-of-factly to verbal hostility. Talk to him in low, calm voice, use clear and direct speech.
- Have sufficient staff to indicate a show of strength to patient if necessary. State limitations and expectations.
- Administer tranquilizing medication; if patient refuses, use of restraints may be necessary. In such a case, explain the reason to the patient.
- Following application of restraints observe patient every 15 minutes.
- Remove restraints gradually once at a time.

### *Nursing Diagnosis III*

Altered nutrition, less than body requirements related to refusal or inability to sit still long enough to eat, evidenced by weight loss, amenorrhea.

*Objective*

Patient will not exhibit signs and symptoms of malnutrition.

*Intervention*

- Provide high-protein, high-caloric, nutritious finger foods and drinks that can be consumed 'on the run.'
- Find out patient's likes and dislikes and provide favorite foods.
- Provide 6–8 glasses of fluids per day. Have juice and snacks on unit at all times.

- Maintain accurate record of intake, output and calorie count. Weigh the patient regularly.
- Supplement diet with vitamins and minerals.
- Walk or sit with patient while he eats.

### Nursing Diagnosis IV

Impaired social interaction related to egocentric and narcissistic behavior, evidenced by inability to develop satisfying relationships and manipulation of others for own desires.

*Objective*

Patient will interact with others in an appropriate manner.

*Intervention*

- Recognize that manipulative behavior helps to decrease feeling of insecurity by increasing feeling of power and control.
- Set limits on manipulative behavior. Explain the consequences if limits are violated.
- Ignore attempts by patient to argue or bargain his way out of the limit setting.
- Give positive reinforcement for non- manipulative bahaviors.
- Discuss consequences of patient's behavior and how attempts are made to attribute them to others.
- Help patient identify positive aspects about self, recognize accomplishment and feel good about them.

### Nursing Diagnosis V

Self-esteem disturbance related to unmet dependency needs, lack of positive feedback, unrealistic self-expectations.

*Objective*

Patient will have realistic expectations about self.

*Intervention*

- Ask how client would like to be addressed. Avoid approaches that imply different perception of the client's importance.
- Explain rationale for requests by staff unit routine, etc. strictly adhere to courteous approaches, matter-of-fact style and friendly attitudes.
- Encourage verbalization and identification of feelings related to issues of chronicity, lack of control over self, etc.
- Offer matter-of-fact feedback regarding unrealistic plans. Help him to set realistic goals for himself.
- Encourage client to view life after discharge and identity aspects over which control is possible. Through role play, practice how he will demonstrate that control.

### Nursing Diagnosis VI

Altered family processes related to euphoric- mood and grandiose ideas, manipulative behavior, refusal to accept responsibility for own actions.

*Objective*

The family members will demonstrate coping ability in dealing with the patient.

*Intervention*

- Determine individual situation and feelings of individual family members like guilt, anger, powerlessness, despair and alienation.
- Assess patterns of communication. For example: Are feelings expressed freely? who makes decisions? What is the interaction between family members? Determine patterns of behavior displayed by patient in his relationships with others, e.g. manipulation of self-esteem of others, limit testing, etc.
- Assess the role of patient in the family, like provider, etc. and how the illness affects the roles of other members.
- Provide information about behavior patterns and expected course of the illness.

*Evaluation*

In this step, the nurse assesses if the goals of care are achieved. The plan may need to be revised or modified in the light of this evaluation.

## DEPRESSIVE EPISODE

Depression is a widespread mental health problem affecting many people. The lifetime risk of depression in males is 8 to 12% and in females it is 20 to 26%. Depression occurs twice as frequently in women as in men.

### Classification of Depression (ICD10)

- Mild depression
- Moderate depression
- Severe depression
- Severe depression with psychotic symptoms.

### Clinical Features

A typical depressive episode is characterized by the following features, which should last for at least two weeks in order to make a diagnosis:

- *Depressed mood:* Sadness of mood or loss of interest and loss of pleasure in almost all activities (pervasive sadness), present throughout the day (persistent sadness).
- *Depressive cognitions:* Hopelessness (a feeling of 'no hope in future' due to pessimism), helplessness (the patient feels that no help is possible), worthlessness (a feeling of inadequacy and inferiority), unreasonable guilt and self-blame over trivial matters in the past.
- *Suicidal thoughts:* Ideas of hopelessness are often accompanied by the thought that life is no longer worth living and that death had come as a welcome release.
- *Psychomotor activity:* Psychomotor retardation is frequent. Slowing of thought is reflected in the patient's speech; questions are often answered after a long delay and in a monotonous voice.
- *Psychotic features:* Some patients have delusions and hallucinations (the disorder may then be termed as psychotic depression); these are often mood congruent, i.e. they are related to depressive themes and reflect the patient's dysphoric mood.
- *Somatic symptoms of depression:* According to ICD10 (these are called as *'melancholic features'* in DSM-IV):
  - Significant decrease in appetite or weight.
  - Early morning awakening, at least 2 or more hours before the usual time of waking up.

- Diurnal variation, with depression being worst in the morning.
- Pervasive lack of interest and lack of reactivity to pleasurable stimuli.
- Psychomotor agitation or retardation.

### Other Features

- Difficulties in thinking and concentration.
- Subjective poor memory.
- Menstrual or sexual disturbances.
- Vague physical symptoms such as fatigue, aching discomfort, constipation, etc.

## Treatment

### Pharmacotherapy

Antidepressants are the treatment of choice for a vast majority of depressive episodes.

## Antidepressants

Antidepressants are those drugs, which are used for the treatment of depressive illness. These are also called as mood elevators or thymoleptics.
*Example:* Imipramine, amitriptyline, isocarboxazid.

### Electroconvulsive Therapy (ECT)

Severe depression with suicidal risk is the most important indication for ECT.

### Psychosocial Treatment

- *Cognitive therapy:* It aims at correcting the depressive negative cognitions like hopelessness, worthlessness, helplessness and pessimistic ideas, and replacing them with new cognitive and behavioral responses.
- *Supportive psychotherapy:* Various techniques are employed to support the patient. They are reassurance, ventilation, occupational therapy, relaxation and other activity therapies.
- *Group therapy:* Group therapy is useful for mild cases of depression. In group therapy negative feelings such as anxiety anger, guilt, despair are recognized and emotional growth is improved through expression of their feelings.
- *Family therapy:* Family therapy is used to decrease intrafamilial and interpersonal difficulties and to reduce or modify stressors, which may help in faster and more complete recovery.
- *Behavior therapy:* It includes social skills training, problem-solving techniques, assertiveness training, self-control therapy, activity scheduling and decision making techniques.

## Bipolar Mood Disorder

This is characterized by recurrent episodes of mania and depression in the same patient at different times.

Bipolar mood disorder is further classified into bipolar I and bipolar II disorder (DSM-IV).

- Bipolar I: Episodes of severe mania and severe depression.
- Bipolar II: Episodes of hypomania and severe depression.

### Recurrent Depressive Disorder

This disorder is characterized by recurrent depressive episodes. The current episode is specified as mild, moderate, severe, severe with psychotic symptoms.

### Persistent Mood Disorder

*Cyclothymia and Dysthymia*

- These disorders are characterized by persistent mood symptoms that last for more than 2 years.
- Cyclothymia refers to a persistent instability in mood in which there are numerous periods of mild elation or mild depression.
- Dysthymia (neurotic/reactive depression) is a chronic, mild depressive state persisting for months or years. It is more common in females with an average age of onset in late third decade. An episode of major depression may sometimes become superimposed on an underlying neurotic depression. This is known as 'double depression.'

## Organic Mental Disorders

Organic mental disorders are behavioral or psychological disorders associated with transient or permanent brain dysfunction.

# CLASSIFICATION OF ORGANIC MENTAL DISORDERS

- Dementia
- Delirium
- Organic amnestic syndrome
- Mental disorders due to brain damage, dysfunction and physical disease
- Personality and behavioral disorders due to brain disease, damage and dysfunction.

# DEMENTIA (CHRONIC ORGANIC BRAIN SYNDROME)

Dementia is an acquired global impairment of intellect, memory and personality but without impairment of consciousness.

## Etiology

### Untreatable and Irreversible Causes

- Degenerating disorders of CNS
- Alzheimer's disease (this is the most common of all dementing illnesses)
- Pick's disease
- Huntington's chorea
- Parkinson's disease.

### Treatable and Reversible Causes

- *Vascular:* Multi-infarct dementia
- Intracranial space occupying lesions
- *Metabolic disorders:* Hepatic failure, renal failure
- *Endocrine disorders:* Myxedema, Addison's disease
- *Infections:* AIDS, meningitis, encephalitis
- *Intoxication:* Alcohol, heavy metals (lead, arsenic), chronic barbiturate poisoning
- *Anoxia:* Anemia, postanesthesia, chronic respiratory failure
- Vitamin deficiency, especially deficiency of thiamine, and nicotine
- *Miscellaneous:* Heatstroke, epilepsy, electric injury.

## Stages of Dementia

### *Stage I: Early Stage (2–4 Years)*

- Forgetfulness
- Declining interest in environment
- Hesitancy in initiating actions
- Poor performance at work.

### *Stage II: Middle Stage (2–12 Years)*

- Progressive memory loss
- Hesitates in response to questions
- Has difficulty in following simple instructions
- Irritable, anxious
- Wandering
- Neglects personal hygiene
- Social isolation.

### *Stage III: Final Stage (up to a Year)*

- Marked loss of weight because of inadequate intake of food
- Unable to communicate
- Does not recognize family
- Incontinence of urine and feces
- Loses the ability to stand and walk
- Death is usually caused by aspiration pneumonia.

## Clinical Features (for Alzheimer's Type)

- *Personality changes:* Lack of interest in day-to-day activities, easy mental fatiguability, self-centered, withdrawn, decreased self-care
- ***Memory impairment:*** Recent memory is prominently affected
- ***Cognitive impairment:*** Disorientation, poor judgment, difficulty in abstraction, decreased attention span
- ***Affective impairment:*** Labile mood, irritableness, depression
- ***Behavioral impairment:*** Stereotyped behavior, alteration in sexual drives and activities, neurotic/psychotic behavior
- ***Neurological impairment:*** Aphasia, apraxia, agnosia, seizures, headache
- ***Catastrophic reaction:*** Agitation, attempt to compensate for defects by using strategies to avoid demonstrating failures in intellectual performances, such as changing the subject, cracking jokes or otherwise diverting the interviewer
- ***Sundown syndrome:*** It is characterized by drowsiness, confusion, ataxia; accidental falls may occur at night when external stimuli such as light and interpersonal orienting cues are diminished.

## Course and Prognosis

Insidious onset but slow progressive deterioration occurs.

### *Treatment*

Until now no specific medicine is available to treat Alzheimer's disease. A drug called 'Tacrine' is being used in Western countries. Tacrine (Tetrahydroaminoacridine) is a long-acting inhibitor of acetylcholine and also delays the progression of the illness. The following drugs may be of some use in causing symptomatic relief:

- Benzodiazepines for insomnia and anxiety
- Antidepressants for depression
- Antipsychotics to alleviate hallucinations and delusions
- Anticonvulsants to control seizures nursing care for patients of Alzheimer's disease is most important. Whether at home, in an acute hospital environment, a day-care center or in a long-term stay institution. Caregivers must be trained to promote the patient's remaining intellectual abilities; help them maintain their independence in attending to their usual functions and avoid injuries; and provide for a good quality of life.

## DELIRIUM (ACUTE ORGANIC BRAIN SYNDROME)

Delirium is an acute organic mental disorder characterized by impairment of consciousness, disorientation and disturbances in perception and restlessness.

### Etiology

- *Vascular:* Hypertensive encephalopathy, cerebral arteriosclerosis, intracranial hemorrhage
- ***Infections:*** Encephalitis, meningitis
- ***Neoplastic:*** Space-occupying lesions
- ***Intoxication:*** Chronic intoxication or withdrawal effect of sedative-hypnotic drugs
- ***Traumatic:*** Subdural and epidural hematoma, contusion, laceration, postoperative, heatstroke
- Vitamin deficiency, e.g. thiamine
- ***Endocrine and metabolic:*** Diabetic coma and shock, uremia, myxedema, hyperthyroidism, hepatic failure
- ***Metals:*** Heavy metals (lead, manganese, mercury), carbon monoxide and toxins
- ***Anoxia:*** Anemia, pulmonary or cardiac failure.

### Clinical Features

- ***Impairment of consciousness:*** Clouding of consciousness ranging from drowsiness to stupor and coma.
- ***Impairment of attention:*** Difficulty in shifting, focusing and sustaining attention.
- ***Perceptual disturbances:*** Illusions and hallucinations, most often visual.
- ***Disturbance of cognition:*** Impairment of abstract thinking and comprehension, impairment of immediate and recent memory, increased reaction time.
- ***Psychomotor disturbance:*** Hypo or hyperactivity, aimless groping or picking at the bedclothes (flocculation), enhanced startle reaction.
- ***Disturbance of the sleep-wake cycle:*** Insomnia or in severe cases total sleep loss or reversal of sleep-wake cycle, daytime drowsiness, nocturnal worsening of symptoms, disturbing dreams or nightmares, which may continue as hallucinations after awakening.
- ***Emotional disturbances:*** Depression, anxiety, fear, irritability, euphoria, apathy or wondering perplexity.

### Treatment

- Identification of cause and its immediate correction, e.g. 50 mg of 50% dextrose IV for hypoglycemia, 02 for hypoxia,

100 mg of B1IV for thiamine deficiency, IV fluids for fluid and electrolyte imbalance.
- *Symptomatic measures:* Benzodiazepines (10 mg diazepam or 2 mg lorazepam IV) or antipsychotics (5 mg haloperidol or 50 mg chlorpromazine IM) may be given.

## ORGANIC AMNESTIC SYNDROME

Organic amnestic syndrome is characterized by impairment of memory and global intellectual functioning due to an underlying organic cause. There is no disturbance of consciousness.

### Etiology

- Thiamine deficiency, the most common cause being chronic alcoholism. It is also called as 'Wernicke-Korsakoff syndrome.' Wernicke's encephalopathy is an acute phase of delirium preceding amnestic syndrome, while Korsakoff's syndrome is a chronic phase of amnestic syndrome
- Head trauma
- Bilateral temporal lobectomy
- Hypoxia
- Brain tumors
- Herpes simplex encephalitis
- Stroke.

### Clinical Features

- Recent memory impairment
- Anterograde and retrograde amnesia
- There is no impairment of immediate memory.

### Management

Treatment for underlying cause.

## MENTAL DISORDERS DUE TO BRAIN DAMAGE, DYSFUNCTION AND PHYSICAL DISEASE

These are mental disorders, which are causally related to brain dysfunction due to primary cerebral disease, systemic disease or toxic substances.

### Primary Cerebral Diseases

Epilepsy, encephalitis, head trauma, brain neoplasms, vascular cerebral disease and cerebral malformations.

### Systemic Diseases

Hypothyroidism, Cushing's disease, hypoxia, hypolycemia, systemic lupus erythematosus and extracranial neoplasms.

### Drugs

Steroids, antihypertensives, antimalarials, alcohol and psychoactive substances. The following mental disorders come under this category:

- Organic hallucinosis
- Organic catatonic disorder
- Organic delusional disorder
- Organic mood disorder
- Organic anxiety disorder.

## PERSONALITY AND BEHAVIORAL DISORDERS DUE TO BRAIN DISEASE, DAMAGE AND DYSFUNCTION

These disorders are characterized by significant alteration of the premorbid personality due to underlying organic cause. There is no disturbance of consciousness and global intellectual function. The personality change may be characterized by emotional lability, poor impulse control, apathy, hostility or accentuation of earlier personality traits.

### Etiology

- Complex partial seizures (temporal lobe seizures)
- Cerebral neoplasms
- Cerebrovascular disease
- Head injury.

### Management

- Treatment for the underlying cause.
- Symptomatic treatment with lithium, carbamazepine or with antipsychotics.

## OBSESSIVE COMPULSIVE DISORDER (OCD)

### Definition

According to ICD9, OCD is a state in which 'the outstanding symptom is a feeling of subjective compulsion which must be resisted to carry out some action, to dwell on an idea, to recall an experience, or ruminate on an abstract topic.

Obsessions and compulsions should have the following characteristics:

- They are ideas, impulses or images, which intrude into conscious awareness repeatedly.
- They are recognized as the individual's own thoughts or impulses.
- They are unpleasant and recognized as irrational.
- Patient tries to resist them but is unable to.
- Failure to resist leads to marked distress.
- Rituals (compulsions) are performed with a sense of subjective compulsion (urge to act).
- They are aimed at either preventing or neutralizing the distress or fear arising out of obsessions.

### Classification (ICD10)

- OCD with predominantly obsessive thoughts or ruminations.
- OCD with predominantly compulsive acts.
- OCD with mixed obsessional thoughts and acts.

### Clinical Picture

- *Obsessional thoughts:* These are words, ideas and, beliefs that intrude forcibly into the patient's mind. They are usually unpleasant and shocking to the patient and may be obscene or blasphemous.
- *Obsessional images:* These are vividly imagined scenes, often of a violent or disgusting kind involving abnormal sexual practices.
- *Obsessional ruminations:* These involve internal debates in which arguments for and against even the simplest everyday actions are reviewed endlessly.

- *Obsessional doubts:* These may concern actions that may not have been completed adequately. The obsession often implies some danger such as forgetting to turn off the stove or not locking a door. It may be followed by a compulsive act such as the person making multiple trips back into the house to check if the stove has been turned off.
- *Obsessive slowness:* Severe obsessive ideas or extensive compulsive rituals characterize obsessional slowness in the relative absence of manifested anxiety. This leads to marked slowness in daily activities.

### Treatment

#### Pharmacotherapy

- Antidepressants (e.g. fluvoxamine, sertraline, etc.)
- Anxiolytics (e.g. benzodiazepines).

#### Behavior Therapy

- Exposure and response prevention
- Thought stoppage
- Desensitization
- Aversive conditioning.

*Exposure and response prevention:* This *in vivo* exposure procedure combined with response prevention techniques.

*Thought stoppage:* Thought stopping is a technique to help an individual to learn to stop thinking unwanted thoughts.

#### Other Therapies

- Supportive psychotherapy
- ECT for patients refractory to other forms of treatment.

## EATING DISORDERS

The two most important eating disorders are:

### Anorexia Nervosa

Anorexia nervosa is characterized by highly specific behavioral and psychopathological symptoms and significant somatic signs. Majority are females and the onset is during adolescence.

The core psychopathological feature is the dread of fatness, weight phobia and a drive for thinness.

#### Clinical Features

- There is an intense fear of becoming obese. This fear does not decrease even if the person loses weight grossly and becomes very thin.
- The body weight is 15% below the standard weight.
- There is a body image disturbance. The patient is unable to perceive the body size accurately.
- The pursuit of thinness may take several forms. Patients generally eat little and set themselves daily calorie limits (often between 600 and 1000 calories). Some try to achieve weight loss by inducing vomiting, excessive exercise, and misusing laxatives.
- Other signs and symptoms are secondary to starvation and include sensitivity to cold, delayed gastric emptying, constipation, low blood pressure, bradycardia, hypothermia and amenorrhea in females.
- Vomiting and abuse of laxatives may lead to a variety of electrolyte disturbances, the most serious being hypokalemia.
- Hormonal abnormalities also may be seen.

#### Treatment

*Pharmacotherapy*

- Neuroleptics
- Appetite stimulants
- Antidepressants.

*Psychological Therapies*

- Individual psychotherapy
- Behavioral therapy
- Cognitive behavior therapy
- Family therapy.

### Bulimia Nervosa

Bulimia nervosa is described as repeated bouts of overeating and a preoccupation with control of weight that leads to self-induced vomiting.

#### Clinical Features

- An irresistible craving for food: There are episodes of overeating in which large amount of food are consumed within short periods of time (eating binges)
- Attempt to counteract the effects of overeating by self-induced vomiting
- There is usually no significant weight loss.

#### Treatment

- Antidepressants, carbamazepine and lithium for patients with comorbid mood disorders
- Group therapy
- Family therapy
- Cognitive behavior therapy.

## ALCOHOL DEPENDENCE SYNDROME

Alcoholism refers to the use of alcoholic beverages to the point of causing damage to the individual, society or both.

### Properties of Alcohol

Alcohol is a clear-colored liquid with a strong burning taste. The rate of absorption of alcohol into the bloodstream is more rapid than its elimination. Absorption of alcohol into the bloodstream is slower when food is present in the stomach. A small amount is excreted through urine and a small amount is exhaled. A concentration of 80 to 100 mg of alcohol per 100 mL of blood is considered intoxication. A person with 200 to 250 mg will be toxic, sleepy, confused and his thought process will be altered. If blood level is 300 mg/100 mL of blood the person may lose consciousness. A concentration of 500 mg/100 mL is fatal. All the symptoms change according to tolerance.

### Medical and Social Complications of Alcohol Dependence

#### Medical Gastrointestinal System

- Gastritis, peptic ulcer, reflux esophagitis, carcinoma of stomach and esophagus

- Fatty liver, cirrhosis of liver, hepatitis, liver cell carcinoma
- Acute and chronic pancreatitis
- Malabsorption syndrome.

*Cardiovascular System*

- Alcoholic cardiomyopathy
- High-risk for myocardial infarction.

*Central Nervous System*

- Peripheral neuropathy
- Epilepsy
- Head injury
- Cerebellar degeneration.

*Miscellaneous*

- Protein malnutrition
- Vitamin deficiency disorder
- Peripheral muscle weakness
- Acne
- Sexual dysfunction in males, failure of ovulation in females.

*Damage to the Fetus*

Fetal alcohol syndrome (facial abnormality, low birth weight, low intelligence), increased stillbirths. Alcohol dependence is responsible for 3% of all cases of mental retardation.

### *Social*

- Marital disharmony
- Occupational problems
- Financial problems
- Criminality
- Accidents.

## PSYCHIATRIC DISORDERS DUE TO ALCOHOL DEPENDENCE

### Acute Intoxication

Acute intoxication develops during or shortly after alcohol ingestion. It is characterized by clinically significant maladaptive behavior or psychological changes, e.g. in appropriate sexual or aggressive behavior, mood lability, impaired judgment, slurred speech, incoordination, unsteady gait, nystagmus, impaired attention and memory finally resulting in stupor or coma.

### Withdrawal Syndrome

In persons who have been drinking heavily over a prolonged period of time, any rapid decrease in the amount of alcohol in the body is likely to produce withdrawal symptoms. These are:

#### *Simple Withdrawal Syndrome*

It is characterized by mild tremors, nausea, vomiting, weakness, irritability, insomnia and anxiety.

#### *Delirium Tremens*

It occurs usually within 2 to 4 days of complete or significant abstinence from heavy alcohol drinking. The course is short, with recovery occurring within 3 to 7 days. It is characterized by:

- A dramatic and rapidly changing picture of disordered mental activity, with clouding of consciousness and disorientation in time and place
- Poor attention span
- Vivid hallucinations which are usually visual; tactile hallucinations can also occur
- Severe psychomotor agitation, shouting and evident fear
- Grossly tremulous hands which sometimes pick up imaginary objects; truncal ataxia
- Autonomic disturbances such as sweating, fever, tachycardia, raised blood pressure, pupillary dilatation
- Dehydration with electrolyte imbalances
- Reversal of sleep-wake pattern or insomnia
- Blood tests reveal leukocytosis and impaired liver function
- Death may occur due to cardiovascular collapse, infection, hyperthermia or selfinflicted injury.

### Alcohol-induced Amnestic Disorders

Chronic alcohol abuse associated with thiamine (vitamin B) deficiency is the most frequent cause of amnestic disorders. This condition is divided into:

#### *Wernicke's Syndrome*

This is characterized by prominent cerebellar ataxia, palsy of the 6th cranial nerve, peripheral neuropathy and mental confusion.

#### *Korsakoff's Syndrome*

The prominent symptom in Korsakoff's syndrome is gross memory disturbance. Other symptoms include:

- Disorientation
- Confusion
- Confabulation
- Poor attention span and distractibility
- Impairment of insight.

### Alcohol-induced Psychiatric Disorders

#### *Alcohol-induced Dementia*

It is a long-term complication of alcohol abuse, characterized by global decrease in cognitive functioning (decreased intellectual functioning and memory). This disorder tends to improve with abstinence, but most of the patients may have permanent disabilities.

#### *Alcohol-induced Mood Disorders*

Excess drinking may induce persistent depression or anxiety.

#### *Suicidal Behavior*

Suicidal rates are higher in alcoholics when compared to nonalcoholics of the same age. The risk factors for suicidal behavior are continued drinking, comorbid major depression, serious medical illness, unemployment and poor social support.

#### *Alcohol-induced Anxiety Disorder*

Alcohol persons report panic attacks during acute withdrawal, similarly during the first 4 to 6 weeks of abstinence.

### *Impaired Psychosexual Function*

Erectile dysfunction and delayed ejaculation are common in chronic alcoholics.

### *Pathological Jealousy*

Excessive drinkers may develop an overvalued idea or delusion that the partner is being unfaithful.

### *Alcoholic Seizures (Rum Fits)*

Generalized tonic clonic seizures occur usually within 12 to 48 hours after a heavy bout of drinking. Sometimes, status epilepticus may be precipitated.

### *Alcoholic Hallucinosis*

This is characterized by the presence of hallucinations (auditory) during abstinence, following regular alcohol intake. Recovery occurs within one month.

## Treatment

- *A full assessment:* Including an appraisal of current medical, psychological and social problems.
- *Goal setting:* Setting up of short-term goals that deal with any accompanying problems in health, marriage, job and social adjustments; long-term goals can be set as treatment progresses, which are concerned with trying to change factors that precipitate or maintain excessive drinking, such as tensions in the family.
- *Treatment of withdrawal from alcohol*
  - *Detoxification:* Detoxification is the treatment for alcohol withdrawal symptoms.
  - The drugs of choice are benzodiazepines.
  - The most commonly used drugs from this class are chlordiazepoxide 80 to 200 mg/day and diazepam 40 to 80 mg/day, in divided doses.
  - *Others:*
  - For vitamin B deficiency a preparation of vitamin B containing 100 mg of thiamine should be administered parenterally, twice daily for 3 to 5 days. This should be followed by oral administration of vitamin B for at least 6 months.
  - Administration of anticonvulsants as necessary, maintaining fluid and electrolyte balance, strict monitoring of vitals, level of consciousness and orientation. Close observation is essential, especially during the first five days.
- *Alcohol deterrent therapy:* Deterrent agents are those which are given to desensitize the individual to the effects of alcohol and maintain abstinence. The most commonly used drug is disulfiram (tetraethylthiuram disulfide) or antabuse.

## Disulfiram

Disulfiram is used to ensure abstinence in the treatment of alcohol dependence. Its main effect is to produce a rapid and violently unpleasant reaction in a person who ingests even a small amount of alcohol while taking disulfiram.

### *Mechanism of Action*

Disulfiram is an aldehyde dehydrogenase inhibitor that interferes with the metabolism of alcohol and produces a marked increase in blood acetaldehyde levels. The accumulation of acetaldehyde (to a level of 10 times more than that which occurs in the normal metabolism of alcohol) produces a wide array of unpleasant reactions called the disulfiram-ethanol reaction (DER), characterized by nausea, throbbing headache, vomiting, hypotension, flushing, sweating, thirst, dyspnea, tachycardia, chest pain, vertigo, blurred vision and a sense of impending doom associated with severe anxiety. The action occurs almost immediately after the ingestion of even one alcoholic drink and may last upto 30 minutes.

### *Therapeutic Indications*

The primary indication for disulfiram use is as an aversive conditioning treatment for alcohol dependence.

### *Side Effects*

The adverse effects of disulfiram in the absence of alcohol consumption include fatigue, dermatitis,. impotence, optic neuritis, mental changes, acute polyneuropathy and hepatic damage. With alcohol consumption the intensity of the disulfiram-alcohol reactions varies with each patient. In extreme cases it is marked by convulsions, respiratory depression, cardiovascular collapse, myocardial infarction and death.

### *Contraindications*

- Pulmonary and cardiovascular disease.
- Disulfiram should be used with caution in patients with nephritis, brain damage, hypothyroidism, diabetes, hepatic disease, seizures, poly-drug dependence or an abnormal electroencephalogram.
- Patients at high risk of alcohol ingestion.

### *Dosage*

Disulfiram is supplied in tablets of 250 and 500 mg. The usual initial dose is 500 mg/day orally for the first 2 weeks, followed by a maintenance dosage of 250 mg/day. The dosage should not exceed 500 mg/day.

## CHILDHOOD PSYCHIATRIC DISORDERS

## Mental Retardation (F7)

### *Definition*

'Mental retardation refers to significantly subaverage general intellectual functioning resulting in or associated with concurrent impairments in adaptive behavior and manifested during the developmental period'. *(American Association on Mental Deficiency, 1983).*

### *Classification*

| | |
|---|---|
| Mild (educable) | IQ 50–70 |
| Moderate (trainable) | IQ 35–50 |
| Severe (dependent retarded) | IQ 20–35 |
| Profound (life support) | IQ < 20 |

## Behavioral Manifestations

### *Mild Retardation (IQ 50–70)*

This is the commonest type of mental retardation accounting for 85 to 90% of all cases. These individuals have minimum retardation in sensory motor areas. They can develop social and communication skills, but have deficits in cognitive function like poor ability for abstraction and egocentric thinking.

### *Moderate Retardation (IQ 35–50)*

About 10% of mentally retarded come under this group. Communication skills develop much slowly in these individuals. They can be trained to support themselves by performing semiskilled or unskilled work under supervision.

### *Severe Retardation (IQ 20–35)*

Severe mental retardation is often recognized early in life with poor motor development and absent or markedly delayed speech and communication skills. There is a possibility of teaching some skills in AOL skills with long-term consistent behavior modification. But most of them require a great deal of assistance and structured living arrangements.

### *Profound Retardation (1.0 < 20)*

This group accounts for 1 to 2% of all mentally retarded. The achievement of developmental milestones is markedly delayed. They require constant nursing care and supervision. Associated physical disorders are common.

## Diagnosis

- History collection from parents and caretakers.
- Physical examination.
- Neurological examination.
- Assessing milestones development.
- Investigations urine and blood examination for metabolic disorders culture for cytogenic and biochemical studies.
- Amniocentesis in infant chromosomal disorders chorionic villi sampling.
- Hearing and speech evaluation.
- EEG,especially if seizures are present.
- CT scan or MRI brain, e.g. in tuberous sclerosis.
- Thyroid function tests when cretinism is suspected.
- Psychological tests like Stanford Binet Intelligence Scale and Wechsler Intelligence Scale For Children (WISC), for categorizing the child's level of disability.

  Through psychological testing the mental age of the child is estimated. The intelligence quotient is then determined using the formula:

$$\frac{\text{Mental age (MA)}}{\text{Chronological age (CA)}} \times 100$$

## Prognosis

The prognosis for children with mental retardation has improved and institutional care is no longer recommended.

## Prevention

### *Primary Prevention*

*Preconception*

- Genetic counseling which is an attempt to determine risks of occurrence or recurrence of specific genetic or chromosomal disorders; parents can then make an informed decision as to the risks of having a retarded child.
- Immunization for maternal rubella.
- Blood tests for marriage licenses can identify the presence of venereal diseases.
- Adequate maternal nutrition can lay a sound metabolic foundation for later childbearing.
- Family planning in terms of size, appropriate spacing, and age of parents can also affect a variety of specific causal agents.

*During Gestation*

Two general approaches to prevention are associated with this period:

- Prenatal care
- Analysis of fetus for possible genetic disorders.

Prenatal Care

- Adequate nutrition, fetal monitoring and protection from disease.
- Avoidance of teratogenic substances like exposure to radiation and consumption of alcohol and drugs.

Analysis of Fetus

By amniocentesis, fetoscopy, fetal biopsy and ultrasound.

## Care and Rehabilitation of the Mentally Retarded

The main elements in a comprehensive service for mentally retarded individuals and their families include:

- The prevention and early detection of mental handicaps.
- Regular assessment of the mentally retarded person's attainments and disabilities.
- Advice, support, and practical measures for families.
- Provision for education, training, occupation, or work appropriate for each handicapped person.
- Housing and social support to enable self-care.
- Medical, nursing, and other services for those who require them as outpatients, day patients, or inpatients.
- Psychiatric and psychological services.

## General Provisions

The general approach to care is educational and psychosocial. The family doctor and pediatrician are mainly responsible for the early detection and assessment of mental retardation. The team providing continuing health care also includes psychologists, speech therapists, nurses, occupational therapists and physic-therapists.

## The Mildly Retarded

A few mildly retarded children require fostering, boarding schools placements or residential care, but usually specialist services are not required. Mildly retarded adults may need help with housing, employment, or with the special problems of old age.

### The Severely Retarded

In case of children some require special services throughout their lives, which may include a sitting service, day respite during school holidays, or overnight stays in a foster family or residential care. In case of adults, provisions are required for work, occupation, housing, adult education, etc.

### Education and Training

The aim is that as many mentally retarded children as possible are educated in ordinary schools either in normal classes or in special classes. There is now an increasing use of more specialist teaching and a variety of innovative procedures for teaching language and other methods of communication.

### Vocational Training

The activities included in vocational training are work preparation, selective placement, post-placement and follow-up.

### Help for Families

Help for families is needed from the time that the diagnosis is first made; adequate time must be allowed to explain the prognosis; indicate what help can be provided, and discuss the part that the parents can play in helping their child to achieve full potential. When the child starts school, the parents should not only be kept informed about his progress, but should feel involved in the planning and provision of care.

#### *Stages in Parent Counseling*

*Stage 1*

Impart information regarding condition of the mentally retarded child. Avoid giving misleading information or building false hopes in the parents.

*Stage 2*

Help the parents develop right attitude towards their mentally retarded child (to prevent overprotection, rejection, pushing the child too hard). Handle guilty feelings in parents.

*Stage 3*

Create awareness in parents regarding their role in training the child. The parents should be made to realize that training a mentally retarded child does not need complex skills and with repeated training in simple steps, the child can learn. Parents are taught behavior modification techniques to decrease or eliminate problematic behavior, increase adaptive behavior and develop new skills. Some of these techniques include positive reinforcement, shaping, prompting, modeling, extinction procedures, etc.

*Residential Care*

Parents should be supported in caring for their retarded children at home, or if they are too heavy a burden for their parents, the child should be cared for in day-care centers, halfway homes, etc.

*Specialist Medical Services*

Retarded children and adults often have physical handicaps or epilepsy for which continuing medical care is needed.

*Psychiatric Services*

Expert psychiatric care is an essential part of a comprehensive community service for the mentally retarded.

## THERAPEUTIC MODALITIES IN PSYCHIATRY

The various treatment modalities in psychiatry are broadly divided as:

- Somatic (physical) therapies
- Psychological therapies.

Other therapies included in this unit are:

- Milieu therapy
- Therapeutic community
- Activity therapy.

### Psychopharmacology

The understanding of the biological regulation of thought, behavior and mood is the basis of all somatic therapies used in modern psychiatry. Psychopharmacological agents are now the first line treatment for almost every psychiatric ailment. With the growing availability of a wide range of drugs to treat mental illness, the nurse practicing in modern psychiatric settings needs to have a sound knowledge of the pharmacokinetics involved, the benefits and potential risks of pharmacotherapy, as well as her own role and responsibility.

## CLASSIFICATION OF PSYCHOTROPIC DRUGS

- Antipsychotics
- Antidepressants
- Mood stabilizing drugs
- Anxiolytics and hypnosedatives
- Antiepileptic drugs
- Antiparkinsonian drugs
- Miscellaneous drugs which include stimulants, drugs used in eating disorders, drugs used in deaddiction, drugs used in child psychiatry, vitamins, calcium channel blockers, etc.

### Antipsychotics

Antipsychotics are those psychotropic drugs, which are used for the treatment of psychotic symptoms. These are also known as neuroleptics (as they produce neurological side effects), major tranquilizers, D2-receptor blockers and antischizophrenic drugs.

#### *Indications*

Organic psychiatric disorders

- Delirium
- Dementia
- Delirium tremens
- Drug-induced psychosis and other organic mental disorders.

*Functional Disorders*

- Schizophrenia
- Schizoaffective disorders
- Paranoid disorders.

*Mood Disorders*

- Mania
- Major depression with psychotic symptoms.

*Childhood Disorders*
- Attention-deficit hyperactivity disorder
- Autism
- Enuresis
- Conduct disorder.

*Neurotic and other Psychiatric Disorders*
- Anorexia nervosa
- Intractable obsessive compulsive disorder
- Severe, intractable and disabling anxiety.

*Medical Disorders*
- Huntington's chorea
- Intractable hiccough
- Nausea and vomiting
- Tic disorder
- Eclampsia
- Heatstroke
- Severe pain in malignancy
- Tetanus.

### Pharmacokinetics

Antipsychotics when administered orally are absorbed variably from the gastrointestinal tract, with uneven blood levels. They are highly bound to plasma as well as tissue proteins. Brain concentration is higher than plasma concentration. They are metabolized in the liver, and excreted mainly through the kidneys. The elimination half-life varies from 10 to 24 hours.

Most of the antipsychotics tend to have a therapeutic window. If the blood level is below this window, the drug is ineffective. If the blood level is higher than the upper limit of the window, there is toxicity or the drug is again ineffective.

### Mechanism of Action

Antipsychotic drugs block D2 receptors in the mesolimbic and mesofrontal systems (concerned with emotional reactions). Sedation is caused by alpha-adrenergic blockade. Antidopaminergic actions on basal ganglia are responsible for causing extrapyramidal symptoms (EPS). Atypical antipsychotics have antiserotonergic (5-hydroxytryptamine or 5-HT) antiadrenergic and antihistaminergic actions.These are therefore called as serotonin-dopamine antagonists.

### Adverse Effects of Antipsychotic Drugs

- ***Extrapyramidal Symptoms (EPS)***
  - ***Neuroleptic-induced parkinsonism:*** Symptoms include rigidity, tremors, bradykinesia, stooped posture, drooling, akinesia, ataxia, etc. The disorder can be treated with anticholinergic agents.
  - ***Acute dystonia:*** Dystonic movements results from a slow sustained muscular spasm that lead to an involuntary movement. Dystonia can involve the neck, jaw, tongue and the entire body (opisthotonos). There is also involvement of eyes leading to upward lateral movement of the eye known as oculogyric crisis. Dystonias can be prevented by anticholinergics, antihistaminergics, dopamine agonists, beta-adrenergic antagonists, benzodiazepines, etc.
  - ***Akathisia:*** Akathisia is a subjective feeling of muscular discomfort that can cause patients to be agitated, restless and feel generally dysphoric. Akathisia can be treated with propranolol, benzodiazepines and clonidine.
  - ***Tardive dyskinesia:*** It is a delayed adverse effect of antipsychotics. It consists of abnormal, irregular choreoathetoid movements of the muscles of the head, limbs and trunk. It is characterized by chewing, sucking, grimacing and perioral movements.
  - ***Neuroleptic malignant syndrome:*** This is a rare but serious disorder occurring in a small minority of patients taking neuroleptics, especially high-potency compounds. The onset is often, but not invariably, in the first 10 days of treatment. The clinical picture includes the rapid onset (usually over 24–72 hours) of severe motor, mental and autonomic disorders. The prominent *motor* symptom is generalized muscular hypertonicity. Stiffness of the muscles in the throat and chest may cause dysphasia, and dyspnea. The *mental* symptoms include akinetic mutism, stupor or impaired consciousness. Hyperpyrexia develops with evidence of *autonomic* disturbances in the form of unstable blood pressure, tachycardia, excessive sweating, salivation, and urinary incontinence. In the blood, creatinine phosphokinase (CPK) levels may be raised to very high levels, and the white cell count may be increased. Secondary features may include pneumonia, thromboembolism, cardiovascular collapse, and renal failure. The syndrome lasts for 1 to 2 weeks after stopping the drug.
- ***Autonomic Side Effects:*** Dry mouth, constipation, cycloplegia, mydriasis, urinary retention, orthostatic hypotension, impotence and impaired ejaculation.
- ***Seizures***
- ***Sedation***
- ***Other Effects***
  - Agranulocytosis (especially for clozapine)
  - Sialorrhea or increased salivation (especially for clozapine)
  - Weight gain
  - Jaundice
  - Dermatological effects (contact dermatitis, photosensitive reaction).

## Antidepressants

Antidepressants are those drugs, which are used for the treatment of depressive illness. These are also called as mood elevators or thymoleptics.

### Indications

*Depression*
- Depressive episode
- Dysthymia
- Reactive depression
- Secondary depression
- Abnormal grief reaction.

*Childhood Psychiatric Disorders*
- Enuresis
- Separation anxiety disorder

- Somnambulism
- School phobia
- Night terrors.

*Other Psychiatric Disorders*
- Panic attack
- Generalized anxiety disorder
- Agoraphobia, social phobia
- OCD with or without depression
- Eating disorder
- Borderline personality disorder
- Post-traumatic stress disorder
- Depersonalization syndrome.

*Medical Disorders*
- Chronic pain
- Migraine
- Peptic ulcer disease.

### Pharmacokinetics

Antidepressants are highly lipophilic and protein-bound. The half-life is long and usually more than 24 hours. It is predominantly metabolized in the liver.

*Mechanism of Action*

The exact mechanism is unknown. The predominant action is by increasing catecholamine levels in the brain. TCAs are also called as monoamine reuptake inhibitors (MARIs). The main mode of action is by blocking the reuptake of norepinephrine (NE) and/or serotonin (5-HT) at the nerve terminals, thus increasing the NE and 5-HT levels at the receptor site. MAO is instead act on MAO (monoamine oxidase),which is responsible for the degradation of catecholamines after reuptake. The final effect is the same, a functional increase in the NE and 5-HT levels at the receptor site. The increase in brain amine levels is probably responsible for the antidepressant action. It takes about 5 to 10 days for MAO is and 2 to 3 weeks for TCAs to bring down depressive symptoms. SSRIs act by inhibiting the reuptake of serotonin and increasing its levels at the receptor site.

*Side Effects*

- ***Autonomic side effects:*** Dry mouth, constipation, cycloplegia, mydriasis, urinary retention, orthostatic hypotension, impotence, impaired ejaculation, delirium and aggravation of glaucoma.
- ***CNS effects:*** Sedation, tremor and other extrapyramidal symptoms, withdrawal syndrome, seizures, jitteriness syndrome, precipitation of mania.
- ***Cardiac side effects:*** Tachycardia, ECG changes, arrhythmias, direct myocardial depression, quinidine-like action (decreased conduction time).
- ***Allergic side effects:*** Agranulocytosis, cholestatic jaundice, skin rashes, systemic vasculitis.
- ***Metabolic and endocrine side effects:*** Weight gain.
- ***Special effects of MAOI drugs:*** Hypertensive crises, severe hepatic necrosis, hyperpyrexia.

## Lithium and other Mood Stabilizing Drugs

Mood stabilizers are used for the treatment of bipolar affective disorders. Some commonly used mood stabilizers are:

- Lithium
- Carbamazepine
- Sodium valproate.

### Lithium

Lithium is an element with atomic number 3 and atomic weight 7. It was discovered by FJ Cade in 1949, and is a most effective and commonly used drug in the treatment of mania.

*Indications*
- Acute mania
- Prophylaxis for bipolar and unipolar mood disorder
- Schizoaffective disorder
- Cyclothymia
- Impulsivity and aggression
- Other disorders:
  - Premenstrual dysphoric disorder
  - Bulimia nervosa
  - Borderline personality disorder
  - Episodes of binge drinking
  - Trichotillomania
  - Cluster headaches.

*Pharmacokinetics*

Lithium is readily absorbed with peak plasma levels occurring 2 to 4 hours after a single oral dose of lithium carbonate. Lithium is distributed rapidly in liver and kidney and more slowly in muscle, brain and bone. Steady state levels are achieved in about 7 days. Elimination is predominantly via kidneys. Lithium is reabsorbed in the proximal tubules and is influenced by sodium balance. Depletion of sodium can precipitate lithium toxicity.

*Mechanism of Action*

The probable mechanisms of action can be:
- It accelerates presynaptic reuptake and destruction of catecholamines, like norepinephrine.
- It inhibits the release of catecholamines at the synapse.
- It decreases postsynaptic serotonin receptor sensitivity.

All these actions result in decreased catecholamine activity, thus ameliorating mania.

*Dosage*

Lithium is available in the market in the form of the following preparations:
- Lithium carbonate: 300 mg tablets (e.g. Licab); 400 mg sustained release tablets (e.g. Lithosun-SR).
- Lithium citrate: 300 mg/5mL liquid.

The usual range of dose per day in acute mania is 900–2100 mg given in 2–3 divided doses.

The treatment is started after serial lithium estimation is done after a loading dose of 600 mg or 900 mg of lithium to determine the pharmacokinetics.

*Blood Lithium Levels*
- Therapeutic levels = 0.8–1.2 mEq/L (for treatment of acute mania)
- Prophylactic levels = 0.6–1.2 mEq/L (for prevention of relapse in bipolar disorder)
- Toxic lithium levels > 2.0 mEq/L.

*Management of Lithium Toxicity*

- Discontinue the drug immediately.
- For significant short-term ingestions, residual gastric content should be removed by induction of emesis, gastric lavage and adsorption with activated charcoal.
- If possible instruct the patient to ingest fluids.
- Assess serum lithium levels, serum electrolytes, renal functions, ECG as soon as possible.
- Maintenance of fluid and electrolyte balance.
- In a patient with serious manifestations of lithium toxicity, hemodialysis should be initiated.

*Contraindications of Lithium Use*

- Cardiac, renal, thyroid or neurological dysfunctions
- Presence of blood dyscrasias
- During first trimester of pregnancy and lactation
- Severe dehydration
- Hypothyroidism
- History of seizures.

### Carbamazepine

It is available in the market under different trade names like Tegretol, Mazetol, Zeptol and Zen Retard.

*Indications*

- ***Seizures:*** Complex partial seizures, GTCS, seizures due to alcohol withdrawal.
- ***Psychiatric disorders:*** Rapid cycling bipolar disorder, acute depression, impulse control disorder, aggression, psychosis with epilepsy, schizoaffective disorders, borderline personality disorder, cocaine withdrawal syndrome.
- ***Paroxysmal pain syndromes:*** Trigeminal neuralgia and phantom limb pain.

*Dosage*

The average daily dose is 600 to 1800 mg orally, in divided doses. The therapeutic blood levels are 6 to 12 µg/mL. Toxic blood levels are attained at more than 15 µg/mL.

*Mechanism of Action*

Its mood stabilizing mechanism is not clearly established. Its anticonvulsant action may however be by decreasing synaptic transmission in the CNS.

*Side Effects*

Drowsiness, confusion, headache, ataxia, hypertension, arrhythmias, skin rashes, Steven-Johnson syndrome, nausea, vomiting, diarrhea, dry mouth, abdominal pain, jaundice, hepatitis, oliguria, leukopenia, thrombocytopenia, bone marrow depression leading to aplastic anemia.

## Sodium Valproate (Encorate Chrono, Valparin, Epilex, Epival)

### Indications

- Acute mania, prophylactic treatment of bipolar I disorder, rapid cycling bipolar disorder
- Schizoaffective disorder
- Seizures
- Other disorders like bulimia nervosa, obsessive compulsive disorder, agitation and PTSD.

### Mechanism of Action

The drug acts on gamma-aminobutyric acid (GABA) an inhibitory amino acid neurotransmitter. GABA receptor activation serves to reduce neuronal excitability.

### Dosage

The usual dose is 15 mg/kg/ day with a maximum of 60 mg/kg/day orally.

*Side Effects*

Nausea, vomiting, diarrhea, sedation, ataxia, dysarthria, tremor, weight gain, loss of hair, thrombocytopenia, platelet dysfunction.

## Anxiolytics (Antianxiety Drugs) and Hypnosedatives

These are also called as minor tranquilizers. Most of them belong to the benzodiazepine group of drugs.

### Classification

- ***Barbiturates:*** Example, phenobarbital, pentobarbital, secobarbital and thiopentone.
- ***Nonbarbiturate nonbenzodiazepine anti-anxiety agents:*** Meprobamate glutethimide, ethanol, diphenhydramine and methaqualone.
- ***Benzodiazepines:*** Presently benzodiazepines are the drugs of first choice in the treatment of anxiety, and for the treatment of insomnia.
  - ***Very short-acting:*** Triazolam, midazolam.
  - ***Short-acting:*** Oxazepam (Serepax), lorazepam (Ativan, Trapex, Larpose), alprazolam (Restyl, Trika, Alzolam, Quiet, Anxit).
  - ***Long-acting:*** Chlordiazepoxide (Librium), diazepam (Valium, Calmpose), clonazepam (Lonazep), Flurazepam (Nindral), nitrazepam (Dormin).

### Indications for Benzodiazepines

- Anxiety disorders
- Insomnia
- Depression
- Panic disorder and social phobia
- Obsessive compulsive disorder
- Post-traumatic stress disorder
- Bipolar I disorder
- Other psychiatric indications include alcohol withdrawal, substance-induced and psychotic agitation.

*Dosage (mg/day)*

| | |
|---|---|
| Alprazolam: | 0.5–6 PO |
| Oxazepam: | 15–120 PO |
| Lorazepam: | 2–6 PO/IV/IM |
| Diazepam: | 2–10 PO/IM/slow IV |
| Clonazepam: | 0.5–20 PO/IM |
| Chlordiazepoxide: | 15–100 PO; 50–100 slow IV |
| Nitrazepam: | 5–20 PO |

### Mechanism of Action

Benzodiazepines bind to specific sites on the GABA receptors and increase GABA level. Since GABA is an inhibitory neurotransmitter, it has a calming effect on the central nervous system, thus reducing anxiety.

### Side Effects

Nausea, vomiting, weakness, vertigo, blurring of vision, body aches, epigastric pain, diarrhea, impotence, sedation, increased reaction time, ataxia, dry mouth, retrograde amnesia, impairment of driving skills, dependence and withdrawal symptoms (the drug should be withdrawn slowly, as a result).

## Antiparkinsonian Agents

In clinical practice anticholinergic drugs, amantadine and the antihistamines have their primary use as treatments for medication-induced movement disorders, particularly neuroleptic-induced parkinsonism, acute dystonia and medication-induced tremor.

### Anticholinergics

- Trihexyphenidyl
- Benztropine
- Biperiden.

### Dopaminergic Agents

- Bromocriptine
- Carbidopa/levodopa.

### Monoamine Oxidase Type B Inhibitors

- Selegiline

### Trihexyphenidyl (Artane, Trihexane, Trihexy, Pacitane)

*Indications*

- Drug-induced parkinsonism
- Adjunct in the management of parkinsonism.

*Mechanism of Action*

It acts by increasing the release of dopamine from presynaptic vesicles, blocking the reuptake of dopamine into presynaptic nerve terminals or by exerting an agonist effect on postsynaptic dopamine receptors.

Trihexyphenidyl reaches peak plasma concentrations in 2–3 hours after oral administration and has a duration of action of upto 12 hours.

*Dosage*

1–2 mg per day orally initially. Maximum dose up to 15 mg/day in divided doses.

*Side Effects*

Dizziness, nervousness, drowsiness, weakness, headache, confusion, blurred vision, mydriasis, tachycardia, orthostatic hypotension, dry mouth, nausea, constipation, vomiting, urinary retention and decreased sweating.

## Drugs Used in Child Psychiatry

### Clonidine

*Indications*

- Control of withdrawal symptoms from opioids
- Tourette's disorder
- Control of aggressive or hyperactive behavior in children
- Autism.

### Mechanism of Action

- Alpha 2-adrenergic receptor agonist.
- The agonist effects of clonidine on presynaptic alpha 2-adrenergic receptors result in a decrease in the amount of neurotransmitter released from the presynaptic nerve terminals. This decrease serves generally to reset the sympathetic tone at a lower level and to decrease arousal.

### Dosage

Usual starting dosage is 0.1 mg orally twice a day; the dosage can be raised by 0.3 mg a day to an appropriate level.

### Side Effects

Dry mouth, dryness of eyes, fatigue, irritability, sedation, dizziness, nausea, vomiting, hypotension and constipation.

## Methylphenidate (Ritalin)

Methylphenidate, dextroamphetamine and pemoline are sympathomimetics.

### Indications

- Attention-deficit hyperactivity disorder
- Narcolepsy
- Depressive disorders
- Obesity.

### Mechanism of Action

Sympathomimetics cause the stimulation of alpha and beta-adrenergic receptors directly as agonists and indirectly by stimulating the release of dopamine and norepinephrine from presynaptic terminals. Dextroamphetamine and methylphenidate are also inhibitors of catecholamine reuptake, especially dopamine reuptake and inhibitors of monoamine oxidase. The net result of these activities is believed to be the stimulation of several brain regions.

### Dosage

Starting dose is 5 to 10 mg per day orally, maximum daily dose is 80 mg/day.

### Side Effects

Anorexia or dyspepsia, weight loss, slowed growth, dizziness, insomnia or nightmares, dysphoric mood, tics and psychosis.

## Electroconvulsive Therapy

Electroconvulsive therapy is a type of somatic treatment first introduced by Bini and Cerletti in April 1938. From 1980 onwards ECT is being considered as a unique psychiatric treatment. Electroconvulsive therapy is the artificial induction of a grand mal seizure through the application of electrical current to the brain. The stimulus is applied through electrodes that are placed either bilaterally in the frontotemporal region, or unilaterally on the nondominant side (right side of head in a right-handed individual).

### Parameters of Electrical Current Applied

Standard dose according to American Psychiatric Association, 1978:

- Voltage: 70 to 120 Volts
- Duration: 0.7 to 1.5 seconds.

### Type of Seizure Produced

- Grand mal seizure—tonic phase lasting for 10 to 15 seconds.
- Clonic phase lasting for 30 to 60 seconds.

### Mechanism of Action

The exact mechanism of action is not known. One hypothesis states that ECT possibly affects the catecholamine pathways between diencephalon (from where seizure generalization occurs) and limbic system (which may be responsible for mood disorders), also involving the hypothalamus.

### Types of ECT

*Direct ECT:* In this, ECT is given in the absence of anesthesia and muscular relaxation. This is not a commonly used method now.
*Modified ECT:* Here ECT is modified by drug- induced muscular relaxation and general anesthesia.

### Frequency and Total Number of ECT

**Frequency:** Three times per week or as indicated.
**Total number:** 6 to 10; upto 25 may be preferred as indicated.

### Application of Electrodes

*Bilateral ECT:* Each electrode is placed 2.5 to 4 cm (1–1½ inch) above the midpoint, on a line joining the tragus of the ear and the lateral canthus of the eye.
*Unilateral ECT:* Electrodes are placed only on one side of head, usually nondominant side (right side of head in a right-handed individual).

Unilateral ECT is safer, with much fewer side effects particularly those of memory impairment.

### Indications

- *Major depression:* With suicidal risk; with stupor; with poor intake of food and fluids; melancholia with psychotic features with unsatisfactory response to drugs or where drugs are contraindicated or have serious side effects.
- *Severe catatonia (functional):* With stupor; with poor intake of food and fluids; with unsatisfactory response to drug therapy, or when drugs are contraindicated or have serious side effects.
- *Severe psychosis (schizophrenia or mania):* With risk of suicide, homicide or danger of physical assault; with depressive features; with unsatisfactory response to drug therapy, or when drugs are contraindicated or have serious side effects.
- *Organic mental disorders:*
  - Organic mood disorders.
  - Organic psychosis.
- *Other indications:* ECT is preferred to antidepressant therapy in some cases, such as for clients with cardiac disease; when tricyclics are contraindicated because of the potential for dysrhythmias and congestive heart failure; and for pregnant women, in whom antidepressants place the fetus at risk for congenital defects.

### Contraindications

*Absolute*

Raised ICP (intracranial pressure).

*Relative*

- Cerebral aneurysm
- Cerebral hemorrhage
- Brain tumor
- Acute myocardial infarction
- Congestive heart failure
- Pneumonia or aortic aneurysm
- Retinal detachment.

### Complications of ECT

Life-threatening complications of ECT are rare. ECT does not cause any brain damage. Fractures can sometimes occur in elderly patients with osteoporosis. In patients with a history of heart disease, dysrhythmias and respiratory arrest may occur.

*Side Effects of ECT*

- Memory impairment.
- Drowsiness, confusion and restlessness.
- Poor concentration, anxiety.
- Headache, weakness/fatigue, backache, muscle aches.
- Dryness of mouth, palpitations, nausea, vomiting.
- Unsteady gait.
- Tongue bite and incontinence.

### ECT Team

Psychiatrist, anesthesiologist, trained nurses and aides should be involved in the administration of ECT.

### Treatment Facilities

There should be a suite of three rooms:

1. A pleasant, comfortable waiting room (pre- ECT room).
2. ECT room, which should be equipped with ECT machine and accessories, an anesthetic appliance, suction apparatus, face masks, oxygen cylinders with adjustable flow valves, curved tongue depressors, mouth gags, resuscitation apparatus and emergency drugs. There should be immediate access to a defibrillator.
3. A well-equipped recovery room.

### Psychosurgery

Psychosurgery is defined by APA's Task Force as 'a surgical intervention, to sever fibers connecting one part of the brain with another, or to remove, destroy, or stimulate brain tissue, with the intent of modifying behavior, thought or mood disturbances, for which there is no underlying organic pathology.'

### Indications

- Severe psychiatric illness
- Chronic duration of illness of about 10 years
- Persistent emotional distress

- Failure to respond to all other therapies
- High-risk of suicide.

### *Major Surgical Procedures*

- Stereotactic subcaudate tractotomy
- Stereotactic limbic leukotomy
- Stereotactic bilateral amygdalotomy.

Nursing care for a patient undergoing psychosurgery is the same as for any neurosurgical procedure.

### Psychological Therapies

There are several kinds of psychological therapies:

- Psychoanalytic therapy
- Behavior therapy
- Cognitive therapy
- Hypnosis
- Abreaction therapy
- Relaxation therapies
- Individual psychotherapy
- Supportive psychotherapy
- Group therapy
- Family and marital therapy.

## LEGAL ASPECTS OF MENTAL HEALTH NURSING

There are two acts concerned with the care and treatment of the mentally ill:

### The Indian Lunacy Act (1912)

It is derived from English Lunacy Act, 1890 and it contains eight Chapters.

#### *Chapter I*

It contains some preliminary information and definitions.

#### *Chapter II*

It contains mainly the procedure to be followed to admit a psychiatric patient into a mental hospital.

#### *Chapter III*

It describes the procedure to be followed for administering care, treatment and discharge. In Chapter III the term 'Parole' refers to the 'permission given to patients to perform certain rituals or atten certain family functions. During parole, the patient can leave the hospital any time and can be brought back forcefully if he does not return within a maximum period of 90 days. The remaining Chapters (IV–VIII) deal with establishment of asylum, expenses of lunatics and the rules to be imposed by the State Government regarding care of lunatics.

### The Indian Mental Health Act (1987)

The Indian Mental Health Act is derived from Mental Health Act of England and Wales (1959 amended in 1982). The Mental Health Bill became the Act 14 of 1987 on 22nd May, 1987.

### *Objectives of the Indian Mental Health Act*

- To regulate admission into psychiatric hospitals and psychiatric nursing homes.
- To protect society from the presence of mentally ill persons.
- To protect citizens from being detained in psychiatric hospitals/nursing homes without sufficient cause.
- To regulate maintenance charges of psychiatric hospitals/ nursing homes.
- To provide facilities for establishing guardianship of mentally ill persons who are incapable of managing their own affairs.
- To establish central and state authorities for mental health services.
- To regulate the powers of the government for establishing, licensing and controlling psychiatric hospitals/nursing homes.
- To provide legal aid to mentally ill persons at state expense in certain cases. The Act contains 10 Chapters.

#### *Chapter I*

It contains preliminary information. Some definitions included in this are:

- ***Psychiatric hospital/nursing home:*** A hospital/nursing home established or maintained by the government or any other person for the care of mentally ill persons.
- ***Mentally ill person:*** A person who is in need of treatment by reason of any mental disorder other than mental retardation.
- ***Psychiatrist:*** A medical practitioner possessing a post-graduate degree or diploma in psychiatry recognized by the MCI (Medical Council of India).
- ***Reception order:*** An order made under the provisions of this Act for the admission and detention of a mentally ill person in a psychiatric hospital/nursing home.

#### *Chapter II*

It deals with establishment of central and state authorities for regulation and coordination of mental health services.

#### *Chapter III*

It provides guidelines for establishment and maintenance of psychiatric hospitals/nursing homes.

#### *Chapter IV*

It deals with the procedures for admission and detention in psychiatric hospitals/nursing homes.

*Admission on Voluntary Basis*

Any person who considers himself to be mentally ill and wishes to be admitted to a psychiatric hospital may apply to the medical officer in-charge, if he is a minor, the guardian can make this application on his behalf.

*Admission under Special Circumstances*

Any mentally ill patient who is unwilling for admission on a voluntary basis may be admitted and kept as an inpatient in a psychiatric hospital/nursing home.

*Admission under Reception Order*

- ***On application:*** Only a relative not other than husband, wife, guardian or a friend can make out an application for the admission of a mentally ill patient. Such an application should be made out to the Magistrate in writing supported by two medical certificates, one of them issued by a gazetted medical officer. However no person being a minor or one who has not seen the mentally ill patient in the last 14 days can make such an application.

- *On production before the Magistrate:* Mentally ill patients exhibiting violent behavior, creating obscene scenes and dangerous to the society can be detained by the police officer and produced in court within 24 hours of such detention, supported by two medical certificates, subsequent to which the Magistrate issues a reception order.

*Admission in Emergencies*

The medical officer in-charge may order the admission of a mentally ill patient if he thinks he is dangerous to himself or others. However the patient should be produced before the Magistrate within 24 hours (maximum time limit is 72 hours, which is exclusive of the examination period), or the Magistrate himself may visit the psychiatric hospital/ nursing home and pass reception order on examination.

*Temporary Treatment Order*

It is an order issued by the Magistrate in cases where the risk is perceived to the patient's life or to that of others. If the medical officer in-charge feels it necessary to bring legal authorities into the picture he can do so by applying to the Magistrate.

### Chapter V

It deals mainly with the procedure to be followed for the *discharge* of mentally ill persons from a mental hospital under different circumstances.

*Discharge of a Patient Admitted on Voluntary Basis*

Medical officer in-charge of psychiatric hospital/nursing home on recommendation from two medical practitioners preferably a psychiatrist, can issue directions for discharge of the patient.

*Discharge of a Patient Admitted under Special Circumstances*

A relative or a friend may make an application to the medical officer for care and custody of the patient. The relatives are required to furnish a bond with or without sureties, along with an undertaking that the mentally ill person shall be prevented from causing injury to self or others.

*Discharge of a Patient Admitted on Reception Order*

An applicant who feels that the patient has recovered from illness may make an application for discharge to the Magistrate. A certificate should accompany such an application from medical officer in-charge of the psychiatric hospital/nursing home. If the Magistrate deems fit he may issue an order for discharge.

*Discharge of a Patient Admitted by Police*

In cases where the police detain the mentally ill individual in hospital, he may be discharged after the family members agree in writing to take proper care, and the medical officer in-charge opines that he is fit to be discharged.

*Discharge of a Mentally Ill Prisoner*

The hospital authorities have to report every 6 months about the person's state of mind to the authority, which had ordered detention. As soon as they find that the person is fit to stand the trial, they have to inform about the same to the authority concerned. The person is then handed over to the prison officer for further legal action.

### Leave of Absence

On application by a relative or others to the medical officer in-charge and a bond duly signed stating that the patient will be taken proper care of and prevented from injuring self or others, leave of absence may be granted (for a period of maximum 60 days).

### Chapter VI

It deals with judicial enquiry regarding mentally ill persons possessing property, their custody and management of property. A guardian may be appointed by court of law on behalf of an alleged mentally ill person incapable of looking after self and property.

### Chapter VII

It deals with ways and means to meet the cost of maintenance of mentally ill persons detained in psychiatric hospital/nursing home.

### Chapter VIII

It is the latest addition to the act, which provides for the protection of human rights of mentally ill person. These rights include:

- No mentally ill person shall be subjected during treatment to any indignity (physical or mental) or cruelty.
- No mentally ill person under treatment shall be used for the purpose of research unless
  - Such research is of direct benefit to him.
  - A consent has been obtained in writing from the person (in voluntary admission) or from the guardian/relative (if admission was involuntary).
- No letter or communication sent by or to a mentally ill person shall be intercepted, detained or destroyed.

### Chapter IX

It deals with procedures to be followed for the establishment and maintenance of psychiatric hospitals/nursing homes, and the penalties, which can be relatively severe and explicit, for contravening them.

### Chapter X

It deals with clarification pertaining to certain procedures to be followed by the medical officer in-charge of the psychiatric hospital/nursing home.

## MULTIPLE CHOICE QUESTIONS

**1. Delirium is an acute organic mental illness in which there is:**
(a) Impairment of consciousness
(b) Psychomotor and perceptual disturbances
(c) Disturbance in sleep
(d) All of the above

**2. Management of stress is extremely important in today's society as:**
(a) Evolution has diminished human capability for fight or flight
(b) The stressor of today tends to be ongoing, resulting in a sustained response
(c) We have stress disorder that did not exist in the time of our ancestors
(d) One never knows when one will have to face giggly bear or sober toothed tiger in today's society

**3. Which of the following is selective serotonin reuptake inhibitors (SSRI):**
(a) Citalopram (b) Trazodone
(c) Mirtazapine (d) Amitriptyline

**4. Dispomania:**
(a) Polydypsia (b) Type of mania
(c) Compulsive drinking (d) Speech disorder

**5. The mental health bill became the act in the year of:**
(a) 1981 (b) 1987
(c) 1912 (d) 1981

**6. The ability to see beyond outward behavior and to understand the situation from the client's point of view is known as:**
(a) Rapport (b) Trust
(c) Respect (d) Empathy

**7. Transfer of feeling from one target to another that is considered less threatening or that is neutral is:**
(a) Displacement (b) Projection
(c) Sublimation (d) Suppression

**8. As per psychodynamic theory, anxiety is usually deal with the defence mechanism of:**
(a) Repression (b) Projection
(c) Displacement (d) Sublimation

**9. A false sense of familiarity with unfamiliar circumstances or scenes is:**
(a) Distractibility (b) Déjà vu
(c) Delusion (d) Disorientation

**10. The optimal number of client in a group therapy would be:**
(a) 4–6 (b) 10–12
(c) 8–10 (d) 3–5

**11. Gross and persistent attitude of irresponsibility and disregard for social norms, rules and obligations is seen in:**
(a) Histrionic personality disorder
(b) Antisocial/dissocial personality disorder
(c) Schizotypal disorder
(d) Narcissistic personality disorder

**12. When fixed goal is never reached and patient loses track of the original question is:**
(a) Incoherence (b) Tangentiality
(c) Circumstantiality (d) Perseveration

**13. The commonest cause of dementia is:**
(a) Alzheimer's disease
(b) AIDS dementia complex
(c) Multi-infarct dementia
(d) Lewy body dementia

**14. With which of the following diagnostic imaging technique can metabolic activity of brain is visualized:**
(a) MRI
(b) EEG
(c) Computerized EEG mapping
(d) PET

**15. The affect most commonly seen in the client with schizophrenia is one of the:**
(a) Happiness and elation
(b) Apathy and emotional blunting
(c) Sadness and depression
(d) Anger and hostility

**16. An extrapyramidal symptoms (EPS) that is potentially irreversible side effect of antipsychotic is:**
(a) Torticollis
(b) Oculogyric crisis
(c) Pseudoparkinsonism
(d) Tardive dyskinesia

**17. Correct assumption regarding the concept of crisis is:**
(a) Crisis occurs only in individual with psycjopathology
(b) The stress event that precipitates crisis is seldom identifiable
(c) A crisis situation contain the potential for psychological growth or deterioration
(d) Crisis is a chronic situation

**18. Biological situations are:**
(a) Genetic and decreased level of serotonin
(b) Heredity and increased level of norepinephrine
(c) Temporal lobe atrophy and decreased level of acetylcholine
(d) Structural alteration of the brain and increased level of dopamine

**19. Hallucination that usually occurs in alcoholic hallucinosis is:**
(a) Auditoy
(b) Visual
(c) Tactile
(d) Olfactory

**20. ICD 10 classification in psychiatry section F20 to F29 includes:**
(a) Schizophrenia, schizotypal and delusional disorder
(b) Mood disorder
(c) Mental retardation
(d) Unspecified mental disorder

**21. Irrational fear of situation is known as:**
(a) Specific phobia (b) Social phobia
(c) Agrophobia (d) Algophobia

**22. Exaggerated concern overly bodily health is seen in:**
(a) Hysterical patient
(b) Hypochondriac patient
(c) Obsessive patient
(d) Paranoid patient

**23. The nurse-patient relationship where most of the problem-solving occurs:**
(a) Orientation phase (b) Working phase
(c) Planning phase (d) Termination phase

**24. Delusion of guilt are common in:**
(a) Depression (b) Mania
(c) OCD (d) Schizophrenia

**25. An obsession is:**
(a) An ideal, impulse (b) A form of behavior
(c) A type of delusion (d) A type of hallucination

**26. In the moderate level of mental retardation, IQ range from:**
(a) 20–35 (b) < 20
(c) 35–50 (d) 50–70

**27. Delusion of double is:**
(a) Reactive psychosis
(b) Capgras' syndrome
(c) Schizo- affective disorder
(d) Induced delusion disorder

**28. Therapeutic serum level of lithium on maintenance is:**
(a) 2.2–2.5 mEq/L (b) 0.8–1.8 mEq/L
(c) 1.8–2.0 mEq/L (d) 0.6–1.2 mEq/L

**29. ECT is most commonly prescribed for:**
(a) Bipolar disorder
(b) Paranoid disorder
(c) Major depression with suicidal ideas
(d) OCD

**30. Attention of client during mental status examination is checked by:**
(a) Digit span test
(b) Subtracting several seven test
(c) Proverb testing
(d) By asking the name of the president

**31. In psychiatric disorder their is impairment of:**
(a) Cognition (b) Conation
(c) Affect (d) All of the above

**32. Agoraphobia is dread of:**
(a) High places (b) Open places
(c) Pain (d) Animal

**33. All of the following are true about dementia EXCEPT:**
(a) Impaired memory
(b) Impaired consciousness
(c) Impaired intellect
(d) Impaired personality

**34. Which of the following is most disturbed in manic-depressive is order psychosis?**
(a) Affect (b) Thought
(c) Behavior (d) Orientation

**35. All of the following are conduct disorder of childhood EXCEPT:**
(a) Truancy (b) Vagrancy
(c) Fire setting (d) Nail biting

**36. Introverted and extroverted personality types were proposed by:**
(a) Jung (b) Freud
(c) Skinner (d) Kretschmer

**37. Onset of delirium tremens is:**
(a) Acute (b) Chronic
(c) Subacute (d) Insidious

**38) Redirection of repressed primitive impulse into socially acceptable and productive channel:**
(a) Displacement
(b) Sublimation
(c) Transferences
(d) Reaction formation

**39. The most common type of neurosis is:**
(a) Hypochondriasis
(b) Obsessive compulsive neurosis
(c) Anxiety neurosis
(d) Phobia

**40. The most probable biochemistry abnormality in schizophrenia is:**
(a) GABA (b) Dopamine
(c) Adrenaline (d) Acetylcholine

**41. McNaughton's rules are meant for:**
(a) Establishing testamentary capacity
(b) Establishing criminal responsibility
(c) Establishing divorce
(d) Proper care of mentally ill

**42. All the following drugs have antidepressant effect EXCEPT:**
(a) Trifluoperazine (b) Amitriptyline
(c) Imipramine (d) MAO inhibitor

**43. Suicide is most common in:**
(a) Alcoholism
(b) Personality disorder
(c) Depression
(d) Obsessive compulsive disorder

**44. Phallic stage of psychosexual development is:**
(a) First 18 month of life
(b) 18 months to 3 years
(c) 3–5 years
(d) 5–11 years

**45. Waxy flexibility is a feature of:**
(a) Paranoid schizophrenia
(b) Catatonic schizophrenia
(c) Hebephrenic schizophrenia
(d) Schizoaffective schizophrenia

**46. Models of normalcy and abnormalcy are all EXCEPT:**
(a) Medical model
(b) Psychoanalytical model
(c) Biological model
(d) Sociocultural model

**47. Injection atropine sulfate is given to patient ½ an hour before ECT:**
(a) To induce anxiety
(b) To induce anesthesia
(c) To relax muscle
(d) To reduce secretion and prevention aspiration

**48. Secondary prevention of mental illness includes:**
(a) Health maintenance (b) Early diagnosis
(c) Specific protection (d) Rehabilitation

**49. Task of preinteraction phase of therapeutic nurse-patient relationship is:**
(a) Assist patient to identify his own problem
(b) Encourage patient to socialize
(c) Nurse explore her own fears and anxiety
(d) Evaluate progress toward the goals

**50. Behavioral psychotherapy includes all EXCEPT:**
(a) Abreaction (b) Aversion therapy
(c) Implosive therapy (d) Assertiveness training

**51. Following are the biological factors causing mental illness EXCEPT:**
(a) Constitutional factor (b) Maternal factor
(c) Genetic factor (d) Physical factor

**52. Inability to experience pleasure in previously pleasurable activities is known as:**
(a) Anergia (b) Anxiety
(c) Anhedonia (d) Withdrawal

**53. Patient says that he is dead or his leg is missing is delusion of:**
(a) Grandeur (b) Nihilistic
(c) Persecution (d) Control

**54. A condition in which activity is carried out without conscious knowledge on the part of patient is:**
(a) Automatism (b) Ecoprexia
(c) Stereotype (d) Negativism

**55. In a therapy when individual is exposed directly to a maximum intensity fear in imagination or real life:**
(a) Cognitive behavior therapy
(b) Implosive therapy
(c) Catharsis
(d) Physical therapy

**56. Pleasurable affect includes all of the following EXCEPT:**
(a) Elation (b) Exaltation
(c) Echolalia (d) Euphoria

**57. Digression into unnecessary details that distract from the central theme but return back to original theme after digression known as:**
(a) Tangentiality (b) Confabulation
(c) Echolalia (d) Circumstantiality

**58. The branch of mental health nursing where application of knowledge of psychiatry nursing preventive, promotive and rehabilitative health of the people is:**
(a) Psychiatric mental health nursing
(b) Community mental health nursing
(c) Curative aspect of psychiatric nursing
(d) None of the above

**59. Factors that comes before the disease has occurred, that condition is called:**
(a) Predisposing factor (b) Primary factor
(c) Precipitatory factor (d) Secondary factor

**60. Fear of embarrassing oneself in public characterizes:**
(a) General anxiety disorder
(b) Panic disorder
(c) Specific phobia
(d) Social phobia

**61. Disturbed client repeat phrases that others have just said is known as:**
(a) Autism (b) Echolalia
(c) Neologism (d) Echopraxia

**62. In ECT the intensity of current varies between:**
(a) 90–140 Volts (b) 100–120 Volts
(c) 70–130 Volts (d) 120–160 Volts

**63. Neurotic depression is also known as:**
(a) Endogenous depression
(b) Psychotic depression
(c) Reactive depression
(d) Major depression

**64. The pathological impulse to wear the clothes and accessories of the opposite sex is called as:**
(a) Transsexuality (b) Transvestism
(c) Machoism (d) Voyeurism

**65. The pleasurable feeling with grandiosity is known as:**
(a) Euophoria (b) Elation
(c) Exhalation (d) Ecstasy

**66. When individual is exposed directly to a minimum intensity fear producing situation is:**
(a) Aversion therapy (b) Systematic desensitization
(c) Flooding (d) Assertiveness training

**67. Abnormal, repetitive, involuntary movement of small group of muscle is called:**
(a) Tardive dyskinesia (b) TIC disorder
(c) Truancy (d) Somnambulism

**68. Feeling of familiarity with unfamiliar situation that a person has experienced is known as:**
(a) Delusion (b) Déjà vu
(c) Selective amentia (d) Confabulation

**69. During nurse-patient relationship, the nurse makes an agreement with patient towards social recovery is:**
(a) Confidentiality (b) Contract
(c) Pact (d) Transference

**70. ECT is not effective in:**
(a) Major depression
(b) Involutional melancholia
(c) Postpartum depression
(d) Neurotic depression

**71. False belief of nonexistence of self or other or world is:**
(a) Delusion of grandure (b) Delusion of persecution
(c) Nihilistics delusion (d) Bizarre delusion

**72. Negativism is a disorder of:**
(a) Thought (b) Affect
(c) Perception (d) Psychomotor activity

**73. Amphetamines can be used in treatment of:**
(a) Obesity
(b) Narcolepsy
(c) Attention deficit hyperactivity disorder
(d) All of the above

**74. National Mental Health Programme was started in year:**
(a) 1980 (b) 1979
(c) 1981 (d) 1982

**75. Tardive kinesia is a complication seen in:**
(a) Extrapyramidal symptom
(b) Parkinsonism
(c) Catatonia
(d) Akathesia

**76. Withdrawal from all pleasurable activities is called:**
(a) Anhedonia (b) Depression
(c) Dysthymia (d) Apathy

**77. Founder of psychoanalysis is:**
(a) Linda Richard (b) Sigmund Freud
(c) Jean Martin (d) Philippe Pinel

**78. Excessive elation, inflated self-esteem and grandiosity is present in:**
(a) Bipolar disease (b) Paranoid schizophrenia
(c) Schizophrenia (d) Mania

**79. Bleuler's 4A are fundamental symptoms in:**
(a) Dementia (b) Agoraphobia
(c) Schizophrenia (d) Depression

**80. Recent intake of heroin is clinically judge by:**
(a) Papillary constriction (b) Sedation
(c) Dry mouth (d) Muscle spasm

**81. Delusion is thought disorder at:**
(a) Formation level (b) Content level
(c) Progression level (d) Fantasy level

**82. Which is the expected outcome when working with a client who has experienced a crises?**
(a) Stabilization of mood with medication and return to previous level of functioning
(b) Recovery from crisis and return to precrisis level
(c) Recovery from crisis with intense outpatient therapy
(d) Recovery from crisis with total adjustment of precrisis event

**83. Exaggerated pathological fear of specific type of stimulus or situation:**
(a) Anxiety (b) Negativism
(c) Phobia (d) Denial

**84. Sudden failure to recall one's own identity and past life without forgetting basic habits and skill is:**
(a) Psychogenic amnesia (b) Multiple personality
(c) Depersonalization (d) Fugue

**85. 'Dyslexia' is a specific disorder of:**
(a) Learning (b) Language
(c) Articulation (d) Calculation and arithmetic

**86. The term 'truancy' in child psychiatry refers to:**
(a) Nail biting
(b) Juvenile delinquency
(c) Assault
(d) Running away from home or school

**87. Community mental health services provided in case of emergency is:**
(a) Hotline (b) Walk in clinic
(c) Home visit (d) All of the above

**88. The primary approach of community mental health is ________ mental health illness.**
(a) To treat (b) To rehabilitate
(c) To detect (d) To prevent

**89. An absolute contraindication of ECT:**
(a) Increased ICP (b) Pulmonary disease
(c) CCF (d) Recent stroke

**90. The commonest cause of recurrent relapse in schizophrenia is:**
(a) Unemployment
(b) Poor social support
(c) Noncompliance to treatment
(d) Genetics

**91. Emotional blunting is a typical clinical manifestation of:**
(a) Mania (b) Delirium
(c) Schizophrenia (d) Amnesia

**92. Pica is disorder:**
(a) Eating (b) Sleeping
(c) Psychomotor activity (d) Speech

**93. ECT is referred as:**
(a) Physical therapy (b) Psyche therapy
(c) Drug therapy (d) Psychological therapy

**94. During ECT current is passed for:**
(a) 5–10 sec (b) 10–30 sec
(c) 1.0–3.0 sec (d) 0.5–1.5 sec

**95. Hallucinations are:**
(a) Feeling of familiarity with unfamiliar things
(b) Alteration of perception of ones reality
(c) Misinterpretation of stimulus
(d) Perception occurring without external stimulus

**96. A patient sees a rope and fears like a snake, is called:**
(a) Illusion
(b) Hallucination
(c) Derealization
(d) Depolarization

**97. Father of psychiatry:**
(a) Hippocrates (b) Aspieprades
(c) Renaissance (d) Aristotle

**98. ECT was introduced in year:**
(a) 1936 (b) 1938
(c) 1948 (d) 1942

**99. Behavior modification is a type of:**
(a) Behavior therapy
(b) Cognitive behavior therapy
(c) Humanistic therapy
(d) Client centered therapy

**100. Grimacing and mannerism is seen in:**
(a) Catatonic schizophrenia
(b) Simple schizophrenia
(c) Hebephrenic schizophrenia
(d) Phobia

**101. Who is the founder of psychoanalytical model:**
(a) Hippocrates (b) Aristotle
(c) Sigmund Freud (d) Eugen Bleuler

**102. Formed visual hallucinations are seen in which lesion:**
(a) Frontal (b) Occipital
(c) Temporal (d) Parietal

**103. Behavior analysis is based upon the principles of:**
(a) Dream analysis (b) Operant conditioning
(c) Classical conditioning (d) All of the above

**104. Id mainly works on principle of:**
(a) Reality (b) Behavior
(c) Pleasure (d) Anxiety

**105. The process of looking within oneself is:**
(a) Observation (b) Consolidation
(c) Introspection (d) Intensation

**106. The brain parts are:**
(a) Forebrain (b) Midbrain
(c) Hindbrain (d) All of the above

**107. Repetitive voiding of urine, either during day or night at inappropriate:**
(a) Ecopresis (b) Enuresis
(c) Echolalia (d) Echopraxia

**108. Sexual arousal occurs either solely predominantly with nonliving object:**
(a) Voyeurism (b) Exhibitionism
(c) Pedophilia (d) Fetishism

**109. Disulfiram therapy is mainly used for patient with:**
(a) Cocaine addiction (b) Alcohol addiction
(c) Heroin addiction (d) None of the above

**110. Drug used for mania EXCEPT:**
(a) Amitriptyline (b) Lithium carbonate
(c) Sodium valproate (d) Carbamazepine

**111. Specifically used psychotherapy for phobias is:**
(a) Flooding
(b) Supportive psychotherapy
(c) Environmental modification
(d) Reassurance

**112. There is no brain in my skull, intestine hane rotated away, world is coming to end:**
(a) Delusion of control (b) Delusion of nihilism
(c) Delusion of reference (d) Delusion of persecution

**113. Specific reading disorder is:**
(a) Dysphasia (b) Dyslexia
(c) Dyscalculia (d) Dyspnea

## ANSWERS

| | | | | | | | | | | | |
|---|---|---|---|---|---|---|---|---|---|---|---|
| **1.** | (a) | **21.** | (d) | **41.** | (b) | **61.** | (b) | **81.** | (b) | **101.** | (c) |
| **2.** | (c) | **22.** | (b) | **42.** | (a) | **62.** | (c) | **82.** | (b) | **102.** | (b) |
| **3.** | (a) | **23.** | (b) | **43.** | (c) | **63.** | (c) | **83.** | (c) | **103.** | (d) |
| **4.** | (c) | **24.** | (a) | **44.** | (c) | **64.** | (a) | **84.** | (c) | **104.** | (c) |
| **5.** | (b) | **25.** | (a) | **45.** | (b) | **65.** | (d) | **85.** | (a) | **105.** | (c) |
| **6.** | (d) | **26.** | (c) | **46.** | (d) | **66.** | (b) | **86.** | (d) | **106.** | (d) |
| **7.** | (a) | **27.** | (b) | **47.** | (d) | **67.** | (b) | **87.** | (d) | **107.** | (b) |
| **8.** | (a) | **28.** | (d) | **48.** | (b) | **68.** | (a) | **88.** | (d) | **108.** | (d) |
| **9.** | (d) | **29.** | (c) | **49.** | (c) | **69.** | (b) | **89.** | (a) | **109.** | (b) |
| **10.** | (c) | **30.** | (a) | **50.** | (a) | **70.** | (c) | **90.** | (b) | **110.** | (a) |
| **11.** | (b) | **31.** | (d) | **51.** | (a) | **71.** | (c) | **91.** | (b) | **111.** | (a) |
| **12.** | (b) | **32.** | (b) | **52.** | (c) | **72.** | (a) | **92.** | (c) | **112.** | (b) |
| **13.** | (a) | **33.** | (b) | **53.** | (b) | **73.** | (a) | **93.** | (a) | **113.** | (b) |
| **14.** | (a) | **34.** | (b) | **54.** | (a) | **74.** | (d) | **94.** | (d) | | |
| **15.** | (a) | **35.** | (d) | **55.** | (b) | **75.** | (a) | **95.** | (d) | | |
| **16.** | (d) | **36.** | (a) | **56.** | (c) | **76.** | (a) | **96.** | (a) | | |
| **17.** | (c) | **37.** | (a) | **57.** | (d) | **77.** | (b) | **97.** | (b) | | |
| **18.** | (b) | **38.** | (d) | **58.** | (d) | **78.** | (b) | **98.** | (b) | | |
| **19.** | (b) | **39.** | (c) | **59.** | (a) | **79.** | (c) | **99.** | (a) | | |
| **20.** | (a) | **40.** | (b) | **60.** | (d) | **80.** | (c) | **100.** | (a) | | |

# QUICK REVIEW

## Community Health Nursing Review and Multiple Choice Questions

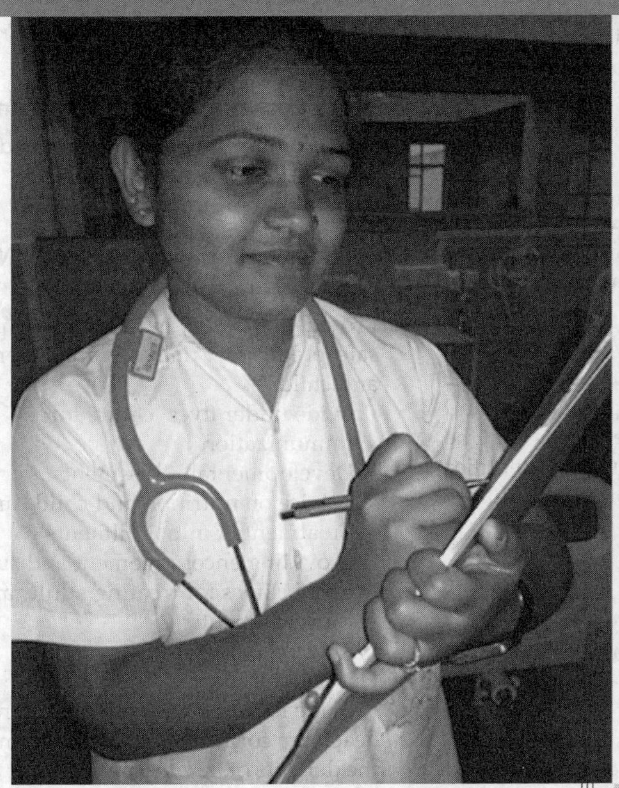

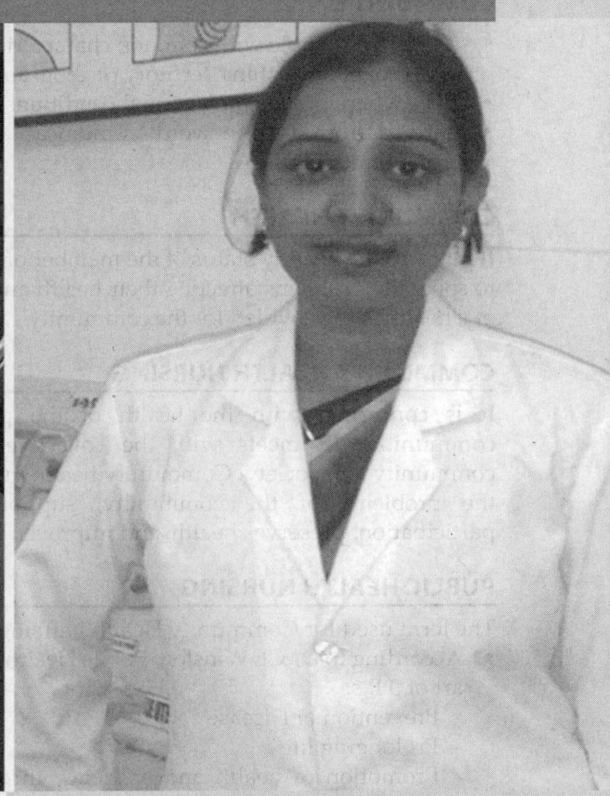

### HIGHLIGHTS

- Community Health and Community Health Nursing
- Epidemiology
- Important Communicable Diseases
- Family Planning Methods
- Primary Health Care
- National Health Programs
- Five Year Plans
- Health Problems in India
- National Health Committees
- Awareness Days/Health Calendar
- Multiple Choice Questions

# Community Health Nursing

## COMMUNITY

- A group of people with common characteristics or interests living together within a territory or geographical boundary.
- Place where people under usual conditions are found.
- Derived from a Latin word 'comunicas' which means a group of people.

## COMMUNITY HEALTH

It refers to the healthy status of the member of the community to solve the problems affecting their health and to the totality of a health care provided for the community'. — WHO

## COMMUNITY HEALTH NURSING

It is concerned with the health of the population and communities. It meets with the collective needs of the community and society. Community health nursing identifies the problems of the community, supports community participation, preserves health, and improves health.

## PUBLIC HEALTH NURSING

The term used for Community Health Nursing.

- According to Dr CE Winslow Public Health is a science and art of 3 P's:
  - Prevention of Disease
  - Prolonging life
  - Promotion of health and efficiency through organized community effort.

### The Key Characteristics of Community Health Nursing

- Caring relationships and partnerships with families and communities.
- People are seen as essential participants in the process of promoting health and preventing illness.
- Participant and facilitator rather than just a dispenser of medications or information.
- Focus on empowerment of families and communities. Allows the communities and families acquire skills and knowledge so that they can participate in decision making about their health.
- Focus on the populations and sub-populations.
- Mutual respect and cooperation from both the giver and the receiver of care to help empower the people.

### Aims of Community Health Nursing

- *Reduction of risk factors:* To reduce morbidity and mortality rate.
- *Strengthening self-care activities:* To promote the health and prevent the occurrence of diseases.
- *Maintain quality of life:* To live productive life.

### Goals of Community Health Nursing

- To prevent, promote, maintain and restore the community health.
- To reduce morbidity and mortality rate among community.

### Objectives of Community Health Nursing

Include the following, to:

- Provide antenatal, maternity and postnatal care to ensure safe pregnancy, delivery and puerperium for the mother and child.
- Provide under fives' clinics for:
  - Immunization
  - Developmental assessment
  - Advice on nutrition and child care
  - Treatment of minor ailments
  - Providing encouragement and support to mothers.
- Provide clinics for treating adults and children for:
  - Minor ailments
  - Referral of major illness
- Health education.
- Provide facilities for family planning.
- Teach the correct use of common medicines and drugs and the dangers of buying medicines at the chemist and market.
- Explain and promote the use of local health services in the community, advising people to seek health care from safe, qualified heath personnel.
- Promote projects in the community that will improve life for the people there, e.g. women's cooperatives, literacy programs, provision of safe water.
- Teach and demonstrate healthy ways of living (health education) according to local needs.
- Assist in the prevention and control of communicable disease.
- Visit people in their own homes and villages to identify health needs and priorities, and deal with them effectively.
- Promote the health of *school children* (through the health service.)
- Promote the health of the worker (occupational health).
- Maintain and promote the health of the elderly and handicapped.
- Work in close cooperation with government and other local organizations to promote health and welfare of individuals, families and communities.

## Scope of Community Health Nursing

The scope of community health nursing includes health promotion, illness prevention and restoration of health of individuals, families and communities.

- The scope of community health nursing is wide, there is still a much wider scope for a nurse.
- Nurses can work in different places.

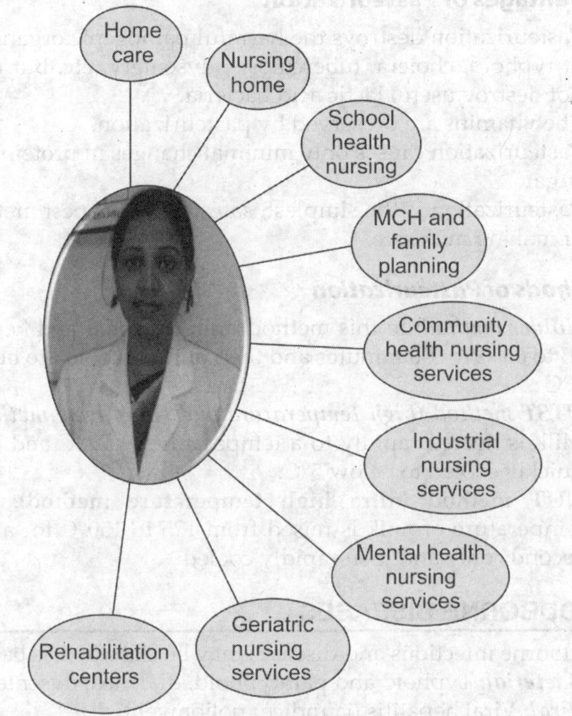


## Functions and Roles of Community Health Nursing

- Collaborator
- Coordinator
- Adviser
- Counselor
- Advocate
- Caregiver
- Communicator
- Trainer
- Investigator
- Promoter of health
- Team leader
- Observer
- Participant practitioner
- Health educator
- Health monitor
- Role model
- Change agent
- Community organizer
- Coordinator of services
- Recorder/reporter/statistician

## HEALTH

*According to WHO:* Health is a state of complete physical, mental, and social well-being, not merely the absence of disease or infirmity.

### Concept of Health

- *Biomedical concept:* Traditionally health has been viewed as an 'absence of disease' and if one was free from disease, then the person was considered healthy. This concept known as the biomedical concept.
- *Ecological concept:* According to this concept, health as a dynamic equilibrium between man and his environment, and disease a maladjustment of the human organism to environment. According to one ecologist, 'Health implies the relative absence of pain and discomfort and a continuous adaptation and adjustment to the environment to ensure optimal function'. This was defined by Dubos.
- *Psychosocial concept:* According to this concept, health is not only a biomedical phenomenon but one which is influenced by social, psychological, culture, economic and political factors of the people concerned. These factors must be taken into consideration in defining and measuring health. Thus, health is both biological and social phenomenon.
- *Holistic concept:* This holistic concept is a synthesis of all above concepts. It recognizes the strength of social, economic, political and environmental influences on health. The holistic approach implies that all sectors of society have an effect on health.

### Dimensions of Health

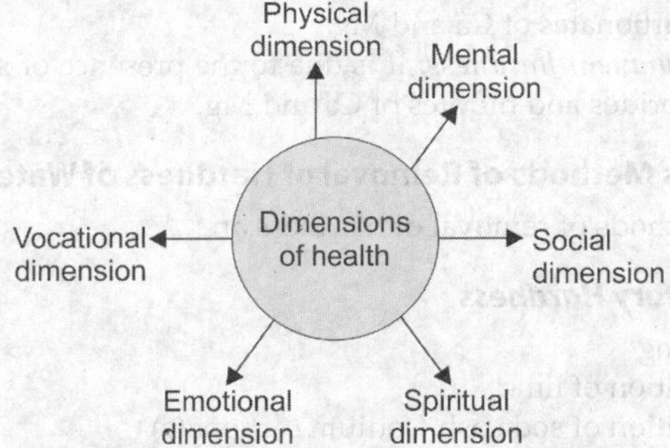


### Health Promotion and Health Maintenance

- *Health promotion:* 'The process of enabling people to increase control over their health and its determinants, and thereby improve their health'. —*WHO*
- *Health maintenance:* 'A systematic program or procedure planned to prevent illness, maintain maximum function, and promote health. It is central to health care, especially to nursing care at all levels (primary, secondary, and tertiary) and in all patterns (preventive, episodic, acute, chronic, and catastrophic)'.

The factors/steps/activities which help to promotion and maintenance of health are:

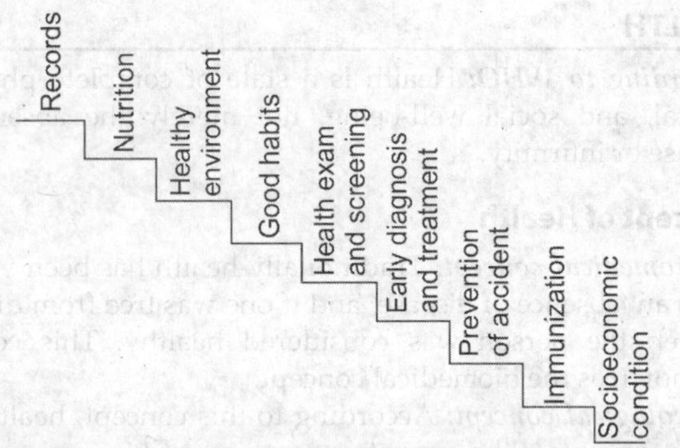


## WATERBORNE DISEASES

| Agent | Diseases |
|---|---|
| Bacterial | Cholera, diarrhea, dysentery, typhoid |
| Virus | Infective hepatitis |
| Helminthic | Roundworm, threadworm, guinea worm infection |
| Protozoa | Amebiasis, giardiasis |
| Spirochetal | Weil's diseases. |

All of these diseases are spread by drinking dirty (unsafe) water, or by washing in dirty (unsafe) water, or by lack of water for washing.

## HARDNESS OF WATER

Presence of impurities such as chloride, sulfates, bicarbonates of calcium and magnesium in water.Hardness is clarified into 2 kinds:

1. *Temporary hardness:* It is due to the presence of bicarbonates of Ca and Mg.
2. *Permanent hardness:* It is due to the presence of sulfates, chlorides and nitrates of Ca and Mg.

### Various Methods of Removal of Hardness of Water

The methods of removal of hardness are:

#### *Temporary Hardness*

- Boiling
- Addition of lime
- Addition of soda ash (sodium carbonate)
- Permutit process.

#### *Permanent Hardness*

- Addition of soda ash (sodium carbonate)
- Permutit process.

## ORTHOTOLIDINE TEST

- This test is used to find out the amount of free residual chlorine.
- In 1 mL of water 0.1 mL of Orthotolidine reagent will be added.
- The solution changed into yellow color means: It indicates chlorine is present in the water.

## PASTEURIZATION OF MILK

**Definition:** According to WHO, Pasteurization may be defined as:

The heating of milk to such temperature and for such periods of time as are required to destroy any pathogens that may be present while causing minimal changes in the composition, flavor and nutritive value.

### Advantages of Pasteurization

- Pasteurization destroys the harmful pathogenic organisms of typhoid, cholera, tuberculosis, dysentery, etc. But does not destroy useful lactic acid bacteria.
- The vitamins are preserved by pasteurization.
- Pasteurization causes only minimal changes in protein and sugar.
- Pasteurization is the simplest, safest and cheapest method of making milk safe.

### *Methods of Pasteurization*

- ***Holder method:*** In this method milk is heated and kept at 63 to 66°C for 30 minutes and then quickly cooled to below 5°C .
- ***HTST method (high temperature and short time method):*** Milk is heated rapidly to a temperature of 72°C and then quickly cooled to below 5°C.
- **UHT method (ultra high temperature method):** The temperature of milk is raised from 125 to 150°C for a few seconds only and then rapidly cooled.

## FOODBORNE DISEASES

Foodborne infections and diseases may be classified as below:

- ***Bacterial:*** Typhoid and paratyphoid, diarrhea; dysentery
- ***Viral:*** Viral hepatitis (jaundice) poliomyelitis.
- ***Protozoal:*** Amebiasis.
- ***Intestinal:*** Tapeworm and roundworm
- ***Others:*** Food poisoning.

## EPIDEMIOLOGY

### Definition

- Epidemiology is the study of the:
  - Frequency
  - Distribution—time, place and person
  - Determinants—physical, biological, social, behavioral and cultural of health problems and health related events and application of this study to control health problems.

Or

- Epidemiology is 'the study of the distribution and determinants of health-related states or events in specified populations, and the application of this study to the prevention and control of health problems'.

### Aims of Epidemiology

According to the *International Epidemiological Association* (IEA), epidemiology has three main aims:

1. To describe the distribution and magnitude of health and disease problems in human population.

2. To identify etiological factors in the pathogenesis of disease.
3. To provide the data essential to the planning, implementation and evaluation of services for the prevention, control and treatment of disease and to the setting up of priorities among those services.

## Modes of Transmission

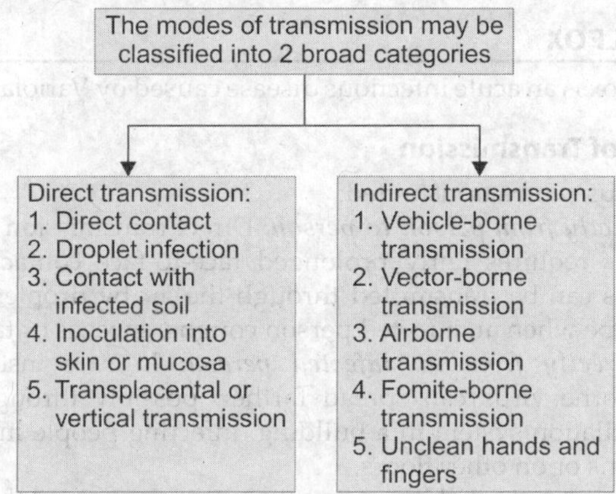


### *Direct Transmission*

- ***Direct contact:*** Some diseases are transmitted from person to person by direct contact, e.g. kissing, sexual contact. Diseases transmitted by direct contact include sexually transmitted diseases. (Syphilis, gonorrhea, leprosy, scabies, skin sepsis).
- ***Droplet infection:*** When a person with respiratory infection coughs, sneezes or even talks loudly, fine droplets of saliva containing millions of bacteria and viruses are blown into the surrounding air. These droplets become sources of infection, when inhaled by susceptible person in the vicinity. This is known as droplet infection, which is the most common mode of spread of disease, e.g. common cold, tuberculosis, measles, whooping cough, diphtheria, etc.
- ***Contact with soil:*** The disease agent may be occurred by direct contact with infected soil, e.g. hookworm larvae and strongyloides.
- ***Inoculation into skin or mucosa:*** The disease agent may be inoculated directly into the skin or mucosa, e.g. rabies virus through dog bite, hepatitis-B virus through contaminated needles and syringes.
- ***Transplacental transmission:*** The disease agents may be transmitted in uterus from the mother to the fetus. This is also known as vertical transmission, e.g. toxoplasmosis, rubella virus, syphilis, hepatitis-B, AIDS, etc.

### *Indirect Transmission*

- ***Vehicle-borne transmission:*** The chief vehicles of transmission are water, milk or food. Other vehicles include blood, serum, plasma and other biological products. This group includes waterborne, milkborne, foodborne and bloodborne infections. Diseases transmitted by water, milk and food include chiefly infection of the alimentary tract such as enteric fever, cholera, diarrhea and dysentery, hepatitis B is the most important diseases transmitted through blood contact.
- ***Vector-borne transmission:*** Malaria, filarial, kala-azar and plagues are transmitted by insects. This mode of transmission is known as vector transmission.
- ***Airborne transmission:*** Airborne transmission includes transmission by droplet nuclei and infected dust.
  - *Droplet nuclei:* These are extremely small infective particle (less than 0.1 mm) which keep floating in the air. These are generated during coughing or sneezing, e.g. influenza, tuberculosis, measles and several other respiratory infections.
  - *Infected dust:* Some of the larger droplets which are expelled during coughing and sneezing settle down on the floor, cloths, linen and become part of the dust. This is known as infected dust. During sweeping, dusting and bed making, the infected dust is released again into the atmosphere and if inhaled is a potential danger, e.g. tuberculosis, pneumonia, strepto and staphylococcal infection.
- ***Fomiteborne transmission:*** Fomites are articles that convey infection to others because they have been contaminated by pathogeneses organism, e.g. handkerchief, drinking glasses, door handles, towels, clothings, toys, etc.

  Fomite plays an important part in indirect infection.
- ***Unclean hands and fingers:*** Hands are the most common medium by which pathogenic agents are transferred, e.g. typhoid, hepatitis A, etc.

## Levels of Prevention

- ***Primordial Prevention:*** Prevention of chronic disease, prevention of the emergence or development of risk factor in countries or population groups in which they have not yet appear, e.g. many adult health problems (e.g. obesity, hypertension (HTN)).

  The main intervention in primordial prevention is through individual and mass education.
- ***Primary prevention:*** It is defined as 'action taken prior to the onset of disease, which removes the possibility that a disease will even occur'. It signifies intervention in the pre-pathogeneses phase of a disease or health problem (e.g. low birth weight) or other departure from health.

### Modes of Intervention in Primary Prevention

- ***Health promotion:*** It is the process of enabling people to control over and to improve health. The well-known intervention in this areas:
  - Health education
  - Environmental modification
  - Nutritional interventions
  - Lifestyle and behavioral changes.
- ***Specific protection:*** The currently available interventions are:
  - Immunization
  - Use of specific nutrients

- Chemoprophylaxis
- Protection against occupational hazards
- Protection against accidents
- Avoidance of allergens, etc.

- *Secondary prevention:* It can be defined as 'the action which halts the progress of a disease at its incipient stage and prevents complications'.
  - It is largely the domain of clinical medicine.
  - It includes the early diagnosis and treatment.
  - The drawback of secondary prevention is that the patient has already been subject to mental anguish, physical pass and the community to loss of productivity.
- *Tertiary prevention:* When the disease process has advanced beyond its early stages. It is still possible to accomplish prevention by what might be called 'Tertiary prevention.' It includes:
  - ***Disability limitation:*** When a patient reports late in the pathogenesis phase, then it is disability limitation.
  - ***Rehabilitation:*** It is a treatment or treatments designed to facilitate the process of recovery from injury, illness, or disease to as normal a condition as possible.

The following areas of concern in rehabilitation have been identified:

- *Medical rehabilitation:* Restoration of function.
- *Vocational rehabilitation:* Restoration of the capacity to earn a livelihood.
- *Social rehabilitation:* Restoration of family and social relationship.
- *Psychological:* Restoration of personal dignity and confidence.

## IMPORTANT COMMUNICABLE DISEASES

### Communicable Diseases

- An illness due to specific infectious agent which is spread from one person to another person.
- Communicable diseases are diseases that are the result of a causative organism spreading from one person to another or from animals to people.

### *Classification of Communicable Diseases*

We shall now focus on the various classes of communicable diseases. There are various ways of classifying communicable diseases. The classification given below is considered to be the most appropriate for ease of understanding.

The classes include:

- ***Contact diseases*** such as scabies, pediculosis, fungal skin infections, trachoma, and acute bacterial conjunctivitis.
- ***Sexually transmitted diseases and HIV/AIDS.***
- ***Vector-borne diseases*** such as relapsing fever, bancroftian filariasis, onchocerciasis, yellow fever, trypanosomiasis, plague, schistosomiasis, dracunculiasis, leishmaniasis and malaria.
- ***Diseases caused by fecal-oral contamination*** such as acute gastroenteritis, bacillary dysentery, ***campylobacter jejuni***, giardiasis, amebiasis, cholera, enteric fevers, food poisoning, poliomyelitis, viral hepatitis.
- ***Helminthic diseases*** such as ascariasis, enterobiasis, trichuriasis, hookworm, strongyloidiasis, taeniasis, hydatidosis.
- ***Airborne diseases*** such as acute respiratory infections, meningitis (bacterial and fungal) tuberculosis and leprosy.
- **Zoonotic diseases (diseases of contact with animals or animal products)** such as anthrax, brucellosis, rabies, hydatidosis, tetanus.

## SMALLPOX

Smallpox is an acute infectious disease caused by Variola virus.

### Mode of Transmission

The virus can be transmitted:

- ***Directly from person to person:*** Direct transmission of the virus requires fairly prolonged face-to-face contact. The virus can be transmitted through the air by droplets that escape when an infected person coughs, sneezes or talks.
- ***Indirectly from an infected person:*** In rare instances, airborne virus can spread farther, possibly through the ventilation system in a building, infecting people in other rooms or on other floors.
- ***Via contaminated items:*** Smallpox can also spread through contact with contaminated clothing and bedding, although the risk of infection from these sources is less common.
- ***As a terrorist weapon, potentially:*** A deliberate release of smallpox is a remote threat. However, because any release of the virus could spread the disease quickly, government officials have taken numerous precautions to protect against this possibility, such as stockpiling smallpox vaccine.

### Incubation Period

7–17 days.

### Symptoms of Smallpox

- The first ***symptoms*** of ***smallpox*** are: *High fever, Fatigue, Malaise, Headache, Backache, Rash*
- A few days later, flat, red spots appear first on your face, hands and forearms, and later on your trunk. Within a day or two, many of these lesions turn into small blisters filled with clear fluid, which then turns into pus. Scabs begin to form eight to nine days later and eventually fall off, leaving deep, pitted scars.
- Lesions also develop in the mucous membranes of your nose and mouth and quickly turn into sores that break open.

### Treatment

- There is no proven treatment for smallpox.
- If an infected person gets the smallpox vaccine within 4 days after exposure to the virus, it may lessen the severity of illness or even prevent it.
- Other than vaccination, treatment of smallpox is primarily supportive, such as wound care and infection control, fluid therapy, and possible ventilator assistance.
- The antiviral drug Cidofovir might be used as a therapeutic agent.

- The majority of people with smallpox recover, but death may occur in up to 30 percent of cases. Those who do recover are often left with disfiguring scars.

### Prevention/Control of Smallpox

To prevent the spread of smallpox, healthcare providers must:
- Isolate infected people
- Vaccinate close contacts of infected people.

### Vaccine

#### *Smallpox Vaccine*

- Vaccinia virus
  - Protects against variola virus
  - Origins unknown
- Live vaccine
  - Used in US until 1972
- Immunity high for 3–5 years
  - Potentially protective much longer

The currently licensed smallpox vaccine, which consists of a laboratory strain of vaccinia virus, is highly effective in preventing infection. Medical experts believe the vaccine may lessen the severity of, or even prevent, illness in unvaccinated people if given within 4 days of exposure to the virus.

The smallpox vaccine helps the body develop immunity to smallpox. The vaccine is made from a 'pox'—type virus related to smallpox. The smallpox vaccine contains live vaccinia virus—unlike many other vaccines that use killed virus. The vaccine does not contain the smallpox virus and cannot transmit smallpox. Learn more about the smallpox vaccine from the Centers for Disease Control and Prevention (CDC).

A few data exist showing just how long vaccinia vaccines protect people against smallpox infection. Therefore, those vaccinated against the smallpox virus before 1972 may be susceptible to the disease. Military and other high-risk groups (for example, scientists who work with vaccinia and other orthopoxviruses related to Variola major) have been getting the vaccine since the United States stopped routine smallpox vaccinations in 1972.

#### *Getting the Vaccine*

Health care providers do not use a hypodermic needle, usually used for vaccinations, to give the smallpox vaccine. Instead, they use a tiny, two-pronged needle that is dipped into the vaccine solution. When removed from the solution, the needle keeps a droplet of the vaccine. The needle is used to prick the skin, usually in the upper arm, a number of times within a few seconds. The pricking is not deep, but it will cause a sore spot and one or two droplets of blood.

If the vaccination is successful, a red and itchy bump develops at the vaccine site in 3 or 4 days.
- In the first week, the bump becomes a large blister, fills with pus, and begins to drain.
- During the second week, the blister begins to dry up and a scab forms.
- In the third week, the scab falls off, leaving a small scar.
- People who get the vaccine for the first time have a stronger reaction than those who are revaccinated.

## CHICKENPOX (VARICELLA)

Chickenpox is an highly contagious disease caused by Varicella Zoster virus which is also called human herpes virus.

### Modes of Transmission

- Chickenpox is transmitted by droplet nuclei.
- Persons get infected by personal contact.
- Portal of entry is respiratory tract.

### Incubation Period

About 7–21 days, usually 15 days.

### Clinical Manifestation

High fever, Cold, Restlessness, Tiredness, Loss of appetite, Backache, after this rashes are found on the body which are less on face and hands and more over the body. Different stages of rashes are macular, popular, vesicular and scabal.

### Prevention and Control/Management

- Provide symptomatic treatment (is started such as tablet paracetamol for fever)
- *Isolation:* Isolation means separating the infected individual from healthy individuals for the period of communicability.
- Disinfect the material contaminated by secretion and wound properly.
- Sterilization of cloths, utensils, fomites must.
- *Quarantine:* All persons living in same place as the patient should vaccinated and kept under daily surveillance, as patient infections.

## MEASLES (RUBEOLA)

Measles is a childhood infectious diseases. Rubella is produced by a virus spreading in the rubeola which means, red spots. This disease can be identified by cold, cough and skin rashes.

Measles or rubeola is an acute and highly communicable disease, and also a specific infections disease effecting children, caused by specific viruses that is group of paramyxovirus.

### Definition

- Measles is a very contagious (easily spread) infection that causes a rash all over your body. It is also called rubeola or red measles.
- *Mode of transmission:* Droplet infection, direct contact with respiratory secretions.
- *Incubation period:* For measles is 10 days to fever onset and 14 days to rash onset.
  - This period may be shorter in infants and longer (upto 3 weeks) in adults.

### Signs and Symptoms

Signs and symptoms appear 10 to 14 days after exposure to the virus. Signs and symptoms of measles typically include: Fever, Dry cough, Runny nose, Sore throat, Inflamed eyes (conjunctivitis), Tiny white spots with bluish-white centers on a red background found inside the mouth on the inner lining of the cheek—also called ***Koplik's spots***, A skin rash made up of large, flat blotches that often flow into one another.

The infection occurs in sequential stages over a period of 2 to 3 weeks.

### Treatment

- There is no specific antiviral therapy for measles.
- Treatment consists of general supportive measures, such as hydration and administration of antipyretic agents.
- Antibiotic therapy for the secondary bacterial infections.
- Vitamin A is effective for the treatment of measles.

### Prevention

- Measles vaccine is given at 9 months of age to all children.
- MMR vaccine is given at 18 months of age.

## MUMPS

Mumps is a contagious disease that is caused by the mumps virus.

### Mode of Transmission

Mumps is spread by droplets of saliva or mucus from the mouth, nose, or throat of an infected person, usually when the person coughs, sneezes, or talks. Items used by an infected person, such as soft drink cans or eating utensils can also be contaminated with the virus, which may spread to others if those items are shared.

In addition, the virus may spread when someone with mumps touches items or surfaces without washing their hands and someone else then touches the same surface and rubs their mouth or nose.

Most mumps transmission likely occurs before the salivary glands begin to swell and up to 5 days after the swelling begins. Therefore, CDC recommends isolation of mumps patients for 5 days after their glands begin to swell.

### Incubation Period

For mumps is between 14 and 18 days.

### Symptoms of Mumps

Inflammation of Parotid Gland in mumps, swollen, painful salivary (parotid) glands on one or both sides of face (parotitis), fever, headache, weakness and fatigue, loss of appetite, pain while chewing or swallowing. The primary—and best known—sign of mumps is swollen salivary glands that cause the cheeks to puff out. In fact, the term 'mumps' is an old expression for lumps or bumps within the cheeks.

### Prevention and Control of Mumps

- Mumps is best prevented by the measles, mumps and rubella (MMR) combination vaccine or the measles, mumps, rubella and Varicella (MMRV) combination vaccine.
- Almost 100% of people who have had 2 doses of a mumps-containing vaccine will be protected against mumps.
- Vaccination after exposure will not stop the infection, though it will protect against future exposures.
- Washing hands well and often with soap, and teaching children to wash their hands too.
- Not sharing eating or drinking utensils.
- Cleaning surfaces that are frequently touched (such as toys, doorknobs, tables, and counters) regularly with soap and water or with cleaning wipes.
- Minimize close contact with other people if you are sick.
- Cover your mouth and nose with a tissue when you cough or sneeze, and put your used tissue in the trash can. If you do not have a tissue, cough or sneeze into your upper sleeve or elbow, not your hands.

## RUBELLA (GERMAN MEASLES)

Rubella—commonly known as German measles or 3-day measles—is an infection that primarily affects the skin and lymph nodes.

It is caused by rubella virus (not the same virus that causes measles).

### Mode of Transmission

It is (spread) transmitted by airborne droplets when infected people sneeze or cough. Humans are the only known host.

### Incubation Period

2–3 weeks.

### Symptoms of Rubella

Microcephaly, Congenital Cataract, Deafness, A red-pink rash is a common symptom of rubella, A red-pink skin rash, it consists of a number of small spots, which may be slightly itchy, A high temperature (fever), which is usually mild (less than 39°C or 102.2°F), but can be more severe in adults, cold-like symptoms, such as a runny nose, watery eyes, sore throat and cough, slightly sore and red eyes (conjunctivitis), aching and painful joints, loss of appetite, tiredness.

The symptoms of rubella usually only last a few days, but your glands may be swollen for several weeks.

### Prevention

There is a safe and effective vaccine to prevent rubella. The rubella vaccine is recommended for all children. It is routinely given when children are 12–15 months old, but is sometimes given earlier during epidemics. A second vaccination (booster) is routinely given to children ages 4–6. MMR is a combination vaccine that protects against measles, mumps, and rubella.

Women of childbearing age usually have a blood test to see if they have immunity to rubella. If they are not immune, women should avoid getting pregnant for 28 days after receiving the vaccine. Those who should not get vaccinated include:

- Women who are pregnant
- Anyone whose immune system is affected by cancer, corticosteroid medications, or radiation treatment.

Great care is taken not to give the vaccine to a woman who is already pregnant. However, in the rare instances when pregnant women have been vaccinated, no problems have been detected in the infants.

## INFLUENZA

- ***Influenza:*** An acute viral disease of the respiratory tract.
- ***Infectious agent:*** Three types of influenza virus (A, B and C)

- ***Mode of transmission:*** Airborne spread predominates among crowded populations in closed places such as school buses.
- ***Incubation period:*** Short, usually 1–3 days
- ***Clinical manifestation:*** Fever, headache, myalgia, prostration, sore throat and cough, cough is often severe and protracted, but other manifestations are self-limited with recovery in 2–7 days.

### Prevention and Control

- Educate the public in basic personal hygiene, especially the danger of unprotected coughs and sneezes and hand to mucus membrane transmission.
- Immunization with available killed virus vaccines may provide 70–80% protection.
- Amantadine hydrochloride is effective in the chemoprophylaxis of type A virus but not others.

## WHOOPING COUGH/PERTUSSIS

Pertussis, or whooping cough, is an upper respiratory infection caused by the *bordetella pertussis* bacteria.

The best way to protect against pertussis is immunization.

### Incubation Period

7–14 days.

### Clinical Manifestation

*Stage 1: Catarrhal Stage*

- Running nose
- Sneezing
- Low grade fever
- Loss of appetite
- Nocturnal cough are found in this stage.

*Stage 2: Paroxysmal Stage*

In this stage bouts cough occurs and each bouts ends in a specific inspirational noise resembling kho-kho, because of mucus blockage, vomiting might occur, cough and the child face turn red.

*Stage 3: Convalescent Stage*

Bouts of cough and vomiting become less during this period. But for months even ordinary respiratory infection can bring about bouts of cough.

*Diagnostic Evaluation*

- Identify with typical type of cough and by examination of nose or throat swabs.
- Sputum culture shows the growth of ***bordetella pertussis***.
  - Encephalitis.

### Prevention and Control Measures/Management

- Admit the patient in hospital
- Provide antibiotic medicine for cough
- Oxygen treatment
- Plenty of fluids and nourishment
- Provide isolation
- Provide quite environment, that will not accelerate cough
- Provide active protection by vaccination.

## DIPHTHERIA

Diphtheria is an infection caused by ***Corynebacterium diphtheriae*** bacteria.

- ***Mode of transmission:*** The disease is spread mainly by droplet infection through coughing and sneezing. It can also be transmitted directly to susceptible persons from infected cutaneous lesions. Transmission by objects (e.g. cups, toys, pencils) contaminated by nasopharyngeal secretions of patient is possible but for only short periods.
- ***Incubation period:*** 2 to 5 days
- ***Clinical manifestations/symptoms of diphtheria:*** A high temperature (fever) of 38°C (100.4°F) or above, chills, formation of grayish yellow membrane over tonsils and throat. Fatigue (extreme tiredness), sore throat, hoarse voice, cough, headache, difficulty in swallowing or pain when swallowing, difficulty in breathing, foul-smelling, bloodstained nasal discharge, swollen glands (nodes) in the neck, pale, blue skin.

### Prevention of Diphtheria

Diphtheria can be prevented by active immunization either by DPT or diphtheria vaccine.

- The current practice is to immunize all infants with DPT starting from age of 6 weeks.
- DPT vaccine protects not only against diphtheria but also against pertussis and tetanus.
- These doses of DPT are recommended at an interval of 1–2 months.
- Universal immunization programme undertakes DPT along with oral polio and BCG when the child is 6 weeks old.
- A booster dose of DPT at age of the 1 1/2–2 years, followed by another dose at 5–6 years of age.
- It should store in a refrigerator between 4–8°C.

### *Schick Test*

- This is an intradermal (skin) test. By this test we can find out those who are immune to diphtheria and those who are not.
- This test is carried out by injecting into the skin of the forearm 0.2 ms of Schick test toxin. Into the opposite arm is injected as a 'control' an equal amount of toxin which has been in activated by heat. The results are read on fourth day.
- If there is no reaction of any kind, the person is considered immune to diphtheria.
- If there is a red flush, the person is considered susceptible to diphtheria. The susceptible person to diphtheria should be actively immunized against diphtheria.

### *Control Measures*

The control measures comprise the following:

- Notification to the local health authority.
- Prompt isolation and treatment of cases.
- Disinfection of all articles and clothes soiled by the patient.
- All children who have been exposed to infection and are not previously immunized should be given a dose of 500–1000 IU diphtheria antitoxin. This should be followed by active immunization with DPT or APT.

## TUBERCULOSIS

### Introduction

Tuberculosis (TB) is known as the White Plague during the 19th century, has inflicted the human race ever since. It is described as a chronic infectious disease caused by an organism called Mycobacterium tuberculosis through droplet transmission, like coughing, sneezing, or if the person inhales the infected droplet.

### Modes of Transmission

- Droplet infection and droplet nuclei generated by an 'open case'.
- Inhalation of fine dust containing tubercle bacilli from infected spectrum.
- Ingestion of contaminated food and milk.

### Incubation Period

The time from recipient of infection to the development of a positive tubercle test ranges from 3 to 6 weeks or more.

### Signs/Symptoms of Tuberculosis

Cough, continuous low grade fever, loss of weight, night sweat, blood stain sputum, chest pain.

### Preventing Tuberculosis

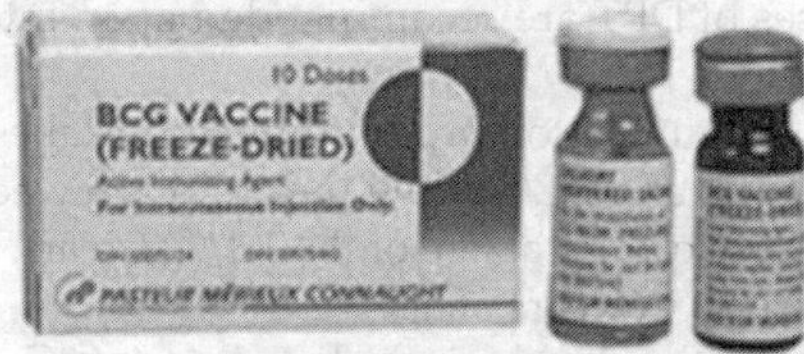

BCG vaccination

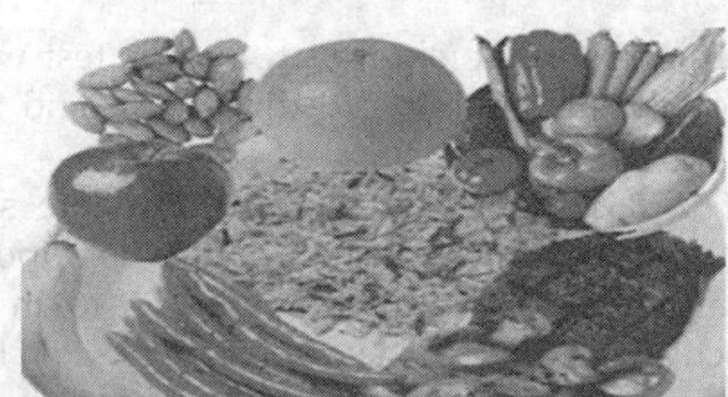
Balanced diet

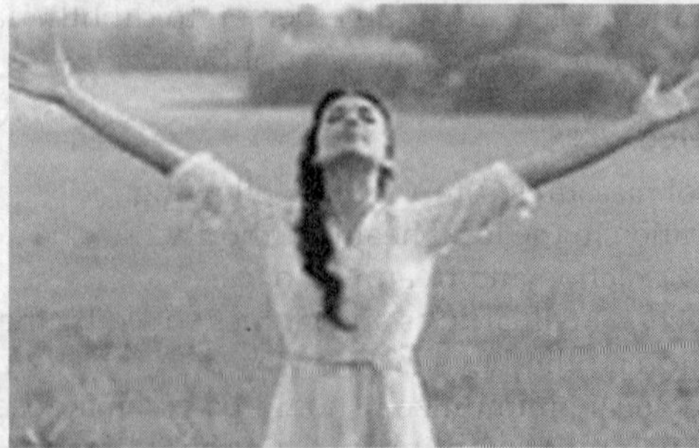
Fresh air

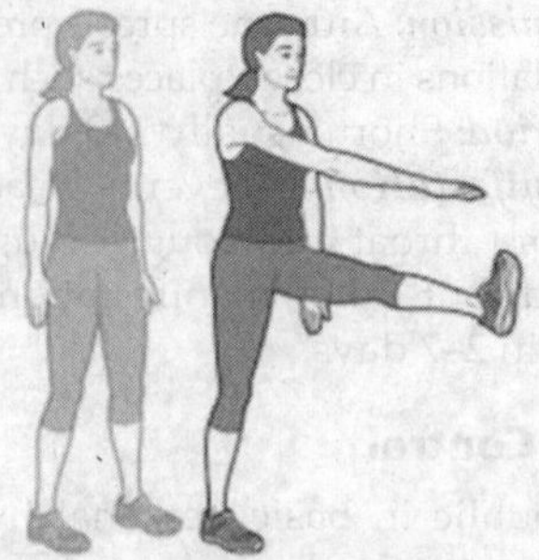
Adequate exercise

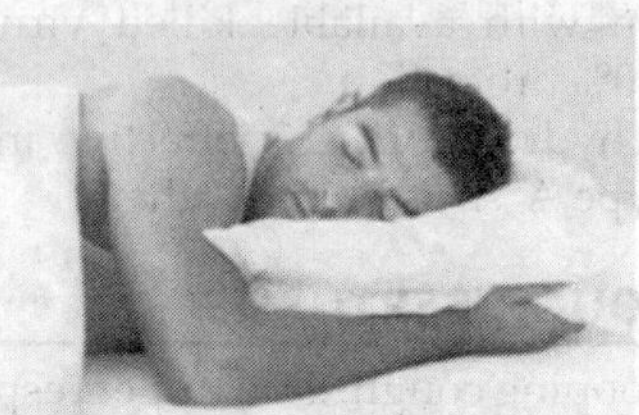
Adequate rest

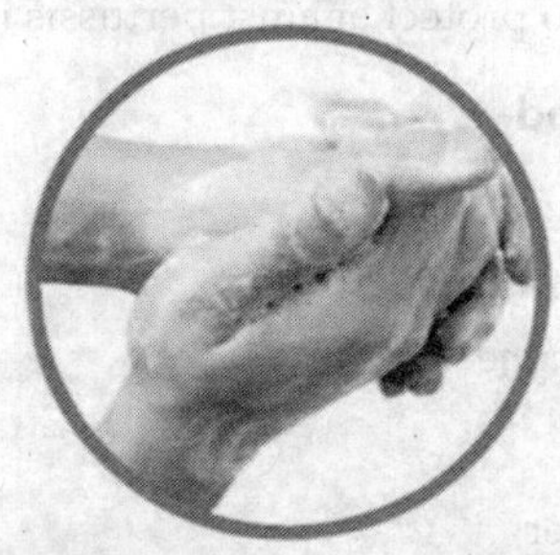

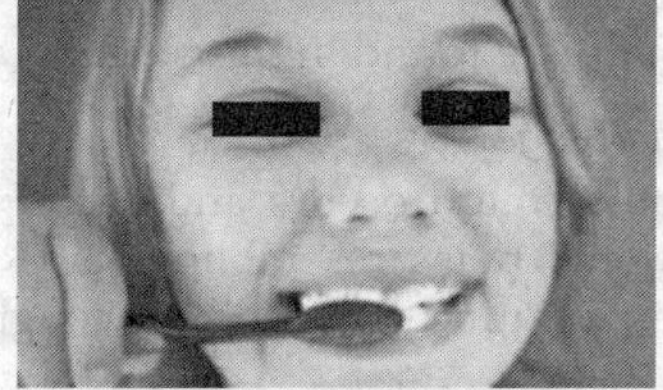
Good personal hygiene

### Prevention and Control of Tuberculosis

- *Early detection of cases:* The first step in TB control programme is early detection of all cases.
  - *Sputum examination:* Sputum should be examined from any patient presenting one or more of the following symptoms of respiratory disease.
    - ➢ Coughing lasting more than 2 weeks.
    - ➢ Continuous fever
    - ➢ Chest pain
    - ➢ Hemoptysis.
- *Mantoux test:* PPD injection results in red papule after 72 hours. Palpable edema or in duration more than 10 mm in the longitudinal diameter is considered acceptable infection with bacilli.
- *Chemotherapy:*
  - Antitubercular drug
  - Thiacetazone 150 mg + 1NH 300 mg

**Direct observed treatment short course:** Comprehensive strategy to detect and cure TB patients.

### DOTS (Direct Observed Treatment Short Course)

- *Category 1:* New TB patients whose sputum is positive; seriously ill patients with severe forms of smear-negative pulmonary tuberculosis (PTB) with extensive parenchymal involvement (moderately- or far advanced) and extra-pulmonary TB (meningitis, pleurisy, etc.)
  - ***Intensive phase*** (given daily for the first 2 months) – rifampicin + isoniazid + pyrazinamide + ethambutol.
  - If sputum result becomes negative after 2 months, maintenance phase starts. But if sputum is still positive in 2 months, all drugs are discontinued from 2–3 days and a sputum specimen is examined for culture and drug sensitivity. The patient resumes taking the 4 drugs for another month and then another smear exam is done at the end of the 3rd month.
  - ***Maintenance phase*** (after 3rd month, regardless of the result of the sputum exam)—INH + rifampicin daily
- *Category 2:* Previously-treated patients with relapses or failures.
  - ***Intensive phase*** (daily for 3 months, month 1, 2 and 3)—isoniazid + rifampicin + pyrazinamide + ethambutol + streptomycin for the first 2 months, streptomycin + rifampicin pyrazinamide + ethambutol on the 3rd month. If sputum is still positive after 3 months, the intensive phase is continued for 1 more month and then another sputum exam is done. If still positive after 4 months, intensive phase is continued for the next 5 months.
  - ***Maintenance phase*** (daily for 5 months, month 4, 5, 6, 7, and 8)—isonazid + rifampicin + ethambutol
- ***Category 3:*** New TB patients whose sputum is smear negative for 3 times and chest X-ray result of PTB minimal
  - ***Intensive phase*** (daily for 2 months)– isoniazid + rifampicin + pyrazinamide
  - ***Maintenance phase*** (daily for the next 2 months)– isoniazid + rifampicin
- ***BCG vaccination:*** It is given soon after birth. The dose of the vaccine is 1 mL. It is administered intradermally using a tuberculin syringe.

## POLIOMYELITIS

Poliomyelitis is also known as infantile paralysis. Poliomyelitis (polio) is a highly infectious viral disease that can affect nerves and can lead to partial or full paralysis.

### Causes

Poliomyelitis is a highly infectious disease caused by polio-virus.

### Mode of Transmission

- Poliovirus is often transmitted from person-to-person through fecal matter.
- People living in areas with limited access to running water or flush toilets often get the virus from drinking water contaminated by human waste that contains the virus.
- In addition, the virus can be spread by contaminated food or water or direct contact with another infected person.
- The virus enters through the mouth and nose, multiplies in the throat and intestinal tract, and then is absorbed and spread through the blood and lymph system.

### People Most at Risk

Polio mainly affects children under 5 years of age.

- ***Incubation period:*** 7–14 days.
- ***Clinical manifestations:*** The responses of polio affected person are:
  - ***Inapperent (sub-clinical) infection:*** This occurs approximately in 95 percent of poliovirus infection. There are no presenting symptoms. Recognition only by isolation.
  - ***Abortive Polio or Minor Illness:*** Occurs approximately in 4–8 percent of the infection. It causes only a mild or self-limiting illness due to viremia. The patient recovers quickly.
  - ***Non-paralytic polio:*** Occurs approximately in one percent of all infections. The presenting features are stiffness and pain in neck and back. The disease lasts for two to ten days. Recovery is rapid.
  - ***Paralytic polio:*** Occurs in less than one percent of infections. The virus enters the brain and causes varying degree of disability.

**Other associated features are:** Fever, headache, fatigue, restlessness, vomiting, diarrhea, cough, cold, muscular weakness, stiffness in neck, pain in the limbs. Paralysis may occur in leg, face, larynx, and esophagus. Many polio patients suffer from paralysis of lower part of the body. They become permanently handicapped.

### Management

- There is no specific treatment for the disease, symptomatic treatment is given.
- Prevention is the best treatment, giving polio drops according to the national immunization scheduled.
- Two types of vaccines are used throughout the world. They are:
  1. *Oral (Sabin) polio vaccine (OPV):* The polio vaccine is the live attenuated Sabin vaccine, commonly known as OPV (oral polio vaccine). It gives nearly 100% protection. It gives gut immunity and prevents spread of wild virus and provides humoral and gut antibodies. It is more convenient to give.

     Storage OPV retains its potency for 3 months if stored at 2 to 10°C for 1 year if stored at –10°C. It should be kept in one of compartments of refrigerator and not in the door shelf, nor in the freezer.
  2. *Inactivated (Salk) polio vaccine (IPV):* It is parenteral, killed vaccine, given intramuscularly. It is given in special circumstances only.

**Schedule:**

| | | |
|---|---|---|
| 1st primary dose | - | 6 to 12 weeks of age. |
| 2nd primary dose | - | 4 to 8 weeks after 1st dose. |
| 3rd Primary dose | - | 4 to 8 weeks after 2nd dose. |
| Booster dose | - | 18 to 24 months of age. |

OPV should not exposed to sunlight, it must be given within 15 minutes after opening the vial. It should not be given to individuals proven or suspected to be immune deficient.

## VIRAL HEPATITIS

Viral Hepatitis is an inflammation of the liver caused by a virus. The condition can be self-limiting or can progress to fibrosis (scarring), cirrhosis or liver cancer. Hepatitis viruses are the most common cause of hepatitis in the world but other infections, toxic substances (e.g. alcohol, certain drugs), and autoimmune diseases can also cause hepatitis.

There are 5 main hepatitis viruses, referred to as types A, B, C, D and E. These 5 types are of greatest concern because of the burden of illness and death they cause and the potential for outbreaks and epidemic spread. In particular, types B and C lead to chronic disease in hundreds of millions of people and, together, are the most common cause of liver cirrhosis and cancer.

**Table:** Hepatitis A, B and C: Learn the differences

| Content | Hepatitis A | Hepatitis B | Hepatitis C |
|---|---|---|---|
| **What is it?** | A liver illness caused by hepatitis A virus. The virus makes people sick but only for 1–3 weeks | A liver illness caused by hepatitis B virus. The virus affects people differently:<br>• Most adults clear their infection and have no further problems.<br>• Many babies and children don't clear it and may have liver problems later in life. | A liver illness caused by hepatitis C virus. Most people don't clear the virus and have the illness for life.<br>The illness can cause liver problems. |
| **Incubation period** | 10–50 days, average age 28 days | 60–150 days, average 90 days. | 14–180 days, average 45 days. |
| **Transmitted by** | Food or water contaminated with sewerage.<br>Anything with human feces (poo) on it that comes in contact with the mouth.<br>Household contact with an infected person.<br>Sexual contact (involving anal sex) with an infected person.<br>Traveling through developing countries. | Blood-to-blood contact. (when one person's blood gets into another person's bloodstream).<br>Sexual contact with an infected person.<br>Sharing needles and syringes when injecting drugs.<br>Sharing other equipment (e.g. spoons, filters, tourniquets) when injecting drugs.<br>Having a needle stick injury.<br>Tattooing or body piercing with contaminated equipment.<br>Medical procedures in developing countries.<br>Mother to baby. | Blood-to-blood contact<br>Sharing needles and syringes when injecting drugs.<br>Sharing other equipment (e.g. spoons, filters, tourniquets) when injecting drugs.<br>Receiving blood products before February 1990 in Australia.<br>Having a needle stick injury.<br>Tattooing or body piercing with contaminated equipment.<br>Medical procedures in developing countries.<br>Mother to baby. |
| **Symptoms in short-term infection** | Feeling unwell, aches and pains, fever, nausea, lack of appetite, abdominal pain, dark urine, followed by jaundice (yellowing of eyes and sometimes skin). Young children usually have no symptoms. | Often no symptoms, but if they do present, they include jaundice (see left), dark urine, fatigue, abdominal pain, loss of appetite, nausea and joint pain. | Often no symptoms, but if they do present, are like having a mild flu.<br>A small number of people may have symptoms similar to hepatitis B (see left). |
| **Symptoms in long-term infection** | No long-term infection. | Fatigue, nausea, muscle aches and pains, abdominal discomfort or jaundice (see above left). | Fatigue, nausea, muscle aches and pains or abdominal discomfort. |
| **Treatment** | Not needed. | Adefovir, entecavir, pegylated interferon, lamivudine and telbivudine.<br>Some people use complementary medicine (e.g. herbalism) to manage their symptoms. | Combination therapy with pegylated interferon and ribavirin.<br>Some people use complementary medicine (e.g. herbalism) to manage their symptoms. |
| **Vaccine** | Yes. It is safe and effective.<br>Get vaccinated. | Yes. It is safe and effective.<br>Part of universal childhood vaccination.<br>Get vaccinated. | None available. |
| **Prevention** | Household contacts and sexual partners of someone with hepatitis A should have an injection of immunoglobulin (drug that provides immediate short-term protection against particular diseases).<br>Wash hands after going to the toilet and before eating.<br>Practice safe sex. | Do not share needles and syringes when injecting drugs.<br>Avoid other blood-to-blood contact.<br>Practice safe sex.<br>Newborn babies should be given an injection of immunoglobulin (see left) within 12 hours of birth. | Do not share needles and syringes when injecting drugs.<br>Do not share other equipment when injecting drugs.<br>Avoid other blood-to-blood contact. |

## CHOLERA

It is an infectious disease caused by *Vibrio Cholerae*.

### Modes of Transmission

- The infection spread through contaminated water, food, drinks, hands, flies, etc.
- In short 5F's, i.e. fingers, flies, fluid, food and fommites are chief modes of transmission.

**Incubation period:** A few hours to 5 days.

**Clinical manifestation:** Painless watery diarrhea.vomiting, dehydration, sunken eyes and cheeks, low BP, shallow rapid respiration, stomach pain, leg cramps, decreased urine output.

**In children:** Fever, convulsions of coma, loss of muscular tone.

### Control and Preventive Measures of Cholera

- Verification of the diagnosis
- Notification
- Early case finding
- Establishment of treatment centers
- Rehydration of therapy (ORS)
- Adjuncts to therapy
- Epidemiological investigations
- Sanitation measures
- Chemoprophylaxis
- Vaccination
- Health education.

## TYPHOID FEVER (ENTERIC FEVER)

### Definition

Typhoid fever is an acute communicable disease caused by ***'Salmonella Typhi'***. This disease is also called enteric fever.

### Mode of Transmission

Typhoid fever is transmitted by feco-oral route or urine-oral routes—either directly through hands soiled with feces or urine of cases or carriers or indirectly by ingestion of contaminated water, milk, food, or through flies. Contaminated ice, ice-creams, and milk products are a rich source of infection.

- ***Incubation period:*** 7–28 days.
- ***Signs and symptoms:*** Prolonged fever with chills, malaise, headache, cough, sore throat, abdominal pain, constipation, swelling occurs in the lymph glands of small intestine, splenomegaly, bradycardia, rose spots on chest wall.

### Prevention and Control of Typhoid Fever/ Enteric Fever

- A complementary approach to prevention is immunization which is the only specific preventive measure likely to yield the highest benefit for the money spent. It does not give 100% protection but definitely lowers the incidence and seriousness of infection. It is recommended to:
  - Those living are endemic areas.
  - Household contacts.
  - Groups at risk of infection such as school children and nurses.
  - Travelers preceding to endemic areas.
  - Those attending meals and yatras.

It was introduced by 'Wright' in 1896. The anti-typhoid vaccine currently available in India are:

- ***Monovalent vaccine:*** The vaccine of choice is monovalent vaccine, which is an agar grown, heat-killed and phenol preserved vaccine containing 1000 mL *S typhi* per mL. It may also be prepared by inactivation of organisms with acetone and the vaccine is known as AKD (Acetone Killed and Dried).
- ***Bivalent vaccine:*** It contains *S typhi* and *S Paratyphi* A is proportion of 1000 million and 500 million organisms respectively. The organisms are killed and preserved by heating at 54 degree for the addition of 0.5% phenol. It can also be prepared by inactivation of organism with acetone in dried form.
- ***TAB vaccine:*** Traditional TAB vaccine contained *S Typhi, S paratyphi* A and *S paratyphi* B. The proteins of paratyphoid A and B enhance the reactions. Therefore WHO recommended that TAB vaccine should be discontinued.

### *Other Preventive Measures*

- Provision of safe water and improvement of sanitation.
- ***Food sanitation:*** Protection of food from flies and dust, preventing carries from handling food. Cooks and food handlers should observe sanitary precautions.
- Detection of typhoid carriers and treating them.
- Human excreta must be collected and disposed of properly.
- Milk should be pasteurized before use.
- The role of fingers, foods, flies, fomites, feces (5 fs) must be explained to the public through health education and see that they practice all instructions which are given to them.

### *Specific Treatment*

- Chloramphenicol 1 gm every 6 hourly is given orally for 2–3 days or until the temperature comes down and then 250 mgm every 8 hourly for 2–3 weeks.
- To lower the fever tepid, cold water sponge or ice bag may be given as per doctor's order.

## DENGUE FEVER

### Definition

Dengue fever is an acute viral infection caused by dengue virus. Which spreads in human being by aedes aegypti and aedes albopictus mosquitoes.

Dengue fever is also called as break bone fever.

*Aedes* mosquito become injective after feeding on infective patient. The incubation period for development of infection via ***aedes*** mosquito is 8–10 days. And once the ***aedes*** mosquito is infective it remains infective for life.

### Clinical Manifestations

- Classical dengue fever:
  - High fever with chills (39 to 90°C)
  - Intense headache
  - Muscle and joint pain
  - Retro-orbital pain
  - Photophobia

- Weakness
- Anorexia
- Constipation
- Altered taste sensation
- Colicky pain
- Abdominal tenderness
- Pain in inguinal region
- Sore throat
- Rash diffuse flushing, mottling
- Fleeting pin point eruptions on face, neck, chest during the first half of febrile period.

- Dengue hemorrhagic fever (DHF).
- Dengue shock syndrome.

### Laboratory Diagnosis

Blood test for platelets and hematocrit platelets less than 100,000/mm$^3$ will be in dengue hemorrhagic fever and hematocrit increased by 20% or more.

### Prevention and Control

Prevention and control of dengue, DHF has become urgent with expanding geographic distribution and increase incidence in the past 20 years. Effective disease prevention program must have several integrated components, including active laboratory based surveillance, emergency, response, and education of medical community to ensure effective case management, community based integrated mosquito control and effective use of vaccines when they become available.

- Active surveillance.
- Mosquito control
- Community participation.
- Prevention of dengue in travelers.
- *Early diagnosis and treatment:* The treatment of dengue fever is symptomatic and supportive treatment includes:
  - Bed rest
  - Antipyretics
  - Hydrotherapy
  - Intravenous/oral fluids. In case of vomiting, diarrhea or excessive sweating.
  - Blood transfusion—In case of resistant shock.
- *Protect yourself:* Wear full sleeves clothes and long dresses to cover as much of your body as possible during 2 hours after sunrise and before sunset as highest biting intensity is during this time.
- *Use repellents:* Use mosquito coils and electric vapor mats during dry times to prevent dengue, use mosquito nets to protect children, older people, etc.

## MALARIA

Malaria is a protozoal infection caused by 'Plasmodium' and transmitted to man by bite of infected female Anopheline mosquito.

### By Vector Transmission

Infected, female, *anopheles* mosquito is responsible for spread of malaria. A single infected vector is able to spread infection to several persons.

### Direct Transmission

Blood transfusion, needle injury.

### Congenital

- Rarely, mother-to-child transmission will occur.
- Thus infected mother can spread disease to child in womb.

### Incubation Period

- ***Plasmodium vivax:*** 8–17 days.
- ***Plasmodium falciparum:*** 9–14 days.
- ***Plasmodium quartan (malaria):*** 18–40 days.
- ***Plasmodium ovale:*** 16 to 18 days.

### Clinical Manifestations

*An attack of malaria has 3 tages,* i.e. cold, hot and sweating stage.

| Cold stage | Hot stage | Sweating stage |
|---|---|---|
| • Headache<br>• Nausea and vomiting<br>• Chills<br>• Fever rises<br>• Tachycardia | • Fever<br>• Eye and face become red<br>• Skin hot dry and red<br>• High pulse rate | • Temperature decreases with sweating<br>• Skin cool and moist |

### Prevention and Control of Malaria

- ***Protection against mosquito:*** Man should protect himself against mosquito by use of:
  - Repellents
  - Protective clothing
  - Bed nets
  - Use mosquito coils
  - Use net in the doors and windows
  - Use mosquito nets
  - Screening of houses
  - Do not sleep in the open places
  - Cover most of the body parts.
- ***Mosquito control measures:***
  - ***Antilarval measures:***
    - ➢ Use of larvicides on the standing water
    - ➢ Oil on stagnant water
    - ➢ Paris green
    - ➢ Temphos.
  - ***Antiadult measures:*** Spraying of DDT powder.
  - ***Mass drug administration:*** Mass drug administration is recommended in highly endemic area.
- ***Reduction of mosquito breeding sites:***
  - Proper drainage system
  - Filling of drains
  - Management of water level
  - Cleaning of water coolers.

## LEPROSY

Leprosy is a chronic communicable disease. This is commonly called as a ***'Social disease'*** because this disease spreading from social factors.

Leprosy ***(Hansen's disease)*** is chronic infections disease caused by ***Mycobacterium leprae.*** This disease affects mainly the peripheral nerves. It also affects the skin, muscles, eyes, bones and internal organs.

### Signs and Symptoms of Leprosy

- Headache
- Malaise
- Chilliness
- Mental depression
- Numbness of body.

### *Main Diagnostic Signs*

- Marks or hypopigmented patches on skin
- Total or partial loss of sensation (pain, touch and temperature) in leprosy affected parts.
- Nerves become thick and starting the hair falling
- Tumors on the skin of face and ears.
- Loss of fingers
- Claw toes
- Loss of sweating or loss of hair over the skin lesion.

### Modes of Transmission

- *Contact transmission:* Lepra bacilli transmitted by direct close contact with families, persons who have infected from leprosy.
- *Droplet infection:* Droplet infection is very common for leprosy through coughing, sneezing.
- *Other route:* Lepra bacilli found in human milk.

**Incubation period:** 3–5 years.

### Role of Community Health Nurse in Leprosy Control

Community nurse plays a major role in the control of leprosy.

The following elements are considered as a minimum requirement for all leprosy control programs.

- Medical measures:
  - Estimation of problem
  - Early case detection
  - Multidrug therapy
  - Surveillance
  - Immunoprophylaixs
  - Chemoprophylaixs
  - Deformities
  - Rehabilitation
  - Health education
  - Others.
- Social support
- Program management
- Evaluation.

As a community health nurse, she has to explain regarding 3 aspects of medical management, they are:

1. About treatment
2. Maintenance of hygiene
3. Loss of sensation includes—care of hands, feet, care of shoes, etc.

## SEXUALLY TRANSMITTED DISEASES (STD)

Diseases which are produced due to sexual contact are called sexually transmitted disease.

The sexual transmitted diseases also known as vulnerable diseases constitute family health and social problems.

STD is transmitted mainly by direct contact of an infected person with a non-infected person. Common STD are:

- Syphilis
- Gonorrhea
- Chancroid
- Granuloma
- Lymphogranuloma venereum
- AIDS.

### AIDS (Acquired Immune Deficiency Syndrome)

- It is an immune-deficiency disorder that is often fatal
- It was first recognized in USA in July 1981.
- In August 1981, it was reported in intravenous users.
- In June 1982, clusters of AIDS patients appeared among homosexual and later in hemophiliacs and blood transfusion associated patients.
- In January 1983, it was reported in heterosexual cases in female.
- First case of HIV infection in India was reported in 1986 and that of HIV-2 in 1991.
- It is caused by a virus known as Human Immunodeficiency Virus (HIV). Once infected, it is probable that a person will be infected for life. AIDS breaks down the body's immune system exposing the individual to numerous life-threatening infections, neurological disorders and malignancies.

'HIV' stands for Human Immunodeficiency Virus. To understand what that means, let's break it down:

- **H**–Human: This particular *virus* can only infect human beings.
- **I**–Immunodeficiency: HIV weakens your *immune system* by destroying important cells that fight disease and infection. A 'deficient' immune system cannot protect you.

HIV can be transmitted through

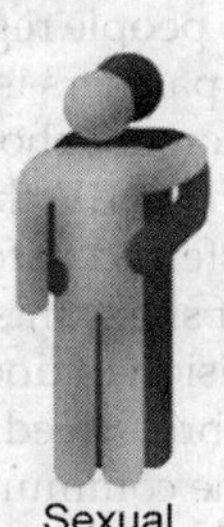
Sexual contact

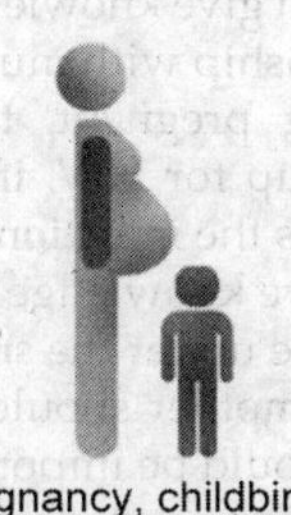
Pregnancy, childbirth and breastfeeding

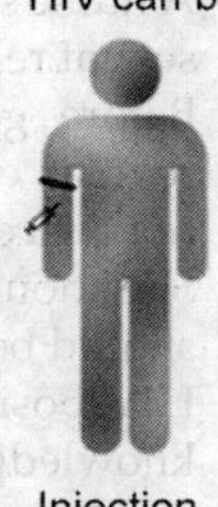
Injection drug use

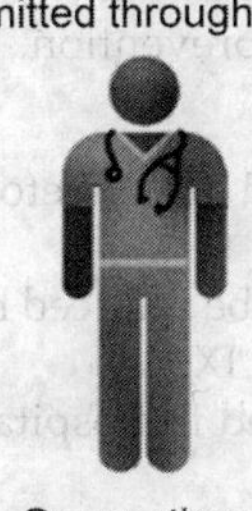
Occupational exposure

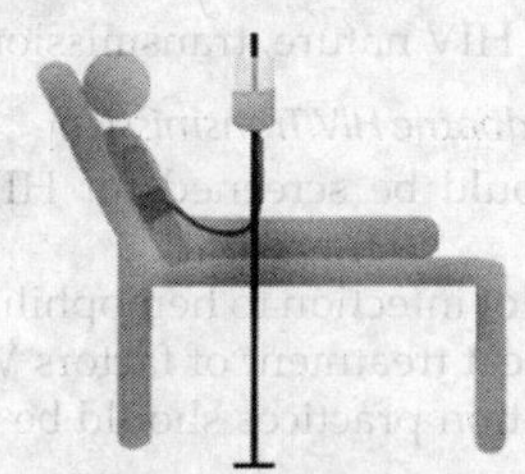
and rearely, Blood transfusion/organ transplant

- V–Virus: A virus can only reproduce itself by taking over a cell in the body of its host.

### Epidemiological Factors

- *Agent:* Human Immunodeficiency Virus (HIV).
- *Source of infection:* HIV Cases and Carriers.
- *Infective material:* Blood and semen of infected persons.
- *Age:* Sexually active persons (20–49 years).
- *High risk groups:* Prostitutes, homosexuals, intravenous drug users, etc.
- *Immunity:* Man has no natural immunity.
- *Incubation Period:* 6 years or more.

### Clinical Features

- *Major signs:* Weight loss, chronic diarrhea for longer than 1 month, prolonged fever for longer than 1 month (intermittent or constant), skin tumors (Kaposi' sarcoma).
- *Minor signs:* Persistent cough, oropharyngeal candidiasis or fungus infection, generalized lymph-adenopathy, intercurrent infections such as pneumonia and tuberculosis.

### Prevention and Control of HIV Infection

Control of HIV infection:

- Prevention
- Antirectroviral treatment
- Specific prophylaxis
- Primary health care.

#### Prevention

- Education
- Prevention of bloodborne HIV transmission.

#### Education

- There is no vaccine or cure for HIV.
- At present, only health education is available which enables the people make life saving choices, e.g. avoiding indiscriminate sex, using condoms.
- There is no guarantee that the use of condom will give full protection.
- One should avoid the use of shared razors and tooth-brushes.
- Intravenous drug users should be informed that the sharing of needles and syringes involves special rile.
- Women suffering from HIV should not be conceived since infection can be transmitted to the newborn.
- Educational material and guidelines for prevention should be made widely available.
- All mass media channels should be involved in educating the people on HIV nature, transmission and prevention.

#### Prevention of Bloodborne HIV Transmission

- All blood should be screened for $HIV_1$ and $HIV_2$ before transmission.
- Transmission of infection to hemophiliac can be reduced by introducing heat treatment of factors VII and IX.
- Strict sterilization practices should be ensured in hospitals and clinics.
- Presterilized disposable syringes and needles should be used as far as possible.
- *Antiretroviral treatment:* At present, there is no vaccine or cure for treatment of HIV. However, the development of drugs that suppress the HIV infection itself rather than its complications has been important development. These drugs help in prolonging the life of severely ill patients. These drugs are:

***Zidovudine (AZT):*** Dose: 600 mg orally daily in two divided doses.

#### Side Effect

- Anemia
- Neutropenia
- Nausea
- Malaise
- Headache
- Insomnia
- Myopathy.

***Lamivudine (3TC) (Epivir):*** Dose; 150 mg orally twice daily.

#### Side Effects

- Rash
- Peripheral neuropathy.

***Tenofovir (viread):*** Dose: 300 mg orally twice daily.

- ***Side effects:*** Gastrointestinal distress

***Amprenavir (Agenerase):*** Dose: 1200 mg orally twice daily

- ***Side effects:*** Gastrointestinal, rash.

***Delavirdine (Rescripter):*** Dose: 400 mg orally 3 times daily.

- **Side effects:** Rash.

#### Specific Prophylaxis

- Primary prophylaxis against *P Carinii* pneumonia should be offered to patient with count below 200 cell/uL. The regimen available are trimethroprim-sulfamethoxazole, aerosolized pentamidine and dapsone.
- Patient who develop *P carinii* infection on a particular prophylactic regimen should be switched to the other drug or should receive combination regimen.
- *M. avium* complex occur in at least one kind of AIDS patients. Rifabutin has been shown in a randomized trial to decrease the incidence of disseminated *M. avium* intracellulare in persons with less than 200 CD4 Cell/uL.
- M tuberculosis is 300 mg isoniazid daily for 9 months to one year should be given to HIV patient with the PPD reaction.

#### Primary Health Care

- A nurse should give knowledge to community people regarding the safe use of razors, syringe, etc.
- She should give knowledge to people that the previously used blades and syringes should never be used again as this disease easily spread by these things.
- A nurse should give knowledge to people regarding having sexual relationship with multiple partners is harmful.
- Before getting pregnant, the women should go under regular checkup for HIV, if she has HIV then she should not conceive as the infection transferred to fetus.
- She should give knowledge that if she wants to conceive, it should be done under the supervision of doctor.
- HIV positive mother should not breastfeed her child, this knowledge should be import to the community people.
- She should give knowledge that during sexual intercourse, the couple should use condoms.

| National Immunization Schedule | | | | |
|---|---|---|---|---|
| Age | Vaccine name | Dosage | Route | Disease prevented |
| At birth | BCG<br>OPV<br>Hepatitis B | 0.05 mL<br>2 drops<br>0.5 mL | Intradermal<br>Oral<br>IM | TB<br>Polio<br>Hepatitis B |
| 1 ½ months | BCG (if not given at birth)<br>DPT-1<br>OPV-1<br>Hepatitis B-1 | 0.5 ml<br>0.5 mL<br>2 drops<br>0.5 mL | Intradermal<br>IM<br>Oral<br>IM | TB<br>Diphtheria, Pertussis, Tetanus<br>Polio<br>Hepatitis B |
| 2 ½ month | DPT-2<br>OPV-2<br>Hepatitis B-2 | 0.5 mL<br>2 drops<br>0.5 mL | IM<br>Oral<br>IM | Diphtheria, Pertussis, Tetanus<br>Polio<br>Hepatitis B |
| 3 ½ months | DPT-3<br>OPV-3<br>Hepatitis B-3 | 0.5 mL<br>2 drops<br>0.5 mL | IM<br>Oral<br>IM | Diphtheria, Pertussis, Tetanus<br>Polio<br>Hepatitis B |
| 9 months | Measles<br>Vit-A | 0.5 mL<br>1 lakh IU | Subcutaneous<br>Oral | Measles<br>Night blindness |
| 16–24 months | DPT (Booster)<br>OPV (Booster)<br>Vit-A (Booster)<br>Measles (Booster) | 0.5 mL<br>2 drops<br>2 lakh<br>0.5 mL | IM<br>Oral<br>Oral<br>Subcutaneous | Diphtheria, Pertussis, Tetanus<br>Polio<br>Night blindness |
| 5 years<br>6 years<br>10 years<br>16 years | DPT-1<br>DPT-2<br>TT<br>TT | 0.5 mL<br>0.5 mL<br>0.5 mL<br>0.5 mL | IM<br>IM<br>IM<br>IM | Diphtheria, Pertussis, Tetanus<br>Tetanus<br>Tetanus |
| Early in pregnancy (Primi) | TT-1 | 0.5 mL | IM | Tetanus |
| One month interval (Para) | TT-2 | 0.5 mL | IM | Tetanus |
| If immunized with TT within 3 years | TT booster dose | 0.5 mL | IM | Tetanus |

- The nurse should educate the people regarding the mode of transmission of HIV and about various measures by which we can prevent this.
- She should educate the people about the disease and should clear all the doubts of people about the disease.

## COLD CHAIN

'Cold Chain' is a system of storage and transport of vaccine at low temperature from the manufacturer to the actual vaccination site.

The cold chain system is necessary because vaccine failure may occur due to failure to store and transport under strict temperature controls.

### Objective of Cold Chain

The main objective of cold chain is to maintain the potency of the vaccine by providing adequate cooling facilities.

### Functions of Cold Chain

- To obtain the vaccines.
- To store the vaccines.
- To supply the vaccines.
- To find out the equipment failure, power failure, etc.

### How to Monitor the Cold Chain?

To avoid the unnecessary accumulation of vaccines the supplies should follow demands and utilization. Storage temperature should be recorded twice in a day. If the temperature rise above +8°C and falls below +2°C an intervention is indicated.

## FAMILY PLANNING METHODS

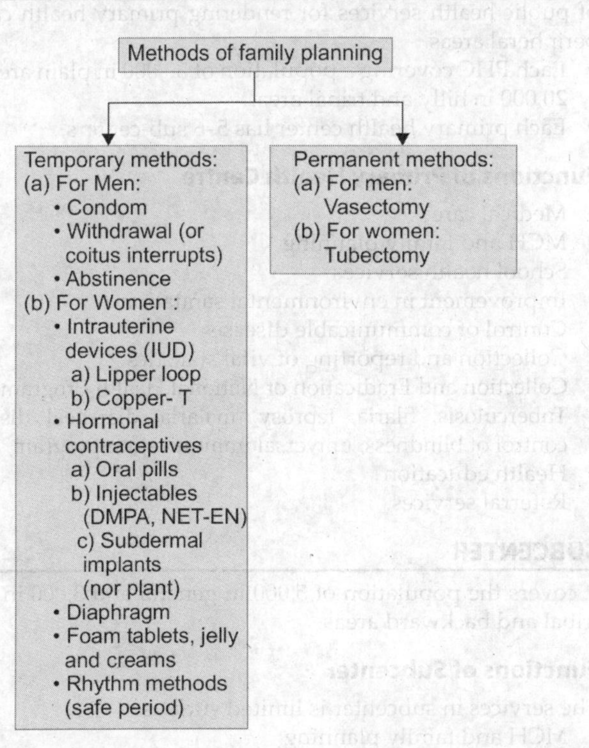

## PRIMARY HEALTH CARE

### Definition

'Primary health care is an essential health care made universally accessible to individuals and acceptable to them through their full participation and at a cost the community and country can afford'. —*WHO*

### Elements of Primary Health Care (PHC)

- **E** – Education for Health.
- **L** – Locally endemic disease control.
- **E** – Expanded program on immunization.
- **M** – Maternal and child health and family planning.
- **E** – Environment sanitation and promotion of safe water supply.
- **N** – Nutrition and Promotion of Adequate Food Supply.
- **T** – Treatment of Communicable Diseases and Common Illness.
- **S** – Supply of Essential Drugs.

### Principles of Primary Health Care

- Equitable distribution.
- Community participation.
- Intersectoral coordination.
- Appropriate technology.
- Focus on prevention.

## PRIMARY HEALTH CENTER

### Definition

Primary health center is the basic structural and functional unit of public health services for rendering primary health care in peripheral areas.

- Each PHC covering a population of 30,000 in plain area and 20,000 in hilly and tribal area.
- Each primary health center has 5–6 sub-centers.

### Functions of Primary Health Centre

- Medical care
- MCH and family planning
- School health services
- Improvement in environmental sanitation
- Control of communicable diseases
- Collection and reporting of vital statistics
- Collection and Eradication of National Health Programs (e.g. Tuberculosis, filaria, leprosy, malaria, diarrheal diseases, control of blindness, universal immunization program, etc.)
- Health education
- Referral services.

## SUBCENTER

It covers the population of 5,000 in general and 3,000 in hilly, tribal and backward areas.

### Functions of Subcenter

The services in subcenter is limited such as:

- MCH and family planning
- Immunization
- Health education
- Training and supervision of Dais, etc.

## COMMUNITY HEALTH CENTER

### Definition

Community health centers (CHC) are the nonprofit community governed health organizations that provide primary health care, health promotion and community development services, using them inter disciplinary terms of health providers.

Each Community Health Center covering a population of 80,000–1,20,000 with 3–4 PHC. Each CHC has 30 sanctioned beds and has facility for specialized services in:

- Surgery, medicine, obstetrics, gynecology, pediatric, dental and ENT. The services are given by a team of Specialists nurses and other personnel.

### Functions of CHC

- Care of routine and emergency cases in surgery.
- Care of routine and emergency cases in medicine.
- 24-hour delivery services including normal and assisted deliveries.
- Essential and emergency obstetric cases including surgical interventions.
- Full range of family planning services including laparoscopic services.
- Safe abortion services.
- Newborn care.
- Routine and emergency care of sick children.
- Other management including nasal packing, tracheotomy, foreign body removal, etc.
- All national health programs should be delivered.
- Blood storage facility.
- Essential laboratory services.
- Referral services.

## HEALTH EDUCATION

### Definition of Health Education

- 'Health education is a process which affects changes in the health practice of people and in the knowledge and attitude related to such changes'. —*WHO*

### Principles of Health Education

Some basic principles that should be followed in imparting health education (It can be summed up using a memories. 'MILKCPRLGCSF')

**M** : Motivation
**I** : Interest
**L** : Learning by doing
**K** : Known to unknown
**C** : Credibility
**P** : Participation
**R** : Reinforcement
**L** : Leader
**G** : Good human relation
**C** : Comprehensive
**S** : Setting an example
**F** : Feedback

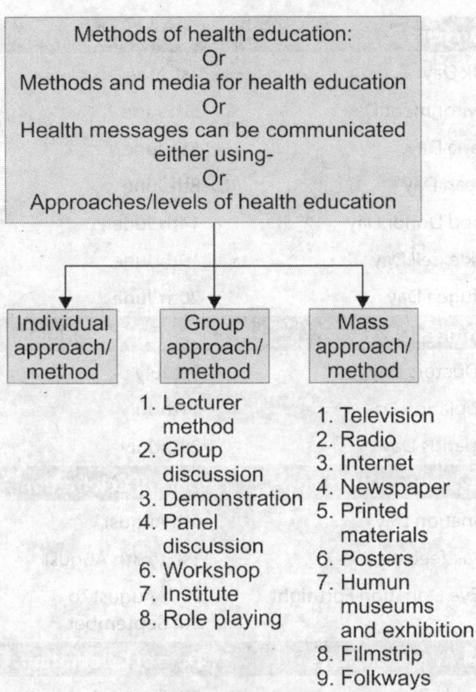


## NATIONAL HEALTH PROGRAMS

| List of national health programs | Year |
|---|---|
| National Tuberculosis Control Programme (NTCP) | 1962 |
| Revised National Tuberculosis Control Programme (RNTCP) | 1997 |
| National Malaria Control Programme (NMCP) | 1953 |
| National Malaria Eradication Programme (NMEP) | 1958 |
| National Anti-Malaria Programme (NAMP) | 1999 |
| National Filaria Control Programme (NFCP) | 1955 |
| National Leprosy Control Programme (NLCP) | 1955 |
| National Leprosy Elimination Programme (NLEP) | 1997 |
| National AIDS Control Programme (NACP) | 1986 |
| National AIDS Control Organization (NACO) | 1992 |
| National Programme for Control of Blindness (NPCB) | 1976 |
| National Cancer Control Programme (NCCP) | 1975 |
| National Diabetes Control Programme (NDCP) | 1987 |
| National Iodine Deficiency Disorders Programme (NIDDP) | 1962 |
| Universal Immunization Programme (UIP) | 1985 |
| Reproductive and Child Health Programme (RCH phase-I) | 1997 |
| Reproductive and Child Health Programme (RCH phase-II) | 2005 |
| National Mental Health Programme (NMHP) | 1982 |
| National Family Welfare Programme (NFWP) | 1952 |
| National Surveillance Programme for Communicable Disease (NSPCD) | 1988 |
| National Water Supply and Sanitation Programme | 1954 |
| Minimum Needs Programme (MNP) | 1974 |
| Child Survival and Safe Motherhood (CSSM) | 1992 |
| National Rural Health Mission (NRHM) | 2005 |

## FIVE YEAR PLANS

In 1950, Planning Commission was constituted to help government to plan out integrated development plan for the entire country within the available resource for a defined period of five years for its socioeconomic progress.

Five years plan is mechanism to bring about uniformity in policy formulation in programs of national importance. The specific objectives of the health program, during five years plan, are as follows:

- Control and eradication of major communicable diseases.
- Strengthening of basic health services through the establishment of the PHC and subenters.
- Population control.
- Development of health manpower resources.

| List of Five Year Plans | Year |
|---|---|
| First Five Year Plan | 1951–1956 |
| Second Five Year Plan | 1956–1961 |
| Third Five Year Plan | 1961–1966 |
| Fourth Five Year Plan | 1969–1974 |
| Fifth Five Year Plan | 1974–1979 |
| Sixth Five Year Plan | 1980–1985 |
| Seventh Five Year Plan | 1985–1990 |
| Eighth Five Year Plan | 1992–1997 |
| Ninth Five Year Plan | 1997–2002 |
| Tenth Five Year Plan | 2002–2007 |
| Eleventh Five Year Plan | 2007–2012 |
| Twelfth Five Year Plan | 2012–2017 |

## HEALTH PROBLEMS IN INDIA

For health problems in India see flowchart.

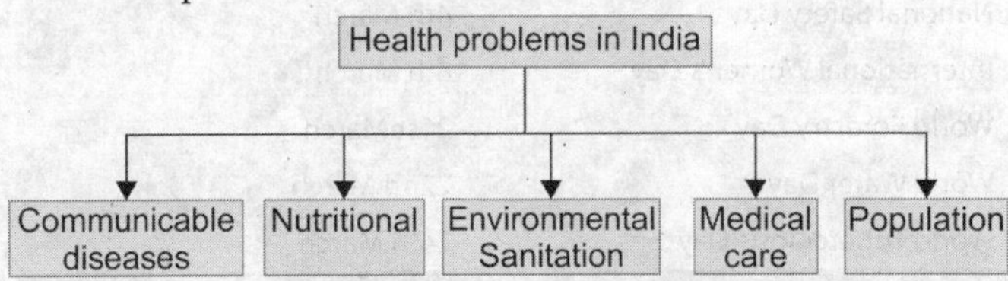


## NATIONAL HEALTH COMMITTEES

| List of various committees | Year |
|---|---|
| Bhore Committee | 1946 |
| Mudaliar Committee | 1962 |
| Chadha Committee | 1963 |
| Mukherjee Committee | 1965 |
| Jungalwalla Committee | 1967 |
| Kartar Singh Committee | 1973 |
| Srivastava Committee | 1975 |
| Balaji Committee | 1986 |

## ORAL REHYDRATION SOLUTION

Oral rehydration therapy (ORT) is a type of fluid replacement used to prevent or treat dehydration especially due to diarrhea.

If the patient is having mild diarrhea with few loose stools, ORS may be given every hour.

### Composition of ORS-bicarbonate

| Ingredient | Quantity |
|---|---|
| Sodium Chloride | 3.5 g |
| Sodium Bicarbonate | 2.5 g |
| Potassium Chloride | 1.5 g |
| Glucose (dextrose) | 20 g |
| Potable water | 1 liter |

### Composition of ORS-citrate

| Ingredient | Quantity |
|---|---|
| Sodium Chloride | 3.5 g |
| Tri-sodium citrate dehydrate | 2.9 g |
| Potassium Chloride | 1.5 g |
| Glucose | 20 g |
| Potable water | 1 liter |

## AWARENESS DAYS/HEALTH CALENDAR

| January Awareness Days | Date of Celebration |
|---|---|
| Road Safety Week | 2nd to the 7th January |
| National Youth Day | 12th January |
| National Girl Child Day | 24th January |
| National Science Day | 28th January |
| Anti-Leprosy Day | 30th January |
| **February Awareness Days** | **Date of Celebration** |
| World Cancer Day | 4th February |
| **March Awareness Days** | **Date of Celebration** |
| National Safety Day | 4th March |
| International Women's Day | 8th March |
| World Forestry Day | 21st March |
| World Water Day | 22nd March |
| World Tuberculosis Day | 24th March |
| **April Awareness Days** | **Date of Celebration** |
| Prevention of Blindness Week | 1st to 7th April |
| World Health Day | 7th April |
| World Earth Day | 22nd April |
| **May Awareness Days** | **Date of Celebration** |
| International Labor Day | 1st May |
| World Asthma Day | 6th May |
| World Thalassemia Day | 8th May |
| World Red Cross Day | 8th May |
| International Nurses Day | 12th May |
| World Hypertension Day | 17th May |
| World No Tobacco Day | 31st May |
| **June Awareness Days** | **Date of Celebration** |
| World Milk Day | 1st June |
| World Environment Day | 5th June |
| World Filaria Day | 5th June |
| World Ocean Day | 8th June |
| World Blood Donor Day | 14th June |
| World Sickle Cell Day | 19th June |
| World Refugee Day | 20th June |
| **July Awareness Days** | **Date of Celebration** |
| National Doctors Day | 1st July |
| World Population Day | 11th July |
| World Hepatitis Day | 28th July |
| **August Awareness Days** | **Date of Celebration** |
| Organ Donation Day | 6th August |
| World Breastfeeding Week | 1st to 7th August |
| National Eye Donation Fortnight | 25th August to 8th September |
| **September Awareness Days** | **Date of Celebration** |
| International Literacy Day | 8th September |
| National Nutrition Week | 1st to 7th September |
| World Alzheimer's Day | 21st September |
| World Deaf Day | 26th September |
| World Heart Day | 29th September |
| **October Awareness Days** | **Date of Celebration** |
| World Mental Health Day | 1st October |
| World Blood Donation Day | 1st October |
| World Geriatric Day | 1st October |
| World Food Day | 16th October |
| World Habitat Day | First Monday of the month of October |
| **November Awareness Days** | **Date of Celebration** |
| Cancer Awareness Day | 7th November |
| World Immunization Day | 10th November |
| National Children's Day | 14th November |
| World Diabetic Day | 14th November |
| **December Awareness Days** | **Date of Celebration** |
| World AIDS Day | 1st December |
| National Pollution Control Day | 2nd December |
| International Day of Disabled Persons | 3rd December |
| International Volunteer Day for Economic and Social Development | 5th December |
| Armed Forces Flag Day | 7th December |
| World Patient Safety Day | 9th December |
| Human Rights Day | 10th December |
| National Energy Conservation Day | 14th December |

## MULTIPLE CHOICE QUESTIONS

**1. Mantoux test is done for:**
(a) Filaria (b) Leprosy
(c) Malaria (d) Tuberculosis

**2. What is the optimal temperature for cold chain maintenance? (AIIMS Bhubaneswar, 2016)**
(a) –20°C (b) +10°C
(c) +2 to + 8°C (d) –18°C

**3. What is pandemic disease? (AIIMS Bhubaneswar, 2016)**
(a) One which is caused by animal bite
(b) One which is found all over world
(c) One which is regularly found among a particular group of people
(d) One which is spreading among a large number of people in the same place for the same time

**4. Causative organisms of AIDS: (ESI, 2009)**
(a) Retrovirus (b) Adenovirus
(c) Orthomyxovirus (d) Rhabdovirus

**5. Causative organism of smallpox:**
(a) Rubella (b) Varicella zoster
(c) Retrovirus (d) Variola virus

**6. Which is the main test for Tuberculosis?**
(a) Coomb's text (b) Mantoux text
(c) Widal test (d) Schick test

**7. What of the following is celebrated on 7th December every year? (AIIMS Bhubaneswar, 2016)**
(a) Armed Forces Flag Day
(b) International Yoga Day
(c) National Science Day
(d) Human Rights Day

**8. Measures taken to stop the progress of disease is called: (RPSC Nursing Grade II Exam, 2010)**
(a) Primary prevention (b) Secondary prevention
(c) Tertiary prevention (d) All of the above

**9. Which of the following is NOT included in the major criteria for the diagnosis of rheumatic fever? (AIIMS Bhubaneswar, 2016)**
(a) Carditis (b) Chorea
(c) Fever (d) Arthritis

**10. _____ is the diseases (or) infections which are naturally transmitted between vertebrate animals and man.**
(a) Communicable disease
(b) Noncommunicable disease
(c) Zoonosis
(d) Malnutrition

**11. Leprosy affects all, except: (CGHS, 2009)**
(a) Ovary (b) Upper respiratory tract
(c) Uterus (d) Skin

**12. Universal immunization program was started in: (ESI, 2009)**
(a) 1992 (b) 1985
(c) 1975 (d) 1982

**13. Which of the following is NOT a barrier method of contraception? (AIIMS Bhubaneswar, 2016)**
(a) Diaphragm
(b) Condom
(c) Oral contraceptive pills
(d) Cervical cap

**14. An anganwadi worker is trained for: (Bihar PSC, 1987)**
(a) 1 month (b) 5 months
(c) 4 months (d) 8 months

**15. Dapsone and Rifampicin drug used for treatment of:**
(a) Cholera (b) Leprosy
(c) Diarrhea (d) Constipation

**16. Health is defined as 'State of complete physical, mental and social well-being and not merely absence of disease or infirmity' by_____.**
(a) Perkin (b) Oxford English Dictionary
(c) WHO (d) Webster

**17. April, 1948 is celebrated every year as:**
(a) Nurses day (b) World Health Day
(c) AIDS day (d) Tuberculosis day

**18. Which is the highly specific test for HIV? (AIIMS Bhubaneswar, 2016)**
(a) Mantoux (b) Widal
(c) ELISA (d) Western blot

**19. Hind Kusht Nivaran Sangh is a voluntary agency related to the disease: (RRB PMJHI, 2012)**
(a) Tuberculosis (b) Leprosy
(c) Malaria (d) Filaria

**20. The concept 'Disease agent man disease' is known as:**
(a) Germ theory of disease
(b) Natural history of disease
(c) Epidemiological triad
(d) All the above

**21. Who is the father of germ theory of disease?**
(a) Louis Pasteur (b) Virginia Apgar
(c) Newton (d) None of the above

**22. The average population of a village in India is estimated to be: (RRB PMJHI, 2012)**
(a) 5000 (b) 2500
(c) 1500 (d) 550

**23. Objective of community health nursing is:**
(a) Restoration of health
(b) Monitoring of health
(c) Maintenance of health
(d) All of the above

**24. In community health nursing focus is on _____.**
(a) Whole community with entire people
(b) Vulnerable groups
(c) Sick people
(d) Mothers and children

**25. Which of the following is the characteristic of community?**
(a) Different language
(b) Different attitude
(c) Common values and interest
(d) None of above

**26. Rice water stools is seen in: (RRB PMJHI, 2012)**
(a) Cholera (b) Typhoid
(c) Salmonellosis (d) Botulism

**27. Keratomalacia is due to deficiency of: ______ (AIIMS Bhubaneswar, 2016)**
(a) Vitamin A (b) Vitamin B12
(c) Vitamin C (d) Vitamin D

**28. Dimension of health is:**
(a) Mental dimension (b) Physical dimension
(c) Social dimension (d) All the above

**29. The determinants of health include______.**
(a) Biological determinants
(b) Behavioral and sociocultural conditions
(c) Environmental
(d) All of the above

**30. BCG vaccination is given to the infant to protect against: (AIIMS Bhubaneswar, 2016)**
(a) Leprosy (b) Tuberculosis
(c) Typhoid (d) Malaria

**31. The Vitamin A supplement administered in 'Prevention of nutritional blindness in children programme' contain:**
(a) 25,000 IU/mL (b) 50,000 IU/mL
(c) 1 lakh IU/mL (d) 2,00,000 IU/mL

**32. In following which disease caused by Varicella Zoster? (ESI Delhi, 2009)**
(a) Syphilis (b) Chickenpox
(c) Smallpox (d) Diphtheria

**33. Health Survey and Planning Committee is popularly known as:**
(a) Mudaliar Commitee (b) Mukherjee Committee
(c) Bhore Committee (d) Kartar Singh Committee

**34. Best test to detect iron deficiency in community is: (Karnataka PSC, 1996)**
(a) RBC test (b) Serum ferritin
(c) Serum iron (d) Transferrin

**35. An infant usually doubles his birth weight by the age of__________months. (AIIMS Bhubaneswar, 2016)**
(a) 10 (b) 8
(c) 3 (d) 5

**36. If cases occur irregularly haphazardly from time to time and generally frequently. It is called as an ______ (AIIMS Bhubaneswar, 2016)**
(a) Pandemic (b) Sporadic
(c) Endemic (d) Epidemic

**37. In India, the Consumer Protection Act came into force in the year:**
(a) 1999 (b) 1986
(c) 1988 (d) 1996

**38. Hygiene aspect of health maintenance includes:**
(a) Personal hygiene (b) Environmental hygiene
(c) Both of above (d) None of above

**39. Health promotion is the process to achieve health by:**
(a) Enabling people to increase control over their health
(b) Improving their health by lifestyle changes
(c) Creating awareness among people
(d) All of above

**40. Which of the following is not a pre-requisite of health promotion?**
(a) Educate (b) Treat
(c) Enable (d) Mediate

**41. Hardness of water can be caused due to: (RRB PMJHI, 2012)**
(a) Chlorides (b) Sulfate
(c) Nitrate (d) All of the above

**42. In India 'Rabies free' zone is: (AIIMS, 1990)**
(a) Manipur (b) Lakshadweep
(c) Goa (d) Rajasthan

**43. Health maintenance requires the measures to achieve health by:**
(a) Unsafe environment (b) Health services
(c) Increasing stress (d) Increasing conditions

**44. According to Holistic concept, health is considered as:**
(a) Absence of disease
(b) Proper adequate environment
(c) Good interpersonal relationship
(d) Sound body with sound mind living in sound family surrounded by sound environment.

**45. Identify the factors which are responsible for health:**
(a) External environment
(b) Genetic inheritance
(c) Social Support system
(d) All of above

**46. Which of the following is not the pre-requisite of health promotion?**
(a) Educate (b) Unhealthy practices
(c) Enable (d) Mediate

**47. _____ is the physiological or psychological dysfunction.**
(a) Illness (b) Sickness
(c) Disease (d) None of the above

**48. Intensity of noise is measured in terms of:**
(a) Decibels (b) Deciliter
(c) Foot candle (d) Centimeters

**49. Hansen's disease is the other name for: (AIIMS Bhubaneswar, 2016)**
(a) Malaria (b) Tuberculosis
(c) Typhoid (d) Leprosy

**50. Environment is classified into:**
(a) Macro and micro (b) Mini and minute
(c) Small and large (d) None of the above

**51. The quantification of the following diseases of health is considered very difficult or impossible ______________**
(a) Physical (b) Social
(c) Mental (d) Spiritual

**52. Sanitation and the national water supply program in India was launched in the year:**
(a) 1954 (b) 1964
(c) 1974 (d) 1984

**53. Message in a poster created for health education should be: (RRB PMJHI, 2012)**
(a) Short (b) Simple
(c) Direct (d) All of the above

**54. As per the ICDS scheme an Anganwadi worker is meant to be these for every ________population. (RRB PMJHI, 2012)**
(a) 500 (b) 1000
(c) 3000 (d) 5000

**55. Which is the most suitable method for disposal of night soil, litter, refuse, etc. in rural area?**
(a) Biogas plant (b) Composting
(c) Dumping (d) Manure pit

**56. Oxidation pond is the method used for:**
(a) Solid waste disposal (b) Sewage treatment
(c) Water purification (d) Sullage disposal

**57. Seullage is ____________.**
(a) Liquid excreta
(b) Waste water from kitchen
(c) By product of chemical industry
(d) Waste water from an industry

**58. Solid waste during the preparation, cooking and consumption of food is known as ________.**
(a) Garbage (b) Refuse
(c) Rubbish (d) Litter

**59. Orthotolidine test is used to determine:**
(a) Nitrates in water
(b) Potassium in water
(c) Ammonia in water
(d) Free combined chlorine in water

**60. Temporary hardness of water can be removed by:**
(a) Filtering (b) Boiling
(c) Disinfecting (d) Chlorination

**61. When chlorine is added to water what will happen?**
(a) Hydrochloric and hypochlorous acid forms
(b) Carbon dioxide is released
(c) $O_2$ and $CO_2$ is released
(d) None of the above

**62. The Greatest advancement in the water purification is ____________.**
(a) Sand bed filtration (b) Disinfection
(c) Chlorination (d) All the above

**63. Which of the following is NOT a live attenuated vaccine? (AIIMS Bhubaneswar, 2016)**
(a) Rabies (b) Chickenpox
(c) Mumps (d) Measles

**64. Which is the most universally accepted indicators of health status of whole population? (AIIMS Bhubaneswar, 2016)**
(a) Crude death rate (b) Infant mortality rate
(c) Adult mortality rate (d) Child mortality rate

**65. Chemical used for purification of water is:**
(a) Potassium permanganate
(b) DDT
(c) Alum
(d) Ammonia

**66. House hold purification of water is:**
(a) Boiling
(b) Mixing of bleaching powder
(c) Double pot method
(d) None of the above

**67. How much mg of calcium carbonate per liter water is considered as hardness of water?**
(a) 100 mg/L (b) 200 mg/L
(c) 300 mg/L (d) 400 mg/L

**68. In standard housing floor space should be at least ____________sq. ft. per person.**
(a) 40 sq. ft. (b) 100 sq. ft.
(c) 120 sq. ft. (d) 60 sq. ft.

**69. Prevention of food adulteration act is enacted by Government of India in ______.**
(a) 1950 (b) 1954
(c) 1960 (d) 1961

**70. On prescription of oral pills to the user, the health worker will ask about the following, except: (DSSSB, 2010)**
(a) Swelling of feet (b) Headache
(c) Calf tenderness (d) Number of death children

**71. Most common cause of blindness in India is: (RRB PMJHI, 2012)**
(a) Cataract (b) Glaucoma
(c) Refractive index (d) Vitamin A deficiency

**72. The best method of refuse disposal is ____________.**
(a) Burning (b) Dumping
(c) Composting (d) None of the above

**73. The tests for the biological examination of water includes______.**
(a) Algae (b) Diatoms
(c) Fungi (d) All

**74. The agent for the dechlorinating is known as________.**
(a) Charcoal (b) Sodium thiosulfate
(c) Sodium fluoride (d) Sodium bicabonate

**75. Which of the following is the natural ways of purification of water?**
(a) Sedimentation (b) Storage
(c) Filtration (d) All

**76. Which one of the following is the most effective disinfectant action after chlorination?**
(a) Sedimentation (b) Storage
(c) Filtration (d) All

**77. MMR vaccine is given at______. (ESI Delhi, 2009)**
(a) 5 years (b) 9 months
(c) 18 months of age (d) Birth

**78. In which year mid-day meal programme was started? (ESI, 2009)**
(a) 1920 (b) 1972
(c) 1961 (d) 1958

**79. The sanitary disposal of excreta is important from the following points of view except:**
(a) Food contamination (b) Water pollution
(c) Air pollution (d) Soil pollution

**80. What is the most hygienic method of disposal of solid wastes?**
(a) Composting (b) Incineration
(c) Burial (d) Manure pits

**81. ________ is receiving special attention in the prevention of chronic disease.**
(a) Primary prevention (b) Secondary prevention
(c) Tertiary prevention (d) Premorbid prevention

**82. The epidemiological triad include___ host and environment.**
(a) Disease (b) Agent
(c) Infection (d) Quarantine

**83. The entry and development (or) multiplication of a disease-producing agent in the body of man (or) animals is called ________.**
(a) Infection (b) Disease
(c) Health (d) Quarantine

**84. Which is the only disease that has been eradicated in India? (AIIMS Bhubaneswar, 2016)**
(a) Measles (b) Cholera
(c) Smallpox (d) Chickenpox

**85. Appearance of Koplik's spots buccal mucosa is pathognomonic of: (AIIMS Bhubaneswar, 2016)**
(a) Chickenpox (b) Smallpox
(c) Measles (d) Mumps

**86. The time interval between the entry of the disease agent into the body and the appearance of the first sign (or) symptom of the disease is called ________.**
(a) Health (b) Infection
(c) Isolation (d) Incubation period

**87. The person who harbor the disease agent without having any outward signs and symptoms is called ____.**
(a) Harbor (b) Carrier
(c) Transmitter (d) Infection

**88. The separation of a person with infectious disease from contact with other human being is called ________.**
(a) Incubation (b) Isolation
(c) Termination (d) Carrier

**89. Vector borne diseases are transmitted by:**
(a) Air (b) Animal
(c) Insects (d) All

**90. Fomites are ________.**
(a) Non-living things (b) Living things
(c) Insects (d) Animals

**91. Diabetes is caused due to deficiency of: (RRB-PMJHI, 2012)**
(a) Insulin (b) Ptyalin
(c) Thyroxin (d) Glucagon

**92. Which following treatment therapy is used for tuberculosis? (DSSSB, 2009)**
(a) Phototherapy (b) PPI
(c) DOTs (d) MDT

**93. To a polio victim during initial hospitalization hydrotherapy is a part of ________.**
(a) Specific protection
(b) Early diagnosis and treatment
(c) Rehabilitation
(d) Disability limitation

**94. Study of place distribution in epidemiology is useful for________.**
(a) Urban rural comparison
(b) Inter country comparison
(c) Intra nation comparison
(d) All the above

**95. The inability to walk without support is known as:**
(a) Handicap (b) Disability
(c) Impairment (d) None of the above

**96. The commonest mode of transmission of hookworm is___.**
(a) Mechanical vector (b) Percutaneous
(c) Feco-oral (d) All the above

**97. What is the leading cause for blindness in India? (AIIMS Bhubaneswar, 2016)**
(a) Refractive error (b) Glaucoma
(c) Corneal opacity (d) Cataract

**98. What does an ORS packet usually contains? (AIIMS Bhubaneswar, 2016)**
(a) Sodium and Glucose
(b) Potassium and Fructose
(c) Glucose and Fructose
(d) Sodium and Fructose

**99. Epidemiology includes the measurement of which of the following?**
(a) Measurement of frequency of disease
(b) Measurement of distribution of disease
(c) Measurement of determinants of disease
(d) All of the above

**100. Primary prevention means measures taken prevent the occurrence of disease.**
(a) After the initiation of disease
(b) Before the occurrence of disease
(c) After the disease is being complicated
(d) None of the above

**101. Primary prevention includes which of the following?**
(a) Health promotion and specific protection
(b) Early diagnosis and treatment
(c) Disability limitation
(d) All of the above

**102. Impairment is defined as any loss or abnormality______.**
(a) Within the range considered normal for a human being
(b) That leads to secondary treatment
(c) In psychological physiological and anatomical structure or function
(d) All of the above

**103. Deficiency of vitamin D causes: (RRB-PMJHI, 2012)**
(a) Rickets (b) Scurvy
(c) Night blindness (d) All of the above

**104. Leptospirosis is transmitted through: (RRB-PMJHI, 2012)**
(a) Rat urine (b) Rat bite
(c) Mosquito (d) Dog bite

**105. Hepatitis A virus is mainly transmitted through: (RRB-PMJHI, 2012)**
(a) Feco-oral route (b) Parental route
(c) Sexual transmission (d) Blood transmission

**106. Medical rehabilitation means:**
(a) Restoring and retaining the functional ability of an individual
(b) Making an individual capable to earn his livelihood.
(c) Restoring family and social relationship
(d) Restoring the dignity and confidence of disabled individual

**107. Descriptive epidemiology is one of the method of epidemiology. It includes:**
(a) The description of the occurrence of a disease in population.
(b) The relationship between the health status and other variables.
(c) The alteration in the program of disease
(d) None of the above

**108. An epidemiologist study the cohort in relation to exposure factor and outcome back in years. Then it is which type of study?**
(a) Retrospective cohort study
(b) Prospective cohort study
(c) Case control study
(d) All of the above

**109. Cross sectional deign is used to measure the disease in population. It is the design which include:**
(a) Repetition of observations in the same population over a prolonged period of time
(b) Single examination of a cross-section of population at one point in time
(c) Comparing the known indices
(d) All of the above

**110. Formulation of hypothesis Primary level of prevention includes all except:**
(a) Health promotion
(b) Specific protection
(c) Early diagnosis and treatment
(d) Immunization

**111. Prevention of coronary artery disease by changing lifestyle by education is referred as:**
(a) Primary prevention (b) Secondary prevention
(c) Tertiary prevention (d) Primordial prevention

**112. What does inhalation of cotton fiber dust over long periods of time cause? (AIIMS Bhubaneswar, 2016)**
(a) Anthracosis (b) Byssinosis
(c) Silicosis (d) Bagassosis

**113. Which of the following is not a zoonotic disease? (AIIMS Bhubaneswar, 2016)**
(a) Yellow fever (b) Plague
(c) Filariasis (d) Rabies

**114. Epidemiology deals with study of:**
(a) All health related events and states in population
(b) Epidemic diseases
(c) Communicable and non-communicable diseases
(d) Study of human population

**115. Levels of health care are:**
(a) Primary health care (b) Secondary health care
(c) Tertiary health care (d) All of the above

**116. Promotion of health is:**
(a) Primary level of health prevention
(b) Secondary level of health prevention
(c) Tertiary level of health prevention
(d) None of the above

**117. Oral polio vaccine is: (RRB-PMJHI, 2012)**
(a) Live vaccine (b) Killed vaccine
(c) Freeze dried vaccine (d) Recombinant vaccine

**118. Calorie intake of infant: (AIIMS, 1991)**
(a) 1600 kcal/day (b) 1200 kcal/day
(c) 1000 kcal/day (d) 800 kcal/day

**119. The most suitable strategy to prevent diabetes is the occurrences of:**
(a) Early diagnosis and treatment
(b) Specific protection
(c) Primordial prevention
(d) Rehabilitation

**120. Level of prevention that includes specific protection is__________.**
(a) Primordial (b) Primary
(c) Secondary (d) Tertiary

**121. Immunization is which level of prevention?**
(a) Primary level prevention
(b) Secondary level prevention
(c) Tertiary level prevention
(d) Primordial level of prevention

**122. Number of new cases occurring in a defined population during a specific period of time is:**
(a) Mortality rate (b) Incidence rate
(c) Prevalence rate (d) Morbidity rate

**123. BCG Vaccine is administered to prevent:**
(a) Tuberculosis (b) Measles
(c) Chickenpox (d) Mumps

**124. Incubation period of measles is:**
(a) 10–14 days (b) 1–3 days
(c) 20–30 days (d) 4–5 days

**125. Whooping cough is caused by:**
(a) Varicella zoster (b) Bordetella pertussis
(c) Peramyxovirus (d) Enterovirus

**126. Chickenpox is caused by:**
(a) Varicella zoster
(b) Bordetella pertussis
(c) Herpes virus varicella
(d) Paramyxovirus

**127. Malaria is caused by: (RRB-PMJHI, 2012)**
(a) Bacteria (b) Protozoa
(c) Virus (d) Fungus

**128. In hospital waste management, plastic bag of which color is not used: (RPSC Nursing Grade II Exam, 2007)**
(a) Yellow (b) Red
(c) Blue (d) Green

**129. National malaria eradication programme launched in the year of:**
(a) 1953 (b) 1982
(c) 1956 (d) 1990

**130. In which year AIDS is detected in India?**
(a) 1984 (b) 1986
(c) 1990 (d) 1956

**131. What is the incubation period of chicken pox?**
(a) 14–17 days (b) 9–10 days
(c) After 21 days (d) 5–7 days

**132. The drug used for tuberculosis includes all except: (RRB-PMJHI, 2012)**
(a) Dapsone (b) Rifampicin
(c) Ethambutol (d) Isoniazid

**133. As per the Mid-day meal programme the meals should supply at least ________ of the total energy requirement. (RRB-PMJHI, 2012)**
(a) 1/3rd (b) 1/4th
(c) 2 1/2 (d) 3/4th

**134. The amount of protein required by an Indian adult is ________ grams protein/kg body weight. (RRB-PMJHI, 2012)**
(a) 0.5 (b) 1
(c) 5 (d) 10

**135. The causative organism of mumps is:**
(a) Varicella zoster (b) Rubeola
(c) Rubella (d) Paramyxovirus

**136. Typhoid fever is otherwise known as ___.**
(a) Chickenpox (b) Enteric fever
(c) Malaria (d) None of the above

**137. What is the major cause of infant mortality in India?**
(a) Hypothermia (b) Jaundice
(c) Neonatal tetanus (d) Birth asphyxia

**138. What is the main clinical manifestation of rabies:**
(a) Photophobia (b) Hydrophobia
(c) Tetanus (d) Neonatal tetanus

**139. Hookworm is the common name for: (AIIMS Bhubaneswar, 2016)**
(a) Ancylostoma deodenale
(b) Enterobius vermicularis
(c) Ascaris lumbricoides
(d) Entamoeba histolytica

**140. In which year was the nationwide family planning programme launched in India? (AIIMS Bhubaneswar, 2016)**
(a) 1972 (b) 1962
(c) 1942 (d) 1952

**141. The causative organism of AIDS:**
(a) Varicella zoster (b) HIV
(c) Rubella (d) Variola

**142. National AIDS control programme launched in the year ______.**
(a) 1990 (b) 1991
(c) 1988 (d) 1987

**143. Poliomyelitis is a ________ infection.**
(a) Fungal (b) Bacterial
(c) Protozoa (d) Viral

**144. Incubation period of the poliomyelitis is:**
(a) 7–21 days (b) 10–20 days
(c) 8–15 days (d) 10–25 days

**145. Hepatitis B is otherwise known as:**
(a) Viral hepatitis (b) Serum hepatitis
(c) Bacterial hepatitis (d) None of this

**146. Which vitamin plays a role in production and release of certain coagulation factors? (AIIMS Bhubaneswar, 2016)**
(a) Vitamin K (b) Vitamin E
(c) Vitamin $B_{12}$ (d) Vitamin D

**147. Which immunization produces a permanent scar?**
(a) DPT (b) BCG
(c) Measles vaccination (d) Hepatitis B vaccination

**148. During the physical examination of a young child, what is the earliest sign of xerophthalmia that may observe?**
(a) Keratomalacia (b) Corneal opacity
(c) Night blindness (d) Conjunctival xerosis

**149. The major sign of iron deficiency anemia is pallor. What part is best examined for pallor?**
(a) Palms (b) Nail beds
(c) Around the lips (d) Lower conjunctival sac

**150. Major symptoms of an AIDS patient is: (RRB-PMJHI, 2012)**
(a) Weight loss (b) Diarrhea
(c) Fever (d) All of the above

**151. In the following which vaccine is not included in the National Immunization Schedule? (ESI, 2009)**
(a) Typhoid (b) DPT
(c) Measles (d) BCG

**152. Which is the most appropriate time of IUD insertion? (RPSC Nursing Grade II Exam, 2010)**
(a) At any time of menstruation
(b) Just before menstruation
(c) About the midst of the cycle
(d) During or within 10 days of menstruation

**153. Administration of readymade antibody creates: (AIIMS, 2010)**
(a) Passive natural immunity
(b) Active natural immunity
(c) Passive acquired immunity
(d) Active acquired immunity

**154. Secondary prevention for malaria includes:**
(a) Planting of neem or eucalyptus trees
(b) Residual spraying of insecticides at night
(c) Determining whether a place is endemic or not
(d) Growing larva-eating fish in mosquito breeding places

**155. Which of the following signs indicates the need for sputum examination for AFB?**
(a) Hematemesis (b) Fever for 1 week
(c) Cough for 3 weeks (d) Chest pain for 1 week

**156. Among the following diseases, which is airborne?**
(a) Viral conjunctivitis
(b) Acute poliomyelitis
(c) Diphtheria
(d) Measles

**157. The causative organism of measles is:**
(a) Variola (b) Rubella
(c) Rubeola (d) None of the above

**158. Measles is a _______ infection.**
(a) Bacterial (b) Viral
(c) Pathogen (d) None of the above

**159. Whooping cough is otherwise called ____.**
(a) Influenza (b) Pertussis
(c) Varicella (d) Rubeola

**160. District TB control programme was started in which year?**
(a) 1986 (b) 1962
(c) 1965 (d) 1974

**161. Complication of smallpox or antirabies vaccine is:**
(a) Encephalopathy and vaccinal encephalitis
(b) Thalassemia
(c) Anemia
(d) All of the above

**162. Which vaccine is given at birth?**
(a) BCG and OPV (b) Measles
(c) DPT (d) Mumps

**163. DPT-1 and OPV-1 vaccine given in which week?**
(a) 6 weeks after birth (b) 5 years
(c) 9 months (d) 2 weeks after birth

**164. Vaccine given at 10–16 years:**
(a) TT (b) DT
(c) DPT (d) OPV

**165. National immunization programme started in the year _______.**
(a) 1978 (b) 1986
(c) 1986 (d) 1972

**166. Incubation period of rubella is:**
(a) 2 to 3 weeks (b) 5 to 6 weeks
(c) 7 to 8 weeks (d) 5 to 7 weeks

**167. Causative organism of diphtheria:**
(a) Corynebacterium diphtheriae
(b) Clostridium tetani
(c) Influenza virus

**168. The Incubation period of whooping cough is:**
(a) 7 to 14 days (b) 10 to 14 days
(c) 5 to 6 days (d) 7 to 10 days

**169. Causative organizm of tuberculosis is:**
(a) Mycobacterium tuberculosis
(b) Clostridium tetani
(c) Influenza virus
(d) All of the above

**170. National filarial control programme started in which year?**
(a) 1955 (b) 1956
(c) 1960 (d) 1962

**171. Incubation period of viral hepatitis:**
(a) 15 to 45 days (b) 20 to 40 days
(c) 10 to 20 days (d) 20 to 30 days

**172. Incubation period of cholera:**
(a) 1 – 2 days (b) 5 – 6 days
(c) 5 – 8 days (d) 3 – 5 days

**173. Rubella is otherwise known as:**
(a) Diphtheria (b) Measles
(c) German measles (d) None of the above

**174. _______ vaccine should not be administered to the persons with immune deficiency disease.**
(a) Inactivated or killed vaccine
(b) Toxoids
(c) Live vaccines
(d) Cellular fractions vaccine

**175. What is the storage temperature of polio vaccine?**
(a) 20°C (b) – 30°C
(c) – 20°C (d) 30°C

**176. _______ is the first step in the control of a communicable disease.**
(a) Early diagnosis (b) Notification
(c) Rapid identification (d) All of the above

**177. The other name for enteric fever is:**
(a) Cholera (b) Typhoid
(c) Malaria (d) Chickenpox

**178. The disease caused by mycobacterium leprae is:**
(a) Leprosy (b) Tuberculosis
(c) AIDS (d) Typhoid

**179. NACO is the program for _______.**
(a) Tuberculosis (b) STD
(c) AIDS (d) Leprosy

**180. Scabies is a skin disease caused by _____.**
(a) Rodents (b) Itch mite
(c) Cats (d) Rabies

**181. The separation of a person with infectious disease from contact with other human being is called _______.**
(a) Incubation (b) Isolation
(c) Termination (d) Infection

**182. Tuberculosis test was discovered in the year_________.**
(a) 1927 (b) 1905
(c) 1907 (d) 1910

**183. Best primary prevention of TB and leprosy is:**
(a) Health education
(b) Isolation
(c) Early diagnosis and treatment
(d) Chemotherapy

**184. Live vaccine is _________.**
(a) BCG, oral polio
(b) Rabies
(c) Tetanus
(d) Plague

**185. Reconstituted measles vaccine should be used within how many hours?**
(a) 1 hour (b) 2 hours
(c) 3 hours (d) 4 hours

**186. Ideally the vaccine in a vaccine carrier can be stored for a minimum period of __________.**
(a) 6 hours (b) 48 hours
(c) 12 hours (d) 24 hours

**187. The polio virus can remain viable in water in cold environment for __________.**
(a) One year (b) One month
(c) 4 weeks (d) 6 weeks

**188. The target by which primary immunization is to be completed, UIP is __________.**
(a) 5 years (b) 3 years
(c) 2 years (d) 1 year

**189. First dose of triple vaccine is given at the age of ______.**
(a) 6 weeks (b) 10 weeks
(c) 14 weeks (d) 18 weeks

**190. Syphilis is caused by __________.**
(a) Spirochetes (b) Virus
(c) Fungus (d) None of the above

**191. The following disease are transmitted by the *Aedes* mosquitoes except:**
(a) Japanese encephalitis
(b) Yellow fever
(c) Dengue fever
(d) Hemorrhagic fever

**192. Megaloblastic anemia is caused due to the deficiency of __________.**
(a) $B_{12}$ (b) $B_2$
(c) $B_6$ (d) $B_1$

**193. TAB vaccine is given for the prevention of:**
(a) Typhoid (b) Cholera
(c) TB (d) None of the above

**194. RNTCP was introduced in__________.**
(a) 1992 (b) 1904
(c) 1980 (d) 1990

**195. Gentian violet solution will be used to mark the children vaccinated for__________.**
(a) BCG (b) Polio
(c) Vit–A (d) Measles

**196. The most common cause of death in children under 5 years of age are __________.**
(a) Diarrhea (b) Measles
(c) Accidents (d) Prematurity

**197. How many doses of hepatitis B vaccine is given to an infant?**
(a) 3 (b) 4
(c) 5 (d) 2

**198. What is VVM?**
(a) Test for vaccine potency
(b) Test for vaccine contamination
(c) Measurement of dosage
(d) All the above

**199. Which of the following is the example of modes of transformation of hepatitis B?**
(a) Blood
(b) Contaminated syringes, needles
(c) Sexual contact
(d) All the above

**200. Hepatitis B is otherwise known as _______.**
(a) Viral hepatitis (b) Serum hepatitis
(c) Bacterial hepatitis (d) None of the above

**201. The toxins that released during the food poisoning is__________.**
(a) Alpha toxin (b) Toxins
(c) Antitoxins (d) All the above

**202. Prevention of food adulteration act started in the year __________.**
(a) 1954 (b) 1964
(c) 1960 (d) 1984

**203. India became smallpox free on __________.**
(a) 5th July 1975 (b) 5th May 1975
(c) 5th April 1975 (d) None of the above

**204. The best medicine used for the syphilis is:**
(a) Inj. procainepenicillin for 10 days (600,000 units)
(b) Inj. penidure for 10 days (6,00,000 units)
(c) Inj. amox for 10 days (600,000 units)
(d) None of the above

**205. The best method of killing the Larva of mosquito is __________.**
(a) Mineral oils (b) Paris Green
(c) Synthetic method (d) All the above

**206. The National Tuberculosis Programme has been in operation since__________.**
(a) 1962 (b) 1960
(c) 1970 (d) None of the above

**207. The Acquired Immunodeficiency Syndrome some time called__________.**
(a) Zoonosis (b) Slim disease
(c) Both (a) and (b) (d) None of the above

**208. Test dose is not necessary before administration of following injection:**
(a) Penicillin (b) Ampicillin
(c) Tetanus toxoi (d) None of the above

**209. Koplik's spots are diagnostic features of:**
(a) Mumps (b) Chickenpox
(c) Measles (d) Cholera

**210. TAB vaccine is given to prevent__________.**
(a) Typhoid (b) Cholera
(c) Tuberculosis (d) Measles

**211. Leprosy is a chronic __________disease.**
(a) Communicable
(b) Noncommunicable
(c) Both (a) and (b)
(d) None

**212. Leprosy is commonly called __________.**
(a) Mental disease (b) Social disease
(c) Physical disease (d) All the above

213. **Causative organism of leprosy is______.**
(a) Staphylococci
(b) Mycobacterium tuberculosis
(c) Mycobacterium leprae
(d) Both (a) and (b)

214. **Incubation period of leprosy is ______.**
(a) 3–5 years (b) 5–15 days
(c) 7–17 days (d) 1–2 years

215. **Lepra bacilli present in ______.**
(a) Animal milk (b) Human milk
(c) Both (a) and (b) (d) None of the above

216. **JE was first identified in______.**
(a) Japan (b) Thailand
(c) India (d) Malaysia

217. **________are the vectors responsible for spread of JE.**
(a) Mosquitoes (b) Pigs
(c) Human being (d) Cattles

218. **The transporting and storing system of vaccine is known as__________.**
(a) Cold chain (b) Refrigerator
(c) Hot chain (d) Chain of infection

219. **What is the causative organism of rabies?**
(a) Lyssa virus type I (b) Rubella
(c) Varicella zoster (d) None of the above

220. **The last case of smallpox was reported in the world in__________.**
(a) 1977 (b) 1978
(c) 1979 (d) 1982

221. **Smallpox was eradicated because of the following factors except:**
(a) Potent vaccine
(b) Easy to recognize
(c) Extra human reservoir control
(d) Long incubation period

222. **Carriers are associated with transmission of disease in all except:**
(a) Typhoid (b) Cholera
(c) Measles (d) Diphtheria

223. **Koplik's spots are seen in:**
(a) Rubella (b) Measles
(c) Typhoid (d) Chickenpox

224. **Which of the following disease gives life-long immunity after an attack?**
(a) Mumps (b) Typhoid
(c) Tetanus (d) Diphtheria

225. **Period of maximum infectivity in mumps is during______.**
(a) Incubation period (b) Onset of swelling
(c) After swelling appeas (d) Prodromal period

226. **Schick test is done in______.**
(a) Meningitis (b) Diphtheria
(c) Pertussis (d) Poliomyelitis

227. **Recommended site of administration of DPT in infants is:**
(a) Gluteal (b) Deltoid
(c) Forearm (d) Lateral aspect of thigh

228. **Measles vaccine is given under the National Immunization Programme:**
(a) 6 weeks (b) 6 months
(c) 9 months (d) 18 months

229. **Modifiable risk factors in case of Hypertension include all, except:**
(a) Age (b) Obesity
(c) Salt intake (d) Alcohol intake

230. **Infections primarily of animals that can be transmitted through milk is all, except:**
(a) Tuberculosis (b) Brucellosis
(c) Q fever (d) Dengue fever

231. **Quickening means:**
(a) Hearing of the fetal heart sound
(b) Sudden cessation of Menstruation
(c) The movement of the fetus in the uterus felt by the mother
(d) Nausea and vomiting in the morning

232. **Discoloration of teeth is caused by a kind of antibiotics called:**
(a) Streptomycin (b) Neomycin
(c) Tetracycline (d) Penicillin

233. **Dengue fever is otherwise called as:**
(a) Enteric fever (b) Break bone fever
(c) Q-fever (d) Brain fever

234. **Ninety percent of the oral cancer in India is due to:**
(a) Spicy food (b) Beedi rolling
(c) Over eating (d) Chewing tobacco

235. **A mentally healthy person________.**
(a) Feels reasonably secure and accepts his short mistake
(b) Is unable to concentrate
(c) Looses temper
(d) None of the above

236. **A spoon shaped nails are seen in:**
(a) Iron deficiency anemia
(b) Megaloblastic anemia
(c) Sickle cell anemia
(d) Pernicious anemia

237. **Megaloblastic anemia is caused due to the deficiency of__________.**
(a) $B_{12}$ (b) $B_2$
(c) $B_6$ (d) $B_1$

238. **PEM can be prevented by__________.**
(a) Adequate nutrition
(b) Treatment of infection
(c) All of the above
(d) Health education

239. **Vitamin A prophylaxis programme advocates the administration of Vitamin A orally in solution form in a dose of:**
(a) 10,000 micrograms
(b) 56,000 micrograms
(c) 66,000 micrograms
(d) 76,000 micrograms

**240. Blindness as defined by WHO is visual acuity is less than________.**
(a) 1/60 (b) 6/18
(c) 6/24 (d) 6/60

**241. ________ is the scientific study of human population.**
(a) Sex ratio (b) Demography
(c) Urbanization (d) Family welfare

**242. What is the major cause of infant mortality in India?**
(a) Hypothermia (b) Jaundice
(c) Neonatal tetanus (d) Birth asphyxia

**243. ________ is the number of deaths per thousand population per year in a given community.**
(a) Crude death rate
(b) Expectation of life
(c) Propositional mortality rate
(d) None of the above

**244. Crude death rate means:**
(a) Death per 1000 population in a year
(b) Death per 1000 population per month
(c) Both (a) and (b)
(d) None of the above

**245. As per birth and death registration act the birth should be registered within:**
(a) 5 days (b) 7 days
(c) 9 days (d) 14 days

**246. The term incidence refers to:**
(a) The number of new cases occurring in a defined population during a specific period of time
(b) The number of old cases seen in area
(c) Both (a) and (b)
(d) None of the above

**247. Prevalence refers to:**
(a) All correct cases (old and new) existing in a given time (or) over a period of time in a given population
(b) Disease rate of the old cases
(c) Both (a) and (b)
(d) None of the above

**248. What is the denomination in general fertility rate?**
(a) Married women
(b) Women in reproductive age group (15–44 years)
(c) Married women in the age of 15–44
(d) All women

**249. The percentage of women in the reproductive age group is ________.**
(a) 15% (b) 22%
(c) 30% (d) 40%

**250. The national policy is to bring the couple protection rate to________.**
(a) 50% (b) 60%
(c) 75% (d) 90%

**251. The highest per capital income in India is in________.**
(a) Kerala (b) Punjab
(c) Haryana (d) Goa

**252. Population count is taken on: ________.**
(a) 1st January (b) 1st March
(c) 1st July (d) 1st August

**253. First 5 years plan in India started at ____.**
(a) 1950 (b) 1951
(c) 1952 (d) 1953

**254. Declining death rate and more declining birth rate, the stage is:**
(a) Late expanding (b) Early expanding
(c) High stationary (d) Declining

**255. Under the national population policy, family size should be brought down to:**
(a) 1 (b) 2.3
(c) 3.2 (d) 4.2

**256. Total fertility rate refers to:**
(a) Number of women between 15–44 years of age
(b) Number of birth/1000 women.
(c) Approximate completed family size
(d) Number of female children/women.

**257. In demographic study of population, a country with low birth rate and a low death rate is in following phases:**
(a) 1st phase (b) 2nd phase
(c) 3rd phase (d) 4th phase

**258. Demographic gap means:**
(a) Difference between birth and death
(b) Difference between age specific birth and death rates
(c) Difference in sex ratio
(d) Difference in child:women ratio

**259. In what stage of demographic cycle is India today?**
(a) Low stationary (b) High stationary
(c) Early expanding (d) Late expanding

**260. Permanent method of family planning in male is:**
(a) Tubectomy (b) Laparoscopy
(c) Vasectomy (d) Appendectomy

**261. Currently one third of the world's population is under the age of:**
(a) 5 years (b) 25 years
(c) 15 years (d) 20 years

**262. The first census of India was conducted in:**
(a) 1872 (b) 1965
(c) 1947 (d) 1951

**263. The state with highest population in India is:**
(a) Uttar Pradesh (b) Maharashtra
(c) Karnataka (d) Andhra Pradesh

**264. Best method of postcoital contraception is:**
(a) Androgens
(b) High Estrogen pills
(c) Menstrual regulation
(d) IUCD
(e) High progestin pills

**265. Best method for spacing is:**
(a) Condom (b) Pessary
(c) IUCD (d) Tubectomy

**266. Family welfare programme's goal is to reach couple protection rate of:**
(a) 20% (b) 40%
(c) 50% (d) 60%

**267. Male contraceptive pill contains:**
(a) Bromocriptine (b) Cyproheptadine
(c) Cyproterone acetate (d) None of the above

**268. The MTP act was passed in:**
(a) 1949 (b) 1962
(c) 1971 (d) 1974

**269. The family planning programme started in:**
(a) 1947 (b) 1950
(c) 1952 (d) 1960

**270. The national family planning programme was started in:**
(a) 1952 (b) 1965
(c) 1955 (d) 1977

**271. DMPA is an injectable contraceptive given every:**
(a) Three weeks (b) Two months
(c) Two years (d) Three months

**272. Which one of the following is a rate complication of the use of hormonal contraceptives?**
(a) Contraceptive failure (b) Cardiovascular effects
(c) Carcinogenesis (d) Metabolic effects

**273. Multiload device refers to:**
(a) First generation IUCD
(b) Second generation IUCD
(c) Oral contraceptive pills
(d) Barrier contraceptives

**274. Mini pill contains:**
(a) Only progesterone in small quantity
(b) Progesterone and estrogen in small quantity
(c) Estrogen in small quantity and progesterone in large quantity

**275. IUCD acts by :**
(a) Increasing cervical mucus
(b) Aseptic inflammation of endometrium
(c) Killing spermatozoa
(d) Preventing the fertilization of ova

**276. An average failure rate in the couple using condom is about:**
(a) 0–5% (b) 10–20%
(c) 30–40% (d) 50% or more

**277. Calendar method was described by:**
(a) Bitings (b) Ogino
(c) Wallace (d) Ogive

**278. Copper T is ideally inserted at:**
(a) Menstruation
(b) Just before Menstruation
(c) Just after Menstruation
(d) On the 14th day

**279. Following vasectomy for family planning, a patient should be advised to use some other method of contraception till:**
(a) Removal of all sutures (b) Pain completely resolved
(c) Two weeks (d) None of above

**280. Copper T 200 need to be replaced after:**
(a) 3 year (b) 2 year
(c) 1 year (d) 5 year

**281. Indian MTP act allows abortions only up to:**
(a) 15 weeks (b) 20 weeks
(c) 24 years (d) 28 weeks

**282. What is the age group of the eligible couple?**
(a) 15 – 50 years (b) 15 – 45 years
(c) 20 – 60 years (d) 18 – 40 years

**283. What is the permanent termination method in males?**
(a) Tubectomy (b) Diaphragm
(c) Vasectomy (d) Condom

**284. What is the permanent termination method in female?**
(a) Vasectomy (b) Copper-T
(c) Tubectomy (d) Diaphragm

**285. The natural contraceptive method is:**
(a) Mala N (b) Mala D
(c) Breastfeeding (d) Withdrawal

**286. Coitus interrupts is otherwise known as:**
(a) Withdrawal (b) IUD
(c) Nirodh (d) Copper-T

**287. The best time for IUD insertion is:**
(a) After 1 week of menstruation
(b) 3–7 days
(c) 3rd day
(d) 14th day

**288. In contraceptives, the spacing method for men:**
(a) Condom (b) Lipper loop
(c) Copper-T (d) Both (a) and (b)

**289. The age of eligible couple is:**
(a) 15–45 years (b) 20–30 years
(c) 25–35 years (d) 20–25 years

**290. Name of the committee who reviewed family planning is:**
(a) Bhore (b) Kartar
(c) Mukharjee (d) Chardah

**291. Oral pills contain a small amounts of:**
(a) Estrogen and progesterone
(b) Norplant
(c) Oxytocin
(d) None of the above

**292. Oral pills mala-N consist of:**
(a) Norgestrel
(b) Ethinyl oestradiol
(c) Both (a) and (b)
(d) None of the above

**293. Give the example for injectable contraceptives:**
(a) DMPA (Depot Medroxyprogesterone acetate)
(b) NET-EN (Norethisterone Enanthate)
(c) Both (a) and (b)
(d) None of the above

**294. One of the following is contraindication for IUD's:**
(a) Previous ectopic pregnancy
(b) Fever
(c) Headache
(d) The mother who wants to practice spacing method

**295. Copper 'T' is contraindicated in:**
(a) Pregnancy (b) Pelvic infections
(c) Heart diseases (d) All of the above

**296. How much population is coming under PHC?**
(a) 5000 (b) 1000
(c) 30000 (d) 25500

**297. Who is the team leader in the health care team?**
(a) Block extension educator
(b) Health guide
(c) Head nurse
(d) Medical office

**298. What is the other name of domiciliary midwifery?**
(a) Home care (b) Home confinement
(c) Home visit (d) Antenatal care

**299. The backbone of all MCH services is:**
(a) Antenatal care (b) Home visiting
(c) *Dais* (d) Health worker

**300. _______ is an essential component of health care system.**
(a) Referral system (b) Drainage system
(c) Health care system (d) None of the above

**301. How much population is coming under one subcenter?**
(a) 5000 (b) 10000
(c) 2000 (d) 2500

**302. The important person in the village is:**
(a) Midwife (b) ANM
(c) *Dai* (d) Female health worker

**303. _______ is intended to deliver health services.**
(a) Health system (b) Health care
(c) Health development (d) Health team concept

**304. Primary health care means:**
(a) First level health care
(b) Second level health care
(c) Tertiary health care
(d) All of the above

**305. The following is the main feature of primary health care:**
(a) Acceptability
(b) Essential health care
(c) Universal accessibility
(d) Physician mediated

**306. The population of municipality is:**
(a) 10,000 to 2 lakhs (b) 5 to 7000
(c) 10 lakhs (d) 5 lakhs

**307. Incharge of community development block is:**
(a) BDO (b) HM
(c) GM (d) PD

**308. Elements of primary healthcare is:**
(a) Promotion of food supply and proper nutrition
(b) Adequate supply of safe water and sanitation
(c) Maternal and child health care
(d) All of the above

**309. The purposes of home visiting are:**
(a) Prevention of diseases
(b) Promotion of health of family members
(c) To carry out simple nursing procedures in the home
(d) All of the above

**310. Elements of primary health care include all of the following except:**
(a) Providing essential drugs
(b) Adequate supply of safe Water and basic sanitation
(c) Sound referral system
(d) Health education

**311. Community health center_______.**
(a) Covers a population of approx one lakh
(b) Has 100 beds
(c) Has X-ray and laboratory facilities
(d) Acts as a referral hospital for the community development block

**312. National Health Policy 2002, includes the following goals to be achieved by 2015 except:**
(a) Eliminate leprosy (b) Eliminate kala-azar
(c) Eliminates TB (d) Eliminate Polio

**313. Chairman of central council of health is:**
(a) Prime Minister (b) Union Health Minister
(c) Health Secretary (d) Finance Minister

**314. The auxiliary midwives to be replaced by the newly designated female health workers was recommended by:**
(a) Shrivastava Committee
(b) Mukherjee Committee
(c) Jungalwalla Committee
(d) Kartar Singh Committee

**315. Concept of comprehensive health care was given by:**
(a) Bhore Committee
(b) Mukherjee Committee
(c) Jangalwalla Committee
(d) Shrivastava Committee

**316. Concept of Multipurpose worker was given by:**
(a) Shrivastava Committee
(b) Kartar Singh Committee
(c) Mukherjee Committee
(d) Bhore Committee

**317. National health policy evolved in the year_______.**
(a) 1983 (b) 1985
(c) 2000 (d) 2002

**318. National Rural Health Mission was launched in the year_______.**
(a) 2005 (b) 2007
(c) 2006 (d) 2004

**319. Protein deficiency in children leads to_______.**
(a) Kwashiorkor (b) Beriberi
(c) Anemia (d) Blindness

**320. National Health Policy, 2002, includes the following goals to be achieved by 2015, except:**
(a) Eliminate leprosy
(b) Eliminate Kala-Azar
(c) Eliminate Tuberculosis
(d) Eradicate Polio

**321. One ASHA worker covers a population of_______.**
(a) 5,000 (b) 1,000
(c) 7,000 (d) 10,000

322. **Following is a first tier in Panchayat Raj System:**
(a) Gram panchayat (b) Panchayat Samiti
(c) Zila Parishad (d) Block

323. **Office responsible to record birth and death in rural area in most of states is:**
(a) Palwari (b) Choukidar
(c) Panchayat member (d) Village health guide

324. **All components of school health program except:**
(a) Health appraisal (b) Nonformal education
(c) Mid-day meal (d) Healthful school event

325. **Currently married couple wherein the wife is in the reproductive age is called __________.**
(a) Target couple (b) Eligible coupe
(c) Young couple (d) Family planning couple

326. **The Trained Dais mainly deals with:**
(a) Child care
(b) Bathing and massaging postnatal mothers
(c) Delivery of mothers
(d) Immunization

327. **The role of community health nurse in small family norm is as follows:**
(a) Motivating couple for permanent method of family planning.
(b) Motivating target couple for self- decision for adopting small family
(c) Explain the methods of contraception
(d) None of the above

328. **_______ hazard in industry center around machinery.**
(a) Mechanical (b) Biological
(c) Chemical (d) Psychological

329. **Mala-D and Mala-N are available in packet of ________ tablets.**
(a) 24 (b) 28
(c) 20 (d) 30

330. **A pregnant women must get 2 injections of TT during the period between_________weeks.**
(a) 16–36 (b) 12–18
(c) 14–20 (d) 16–20

331. **Which of the following epidemiological measurement is normally expressed as a percent?**
(a) Rate (b) Ratio
(c) Proportion (d) Standardized rate

332. **Byssinosis is caused due to inhalation of ________.**
(a) Free Silica (b) Sugar cane dust
(c) Saw Dust (d) Cotton fiber dust

333. **The executive organ of the gram sabha is _______.**
(a) Nyay sabha (b) Gram panchayat
(c) Khap panchayat (d) Zila parishad

334. **Census in India takes place after every ________ years.**
(a) 5 (b) 10
(c) 10 (d) 20

335. **The Indian Factories act was passed in the year_____.**
(a) 1946 (b) 1881
(c) 1981 (d) 1952

336. **The key person in the village who is responsible for transforming the economic and social life of the people are________________.**
(a) Local *dais* (b) Health guides
(c) Gram sevak (d) Female health workers

337. **Size of respirable dust is below _______.**
(a) 0.1 micron (b) 1 micron
(c) 5 micron (d) 10 micron

338. **To calculate vital statistics the populations is as ______.**
(a) January 1 (b) April 1
(c) July 1 (d) October 1

339. **In 1992, a program was implemented to improve the health of the mother:**
(a) ICDS (b) CSSM
(c) RCH (d) Rural Health Mission

340. **Disease that lead to morbidity and mortality in children below 5 yrs of age is:**
(a) Tuberculosis (b) Malaria
(c) Meningitis (d) Diarrheal disease

341. **Currently married couple wherein the wife is in the reproductive age is called __________.**
(a) Eligible couple (b) Family planning couple
(c) Target couple (d) Young couple

342. **ESI Act was passed in___________:**
(a) 1975 (b) 1948
(c) 1984 (d) 1988

343. **The time limit for the registration of death is ____days.**
(a) 7 days (b) 8 days
(c) 6 days (d) 9 days

344. **Which of the following is tertiary level of prevention?**
(a) Rehabilitation (b) Health promotion
(c) Chemoprophylaxis (d) Specific protection

345. **Effective method of health education to bring change in health behavior is _____________.**
(a) Symposium (b) Group discussion
(c) Panel discussion (d) Workshop

346. **Most appropriate time for IUD insertion is___________.**
(a) Mid cycle menstruation
(b) Within 10 days of menstruation (last day)
(c) Any time of menstrual cycle
(d) Just immediate after menstruation

347. **Disease that lead to morbidity and mortality in children below 5 years of age:**
(a) Diarrheal diseases (b) Tuberculosis
(c) Meningitis (d) Malaria

348. **Health education is a major means for achieving change except:**
(a) Motivation (b) Indifference
(c) Communication (d) Decision making

349. **Byssinosis is caused due to inhalation of ________.**
(a) Free silica (b) Sugar cane dust
(c) Saw dust (d) Cotton fiber dust

350. **_________ is component of MCH program.**
(a) Adolescent health (b) Family planning
(c) Maternal health (d) Child health

**351. Janani Suraksha Yojna is the version of national _____ benefit scheme.**
(a) Female
(b) Girl child
(c) Maternity
(d) Old age

**352. Condoms are effective in preventing ________.**
(a) Sexually transmitted Infections
(b) Pregnancy
(c) Sexual transmission of HIV infection
(d) All of the above

**353. The CSSM program was launched on ____.**
(a) 1992
(b) 1994
(c) 1996
(d) 1997

**354. Which of the following is tertiary level prevention?**
(a) Health promotion
(b) Chemoprophylaxis
(c) Rehabilitation
(d) Immunization

**355. Population strategy is the appropriate recommendation by WHO for________.**
(a) Primordial prevention
(b) Primary prevention
(c) Secondary prevention
(d) Tertiary prevention

**356. As per the National Health Plan, 1983 a Primary Health Center covers a rural population of________.**
(a) 30,000
(b) 25,000
(c) 5,000
(d) 1,80,000

**357. Which of the following early detection is level of prevention?**
(a) Primary
(b) Secondary
(c) Tertiary
(d) Primordial

**358. The record of individual family is called________.**
(a) Family record
(b) Cumulative record
(c) Clinical record
(d) Anecdotal record

**359. Epidemiological triangle is ________.**
(a) Agent, host, environment
(b) Agent, host, treatment
(c) Host, Environment, treatment
(d) Environment, agent, germs

**360. The authoritative direction of the work of one's subordinate is called ________.**
(a) Evaluation
(b) Administration
(c) Management
(d) Supervision

**361. A clinical, scientific, administrative and legal document relating to the nursing care given to individual and family or community is known as________.**
(a) Nursing report
(b) Nursing record
(c) Nursing diaries
(d) Nursing audit

**362. A permanent written communication of a patient's health status is a________**
(a) Report
(b) Record
(c) Assignment
(d) Care plan

**363. Records and reports are important in nursing service as they________.**
(a) Serve as documents of patients history of illness
(b) Assist in the continuity of rendering care
(c) Serve as evidence to support legal implications
(d) All of the above

**364. What protects the doctors and nurses in case of legal issues?**
(a) Notes
(b) Books
(c) Records
(d) Diaries

**365. Which among these reports are not permanent?**
(a) Oral reports
(b) Written reports
(c) Service reports
(d) Night reports

**366. Antimalaria month is observed every year during ________ month in India.**
(a) July (b) September
(c) August (d) June

**367. In nutrition survey anthropometric measurements includes________.**
(a) Arm circumference
(b) Height and weight
(c) Skin fold thickness
(d) All of the above

**368. The pulse polio immunization days selected fall between Nov–Feb because:**
(a) Assurance of availability of children
(b) Low transmission season
(c) Coverage of two doses in consecutive years
(d) Winter seasons in India

**369. Short-term objective of national tuberculosis programme is________.**
(a) Detect Maximum number of TB Cases
(b) Vaccine newborn and infant with BCG
(c) Treatment of the patient of TB
(d) All of the above

**370. National programme of control of blindness was launched in________.**
(a) 1971 (b) 1976
(c) 1973 (d) 1977

**371. Following are the components of minimum need programme except:**
(a) Rural health (b) Rural Industry
(c) Rural electrification (d) Rural water supply

**372. First dose of 'Vit A' is ________.**
(a) 1 lakh IU (b) 2 lakh IU
(c) 4 lakh IU (d) 5 lakh IU

**373. Drugs used in treatment of leprosy:**
(a) Hetrazan (b) Clomiphene
(c) Tetracycline (d) Dapsone and Rifampicin

**374. Main aim of tuberculosis treatment is:**
(a) Radiological cure
(b) Contact tracing
(c) Bacteriological cure
(d) Prevention of complication

**375. In India, antimalaria month is observed every year during ________.**
(a) July (b) September
(c) August (d) June

**376. In DOTS therapy, category III medications does not include________.**
(a) Isoniazid (b) Rifampicin
(c) Ethambutol (d) Pyrazinamide

**377. A mid-day meal program must provide a minimum of________.**
(a) 400 cal (b) 300 cal
(c) 350 cal (d) 500 cal

**378. National AIDS Control Programme launched in the year ________.**
(a) 1990 (b) 1991
(c) 1988 (d) 1987

**379. Revised National Tuberculosis Control Programme launched in the year ________.**
(a) 1992
(b) 1997
(c) 1987
(d) 1988

**380. Under the ICDS scheme, each child up to 6 years of age should get ______ gms of proteins.**
(a) 2–4 (b) 8–10
(c) 10–20 (d) 4–8

**381. GOBI campaign is promoted by:**
(a) UNICEF
(b) WHO
(c) FAO
(d) UNDP

**382. Food and Agriculture Organization (FAO) was formed in________.**
(a) 1920 (b) 1930
(c) 1935 (d) 1945

**383. International Agency concern for children health and welfare is________.**
(a) UNICEF
(b) WHO
(c) FAO
(d) UNESCO

**384. Which of the following voluntary agency involved actively in relief work in India?**
(a) Bharat Sevak Samaj
(b) Kasturba Memorial Fund
(c) Indian Red Cross Society
(d) Central Social Welfare Board

**385. TNAI organization was established in the year ______.**
(a) 1922
(b) 1923
(c) 1932
(d) 1930

**386. UNICEF is established in the year ______.**
(a) 1945
(b) 1947
(c) 1948
(d) 1946

**387. DOTS is used in the treatment of: (MSc AIIMS, 1996)**
(a) Diphtheria
(b) Malaria
(c) Leprosy
(d) Tuberculosis

**388. Which of the following communicable disease is eradicated in our country?**
(a) Filariasis
(b) Poliomyelitis
(c) Tuberculosis
(d) Smallpox

**389. Coma vigil is seen in:**
(a) Hyperosmolar state
(b) Enteric fever
(c) Myxoedema coma
(d) Head Injury

**390. Mid-day meal programme provides how many calories and proteins per day? (RPSC, 2010)**
(a) 300 calories and 6–12 gms of protein
(b) 200 calories and 6–12 gms of protein
(c) 300 calories and 8–12 gms of protein
(d) 200 calories and 8–12 gms of protein

**391. The most common cause of Blindness in India is: (MSc RAK, 2010)**
(a) Cataract
(b) Trachoma
(c) Refractive errors
(d) Vitamin A deficiency

## ANSWERS

| **1.** | (d) | **41.** | (d) | **81.** | (a) | **121.** | (d) | **161.** | (b) |
|---|---|---|---|---|---|---|---|---|---|
| **2.** | (c) | **42.** | (b) | **82.** | (b) | **122.** | (b) | **162.** | (a) |
| **3.** | (b) | **43.** | (b) | **83.** | (a) | **123.** | (a) | **163.** | (a) |
| **4.** | (a) | **44.** | (d) | **84.** | (c) | **124.** | (a) | **164.** | (a) |
| **5.** | (d) | **45.** | (d) | **85.** | (c) | **125.** | (b) | **165.** | (a) |
| **6.** | (b) | **46.** | (b) | **86.** | (d) | **126.** | (c) | **166.** | (a) |
| **7.** | (a) | **47.** | (c) | **87.** | (b) | **127.** | (b) | **167.** | (a) |
| **8.** | (b) | **48.** | (a) | **88.** | (b) | **128.** | (d) | **168.** | (c) |
| **9.** | (c) | **49.** | (d) | **89.** | (c) | **129.** | (a) | **169.** | (a) |
| **10.** | (c) | **50.** | (a) | **90.** | (a) | **130.** | (b) | **170.** | (a) |
| **11.** | (c) | **51.** | (d) | **91.** | (a) | **131.** | (a) | **171.** | (a) |
| **12.** | (b) | **52.** | (a) | **92.** | (c) | **132.** | (a) | **172.** | (a) |
| **13.** | (c) | **53.** | (d) | **93.** | (d) | **133.** | (a) | **173.** | (c) |
| **14.** | (c) | **54.** | (b) | **94.** | (d) | **134.** | (b) | **174.** | (c) |
| **15.** | (c) | **55.** | (a) | **95.** | (b) | **135.** | (d) | **175.** | (c) |
| **16.** | (c) | **56.** | (c) | **96.** | (b) | **136.** | (b) | **176.** | (c) |
| **17.** | (b) | **57.** | (b) | **97.** | (d) | **137.** | (c) | **177.** | (b) |
| **18.** | (d) | **58.** | (d) | **98.** | (a) | **138.** | (b) | **178.** | (a) |
| **19.** | (b) | **59.** | (d) | **99.** | (d) | **139.** | (a) | **179.** | (b) |
| **20.** | (a) | **60.** | (b) | **100.** | (b) | **140.** | (d) | **180.** | (b) |
| **21.** | (a) | **61.** | (a) | **101.** | (a) | **141.** | (b) | **181.** | (b) |
| **22.** | (d) | **62.** | (c) | **102.** | (c) | **142.** | (d) | **182.** | (c) |
| **23.** | (d) | **63.** | (a) | **103.** | (a) | **143.** | (d) | **183.** | (c) |
| **24.** | (a) | **64.** | (b) | **104.** | (a) | **144.** | (a) | **184.** | (a) |
| **25.** | (c) | **65.** | (c) | **105.** | (a) | **145.** | (b) | **185.** | (a) |
| **26.** | (a) | **66.** | (a) | **106.** | (a) | **146.** | (a) | **186.** | (a) |
| **27.** | (a) | **67.** | (c) | **107.** | (a) | **147.** | (b) | **187.** | (d) |
| **28.** | (d) | **68.** | (b) | **108.** | (a) | **148.** | (d) | **188.** | (b) |
| **29.** | (d) | **69.** | (b) | **109.** | (b) | **149.** | (a) | **189.** | (d) |
| **30.** | (b) | **70.** | (d) | **110.** | (c) | **150.** | (d) | **190.** | (a) |
| **31.** | (c) | **71.** | (a) | **111.** | (d) | **151.** | (a) | **191.** | (a) |
| **32.** | (b) | **72.** | (c) | **112.** | (b) | **152.** | (d) | **192.** | (a) |
| **33.** | (c) | **73.** | (d) | **113.** | (c) | **153.** | (c) | **193.** | (a) |
| **34.** | (b) | **74.** | (b) | **114.** | (a) | **154.** | (c) | **194.** | (a) |
| **35.** | (d) | **75.** | (d) | **115.** | (d) | **155.** | (c) | **195.** | (a) |
| **36.** | (b) | **76.** | (c) | **116.** | (a) | **156.** | (d) | **196.** | (a) |
| **37.** | (b) | **77.** | (c) | **117.** | (a) | **157.** | (c) | **197.** | (a) |
| **38.** | (c) | **78.** | (c) | **118.** | (c) | **158.** | (b) | **198.** | (a) |
| **39.** | (d) | **79.** | (r) | **119.** | (c) | **159.** | (b) | **199.** | (b) |
| **40.** | (b) | **80.** | (b) | **120.** | (b) | **160.** | (a) | **200.** | (b) |

| 201. | (a) | 241. | (b) | 281. | (b) | 321. | (b) | 361. | (b) |
|---|---|---|---|---|---|---|---|---|---|
| 202. | (a) | 242. | (c) | 282. | (b) | 322. | (a) | 362. | (b) |
| 203. | (a) | 243. | (a) | 283. | (c) | 323. | (d) | 363. | (d) |
| 204. | (a) | 244. | (a) | 284. | (c) | 324. | (b) | 364. | (c) |
| 205. | (d) | 245. | (d) | 285. | (c) | 325. | (b) | 365. | (a) |
| 206. | (a) | 246. | (a) | 286. | (a) | 326. | (c) | 366. | (d) |
| 207. | (b) | 247. | (a) | 287. | (b) | 327. | (b) | 367. | (d) |
| 208. | (c) | 248. | (b) | 288. | (a) | 328. | (a) | 368. | (c) |
| 209. | (c) | 249. | (b) | 289. | (a) | 329. | (b) | 369. | (d) |
| 210. | (a) | 250. | (b) | 290. | (c) | 330. | (d) | 370. | (b) |
| 211. | (a) | 251. | (c) | 291. | (a) | 331. | (d) | 371. | (b) |
| 212. | (b) | 252. | (c) | 292. | (c) | 332. | (d) | 372. | (a) |
| 213. | (c) | 253. | (b) | 293. | (c) | 333. | (b) | 373. | (d) |
| 214. | (a) | 254. | (d) | 294. | (c) | 334. | (b) | 374. | (c) |
| 215. | (b) | 255. | (b) | 295. | (d) | 335. | (b) | 375. | (d) |
| 216. | (a) | 256. | (c) | 296. | (c) | 336. | (a) | 376. | (c) |
| 217. | (a) | 257. | (d) | 297. | (d) | 337. | (b) | 377. | (b) |
| 218. | (a) | 258. | (a) | 298. | (b) | 338. | (c) | 378. | (d) |
| 219. | (a) | 259. | (d) | 299. | (b) | 339. | (b) | 379. | (a) |
| 220. | (a) | 260. | (c) | 300. | (a) | 340. | (d) | 380. | (b) |
| 221. | (c) | 261. | (b) | 301. | (a) | 341. | (a) | 381. | (a) |
| 222. | (c) | 262. | (c) | 302. | (c) | 342. | (b) | 382. | (d) |
| 223. | (b) | 263. | (a) | 303. | (a) | 343. | (a) | 383. | (a) |
| 224. | (b) | 264. | (d) | 304. | (a) | 344. | (a) | 384. | (c) |
| 225. | (b) | 265. | (c) | 305. | (d) | 345. | (b) | 385. | (a) |
| 226. | (b) | 266. | (c) | 306. | (a) | 346. | (b) | 386. | (d) |
| 227. | (b) | 267. | (d) | 307. | (a) | 347. | (a) | 387. | (d) |
| 228. | (c) | 268. | (c) | 308. | (d) | 348. | (b) | 388. | (d) |
| 229. | (a) | 269. | (c) | 309. | (d) | 349. | (d) | 389. | (b) |
| 230. | (d) | 270. | (a) | 310. | (c) | 350. | (a) | 390. | (d) |
| 231. | (d) | 271. | (d) | 311. | (a) | 351. | (c) | 391. | (a) |
| 232. | (c) | 272. | (a) | 312. | (c) | 352. | (d) | | |
| 233. | (b) | 273. | (b) | 313. | (b) | 353. | (a) | | |
| 234. | (d) | 274. | (a) | 314. | (d) | 354. | (c) | | |
| 235. | (a) | 275. | (a) | 315. | (a) | 355. | (a) | | |
| 236. | (a) | 276. | (b) | 316. | (b) | 356. | (a) | | |
| 237. | (a) | 277. | (b) | 317. | (a) | 357. | (b) | | |
| 238. | (d) | 278. | (a), (c) | 318. | (a) | 358. | (a) | | |
| 239. | (c) | 279. | (b) | 319. | (a) | 359. | (a) | | |
| 240. | (a) | 280. | (a) | 320. | (c) | 360. | (d) | | |

# QUICK REVIEW

# Administration and Management Review and Multiple Choice Questions

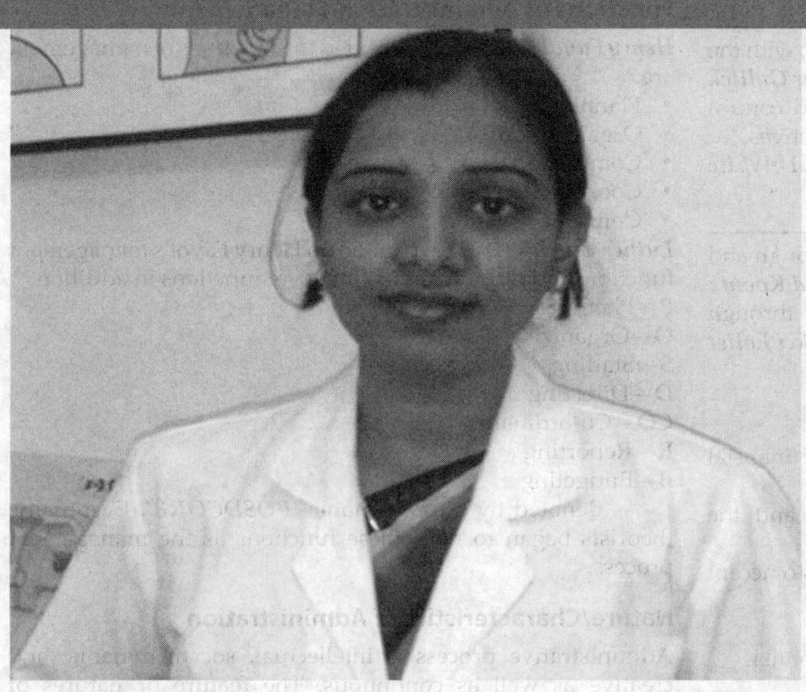

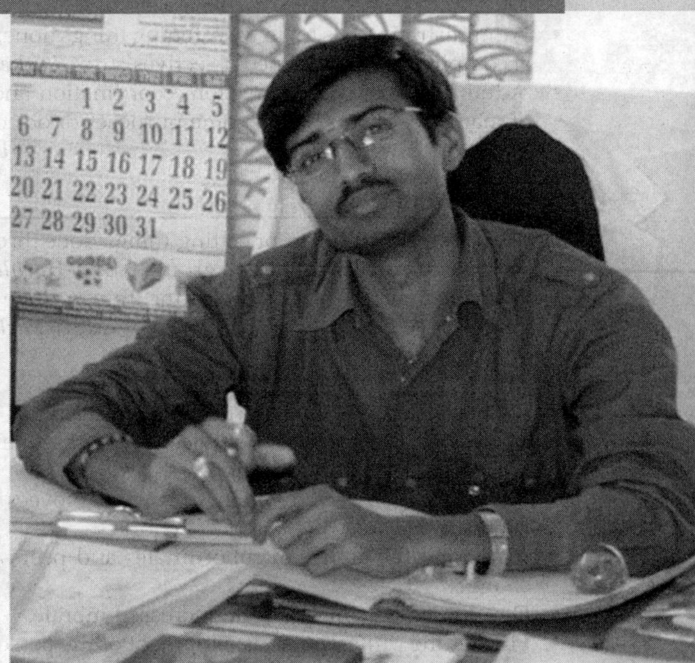

## HIGHLIGHTS

- Administration
- Management
- Material Management
- Quality Assurance
- Hospital
- Staff Development
- Supervision
- Nursing Rounds
- Performance Appraisal
- Communication
- Leadership
- Multiple Choice Questions

# Administration and Management

## ADMINISTRATION

- 'Administration has to do with getting things done; with the accomplishment of defined objectives'. —*Luther Gullick*
- 'Administration is the direction, coordination and control of many people to achieve some purposes or objectives.' —*LD White*

## MANAGEMENT

- 'Management is the art of getting things done through and with an informally organized group.' —*Harold Koontz*
- 'Management is the art of getting things done through people'. —*Mary Parker Follet*

### Importance/Purposes of Administration

- Accomplishing the goals of the organizations.
- Maintaining the quality of service/care within the financial limitations of the organization.
- Encouraging the motivation of the employees and the clients in the area.
- Increasing the ability of subordinates and peers to accept change.
- Developing a team spirit and increased morale.
- Further the professional development of the personnel.

### Principles of Administration/Management

**According to Henry Fayol:**

- ***Division of work:*** Depending on knowledge and skills available with personnel.
- ***Authority and responsibility:*** Authority bestowed should be in accordance to responsibility.
- ***Discipline:*** Maintenance or rules and regulations, punctuality etc.
- ***Unity of command:*** One person commands order.
- ***Unity of direction:*** One person gives direction.
- ***Subordination of individual to general interest:*** Individual interest must be subordinated to general interest when there is conflict between two.
- ***Centralization of authority:*** Refers to greater and larger authority resting with the top management level.
- ***Scalar chain:*** Authority from highest to lowest position.
- ***Remuneration of personnel:*** Salary for all staffs.
- ***Stability to tenure:*** Job security.
- ***Order:*** People and materials should be in the right place at the right time.
- ***Equity:*** justice and kindliness.
- ***Initiative:*** Within the limits of authority and discipline, managers should encourage their employees to take initiative.
- ***Espirit de corps:*** Unity is strength. Team work.

### Functions of Administration/Management

***Henry Fayol (1925)*** first identified the functions of management are:

- Planning
- Organization
- Command
- Coordination
- Control

***Luther Gullick (1937)*** expanded on Henry Fayol's management functions by introducing two or more functions in addition.

**P**—Planning
**O**—Organizing
**S**—Staffing
**D**—Directing
**CO**—Co-ordinating
**R**—Reporting
**B**—Budgeting

As denoted by the Mnemonic ***'POSDCORB'***. Eventually, theorists began to refer these functions as the management process.

### Nature/Characteristics of Administration

Administrative process is intellectual, social, dynamic and creative as well as continuous. The feature or natures of administration are:

- ***It is universal:*** Because irrespective of nature and objectives of the organization, all basic elements of administration such as planning, organizing, staffing, directing, coordinating, reporting, budgeting can apply for its effective achievement of goals.
- ***It is holistic:*** The whole process of administration embraces the organization and its function in entirely, i.e. involve total activities of the organizations.
- ***It is intangible:*** Since administration is visualized as abstract. It cannot be transferable to anywhere. So, every organization has to develop its own administrative style within the contact of functional elements of administration.
- ***It is continuous and ongoing process:*** The cycle of administration goes on continuously.
- ***It is goal oriented:*** Administration is always struggling to achieve the laid down goals and objectives of the organizations.
- ***It is social and human:*** Usually in administration group of people are there to achieve the objective. It needs good social and interpersonal contact or relationship to achieve the goal.
- ***It is dynamic:*** Administration has the elements of flexibility and adaptability and adjustability rising to the needs and demands of different situation.

- *It is creative or innovative:* To have an effective administration existed administration provides innovation, offers and invites creative ideas to its organizational teams.

## Levels of Management

### Levels of Management/Types of Managers, Managerial Skills

Nursing service managers are people who appointed to positions of authority, which enable others to perform their work effectively, who have responsibility for resource utilization and who are accountable for work results and can be proud of their organizations and what they do.

Traditionally classifications of managers are by level in the organizational hierarchy, common nomenclature is:

- Top level management—such as board of directors, presidents and vice presidents
- Middle level management—such as directors of nursing, supervisory staffs and department heads
- First line/front line/or supervisory management—such as head nurses and staffs.

Regardless of level, managers have several common attributes, they are:

- Formally appointed to positions of authority
- Charged with directing and enabling others to do their work effectively
- Responsible for utilizing resources
- Accountable to superiors for results.

The primary differences between levels of managers are the degree of authority and the scope of responsibility and organizational activity at each level.

*Example*

- ***Top-level managers*** such as nursing administrators have authority over and responsibility for the entire organization.
- ***Middle level managers*** such as department heads and heads of services have authority over and responsibility for a specific segment, in contrast to the organization as a whole and act as a liaison between top-level managers and first level managers.
- ***First line managers,*** who generally report to middle level managers have authority over and are responsible for overseeing specific work for a particular group of works.

### Management Skills or Skills Required in Management

At all the three levels of management, every manager requires certain skills. They are:

1. Human relation skills
2. Conceptual skills
3. Technical skills

## PLANNING

- According to ***Koontz and O'Donnell*** 'planning is deciding in advance. What to do? (aim), how to do? (practice), when to do? (Time), who is to do? (workers). It bridges the gap from where we are to, where we want to go'.
- Planning is deciding in advance what is to be done. It involves the selection of objectives, policies, procedures and programmes from among alternatives. —*ME Hurley*

### Types of Planning

- *Strategic planning* is long-term planning for achievement of goals.
- *Operational or tactical planning* is short-term planning for operations of the activities.

### Importance of Planning/Purposes/ Advantages

- Planning is the first function of administration and management. It precedes all other functions. Therefore, the success of the organizational activities depends on the planning.
- It helps to eliminate or reduce the chances of uncertainty.
- It avoids overlapping of activities.
- It helps to set standards and targets.
- It helps in co-ordination
- It gives direction to the organization.
- It improves efficiency.
- It eliminates duplication of efforts.
- It concentrates resources on important services.
- It improves communication and co-ordination of activities.
- Planning is looking ahead, determining goals, objectives, policies, procedures and methods, considering various alternatives.
- Planning assures the best utilization of resources and economy of performance.
- Planning is a continuous process, affecting improvements in the services and solving problems encountered or likely to be encountered.
- It ensures order and control.
- Servers as an integral part of other administrative functions. (i.e. POSDCORB: Planning, Organizing, Staffing, Directing, Coordinating, Reporting, and Budgeting.)
- It leads to effectiveness and efficiency.
- Provides flexibility and makes provision for future growth and development.
- It also helps in decision-making.
- It reduces the cost of performance.
- It makes control effective.

### Elements of Planning or Components of Planning

- Objectives
- Policies
- Procedures
- Programmes
- Budget

## STAFFING

### Definition of Staffing

- *Theo Haimann*, 'Staffing pertains to recruitment, selection, development and compensation of subordinates.'
- *Luther Gidick* 'Staffing is the whole personnel function of bringing in and training the staff and maintaining favorable conditions of work'.

### Nature of Staffing Function

- Staffing is an important managerial function
- Staffing is a pervasive activity
- Staffing is a continuous activity

- The basis of staffing function is efficient management of personnels
- Staffing helps in placing right men at the right job
- Staffing is performed by all managers.

## COST ANALYSIS

It is the system of analyzing the relationship between the fixed and the variable cost.

### Purposes of Cost Analysis

- The administrator utilizes data provided by a cost study to interpret the needs of the nursing units and to gain financial support for the unit.
- It can be used to show the portion of the requested funds being used for research programs.
- It will show the relationship of the faculty salaries to the cost per student.
- It assists the administrator in measuring change and provides the necessary data which can serve as a guide in modifying the program.
- It gives the supporting data when the board of trustees, central administrators, legislators, foundations and other groups question the high cost of nursing education.
- It provides valuable information for institutions questions of higher learning that wish to establish a new baccalaureate program.

### Types of Cost Analysis

- Cost benefit analysis (CBA)
- Cost effectiveness analysis (CEA)
- Cost benefit ratio (CBR)
- Cost-of-illness analysis
- Cost-minimization analysis
- Cost utilization analysis
- Cost consequences analysis

## INVENTORY CONTROL

### Definition

Inventory control means stocking adequate number and kind of materials are available whenever and wherever is required. This has to be done at an optimum outlay of financial and human resources.

### Functions of Inventory Control

- To protect against stock-outs
- To smooth production requirement
- To meet anticipated demand
- To order sufficient quantity per order to reduce order cost
- To stock just sufficient quantity to minimize inventory carrying cost
- To take advantage of seasonal cyclic variation on availability of materials to order the right quantity at the right time.
- To provide safety stock to take care of fluctuation in demand/consumption during lead time.
- To ensure optimum level of inventory holding to minimize the total inventory cost.
- To take advantage of quality discounts.

### Classification of Inventory Control

- *Official inventory:* It is one in which brought to the unit, counted and controlled until it is dispensed to a using department, e.g. medical surgical items, dressings, linens, X-ray supplies, laboratory supplies, housekeeping items, all processed sterile supplies, pharmaceutical items-fluids, dietary items like cereals, pulses, etc.
- *Unofficial inventory:* It is one in which have been expensed and dispensed from the central stores to the various departments and units where they are stored until used, e.g. nursing departments, emergency rooms, radiology department, maintenance, physicians office, recovery room.

### Other Classifications

- *Raw materials inventories:* Iron, steel.
- *Finished goods inventories:* Utensils, garments.

### Techniques/Methods in Inventory Control

- ABC Analysis (Always Better Control)
- FSN Analysis (Fast, Slow moving and Non-moving)
- VED Analysis (Vital, Essential, Desirable)
- SDE Analysis (Scarce, Difficult, Easy)
- GOLF Analysis (Government suppliers, ordinary suppliers, local suppliers, foreing suppliers)
- SOS Analysis (Seasonal or off season items)

### *ABC Analysis*

- ABC analysis are the analysis of the store items and are based on cost criteria.
- It is a simple approach, which avoids being money wise.
- The cost of each item is multiplied by the number used in a given period and then these items are tabulated in descending numerical value order.
- It will be seen that first 10% of items approximately account for 70%, the next 20% for 20% of value and the last 70% account for 10% of value.
- It has been seen that a large number of items consume only a small percentage of resources and vice-versa.
- A–Items represent the high cost center, B–items represent the immediate cost centers, and C–items represent low cost centers.
- A very close control is exercised over A–items while less stringent control is adequate for those in the category B, and less attention for category C.

*A—Items*

- Tight controls
- Rigid estimates of requirements
- Strict and close watch
- Safety stocks should be low
- Management of items should be done at top management level.

*B—Items*

- Moderate control
- Purchase based on rigid requirements
- Reasonably strict watch and control
- Safety stocks moderate
- Management be done at middle level.

*C—Items*

- Ordinary control measure
- Purchase based on usage estimates
- Controls exercises by store keeper.
- Safety stocks high.
- Management be done at lower levels.

| Class | Number of items | Rupee value in items |
|---|---|---|
| A | 10% of total items | 70% |
| B | 20% of total items | 20% |
| C | 70% of total items | 10% |

### *FSN Analysis*

- It is based on rate of consumption.
- The items can be classified into:
  - Fast moving
  - Slow moving
  - Non-moving
  - Obsolete

An understanding of the movement of items helps to keep proper levels of inventories by deciding a rational policy or reordering. This method is based on the fact that some stock items have a much higher annual usage value than others. This after doing a cost analysis, stock items are separated into three classes with the following characteristics.

### *VED Analysis*

The stores when subjected to analysis based on their criticality can be classified into vital, essential and desirable stores. This analysis is termed as VED analysis.

- *Vital:* Items without which treatment comes to standstill: i.e. non-availability cannot be tolerated.
- *Essential:* Items whose non-availability can be tolerated for 2–3 days, because similar or alternative items are available.
- *Desirable:* Items whose non-availability can be tolerated for a long-period. Although the proportion of vital, essential and desirable items varies from hospital to hospital depending on the type and quantity of workload, on an average vital items are 10%, essential items are 40% and desirable items make 50% of total items available.

Although not included in scientific VED analysis, in some public organizations which are static or inefficiently managed, there is a peculiar category of 'U' items which can be grouped as unnecessary. These unnecessary items get purchased due to the following reasons.

- Thoughtless continuation of previous purchase.
- Indifferent attitude towards hospital formulary
- Fear of change
- Poor supervision and control
- Unfair practice due to vested interest.
  - The vital items are stocked in abundance, essential items are stocked in medium amounts and desirable items we stocked in small amounts.
  - By stocking the items in order of priority, vital and essential items are always in stock which means a minimum disruption in the services offered to the people.

### *SDE Analysis*

Classification of methods based on source of supply, SDE classification is a system where materials are sorted out as scare to obtain, difficult to obtain and easy to obtain.

### *GOLF Analysis*

In the GOLF system, classification is based on the availability and nature of supplies. Government suppliers, ordinary suppliers, local suppliers and foreign suppliers.

### *SOS Analysis*

Raw materials can be classified into seasonal or off season items.

## MANAGEMENT BY OBJECTIVES (MBO)

### Definition

'Each and Every employee of an organisation works whole heartedly towards the attainment of the objectives of an organisation is known as management by objectives.

*—Peter F Drucker*

### Purposes/Needs for Management by Objectives

- The management by objectives process helps the employees to understand their duties at the workplace.
- The employees are clear as to what is expected out of them.
- Management by objectives process leads to satisfied employees. It avoids job mismatch and unnecessary confusions later on.
- Employees in their own way contribute to the achievement of the goals and objectives of the organization.

Every employee has his own role at the workplace. Each one feels indispensable for the organization and eventually develops a feeling of loyalty towards the organization. They tend to stick to the organization for a longer span of time and contribute effectively. They enjoy at the workplace and do not treat work as a burden.

- Management by objectives ensures effective communication amongst the employees. It leads to a positive ambience at the workplace.
- Management by objectives leads to well defined hierarchies at the workplace. It ensures transparency at all levels.

A supervisor of any organization would never directly interact with the managing director in case of queries. He would first meet his reporting boss who would then pass on the message to his senior and so on. Everyone is clear about his position in the organization.

- The MBO process leads to highly motivated and committed employees.
- The MBO process sets a benchmark for every employee. The superiors set targets for each of the team members. Each employee is given a list of specific tasks.

### MBO Process Steps

- Setting objectives
- Action planning
- Performance review

## PROGRAM EVALUATION AND REVIEWING TECHNIQUE (PERT)

### Definition

'Program evaluation and reviewing technique (PERT) is a project management tool used to schedule, organize and coordinate tasks within a project. It is basically a method to analyze the tasks involved in completing a giving project, especially the time needed to complete each task and to identify the minimum time needed to complete the total project. The main objective of PERT is to facilitate decision making and to reduce both the time and cost required to complete a project'.

### Uses of PERT

- Useful management tool for planning, coordinating, and controlling large, complex projects such as formulation of a master budget, construction of buildings, installation of computers, and scheduling of the closing of books.
- Used to plan the scheduling of individual activities that make up a project
- They can be used to determine the earliest/latest start and finish times for each activity.

### Advantages of PERT

*Modern and Philips* enlists the following advantages of PERT.

- It encourages logical discipline in planning, scheduling and control of project.
- It encourages more long-range and detailed project planning.
- It provides a standard method of documenting and communicating project plans, schedules, and time and cost performance.
- It identifies the most critical elements in the plan thus focusing management attention on the 10–20% of the project, i.e. most constraining on the schedule.
- It illustrates the effect of technical and procedural changes or overall schedules.

### Benefits of PERT

PERT is useful because it provides the following information:

- Expected project completion time
- Probability of completion before a specified date
- The critical path activities that directly impact the completion time
- The activities that have slack time and that can be lend resources to critical path activities
- Activity start and end date.

## BENCH MARKING

### Definition

- Bench marking is a management technique to evaluate the performance.
- Bench marking is a systematic process for identifying and implementing best or better practices.

### Bench Marking in Nursing

Nurses are the backbone of health care delivery system. Due to the modern technique or technology, nurses require skills to cope up the situations to face the challenges. It is necessary for the manager/administrator of nursing to provide quality of health care to their clients. To provide quality of care, to meet the health needs of clients, it is necessary to establish the standard of education and practice.

### Benefits of Bench Marking

- Prevent unfair means during evaluation
- Maintain the standards/quality
- Save time
- Enhance satisfaction.

### Principles of Bench Marking

According to Watson, 1993, there are three principles of bench marking:

1. Maintaining quality
2. Customer satisfaction
3. Continuous improvement.

## BUDGET

### Definition

'Budget is a balance estimated expenditure and receipts for a given period of time. In the hands of the administrator the budget is the record of the past performance, a method of current control and projection of future pans'. *—Dimock*

### Importance/Purposes/Objectives of Budget

- To provide definite targets for income and expenditure of the department
- To co-ordinate the activities of the different functional heads in the working of these departmental budget
- To enable a cash flow statement prepared month by month
- To aid management in formulating future policy decision to promote the growth and welfare of the organizations
- To provide useful tool for the control of costs
- To provide a tool for communication and co-ordination within the organization
- To improve financial planning and decision making
- To identify controllable and uncontrollable cost area.

### Features of Budget

- Should be flexible.
- Should be synthesis of past, present and future.
- Should be product of joint venture and cooperation of executives/department heads at different levels of management.
- It should be clearly defined.
- It should be in the form of statistical standard laid down in specific numerical terms.
- It should have support of top management throughout the period of its planning and supplementation
- It should facilitate goal achievement.
- It should be in a time period. This is usually annual.
- It should be based on specific concepts of financial management.
- It should estimate revenues and expenditures as accurately as possible.
- It should focus on objectives and policies of organization.

### Classification/Types of Budget

Budget consists mainly three sections, i.e.

1. *Manpower budget:* The manpower budget includes wages and other benefits provided for regular and temporary workers.
2. *Capital expenditure budget:* It is for long life, e.g. purchase of buildings, major equipment.
3. *Operating/recurrent budget:* It includes daily expenditure, e.g. personnel salaries, light, water, drugs, repairs and maintenance, etc.

### Other Types of Budget

- According to time
  - Long-term budget
  - Short-term budget
  - Current budget
- According to function
  - Sales budget
  - Production budget
  - Cost of production area
  - Purchase budget
  - Personal budget
  - Research budget
  - Capital budget
  - Cash budget
  - Master budget
- According to flexibility
  - Fixed budget
  - Flexible budget
  - Operating budget
  - Performance budget
  - Programme budget
  - Special purpose budget.

## NURSING AUDIT

### Definition

Assessment of the quality of nursing care or evaluation of the quality of patient care.

### Purposes of Nursing Audit

- Evaluating nursing care given
- Achieves deserved and feasible quality of nursing care
- Stimulant to better records.
- Focuses on care provided and not on care provider
- Contributes to research
- Quality of nursing care
- Cost effectiveness.

### Types/Method of Nursing Audit

#### *Concurrent Audit*

It is a method for evaluating quality of ongoing care through appraisal of nursing process. It is done while the patient is still in the ward.

*Advantages*

- Identification of problems at the time care is given.
- Provision of mechanism for identifying and meeting clients' needs during care.
- Implementation of measures to fulfil professional responsibilities.
- Provision of a mechanism for communicating on behalf of client.

#### *Retrospective Audit*

- It evaluates quality of care through appraisal of the nursing process after the clients discharge from health care system.
- The patient is evaluated after the patients discharge from the hospital.

*Advantages*

- Comparison of actual practice to standards of care.
- Analysis of actual practice to standards of care.
- It gives total picture of care given.
- More accurate data for planning corrective action.

## MATERIAL MANAGEMENT

### Definition

Material management is concerned with providing the drugs, supplies and equipment needed by the health personnel to deliver health services.

### Purposes/Importance of Material Management

It very important in nursing. All the nursing procedures starting from simple to complex, non-invasive techniques require materials. In other words, no nursing procedures can be done in a scientific way without adequate and appropriate materials.

- To gain economy in purchasing.
- To satisfy the demand during period of replenishment
- To carry reserve stock to avoid stock out.
- To stabilize fluctuations in consumption.
- To provide reasonable level of client services.
- Increase efficiency of health care systems.
- Develop knowledge and skills of health care.
- Provide materials in required quantity and quality as when required.

### Functions of Material Management

- Material planning and budgeting
- Purchasing of material
- Inventory control
- Cost reduction
- Value analysis
- Store administration
- Quality control for inspection
- Stocking and distribution
- Disposal of scrap surplus and obsolete materials.
- Simplification, product development.

### Elements of Material Management Planning

- Demand estimation
- Procurement
- Receipt and inspection
- Storage
- Issue and use

- Maintenance and Repair
- Disposal
- Accounting and information system.

## QUALITY ASSURANCE

### Definition

Quality assurance is a general term for all arrangements and activities that are meant to safeguard, maintain and promote quality of care. —*Dr Aredis Dona Bedian*

### Goals of Quality Assurance

The major goal of quality assurance is to identify areas where standards have not been met and correct them, or in other terms quality assurance are:

- To ensure the delivery or quality care
- To evaluate the efforts of the health care provider to provide best possible result.

### The Quality Assurance Methods/Activities in Hospital

#### *Nursing Audit*

It is a method for evaluating quality of nursing care through the appraisal of the nursing process or customers of care as it is reflected in the patient care records. There are two types of audit:

1. ***Concurrent audit:*** It is one in which the patient care is observed and evaluated as it is given.
2. ***Retrospective audit:*** The patient is evaluated after the patients discharge from the hospital.

#### *Peer Review*

It is a process by which nurses evaluate one another's job performance against accepted standards.

#### *Patient Care Profiles Analysis*

The analysis of longitudinal or cross-sectional complications of data about patients with a particular diagnosis or problem.

#### *Quality Circles*

A quality circle is a small group of 5 to 15 employees who perform similar work and meet for 1 hour each week to solve problems related to their work.

#### *Patient Satisfaction Studies/Patients Opinion Studies*

The patients are interviewed or they are given a set of questions to answer in which the patients state how they experienced the hospital stay.

#### *Control Committees*

Committees may be set up in hospitals to evaluate a particular problem and to take corrective measures. Examples are infection control committee, safety committee etc.

### Quality Assurance Process

It is the process of evaluating the outcomes of care and ensuring that each patient receives a predetermined high standard of care, by:

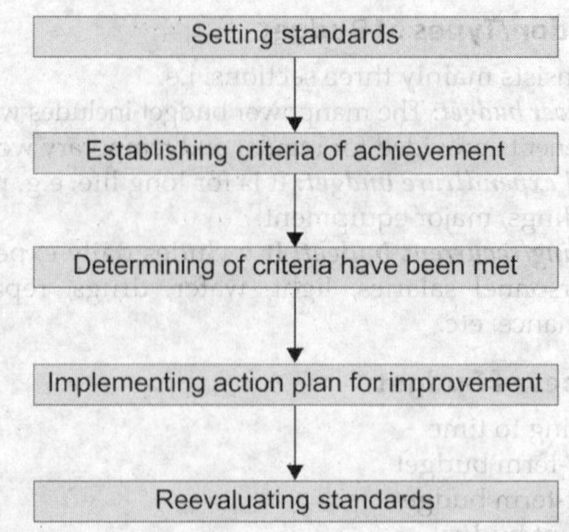


### Factors Affecting Quality Assurance in Nursing Care

- Lack of resources
- Lack of qualified nursing personnel
- Improper maintenance
- Unreasonable patients and relatives
- Absence of well informed population
- Absence of accreditation laws
- Lack of incident review procedures
- Lack of good and Hospital Information System (HIS)
- Absence of patient satisfaction surveys
- Lack of nursing care records
- Miscellaneous factors:
  - Lack of good supervision
  - Absence of knowledge about philosophy of nursing care
  - Lack of policy and administrative manuals.
  - Shortage of trained nurses in hospital
  - Lack of adequate nurse administrator
  - Lack of written job description and job specifications
  - Lack of in-service and continuing educational program
  - Lack of evaluation technique
  - Lack of supplies and equipment in hospital.

## ORGANIZATION

### Definition

'Organization is a group of people whose activities are consciously co-ordinated towards common objective or objectives'. —*Chester Bernard*

### Types/Classification of Organization

- Formal organization
- Informal organization.

### Principles of Organization

According to *Henry Fayol:*

- Hierarchy
- Division of work
- Unity of command
- Centralization vs decentralization

- Span of control
- Delegation.

## Organization Chart

Organization chart is one of the visual which helps any visitor to get an understanding of an organization at a glance.

### *Types of Organizational Chart*

- Vertical chart (i.e. from top to bottom)
- Horizontal charts (i.e. from left-to-right)
- Circular chart
- Departmental chart.

## SPAN OF CONTROL

It is the number of subordinates that a manager or a supervisor can effectively supervise. This is also known as *span of supervision or span of management.*

The span of control will depends upon:

- Unity of objectives
- Division of work and specialization
- Job description
- Unity of command
- Principle of adequate authority
- Span of supervision.

### Factors Affecting Span of Control or Span of Management

- Qualification and qualities
- Level of management
- Nature of work
- Superior-subordinates relationship
- Degree of centralization
- Use of communication technology
- Financial position of the organization
- Clarity of plans and responsibilities
- Time available for subordinates
- Faith and trust in subordinates.

## HOSPITAL

- According to WHO, 'the hospital is an integral part of a social and medical organization, the function of which is to provide for the population complete health care-both curative and preventive, and whose outpatient services reach out to the family and its environment. The hospital is also a center for the training of health workers and biosocial workers.'
- A hospital is a health care institution providing medical and surgical treatment and nursing care for sick or injured people.

### Classification of Hospital

Hospitals have been classified in many ways.

| Classification according to: Clinical basis | Classification according to: Ownership/control | Classification according to: Teaching or non-teaching status | Classification according to: Size | Classification according to: System of medicine |
|---|---|---|---|---|
| **General hospital:** Patients treated in general hospitals are with all kinds of diseases such as pneumonitis, typhoid, fever, etc. | **Public hospitals:** Public hospitals are those run by the central government, state government or local bodies on non-commercial lines. These hospitals may be general hospitals or specialized or both | **Teaching hospital:** A hospital may have a medical college attached to it, when it is called as a teaching hospital | **Teaching hospitals:** Bed strength 500. (It is to be increased according to the number of students) | Allopathic hospitals |
| **Specialized hospitals:** Here patients are treated for those diseases for which that hospital has been setup such as heart diseases, tuberculosis, cancer, maternity, etc. | **Voluntary hospitals:** Voluntary hospitals are those which are established and incorporated under the societies registration act, 1860 or public trust act, 1882 or any other appropriate act of the central or state government. They are run with public or private funds on a non commercial basis | **Non-Teaching hospital:** A hospital without a medical college is termed as a non–teaching hospital | **District hospitals:** Bed strength 200. (It may be raised up to 300 beds depending upon the population) | Ayurvedic hospitals |
| **Isolation hospital:** This is a hospital in which the person is suffering from infection or communicable diseases requiring isolation are treated, e.g. epidemic disease hospital, Bengaluru | **Private nursing homes:** They are generally owned by an individual doctor or a group of doctors. They accept patients suffering from infirmity, advanced age, illness, injury, chronic disability etc. or those who are convalescing, Nursing homes are run on a commercial basis. Naturally ordinary citizens cannot afford medical treatment there | | **Taluk hospitals:** Bed strength 50 (it can be raised depending upon the population to be served | Homeopathic hospitals |
| | **Corporate hospitals:** The latest concept is of corporate hospitals, which are public limited companies formed under the companies act. They are normally run on commercial lines. They can be either general or specialized or both | | **Primary health centers:** Bed strength 6 (it may be increased upto 10 depending upon the needs | Unani hospitals |
| | | | | Naturopathy hospitals |

## Functions of Hospital

### *Intramural Functions*

- OPD (Out Patient Department)
- IPD (In Patient Department)
- Diagnostics
- Emergency services
- Teaching and Education.

### *Extramural Functions*

- Home Care Services
- Health Camps
- Health Promotion
- Day Care Centers.

## STAFF DEVELOPMENT

*According to American Nurses Association (ANA):* 'Staff development programme is a process consisting of orientation, in-service education and continuing education for the purpose of promoting the development of personal, within any employment setting 'consistent with the goals and responsibilities of the employer'.

### Need/Purposes/Importance of Staff Development

- Societal change and scientific advancement.
- Need to increase productivity and quality of work.
- Preparing nurse leaders.
- Personal growth.
- Improved organizational climate.
- Motivating staff nurses to continue to learn through their own efforts.
- Upgrading the competencies of those who have been inadequately prepared.
- Updating the knowledge and skills of those who are behind or those who would like to assume new tasks or go further in their position.
- Provision of opportunity for nurses to continually acquire and implement for maintenance of high quality of nursing care.
- As a part of individual's long term career growth.
- To add or the knowledge, skills, attitude, ideals and valued essentials improve skills.
- Fill the gap in the past performance.
- Change or correct long held attitudes of the employee.
- To move ahead and keep up the change.
- Fast changing technologies.
- To motivate employees and promote employee loyalty.
- Fast growing organization.

### Types/Areas of Staff Development Program/Faculty Development Process

Faculty development is a comprehensive program and includes:

### *Induction Training*

- First phase of staff development
- Carried out after the employee has been selected, but prior to performing the job role.
- Includes all the activities that educate the new employee (during his/her first 2–3 days of employment) about the organization as well as employment personal policies and procedures.

### *Orientation*

- Introduces employees to new situations.
- Includes contents related to philosophy, goals, procedures, role expectations and physical facilities.
- Orientation is required whenever the employees have a role change.

### *In-Service Education*

- Provides learning experiences in the work setting for the purpose of refining and developing new skills and knowledge related to job performance
- Usually narrow in scope because
- The learning experiences are brief as they are aimed at only one competency or knowledge area.

### *Continuing Education*

- Planned and organized learning experiences which focus on competencies and knowledge.
- Employees can use in a variety of settings instead of just a particular area.

### *Job Related Counseling*

- Involves promoting professional growth of employees by helping them to give their best job performance
- Also involves counseling on promotion, possibilities and assistance in obtaining formal training.

## SUPERVISION

### Concept of Supervision

The word supervision is derived from two words 'super' means above or over and 'vision' means seeing. Hence the word supervision means overseeing which means that 'supervision' is an act of a superior person to see the work of the personnel working under him or her. This overseeing also means directing, investigating, guiding, helping and advising the subordinates in their performance with the purpose of achieving the essential objectives. Thus supervision is the art of overseeing, watching and directing with authority, the work and behavior of other. The concept of supervision is to guide and help the subordinates in their:

- Duties
- Work
- Activities.

The main components of supervision are:

- Training
- Guidance
- Demonstration
- Counseling of an individual and checking.

## Definition of Supervision

- Supervision is defined as 'guiding and directing efforts of the employees and other resources to accomplish stated work outputs' —*Terry and Franklin*
- Supervision is the art of overseeing, watching and directing with authority, the work and behavior of other.

## Types of Supervision

Generally there are two types of supervision:

1. ***Direct supervision:*** This is done through face to face talk with the workers or supervision is to observe subordinates concurrently how they are working. This can be exercised at the ward/unit level in the hospital or PHC or sub centre of the community setting.
2. ***Indirect supervision:*** It is done with the help of records and reports of the workers and through written instructions or through some agency between the supervisor and supervisee or indirect supervision is to go after the subordinates have performed and check in the hospital or in the community as to what has been done. Reviewing records and reports are indirect supervision.

## Factors Essential for Good Supervision

The factors governing the effectiveness of supervision are:

- Human relationship
- Technical job knowledge skills
- Knowledge of organization
- Proper leadership
- Favorable work climate.

## Methods of Supervision

- Technical vs creative supervision
- Cooperative vs authoritarian supervision
- Scientific vs intuitive supervision.

## Techniques and Tools Used for Supervision

- Observation, e.g. ward rounds
- Individual and group conferences
- Initial conference
- Check list
- Rating scale
- Performance evaluation—self evaluation, peer evaluation, supervisor's evaluation, evaluation by general public.
- Verbal and written reports—anecdotal reports, critical incident reports, confidential reports, etc.
- Orientation and guided experience
- Manuals and protocols
- Staff meetings
- In-service education program
- Continuing education.

# NURSING ROUNDS

## Definition

'Nursing rounds are conducted by the head nurse/nurse teacher for the members of her staff/students for a clear understanding of the disease process and the effect of nursing care for each patient.' —*Jean Barett*

## Purposes of Nursing Rounds

- ***To demonstrate***
  - Important clinical manifestations in client.
  - Effects of drugs, i.e. indication, action, reaction of drugs.
- ***To clarify:*** Terminologies used and studied.
- ***To compare***
  - Patient's reaction to disease and study the disease's condition.
  - Method of meeting nursing needs and to have better understanding
- ***To illustrate:*** Skilful nursing care.
- ***To give:*** More purposeful care to the patient.
- ***To observe***
  - The physical and mental condition of the patient.
  - The work of staff.
  - The result of the treatment.
- ***To make:*** Specific observation of the patient and to give report to the doctor.
- ***To carryout plan:*** Made for the care of the patient.

# EVALUATION

## Definition

'Evaluation or assessment in education is a process of judging the effective of educational experiences through careful appraisal'. —*LE Hidgerken*

## Types of Evaluation

### *Formative Evaluation*

The ongoing or systematic assessment of students' achievement during the curricular program or it determines the strength and weakness at each stage of the program.

### *Summative Evaluation*

An evaluation done at the end to assess the outcome of the program or it determines the strength and weakness at the end of the program.

## Importance/Purposes of Evaluation

- To determine the level of knowledge and understanding of the student.
- To determine the level of knowledge and understanding of the student's clinical performance.
- To find out the weakness and strength of students in different areas.
- To improve self-directed knowledge.
- To check effectiveness of teaching.
- To improve teaching methods.
- It helps in the improvement of the curriculum.
- It helps the students to identify their difficulties and problems in learning and know the progress they make.
- To guide the teacher and students in selecting of future learning.
- To provide guidance counseling to the students related to learning.
- To decide promotion and placement etc.
- To reports to the parents the achievement of students.
- To motivate and encourage students to learn.

## Methods of Evaluation

Learning objectives are based on three domains
1. Assessment of knowledge (cognitive domain)
2. Assessment of skill (psychomotor domain)
3. Assessment of attitude (affective domain).

So these domains can be evaluated by following tools:

### *Assessment/Evaluation of Knowledge (Cognitive Domain)*

The tools used for assessment/evaluation of knowledge are:
- Essay type questions.
- Short answer questions (SAQ)
- Multiple choice questions (MCQ)
- True and false.
- Fill in the blanks.

#### *Essay Type Questions*

Essay type test consists of questions for which the students prepares her own answers and it evaluates the points like handwriting, spelling, neatness, organization, ways of expressing ideas may be considered in scoring the items.

#### Advantages of Essay Type Questions

- It requires short time for the teacher to prepare the test.
- Increases the ability to recall by students.
- Give degree knowledge in that subject.
- Students get an opportunity to answer questions without any binding or instruction.
- Students get a good opportunity to express their individual ideas and talents.

#### *Short Answer Questions (SAQ)*

The student responds by selection of one or more of several given alternatives by giving or filling in a word or phrase. It does not call for an extensive written response.

Questions should be drafted in such a way that, the answer calls for a predetermined and precise concept. The answer is expected in short answer can be expressed in different forms. Ideally, only one answer is acceptable.

#### Advantages of Short Answer Questions

- Easy to score
- Reliability of score is improved, quick response.

#### *Multiple Choice Questions (MCQ)*

A MCQ consists of a problem and a list of suggested solutions. The problem may be stated in the form of a question or an incomplete statement called stem of the item. The list possible/correct answer /list of possible distracters are called alternatives also called options. The students are requested to select one correct answer or the best answer.

#### Advantages of MCQ

- It can measure effectively the learning outcomes.
- High quality and feasibility.
- Free from ambiguity and vagueness.
- Ensure objectivity, reliability and validity.
- Easy and rapid to score.
- Saves time of teacher as computers can correct them.
- Provides detailed feedback for both students and teachers.
- Provide constructive criticism.

### *Assessment/Evaluation of Skills (Psychomotor Domain)*

The tools used for assessment of skills are:
- Observation
- Practical exam
- Oral/viva examination
- Objective structured clinical examination (OSCE).

#### *Observation*

- Observation has been defined as a measurement without instrument.
- Observation is a method of data gathering by recognizing and nothing facts or occurrence.
- Accurate watching and nothing of phenomenon.

***The observational technique or qualitative techniques*** are systematic methods of recording the observations of students for the purposes of evaluation.

The following tools are used for ***observation techniques***.
- Anecdotal records
- Check lists
- Rating scale
- Sociometric.

#### *Anecdotal Records*

An anecdotal record is a disruption of what an individual does or says. Anecdotal records are factual description of the meaningful incidents and events which the teacher has observed in the lives of pupils.

#### Advantages

- Helpful for counseling the weak individual or the needed individual.
- Easy for the evaluators to interpret.
- It gives the entire course performance of an individual and determination of the progress easy.
- Use of formative feedback.
- Economical and easy to develop.

#### *Check List*

It is a form of list containing number of items which the respondent has to check or mark. The respondent can be a teacher or a student. This can be used to report the students about their performance or to their parents.

#### Advantages of Check List

- Clearly specified characteristics to be observed
- They are adoptable to most subject matter area
- They provide simple method to record observation
- It can be applied on an individual at a time.

#### *Rating Scale*

- Rating scale are devices by which the judgment may be qualified
- Rating is a term use to express an opinion or judgment regarding some situation, object or character. Opinions are expressed on a scale of values.

#### Types of Rating Scale

- Descriptive rating scale
- Numerical rating scale
- Graphic rating scale

Advantages

- Easy to administer and score
- Act as an instrument to find out the students need
- Help to recognize the individual talents and difference
- Can be use for large group of students.

*Practical Exam*

The practical examinations are conducted to evaluated the nursing competence or practical skills of students.

Purposes of Practical Exam

- To assess the ability of students to give care in a practical situation.
- The attitude of the student towards client.
- Able to meet the need of the client and work to allow with other.
- Ability to give need based health education.

Advantages

- Possibility of performance evaluation in clinical situation.
- Attitudes of the students can be observed and tested including the responsiveness to a complex situation
- Provides the opportunity to test all the senses in a realistic situation.

*Oral (Viva) Examination*

Oral examination is a face to face question answer activity between the examiner and the examinee. The examiner ask questions and the examinee attempts to answer them. Finally the examiner judges the quality of the answers and grades the examinee accordingly.

Advantages

- Provides direct personal contact with the candidates.
- Provides opportunity of students for calcifying answers and doubts.
- Require the student to formulate her own answers.
- Provides flexibility in moving from strong point to weak point.

*Objective Structured Clinical Examination (OSCE)*

In OSCE each component of clinical competence is tested uniformly and objectively for all the students who are taking up a practical examination at a given place.

Through OSCE one gets a reasonable idea of the extent of achievement of each student in every practical skill related to a particular discipline. It can be used for formative and summative evaluation.

Advantages

- It helps us to observe and assess student for different professional and technical skills in real life situation.
- It enables us to have an overall view of the students performance.

### *Assessment/Evaluation of Attitude (Affective Domain)*

The tools used for assessment of attitude are:

*Attitude Scales*

- Attitude scales are used for measuring the social attitudes.
- Questionnaire is prepared by the items in the questionnaire are the attitudes of an individual towards a matter things, and or object or system and score will be allotted for each item.
- We will ask the individual to express his response towards an object or system, on the basis of his responses; he is assigned a score which indicates the position.
- Some relevant and indirect statements will also be used to reveal the attitude.
- The scale also specifies the crucial shades of opinions.

Types of Attitude Scales

- Point scale
- Differential scale: LL Thurstone scale
- Summated scale.

## PERFORMANCE APPRAISAL

### Definition

'Performance appraisal is the process by which organizations evaluate individual job performance'. —*Werther and Davis*

### Importance/Need/Purposes of Performance Appraisal

- Performance appraisal helps the management to take decisions about the salary increase of an employee.
- The continuous evaluation of an employee helps in improving the quality of an employee in job performance.
- It minimizes the communication gap between the employee and employer.
- Promotion is given to an employee on the basis of performance appraisal.
- The training needs of an employee can be identified through performance appraisal.
- The decision for discharging an employee from the job is also taken on the basis of performance appraisal.
- Performance appraisal is used to transfer a person is misfit for job to the right placement.
- It helps to improve the employer and employee relationship.

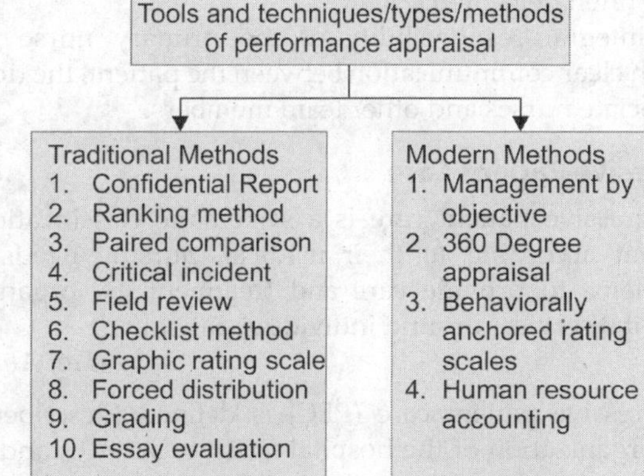


## METHODS OF PATIENT CARE ASSIGNMENT

The following are the methods of patient care assignments in the ward/clinical set up.

### The Patient Method (Case Method/Total Patient Care)

Total patient care nursing is sometimes referred to as the case method of assignment because patients were assigned as cases, much like contemporary private duty nursing is carried out. In the patient method of assignment:

- A nurse is expected to give complete nursing care to one or more patents.
- The care includes general nursing measures, treatments, administering medications, taking temperature, pulse, and respiration, serving food and giving health instructions.
- If the primary nurse goes 'off duty', her group of patients will be taken over by another nurse in her absence in order that the patients may still receive individualized care.

### The Functional Method

When functional method is used, nurses are assigned to specific functions in the ward such as giving medications or treatment to all patients, taking the temperature of all or giving general nursing care to a group of individuals.

The functional method may be used at some period of the day such as evenings and nights when a few nurses are on duty.

### Team Method/Nursing (Modular Nursing)

'Team nursing is the one in which a team leader is responsible for co-coordinating a small group of licensed and unlicensed personnel to provide patient care to a small group of a patients'.

### Primary Nursing

It involves total nursing care, directed by a nurse on a 24 hours basis as long as the client is under care.

The primary nurse assumes 24 hours responsibility for planning the care of one or more patient from admittance or the start of treatment to discharge or the treatment's end. During working hours the primary nurse provides total direct care for that patient, when the primary nurse is not on duty, care is provided by other junior nurses who follow the care plan established by the primary nurse, that means, even though the primary nurse is the director of care for client, segments of care are often delegated.

An integral responsibility of the primary nurse is to establish clear communication between the patient, the doctor, the associate nurses and other team members.

### Progressive Patient Care

- 'Progressive patient care is a systematic classification of patient according to their medical, nursing needs and problems to provide care and treatment, by organizing hospital services around individual patient'

  —*Fay Abdulla*

- Progressive patient care (PPC) is defined (described) as the organization of the hospital facilities services and staff around the changing medical and nursing needs of the patient. —*Promise and Pitfulls*

## COMMUNICATION

### Definition

Communication is the process of passing message, ideas, facts, opinions, attitudes, information and understanding from one person to another.

### Importance/Purposes/Needs of Communication

- Communication is important for the nurse to understand and to exchange ideas to the client and their relatives, the doctors and other members of the health team.
- Poor communication results in poor patient care and poor interpersonal relationship.
- Good communication helps the nurses to improve quality care for the patients.
- Delegate authority and responsibility.
- It reduces the interpersonal tension and improves the interpersonal relationship.
- Good communication prevents disorders in the ward and hospital organization.
- Recruit, select, train and develop the personnel in the organization.
- It also helps to improve employer- employee relationship.
- Good communication helps the nurse to change or modify her behavior and at the same time, she will be able to influence the behavior of co-workers or subordinators.
- Encourage the participation in decision making.
- It helps in the grievance procedure and disciplinary actions.
- Ensures job satisfaction.
- Improve public relation with government and other agencies.
- Include motivation, cooperation and coordination of the employees.
- Better understanding of the organization's role and policies.
- Better relationships between management, staff and clients.

### Types/Methods/Forms of Communication

- One-way communication
- Two-way communication
- Verbal Communication
- Non-Verbal communication
- Formal and informal communication
- Visual communication
- Telecommunication and internet.

### Communication Process

Communication between two or more persons involves a series of elements. This is called communication process. We shall now see the elements of communication, steps in the process of communication and the process of communication itself.

### Elements of Communication

In order to communicate, we should have to have the following basic elements.

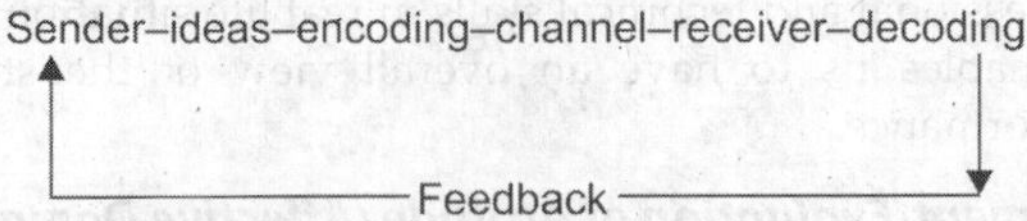


- ***Sender or the communicator or source:*** The person which passes information's or ideas to another person is known of sender.
- ***Ideas:*** This is the subject matter of communication. This might be opinions, attitudes, feelings, views, suggestions, orders, etc.

- *Encoding:* The process of transmission of message to symbols (words, actions, pictures etc.) is called encoding. Symbols are transmitted from the sender to the receiver.
- *Channel:* The symbols are transmitted through certain channels, e.g. radio, telephone, speech, written message etc., the choice of channel usually depends upon the nature, importance and urgency of the message.
- *Receiver:* It is the listener or the one who receive the message.
- *Decoding:* Receiver converts the symbols received from the sender to give him the meaning of the message.
- *Response or feedback:* It is the message that the receiver returns to the sender.

### Barriers of Communication

There are several factors that can:

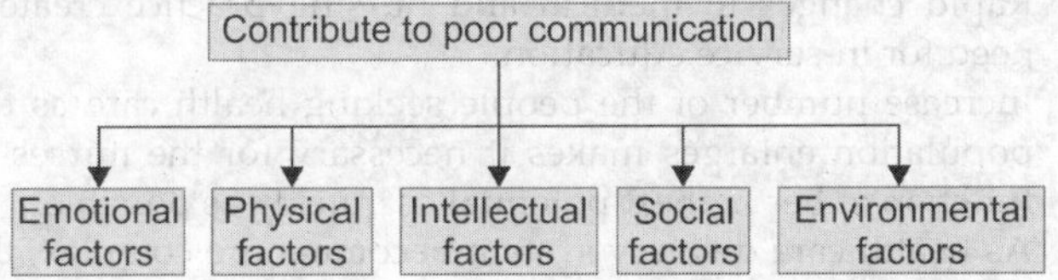


### Techniques of Communication

The following are the techniques of communication:

- Observation
- Listening
- Restating
- Validating
- Providing information
- Clarifying
- Paraphrasing
- Pinpointing
- Linking
- Questioning
- Focusing
- Sharing
- Summarizing.

## LEADERSHIP

### Definition

- Leadership is defined as the 'Process of influencing others towards a goal'. —*Bennie and Nanas*
- Leadership is the art of motivating a group of people to act towards achieving a common goal.

### Leadership Style

Leadership style is how a leader uses interpersonal influence to accomplish goals of an organization.

### Types of Leadership Styles

#### *Autocratic (Directive) Leadership*

- The leader assumes complete control over the decision and activities of group.
- The authority for decision-making is not delegated to persons in lower level positions.
- This type of leadership is useful in emergency situations, when the leader has to take immediate action without consulting subordinates.

#### *Democratic (Participative) or Creative Leadership*

The leader delegates authority to subordinate employees.

#### *Laissez-faire (Abdicratic) Leadership*

The leader gives up all power to the group.

#### *Bureaucratic Style of Leadership*

- The leader functions only in lines with rules and regulations.
- The leader cannot be flexible and does not like to take any risk out of the rules.

### Techniques of Effective Leadership in Nursing

The following are the techniques which can be applied by the nurse administrators to be an effective leader.

- Planning and organizing
- Division of labor
- Guidance
- Effective communications
- Cooperation and coordination
- Encouraging participation
- Supervision
- Evaluation

### Leadership Theories

#### *Trait Theory/Great Man Theory*

This theory believed that the leaders are born, and not made. They have certain set of characteristics that are crucial for inspiring others towards a common goal.

A successful leader may have the following traits:

- Good personality
- Tirelessness
- Capacity to read others mind
- Ability to make quick decision
- Courage, persuasion
- Reliability
- Self-confidence
- Cheerfulness
- Imagination
- Ambition
- Communication
- Teaching skills
- Self-assurance.

*Common Leadership Traits*

- *Knowledge:* Leaders need to be more knowledge of self, i.e. self-awareness.
- *Personal qualifications:* Leaders must have personal qualification like integrity, honesty, ability to cooperate, ability to attract, motivate, enthusiasm and unite others to work.

- ***Initiative qualities:*** Leaders must have initiative qualities like willingness to come forward to help and assist, self-confidence, courage and decisiveness.
- ***Teaching mastery:*** Leaders must have teaching mastery, i.e. expert knowledge and expertize to work.
- ***Teaching abilities:*** Leaders must have teaching abilities, i.e. ability to communicate.
- ***Administrative abilities:*** Leaders must have administrative abilities, i.e. abilities to manage, organize and co-ordinate.

### *Behavioral Theory*

Behavioral theory believed that good leaders are not born, but can be trained to be effective. It is believed that what makes the leaders effective is what they do, such as how they communicate, give direction, motivate their followers, delegate, plan the activities, etc.

Behavioral approach has led to the development of a classification of leadership styles.

- *Autocratic:* Takes all decisions and assigns all responsibility to himself . —*Aurangzeb, Tipu, Shahjahan*
- *Democratic:* The leader is catalyst for group decision-making and shared responsibility. —*Lal Bahadur Shastri*
- *Laissez faire:* The leader leaves all decision making and responsibility to the group uninvolved. —*King Farouk*
- *Benevolent autocratic:* A paternalistic leader. 'You do what I say, I know what is best for you'.

The behavioral theory takes into consideration not only the leader's qualities but also the leaders activities and response to the group's needs and expectations. However, this theory was also found wanting in that it did not consider how the followers perceive the leader's attitudes and his responses, nor the effect of the environment which is unique to each situation.

### *Situational Theory*

- In this theory, a leader is the product of a given situation and his behavior may in fact, vary from one situation to another.
- There are four situational variables that affect the performance of leadership. They are:
  1. Difference between culture.
  2. Difference between individuals.
  3. Difference between jobs.
  4. Difference between organizations.
- A person may be a leader in one situations and a follower in other situations because the type leadership required–depends on the situation.
- The situational theory states that the leader must have insight and flexibility. She/he must be aware of and assess the force in herself/himself the group members and the situation.

### *Transactional/Transformational Theory*

- This theory describes the relationship between leaders and followers.
- New concepts such as empowerment, inspiration, motivation and social learning are present.
- This refers to a process whereby the leader attends to the needs and motives of followers so that interaction raises to high levels of motivation and morality.

## IN-SERVICE EDUCATION

### Definition

*'In-service education* is a planned educational experience provided in the job setting and closely identified with services in order to help person perform more effectively as a person and as a worker'.

### Needs/Purposes/Importance of In-service Education

- Social changes and scientific advancement.
- Changes and advancement in the field of service.
- Increased the demand of nursing services.
- Consumer demand quality care.
- Rapid changes in medical and nursing practice create a need for in-service education.
- Increase number of the people seeking health care as the population enlarges makes it necessary for the nurses to function at her highest potential as quickly as possible.
- As health care delivery system become more complex, the need for continues skill training also increased.

### Types of In-service Education/Approaches to In-service Education

- Centralized approach
- Decentralized approach
- Combined or coordinated approach

### Components/Organization of In-service Education or Different Areas of In-service Education Programs

These areas are:

### *Orientation*

This introduces a new employee to the basic aspects of her/his job. If a new staff is appointed, the supervisor will discuss with her/his, the policies, procedures, objectives, standing orders, etc.

- By orientation, an employee should become familiar with the department or unit where he/she will be working. He should be made familiar with the routines of the unit, his responsibilities to carry out his functions, the line of communication, his place in the organizational structure, the organizational policies, operation of any equipment that he has to handle while on duty etc. In many instances, a printed booklet containing all the relevant information's is given to the new employee.

### *Skill Training*

- Skill are a level of proficiency. Skill training may range from known to unknown, simple to complex or general to specific. It provides close relationship between good nursing care and good ward management. It helps the new employee to develop knowledge and skill to do a particular task. And also fills any gap in her/his knowledge of total patient care by keeping her aware of changing methods and new techniques through instruction, demonstration and supervized practice.

- This is concerned with developing expert technical or manual skills, communication and helps the personnel to perform their functions effectively.

*Types of Skills*

- Psychomotor skill
- Cognitive skill
- Teaching skills
- Affective skill
- Communication skill
- Supervisory skills

### Leadership and Management Development

The staff should have skills in leadership and management in order to guide a new employee in caring outpatient care activities. At present the hospitals are recognizing the development of leadership and management qualities among the staff members.

### Continuing Education

In-service education is a part of continuing education, it is defined as those activities which contribute to the nurse's development in the areas of knowledge, skills and attitudes.

- Continuing education helps in the development of the three domains (cognitive, affective, and psychomotor) as well as leadership and management skills. This is especially helpful since the nurse is an auxiliary personnel working under her.

*Need of Continuing Education*

- To ensure safe and effective nursing care
- Changing health care delivery system
- Development of nurses by updating their knowledge
- For career advancement
- Professional are altered as society changes and as technologies emerge
- To acquire specialized skill for professional
- Meet the need of the population
- Acquire specialized skills of personnel and meet technologic adjuncts
- Prepare in administrative and leadership positions
- Shape their own destiny.

### Methods of In-service Education

- Ward teaching
- Discussion
- Demonstration
- Health team conference
- Individual conference
- Workshop
- Seminars
- Panel discussion
- Field trips

## MULTIPLE CHOICE QUESTIONS

**1. Characteristics of administration EXCEPT:**
(a) It is a profession (b) It is social and dynamic
(c) It is universal (d) It is continuous process

**2. The principle of unity of command implies ______.**
(a) Employees should receive orders from one superior only
(b) Authority from the highest executive to the lowest one
(c) Scale to measure productivity
(d) In union is strength

**3. Who is known as the 'Father of Scientific Management'?**
(a) Henry Fayol (b) FW Taylor
(c) Peter F Drucker (d) Philip Kotler

**4. Who is known as the 'Spiritual father' of behavioral science?**
(a) McGregor (b) FW Taylor
(c) Peter F Drucker (d) Chester I Barnard

**5. Henry Fayol suggested the following principles of administration EXCEPT:**
(a) Authority and responsibility
(b) Scalar chain
(c) Division of work
(d) Delegation

**6. Scalar chain denotes______.**
(a) A process of production
(b) Authority from the highest executive to the lowest one
(c) Scale to measure productivity
(d) Emphasizes the need for teamwork

**7. Unity of command implies ______.**
(a) In union there is strength
(b) Each employee/worker should receive orders from only one superior or manager.
(c) Group to be assigned the responsibility of commanding
(d) None

**8. Collaboration in providing care to a group of patients under the direction of a professional nurse is:**
(a) Case method
(b) Primary method
(c) Team method
(d) Modular method

**9. One of the following is not a tool used for supervision:**
(a) Listening
(b) Staff meetings
(c) In-service education program
(d) Rating scale

10. **Negotiation between employer and employee is called:**
(a) Checklist (b) Nursing round
(c) Modular method (d) Collective bargaining

11. **'Management is the art of getting things done through and with people in formally organized groups' is stated by__________.**
(a) Kimball (b) Harold D Koontz
(c) S Vance (d) Theo Haimann

12. **Which of the following has not been included in Fayol's principles of management?**
(a) Division of labor (b) Scalar chain
(c) Espirit de Corps (d) MBO

13. **Authority refers to the____________.**
(a) Right to use power
(b) Right to command
(c) Right to perform duty
(d) Right to grant orders

14. **Philosophy is a Greek word which means:**
(a) Understanding nature
(b) A way of thinking
(c) A set of standards
(d) Love of wisdom

15. **Concentration of authority at or near the top level is called ______________.**
(a) Span of control (b) Hierarchy
(c) Centralization (d) Decentralization

16. **Fourteen principles of administration were identified by________________.**
(a) Frederic Winslow Taylor
(b) Henry Fayol
(c) Luther Gullick
(d) Lyndal Urwick

17. **Espirit de corps refers to____________.**
(a) Sense of belonging
(b) Security
(c) Promotion of production
(d) Unity of direction

18. **Professor Luther Gullick summed up certain principles or elements of administration in the word:**
(a) POSTCORB (b) POSDOORD
(c) POSDCORB (d) POSDCARB

19. **The right to decide, command and perform the assigned responsibility is:**
(a) Command (b) Authority
(c) Ability (d) Responsibility

20. **The famous acronym 'POSDCORD' was condensed by___________.**
(a) Luther Gullick (b) Henry Fayol
(c) Max Weber (d) Mary Follett

21. **Eight types of standards of management have been identified by__________.**
(a) Koont and Weitrich
(b) Edward Deming
(c) Glasser
(d) George

22. **The most important function of administration is____.**
(a) Commanding (b) Controlling
(c) Coordinating (d) Planning

23. **Management means____________.**
(a) Designing
(b) Maintaining the environment
(c) Getting the job done by people
(d) Taking disciplinary action

24. **Nursing philosophy is a statement of______.**
(a) Objectives of nursing program
(b) Institution's mission, vision and policies
(c) Long-term goals
(d) Values and beliefs of nurse

25. **The word administration is derived from the Latin word______________.**
(a) admin+ister (b) ad+minister
(c) ad+ministraire (d) adam+stir

26. **Administrators who are 'Hollowmen' use the following principle of administration:**
(a) Bureaucracy (b) Morale
(c) Specialism (d) Self-administration

27. **Administraire means______________.**
(a) Care (b) 'Look after'
(c) 'Manage' (d) 'Serve'

28. **Management means__________.**
(a) Designing
(b) Maintaining the environment
(c) Decision-making
(d) Getting job through people

29. **Management is inclusive of__________.**
(a) People (b) Money
(c) Material (d) Man, money and material

30. **Administrative functions of organization deals with:**
(a) Planning and organization
(b) POSDCORB
(c) Directing and leading
(d) Planning only

31. **Persons right to make decisions and take action without approval by higher administration is:**
(a) Status (b) Authority
(c) Power (d) Leader

32. **'Best management' is a true science was believed by___.**
(a) FW Taylor (b) Henry Fayol
(c) Max Weber (d) Mary Elton

33. **Administraire in Latin means to_______.**
(a) Feel for people
(b) Care for people
(c) Deal with people
(d) Mix with people

34. **Administration has to do with getting things done with defined objectives is stated by:**
(a) Luther Gullick
(b) Goel
(c) Pfiffner
(d) Nigro

**35. An employee should receive orders from one superior only, this is known as______.**
(a) Centralization (b) Unity of command
(c) Delegation (d) Authority

**36. Administration is defined as________.**
(a) Enabling process (b) Controlling
(c) Managerial (d) Evaluating

**37. The principle process of task planning, coordinating, motivating and controlling others towards a specific objective is called________.**
(a) Organization (b) Planning
(c) Management (d) Budgeting

**38. Sound decision-making requires all of the skills excepts:**
(a) Critical thinking skills
(b) Interpersonal skills
(c) Judgmental skills
(d) Technical skills

**39. The management theory which focuses on division of work and task specialization is given by:**
(a) Frederick Taylor (b) Henry Fayol
(c) Herbert Simon (d) Alvin Toffler

**40. 'Espirit de corps' refers to________.**
(a) Sense of achievement
(b) Sense of humor
(c) Sense of belonging
(d) Sense of morality

**41. Nature of administration is________.**
(a) Universal (b) Transferable
(c) Personal (d) None of the above

**42. Father of modern management is________.**
(a) McGregor (b) Elton Mayo
(c) FW Taylor (d) Henry Fayol

**43. Max Weber proposed the following word for ideal organization.**
(a) Bureaucracy (b) Leadership
(c) POSDCARB (d) Organization

**44. The father of nuclear management theory is:**
(a) Henry Fayol (b) Elton Mayo
(c) McGregor (d) FW Taylor

**45. Management skills are essential for viability of modern day organizations. Which of the following is not a managerial skill?**
(a) Human (b) Technical
(c) Conceptual (d) Feedback

**46. Who is acknowledge as 'Father of Modern Management' theory?**
(a) Henry Fayol (b) Elton Mayo
(c) McGregor (d) FW Taylor

**47. For smooth functioning of nursing service in the hospital, the top level nurse manager requires more of________.**
(a) Technical skill
(b) Social skill
(c) Decision-making skill
(d) Political skill

**48. All are characteristics of Management EXCEPT:**
(a) It is a science and art
(b) Is not distinct from ownership
(c) Has techniques that are universally applicable
(d) Is a profession

**49. The management theory which focuses on division of work and task specialization is given by:**
(a) Frederick Taylor (b) Henry Fayol
(c) Herbert Simon (d) Alvin Toffler

**50. Authority refers to the________.**
(a) Right to use and abuse power
(b) Right to command
(c) Right to perform duty
(d) Right to grant rewards

**51. At the top level of management which of the following skills are specially valuable?**
(a) Technical (b) Human
(c) Conceptual (d) Design

**52. ERT is a________.**
(a) Non-budgetary control method
(b) Budgetary control method
(c) Motivational technique
(d) None of the above

**53. Process involved in staffing are________.**
(a) Manpower planning
(b) Recruitment and selection
(c) Job analysis
(d) All of the above

**54. Assessment of the quality of nursing care or evaluation of the quality of patient care is:**
(a) Organization (b) Training
(c) Evaluation (d) Nursing audit

**55. The term MBO, i.e. management by objectives was coined by:**
(a) Elton Mayo (b) Henry Fayol
(c) Peter F Drucker (d) FW Taylor

**56. Scheduling can be best described as:**
(a) Process of formulating goals and objectives
(b) Calculation of breakeven point
(c) Evaluation of alternate course of action
(d) As a patterns of on-off duty hours for employees in a particular unit.

**57. Daily balance sheet chart is also known as________.**
(a) Gantt Chart (b) Standard Control Chart
(c) Break even chart (d) None

**58. Who coined the phrase 'management by objectives'?**
(a) Henry Fayol
(b) Prof Peter F Drucker
(c) BO Smith
(d) JJ Gilbert

**59. The nursing superintendent of a hospital will be considered a________.**
(a) Top level manager
(b) First level manager
(c) Middle level manager
(d) Intermediate level manager

60. **Executive functions are basically related to________.**
(a) Planning (b) Reporting
(c) Implementing (d) All of the above

61. **The INC recommendations for clinical supervision of students in a ward by a clinical instructor is________.**
(a) 1:10 (b) 1:15
(c) 1:20 (d) 1:5

62. **Quality assurance refers to________.**
(a) Standards of practice (b) Adequacy of care
(c) Rating (d) Measurement scale

63. **A written order for supplies and equipment or for their repair is______.**
(a) Inventory (b) Indent
(c) Requisition (d) quotation

64. **Permanent articles or items are called as________.**
(a) Supplies (b) Stock
(c) Equipment (d) Resources

65. **Which of the following is a principle in planning duty roster?**
(a) Consider staff's need as top priority
(b) Distribute equal number of staff in a shift
(c) Balance junior and senior staff
(d) List names in alphabetic order

66. **The essential feature of a budget are_____.**
(a) Flexibility
(b) Support of top management
(c) Product of joint venture
(d) All the above

67. **A process of securing application to fill vacant position is called________**
(a) Appointment (b) Recruitment
(c) Interview (d) Selection

68. **An itemized list of available supplies is known as_____.**
(a) Value analysis (b) Inventory
(c) Cost analysis (d) Storage

69. **Objective description of behavior of an employee recorded on a form is known as________**
(a) Inventory (b) Management report
(c) Confidential report (d) Anecdotal record

70. **Monitoring of the budget process is referred as______.**
(a) Audit (b) Cost analysis
(c) Cost expenditure (d) Inventory record

71. **Manpower planning include:**
(a) Labor relations (b) Gratuity benefits
(c) Placement (d) Health services

72. **Nursing audit are all EXCEPT:**
(a) Retrospective analysis
(b) Concurrent audit
(c) Prospective approach
(d) Reviewing the patients record and care plan

73. **Analytical decision involves a problem with________.**
(a) A large number of decision variables
(b) A limited number of decision variables where the outcome of each alternative is known
(c) A limited number of decision variables
(d) None of the above

74. **Performance of a job by a competent and best suited person based on his specialization is:**
(a) Job performance (b) Quality assurance
(c) Division of labor (d) Job detailment

75. **A plan that uses numerical data and predicts an organizations activities for a set time is known as:**
(a) Income (b) Expenditure
(c) Audit (d) Budget

76. **The main objectives of staffing is:**
(a) To provide continuous quality of nursing care
(b) Utilize talents and skill
(c) To recruit staff
(d) To promote orientation to new employee

77. **Quality control process has specific steps:**
(a) Establishment of control standards or criteria
(b) Determine ways to collect information
(c) Collect and analyze the information
(d) All of the above

78. **A Budget is:**
(a) An element of management
(b) A plan for allocation of resources
(c) A blueprint of finance resources
(d) A control of financial expenditure

79. **Inventory refers to:**
(a) List of articles borrowed from central supply
(b) List of articles for repair or replacement
(c) Detailed list of all articles in the ward
(d) List of obsolete materials

80. **Source of income in budgeting term is called:**
(a) Capitation (b) Cash flow
(c) Profit (d) Revenue

81. **The factor which influence quality of nursing care are:**
(a) Quantity of influence and type of hospital
(b) Type of service, turnover of patient
(c) Quality of supervision and experience of nurses
(d) (a) and (c)

82. **The process by which actual performance of staff and people is guided towards organization goal is:**
(a) Directing (b) Supervising
(c) Co-coordinating (d) Performing

83. **The word 'budget' literally means:**
(a) Cloth (b) Leather bag
(c) Book (d) Accounts

84. **An operational plan for a definite period is:**
(a) Staffing (b) Planning
(c) Co-ordination (d) Budget

85. **Material management means:**
(a) Management of supplies and equipments
(b) Storage of supplies
(c) Indenting of equipments
(d) Using equipments during inspection

86. **The purpose of staffing is to:**
(a) Utilize talents and skills
(b) Recruit many staff to work
(c) Provide continuous quality care
(d) Provide orientation to staff

**87. Advantages of nursing audit are all EXCEPT:**
(a) It can be used as a method of measurement in all areas of nursing
(b) It is a simple scoring system
(c) Assess the quality of nursing care rendered
(d) It can be used for judging personal qualities of a person

**88. The most effective skill needed for planning is:**
(a) Application of strategies
(b) Decision-making
(c) Setting objectives
(d) Using cognitive process

**89. Characteristics of planning is all of the following EXCEPT:**
(a) Primary and futuristic
(b) Flexibility
(c) Rigidity
(d) Dynamism and unity

**90. Steps of staffing includes all EXCEPT:**
(a) Planning for staff
(b) Recruitment and selection
(c) Placement of staff, training and development
(d) Counseling and guidance

**91. Directing means:**
(a) Telling people what to do the best
(b) Seeing the ability of a person
(c) Assigning the task
(d) Corresponding procedures

**92. Who coined the phrase 'management by objective (MBO)?**
(a) Wendell L (b) Henry Fayol
(c) Elton Mayo (d) P Drucker

**93. The nurse patient ratio in intensive care unit is:**
(a) 1:1 (b) 1:2
(c) 1:3 (d) 1:4

**94. Choosing a course of action from all available alternatives for accomplishing the desired result is:**
(a) Directing (b) Decision
(c) Planning (d) Analyzing

**95. Steps in managerial decision making process is:**
(a) Conduct meeting (b) Define problem
(c) Evaluate (d) Counsel

**96. Budget is a formal expression of:**
(a) Implemented plan (b) Anticipatory plan
(c) Policies/objectives (d) Strategic plan

**97. Systematic and official examination of records and processes to evaluate performance is known as:**
(a) Accounts (b) Audit
(c) Standards (d) Examination

**98. The unserviceable equipment which is certified beyond repair is disposed off by:**
(a) Local destruction (b) Auction
(c) Condemnation (d) Selling

**99. The technique that involves analyzing all items in inventory on the basis of annual usage time cost is:**
(a) ABC Analysis (b) VED Analysis
(c) XYZ Analysis (d) FSN Analysis

**100. Inventory control is an element of:**
(a) Personnel management
(b) Financial management
(c) Material management
(d) Institutional management

**101. Source of income in budgeting terms is called as:**
(a) Capitation (b) Cash flow
(c) Profit (d) Revenue

**102. Permanent articles or items are called as:**
(a) Supplies (b) Equipment
(c) Stock (d) Resources

**103. Inventory refers to:**
(a) List of articles borrowed from a central supply
(b) List of articles for repair or replacement
(c) Detailed list of all articles on the ward, their specifications and standard quality
(d) Lists of obsolete materials

**104. A written order for supplies and equipment or for their repair is:**
(a) Inventory (b) Indent
(c) Requisition (d) Quotation

**105. The budget which estimates the cost of direct labor necessary to meet the agency's objective is known as:**
(a) Cash budget (b) Personnel budget
(c) Flexible budget (d) Operating budget

**106. The budget which is organized in terms of functions rather than items of expenditure is known as:**
(a) Performance budget (b) Cash budget
(c) Flexible budget (d) Zero budget

**107. Quality assurance refers to:**
(a) Standards of practice (b) Measurement scales
(c) Ratings (d) Adequacy of care

**108. The team 'JCAHO' stands for:**
(a) Joint commission and association of health care organization
(b) Joint-commission for accreditation of health care organization
(c) Joint council on accreditation of health care organization
(d) Join council for academy of hospitals

**109. A systematic, sequential process of choosing among alternatives and putting choice into action is:**
(a) Creativity (b) Decision-making
(c) Linear programming (d) Innovation

**110. MBO—management by objective is an excellent tool that can be used in:**
(a) Managerial supervision
(b) Organizational review
(c) Quality and standards
(d) Performance appraisal

**111. Daily balance sheet chart is also known as:**
(a) Gantt chart
(b) Growth chart
(c) Standard control chart
(d) None

**112. Process of setting formal guidelines and constraints for the behavior of the firm is known as:**
(a) Organizing (b) Planning
(c) Recording (d) Directing

**113. MBO stands for:**
(a) Management budget organisation
(b) Management by objective
(c) Management because objectives
(d) None of the above

**114. PERT Stands for:**
(a) Program evaluation and review technique
(b) Program experiment and relation technique
(c) Program evaluation and rotation technique
(d) None of the above

**115. VED Stand for:**
(a) Vital, estimated, desirable
(b) Valuable estimated, desirable
(c) Vital, essential, desirable
(d) Valuable, essential, desirable

**116. ABC method of inventory control stands for:**
(a) Always, behind, central
(b) Always, better, control
(c) Always, better, central
(d) None of the above

**117. First in–First out is a method in:**
(a) Budgeting (b) Inventory control
(c) Directing (d) Organizing

**118. For controlling the quality of nursing care this is essential:**
(a) Audit (b) Nursing audit
(c) PERT (d) MBO

**119. Activities which have distinctive mission and time schedule are known as:**
(a) Policy's (b) Procedures
(c) Programs (d) Rules

**120. Items based on controls can be monitored by the _____ analysis.**
(a) VED (b) SDE
(c) ABC (d) FSN

**121. Planning is_____________oriented.**
(a) Past (b) Future
(c) Present (d) None of the above

**122. Planning makes it possible to make optimum use of the available resources of:**
(a) Money (b) Materials
(c) Machines (d) All the above

**123. Planning provides for ___________.**
(a) Co-ordination (b) Co-operation
(c) Motivation (d) Organization

**124. ___________helps the enterprize to know whether the plan has been successfully implemented.**
(a) Control
(b) Motivation
(c) Decision-making
(d) None of the above

**125. The various elements of planning are____.**
(a) Policy (b) Procedures
(c) Rules (d) All the above

**126. ___________specifies time limits within which activities are to be completed.**
(a) Schedule (b) Budgets
(c) Projects (d) None of the above

**127. ___________ is a process of selection from a set of alternative courses of action.**
(a) Communication (b) Decision-making
(c) Planning (d) Staffing

**128. Decisions taken by single individual is known as ___________.**
(a) Individual decision (b) Group decision
(c) Policy decision (d) Operating decision

**129. Span of supervision:**
(a) Authority and responsibility
(b) Emphasizes the need for teamwork
(c) Each employee should receive orders from only one superior or manager
(d) It is the number of subordinates that a manager or a supervisor can effectively supervise.

**130. Hierarchy denotes:**
(a) In union is strength
(b) Rule or control of higher to lower
(c) Technique for maintaining security in an organization
(d) Scales to measure productivity

**131. Delegation denotes:**
(a) Concentration of authority at or near the top level
(b) Assigning responsibility and authority to a co-workers
(c) Emphasizes the need for teamwork
(d) As a patterns of on-off duty hours for employees in a particular unit

**132. One of them is a extra neural function of a hospital:**
(a) Restoration
(b) Education
(c) In patient services
(d) Mobile clinic service

**133. Effective use of hospital infection control will include all EXCEPT:**
(a) Good handwashing
(b) Visitors should be allowed freely
(c) Good dietary services
(d) Developing sense of awareness in patients

**134. The minimum number of beds prescribed for a district hospital is:**
(a) 500 (b) 200
(c) 50 (d) 6

**135. The hospitals run by State or Central Government are come under the category of:**
(a) Voluntary hospital
(b) Public hospital
(c) Private hospital
(d) Trust hospital

**136. An organizational chart provides:**
(a) Information about hospital activities
(b) Information about various departments of the hospital
(c) Lines of authority and channels of communication
(d) Activities of the Managing Director

**137. The ward supervisor is directly responsible to:**
(a) The Medical Director
(b) The Ward Incharge
(c) The Nursing Superintendent
(d) The Finance Manager

**138. Nursing superintendent is responsible for:**
(a) Maintaining ward inventory
(b) Assisting in various ward procedures
(c) Cleanliness of the ward
(d) Administration of the nursing personnel in the hospital

**139. The formal line of authority and communication in an organization is called:**
(a) Responsibility (b) Chain of command
(c) Unity of control (d) Unity of direction

**140. The hospital infection can be best controlled by:**
(a) Maintaining good hospital hygiene and following aseptic techniques
(b) Increasing class IV staff
(c) Increasing supply of phenol
(d) Conduct surveys

**141. Functions of the hospital include all EXCEPT:**
(a) Patient Care
(b) Diagnosis and treatment
(c) Increasing the death census
(d) Medical and nursing research

**142. Any organization broadest at the base and tapering towards the top is known as:**
(a) Direction (b) Hierarchy
(c) Structure (d) Pointer

**143. The number of subordinates a supervisor can effectively supervise is known as:**
(a) Span of control (b) Commanding
(c) Directing (d) Leading

**144. The standard of a hospital can be measured by ______.**
(a) Number of staff
(b) Number of specialized services
(c) Interpersonal relationships
(d) Quality of care received by the patients

**145. Reviewing the sterilization techniques in the hospital setting is the responsibility of:**
(a) Discipline Control Committee
(b) Infection
(c) Welfare Committee
(d) Waste Management Committee

**146. The formal line of authority and communication in an organization is called:**
(a) Chain of command (b) Responsibility
(c) Unity of command (d) Unity of direction

**147. The number of people directly reporting to any one manager or officer is known as:**
(a) Span of control (b) Staffing
(c) Scalar chain (d) Line organization

**148. The number of people directly reporting to any one manager or officer is known as:**
(a) Span of control (b) Staffing
(c) Scalar chain (d) Line organization

**149. Formal relationship in an organization is based on:**
(a) Friendship
(b) Peer groups
(c) Authority on subordinates
(d) Rules and regulations

**150. Teaching hospital's bed strength is:**
(a) 500 and above (b) 200–300
(c) 50 and above (d) 30–50

**151. What is the process of assessing staff members?**
(a) Peer review
(b) Re-evaluation
(c) Performance appraisal
(d) Evaluation

**152. Use of unskilled personal to deliver the nursing care by allotting specific nursing skills is known as ______.**
(a) Case method (b) Functional nursing
(c) Team nursing (d) None of the above

**153. Assignment of one or two patients in a specified period of time to a nurse is called______.**
(a) Case method (b) Functional method
(c) Primary nursing (d) None of the above

**154. The word 'discipline' come from the ______ term 'disciplina' which means teaching, learning and growing.**
(a) Greek (b) Latin
(c) English (d) French

**155. The authoritative direction of the work of one's subordinate is called______.**
(a) Evaluation (b) Administration
(c) Management (d) Supervision

**156. Each nurse is given total responsibility for planning, execution and evaluation of nursing services for a small case load of 4–6 patients is known as:**
(a) Functional method (b) Team method
(c) Primary nursing (d) Case method of nursing

**157. Acquainting staff with the existing work environment is known as ______.**
(a) Orientation (b) Continuing education
(c) Skill training (d) Leadership training

**158. Orientation programs are conducted during the ______ phase of workers.**
(a) Working (b) Beginning
(c) Leaving (d) Concluding

**159. The activities of staff development are all EXCEPT:**
(a) Recruitment (b) Induction training
(c) Job orientation (d) In-service education

**160. A factor causing in-effective supervision is ______.**
(a) Listening carefully
(b) Possessing leadership
(c) Failure to understand policies
(d) General and loose supervision

**161. In-service education refers to ______.**
(a) An individual training program
(b) Planned education program provided in the job setting
(c) Continued program of education
(d) Planned instructional training program

**162. Sources of nursing care standards are:**
(a) Professional organization
(b) Licensing bodies
(c) Health care agencies
(d) All of the above

**163. The planned educational experience provided in a job setting is:**
(a) Curricular education (b) In-service education
(c) Primary education (d) Specialized education

**164. Halo effect, central tendency error and self-aggrandizing effect are some of the ______ of performance appraisals.**
(a) Nature (b) Philosophy
(c) Problems (d) Benefits

**165. Continuous evaluation of nursing care can be achieved by:**
(a) Promotion
(b) Transfer
(c) Analysis of accidental report
(d) Orientation of staff

**166. A clinical, scientific, administrative and legal document relating to the nursing care given to individual and family or community is known as:**
(a) Nursing report (b) Nursing record
(c) Nursing diaries (d) Nursing audit

**167. The activities of staff development are all EXCEPT:**
(a) Recruitment (b) Induction training
(c) Job orientation (d) In-service education

**168. The records maintained by the nursing colleges are all these EXCEPT:**
(a) Admission (b) Patient record
(c) Leave record (d) Academic record

**169. A process of securing application to fill vacant position is the hospital:**
(a) Appointment
(b) Recruitment
(c) Interview
(d) Selection

**170. Nursing rounds are done to:**
(a) Introduce the nursing superintended to all patients
(b) Make specific observation of patient care and maintain high standard of care
(c) Visit a few patients in the hospital
(d) Observe the cleanliness of the ward

**171. Important advantages of staff development program is:**
(a) Development talents and abilities in an individual
(b) Increasing skill
(c) Giving orientation
(d) Have continuous education

**172. Purposes of evaluation:**
(a) Define objectives
(b) Develop more reliable and valid instrument for measurement
(c) Give direction
(d) (a) and (b)

**173. Staff development activities include the following EXCEPT:**
(a) Job orientation
(b) In-service education
(c) Continuing education
(d) Performance evaluation

**174. Employee referrals may be used for ______.**
(a) Clinical teaching assignment
(b) Recruitment
(c) Hospital organization
(d) Budgeting

**175. An evaluative instrument should have all the following EXCEPT:**
(a) Objectivity (b) Validity
(c) Reliability (d) Transparency

**176. Nursing Audit is done by:**
(a) Checking records of patients maintained by nurses
(b) Patient turnover and mortality statistics
(c) Length of stay of patients
(d) Checking manpower supply

**177. Delegation of duties and responsibilities is effective when it is:**
(a) From senior to subordinate
(b) In accordance with staff position
(c) Needed only
(d) In accordance with experience and ability of individual

**178. Attitude of a student is assessed by:**
(a) Check list (b) Analogy
(c) Rating scale (d) Assignment

**179. Progress or gains made by the participant and the program is measured using the technique of:**
(a) Summative evaluation
(b) Formative evaluation
(c) Diagnostic evaluation
(d) Test evaluation

**180. An agency record of an accident or unusual occurrence is an:**
(a) Unusual report (b) Accident report
(c) Incident report (d) Agency report

**181. Showcase of open a new service or program is one method of recruitment. It is known as:**
(a) Employee referral (b) Open house
(c) Career-day program (d) Interviewing

**182. Pre-employment tests includes tests in all EXCEPT:**
(a) General ability (b) Personality
(c) Trade (d) Socialization

**183. Delivery of individualized nursing care to clients by a group of nurses led by a professional nurse is known as______.**
(a) Primary nursing
(b) Team nursing
(c) Group nursing
(d) Case management

**184. A permanent written communication of a patient's health status is a:**
(a) Report (b) Record
(c) Assignment (d) Care plan

**185. Major responsibilities connected with nursing service administration are all EXCEPT:**
(a) Planning total patient care
(b) General supervision
(c) Treatment
(d) Public relations maintenance

**186. All types of evaluation methods EXCEPT:**
(a) Eye wash evaluation
(b) White wash evaluation
(c) Sub-merged evaluation
(d) Sub-total evaluation

**187. Types of control in administration implies all EXCEPT:**
(a) Primary (b) Secondary
(c) Concurrent (d) Post-action

**188. The ward supervisor is directly responsible to the:**
(a) Director
(b) Medical superintendant
(c) Nursing superintendant
(d) Hospital trustee

**189. Records and reports are important in nursing service as they:**
(a) Serve as documents of patients history of illness
(b) Assist in the continuity of rendering care
(c) Serve as evidence to support legal implications
(d) All of the above

**190. The purpose of evaluating a student nurse is:**
(a) To clarify and define educational objectives
(b) To facilitate learning in clinical practice
(c) To assist the student in work
(d) To provide a sense of accomplishment

**191. One of the pre-requisites in ward management is:**
(a) Knowledge of the ward
(b) Knowledge of names of machines
(c) Knowledge of all investigations
(d) Knowledge of research process

**192. When the appraisal allows one or two positive aspects of assessment of the employee unduly influence all other aspects of employees performance, this is:**
(a) Horn effect
(b) Halo effect
(c) Average effect
(d) Central tendency trap

**193. An evaluation done at the end to assess the outcome of the program is called:**
(a) Formative evaluation
(b) Summative evaluation
(c) Facilitative evaluation
(d) Critical evaluation

**194. What protects the doctors and nurses in case of legal issues?**
(a) Notes (b) Books
(c) Records (d) Diaries

**195. The process of acquainting a new worker with work environment so that she can relate quickly to new surrounding is:**
(a) Orientation (b) Education
(c) Promotion (d) Introduction

**196. The process of filling up new post and replacement of previously established post which fall vacant is called:**
(a) Appointment (b) Recruitment
(c) Placement (d) Promotion

**197. Penalty for minor misconduct includes all of the following, EXCEPT:**
(a) Warning (b) Demotion to lower post
(c) Fine (d) Suspension up to 4 days

**198. The functional method of patient assignment is advantageous because it enhances:**
(a) Technical skill (b) Patient interaction
(c) Continuous care (d) Relationships

**199. Staff development activities includes all from the following EXCEPT:**
(a) Promotion (b) In-service education
(c) Induction training (d) Continuing education

**200. Absence without permission from the place of work is an act of:**
(a) Misconduct (b) Disobedience
(c) Carelessness (d) Ignorance

**201. Purpose of hospital report is to:**
(a) Evaluate employee (b) Satisfy employee
(c) Satisfy patients (d) Give factual information

**202. Bedside performance of a student nurse can be best assessed by:**
(a) Check list (b) Rating scale
(c) Anecdotal (d) Peer review

**203. In an organization, retirement plans are part of:**
(a) Education (b) Personnel management
(c) Rehabilitation (d) Welfare

**204. Objective of Nursing Service Department is to maintain:**
(a) Conducive environment
(b) Highest quality care
(c) Economy
(d) Relationships

**205. The types of 'control' are all from the followings, EXCEPT:**
(a) Decentralized control
(b) Preliminary control
(c) Concurrent control
(d) Post action control

**206. Rating scales are best used as a tool for:**
(a) Teaching (b) Performance appraisal
(c) Supervising (d) Evaluating

**207. Anecdotal record means ________.**
(a) Legal record
(b) Brief description and incident
(c) Ward teaching record
(d) Research record

**208. Acknowledging the performance of an employee is through the way of:**
(a) Self assessment (b) Performance appraisal
(c) Rewards (d) Appreciation

**209. The conflict which occurs when new values are imposed on the group from outside refers to:**
(a) Interpersonal conflict (b) Intergroup conflict
(c) Intragroup conflict (d) Inter-role conflict

**210. The conflict which occur when an individual belongs to more than one group is:**
(a) Intersender conflict (b) Inter-role conflict
(c) Person-role conflict (d) Intra-sender conflict

**211. Performance budgeting is based on:**
(a) Items of expenditure
(b) Items of investment
(c) Objectives of expenditure
(d) Plan of implementation

**212. Mini-team nursing approach which involves 2–3 members and allows professional nurse planning and co-ordination is:**
(a) Modular nursing (b) Case management
(c) Primary nursing (d) Managed care

**213. Free form review of employee appraisal is otherwise called as:**
(a) Essay appraisal (b) Checklist appraisal
(c) Simple appraisal (d) Forced appraisal

**214. A systematic appraisal of the work of a particular jobs in relation to all jobs in the agency is known as job:**
(a) Summary (b) Evaluation
(c) Description (d) Specification

**215. Which among these reports are not permanent?**
(a) Oral reports (b) Written reports
(c) Service reports (d) Night reports

**216. The principal tool of performance evaluation is:**
(a) Check list (b) Rating scale
(c) Direct observation (d) Anecdotal record

**217. The process directed towards the personal and professional growth of the nurses is:**
(a) In-service education (b) Learning
(c) Induction training (d) Staff development

**218. The optimum (time period) duration for induction training is:**
(a) 7 days (b) 7–10 days
(c) 2–3 days (d) 10–15 days

**219. The theory of human motivation was outlined by:**
(a) Abraham Maslow (b) Kurt Lewin
(c) Elton Mayo (d) Douglas McGregor

**220. The trait theory of leadership was developed by:**
(a) McGregor (b) Kelly
(c) FW Taylor (d) Elton Mayo

**221. Employee motivation is done by:**
(a) Rewarding praise and giving incentives
(b) Stress management
(c) Conflict management
(d) Promotion

**222. The basic purpose of public relation is:**
(a) Students are prepared with adequate skill
(b) Establishment and maintenance of good will
(c) To develop attitude
(d) To have community orientation

**223. Most important aspect of communication is:**
(a) Hearing
(b) Passing on information
(c) Exchange of thoughts, ideas and information
(d) Sending messages

**224. In communication process the sender is called as______.**
(a) Encoder (b) Decoder
(c) Channel (d) Receiver

**225. Downward oral communication includes all EXCEPT:**
(a) Personal instruction (b) Wall posters
(c) Verbal orders (d) Counseling

**226. In democratic leadership, the leader:**
(a) Values individual characteristics and abilities of subordinate
(b) Takes decision and assign all responsibility to himself
(c) Denies responsibility and abdicates authority to the group
(d) Leaves all decision-making to the group

**227. Which of the following type of leadership will the leader dominate and members are submissive?**
(a) Democratic (b) Autocratic
(c) Laissez faire (d) All the above

**228. In communication process the sender is called:**
(a) Encoder (b) Decoder
(c) Channel (d) Receiver

**229. Leadership style characterized by moderate control, motivation, awards, interactive communication, group decision-making and constructive criticism is:**
(a) Automatic (b) Democratic
(c) Laissez-faire (d) Authoritarian

**230. 'Leaders are born, not made' this argument is supported by:**
(a) Situational theory
(b) Leadership contingency model
(c) Managerial grid
(d) Trait theory

**231. The author of motivation-hygiene theory or two factor theory is one among the given motivational theorist. Identify the theorist:**
(a) Victor Vroom (b) Frederick Herzberg
(c) BF Skinner (d) Abraham Maslow

**232. The process of arousing and stimulating interest in the learning activities is known as:**
(a) Cognition (b) Motivation
(c) Participation (d) Interaction

**233. Knowledge is the objective of:**
(a) Psychomotor domain
(b) Cognitive domain
(c) Affective domain
(d) None of the above

**234. An individualized training program planned for a newly appointed employee to acquaint with job responsibility, work place, clients and co-workers is known as:**
(a) Induction training (b) Job orientation
(c) In-service education (d) Legislation

**235. Attitude of a student is assessed by:**
(a) Checklist (b) Analogy
(c) Rating scale (d) Assignment

**236. An activity or performance that requires continuous practice for effective organization of learning experience is:**
(a) Concepts (b) Values
(c) Ideas (d) Skill

**237. The judgmental statement given on the performance of a student is known as________.**
(a) Feedback (b) Assessment
(c) Ongoing assessment (d) Evaluation

**238. The method of evaluation which assess the organization and comprehensive ability of the student is:**
(a) Essay type tests (b) Short answer tests
(c) Objective type tests (d) Multiple choice tests

**239. The main disadvantages of essay type test is__________.**
(a) Objectivity
(b) Subjectivity
(c) Partiality
(d) Halo effect

**240. Evaluation in nursing helps to determine the__________.**
(a) Level of knowledge and comprehension
(b) Level of clinical performance
(c) Level of self-direction in the students
(d) Level of overall development in the students

**241. Which among the following is not a characteristic feature of evaluation in education?**
(a) Evaluation is continuous process
(b) Evaluation is applied to academic and non-academic subjects
(c) Evaluation helps in planning
(d) Evaluation does not include non-academic subjects

**242. The ongoing or systematic assessment of students achievement during the curricular program is known as:**
(a) Summative evaluation
(b) Formative evaluation
(c) Intermittent evaluation
(d) None of the above

**243. Summative evaluation is for the benefit of:**
(a) Current students (b) Current teachers
(c) Future students (d) Future teachers

**244. The planned educational experiences provided in a job setting is:**
(a) Curriculum education
(b) Primary education
(c) In-service education
(d) Specialized education

**245. Acquainting staff with the existing work environment is known as__________.**
(a) Orientation (b) Continuing education
(c) Skill training (d) Leadership training

**246. Orientation programs are conducted during the ________ phase of workers.**
(a) Working (b) Beginning
(c) Leaving (d) Concluding

**247. In-service education refers to________.**
(a) An individual training program
(b) Planned education program provided in the job setting
(c) Continued program of education
(d) Planned instructional training program

**248. Progress or gains made by the participant and the program is measured using the technique of:**
(a) Summative evaluation
(b) Formative evaluation
(c) Diagnostic evaluation
(d) Test evaluation

**249. An evaluation done at the end to assess the outcome of the program is called:**
(a) Formative evaluation
(b) Summative evaluation
(c) Facilitative evaluation
(d) Critical evaluation

**250. Anecdotal record means________.**
(a) Legal record
(b) Brief description and incident
(c) Ward teaching record
(d) Research record

**251. The writing of job description should include:**
(a) Policies (b) Job title
(c) Opinions (d) Grievances

**252. Integration of several parts of an information into an orderly whole to meet an organization goal is:**
(a) Co-operation (b) Organization
(c) Co-ordination (d) Planning

**253. A written record of principal duties and scope of responsibility is:**
(a) Job description (b) Job specification
(c) Job evaluation (d) Job analysis

**254. The first step of job evaluation is:**
(a) Job description
(b) Job analysis
(c) Job specification
(d) Job evaluation

**255. A written statement of the main duties and responsibilities which a job entails is called:**
(a) Job analysis (b) Job description
(c) Job specification (d) Job evaluation

**256. The act of synchronizing people and activities so that they function smoothly in the attainment of organization objective is called:**
(a) Planning (b) Organizing
(c) Co-coordinating (d) Leading

**257. A written record of principle duties and scope of responsibility for a particular job together with the required employee characteristics is called as:**
(a) Job description (b) Job evaluation
(c) Supervision (d) Management

**258. Administrative head of the school of nursing is:**
(a) Medical superintendent
(b) Nursing superintendent
(c) Matron
(d) Principal

**259. Accreditation of a College of Nursing refers to:**
(a) Establishing standards of education
(b) Inspection of the college
(c) Voluntary review process by a professional organization
(d) Quality assurance

**260. A written statement of the main duties and responsibilities which a job entails is called________.**
(a) Job analysis (b) Job description
(c) Job evaluation (d) Job specification

**261. Job description denotes:**
(a) Written statement of the main duties and responsibilities which a job entails
(b) Assigning responsibility and authority to a co-workers
(c) Process that ensures that right kind of people at right places at the right time do things for which they are economically most useful
(d) None of the above

**262. Job specification denotes:**
(a) Personal capacities and inclinations deemed necessary for successful job performance
(b) Written statement of the main duties and responsibilities which a job entails
(c) (a) and (b)
(d) None of the above

**263. The process of determining significant information about the duties, responsibilities and conditions of a specific job is:**
(a) Job analysis (b) Job description
(c) Job specification (d) Job evaluation

**264. The first step in job evaluation is:**
(a) Job description (b) Job analysis
(c) Job specification (d) Job evaluation

**265. TNAI organization, was established in the year _____.**
(a) 1922 (b) 1923
(c) 1932 (d) 1930

**266. UNICEF is established in the year _____.**
(a) 1945 (b) 1947
(c) 1948 (d) 1946

**267. TNAI stands for:**
(a) Trained nurses association of India
(b) Trained nurses agents of India
(c) Trained nurses association of Indonesia
(d) Trained nurses association of America

**268. Which is an important component to carry the nursing profession in a safe and qualitative manner legally?**
(a) Good raport
(b) Standards
(c) Licensure
(d) None of the above

**269. Written oral agreement between two people is called________.**
(a) Agreement (b) Contract
(c) Law suit (d) All of the above

**270. Actions that one should take to promote good is called ________.**
(a) Beneficence (b) Autonomy
(c) Justice (d) Neglect

**271. Keeping one's promise or commitment is called______.**
(a) Beneficence (b) Fidelity
(c) Justice (d) Verocity

**272. Involvement of nurse in handling a non-cooperative patient will result in following________.**
(a) Battery (b) Assault
(c) Defamations (d) Invasion of privacy

**273. Touching a patient or holding a patient without consent is called________.**
(a) Battery (b) Assault
(c) Defamation (d) Meal practice

**274. Fidelity means to keep one's________**
(a) Promises or commitments
(b) Values
(c) Morals
(d) Dignity

**275. The ratio of teacher to student as per Indian Nursing Council for Basic Nursing Course (GNM or BSc Nsg.):**
(a) 10:1 (b) 5:1
(c) 1:10 (d) 1:5

**276. After completion of the course the graduate nurse is expected to register her name is:**
(a) State Nursing Council
(b) Indian Nursing Council
(c) International Nursing Council
(d) Respective Universities

**277. The regulatory body responsible for maintaining standards of nursing education in India is________.**
(a) Trained Nurses Association of India
(b) Indian Nursing Council
(c) Red Cross Society of India
(d) Nursing Department in the University of Health

**278. The licensing board granting nursing registration to trained nurses is:**
(a) Indian Nursing Council
(b) State Nursing Council
(c) Respective Specialty Association
(d) TNAI

**279. A set of ethical principles accepted by all members of a profession for practice is__________.**
(a) Bioethics
(b) Code of ethics
(c) Law
(d) Regulations

**280. Nursing profession till today is not a 100% profession because it lacks one of the following components in its practice. Name the factor lacking:**
(a) Autonomy
(b) Code of ethics
(c) Inadequate personnel
(d) Job satisfaction

**281. 'Consumer Protection Act' came into existence in the year__________.**
(a) 1974 (b) 1980
(c) 1986 (d) 1992

**282. Professional negligence is legally termed as__________.**
(a) Crime (b) Assault
(c) Malpractice (d) Slander

**283. Consent used in an emergency situation when it is impossible to gain informed consent is known as ______.**
(a) Minor consent
(b) Emergency consent
(c) Implied consent
(d) Ordinary consent

**284. The main objectives of the International Council of Nursing__________**
(a) To assist national nurses association
(b) To take up individual nursing matters
(c) To assist nation
(d) To promote the development of strong national nurses association

**285. Which of the following is an example of negligence?**
(a) Medical superintendent
(b) Inadequate staff
(c) Inadequate accreditation
(d) Failure to use aseptic technique

**286. SNA membership is open to all student nurses EXCEPT:**
(a) ANM
(b) Multipurpose health workers (female)
(c) GNM and BSc
(d) Nursing volunteers

**287. Assessment of the quality of nursing care or evaluation of the quality of patient care is called__________.**
(a) In-service education program
(b) Budget
(c) Nursing audit
(d) Collective bargaining

**288. Continuation of education while on service is called __________.**
(a) Planning
(b) Budget
(c) In-service education
(d) Summative evaluation

**289. Implied consent is a consent required in relation to:**
(a) Emergency situation
(b) Physician's performance
(c) Minor client
(d) Routine treatment

**290. The process of determining and maintaining competence in nursing practice to uphold the standard of nursing profession is called:**
(a) Licensure
(b) Registration
(c) Credentialing
(d) Certification

**291. What helps the nurses for promotion avenues, vertical and horizontal mobility in professional life?**
(a) Physical development
(b) Emotional development
(c) Financial development
(d) Career development

**292. Collective bargaining is the negotiation about working conditions and term of employment between:**
(a) Rich and poor
(b) Teacher and student
(c) Principal and teachers
(d) Employer and employee

**293. One of the objectives of collective bargaining is_______**
(a) Giving warning to the authorities
(b) Harmonize labor relationship
(c) Begin strike in an organization
(d) Notifying the authorities that employees began the action

**294. The nurse practitioners role may be categorized in all of the following except: (RPSC 2009)**
(a) Traditional (b) Extended
(c) Expanded (d) Evaluative

**295. The physician fails to inform the patient about the surgical operation and the nurse did not obtained an informed consent before the surgical procedure is done. The acts of the medical team are considered are: (RPSC 2001)**
(a) Malpractice (b) Assault
(c) Breach of duty (d) Battery

**296. __________ is the heart of administrative management.**
(a) Anecdotal record (b) Budget
(c) Planning (d) Nursing audit

**297. Span of control is also called as span of:**
(a) Delegation
(b) Evaluation
(c) Supervision
(d) Nursing audit

## ANSWERS

| 1. | (a) | 41. | (a) | 81. | (d) | 121. | (b) | 161. | (b) | 201. | (d) | 241. | (d) | 281. | (c) |
|---|---|---|---|---|---|---|---|---|---|---|---|---|---|---|---|
| 2. | (a) | 42. | (d) | 82. | (a) | 122. | (d) | 162. | (d) | 202. | (c) | 242. | (b) | 282. | (c) |
| 3. | (b) | 43. | (a) | 83. | (b) | 123. | (a) | 163. | (b) | 203. | (b) | 243. | (c) | 283. | (b) |
| 4. | (d) | 44. | (a) | 84. | (b) | 124. | (a) | 164. | (c) | 204. | (b) | 244. | (c) | 284. | (d) |
| 5. | (d) | 45. | (d) | 85. | (d) | 125. | (d) | 165. | (c) | 205. | (a) | 245. | (a) | 285. | (d) |
| 6. | (b) | 46. | (a) | 86. | (c) | 126. | (a) | 166. | (b) | 206. | (d) | 246. | (b) | 286. | (d) |
| 7. | (b) | 47. | (a) | 87. | (d) | 127. | (b) | 167. | (a) | 207. | (b) | 247. | (b) | 287. | (c) |
| 8. | (c) | 48. | (b) | 88. | (b) | 128. | (a) | 168. | (b) | 208. | (b) | 248. | (b) | 288. | (c) |
| 9. | (a) | 49. | (b) | 89. | (c) | 129. | (d) | 169. | (b) | 209. | (c) | 249. | (b) | 289. | (a) |
| 10. | (d) | 50. | (b) | 90. | (d) | 130. | (b) | 170. | (b) | 210. | (b) | 250. | (b) | 290. | (c) |
| 11. | (b) | 51. | (c) | 91. | (c) | 131. | (b) | 171. | (b) | 211. | (c) | 251. | (b) | 291. | (d) |
| 12. | (d) | 52. | (a) | 92. | (a) | 132. | (d) | 172. | (c) | 212. | (a) | 252. | (c) | 292. | (d) |
| 13. | (c) | 53. | (d) | 93. | (a) | 133. | (b) | 173. | (d) | 213. | (a) | 253. | (a) | 293 | (b) |
| 14. | (b) | 54. | (d) | 94. | (c) | 134. | (b) | 174. | (b) | 214. | (b) | 254. | (b) | 294. | (b) |
| 15. | (c) | 55. | (c) | 95. | (c) | 135. | (b) | 175. | (d) | 215. | (a) | 255. | (b) | 295. | (c) |
| 16. | (b) | 56. | (d) | 96. | (a) | 136. | (c) | 176. | (a) | 216. | (a) | 256. | (c) | 296. | (b) |
| 17. | (a) | 57. | (a) | 97. | (b) | 137. | (b) | 177. | (a) | 217. | (d) | 257. | (a) | 297. | (c) |
| 18. | (c) | 58. | (b) | 98. | (c) | 138. | (d) | 178. | (a) | 218. | (c) | 258. | (d) | | |
| 19. | (b) | 59. | (a) | 99. | (a) | 139. | (b) | 179. | (b) | 219. | (a) | 259. | (a) | | |
| 20. | (a) | 60. | (a) | 100. | (c) | 140. | (a) | 180. | (b) | 220. | (b) | 260. | (b) | | |
| 21. | (d) | 61. | (a) | 101. | (d) | 141. | (c) | 181. | (b) | 221. | (a) | 261. | (a) | | |
| 22. | (c) | 62. | (a) | 102. | (c) | 142. | (b) | 182. | (c) | 222. | (c) | 262. | (a) | | |
| 23. | (c) | 63. | (a) | 103. | (c) | 143. | (a) | 183. | (b) | 223. | (c) | 263. | (a) | | |
| 24. | (d) | 64. | (b) | 104. | (c) | 144. | (d) | 184. | (b) | 224. | (a) | 264. | (b) | | |
| 25. | (c) | 65. | (b) | 105. | (c) | 145. | (a) | 185. | (c) | 225. | (b) | 265. | (a) | | |
| 26. | (a) | 66. | (d) | 106. | (a) | 146. | (a) | 186. | (b) | 226. | (a) | 266. | (d) | | |
| 27. | (d) | 67. | (b) | 107. | (a) | 147. | (d) | 187. | (d) | 227. | (b) | 267. | (a) | | |
| 28. | (d) | 68. | (b) | 108. | (b) | 148. | (d) | 188. | (c) | 228. | (a) | 268. | (c) | | |
| 29. | (d) | 69. | (c) | 109. | (b) | 149. | (d) | 189. | (d) | 229. | (b) | 269. | (b) | | |
| 30. | (b) | 70. | (a) | 110. | (d) | 150. | (a) | 190. | (c) | 230. | (d) | 270. | (a) | | |
| 31. | (b) | 71. | (c) | 111. | (a) | 151. | (c) | 191. | (a) | 231. | (b) | 271. | (b) | | |
| 32. | (a) | 72. | (d) | 112. | (b) | 152. | (b) | 192. | (b) | 232. | (b) | 272. | (b) | | |
| 33. | (b) | 73. | (b) | 113. | (b) | 153. | (a) | 193. | (b) | 233. | (b) | 273. | (a) | | |
| 34. | (a) | 74. | (b) | 114. | (a) | 154. | (b) | 194. | (c) | 234. | (b) | 274. | (a) | | |
| 35. | (b) | 75. | (d) | 115. | (c) | 155. | (d) | 195. | (a) | 235. | (c) | 275. | (c) | | |
| 36. | (c) | 76. | (a) | 116. | (b) | 156. | (c) | 196. | (b) | 236. | (d) | 276. | (a) | | |
| 37. | (c) | 77. | (d) | 117. | (b) | 157. | (a) | 197. | (b) | 237. | (a) | 277. | (b) | | |
| 38. | (d) | 78. | (d) | 118. | (b) | 158. | (b) | 198. | (c) | 238. | (a) | 278. | (d) | | |
| 39. | (b) | 79. | (d) | 119. | (a) | 159. | (a) | 199. | (a) | 239. | (b) | 279 | (d) | | |
| 40. | (c) | 80. | (d) | 120. | (c) | 160. | (d) | 200. | (a) | 240. | (d) | 280. | (d) | | |

# QUICK REVIEW

## Nursing Education Review and Multiple Choice Questions

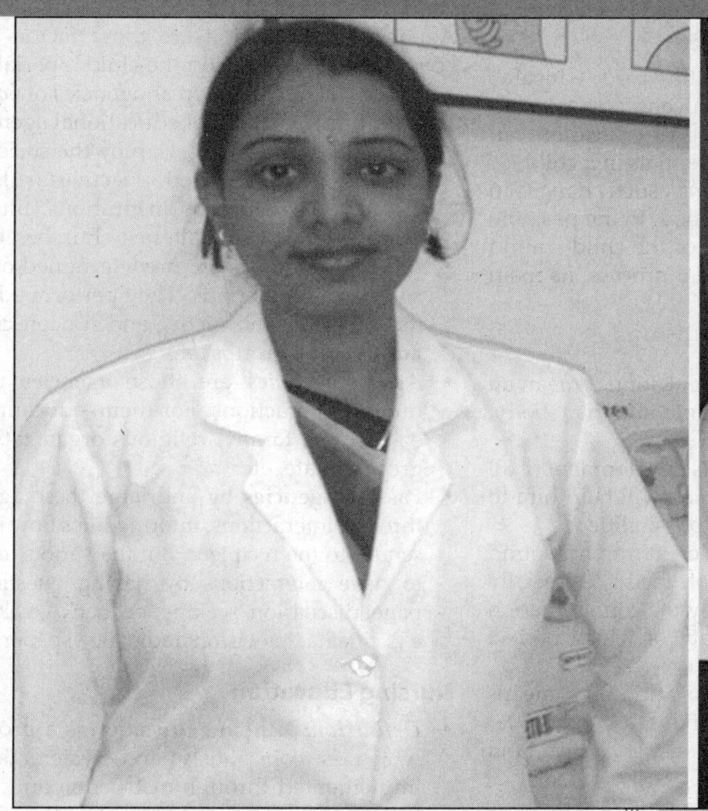

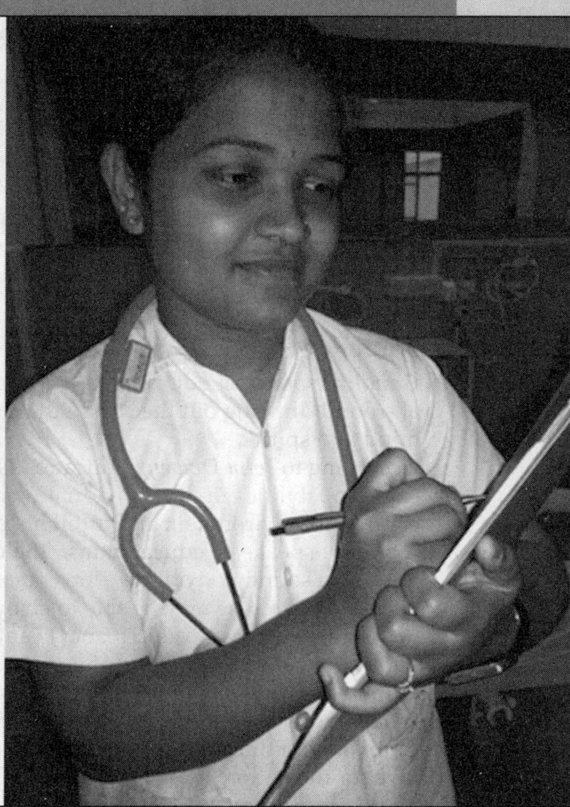

### HIGHLIGHTS

- Education
- Nursing Education
- Learning
- Exhibition
- Programed Instruction/Learning
- Microteaching
- Simulation
- Clinical Teaching Methods
- Brainstorming
- Problem-Based Learning
- Educational Communication Media
- Multiple Choice Questions

# Nursing Education

## EDUCATION

### Meaning

The word education derived from the Latin word 'educate', which means to 'lead out'. The derivation can notes 'growth from the within'. Thus, the roof meaning of education can given as making manifest the inherent potentials in a child.

Education modifies the behavior. It brings such changes in the behavior of the child which is for his good. In the past, the education of a child meant the filling up of the child's mind with stuffed knowledge. Education is social process, its main concern is the modification of behavior.

### Definition

- ***Gandhiji*** speaks of education as, 'By education, I mean an all-round drawing out the best in the child and man–body, mind and spirit'.
- According to ***John Dewey***, 'Education is development of all those capabilities in the individual which will help him to control his environment and fulfill his possibilities'.
- ***Aristotle*** speaks of education as, 'the creation of a sound mind in a sound body. It develops man's faculty especially his mind so that he may be able to enjoy the contemplation of supreme truth, goodness and beauty of which perfect happiness essentially consists.'
- ***Saraswati Dayananda*** considered education as a means for character formation and righteous living.
- ***Chanakya:*** 'Education means training for the country and love for the nation'.
- ***Shankaracharya:*** 'Education is the realization of self'.
- ***Vivekananda:*** 'Education is the manifestation of divine perfection already existing in man'.

### General Aims of Education

- Vocational efficiency
- Knowledge
- Complete living
- Harmonious personality development
- Self-realization
- Cultural development
- Citizenship
- Leisure
- Develop of leadership
- Social and national integration
- Education for modernization
- Education for social, moral and spiritual values
- For scientific temper
- For national cohesion, socialism, secularism and democracy
- Fostering research in all areas of development
- Education for equity.

### Agencies of Education

Agencies of education are those factors which exercise an educational influence on the child. Specialized institutions of education are also known as agencies of education.

Classification/types of educational agencies are as follows:

- ***Formal agencies*** are set up by the society. They have their specific, predetermined objectives, rules and regulations, e.g. schools, religious institutions, museum, recreational centers, library, art galleries, churches, etc.
- ***Informal agencies*** are predetermined objectives, no formal rules and regulations. They perform educational functions incidentally, indirectly and unconsciously, e.g. home, family, play groups, etc.
- ***Active agencies*** are those agencies that work through human interactions. For them, education is a two process, e.g. school, family, religious organizations, society, youth groups, state, etc.
- **Passive agencies** by and large these agencies do not work through interactions. Information's flow in one direction from sender to the recipient. But the various methods are adopted to have interactions by having question-answer sessions, panel discussion, seeking feedback, etc. It is one-way process, e.g. cinema, television, radio, newspapers, magazines, etc.

### Nursing Education

- *Definition:* Nursing education is a professional education which is consciously and systematically planned and implemented through instruction and discipline and aims the harmonious development of the physical, intellectual, social, emotional, spiritual, and esthetic powers or abilities of the student in order to render professional nursing care to people of all ages, in all phases of health and illness, in a variety of settings, in the best or highest possible manner.
- *Meaning:* Nursing education is the 'production aspect' of nursing manpower development and is coordinated with planning and management aspects of nursing manpower, nursing education is also coordinated. The education of professionals in allied sectors of health and development.

Health care personnel of which nursing is usually the largest group, is developed to meet the requirement of the health care system for meeting the health needs of the populations.

#### *Factors Influencing Nursing Education*

- Health needs of the people in the society
- Needs of the student and time
- Philosophy of nursing
- Current trends in general and professional education
- Advances in sciences and technology.

### Objectives of Nursing Education

- To provide nursing who will give expert bedside nursing care in the hospital and home.
- To provide integration of health and social aspects, theory and practice in generalized public health nursing.
- To provide an adequate, sound scientific foundation, intelligent nursing to understand the functioning of body and mind in health and disease.
- To prepare nurses who will be able to work cooperatively with team members who are engaged in health and welfare work.
- To provide opportunities through curricular and extracurricular activities for the full development of the personalities of each individual student.

### Purpose of Nursing Education

- To prepare the nurse who after completion of the educational program is able to plan for and give nursing care and health guidance to individuals and families according to their needs.
- To prepare intellectually enlightened and technically proficient.
- Nurse should be competent in teaching, oriented to community health and research minded.
- Nurse must have the necessary knowledge, principles, skills, and attitudes which are essential to professional nursing practices.
- To develop competent health team members with sound judgment and intellectual and moral enlightenment, profession competence and expertise.

### Historical Development of Nursing Education in India

- In 1871, training for midwives was given for a period of six months with supervised nursing practice.
- In 1918, first lady health visitor course was started in Lady Reading Health School, Mumbai.
- In 1946, 4 years basic nursing training program started at RAK College, New Delhi and CMC Vellore.
- In 1953, postbasic degree program was started in Thiruvananthapuram.
- In 1959, the first master program was started at RAK College of Nursing, New Delhi.
- In 1986, Phil at RAK College of Nursing, New Delhi was started.
- In 1991, the first doctoral program in nursing was established in Institute of Nursing Sciences, MV Shetty Memorial College, Mangalore.

### Traditional Philosophies of Education

The following are the traditional philosophies of education:

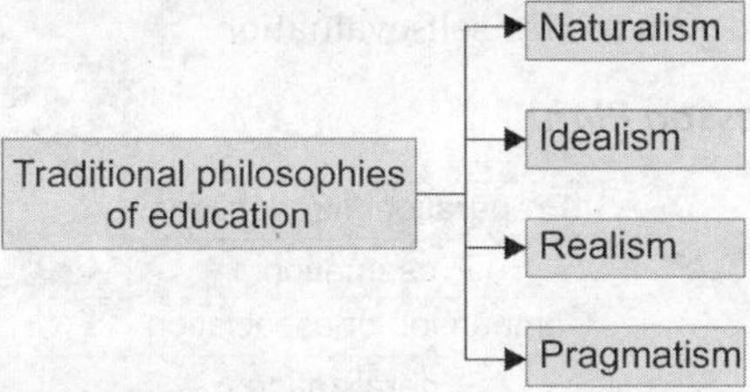


### Modern Contemporary Philosophies of Education

The following are the modern contemporary philosophies of education:

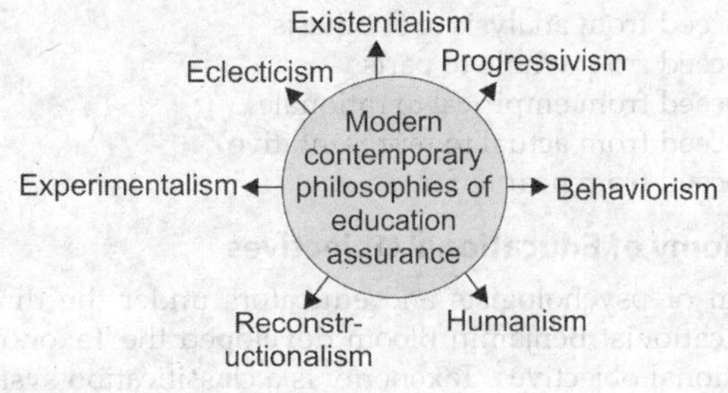


## LEARNING

### Definitions

- Learning is the acquisition of habits, knowledge and attitude. —*Crow and Crow*
- Process of acquiring new knowledge and new responses is the process of learning. —*Woodworth*
- Learning is the acquisition of new behavior or strengthening or weakening of old behavior as the result of experience. —*HP Smith*

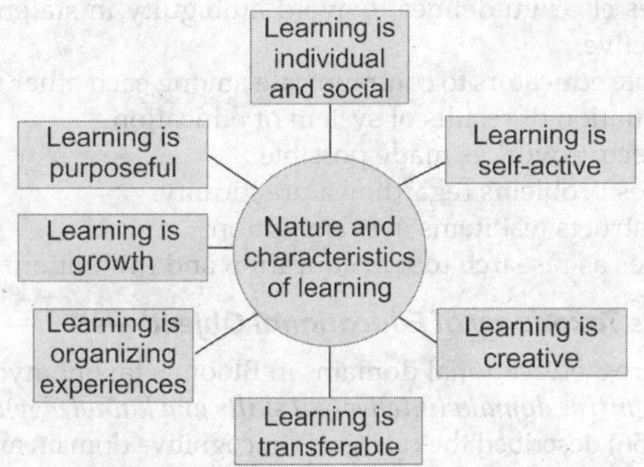


### Nature and Characteristics of Learning

#### Laws of Learning

- Law of readiness
- Law of effect
- Law of exercise.

### General Principles of Teaching

The successful teaching is based on following principles.

- Principle of aim
- Principle of activity or learning by doing
- Principle of interest or motivation
- Principle of sympathy and kind atmosphere
- Principle of flexibility and cooperation
- Principle of looking ahead
- Principle of creativity
- Principle of individual difference
- Principle of revision and practice.

### Maxims of Teaching

- Proceed from known to unknown
- Proceed from easy to difficult
- Proceed from simple to complex
- Proceed from concrete to abstract
- Proceed from particular to general

- Proceed from analysis to synthesis
- Proceed from whole to parts
- Proceed from empirical to rationale
- Proceed from actual to representative
- Proceed from near to far.

## Taxonomy of Educational Objectives

A team of psychologists and educators under the direction of educationist Benjamin Bloom developed the Taxonomy of educational objectives. Taxonomy is a classification system or principles of classification. In educational context, taxonomy refers to hierarchical classification.

When Bloom's taxonomy as applied to educational objectives a nursing educators will keep in their mind that how much of the learner's learning is limited to memorizing factual knowledge and how much is at the level of higher mental abilities.

### *Advantages of Taxonomy*

- Help teachers to formulate educational objectives clearly.
- Gives clear guidelines to avoid ambiguity in statement of objective.
- Enable educators to communicate among each other's goals.
- Evaluation of results of system of education.
- Collective work is made possible.
- Solves problems regarding a practicality.
- Constructs test items in examination.
- Serves as research tool in education and evaluation.

### *Bloom's Taxonomy of Educational Objectives*

There are 3 educational domains in Bloom's taxonomy:

1. *Cognitive domain (intellectual skills and knowledge):* Bloom (1956) described the categories in cognitive domain are:
   - Knowledge
   - Comprehension
   - Application
   - Analysis
   - Synthesis
   - Evaluation.
2. *Affective domain (communication skills):* Attitude means behavior representative of feeling are conviction; three levels are identified: i. Receptivity or attention ii. responses, iii. Internalization.
3. *Psychomotor domain (practical skills):* Three levels are included: i. Imitation, ii. control, iii. Automatism (naturalization).

## Lesson Planning

### *Definition*

- Lesson plan is a plan prepared by teacher to teach a lesson in organized manner.
- It is a plan of action calls for an understanding on teachers' part about the students' knowledge and expertise about the topic being thought and the ability to use effective method.

### *Purposes/Needs/Importance of Lesson Plan*

- It helps the teacher to be systematic orderly in teaching a subject manner.
- It provides confident and self-reliance to the teacher.
- She sets the objective that she is developed in students through certain activities.
- It encourages continuity in teaching process and avoid repetition.
- The interest of the students can be maintained throughout lesson plan.
- It ensures a definite objective the day's work and a clear visualization of that objective.
- It helps to clarify the ideas.
- It helps the teacher to delimit the teaching field, keeps boundaries within which the teacher has to work, and thereby saves the time and labor.
- It is a best technique to judge the outcome of instruction.
- Provides guidelines for the teacher in teaching-learning process.
- Provides awareness of structure, content with which the teacher is involved in the direction to achieve the objectives.
- Develops the reasoning, imagination and decision-making ability of the teacher.
- Facilitates microteaching.
- It is essential for effective teaching.
- It prevents waste of time-help teacher to be systematic and orderly. It encourages organization of subject matter and activities and prevent haphazard teaching and minimize chance of omitting some vital part of the lesson.
- Planning encourage the teacher to consider the need and level of understanding of students.

### *Essentials of Good Lesson Plan*

Successful teaching depends upon:

- It should be written
- It should have a clear aims
- It should be linked with previous knowledge
- It should show techniques of teaching
- It should cover the exact scope
- It should show illustrative ideas
- It should contain suitable subject matter
- It should be divided into units
- It should provide for activity
- It should provide the continuity in the teaching process
- It should provide for individual difference
- It should be flexible
- It should include the summary
- It should refer to reference material
- It should include assignments for students
- It should provide for self-evaluation.

### *Steps of Lesson Plan*

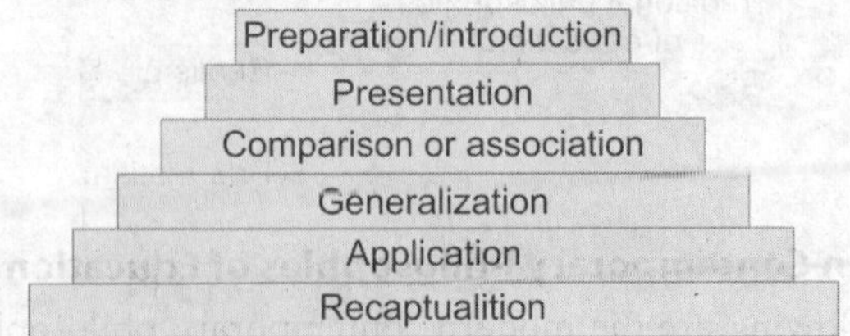

### *Format of Lesson Plan*

Name of the student teacher:
Subject:
Unit:
Topic:
Date:
Time:
Place:
Group and number of students:
Previous knowledge:
Method of teaching:
Audiovisual aids:
General objectives:
Specific objectives:

| Time | Specific objective | Content | Teacher activities | Student activities | AV aids | Method of evaluation |
|---|---|---|---|---|---|---|
| | | | | | | |

Assignment with date of submission:
Teachers references:
Students references:

## Course Planning

### *Definition*

- A course outline is a combination of various topics but interleafs unit.
- A course plan may be defined as a complete series of studies leading to graduation or a degree as in the case of BSc. Nursing course requiring completion of several short courses.

### *Purposes of Course Planning*

- To ensure autonomy
- It gives stability
- It helps to solve the problem
- It supports the curriculum process
- It secures future progress
- It brings about improvements
- It promotes utilization of resources
- It contributes to general planning.

### *Format of Course Plan*

| S. no. | Unit | Content | Time allotted | Faculty in-charge | Teaching method | Learning experience | AV aids used | Evaluation |
|---|---|---|---|---|---|---|---|---|
| | | | | | | | | |

## Unit Planning

### *Definition*

- 'A large subdivision of the subject matter, wherein a principle of a topic or a property is central to the well-organized matter'.
- 'Planning the unit is known as unit planning'.

### *Characteristics of Unit Plan*

- It needs capability and interest to the students.
- A variety of experience like field trips experiences and demonstration, classroom exercises should be planned for better learning.
- The previous experience and background of the students should be taken into an account.
- The length of unit is in such that it should maintain the interest to the students upto the last.
- The teacher should give new experiences to the students.
- Familiar and related topics should be included in the unit.
- The unit should be a part of sequence that permits growth from year-to-year.

### *Unit Plan Format*

Year:
Subject:
Unit:
Time allowed:
Method of teaching:
Evaluation:

| S. no. | Unit | Name the unit | Objective | Context and sub-content | Time | Teaching-learning experiences | Evaluations | References |
|---|---|---|---|---|---|---|---|---|
| | | | | | | | | |

## Interpersonal Relations

Nursing is a personal relationship between the nurse and patient. The relationships of the nurse are reciprocal with patient, the physician, the family of the patient, the hospital and its workers and the nursing profession. Nurse-client relationship is a helping relationship that is therapeutic in nature, is established to meet the needs of clients and is based upon trust and respect.

### *Purposes of Interpersonal Relations*

- Helping the client to identify what is troubling the client.
- To maintain the dignity of the profession.
- It reduces interpersonal tensions.
- Encourage to discuss about the changes needed to make in the client.
- Encourage the client to implement the changes.
- It helps to fulfill the authority and responsibilities in the community.
- To demonstrate personal integrity.
- To provide care for clients in need psychological interventions.
- To meet the needs of clients and is based on trust and respect.

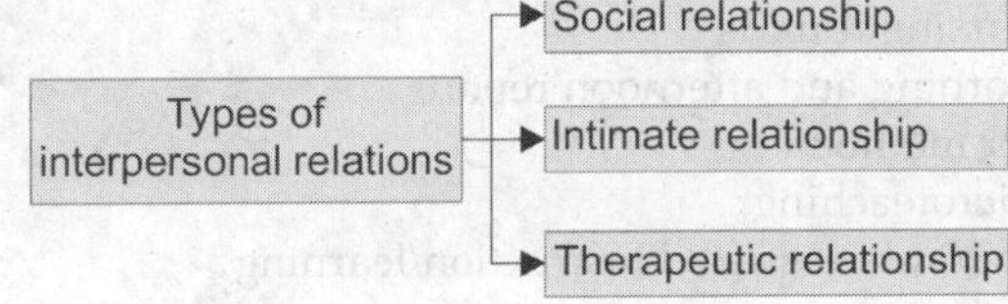

### Phases of Interpersonal Relations

Nurses can identify the progress of a relationship by understanding four phases:

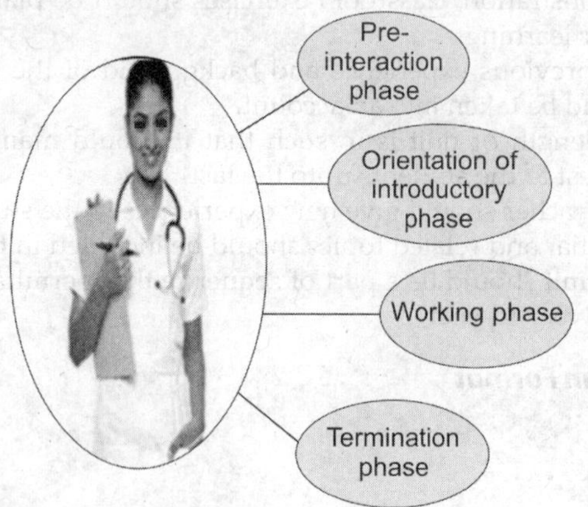


### Various Methods of Teaching

Teaching method is the stimulation, guidance, direction and encouragement for learning. Effective transfer of knowledge can be achieved by employing various student-friendly teaching- learning methods. Progressive method of teaching provide suitable opportunities for effective teaching-learning process. A teaching-learning method will help the teacher to conduct teaching in an agreeable, student-friendly and successful manner by maintaining link between the subject matter and the student.

The various teaching methods are as follows:

- Lecture method
- Demonstration method
- Discussion
  - Group discussion
  - Seminar
  - Symposium
  - Panel discussion
  - Workshops
  - Conference.
- Role play
- Project method
- Field trips (observational visit)
- Exhibition
- Programed instruction/learning
- Self-instructional module
- Simulation
- Process recording
- Clinical teaching methods
  - Bedside clinics/nursing clinics
  - Case methods
  - Nursing rounds
  - Morning and afternoon reports
- Other methods
  - Microteaching
  - Computer-assisted instruction/learning
  - Brainstorming.

### *Lecture Method*

*Definition:* The lecture is an excellent method for presenting information to a large number of persons in a short-period of time. —*A Adivi Reddy*

*Purpose of Lecture Method*

- It stimulates thinking.
- It provides relevant knowledge.
- It provides critical thinking.
- It motivates student to gain knowledge.
- It helps to promote the students with factual basis from which to build concept by concrete examples.
- It is only appropriate method for making available to a large class.
- It arouse students interest in a subject.
- It clarify difficult concepts.
- It draws the attention of the student in it's vital elements and bring student abstract of development in the forefront of research.

*Advantages*

- It presents information in a formal and direct manner.
- The material can be presented to a large group at one time.
- Interruptions and distractions are avoided.
- Many facts can be presented in a short time in an impressive way.
- In a very short time knowledge can be given.
- Covers a large group of students.
- Presence of students.
- It gives a feeling of security to the teacher.

### *Demonstration*

*Definition*

- Demonstration is defined as a method of teaching by exhibition and explanation.
- Demonstration is an activity that describes or illustrates by experiment or practical application, during which one display, operates and explains.
- Demonstration gives a visual representation of ideas, facts or process.

*Purposes of Demonstration*

- To teach psychomotor skill.
- To orient a new equipment/procedure.
- To demonstrate nursing procedure in the classroom and clinical settings.
- To demonstrate the skill in patients and family members to learn how to take care of themselves.
- To educate the patients.
- To promote learning by doing/imitation.
- To utilize the sense of sight and touch.
- To present the procedure with skill.

*Types*

- Individual demonstration, e.g. TPR.
- Group demonstration, e.g. lifting and transportation.
- Lecture-cum-demonstration, e.g. CPR television teaching.
- Demonstration-cum-practice, e.g. TPR in ward or demonstration room.

*Phases of Demonstration*

- Introductory period/preparatory phase
- Working period/phase
- Culminating phase/conclusion.

Advantages

- It activates several senses-provides better learning opportunity.
- It provides opportunities for developing observational skills.
- It uses all teaching approaches like telling, selling, participating, entrusting and reinforcing.
- It motivates to learn.
- It improves physical and cognitive level.
- Student is learning by doing.
- It helps student to retain the lesson better.
- It correlates theory into practice.
- It encourages student attention.
- Opportunity to evaluate the student knowledge.
- It commands interest by use of concrete illustration.

## Group Discussion

**Definition:** 'A discussion in a joint efforts by a group of people to achieve art and understanding of some problem about which they have some previous knowledge, feeling or idea'.

*Reasons for having a Group Discussion*

- It helps you to understand a subject more deeply.
- It improves your ability to think critically.
- It helps in solving a particular problem.
- It helps the group to make a particular decision.
- It gives you the chance to hear other students' ideas.
- It improves your listening skills.
- It increases your confidence in speaking.

*Advantages of Group Discussion*

- Development of skill in speaking in front of the group.
- Acquiring new knowledge about given subject.
- It is beneficial to both the individual participate and to members of the group.
- Self-activity is increased because student participation is provide.
- It gives the student an opportunity to learn how to adjust to social situation.
- It prepares the students to take an active role.
- Two-way communication.
- Direct for self-study.

## Seminar

**Definition:** Seminar is a discussion method of teaching in which informal group 10 to 15 students (not more than 25) participate to solve the problem in a scientific approach and analysis.

*Purposes of Seminar*

- It helps the students to study the subjects matter.
- It helps in problem-solving skills.
- It helps the students to increasing their responsibilities.
- It helps the students to change their attitudes and values.
- It helps the students to participate to method of scientific analysis and research procedures.

*Requirements of Seminar*

- Teacher is a leader (student can also function as leader).
- 10–15 members are participants.
- The topic is presented by the students taking 15–20 minutes-time.
- Duration is 1 to 2 hours.
- Leader should keep the discussion within the limits of the problem discussed.
- Students present their data in an informal way under the leadership of the teacher.
- Care should be taken to avoid stereotype.
- All the members take part in discussion in an informal way but orderly in manner.
- The Chairman should be skilled in encouraging the timid participants.
- A student secretary should record the problems which arise and the solution given.

## Symposium

**Definition:** Symposium is a method of group discussion in which two or more persons under the direction of Chairman present separate speeches which gives several aspects of one question.

*Purposes of Symposium*

- To investigate a problem from several points of view.
- To boost students ability to speak in group.
- To make the students to study independently.

*Members Involved in Symposium*

- Chairman
- Speaker
- Audience.

Role of Chairman

- Selection of topic
- Distribution of topic
- Guide the speaker towards goal
- Control over the group
- Summarizing and giving conclusions.

Qualities of Chairman

- Responsible for planning and coordinating the program
- Good counselor
- A researcher
- A resource person
- A representative to professional nursing organization.

Role of a Speaker

- Preparations of the topics
- Presentation of the topic.

Role of Audience

- Listen over the program
- Arising question and clarifying the doubts during the end.

*Advantages*

- It is suited to a large group or classes.
- This method can be frequently used to present broad topics for discussions a conventions and organization meetings.
- Organization is good because of the set speeches prepared before hand.

- Gives deeper inside into the topics.
- Directs students to continuous and independent study.
- This can be used in political meetings.

## Panel Discussion

**Definition:** Panel is a discussion in which a few persons carry on a conversation in front of an audience.

*Purposes of Panel Discussion*

- The main purpose is to reproduce the features of a small discussion group for the benefit of a large group.
- To promote socialized group conversation in which different points of view are presented.
- To stimulate thoughts, discussion to clarify thinking.
- To develop more critical attitudes and better judgment.

## Role Play

*Definition*

- 'Role play is spontaneous acting out of roles in the context of human relation situations.'
- Role playing is a dramatization along with verbalization.

*Types*

- ***Sociodrama:*** Deals with the interactions of people with other individual or groups as represented in some cultural role.
- ***Psychodrama*** Deals within a group setting, but is mainly concerned with the unique problems of a particular individual.

*Purposes*

- To convey information
- To develop specific skills
- To develop a situation for analysis
- To prevent alternative course of action
- To prepare for meeting future situations
- To develop understanding of points of view of other
- Increasing their insight into typical ways of dealing with them.
- To develop understanding of points of views of other.
- To encourage thinking and creativity.

## Project Method

**Definition:** A project is a bit of real life that has been imparted into school, in project method learning by living, this life has spontaneity, purpose, significance and interest, freedom.

***—Dr Williams, H Kilpatrick***

*Types of Project Method*

- Individual project
- Group project.

***According to Dr Kilpatrick:***

- Producer type
- Consumer type
- Problem type
- Drill type.

*Advantages of Project Method*

- It arouses and maintains interest of the student.
- It keeps student on freedom of thought and action while doing the work.
- It provides more creative constructive thinking of the students.
- It helps the student to think logically and scientifically before starting the project.
- It facilities for development of doing ability, and related learning are coordinated by putting them into practice.
- It provides the growth of individual through activity.
- It teaches the student to evaluate and judge his finished work by comparing.
- It provides for the student to compare with his own previous performance.
- It provides whole hearted purposeful activity of the students.
- Group project develops team spirit and cooperation.

## Field Trip/Field Visit

**Definition:** 'Field trip is defined as an educational procedure by which the student studies first hand objectives and materials in the natural environment'. ***—Heidgerken***

*Purposes of Field Trip*

- It helps to furnish first-hand information to supplement and enrich the classroom teaching.
- It helps to correlate and blend school life without side world by providing a direct touch with community situation.
- It helps to distinguish, differentiate and develop better understanding of housing, sanitation, economic condition, etiology factors of disease.
- It helps to develop keenness and observational skills.
- Field trip provides actual source material for study.
- Field trip provides vitalized instruction which help to arouse interest and motivation.
- Field trip affords an opportunity to solve problems arising from individual and group in a natural situation.
- Field trip serves in an effective means of correlating the subjects of curriculum.
- Field trip helps to develop leadership qualities.

## Workshop

**Definition:** Workshop is a meeting at which a group engages in intensive discussion and activity on a particular subject or project.

*Advantages of Workshop*

- It improves learning activities.
- It helps to improve the knowledge.
- It helps people with previous experience on subject especially departments, institutions and community.
- It provides more interactions and discussion from the participants.
- It helps in evolving policies, programs and methodologies.
- It helps participants to express freely and exchange ideas.
- It is introducing participant to a systematic approach to educational problems.
- It is collective thinking process to solve the problems.

## Exhibition

**Definition:** Exhibition or exhibitions are planned display of models, specimens, charts, posters, etc. presented the public view for instruction, judging in a competition, advertising or entertainment. ***—A Adivi Reddy***

*Purposes*

- To introduce students to a new unit of work.
- To develop creative thinking.
- To evaluate students through courses or units.
- To give recognition to people or institutions by enabling them to display.
- To influence people to adopt better practices by arousing interest.

*Type of Exhibits*

There are two types of exhibits, these are:

1. Simple exhibits
2. Complex exhibits.

*Advantages*

- Exhibition inspires the students to learn by doing things themselves and they get a sense of involvement.
- It gives a sense of accomplishment and achievement.
- It develops social skills of communication, co-operation and achievement.
- It fosters better school-community relations and make community members conscious about the school.
- It diffuses and disseminates interesting new work among students.
- It fosters creativity among students.

## Programed Instruction/Learning

**Definition:** 'Program learning is a systematic, step-by-step, self-instructional program aimed to ensure the learning by stated behavior'. —*Edgar Dale*

*Advantages of Programed Instruction*

- Student is kept active and alert.
- The teacher gets relieved of doing ordinary jobs and she can play the important role of a guide, counselor, motivator, organizer.
- Social and emotional problems can be eliminated.
- The problems of discipline have been automatically solved by the use of self-instructional material.
- Programed instruction makes learning interesting.
- Every student can work at his own place.
- Programed instructions is useful in situations where the human instructions are not available.
- Intellectual and some motor skills will be taught more efficiently.
- More complex of the concepts can be known.

## Microteaching

**Definition:** 'A system of controlled practice that makes it possible to concentrate on specific teaching behavior and to practice teaching under controlled condition'.

## Microteaching Cycle

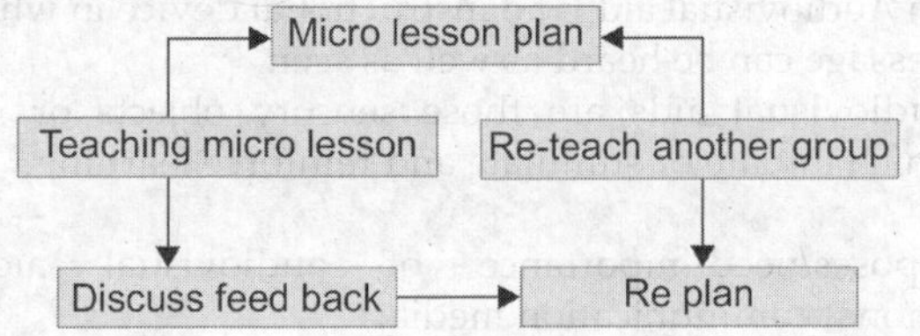


## Microteaching

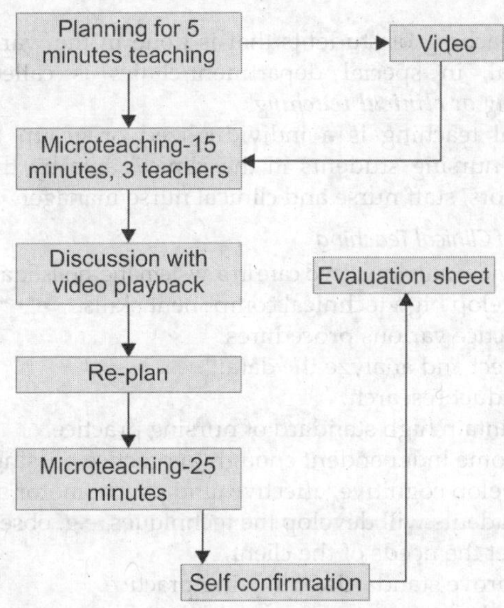


*Advantages of Microteaching*

- Teacher can control the group.
- It enables understanding of behavior.
- It increases the confidence of the learner teacher.
- It is a vehicle of continuous training.
- It enables projection of model instructional skill.
- It provides expert supervision and constructive feedback.
- It helps student teachers to acquire hard-to-attain teaching skills by providing a real situation for practicing skills.
- Since microteaching focuses on a particular skill at a time, student teachers can attain proficiency in teaching skills in a phased manner.
- Provision of immediate feedback makes microteaching more interesting and reliable.
- Since main role is played by the student teacher, it is regarded as a student-centered method.

## Simulation

*Definition*

- Simulations contain the important parts of, but all of reality. Simulation does not have to look like the real life counterpart, but they do not have to act like the real thing.
- A simulation is an actual enactment of a real life situation.

*Purpose of Simulation*

- It is intended to help students practice decision-making and problem-solving skills.
- It helps the student to achieve cognitive, affective and psychomotor outcomes.
- Simulation provides a chance to apply principles and practice theories in learning activity of the students.
- Student can learn how to learn and test various approaches in a setting where patients cannot be hurt and where wrong decisions can always be reminded.

### Clinical Teaching Methods

*Definition*

- 'The teaching of students that is done in the ward of the hospital, in special department/clinics is called *ward teaching or clinical teaching*'.
- Clinical teaching is a individualized or group teaching to the nursing students in the clinical area by the nurse educators, staff nurse and clinical nurse manager.

*Purposes of Clinical Teaching*

- To provide individualized care in a systematic, holistic approach.
- To develop high technical component skills.
- To practice various procedures.
- To collect and analyze the data.
- To conduct research.
- To maintain high standard of nursing practice.
- To become independent enough to practice nursing.
- To develop cognitive, affective, and psychomotor skills.
- The students will develop the techniques, e.g. observation.
- To meet the needs of the client.
- To improve standards of nursing practice.
- To develop various methods in delivering care.
- To identify the problems of the clients.
- To learn various diagnostic procedures.
- To learn various skills in giving health education techniques to clients and significant others.
- To develop communication skills and to maintain interpersonal relationship.
- To develop proficiency and efficiency in carrying out various nursing procedures.
- To assist physician in assisting procedures.
- To learn managerial skills.
- To become professionally active member.

The following are the clinical teaching methods:

1. Beside clinics
2. Case methods
3. Nursing rounds
4. Morning and afternoon reports.

### Brainstorming

Brainstorming is a type of small group interaction designed to encourage the free introduction of ideas on an unrestricted basis and without any limitations as to feasibility.

Brainstorming can be an effective way to generate ideas on a specific issue and then to determine which idea or ideas is the best solution. Brain storming is most effective with groups of 8 to 12 people and should be performed in a relaxed environment. It works best with a varied group of people.

There are various approaches to brain storming. The traditional method is generally the most effective because it openly collaborative allowing participants to build on each other's ideas.

Creativity exercises, relaxation exercises or other activities before the brainstorming session can help participants relax their minds, so that they can be more creative during the session.

There are ***several key factors*** for a successful brainstorming session.

1. ***State your challenge correctly:*** The brainstorming sessions participants need to be given the right challenge to solve the problem.
2. ***Avoid criticizing an idea or a person contributing the idea:*** Criticism makes the person who contributes the idea feel bad and it also tells others that unusual ideas are not welcome.
3. Have mixed participants.This will help in generating creative ideas. Have an enthusiastic facilitator who compliments ideas, gives high praise to the most outrageous ideas.
4. ***Good environment with no disturbances:*** Avoid an uncomfortable environment. Very small room, telephone calls or any other kind of interruption.The facilitator need to insist that the participants are not to be disturbed.

*Advantages*

- It is informal.
- It allows for maximum creativity and inter-stimulation.
- It makes certain that no aspect of a problem has been overlooked.

## PROBLEM-BASED LEARNING

Barrows (1985) describes 'The basic outline of PBL process is encountering the problem first, problem-solving with clinical skills and identifying learning needs in an interactive process, self-study, applying newly gained knowledge to the problem and summarizing what has been learned'.

### Advantages of Problem-based Learning

- Development of an effective and efficient clinical reasoning process.
- Increased retention of data.
- Development of effective self-directed learning skills.
- Increased student-faculty interaction.
- Increased motivation for learning.

## EDUCATIONAL COMMUNICATION MEDIA

Educational communication media is also known as audiovisual media. Audiovisual aids, audio-visual material, communication technology, instructional media and learning resources are broadly meant by the same. Audiovisual aids provides significant gains in the informational learning, retention and recall, thinking and reasoning, activity, interest, imagination, attention, concentration, better assimilation and the personal involvement (growth and development) of the student in active learning and meet individual needs of the learners.

### Definitions of Audiovisual Aids

1. An Audiovisual aid is an instructional device in which the message can be heard as well as seen.
2. Audiovisual aids are those sensory objects or images which initiate or stimulate and reinforce learning.

—***Burton***

Purposes/need/importance of audiovisual aids or educational communication media:

- Improve and make teaching effective.
- Enable audience to look, listen and learn.
- Make learning interesting and profitable.
- Quicken the phase of learning.
- Stimulate curiosity.
- Stimulate thinking and motivate action.
- Economies teacher's effort.
- Foster/develop the knowledge.
- Develop continuity of thought.
- Provide a basis for more effective perceptual and conceptual learning.
- The student acquires clear, accurate and vivid image during the process of learning.
- Increase and sustain attention and concentration.
- Make the personal involvement of the student in active learning and meet individual needs of the learners.
- Provide an opportunity for situational type of learning, e.g. field trips.
- Positive transfer of learning and training and positive environment for creative discipline.
- Audiovisual aids educate children for life, promotes international understanding.
- Save time and energy.
- Change attitude or point of view of learners.

## Principles of Audiovisual Aids

The following are the principles in the use of teaching aids:

- Principle of selection
- Principle of preparation
- Principle of proper presentation.

*Other principles are:*

- Principle of physical control
- Principle of response
- Principle of evaluation.

*Characteristics of good teaching aids*

- The aid must be adapted to the intellectual maturity of the pupils and the nature and extent of their previous experience.
- They should be meaningful and purposeful.
- As far as possible, they should be improvised, i.e. locally available materials should be used in the preparation of audiovisual aids by the teacher.
- They should be simple.
- They should be cost-effective as well as cheap.
- They should be large enough to be properly seen by the whole students in the class.
- They should be up-to-date.
- They should be easily portable.

Above all, they should supplement the instruction properly and motivate the learners.

## Sources of Audiovisual Aids

- Government
- Educational institutions
- Professional organizations
- Nongovernment organizations
- National and international voluntary organizations
- Commercial producers of educational material.

## *Types/Classification of Audiovisual Aids*

The classification of teaching aids/audiovisual aids are as follows:

*Audio Aids*

- Radio
- Tape recorder
- Central sound system
- Megaphone
- Microphone
- Gramaphone
- Mike.

*Visual Aids*

Projected Aids

- Films
- Films strips
- Overhead Projector (OHP)
- Slide projector

Nonprojected Aids

- Graphic aids
  - Cartoons
  - Charts
  - Flash cards
  - Graphs
  - Maps
  - Pictures
  - Photographs
  - Drawings.
- Printed aids
  - Books
  - Newspapers
  - Magazine
  - Pamphlets
  - Leaflets.
- Display–boards
  - Blackboard
  - Bulletin board
  - Flannel board
  - Magnetic board
  - Pegboard.
- 3-dimensional aids
  - Models
  - Specimens
  - Puppets
  - Exhibits
  - Diagrams.

Activity Aids

- Field trips
- Demonstration
- Drama
- Computer-assisted institution
- Folk dance
- Experimentation.

*Audiovisual Aids*

- Television
- Computer
- Demonstration
- Films
- Videotapes.

## MULTIPLE CHOICE QUESTIONS

1. **Education is the creation of a sound mind in a sound body is stated by:**
(a) Mahatma Gandhi (b) Aristotle
(c) Rig Veda (d) Pestalozzi

2. **Idealism believes in :**
(a) Universal mind or god
(b) Curriculum
(c) Environment
(d) Physical set up

3. **Aim of education according to realism is:**
(a) Universal education
(b) Enrichment of cultural environment
(c) Cultivation of moral values
(d) Giving knowledge and understanding of human society

4. **Aim of education according to idealism is:**
(a) Exaltation of human personality
(b) Activities concerned with language
(c) Religious activities
(d) Activities concerned with hygiene

5. **'Exaltation of human personality' was propounded by:**
(a) Naturalism (b) Pragmatism
(c) Idealism (d) Realism

6. **Nursing philosophy is a statement of:**
(a) Objectives of nursing program
(b) Institution's mission, vision and policies
(c) Long-term goals
(d) Values and beliefs of nurse

7. **Who is the father of idealism?**
(a) Hegel (b) Rusk
(c) Frobel (d) Plato

8. **Pragmatism is also known as:**
(a) Idealism (b) Naturalism
(c) Realism (d) Instrumentalism

9. **According to Mahatma Gandhi, the education means:**
(a) The development of all these capacities in the individual which will enable him to control his environment
(b) An all-round drawing out of the best in child and man—body, mind and spirit
(c) The culture which each generation purposely gives to those who are to be its successors
(d) Manifestation of divine perfection already existing in man

10. **According to Swami Vivekananda the education means:**
(a) The development of all these capacities in the individual which will enable him to control his environment
(b) An all-round drawing out of the best in child and man—body, mind and spirit
(c) Manifestation of divine perfection already existing in man
(d) Education is the realization of self

11. **Following factors are closely linked with each other for formulation of philosophy of life:**
(a) Society (b) Education
(c) Religion (d) Wisdom

12. **'Education' word derived from Latin word 'Educate' means:**
(a) Lead (b) Communicate
(c) Stop (d) Transmit

13. **In Rig Veda regards education as a force which makes an individual:**
(a) More religious (b) Self-reliant and selfless
(c) More humble (d) All of the above

14. **Which one of the following statements describes teaching in the most appropriate way?**
(a) Teaching is a skilled occupation
(b) It is a process of giving information
(c) It is an art
(d) It is establishing a relationship between student, teacher and subject

15. **The word 'Educare' means:**
(a) To lead out (b) To bring up
(c) To grow (d) Act of teaching

16. **Self-expression and self-preservation is the philosophy of:**
(a) Naturalism (b) Pragmatism
(c) Idealism (d) Spiritualism

17. **In a philosophy of nursing education the emphasis is placed on:**
(a) Matter and method of education
(b) The patient
(c) The doctor
(d) The nurse

18. **The backbone of entire process of education is:**
(a) Student (b) Teacher
(c) Curriculum (d) Society

19. **He is generally known as 'Father of Realism':**
(a) Plauto (b) Aristotle
(c) Socrates (d) Julius Caesar

20. **Modern concept of education is:**
(a) Bilateral process (b) Unipolar process
(c) Tripolar process (d) Multipolar process

21. **Aims of nursing education are all except:**
(a) Leadership aim
(b) Nursing research
(c) Democratic citizenship
(d) Leisure aim

22. **The formal agency of education is ______.**
(a) School (b) Press
(c) Radio (d) Newspaper

23. **Informal education is __________.**
(a) Preplanned (b) Not-planned
(c) Short-term (d) Private

24. **Philosophy means love for________**
(a) Money (b) Truth
(c) Freedom (d) Wisdom

25. **Following are the primary law of learning except:**
(a) Law of effect (b) Law of exercise
(c) Law of gravity (d) Law of readiness

26. **The philosophy which believes in universal mind is known as________.**
(a) Idealism (b) Nationalism
(c) Pragmatism (d) Realism

27. **The cognitive domain in educational objectives refers to________.**
(a) Knowledge (b) Attitude
(c) Skills (d) Behavior

28. **The best method of assessment of student is by paper-pencil test for________.**
(a) Skill observation (b) Behavioral observation
(c) Knowledge (d) Communication

29. **Knowledge is the objective of________.**
(a) Psychomotor domain
(b) Affective domain
(c) Cognitive domain
(d) None of the above

30. **A lesson plan________.**
(a) Is a guide to the teacher
(b) Contains only few points
(c) Describes method of teaching
(d) Gives the detailed description of content

31. **Teaching should start from________.**
(a) Abstract to concrete (b) Unknown to known
(c) Synthesis to analysis (d) Easy to difficult

32. **Teaching is________.**
(a) An art and science (b) A science
(c) Activity (d) An art

33. **Cognitive domain of learning refers to:**
(a) Communication skills
(b) Intellectual skills and knowledge
(c) Practical skills
(d) Learning to adjust

34. **In educational objectives the psychomotor domain refers to________.**
(a) Knowledge (b) Psychology
(c) Attitude (d) Skill

35. **Words open to fever interpretations are all except:**
(a) To write (b) To identify
(c) To understand (d) To compare

36. **Who classified educational objectives as cognitive, affective and psychomotor domain?**
(a) Adam Smith (b) JJ Gilbert
(c) BS Bloom (d) John Dewey

37. **Which domain of objective is concerned with attitude, value and appreciation?**
(a) Psychomotor domain
(b) Affective domain
(c) Cognitive domain
(d) Gross motor domain

38. **Qualities of instructional objectives are all of the following except:**
(a) Equivocal (b) Relevant
(c) Feasible (d) Measurable

39. **Characteristics of learning include all of the following except:**
(a) Unitary (b) Purposive
(c) Creative (d) Nontransferable

40. **In the psychomotor domain of learning, a person achieves________.**
(a) Knowledge
(b) Attitude which is positive
(c) Attitude which is negative
(d) Skill

41. **The plan of action prepared by a teacher before class is known as________.**
(a) Syllabus (b) Unit plan
(c) Course plan (d) Lesson plan

42. **The basic level of cognitive domain is____**
(a) Analysis (b) Comprehensive
(c) Knowledge (d) Synthesis

43. **Content analysis of the subject matter is essential for________.**
(a) Unit planning (b) Lesson planning
(c) Course planning (d) None of the above

44. **Maxims of teaching are all except:**
(a) Known to unknown (b) Complex to simple
(c) Easy to difficult (d) Whole to parts

45. **One of the characteristics of learning is that it is________.**
(a) Purposive (b) Knowledge
(c) Doing (d) Acquiring

46. **Taxonomy of objectives is given by________.**
(a) R Tagore (b) Gandhiji
(c) BS Bloom (d) John Dewey

47. **The teacher's role regarding the pupil is to except:**
(a) Stimulate
(b) Guide
(c) Direct
(d) Provide ready-made material/subject matter

48. **It is the exact written report of the conversation between the nurse and patient________.**
(a) Process recording
(b) Case analysis
(c) Anecdotal
(d) Nurse record

49. **A method of group discussion in which two or more persons under the direction of Chairperson present separate speeches is called as:**
(a) Seminar (b) Panel discussion
(c) Symposium (d) Workshop

50. **When few persons carry on a conversation in front of an audience where different points of view are presented, is called as________.**
(a) Presentation (b) Demonstration
(c) Panel (d) Lecture

**51. The method of teaching which emphasizes on one-way communication is ________.**
(a) Role playing (b) Discussion
(c) Demonstration (d) Lecture

**52. A study of first hand objects with material in its environment is possible only in case of:**
(a) Field trip (b) Demonstration
(c) Clinics (d) Workshop

**53. It is one type of method teaching which we use in the form of drama________.**
(a) Puppet show (b) Role play
(c) Fancy dress (d) None of these

**54. These are the phases of demonstration except:**
(a) Planning (b) Assessment
(c) Evaluation (d) Performance

**55. It is an exact report of the conversation between the nurse and patient________.**
(a) Programed instruction
(b) Nursing case study
(c) Process recording
(d) Nurses report

**56. The number of members the panel is ______.**
(a) 4–8 (b) 10–12
(c) 12–15 (d) 15–20

**57. Demonstration and return demonstration are essential for acquisition of ________.**
(a) Knowledge (b) Skill
(c) Attitude (d) Aptitude

**58. Following method is the suitable/appropriate to teach mothers to prepare ORS solution ________.**
(a) Role play (b) Discussion
(c) Lecture (d) Demonstration

**59. The advantage of demonstration method is that________.**
(a) It gives more emphasis on knowledge
(b) It activates several senses
(c) It is a substitute to lecture method
(d) It is easier than other methods

**60. The type of discussion where a group of 6–8 qualified experts discuss a topic in front of an audience is called:**
(a) Group discussion (b) Symposium
(c) Panel discussion (d) Workshop

**61. One of the limitation of simulation technique is that it is________.**
(a) Time consuming
(b) One-way communication
(c) Containing of too much of participation
(d) Very expensive

**62. Combination of theory classes and clinical experience as teaching-learning schedule is called as________.**
(a) Exclusive teaching theory block
(b) Partial teaching learning block
(c) Complete study block
(d) Daily routine class block

**63. In microteaching, the class size consists of how many students?**
(a) 5–10 (b) 15–20
(c) 25–30 (d) 35–40

**64. Written report of conversation between nurse and patient________.**
(a) Process recording (b) Progress recording
(c) Outcome recording (d) Clinical recording

**65. The method for presenting several aspects of a subject is called________.**
(a) Symposium (b) Panel discussion
(c) Seminar (d) Workshop

**66. The panel method was originated by____.**
(a) Dr H Kilpatrick (b) Prof Harry A Overstreet
(c) Campbell (d) Froebel

**67. The teaching method that enable to develop insight into real life problems and problem-solving is________.**
(a) Discussion (b) Roleplaying
(c) Lecture (d) Demonstration

**68. In an education programme, a group of 10 people are speaking on a topic of common interest is called as:**
(a) Group discussion (b) Panel discussion
(c) Workshop (d) Seminar

**69. The most teacher active method of teaching is________.**
(a) Lecture demonstration
(b) Lecture discussion
(c) Lecture method
(d) Group discussion

**70. Principlesofprogramedinstructionare________.**
(a) Principle of small step
(b) Principle of active responding
(c) Principle of self-pacing
(d) All of the above

**71. Clinical teaching methods used in nursing are all except:**
(a) Bedside clinic (b) Field visit
(c) Process recording (d) Model simulation

**72. Activity aids are:**
(a) Leaflets (b) Bulletins
(c) Models (d) Puppet shows

**73. The normal size of flash card is ____.**
(a) 25 × 30 cm (b) 32 × 35 cm
(c) 43 × 44 cm (d) 15 × 20 cm

**74. A puppet actions should be accompanied by:**
(a) Claps (b) Dialogues
(c) Charts (d) Models

**75. Nowadays most commonly used teaching aid which has replaced chalkboard in the classroom is ________.**
(a) Overhead projector
(b) Slide projector
(c) LCD projector
(d) Microprojector

76. **Collection of real things for instructional use is called as________.**
(a) Demonstration (b) Objects
(c) Model (d) Exhibition

77. **Collection of real objects for instruction use are______.**
(a) Specimens (b) Model
(c) Objects (d) Exhibits

78. **Nonprojected aid is____________.**
(a) Film (b) Slide
(c) Model (d) Film strips

79. **Audiovisual aids are used to__________.**
(a) Reduce the time of the class
(b) Help the unexperienced teachers
(c) Improve teaching learning
(d) Teach primary education

80. **Which of the following is NOT a graphic aid?**
(a) Model (b) Charts
(c) Flash cards (d) Pamphlets

81. **The size of flash card is__________.**
(a) 22 × 30 inches (b) 10 × 12 inches
(c) 7 × 10 inches (d) 5 × 10 inches

82. **The method of evaluation which assess the organization and comprehensive ability of the student is:**
(a) Essay type tests
(b) Short answer tests
(c) Objective type tests
(d) Multiple choice tests

83. **The main disadvantages of essay type test is______.**
(a) Objectivity (b) Subjectivity
(c) Partiality (d) Halo effect

84. **Evaluation in nursing helps to determine the______.**
(a) Level of knowledge and comprehension
(b) Level of clinical performance
(c) Level of self-direction in the students
(d) Level of overall development in the students

85. **Which among the following is not a characteristic feature of evaluation in education?**
(a) Evaluation is continuous process
(b) Evaluation is applied to academic and nonacademic subjects
(c) Evaluation helps in planning
(d) Evaluation does not include non-academic subjects

86. **The ongoing or systematic assessment of students' achievement during the curricular program is known as:**
(a) Summative evaluation
(b) Formative evaluation
(c) Intermittent evaluation
(d) None of the above

87. **Summative evaluation is for the benefit of______.**
(a) Current students (b) Current teachers
(c) Future students (d) Future teachers

88. **Progress or gains made by the participant and the program is measured using the technique of:**
(a) Summative evaluation (b) Formative evaluation
(c) Diagnostic evaluation (d) Test evaluation

89. **An evaluation done at the end to assess the outcome of the program is called____________.**
(a) Formative evaluation
(b) Summative evaluation
(c) Facilitative evaluation
(d) Critical evaluation

90. **Anecdotal record means__________.**
(a) Legal record
(b) Brief description and incident
(c) Ward teaching record
(d) Research record

91. **The type of oral examination is________.**
(a) Interview (b) Lecture method
(c) Viva-voice (d) Seminar

92. **The questions which are easier to prepare and administer are__________.**
(a) Essay type
(b) MCQ type
(c) Alternate response type
(d) Objective type

93. **The tool which used for observation is__________.**
(a) Anecdotal record (b) Open-ended questions
(c) Checklist (d) Questionnaire

94. **Essay types questions are__________.**
(a) Easy to prepare
(b) Difficult to prepare
(c) Objectivity is uncertain
(d) All of the above

95. **Advantage of essay type test is________.**
(a) Easy to score (b) Easy to construct
(c) Easy to evaluate (d) None of the above

96. **Assessment of skill in procedure is done by________.**
(a) Observation checklist
(b) Multiple choice
(c) Essay type
(d) All of the above

97. **These are the factual description of meaningful incidents and events that the teacher has observed in students lives:**
(a) Cumulative (b) Anecdotal
(c) Attitude scale (d) Rating scale

98. **Which of the following tools use to measure the students' procedure performance**
(a) Rating scale (b) Anecdotal record
(c) Attitude scale (d) Checklist

99. **Which of the following test emphasis more on recall rather recognition to correct answer________.**
(a) MCQs (b) SAQ's
(c) Essay type test (d) Oral examination

100. **These are the tools of evaluation except:**
(a) Checklist
(b) Questionnaire
(c) Interview schedule
(d) Written examination

**101. Viva-voce is the part of__________.**
(a) Quiz
(b) Oral examination
(c) Demonstration
(d) Written examination

**102. Which device will use to measure the student procedure performance __________.**
(a) Anecdotal record (b) Checklist
(c) Rating scale (d) Attitude scale

**103. The degree of the test to which it measures what it is intended to measure is called as __________.**
(a) Reliability (b) Specificity
(c) Validity (d) Practicality

**104. In techniques of evaluation, observation is the example of__________.**
(a) Qualitative type
(b) Quantitative type
(c) Visual type
(d) Audiovisual type

**105. Validity of the test is__________.**
(a) It measures what it intends to measure
(b) It permits quick analysis
(c) Directly related to objectives of the course
(d) It allows summative evaluation

**106. 'Accuracy' measuring the 'intended measure' of test is called as __________.**
(a) Objectivity
(b) Reliability
(c) Validity
(d) Subjectivity

**107. A question is a request for information in the form of __________.**
(a) Opinion (b) Answer
(c) View (d) Expression

**108. The stem of MCQ should be __________.**
(a) As short as possible
(b) Inclusive of answers
(c) Give clue for answer
(d) Included with clearly-stated problem

**109. The writing of job description should include:**
(a) Policies
(b) Job title
(c) Opinions
(d) Grievances

**110. Integration of several parts of an information into an orderly whole to meet an organization goal is:**
(a) Cooperation
(b) Organization
(c) Coordination
(d) Planning

**111. A written record of principal duties and scope of responsibility is:**
(a) Job description
(b) Job specification
(c) Job evaluation
(d) Job analysis

**112. The first step of job evaluation is:**
(a) Job description
(b) Job analysis
(c) Job specification
(d) Job evaluation

**113. A written statement of the main duties and responsibilities which a job entails is called**
(a) Job analysis
(b) Job description
(c) Job specification
(d) Job evaluation

**114. The act of synchronizing people and activities so that they function smoothly in the attainment of organization objective is called:**
(a) Planning
(b) Organizing
(c) Coordinating
(d) Leading

**115. A written record of principal duties and scope of responsibilities for a particular job together with the required employee characteristics is called as:**
(a) Job description
(b) Job evaluation
(c) Supervision
(d) Management

**116. Administrative head of the school of Nursing is:**
(a) Medical Superintendent
(b) Nursing Superintendent
(c) Matron
(d) Principal

**117. Accreditation of a College of Nursing refers to:**
(a) Establishing standards of education
(b) Inspection of the college
(c) Voluntary review process by a professional organization
(d) Quality assurance

**118. In India, the first four year basic Bachelor Degree nursing program was established in:**
(a) 1910 (b) 1880
(c) 1946 (d) 1940

**119. Job description denotes:**
(a) Written statement of the main duties and responsibilities which a job entails
(b) Assigning responsibility and authority to a coworkers
(c) Process that ensures that right kind of people at right places at the right time do things for which they are economically most useful
(d) None of the above

**120. Job specification denotes:**
(a) Personal capacities and inclinations deemed necessary for successful job performance
(b) Written statement of the main duties and responsibilities which a job entails
(c) (a) and (b)
(d) None of the above

121. **The process of determining significant information about the duties, responsibilities and conditions of a specific job is:**
(a) Job analysis
(b) Job description
(c) Job specification
(d) Job evaluation

122. **In India, first MSc Nursing programme was started in RAK College in the year:**
(a) 1947 (b) 1959
(c) 1946 (d) 1968

123. **What is the process of assessing staff members?**
(a) Peer review
(b) Reevaluation
(c) Performance appraisal
(d) Evaluation

124. **Halo effect, central tendency error and self-aggrandizing effect are some of the ____________ of performance appraisals.**
(a) Nature (b) Philosophy
(c) Problems (d) Benefits

125. **A process of securing application to fill vacant position is the hospital__________**
(a) Appointment
(b) Recruitment
(c) Interview
(d) Selection

126. **Employee referrals may be used for_________.**
(a) Clinical teaching assignment
(b) Recruitment
(c) Hospital organization
(d) Budgeting

127. **When the appraiser allows one or two positive aspects of assessment of the employee unduly influence all other aspects of employees performance, this is ________.**
(a) Horn effect
(b) Halo effect
(c) Average effect
(d) Central tendency trap

128. **The principal tool of performance evaluation is_______.**
(a) Checklist
(b) Rating scale
(c) Direct observation
(d) Anecdotal record

129. **The first phase in counseling process is:**
(a) Assessment
(b) Establishing relationship
(c) Selling goals
(d) Making family aware of the goals

130. **The process of guidance and counseling is __________.**
(a) Continuous (b) Concurrent
(c) Terminal (d) Episodic

131. **Guidance and counseling process is _____**
(a) One time required
(b) Continuously required
(c) Intermittently required
(d) Episodic required

132. **A process of enabling the individual to know himself is the_______________.**
(a) Guidance
(b) Counseling
(c) Testing
(d) Advice

133. **An internal disturbance that results from a stressful event or a perceived threat to self is called as_________.**
(a) Discipline
(b) Counseling
(c) Crisis
(d) Guidance

134. **An individualized training program planned for a newly appointed employee to acquaint with job responsibilities, work-place, clients and coworkers is known as:**
(a) Induction training
(b) Job orientation
(c) In-service education
(d) Legislation

135. **The planned educational experiences provided in a job setting is____________.**
(a) Curriculum education
(b) Primary education
(c) In-service education
(d) Specialized education

136. **Acquainting staff with the existing work environment is known as_____________.**
(a) Orientation
(b) Continuing education
(c) Skill training
(d) Leadership training

137. **Orientation programs are conducted during the __________ phase of workers.**
(a) Working (b) Beginning
(c) Leaving (d) Concluding

138. **In-service education refers to___________.**
(a) An individual training program
(b) Planned education program provided in the job setting
(c) Continued program of education
(d) Planned instructional training program

## ANSWERS

| 1. | (b) | 21. | (b) | 41. | (d) | 61. | (d) | 81. | (b) | 101. | (b) | 121. | (a) |
|---|---|---|---|---|---|---|---|---|---|---|---|---|---|
| 2. | (a) | 22. | (a) | 42. | (c) | 62. | (b) | 82. | (a) | 102. | (b) | 122. | (b) |
| 3. | (d) | 23. | (b) | 43. | (b) | 63. | (a) | 83. | (b) | 103. | (c) | 123. | (c) |
| 4. | (a) | 24. | (d) | 44. | (b) | 64. | (a) | 84. | (d) | 104. | (a) | 124. | (c) |
| 5. | (c) | 25. | (c) | 45. | (a) | 65. | (a) | 85. | (d) | 105. | (a) | 125. | (b) |
| 6. | (d) | 26. | (a) | 46. | (c) | 66. | (b) | 86. | (b) | 106. | (c) | 126. | (b) |
| 7. | (d) | 27. | (a) | 47. | (d) | 67. | (a) | 87. | (c) | 107. | (b) | 127. | (b) |
| 8. | (d) | 28. | (c) | 48. | (a) | 68. | (a) | 88. | (b) | 108. | (c) | 128. | (a) |
| 9. | (a) | 29. | (c) | 49. | (c) | 69. | (c) | 89. | (b) | 109. | (b) | 129. | (b) |
| 10. | (c) | 30. | (d) | 50. | (c) | 70. | (c) | 90. | (b) | 110. | (c) | 130. | (a) |
| 11. | (b) | 31. | (d) | 51. | (a) | 71. | (a) | 91. | (c) | 111. | (a) | 131. | (b) |
| 12. | (a) | 32. | (a) | 52. | (a) | 72. | (b) | 92. | (a) | 112. | (b) | 132. | (a) |
| 13. | (c) | 33. | (b) | 53. | (b) | 73. | (a) | 93. | (a) | 113. | (b) | 133. | (c) |
| 14. | (d) | 34. | (d) | 54. | (b) | 74. | (b) | 94. | (a) | 114. | (c) | 134. | (b) |
| 15. | (a) | 35. | (c) | 55. | (c) | 75. | (a) | 95. | (a) | 115. | (a) | 135. | (c) |
| 16. | (a) | 36. | (c) | 56. | (a) | 76. | (b) | 96. | (a) | 116. | (d) | 136. | (a) |
| 17. | (a) | 37. | (b) | 57. | (b) | 77. | (a) | 97. | (b) | 117. | (a) | 137. | (b) |
| 18. | (c) | 38. | (a) | 58. | (d) | 78. | (c) | 98. | (d) | 118. | (b) | 138. | (b) |
| 19. | (b) | 39. | (d) | 59. | (b) | 79. | (c) | 99. | (b) | 119. | (a) | | |
| 20. | (c) | 40. | (d) | 60. | (c) | 80. | (d) | 100. | (d) | 120. | (a) | | |

# QUICK REVIEW

# Obstetrics and Gynecological Nursing

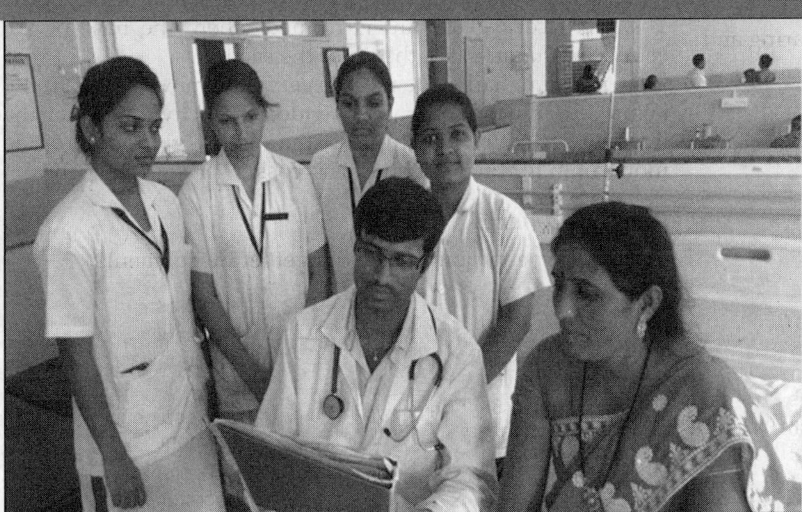

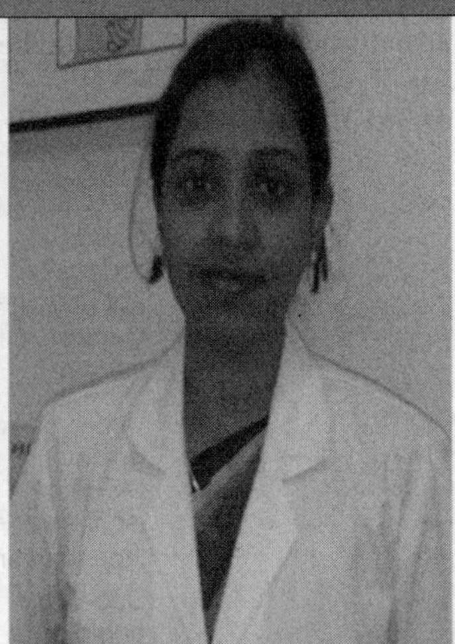

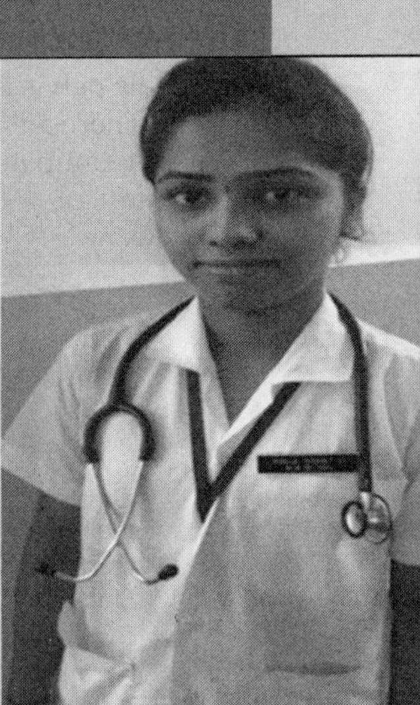

## HIGHLIGHTS

- Female Pelvic Bones
- The Fetal Skull
- Normal Pregnancy
- Minor Disorders of Pregnancy
- Diagnosis of Pregnancy
- Stages of Normal Labor
- Normal Postpartum
- Normal Menstruation
- Amenorrhea
- Menopause
- Episiotomy
- Multiple Choice Questions

# Obstetrics and Gynecological Nursing

## FEMALE PELVIC BONES

The female pelvis is structurally adapted for child bearing and delivery.There are four pelvic bones

- Two innominate or hip bones
- Sacrum
- Coccyx

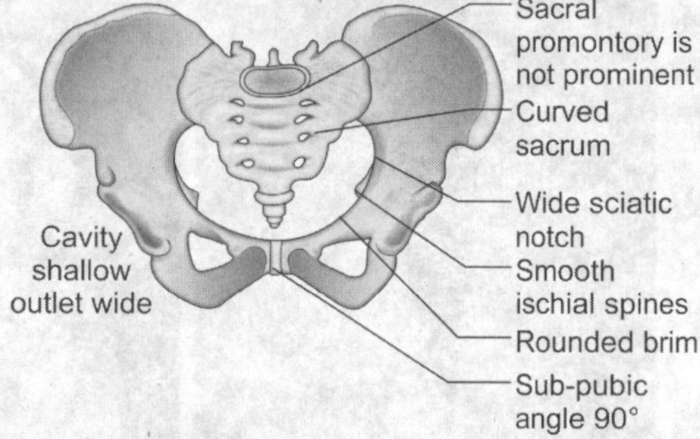


**Fig.:** Structure of the pelvis (Adele Pilliter, 1995)

### Innominate Bones

Each innominate bone is composed of three parts.

1. The ilium the large flared out part
2. The ischium the thick lower part. It has a large prominance known as the ischial tuberosity on which the body rests when sitting behind and a little above the tuberosity is an inward projection, the ischial spine. In labor the station of the fetal head is estimated in relation to ischial spines.
3. *The pubis:* The pubic bone forms the anterior part. The space enclosed by the body of the pubic bone the rami and the ischium is called the obturator foramen.

### Sacrum

*The sacrum:* A wedge shaped bone consisting of five fused vertebra. The upper border of the first sacral vertebra is known as the sacral promontory. The anterior surface of the sacrum is concave and is referred to as the shallow of the sacrum.

### Coccyx

*The coccyx:* is avestigial tail. It consists of four fused vertebra forming a small triangular bone.

#### *Pelvic Joints*

There are four pelvic joints

- One Symphysis pubis
- Two Sacro illiac joint
- One Sacro coccygeal joint
- The symphysis pubis is a cartilaginous joint formed by junction of the two pubic bones along the midline.

The sacro iliac joints are the strongest joints in the body. The sacro coccygeal joint is formed where the base of the coccyx articulates with the tip of the sacrum.

In non-pregnant state there is very little movement in these joints, but during pregnancy endocrine activity causes the ligaments to soften which allows the joints to give and provide more room for the fetal head as it passes through the pelvis.

#### *Pelvic Ligaments*

Each of the pelvic joints is held together by ligaments

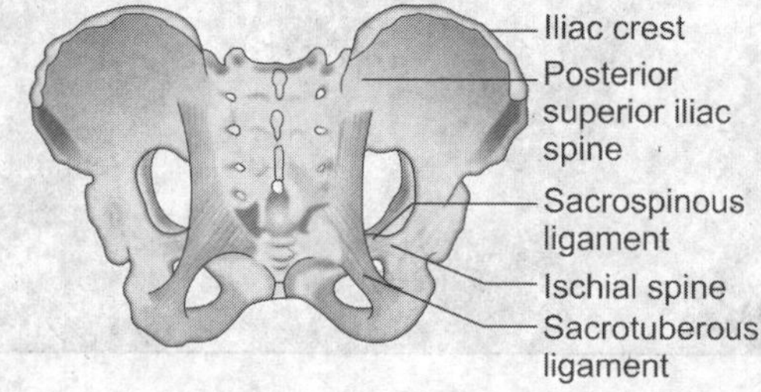


**Fig.:** Pelvic Ligaments on posterior view (Derexllewllyn, 1990)

- Interpubic ligaments at the symphysis pubis (1)
- Sacro iliac ligaments (2)
- Sacro coccygeal ligaments (1)
- Sacro tuberous ligament (2)
- Sacro spinous ligament (2)

### The True Pelvis

The true pelvis is the bony canal through which the fetus must pass during birth. It has a brim, mid cavity and an outlet. The pelvic brim is rounded except where the sacral promontory projects into it. The pelvic cavity is extends from the brim above to the outlet below. The pelvic outlet are two and described as the anatomical and the obstetrical. The anatomical outlet is formed by the lower borders of each of the bones together with the sacrotuberous ligament. It is diamond in shape. The obstetrical outlet is of the space between the narrow pelvic strait and the anatomical outlet.

### Important Landmarks of Female Pelvis

#### *Pelvic Brim*

- Sacral promontary posteriorly
- Superior ramus of the pubic bone anterolateral
- Upper inner border of the body of the pubic bone
- Upper inner border of the symphysis pubis anteriorly

#### *Mid Pelvis*

Ischial spine

### *Outlet*

- Inferior pubic rami antero laterally
- Sacrotuberous ligament postro laterally
- Ischial tuberosity laterally
- Inferior border of symphysis pubis anteriorly
- Tip of coccyx.

## Important Diameters of the Pelvis

### *Inlet*

Diagonal conjugate—a line from the sacral promontory toward the lower border of the symphysis pubis and measures 12.5 centimeter. It is measured by pelvic examination.

### *Mid Cavity*

Interspinous diameter-a line between the two ischial spines and measures 11 centimeter.

### *The Pelvic Outlet*

- Pubic arch
- Intertuberous diameter.

**Table:** Measurements of the pelvic canal in centimeters

| | Anteroposterior | Oblique | Transverse |
|---|---|---|---|
| Brim | 11 | 12 | 13 |
| Cavity | 12 | 12 | 12 |
| Outlet | 13 | 12 | 11 |

*The Four Types of Female Pelvis*

- The gynecoid pelvis (female type)
- The android pelvis (male type)
- The anthropoid pelvis
- The platypelloid pelvis

**Table:** Features of the four types of female pelvis

| Features | Gynecoid | Android | Anthro-poid | Platypelloid |
|---|---|---|---|---|
| Brim | Round | Heart shaped | Long oval | Kidney shaped |
| Fore-pelvis | Generous | Narrow | Narrowed | Wide |
| Side walls | Straight | Convergent | Divergent | Divergent |
| Ischial spines | Blunt | Prominent | Blunt | Blunt |
| Sciatic notch | Rounded | Narrow | Wide | Wide |
| Sub-pubic angle | 900 | < 900 | > 900 | > 900 |
| Incidence | 50% | 20% | 25% | 5% |

## Pelvic Floor or Pelvic Diaphragm

The pelvic floor or diaphragm is amuscular floor that demarcates the pelvic cavity and perineum. Its strength is enforced by its associated condesed pelvic fascia, therefore, it is important for pelvic organs protection.

### *Functions*

- It supports the weight of the abdominal and pelvic organs.
- The muscles are responsible for the voluntary control of micturation, defication and play an important part in sexual intercourse.
- It influences the passive movement of the fetus through the birth canal and relaxes to allow its exit from the pelvis.

The main important muscles of pelivic floor are:

- Levator ani muscles are arising from the lateral pelvic wall and decussate in the mid-line between the urethra, the vagina and rectum. It contains pubococcygeous muscle, ileo coccygeus and pubo rectalis.
- Pubococcygeous muscle is constructed in such a way that it can expand enough for child-birth and contract the pelvis supported.

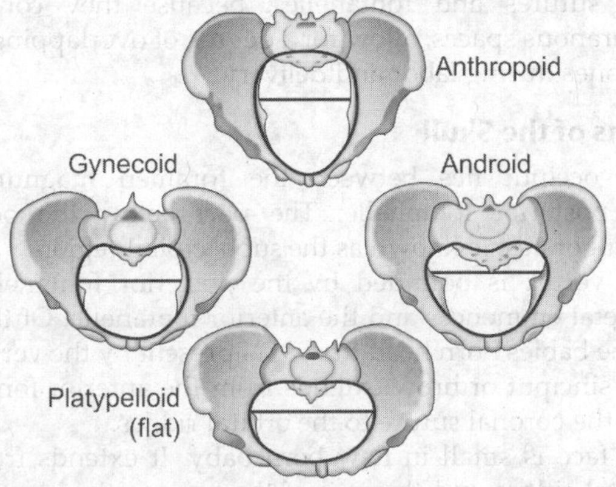


**Fig.:** Types of female pelvis (Alan H Decherney I pemoll, 1994)

## THE FETAL SKULL

The fetal head is the most difficult part to deliver whether it comes first or last. It is large in comparison with the true pelvis and some adptation between skull and pelvis must take place during labor. An understanding of the landmarks and measurements of the fetal skull enables to recognize normal presentation and positions and to facilitate delivery with the least possible trauma to mother and child. The skull is divided into the vault, the base and the face. The vault is the large dome shaped part above the imaginary line drowns between the orbital ridges and the nape of the neck. The base is composed of bones which are firmly united to protect the vital centers in the medulla. The face is composed of 14 small bones which are also firmly united and non-compressible

### Bones of the Vault

There are five main bones in the vault of the fetal skull.

- The occipital bone lies at the back of the head and forms the region of the occiput.
- The two parietal bones lie on either side of the skull.
- The two frontal bones from the forehead or sinciput.

### Sutures and Fontanelles

Sutures are cranial joints and are formed where two bones adjoin. Where two or more sutures meet, a fontanell is formed.

### Types of Sutures

- The lambdoidal suture is shaped like the Greek letter lambda and separates the occipital bone from the two parietal bones.
- The sagittal suture lies between the parittal bones
- The coronal suture separates the frontal bones from the parietal bones, passing from one temple to the other.

- The frontal suture runs between the two halves of the frontal bone.

### Types of Fontanelle

- The posterior fontanelle or lambda is situated at the junction of the lambdoid and sagittal sutures. It is small and triangular in shape and can be recognized vaginally.
- The anterior fontanelle or bregma is found at the junction of the sagittal, coronal and frontal sutures and recognized vaginally.

The sutures and fontanelles, because they consist of memberanous spaces, allow for a degree of overlapping of the skull bones during labor and delivery.

### Regions of the Skull

- The occiput lies between the foramen magnum and the posterior fontanelle. The part below the occipital protuberance is known as the suboccipital region.
- The vertex is bounded by the posterior fontanelle, the parietal eminences and the anterior fontanelle. Of the 96% of the babies born head first, 95% present by the vertex.
- The sinciput or brow extends from the anterior fontanelle and the coronal suture to the orbital ridges.
- The face is small in new born baby. It extends from the orbital ridges and the root of the nose to the junctions of the chin and the neck. The point between the eye brows is known as the glabella. The chin termed as the mentum and it is an important landmark.

### Landmarks of the Fetal Skull

- Sinciput
- Occiput
- Glabella
- Anterior fontanelle
- The vertex
- Posterior fontanelle
- Occipital protuberance
- The mentum

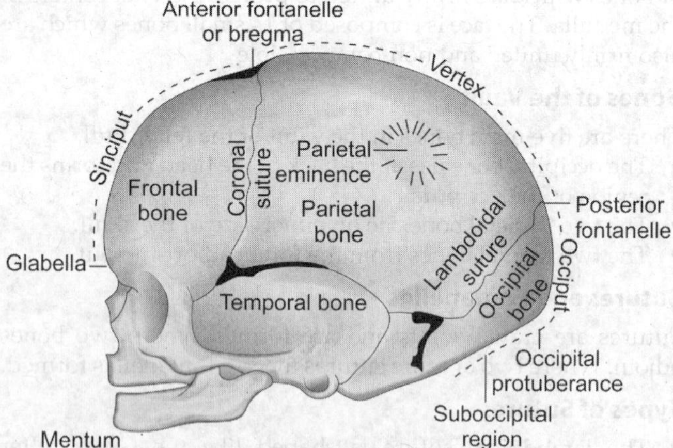


Fig.: Fetal skull (V Ruth Bennett, Linda K Brown, 1993)

### Diameters of the Fetal Skull

The measurement of the skulls are transverse, anteroposterior or longitudinal.

- Transverse diameter
- Biparietal diameter 9.5 cm between the parietal eminence
- Bitemporal diameter 8.2 cm between the furthers points of the coronal suture at the temples.
- Anteroposterior or longitudinal diameters
- Suboccipitobregmatic 9.5 cm from below the occipital protuberance to the center of the anterior fontanelle or bregma.
- Suboccipitofrontal 10 cm from below occipital protuberance to the center of the frontal suture.
- Occipitofrontal 11.5 cm from the occipital protuberance to the glabella.
- Mentovertical 13.5 cm from the point of the chin to the highest point on the vertex sightly nearer to the posterior than to the anterior fontanelle.
- 'Submentovertical 11.5 cm from the point where the chin joins the neck to the highest point on the vertex.
- Submentobregmatic 9.5 cm from the point where the chin joins the neck to the center of the bregma.

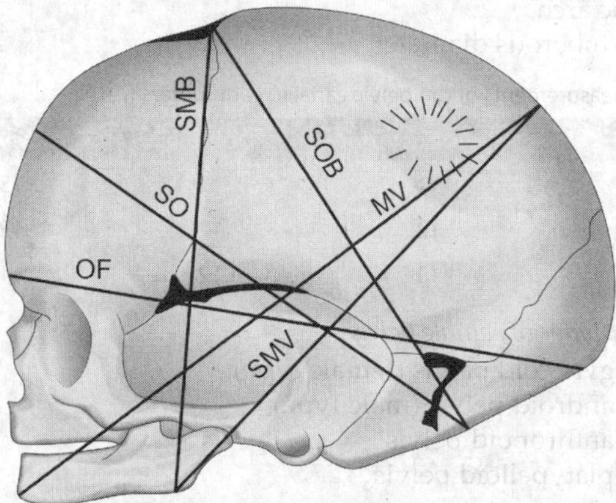


Fig.: Anteroposterior or longitudinal Diameters of Fetal Skull (V Ruth Bennett, Linda K Brown, 1993)

## NORMAL PREGNANCY

Normal pregnancy lasts for 280 days or 40 weeks. A baby who is born after 42 weeks is termed as a postmature baby and one who is born before 37 weeks is a preterm baby.

Pregnancy is divided into three, more or less equal stages, known as trimesters. Each of these trimesters correlate with different stages of fetal development—the first trimester is associated more with development of the fetal organs, the second trimester is associated with growth and enlargement of the developed organs and the third trimester is associated with growth plus physiological maturity. Physiological maturity means that the organs can now function more or less like an adult's—releasing enzymes or hormones, etc.

- The first trimester lasts from the first day of the last missed period to the end of 13 weeks.
- The second trimester lasts from the beginning of the 14th week to the end of the 27th week
- The third trimester lasts from the beginning of the 28th week to the end of the 40th week of pregnancy.
- The expected date of delivery or the expected due date (EDD) is the date when the baby is expected to deliver. It is

calculated by counting 9 months plus 7 days from the first day of the last missed period. This calculation is accurate only if a woman has a regular menstrual cycle of 28 +/- 2 days. If the cycle is longer, the extra days need to be added to the total duration.

## MINOR DISORDERS OF PREGNANCY

Minor disorders are only disorders that occur during pregnancy and are not life-threatening.

### Nausea and Vomiting

This presents between 4 and 12 weeks gestation. Hormonal influences are listed as the most likely causes. It is usually occurs in the morning but can occur any time during the day, aggravated by smelling of food.

#### *Management*

- Reassure the mother
- Small frequent meals (dry meals)
- Reduce fatty and fried containing foods.
- Rest

### Heart Burn

It is a burning sensation in the mid chest region. Progesterone relaxes the cardiac sphincter of the stomach and allows reflex of gastric contents into esophagus. Heart burn is most troublesome at 30–40 weeks gestation because at this moment stage is under pressure from the growing uterus.

#### *Management*

- Small and frequent meal, sleeping with more pillows than usual.
- For persistence/severe case/prescribed antacids.

### Pica

This is the term used when mother craves certain foods of unnatural substances such as coal, soil. etc. The cause is unknown but hormones and changes in metabolism are blamed.

#### *Management*

Seek medical advice if the substance craved is potentially harmful to the unborn baby.

### Constipation

Progestrone causes relaxation and decreased peristaltic activity of the gut, which is also displaced by the growing uterus.

#### *Management*

- Increase the intake of water, fresh fruit, vegetables and ruphages in the diet.
- Exercise is helpful especially walking.

### Backache

The hormones sometime soften the segments to such a degree that some support is needed.

#### *Management*

- Advice the mother to sleep on firm bed.
- Advice support mechanisms of the back.

### Fainting

In early pregnancy fainting may be due to the vasodilation occuring under the influence of progesterone before there has been a compensatory increase in blood volume. The weight of the uterine contents presses on the inferior vena cava and slows the return of blood to the heart.

#### *Management*

Avoid long period of standing:
- Sit or lie down when she feels slight dizziness
- She would be wise not to lie on her back except during abdominal examination.

### Varicositis

Progesterone relaxes the smooth muscles of the veins and result in sluggish circulation. The valves of the dilated veins become insufficent and varicositis result. It occurs in legs, anus (hemorrhoids) and vulva.

#### *Management*

- Exercising the calf muscles by rising on the toes
- Elevate the leg and rest on the table
- Support thighs and legs
- Avoid constipation and advise adequate fluid intake.
- Sanitary pad give support for vulva varicositis

Most minor disorders can be advanced into a more serious complication of pregnancy. The disorders require immediate actions are as follows (danger signals of pregnancy).
- Vaginal bleeding
- Reduced fetal movements
- Frontal or recurring headaches
- Sudden swelling
- Rupture of the membrane
- Premature onset of contractions
- Maternal anxiety for whatever reason.

## DIAGNOSIS OF PREGNANCY

Pregnancy is mainly diagnosed on the symptoms reported by the woman and signs elicited by a healthcare provider.

### Signs and Symptoms of Pregnancy

These signs and symptoms are divided into three classifications; presumptive, probable, and positive.

### Possible (Presumptive) Signs

- Early breast changes-increase in size, darkening of areola, Montgomery's tubercles
- Amenorrhea—a women having regular cycle without the use of hormonal contraceptives
- Morning sickness
- Bladder irritability like frequency of micturation
- Quickening—the date of the first fetal movement felt by the mother provides an indicator of pregnancy. A primigravid women feels it at 18–20 weeks, the multigravida at 14–16 weeks.

### Probable Signs

- Presence of HCG in:
  - Blood
  - Urine
- Uterine growth
- Braxton Hicks contractions
- Ballottement.

### Positive Signs

Visualization of fetus by:
- Ultrasound 6 weeks of gestation
- X-ray after 12 weeks of gestation

Fetal heart sounds by:
- Ultrasound
- Fetal stethoscope or fetoscope (20th to 24th weeks of gestation)

Fetal movements by:
- Palpation
- Visible.

## NORMAL LABOR

Normal Labor or ***eutocia*** is a physiologic process during which the products of conception (i.e. the fetus, membranes, umbilical cord, and placenta) are expelled from the uterus. Labor is said to be normal only when the fetus is mature and the process is spontaneous and uncomplicated.

Abnormal labor or complicated labor is known as ***dystocia***.

Although the terms 'labor' and 'delivery' are used as synonyms, they really describe two different processes. Labor is the process by which a baby is delivered. Delivery is the actual birth of the baby and does not include the labor pains, uterine contractions, etc. which make up the process of labor.

Normal labor can vary from woman to woman and even between pregnancy to pregnancy in the same woman.

The normal duration of active labor is 8–10 hours in the first pregnancy and 6–8 hours in later pregnancies.

The first labor in a woman is usually more difficult than subsequent labors.

Age of the pregnant woman is also a determinant in the type of labor. Labor is easiest when the woman is between 18–25 years of age. Risk of maternal injuries is highest in a woman in her first labor when she is below 18 years or above 35 years.

Risk of maternal injuries also increases in woman who is in labor for the 5th time or higher.

Many women start to get uterine pains in the later stage of pregnancy. These are false labor pains and need to be differentiated from true labor pains.

| True labor pains | False labor pains |
|---|---|
| Regular | Irregular |
| Increases progressively in frequency, duration and intensity | Does not do so |
| Pain in abdomen radiates to back | Pain is mainly in the abdomen |
| Progressive dilation and effacement of cervix | No effect on cervix |
| Cannot be relieved by painkillers or sedatives | Can be relieved by painkillers or sedatives |

## PRODROMAL STAGE OF LABOR

Normal labor is usually preceded by a stage of pre-labor in the last weeks of pregnancy in which clinical symptoms known as Prodromal Symptoms occur. These are:

- ***Lightening:*** Lightening is a sensation of relief in the upper abdomen due to descent of the fetal head into the pelvis. Pressure symptoms like difficulty in breathing, acid reflux and palpitation decreases.
- ***Pelvic pressure symptoms:*** The engagement of the fetal head puts pressure on the surrounding pelvic organs like the bladder and the rectum. This causes increased frequency of urine and a feeling of fullness in the rectum with an increased tendency of wanting to pass stools. Pressure on the hip joints can cause difficulty in walking.
- ***Increased vaginal discharge:*** Pressure on the cervix causes increased secretion of discharge. The cervical mucus plug may also get disturbed and come out in bits to cause increased vaginal discharge.
- ***False labor pain*** False Labor Pains occur in the last few weeks of pregnancy.

## STAGES OF NORMAL LABOR

Normal labor is a physiologic process during which the products of conception (i.e. the fetus, membranes, umbilical cord, and placenta) are expelled outside the uterus. Labor is said to be normal only when the fetus is mature and the process is spontaneous and uncomplicated.

The normal duration of active labor is 8–10 hours in the first pregnancy and 6–8 hours in later pregnancies.

It is difficult to determine exactly when normal labor starts. This is because, very often, a woman may have uterine contractions which are due to false labor pains. False labor pains are not regular, and can be controlled by painkillers and antispasmodic medicines.

True labor is regular, the intensity and number of contractions increases gradually and it is accompanied by passage of mucus and blood. Rupture of the membranes can also occur at the onset of labor and is marked by a gush of clear liquid.

### Onset of Labor

The start of true labor is characterized by:

***True labor pains:*** Normal labor is divided into three stages: Regular pains in the abdomen which gradually increase in intensity and which radiates to the back and to the legs are true labor pains. The duration and number of contractions increases over time.

***Show:*** Show is the passage of blood stained mucus due to the expelled cervical mucus plug. The bleeding occurs from ruptured small vessels as a result of separation of the membranes from the lower uterine segment.

***Dilation of the cervix:*** A dilating cervix is a definite sign of the start of labor, especially in primigradias. In a multigravida, the cervix may admit the tip of the finger even before labor starts.

***Formation of the bag of waters:*** The bag of waters can be felt through the partially dilated cervix at the start of labor.

### First Stage of Normal Labor

Stage I lasts from the onset of labor to full dilation of the cervix. In a woman in her first pregnancy, this stage lasts for about 10 to 12 hours. In a woman who has delivered earlier, it lasts from 6 to 8 hours. The first stage is again divided into three phases:

#### *Phase I*

This is the longest and least painful phase of the entire duration of labor. It starts from the time when the cervix first starts to dilate to the time when the cervix is 4 cm dilated. It is also called the 'Latent phase' of labor or the 'Early phase' of labor. It can last for days and can occur with only the mildest discomfort to the pregnant woman.

#### *Phase II*

This is a more active phase of labor. The cervix dilates from 4 cm to 8 cm during this phase.

The contractions are more painful, of longer duration and come more regularly. It is also called the 'middle phase' of labor.

#### *Phase III*

During this phase, the cervix dilates from 8 cm to 10 cm. At 10 cms, the cervix is fully dilated and the baby's head can come out of the uterus safely and easily.

This phase is also called the 'transition phase' of labor since it marks the transition of the first stage of labor to the second stage of labor.

### Second Stage of Labor

Second stage lasts from the full dilatation of the cervix to the expulsion of the baby. In a first pregnancy, it lasts for about 1–2 hour, in subsequent pregnancies, it lasts for about 1/2 hour.

This stage (second stage) is the stage when the baby's head is travelling down the vaginal canal to be delivered. The contractions are very painful and run into each other, appearing to produce almost continuous pain.

### Third Stage of Labor

Stage III lasts from the birth of the baby to the expulsion of the placenta and the membranes. It lasts for about 15–20 minutes in both first and later pregnancies. The third stage is comparatively less painful and is characterized by a gush of bleeding at the time the placenta separates from the uterus.

## NORMAL POSTPARTUM

The puerperium or the postpartum period is the period of time following the delivery of the child during which the body tissues, especially the reproductive system reverts back to the pre-pregnant state, both anatomically and physiologically.

The process of reversion of the genital organs is called 'involution'.

The puerperium or the postpartum period lasts for 6 weeks. It is divided into three phases:

- ***Immediate postpartum:*** The 24-hour period immediately following delivery.
- ***Early postpartum or puerperium:*** Upto 7 days.
- ***Remote postpartum or puerperium:*** Upto 6 weeks.

### Immediately After Delivery

Immediately after delivery, the body goes into a few hours of stress before it begins to settle down to a normal state again. During these hours, the pulse rate remains high, usually due to the stress of giving birth but also due to a loss of blood during the childbirth. The body temperature may decrease and there may be retention of urine.

### Care in the Postpartum Period

Just after the delivery, the woman is exhausted from the process of childbirth. She should be allowed to rest for a few hours to recuperate and then encouraged to sit up and walk if she has had a normal vaginal childbirth. This helps drainage of lochia and encourages uterine involution. The perineum and the vulva should be checked and the breasts examined to initiate breastfeeding.

### Breastfeeding

Breastfeeding should be initiated within 1 hour of birth—this helps in psychological support of the baby, easy latching of the baby to the breast and in creating the mother-baby bond. The milk secreted in the first few days is thin and whitish and is known as colostrum. It is rich in immunoglobulins which pass from the mother to the child and increases the baby's resistance to various diseases.

### Involution

Involution is the process by which the reproductive organs revert back to the normal pre-pregnant state in about 6 weeks. The uterus not only returns to its pre-pregnant size, but it also returns to its normal position in the pelvic cavity and regains its muscular tone. The vagina, uterine ligaments and muscles of the pelvic floor all revert back to the pre-pregnant state.

### Lochia

Lochia is the vaginal discharge which occurs in the 4-6 weeks after childbirth. In the first week, it is red in color with large amounts of blood and blood clots and is known as the lochia rubra. The color changes to a lighter pinkish to brownish as the amount of blood decreases at this stage it is known as lochia serosa. In the later weeks, it is yellowish to whitish, and is then known as the lochia alba.

### Birth Control in the Postpartum Period

Sex is not advisable for at least 6 weeks after delivery, i.e. in the postpartum period, as the tissues are fragile at this time and need time to recover. But, if necessary, barrier contraceptives like condoms should be used.

Condoms have the advantage of being readily available, of not containing any hormones and being cheap. They have no effect on breastfeeding and have no risks to the mother or child. But they can irritate the vaginal tissues. Other birth control measures which can be used are the hormonal pills, the intrauterine contraceptive device, the rhythm method etc.

### Return of the Period after Childbirth

In women who are breastfeeding exclusively and where the baby gets its entire nutritional needs from the mother's breast, the menstrual period may return only 6 months after the childbirth. But if a woman is bottle-feeding, or combining breast and bottle, the periods may return as early as 1 month after birth. in most cases, it returns after about 3 months.

### Postpartum Exercise

Regular exercise after childbirth helps the body to regain its pre-pregnancy shape and size. Decrease in weight increases energy levels, stimulates appetite and helps a new mother cope with the demands of looking after a newborn. The exercises also help to tone up the pelvic and abdominal walls and to correct postural defects.

### Postpartum Posture

The postpartum period is the time when the woman has not totally recovered from the stress and strain placed on her body by pregnancy and labor. Yet, this is the time when she has to look after her baby-feed, bathe, lift and take care of everything else as well. Wrong posture can cause back pain, knee pain and pain at various parts of the body. The correct postures as shown here, can help decrease many of the aches and pains which occur during the postpartum period.

## NORMAL MENSTRUATION

Menstruation or 'the period' is defined as the spontaneous, monthly, cyclical, bloody vaginal discharge that represents shedding of the endometrium (inner lining of the uterus) every month. Once shedding is complete, it stops spontaneously. The term 'menstruation' comes from the Greek word 'men' meaning month.

Menstruation does not occur during pregnancy, before puberty and after the menopause.

## AMENORRHEA

Amenorrhea (loss of periods) can be:

- Physiological (i.e. in the normal course of life)
- Pathological (i.e. due to some abnormalities).

***Physiological amenorrhea (loss of periods):*** Amenorrhea may be normal at certain periods in a woman's life, for example, during pregnancy, during breastfeeding, before attaining puberty and after the menopause.

***Pathological amenorrhea (loss of periods):*** Pathological Amenorrhea or loss of periods is amenorrhea that occurs as a symptom of an underlying disease. It is not a disease process in itself. There are two types of pathological amenorrhea.

### Primary Amenorrhea

When a girl has never experienced menarche and menses, she is said to be suffering from primary amenorrhea or primary lack of menses. The cause is usually congenital, i.e. from birth, and can be due to genetic or chromosomal abnormalities or due to a defect in the development of the reproductive tract. Treatment of this condition is very difficult.

### Secondary Amenorrhea

When the patient has had at least one episode of spontaneous menses before the loss of her periods, she is said to suffer from secondary amenorrhea. This is the commonest form of amenorrhea. The problem may lie in the hypothalamus and the pituitary, or the uterus or the ovary. Other endocrine glands like the thyroid, the pancreas and the adrenal cortex also have a role to play in causing amenorrhea.

## MENOPAUSE

The term, '**menopause**' refers to the physiological cessation of menstruation at a certain age, usually between 45–55 years, in life. Although the term is used to describe all the various symptoms that occur at this stage, the actual meaning of the word is just what it says - 'pause of menstruation'.

The right term for all the menopausal symptoms as well as menopause itself is 'Climacteric'. Climacteric is the transitional phase lasting for 1–5 years during which the reproductive tract changes in response to the decreasing activity of the ovaries.

The pre-menopause is the 3 to 5 year period before the menopause when a woman's estrogen levels begin to drop.

## EPISIOTOMY

***Definition:*** The making of an incision into the prenium to enlarge the vaginal orifice.

### Indications for Episiotomy

- Delay due to rigid perineum, disproportion between fetus and vaginal orifice.
- Fetal distress due to prolapsed cord in second stage.
- To facilitate vaginal or intrauterine manipulation, eg. forceps, breech delivery.
- Preterm baby in order to avoid intracranial damage.
- Previous 3rd degree repaired on the perineum.

### Advantages of Episiotomy

- Fetal acidosis and hypoxia are reduced
- Over stretching of the pelvic floor is lessened
- Bruising of the urethra is avoided.
- In severe pre-eclampsia or cardiac disease to reduce the effort bearing down.
- A previous third degree tear which may occur again because of the scar tissue which does not stretch well is prevented.

### Types of Episiotomy

- Mediolateral
- Median
- J-shaped
- Lateral

### Local Analgesia for Episiotomy

Lignocaine/lidocaine/0.5 percent of 10 mL is safe and efficient.

It takes effect rapidly within 1 and 2 minutes.

### Timing of the Incision

- The head should be well down on the perineum, low enough to keep it stretched and thinned
- In breech presentation the posterior buttock would be distending the perineum
- It must be made neither too soon nor too late.

## MULTIPLE CHOICE QUESTIONS

**1. Puerperium period lasts for how many weeks?**
(a) 1 week (b) 2 weeks
(c) 3 weeks (d) 6 weeks

**2. What is the commonest cause of PPH? (AIIMS 2010)**
(a) Puerperial sepsis (b) Birth injury
(c) ADH (d) Atonicity of uterus

**3. The relationship of fetal head and limbs to trunk is known as:**
(a) Position (b) Attitude
(c) Lie (d) Presentation

**4. Which uterine layer changed into deciduas during pregnancy?**
(a) Perimetrium (b) Myometrium
(c) Endocardium (d) Endometrium

**5. Three or more consecutive spontaneous abortion is termed as:**
(a) Habitual (b) Threatened
(c) Spontaneous (d) Complete

**6. What is the meaning of term 'Eutocia'?**
(a) Obstructed labor (b) Instrumental labor
(c) Normal labor (d) Surgical labor

**7. What is the color of amniotic fluid in 'Postmaturity'?**
(a) Green (b) Golden
(c) Saffron (d) Grey

**8. Progesterone is normally secreted in relatively large quantity by the:**
(a) Endometrium
(b) Corpus luteum
(c) Adrenal cortex
(d) Pituitary gland

**9. The perception of active fetal movements by the mother at about 18th week is termed as:**
(a) Lightening (b) Tightening
(c) Quickening (d) Kicking

**10. Aspermia is the term used to describe: (PGIMER 2000)**
(a) Absence of semen
(b) Absence of sperm motility
(c) Absence of sperm in ejaculate
(d) None of the above

**11. Which diameter gets engaged when head is fully flexed in vertex presentation?**
(a) Suboccipitobregmatic
(b) Occipitobregmatic
(c) Occipitofrontal
(d) Suboccipitofrontal

**12. What is the approximate weight gain during pregnancy?**
(a) 11–12 kg (b) 13–14 kg
(c) 16–18 kg (d) 19–20 kg

**13. What is the normal ratio of lecithin-sphingomyelin (surfactant) in full mature fetus?**
(a) 1:2 (b) 2:1
(c) 2:2 (d) 1:3

**14. The temporary opening between the two atria in fetal heart is known as:**
(a) Ductus venosus (b) Ductus arteriosus
(c) Foramen ovale (d) Umbilical vein

**15. What do you mean by oligohydramnios? (ESI 2010)**
(a) When amount of amniotic fluid is more than 1200 mL
(b) When amount of amniotic fluid is more than 1000 mL
(c) When amount of amniotic fluid is less than 500 mL
(d) When amount of amniotic fluid is less than 200 mL

**16. The organ which provides nutrition to fetus is: (ESIC 2016)**
(a) Uterus (b) Liver
(c) Placenta (d) Ovary

**17. Which vitamin deficiency results in defective synthesis of RNA and DNA?**
(a) Vitamin B1 (b) Vitamin B2
(c) Vitamin B6 (d) Vitamin B12

**18. Mother who is pregnant second time and undergone spontaneous abortion, it is written as:**
(a) G1A1 (b) G2A1
(c) G2P1 (d) G2A0

**19. The effect of ovarian tumor on labor is:**
(a) Obstructed labor (b) Mechanical distress
(c) Infection (d) Non-engagement of head

**20. Which of the following urinary symptoms does the pregnant lady most frequently experience during the first trimester? (RRB 2006)**
(a) Burning micturition (b) Frequency
(c) Incontinence (d) Dysuria

**21. Hormone essential for milk ejection is: (ESIC 2016)**
(a) Progesterone (b) Estrogen
(c) Prolactin (d) Oxytocin

**22. The 'MTP' Act was enforced in the year:**
(a) 1970 (b) 1972
(c) 1974 (d) 1976

**23. Oxytocin acts directly on:**
(a) Endometrium (b) Myometrium
(c) Perimetrium (d) Myocardium

**24. Primary feature of cervical cancer includes: (ESIC 2009)**
(a) Abdominal pain (b) Irregular menstruation
(c) Anorexia (d) Polyuria

**25. About 25% of maternal deaths are due to: (RPSC Nsg. Tutor 2009)**
(a) Eclampsia (b) Abortion
(c) Infection (d) Obstetric hemorrhage

**26. The diameter of human placenta at term is:**
(a) 2–8 cm (b) 9–14 cm
(c) 15–20 cm (d) 21–27 cm

**27. Which type of episiotomy has more chances of injury to 'Bartholin's duct'?**
(a) Lateral (b) Mediolateral
(c) Median (d) 'J' Shape

**28. What is formed in fetal neck during internal rotation of head in normal labor?**
(a) Crowning (b) Extension
(c) Molding (d) Twist

**29. The process of rupture of mature griffin follicle and egg is shed from ovary is termed as:**
(a) Gematogenesis (b) Oogenesis
(c) Ovulation (d) Spermatogenesis

**30. What is called when the involution of uterus is impaired during puerperium?**
(a) Sub-involution (b) Supra-involution
(c) Super-involution (d) Un-involution

**31. How many arteries are present in umbilical cord?**
(a) One (b) Two
(c) Three (d) Four

**32. Which type of lochia should the nurse expect find in a mother of 2 days postpartum?**
(a) Foul smell (b) Lochia serosa
(c) Lochia alba (d) Lochia rubra

**33. Which obstetrical instrument is invented by 'Peter-2 of chamberlen family' around 1600 AD?**
(a) Ventouse b) Forceps
(c) Spectrum (d) Dialators

**34. The average weight gain during pregnancy is: (ESIC 2006)**
(a) 19–20 kg (b) 15–16 kg
(c) 12–13 kg (d) 5–6 kg

**35. Immediately before expulsion, which of the following cardinal movements occu? (AIIMS 2009)**
(a) External rotation (b) Restitution
(c) Flexion (d) Descent

**36. Which of the following tests should be ordered to confirm diagnosis of beta thalassemia?**
(a) Complete blood count
(b) Hemoglobin A
(c) Hemoglobin electrophoresis
(d) Iron level

**37. The additional contraceptive protection needed after vasectomy is for:**
(a) 1–2 months (b) 2–3 months
(c) 3–4 months (d) 4–5 months

**38. Which antiretroviral treatment is used for pregnant mother?**
(a) Zidovudine (b) Lamuvudine
(c) Efavirenze (d) Nevirapine

**39. Hydatidiform mole is principally a disease of:**
(a) Amnion (b) Chorion
(c) Endometrium (d) Ovary

**40. The commonest site for ectopic pregnancy is:**
(a) Ovary (b) Abdomen
(c) Fallopian tube (d) Peritoneum

**41. The natural method of contraception in postpartum period for a female is:**
(a) Use of OC Pills (b) Barrier method
(c) Cu T Insertion (d) Exclusive breastfeeding

**42. The important landmark in pelvic outlet which is of obstetric importance is:**
(a) Ischial tuberosity (b) Symphysis pubis
(c) Coccyx (d) Ischial spines

**43. In physiological basis of lactation, the phase which deals with preparation of breast is:**
(a) Mammogenesis (b) Lactogenesis
(c) Galactopoiesis (d) Galactokinesis

**44. A primigravida in active stage of labor is noted pushing down continuously. The midwife should:**
(a) Encourage her to pushdown
(b) Ask her not to push down
(c) Ask her to work around
(d) Apply fundal pressure during pushing

**45. A midwife knows that a woman receiving $MgSO_4$, has developed sign of drug toxicity when it shows:**
(a) Presence of patellar reflex
(b) Urine output > 30 mL/hour
(c) Respiratory rate < 14/minute
(d) Eclamptic attack

**46. Before administering in methergine to postnatal woman, who complaints of excessive lochia rubra, the nurse should first assess for:**
(a) Temperature (b) Pulse rate
(c) Respiratory rate (d) Blood pressure

**47. Colostrum has the highest quantity of the following as compared to breast milk:**
(a) Immunoglobulins (b) CHO
(c) Fat (d) Sodium

**48. Out of the following which is NOT cut in episiotomy?**
(a) Skin and superficial perineal muscles
(b) Levator ani muscles
(c) Posterior vaginal wall
(d) Anterior vaginal wall

**49. The best primary action by a midwife, who comes across a woman with APH at home is:**
(a) Shift the woman to hospital
(b) Arrange for intravenous infusion
(c) Give psychological support
(d) Do detail history collection

**50. Out of the following in which state in India has lowest MMR?**
(a) Maharashtra (b) Uttar Pradesh
(c) Bihar (d) Karnataka

**51. With the first half an hour of birth after full term normal delivery, the nurse should encourage the mother to:**
(a) Breastfed the neonate
(b) Allow the neonate to sleep
(c) Bathe the neonate
(d) Handle the neonate

**52. In concealed abruption placenta, the blood may collect in all except:**
(a) Behind membrance and uterine wall
(b) Behind placenta
(c) Myometrium
(d) Amniotic cavity

**53. Buddha's sign is a diagnostic posture in:**
(a) IUGR (b) IUD
(c) Twin pregnancy (d) Hydatidiform mole

**54. Out of the following which is NOT an absolute indication for cesarian section?**
(a) Vaginal atresia (b) Severe contracted pelvis
(c) Ca cervix (d) Fetal distress

**55. In menstrual cycle, the phase which deals with thickening of endometrium is termed as:**
(a) Bleeding phase
(b) Regenerative phase
(c) Proliferative phase
(d) Ovulatory phase

**56. The first line screening test both for high risk and low risk fetus is:**
(a) Fetal movement count
(b) Non stress test
(c) Vibroacoustic stimulation
(d) Carditocography

**57. In which of the following placental abnormality the cord is inserted at the edge of the placenta?**
(a) Placenta acreta
(b) Placenta bipertita
(c) Velamentous
(d) Bettledose

**58. Snow storm appearance on USG is characteristic finding in case of:**
(a) Hydatidiform mole
(b) Twin pregnancy
(c) Intrauterine growth retardation
(d) Normal singleton pregnancy

**59. A midwife is sure that in early diagnosis of pregnancy, among the following the most reliable findings are:**
(a) Subjective symptoms
(b) Clinical symptoms
(c) Immunological test
(d) None of the above

**60. According to WHO, the pregnant woman should visit antenatal clinic at least:**
(a) Once only (b) 4 times
(c) 8 times (d) Every monthly

**61. After the delivery of lower extremities and trunk in breech presentation, the next best action by a midwife is:**
(a) Follow wait and watch policy
(b) Wrap the baby in warm sterile towel
(c) Attempt immediate vaginal delivery
(d) Inform about sex of the child to mother

**62. A nulligravida client diagnosed with probable ruptured ectopic pregnancy is scheduled for emergency surgery the most important assessment is:**
(a) Abdominal distention
(b) Blood pressure and pulse rate
(c) Hemogram
(d) Uterine cramps

**63. In classification of abnormal uterine action, uterine inertia is grouped under:**
(a) Inefficient uterine action
(b) Excessive uterine action
(c) Abnormal pattern of uterine action
(d) Cervical dystocia

**64. Out of the following which sense is believed to be the most highly developed sense at birth for newborn?**
(a) Taste (b) Touch
(c) Hearing (d) Vision

**65. A primigravida with 38 weeks of pregnancy reports with bleeding PV, USG reveals type IV placenta previa. The midwife knows that the line of treatment is:**
(a) Immediate vaginal delivery
(b) Emergency cesarian section
(c) Complete bed rest in hospital
(d) Termination of pregnancy after 1 week

**66. In which type of abortion, the abortion process is started but not reached up to the stage from which recovery is not possible?**
(a) Missed (b) Complete
(c) Threatened (d) Septic

**67. Out of the following which sign and symptoms is present throughout the three trimisters of pregnancy?**
(a) Amenorrhea
(b) Quickening
(c) Lightening
(d) Cholostrum secretion from breast

**68. After full term normal delivery with episiotomy, woman complaints of pain and swelling at episiotomy site. The best action by midwife is:**
(a) Give perineal care
(b) Tell her it is normal response
(c) Apply cold compression
(d) Apply hot pack

**69. In case of Hydatidiform mole, in follow up period after treatment, the woman is monitored regularly for:**
(a) Serum hCG level
(b) Estrogen and progesterone level
(c) Hematocrit
(d) Pervaginal bleeding

**70. In routine antenatal exam, midwife is sure that uterine fundus can be felt at the level of umbilicus at following weeks of gestation:**
(a) 12 weeks (b) 16 weeks
(c) 20 weeks (d) 24 weeks

**71. Which of the following is the direct cause of maternal mortality?**
(a) Accident (b) Anemia
(c) Abortion (d) Diabetes

**72. Hormone responsible for ovulation:**
(a) Estrogen
(b) Follicular stimulating hormone
(c) Leutinizing hormone
(d) Human chorionic gonadotropin

**73. Ectodermal layer of the embryonic disc forms:**
(a) Bones (b) Cartilage
(c) Gallbladder (d) Epidermis of skin

**74. Term placenta weights about:**
(a) 500 gm (b) 1000 gm
(c) 1500 gm (d) 2000 gm

**75. The fertilizable life span of oocyte ranges:**
(a) from 6–11 hrs (b) from 12–24 hrs
(c) from 25–46 hrs (d) from 48–72 hrs

**76. Inner cell mass gives rise to:**
(a) Amnion (b) Chorion
(c) Fetus (d) Placenta

**77. When the cord is attached to the membranes, the placenta is called:**
(a) Circumvallata Placenta
(b) Battledose Placenta
(c) Placenta Marginata
(d) Velamentous Placenta

**78. In a well flexed head of fetus, the engaging transverse diameter:**
(a) Bi-Temporal (b) Bi-Parietal
(c) Occipitofrontal (d) Suboccipito Bregmatic

**79. Lochia serosa is seen on the following:**
(a) 1–4 days (b) 5–9 days
(c) 10–15 days (d) 16–20 days

**80. Prophylactic treatment for prevention of Hyaline membrane disease:**
(a) Fluid therapy (b) Surfactant
(c) Steroids (d) Oxygen

**81. Usually postnatal breast engorgement is seen on the following postpartum days:**
(a) 1 to 2 days (b) 3 to 4 days
(c) 5 to 6 days (d) 7 to 8 days

**82. Methergin is contraindicated for the following condition:**
(a) Abortion
(b) Cardiac condition
(c) Hydatidiform mole
(d) Hemorrhage

**83. The following is a natural method of contraception:**
(a) Billings (b) Condoms
(c) Diaphragm (d) Implants

**84. The largest diameter of the fetal skull:**
(a) Suboccipito bregmatic
(b) Occipito frontal
(c) Suboccipito vertical
(d) Mentovertical

**85. Following fertilization, on which day does the implementation of blastocyst occur?**
(a) 1st (b) 3rd
(c) 6th (d) 10th

**86. The isthmus in non-pregnant uterus is measuring about:**
(a) 0.5 cm (b) 2.5 cm
(c) 5 cm (d) 7 cm

**87. In fetal circulation 80% of oxygenated blood gets mixed up with deoxygenated blood via:**
(a) Ductous venosus (b) Ductous arteriosus
(c) Foramen ovale (d) Umbilical arteries

**88. The number of blood vessels present in umbilical cord:**
(a) 2 arteries 2 veins (b) 2 arteries 1 vein
(c) 1 artery 1 vein (d) 1 artery 2 veins

**89. Blotchy mark of pregnancy called as:**
(a) Chlosma (b) Linea Nigra
(c) Spider Navi (d) Striae gravidarum

**90. Lightening takes place at:**
(a) 16 to 20 weeks (b) 24 to 28 weeks
(c) 30 to 34 weeks (d) 38 to 40 weeks

**91. The discomfort 'Pyrosis' is caused due to the effect of hormone:**
(a) Estrogen
(b) Prolactin
(c) Progesterone
(d) Human chorionic gonadotropin

**92. In breech presentation, the denominator is:**
(a) Acromion (b) Buttocks
(c) Occiput (d) Sacrum

**93. The obstetric score of an antenatal mother with 30 weeks of twin gestation, history of a previous living child:**
(a) G2P1A0L1 (b) G2P2A0L1
(c) G3P2A0L1 (d) G2P3A0L1

**94. Immediately before expulsion, which of the following cardinal movements occur? (AIIMS 2009)**
(a) Descent (b) Flexion
(c) Extension (d) External rotation

**95. What is the principal carbohydrate present in amniotic fluid? (CMC Vellore 98)**
(a) Glucose (b) Fructose
(c) Maltose (d) Galactose

**96. During which of the following stages of labor would the nurse assess 'crowning'? (DSSSB)**
(a) First stage (b) Second stage
(c) Third stage (d) Fourth stage

**97. In placenta previa the blood is:**
(a) Dark red (b) Bright red
(c) Clotted (d) Thick mixed with mucus

**98. Commonest complication of heart disease in pregnancy:**
(a) Arrhythmia (b) Bacterial endocarditis
(c) Pulmonary Edema (d) Pulmonary Embolism

**99. Preterm labor is defined as:**
(a) Labor starts before 37 weeks
(b) Labor starts before 38 weeks
(c) Labor starts before 36 weeks
(d) Labor starts before 35 weeks

**100. Advantages of lower segment cesarean section:**
(a) Delay healing scar
(b) Low chances of rupture
(c) Maternal risk for death
(d) Abdominal distension

**101. Frank breech refers to:**
(a) Breech with flexed leg
(b) Breech with extended head
(c) Breech with extended leg
(d) All of the above

**102. The definitive sign indicating labor has begun would be:**
(a) Progressive uterine contraction
(b) Lightening
(c) Rupture of membranes
(d) Passage of the mucus plug

**103. Secondary PPH occurs due to:**
(a) Retained membrane (b) Sub-involution
(c) Low grade infection (d) All of the above

**104. Ultrasound sonography shows 'Snowstorm' appearance in case of:**
(a) Hydatidiform mole (b) Anencephaly
(c) Fibroid uterus (d) Multiple pregnancy

**105. Assessment of gestational age at birth is done using:**
(a) New Ballard score (b) APGAR score
(c) Bhakoo score (d) Downe score

**106. About 25% of maternal death are due to: (ESI 2004)**
(a) Infection
(b) Obstetric hemorrhage
(c) Unsafe abortion
(d) Eclampsia

**107. When bleeding after 24 hours of delivery is considered as postpartum hemorrhage? (RPSC 2010)**
(a) Blood loss of more than 500 mL
(b) Blood loss of more than 700 mL
(c) Blood loss of more than 100 mL
(d) Blood loss of more than 200 mL

**108. Baby weighing 1000 gm showing no signs of life after delivery.**
(a) Abortus (b) Neonatal death
(c) Perinatal death (d) Stillbirth

## ANSWERS

| | | | | | | | | | | | |
|---|---|---|---|---|---|---|---|---|---|---|---|
| **1.** | (d) | **21.** | (d) | **41.** | (d) | **61.** | (a) | **81.** | (b) | **101.** | (c) |
| **2.** | (d) | **22.** | (b) | **42.** | (a) | **62.** | (c) | **82.** | (b) | **102.** | (a) |
| **3.** | (b) | **23.** | (b) | **43.** | (b) | **63.** | (a) | **83.** | (a) | **103.** | (d) |
| **4.** | (d) | **24.** | (d) | **44.** | (a) | **64.** | (b) | **84.** | (d) | **104.** | (a) |
| **5.** | (a) | **25.** | (b) | **45.** | (d) | **65.** | (b) | **85** | (d) | **105.** | (a) |
| **6.** | (c) | **26.** | (c) | **46.** | (d) | **66.** | (c) | **86.** | (a) | **106.** | (a) |
| **7.** | (c) | **27.** | (b) | **47.** | (a) | **67.** | (a) | **87.** | (a) | **107.** | (a) |
| **8.** | (b) | **28.** | (d) | **48.** | (d) | **68.** | (a) | **88.** | (b) | **108.** | (d) |
| **9.** | (c) | **29.** | (c) | **49.** | (a) | **69.** | (a) | **89.** | (a) | | |
| **10.** | (d) | **30.** | (a) | **50.** | (c) | **70.** | (d) | **90.** | (d) | | |
| **11.** | (a) | **31.** | (b) | **51.** | (a) | **71.** | (c) | **91.** | (c) | | |
| **12.** | (a) | **32.** | (d) | **52.** | (b) | **72.** | (b) | **92.** | (d) | | |
| **13.** | (b) | **33.** | (b) | **53.** | (c) | **73.** | (d) | **93.** | (a) | | |
| **14.** | (c) | **34.** | (c) | **54.** | (a) | **74.** | (a) | **94.** | (d) | | |
| **15** | (d) | **35** | (b) | **55** | (b) | **75** | (b) | **95** | (a) | | |
| **16.** | (c) | **36.** | (d) | **56.** | (c) | **76.** | (c) | **96.** | (b) | | |
| **17.** | (d) | **37.** | (b) | **57.** | (d) | **77.** | (d) | **97.** | (b) | | |
| **18.** | (b) | **38.** | (a) | **58.** | (a) | **78.** | (b) | **98.** | (a) | | |
| **19.** | (b) | **39.** | (b) | **59.** | (c) | **79.** | (b) | **99.** | (a) | | |
| **20.** | (c) | **40.** | (c) | **60.** | (b) | **80.** | (b) | **100.** | (b) | | |

# QUICK REVIEW

## Normal Lab Values for Adults

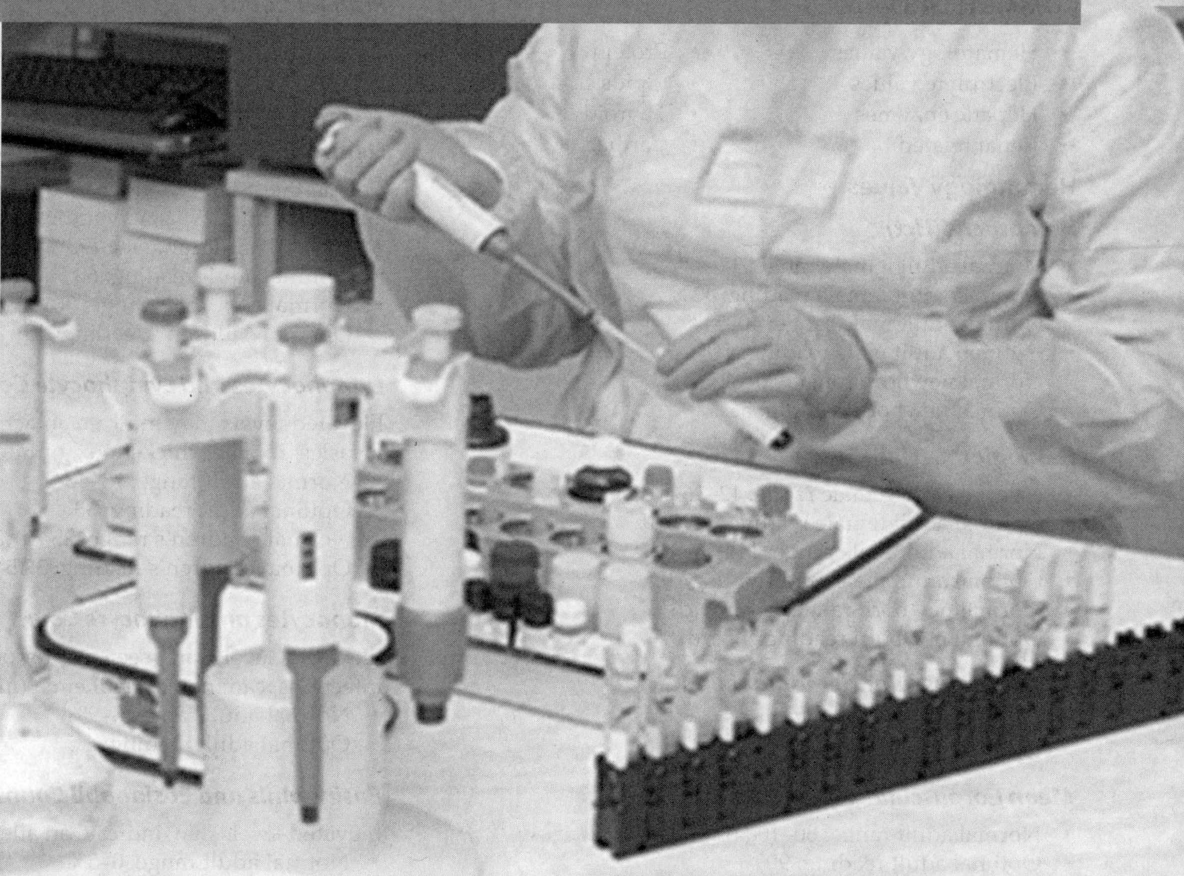

### HIGHLIGHTS

- Common Lab Values
- Something Extra for Your Knowledge

# Normal Lab Values for Adults

## COMMON LAB VALUES

- Hematology values
- Electrolyte values
- Hepatic enzymes
- Renal related
- Protein
- Lipids
- Thyroid
- Cardiac

### Hematology Values

#### *Hematocrit (Hct)*

- Normal adult female range: 37–47%
- Optimal adult female reading: 42%
- Normal adult male range: 40–54%
- Optimal adult male reading: 47%
- Normal newborn range: 50–62%
- Optimal newborn reading: 56%

#### *Hemoglobin (Hgb)*

- Normal adult female range: 12–16 g/dL
- Optimal adult female reading: 14 g/dL
- Normal adult male range: 14–18 g/dL
- Optimal adult male reading: 16 g/dL
- Normal newborn range: 14–20 g/dL
- Optimal newborn reading: 17 g/dL

#### *Mean Corpuscular Hemoglobin (MCH)*

- Normal adult range: 27–33 pg
- Optimal adult reading: 30

#### *Mean Corpuscular Volume (MCV)*

- Normal adult range: 80–100 fL
- Optimal adult reading: 90
- Higher ranges are found in newborns and infants.

#### *Mean Corpuscular Hemoglobin Concentration (MCHC)*

- Normal Adult range: 32–36%
- Optimal adult reading: 34
- Higher ranges are found in newborns and infants.

#### *Red Blood Cell Count (RBC)*

- Normal adult female range: 3.9–5.2 mill/mcL
- Optimal adult female reading: 4.55
- Normal adult male range: 4.2–5.6 mill/mcL
- Optimal adult male reading: 4.9
- Lower ranges are found in children, newborns and infants.

#### *White Blood Cell Count (WBC)*

- Normal adult range: 3.8–10.8 thous/mcL
- Optimal adult reading: 7.3
- Higher ranges are found in children, newborns and infants.

#### *Platelet Count*

- Normal adult range: 130–400 thous/mcL
- Optimal adult reading: 265
- Higher ranges are found in children, newborns and infants.

#### *Neutrophils and Neutrophil Count*

This is the main defender of the body against infection and antigens. High levels may indicate an active infection.

- Normal adult range: 48–73%
- Optimal adult reading: 60.5
- Normal children's range: 30–60%
- Optimal children's reading: 45

#### *Lymphocytes and Lymphocyte Count*

Elevated levels may indicate an active viral infections such as measles, rubella, chickenpox, or infectious mononucleosis.

- Normal adult range: 18–48%
- Optimal adult reading: 33
- Normal children's range: 25–50%
- Optimal children's reading: 37.5

#### *Monocytes and Monocyte Count*

Elevated levels are seen in tissue breakdown or chronic infections, carcinomas, leukemia (monocytic) or lymphomas.

- Normal adult range: 0–9%
- Optimal adult reading: 4.5

#### *Eosinophils and Eosinophil Count*

Elevated levels may indicate an allergic reactions or parasites.

- Normal adult range: 0–5%
- Optimal adult reading: 2.5

#### *Basophils and Basophil Count*

Basophilic activity is not fully understood but it is known to carry histamine, heparin and serotonin. High levels are found in allergic reactions.

- Normal adult range: 0–2%
- Optimal adult reading: 1

### Electrolyte Values

#### *Sodium*

Sodium is the most abundant cation in the blood and its chief base. It functions in the body to maintain osmotic pressure, acid-base balance and to transmit nerve impulses. Very low value: seizure and neurologic Sx.

- Normal adult range: 135–146 mEq/L
- Optimal adult reading: 140.5

### Potassium

Potassium is the major intracellular cation. Very low value: Cardiac arythemia.

- Normal range: 3.5–5.5 mEq/L
- Optimal adult reading: 4.5

### Chloride

Elevated levels are related to acidosis as well as too much water crossing the cell membrane. Decreased levels with decreased serum albumin may indicate water deficiency crossing the cell membrane (edema).

- Normal adult range: 95–112 mEq/L
- Optimal adult reading: 103

### $CO_2$ (Carbon Dioxide)

The $CO_2$ level is related to the respiratory exchange of carbon dioxide in the lungs and is part of the bodies buffering system. Generally when used with the other electrolytes, it is a good indicator of acidosis and alkalinity.

- Normal adult range: 22–32 mEq/L
- Optimal adult reading: 27
- Normal children range: 20–28 mEq/L
- Optimal children reading: 24

### Calcium

Involved in bone metabolism, protein absorption, fat transfer muscular contraction, transmission of nerve impulses, blood clotting and cardiac function. Regulated by parathyroid.

- Normal adult range: 8.5–10.3 mEq/dL
- Optimal adult reading: 9.4

### Phosphorus

Generally inverse with calcium.

- Normal adult range: 2.5–4.5 mEq/dL
- Optimal adult reading: 3.5
- Normal children range: 3–6 mEq/dL
- Optimal children range: 4.5

### Anion Gap (Sodium + Potassium–$CO_2$ + Chloride)

An increased measurement is associated with metabolic acidosis due to the overproduction of acids (a state of alkalinity is in effect). Decreased levels may indicate metabolic alkalosis due to the overproduction of alkaloids (a state of acidosis is in effect).

- Normal adult range: 4–14 (calculated)
- Optimal adult reading: 9

### Calcium/Phosphorus Ratio

- Normal adult range: 2.3–3.3 (calculated)
- Optimal adult reading: 2.8
- Normal children's range: 1.3–3.3 (calculated)
- Optimal children's reading: 2.3

### Sodium/Potassium

- Normal adult range: 26–38 (calculated)
- Optimal adult reading: 32

## Hepatic Enzymes

### AST (Serum Glutamic-Oxalocetic Transaminase-SGOT)

Found primarily in the liver, heart, kidney, pancreas and muscles. Seen in tissue damage, especially heart and liver.

- Normal adult range: 0–42 U/L
- Optimal adult reading: 21

### ALT (Serum Glutamic-Pyruvic Transaminase-SGPT)

Decreased SGPT in combination with increased cholesterol levels is seen in cases of a congested liver. We also see increased levels in mononucleosis, alcoholism, liver damage, kidney infection, chemical pollutants or myocardial infarction.

- Normal adult range: 0–48 U/L
- Optimal adult reading: 24

### Alkaline Phosphatase

Used extensively as a tumor marker it is also present in bone injury, pregnancy or skeletal growth (elevated readings). Low levels are sometimes found in hypoadrenia, protein deficiency, malnutrition and a number of vitamin deficiencies.

- Normal adult range: 20–125 U/L
- Optimal adult reading: 72.5
- Normal children range: 40–400 U/L
- Optimal children reading: 220

### GGT (Gamma-Glutamyl Transpeptidase)

Elevated levels may be found in liver disease, alcoholism, bile-duct obstruction, cholangitis, drug abuse, and in some cases excessive magnesium ingestion. Decreased levels can be found in hypothyroidism, hypothalamic malfunction and low levels of magnesium.

- Normal adult female range: 0–45 U/L
- Optimal female reading: 22.5
- Normal adult male range: 0–65 U/L
- Optimal male reading: 32.5

### LDH (Lactic Acid Dehydrogenase)

Increases are usually found in cellular death and/or leakage from the cell or in some cases it can be useful in confirming myocardial or pulmonary infarction (only in relation to other tests). Decreased levels of the enzyme may be seen in cases of malnutrition, hypoglycemia, adrenal exhaustion or low tissue or organ activity.

- Normal adult range: 0–250 U/L
- Optimal adult reading: 125

### Bilirubin, Total

Elevated in liver disease, mononucleosis, hemolytic anemia, low levels of exposure to the sun, and toxic effects to some drugs, decreased levels are seen in people with an inefficient liver, excessive fat digestion, and possibly a diet low in nitrogen bearing foods.

- Normal adult range: 0–1.3 mg/dL
- Optimal adult reading: .65

## Renal Related

### *BUN (Blood Urea Nitrogen)*

Increases can be caused by excessive protein intake, kidney damage, certain drugs, low fluid intake, intestinal bleeding, exercise or heart failure. Decreased levels may be due to a poor diet, malabsorption, liver damage or low nitrogen intake.

- Normal adult range: 7–25 mg/dL
- Optimal adult reading: 16

### *Creatinine*

Low levels are sometimes seen in kidney damage, protein starvation, liver disease or pregnancy. Elevated levels are sometimes seen in kidney disease due to the kidneys job of excreting creatinine, muscle degeneration, and some drugs involved in impairment of kidney function.

- Normal adult range: .7–1.4 mg/dL
- Optimal adult reading: 1.05

### *Uric Acid*

High levels are noted in gout, infections, kidney disease, alcoholism, high protein diets, and with toxemia in pregnancy. Low levels may be indicative of kidney disease, malabsorption, poor diet, liver damage or an overly acid kidney.

- Normal adult female range: 2.5–7.5 mg/dL
- Optimal adult female reading: 5.0
- Normal adult male range: 3.5–7.5 mg/dL
- Optimal adult male reading: 5.5

### *BUN/Creatinine*

This calculation is a good measurement of kidney and liver function.

- Normal adult range: 6–25 (calculated)
- Optimal adult reading: 15.5

## Protein

### *Protein, Total*

Decreased levels may be due to poor nutrition, liver disease, malabsorption, diarrhea or severe burns. Increased levels are seen in lupus, liver disease, chronic infections, alcoholism, leukemia, tuberculosis amongst many others.

- Normal adult range: 6.0–8.5 g/dL
- Optimal adult reading: 7.25

### *Albumin*

Major constituent of serum protein (usually over 50%). High levels are seen in liver disease (rarely), shock, dehydration or multiple myeloma. Lower levels are seen in poor diets, diarrhea, fever, infection, liver disease, inadequate iron intake, third-degree burns and edemas or hypocalcemia.

- Normal adult range: 3.2–5.0 g/dL
- Optimal adult reading: 4.1

### *Globulin*

Globulins have many diverse functions such as, the carrier of some hormones, lipids, metals and antibodies (IgA, IgG, IgM and IgE). Elevated levels are seen with chronic infections, liver disease, rheumatoid arthritis, myelomas and lupus are present. Lower levels in immune compromised patients, poor dietary habits, malabsorption and liver or kidney disease.

- Normal adult range: 2.2–4.2 g/dL (calculated)
- Optimal adult reading: 3.2
- A/g ratio (albumin/globulin ratio)
- Normal adult range: 0.8–2.0 (calculated)
- Optimal adult reading: 1.9

## Lipids

### *Cholesterol*

High-density lipoproteins (HDL) is desired as opposed to the low-density lipoproteins (LDL), two types of cholesterol. Elevated cholesterol has been seen in artherosclerosis, diabetes, hypothyroidism and pregnancy. Low levels are seen in depression, malnutrition, liver insufficiency, malignancies, anemia and infection.

- Normal adult range: 120–240 mg/dL
- Optimal adult reading: 180

### *LDL (Low-density Lipoprotein)*

Studies correlate the association between high levels of LDL and arterial artherosclerosis.

- Normal adult range: 62–130 mg/dL
- Optimal adult reading: 81 mg/dL

### *HDL (High-density Lipoprotein)*

A high level of HDL is an indication of a healthy metabolic system if there is no sign of liver disease or intoxication.

- Normal adult range: 35–135 mg/dL
- Optimal adult reading: +85 mg/dL

### *Triglycerides*

Increased levels may be present in artherosclerosis, hypothyroidism, liver disease, pancreatitis, myocardial infarction, metabolic disorders, toxemia and nephrotic syndrome. Decreased levels may be present in chronic obstructive pulmonary disease, brain infarction, hyperthyroidism, malnutrition and malabsorption.

- Normal adult range: 0–200 mg/dL
- Optimal adult reading: 100

### *Cholesterol/LDL Ratio*

- Normal adult range: 1–6
- Optimal adult reading: 3.5

## Thyroid

### *Thyroxine (T4)*

Increased levels are found in hyperthyroidism, acute thyroiditis and hepatitis. Low levels can be found in cretinism, hypothyroidism, cirrhosis, malnutrition and chronic thyroiditis.

- Normal adult range: 4–12 ug/dL
- Optimal adult reading: 8 ug/dL

### T3-Uptake

Increased levels are found in hyperthyroidism, severe liver disease, metastatic malignancy and pulmonary insufficiency. Decreased levels are found in hypothyroidism, normal pregnancy, and hyperestrogenis status.
- Normal adult range: 27–47%
- Optimal adult reading: 37%

### Free T4 Index (T7)

- Normal adult range: 4–12
- Optimal adult reading: 8

### Thyroid-stimulating Hormone (TSH)

Produced by the anterior pituitary gland, causes the release and distribution of stored thyroid hormones. When T4 and T3 are too high, TSH secretion decreases, when T4 and T3 are low, TSH secretion increases.
- Normal adult range: .5–6 mili IU/L

## Cardiac

### Creatine Phosphokinase (CPK)

Levels rise 4 to 8 hrs after an acute MI, peaking at 16 to 30 hrs and returning to baseline within 4 days.
- 25–200 U/L
- 32–150 U/L

### CK-MB CK Isoenzyme

It begins to increase 6 to 10 hours after an acute MI, peaks in 24 hours, and remains elevated for up to 72 hours.
- < 12 IU/L if total CK is < 400 IU/L
- < 3.5% of total CK if total CK is > 400 IU/L

### (LDH) Lactate Dehydrogenase

Total LDH will begin to rise 2 to 5 days after an MI; the elevation can last 10 days.
- 140–280 U/L

### LDH-1 and LDH-2 LDH Isoenzymes

Compare LDH-1 and LDH-2 levels. Normally, the LDH-1 value will be less than the LDH-2. In the acute MI, however, the LDH-2 remains constant, while LDH-1 rises. When the LDH-1 is higher than LDH-2, the LDH is said to be flipped, which is highly suggestive of an MI. A flipped pattern appears 12–24 hours post MI and persists for 48 hours.
- LDH-1: 18–33%
- LDH-2: 28–40%

### SGOT (Serum Glutamic-oxaloacetic Transaminase

It will begin to rise in 8–12 hours and peak in 18–30 hours.
- 10–42 U/L

### Myoglobin

Early and sensitive diagnosis of myocardial infarction in the emergency department This small heme protein becomes abnormal within 1 to 2 hours of necrosis, peaks in 4–8 hours, and drops to normal in about 12 hours.
- < 1

### Troponin Complex

Peaks in 10–24 hours, begins to fall off after 1–2 weeks.
- < 0.4

### Table of Cardiac Markers

| Serum markers of myocardial injury | Detected | Peak | Falls |
|---|---|---|---|
| Myoglobin | 1–3 | 1–8 | 12–18 |
| CK/CK-MB | 3–8 | 12–16 | 24–48 |
| MB isoforms | 1–6 | 4–8 | 12–48 |
| Troponin complex | 3–6 | 10–24 | cTnI: 5–9 days cTnT: 7–14 days |

## SOMETHING EXTRA FOR YOUR KNOWLEDGE

### Electrolytes

See the list below:
- Ammonia: 15–50 µmol/L
- Ceruloplasmin: 15–60 mg/dL
- Chloride: 95–105 mmol/L
- Copper: 70–150 µg/dL
- Creatinine: 0.8–1.3 mg/dL
- Blood urea nitrogen: 8–21 mg/dL
- Ferritin: 12–300 ng/mL (men), 12–150 ng/mL (women)
- Glucose: 65–110 mg/dL
- Inorganic phosphorous: 1–1.5 mmol/L
- Ionized calcium: 1.03–1.23 mmol/L
- Magnesium: 1.5–2 mEq/L
- Phosphate: 0.8–1.5 mmol/L
- Potassium: 3.5–5 mmol/L
- Pyruvate: 300–900 µg/dL
- Sodium: 135–145 mmol/L
- Total calcium: 2–2.6 mmol/L
- Total iron-binding capacity: 45–85 µmol/L
- Total serum iron: 65–180 µg/dL (men), 30–170 µg/dL (women)
- Transferrin: 200–350 mg/dL
- Urea: 1.2–3 mmol/L
- Uric acid: 0.18–0.48 mmol/L
- Zinc: 70–100 µmol/L

### Hematology

See the list below:
- Hemoglobin: 13–17 g/dL (men), 12–15 g/dL (women)
- Hematocrit: 40–52% (men), 36–47% (women)
- Glycosylated hemoglobin: 4–6%
- Mean corpuscular volume (MCV): 80–100 fL
- Red blood cell distribution width (RDW): 11.5–14.5%
- Mean corpuscular hemoglobin (MCH): 0.4–0.5 fmoL/cell
- Mean corpuscular hemoglobin concentration (MCHC): 30–35 g/dL
- Reticulocytes: 0.5–1.5%
- White blood cells (WBC): 4–10 × $10^9$/L
- Neutrophils: 2–8 × $10^9$/L
- Bands: < 1 × $10^9$/L
- Lymphocytes: 1–4 × $10^9$/L
- Monocytes: 0.2–0.8 × $10^9$/L
- Eosinophils: < 0.5 × $10^9$/L

- Platelets: 150–400 × $10^9$/L
- Prothrombin time: 11–14 sec
- International normalized ratio (INR): 0.9–1.2
- Activated partial thromboplastin time (aPTT): 20–40 sec
- Fibrinogen: 1.8–4 g/L
- Bleeding time: 2–9 min

### Lipids

See the list below:
- Triglycerides: 50–150 mg/dL
- Total cholesterol: 3–5.5 mmol/L
- High-density lipoprotein (HDL): 40–80 mg/dL
- Low-density lipoprotein (LDL): 85–125 mg/dL

### Acid-base

See the list below:
- pH: 7.35–7.45
- Base excess: (–3)–(+3)
- $H^+$: 36–44 nmol/L
- Partial pressure of oxygen ($pO_2$): 75–100 mm Hg
- Oxygen saturation: 96–100%
- Partial pressure of carbon dioxide ($pCO_2$): 35–45 mm Hg
- Bicarbonate ($HCO_3$): 18–22 mmol/L

### Gastrointestinal Function

See the list below:
- Albumin: 35–50 g/L
- Alkaline phosphatase: 50–100 U/L
- Alanine aminotransferase (ALT): 5–30 U/L
- Amylase: 30–125 U/L
- Aspartate aminotransferase (AST): 5–30 U/L
- Direct bilirubin: 0–6 μmol/L
- Gamma glutamyl transferase: 6–50 U/L
- Lipase: 10–150 U/L
- Total bilirubin: 2–20 μmol/L
- Total protein: 60–80 g/L

### Cardiac Enzymes

See the list below:
- Creatine kinase: 25–200 U/L
- Creatine kinase MB (CKMB): 0–4 ng/mL
- Troponin: 0–0.4 ng/mL

### Hormones

See the list below:
- 17 hydroxyprogesterone (female, follicular): 0.2–1 mg/L
- Adrenocorticotropic hormone (ACTH): 4.5–20 pmol/L
- Estradiol: 1.5–5 ng/dL (male), 2–14 ng/dL (female, follicular), 2–16 ng/dL (female, luteal), < 3.5 ng/dL (postmenopausal)
- Free T3: 0.2–0.5 ng/dL
- Free T4: 10–20 pmol/L
- Follicle-stimulating hormone (FSH): 1–10 IU/L (male), 1–10 IU/L (female, follicular/luteal), 5–25 IU/L (female, ovulation), 30–110 IU/L (postmenopause)
- Growth hormone (fasting) : 0–5 ng/mL
- Progesterone: 70–280 (ovulation), ng/dL
- Prolactin: < 14 ng/mL
- Testosterone (male): 10–25 nmol/L
- Thyroxine-binding globulin: 12–30 mg/L
- Thyroid-stimulating hormone (TSH): 0.5–5 mIU/L
- Total T4: 4.9–11.7 mg/dL
- Total T3: 0.7–1.5 ng/dL
- Free T3: 0.6–1.6 ng/mL

### Vitamins

See the list below:
- Folate (serum): 7–36 nmol/L
- Vitamin A: 30–65 μg/dL
- Vitamin $B_{12}$: 130–700 ng/L
- Vitamin C: 0.4–1.5 mg/dL
- Vitamin D: 5–75 ng/mL

### Tumor Markers

See the list below:
- Alpha fetoprotein: 0–44 ng/mL
- Beta-human chorionic gonadotropin (β–hCG): < 5 IU/l
- CA19.9: < 40 U/mL
- Carcinoembryonic antigen (CEA): < 4 ug/L
- Prostatic acid phosphatase (PAP): 0–3 U/dL
- Prostate-specific antigen (PSA): < 4 ug/L

### Miscellaneous

See the list below:
- Alpha 1–antitrypsin: 20–50 μmol/L
- Angiotensin–converting enzyme: 23–57 U/L
- C–reactive protein: < 5 mg/L
- D–dimer: < 500 ng/mL
- Erythrocyte sedimentation rate (ESR): Less than age/2 mm/hour
- Lactate dehydrogenase (LDH): 50–150 U/L
- Lead: < 40 μg/dL
- Rheumatoid factor: < 25 IU/mL

### Cerebrospinal Fluid

#### *Reference Range*

Characteristics of normal spinal fluid are below:
- Total volume: 150 mL
- Color: Colorless, clear, like water
- Opening pressure: 90–180 mm $H_2O$ (with patient lying in lateral position)
- Osmolarity at 37°C: 281 mOsm/L
- Specific gravity: 1.006 to 1.008
- Acid–base balance:
  - pH: 7.28–7.32
  - $PCO_2$: 47.9 mm Hg
  - $HCO_3^-$: 22.9 mEq/L
- Sodium: 135–150 mmol/L
- Potassium: 2.7–3.9 mmol/L
- Chloride: 116–127 mmol/L
- Calcium: 2.0–2.5 mEq/L (4.0 to 5.0 mg/dL)
- Magnesium: 2.0–2.5 mEq/L (2.4 to 3.1 mg/dL)
- Lactic acid: 1.1–2.8 mmol/L
- Lactate dehydrogenase: Absolute activity depends on testing method, approximately 10% of serum value

- Glucose: 45–80 mg/dL
- Glutamine: 8–18 mg/dL
- Lactate dehydrogenase (LDH): < 2.0–7.2 U/mL
- Proteins: 20–40 mg/dL:
  - At different levels of spinal tap:
    - Lumbar: 20–40 mg/dL
    - Cisternal: 15–25 mg/dL
    - Ventricular: 15–10 mg/dL
  - Normal CSF proteins concentration in children:
    - Up to 6 days of age: 70 mg/dL
    - Up to 4 years of age: 24 mg/dL
- Electrophoretic separation of spinal fluid proteins (% of total protein concentrations)
  - Pre-albumin: 2–7%
  - Albumin: 56–76%
  - a1–globulin: 2–7%
  - a2–globulin: 3.5–12%
  - b–and g–globulin: 8–18%
  - g–globulin: 7–12%
- Oligoclonal bands–absent
- Immunoglobulins
  - IgG: 10–40 mg/L
  - IgA: 0–0.2 mg/L
  - IgM: 0–0.6 mg/L
  - k/L ratio: 1
- Erythrocyte count:
  - Newborn: 0–675/$mm^3$
  - Adult: 0–10/$mm^3$
- Leukocyte count:
  - Children:
    - Younger than 1 year: 0–30/$mm^3$
    - Age 1–4 years: 0–20/$mm^3$
    - Age 5 years to puberty: 0–10/$mm^3$
  - Adult: 0–5/$mm^3$
- Antibodies, viral DNA—none
- Bacteria (gram stain, culture, VDRL)—negative
- Cancerous cells—none
- Cryptococcal antigen—none.

# Solved Previous Year Question Papers

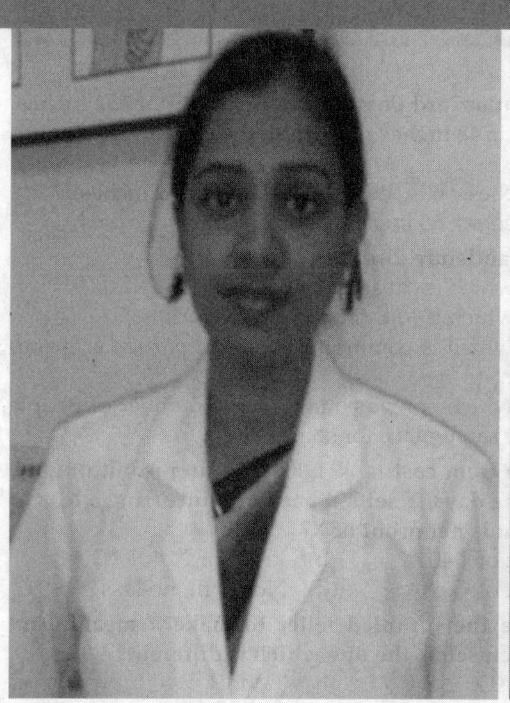

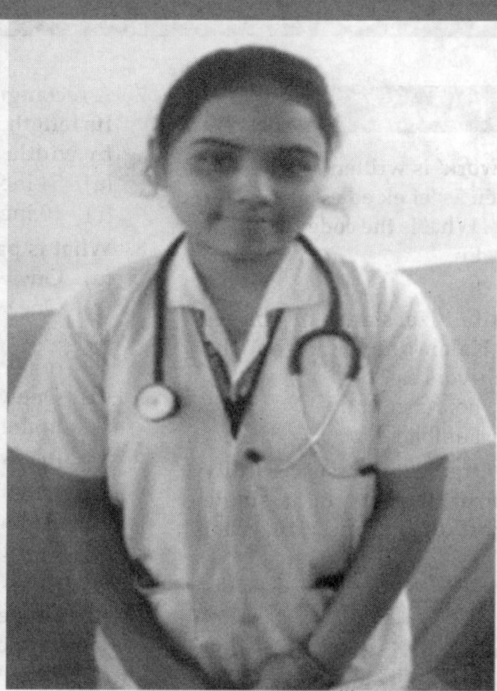

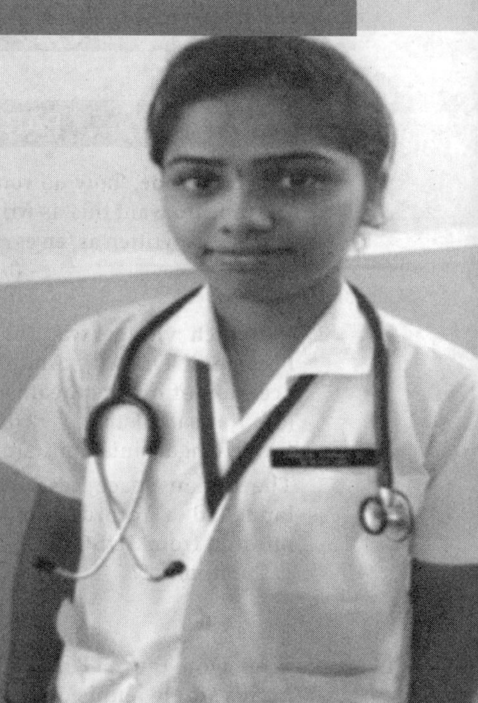

## HIGHLIGHTS

- AIIMS 2016 (Bhubaneshwar)
- PGIMER 2016 (Chandigarh)
- DSSSB 2016 (Delhi)
- RRB 2015 (Secundarabad)
- RRB 2015 (Mumbai)
- MPPEB 2015 (Bhopal)
- RUHS 2014 (Jaipur) (PB BSc Nursing)
- RUHS 2014 (Jaipur) (Medical College Recruitment Exam, Nurse Grade II)
- KEA 2013 (Bangalore Medical College and Research Institute)
- Questions Frequently Asked in All Different Examinations

# AIIMS 2016 (Bhubaneshwar)

## MULTIPLE CHOICE QUESTIONS

### PART I

**1. In certain code, 'how do you work' is written as 'ej ep ed ek', 'do you want this' is written as 'ef ek ed es' and 'want to work' is written as 'en es ep'. What is the code for 'this'?**
(a) Ej (b) En
(c) Ep (d) Es

**2. In which village was the life size statue of former President Dr APJ Abdul Kalam unveiled on the occasion of his first death anniversary?**
(a) Karisalkulam (b) Pei Karumbu
(c) Thangachimadam (d) Pamban

**3. The Indian Space Research Organization successfully launched a record number of satellite in a single mission from SDSC in Shriharikota in June 2016. What is the number?**
(a) 19 (b) 20
(c) 17 (d) 15

**4. Who won the ATP 2016 Toronto Master title in the Men's single tennis category?**
(a) Kei Nishikori (b) Novak Djokovic
(c) Marcelo Melo (d) Ivan Dodig

**5. Some statements followed by some conclusion are given below:**
**Statement:**
1. All crows are birds
2. No bird is human
3. All humans are males
4. Some birds are male

**Conclusion:**
I. Some crows are males
II. No crow is human

**Which of the given conclusion logically follow(s) from the given statement?**
(a) Both I and II
(b) Only conclusion II follows
(c) Neither I nor II follows
(d) Only conclusion I follows

**6. Karan borrowed a certain sum at a simple interest of 6.5% from Payal. He returned ₹ 16,380 to Payal after 4 years. How much did Karan borrow?**
(a) ₹ 13,000 (b) ₹ 12,500
(c) ₹ 13,500 (d) ₹ 11,000

**7. A rectangular card board has a perimeter of 132 inches. Its length is 48 inches more than the width. Find length by width:**
(a) 54 inches × 6 inches (b) 57 inches × 9 inches
(c) 10 inches × 58 inches (d) 59 inches × 7 inches

**8. What is pandemic disease?**
(a) One which is caused by animal bite
(b) One which is found all over the world
(c) One which is commonly found in particular group of people
(d) One which spreads among large number of people in the same place for some time

**9. X sells an item costing ₹ 1,000 to Y at a profit of 20%. After some days, Y sells it back to X incurring a loss of 20%. What is net profit of X?**
(a) Profit of ₹ 40 (b) Profit of ₹ 240
(c) Profit of ₹ 220 (d) No profit, no loss

**10. Rearrange the jumbled letter to make a meaningful word. Then select the one which is different?**
(a) RBDAO (b) TWEIR
(c) LCKAH (d) MSPAT

**11. ________ of hard disk is done to boost the performance of computer.**
(a) Recursion (b) Kerning
(c) Debugging (d) Defragmenting

**12. '>' means taller than and '<' means shorter than. If X>S>Y and T<R>X and S>T, then who is second from the top?**
(a) X (b) R
(c) T (d) S

**13. Which of the following term is NOT associated with the game of cricket?**
(a) Bumper (b) Blue line
(c) Loop (d) Carrom ball

**14. Complete the analogy:**
**31: 69 :: 131:**
(a) 239 (b) 223
(c) 186 (d) 200

**15. Find the 21st term of the given series:**
**7, 16, 25, ..........**
(a) 195 (b) 187
(c) 213 (d) 201

**16. Which of the following day is celebrated on 7th December every year?**
(a) Armed Force Flag Day
(b) International Yoga Day
(c) National Science Day
(d) Human Rights Day

**17. What does CRZ stands for?**
(a) Coastal regulatory zone
(b) Coastal regulation zone
(c) Costal redefined zone
(d) Coastal region zone

**18. The Battle of Waterloo took place in the present day ____.**
(a) Belgium (b) Germany
(c) France (d) Netherland

**19. Find the largest 4 digit number exactly divisible by 77.**
(a) 9944 (b) 9966
(c) 9922 (d) 9933

**20. Milk is ____ to ensure consistency of contents like fat, protein, etc.**
(a) Pasteurized (b) Fortified
(c) Homogenized (d) Standardized

## PART II

**1. Which of the following is not a parameter to assess progress of labor?**
(a) Cervical dilation (b) Fetal heart rate
(c) Descent of fetus (d) Uterine contraction

**2. An infant usually doubles his weight by the age of ____ months.**
(a) 10 (b) 8
(c) 3 (d) 5

**3. Hansen's disease is other name for:**
(a) Malaria (b) Tuberculosis
(c) Typhoid (d) Leprosy

**4. If Frank bleeding occurs at the time of injury or operation, it is called ____ hemorrhage.**
(a) Secondary (b) Reactionary
(c) Concealed (d) Primary

**5. If cases occur irregularly haphazardly from time to time and generally infrequently it is called:**
(a) Pandemic (b) Sporadic
(c) Endemic (d) Epidemic

**6. Which vitamin plays role in production and release of certain coagulation factors?**
(a) Vitamin K (b) Vitamin E
(c) Vitamin $B_{12}$ (d) Vitamin D

**7. Which is the only hormone which lowers blood sugar level?**
(a) Insulin (b) Adrenaline
(c) Cortisol (d) Glucagon

**8. Urinary tract is lined by ____ epithelium.**
(a) Columnar (b) Stratified squamous
(c) Transitional (d) Cuboidal

**9. Which is the most common site of ectopic gestation?**
(a) Abdominal (b) Ovarian
(c) Cervical (d) Tubal

**10. The pacemaker of heart is:**
(a) Purkinje fibers (b) AV node
(c) Bundle of His (d) SA node

**11. Bell's palsy is lesion involving:**
(a) Abducens nerve (b) Olfactory nerve
(c) Optic nerve (d) Facial nerve

**12. Spirometer is used to assess ____ function.**
(a) Gastric (b) Cardiac
(c) Lung (d) Liver

**13. For exchange of gases, the fetus is dependent on ____ circulation.**
(a) Coronary (b) Placental
(c) Pulmonary (d) Hepatic

**14. APGAR scoring involve all of the following except:**
(a) Muscle tone (b) Heart tone
(c) Color (d) Temperature

**15. Keratomalacia is due to deficiency of:**
(a) Vitamin A (b) Vitamin $B_{12}$
(c) Vitamin C (d) Vitamin D

**16. Which of the following is not a live attenuated vaccine?**
(a) Rabies (b) Chickenpox
(c) Mumps (d) Measles

**17. The subjective state of the person who feels aware of not being well is called:**
(a) Sickness (b) Disease
(c) Illness (d) Disability

**18. Which of the most universally accepted health status of whole population?**
(a) Crude death rate
(b) Infant mortality rate
(c) Adult mortality rate
(d) Child mortality rate

**19. Hookworm is the common name for:**
(a) Ancylostoma duodenale
(b) Enterobius vermicularis
(c) Ascaris lumbricoides
(d) Entamoeba histolytica

**20. Hormone synthesized from ovary includes all except:**
(a) Progesterone (b) TSH
(c) Relaxin (d) Estrogen

**21. Which is the best way of estimating the prevalence of tuberculosis in a population?**
(a) Sputum examination (b) Blood culture
(c) Chest X-ray (d) Mantoux test

**22. What is the daily calories intake for women during 3rd trimester of pregnancy?**
(a) 2600 kilocalories (b) 1800 kilocalories
(c) 1500 kilocalories (d) 2000 kilocalories

**23. What is the average of normal pH of blood?**
(a) 7.4 (b) 7.8
(c) 7.0 (d) 8.0

**24. Which of the following is 'Neonatal period'?**
(a) From 28 days to 1 yr of age
(b) From 1 yr to 6 yrs of age
(c) From 3 yrs to 6 yrs of age
(d) From birth to 28 days of age

**25. 'PAP' smear is the screening test commonly used for:**
(a) Cervical cancer (b) Vaginal cancer
(c) Endometrial cancer (d) Ovarian cancer

**26. Which is the most common organism that causes urinary tract infection in community?**
(a) Proteus (b) Escherichia coli
(c) Pseudomonas (d) Streptococci

**27. What is regular bleeding between the cycles termed as?**
(a) Polymenorrhea (b) Oligomenorrhea
(c) Metrorrhagia (d) Menorrhagia

**28. Perception with external stimuli are called:**
(a) Depression (b) Confusion
(c) Hallucination (d) Delusion

**29. Nosocomial infection means infection acquired from:**
(a) Hill station (b) Market place
(c) School (d) Hospital

**30. Vitamin $B_{12}$ is maximally absorbed in:**
(a) Ileum (b) Jejunum
(c) Large intestine (d) Duodenum

**31. The range of Intelligence Quotient (IQ) which can be termed normal is between:**
(a) 50–70 (b) 70–80
(c) 90–100 (d) 80–90

**32. Which drug is commonly used as an antiemetic?**
(a) Metronidazole (b) Domperidone
(c) Dicyclomine (d) Omeprazole

**33. Percentage of saturated fatty acid is maximum in:**
(a) Groundnut oil (b) Sunflower oil
(c) Coconut oil (d) Mustard oil

**34. Barium studied are useful in detecting defect in:**
(a) Respiratory tract (b) Gastrointestinal tract
(c) Urinary tract (d) Respiratory tract

**35. Contaminated dressing are best disposed by:**
(a) Burning (b) Radiation
(c) Autoclaving (d) Boiling

**36. Which of the following is a posterior pituitary hormone?**
(a) Oxytocin (b) Prolactin
(c) Growth hormone (d) Calcitonin

**37. Which is the commonest chromosomal disorder in newborn?**
(a) Turner's syndrome (b) Marfan syndrome
(c) Down syndrome (d) Klinefelter syndrome

**38. What is the normal hemoglobin level in women?**
(a) 8 to 10 g/dL (b) 10 to 12 g/dL
(c) 18 to 20 g/dL (d) 14 to 16 g/dL

**39. What is the first drug of choice for induction of ovulation?**
(a) Mifepristone (b) Clomiphene citrate
(c) Cyproterone acetate (d) Tamoxifen

**40. What does hyperventilation at high altitude cause?**
(a) Respiratory acidosis
(b) Metabolic acidosis
(c) Respiratory alkalosis
(d) Metabolic alkalosis

**41. The third stage of labor is:**
(a) Sage of myometrial contraction and retraction
(b) Stage of expulsion
(c) Stage of placenta; delivery
(d) Stage of dilatation

**42. What does oliguria mean?**
(a) Lack of urine output
(b) Difficulty in passing urine
(c) Decreased urine output
(d) Increased urine output

**43. The vitamin rich food of animal origin mostly is:**
(a) Vitamin C (b) Vitamin A
(c) Vitamin D (d) Vitamin $B_{12}$

**44. The maximum number of oocytes are seen at:**
(a) 20 weeks of gestation
(b) 20 years of age
(c) Puberty
(d) Birth

**45. Which of the following is not absorbable suture material?**
(a) Catgut
(b) Polyamide
(c) Homopolymer of glycolide
(d) Collagen

**46. Which of the following disease that has been eradicated in India?**
(a) Measles (b) Cholera
(c) Smallpox (d) Chickenpox

**47. In which of the following sites is single unit smooth muscle not present?**
(a) Ureter (b) Uterus
(c) Iris (d) GIT

**48. What is the most common cause of secondary postpartum hemorrhage?**
(a) Rupture uterus (b) Uterine atony
(c) Vaginal laceration (d) Retained placenta

**49. What is recommended frequency and timing of administration of glucocorticoids?**
(a) Once at night (b) Once in afternoon
(c) Once in morning (d) Several times a day

**50. Secondary prevention of Rheumatic fever is:**
(a) Treating sore throat early
(b) Giving steroid as suppressive therapy
(c) Giving long acting Benzathine penicillin
(d) A nutritious diet with vitamin supplement

**51. Ascites is best confirmed by:**
(a) Liver function test
(b) Ultrasound
(c) Barium meal studies
(d) Plain X-ray

**52. Which is the most commonly occurring value in a distribution of data?**
(a) Median (b) Mode
(c) Range (d) Mean

**53. Appearance of Koplik's spot in the buccal mucosa is pathognomonic of:**
(a) Chickenpox (b) Smallpox
(c) Measles (d) Mumps

**54. Which electrolyte imbalance is common in patients on insulin therapy?**
(a) Hypokalemia (b) Hyponatremia
(c) Hypernatremia (d) Hyperkalemia

**55. A blood clot of the size of a clenched fist is roughly equal to:**
(a) 500 mL (b) 100 mL
(c) 750 mL (d) 250 mL

**56. Which of the following is not included in TORCH infection in pregnancy?**
(a) Rubella (b) Hepatitis
(c) Cytomegalovirus (d) Toxoplasmosis

**57. What is the leading cause for blindness in India?**
(a) Refractive error (b) Glaucoma
(c) Corneal opacity (d) Cataract

**58. What does carpal tunnel syndrome commonly involve?**
(a) Ulnar N (b) Femoral N
(c) Median N (d) Radial N

**59. Vulsellum forceps is used to hold:**
(a) Cervix (b) Fallopian tube
(c) Uterus (d) Ovary

**60. What is Menghini needle used for?**
(a) Blood transfusion (b) Liver biopsy
(c) Angioplasty (d) Intravenous pyelography

**61. Which vaccine is to be administered immediately after splenectomy?**
(a) Staphylococcal (b) Streptococcal
(c) Pneumococcal (d) Polio

**62. Which mineral prevent dental caries?**
(a) Fluorine (b) Copper
(c) Iodine (d) Zinc

**63. All of the following types of WBCs are granulocytes except?**
(a) Eosinophil (b) Basophil
(c) Monocytes (d) Neutrophil

**64. Milk ejection reflex is due to secretion of :**
(a) Thyroxine (b) Vasopressin
(c) Oxytocin (d) Prolactin

**65. What does an ORS packet usually contain?**
(a) Sodium and glucose
(b) Potassium and fructose
(c) Glucose and fructose
(d) Sodium and fructose

**66. Spontaneous corrections of malpresentations are rare after __________ weeks.**
(a) 20 (b) 34
(c) 28 (d) 24

**67. Ketone bodied in urine are found in all of the following condition except:**
(a) People on high carbohydrate diet
(b) People on prolonged fasting
(c) People on strenuous exercise
(d) Diabetic ketoacidosis

**68. What is the strength of isotonic saline?**
(a) 0.1% (b) 1%
(c) 0.9% (d) 9%

**69. Peripheral tissue are graded against excessive cholesterol accumulation by:**
(a) Low-density lipoprotein
(b) High-density lipoprotein
(c) Very low density lipoprotein
(d) Triglycerides

**70. Incubation period is shortest for:**
(a) Botulism
(b) Salmonella food poisoning
(c) Staphylococcal food poisoning
(d) Perfringens food poisoning

**71. The sphygmomanometer is used to record:**
(a) Temperature (b) Blood pressure
(c) Pulse rate (d) Respiratory rate

**72. Hegar's sign is noticed in:**
(a) Vagina (b) Low uterine segment
(c) Fallopian tube (d) Body of uterus

**73. What is colles fracture?**
(a) Fractured distal end of radius
(b) Fractured proximal end of radius
(c) Fractured distal end of ulna
(d) Fractured shaft of humerus

**74. Elevated serum amylase level is marker of:**
(a) Acute gastritis (b) Acute pancreatitis
(c) Hepatitis (d) Acute appendicitis

**75. A woman who is pregnant for first time is called:**
(a) Nullipara (b) Primipara
(c) Primigravida (d) Nulligravida

**76. What does epistaxis mean?**
(a) Blood in stool (b) Vomiting of blood
(c) Bleeding from nose (d) Coughing of blood

**77. Conjugated bilirubin level alone is raised in:**
(a) Hemolytic jaundice
(b) Obstructive jaundice
(c) Rh incompatibility
(d) Hepatocellular jaundice

**78. What does inhalation of cotton dust fiber over a long-period of time cause?**
(a) Antracosis (b) Byssinosis
(c) Silicosis (d) Bagassosis

**79. Which of the following is not a zoonotic disease?**
(a) Yellow fever (b) Plague
(c) Filariasis (d) Rabies

**80. Which is the only class of immunoglobulin that is transported across the placenta?**
(a) IgA (b) IgD
(c) IgM (d) IgG

**81. Breathlessness on lying down is called:**
(a) Orthopnea
(b) Cyanosis
(c) Dyspnea
(d) Tachycardia

**82. Preterm is defined as babies born alive before _____ weeks of pregnancy.**
(a) 38
(b) 37
(c) 40
(d) 39

**83. Haustral folds are present in:**
(a) Duodenum
(b) Large intestine
(c) Jejunum
(d) Ileum

**84. What is the optimal temperature of cold chain maintenance?**
(a) – 20°C
(b) + 10°C
(c) + 2°C to + 8°C
(d) – 18°C

**85. Which of the following is not included in the major criteria for diagnosis of rheumatic fever?**
(a) Cardiatis
(b) Chorea
(c) Fever
(d) Arthritis

**86. What is the normal duration of puerperium?**
(a) 8 weeks
(b) 6 weeks
(c) 4 weeks
(d) 12 weeks

**87. What does 'thrombocytopenia' means?**
(a) Increased platelet count
(b) Decreased neutrophil count
(c) Decreased platelet count
(d) Decreased RBC count

**88. Lateral curvature of spine is called:**
(a) Scoliosis
(b) Kyphosis
(c) Pes cavus
(d) Hallux valgus

**89. Which of the following is not a barrier method of contraception?**
(a) Diaphragm
(b) Condom
(c) Oral contraceptive pills
(d) Cervical cap

**90. When does ovulation most commonly occur?**
(a) 10 days after the onset of next period
(b) 14 days after the onset of next period
(c) 10 days before the onset of next period
(d) 14 days before the onset of next period

**91. BCG vaccination is given to the infant to protect against:**
(a) Leprosy
(b) Tuberculosis
(c) Typhoid
(d) Malaria

**92. In which year was the nationwide family planning programme launched in India?**
(a) 1972
(b) 1962
(c) 1942
(d) 1952

**93. Anaphylactic reaction to drugs is an example for _____ hypersensitivity reaction.**
(a) Type III
(b) Type II
(c) Type I
(d) Type IV

**94. The concentration of HCG is maximum at:**
(a) 20 weeks of gestation
(b) 10 weeks of gestation
(c) 3 weeks of gestation
(d) Term

**95. Wide separation of eyes seen in Down's Syndrome is called:**
(a) Hypertelorism
(b) Exophthalmos
(c) Enophthalmos
(d) Enophthalmos

**96. Which is the highly specific test for HIV:**
(a) Mantoux
(b) Widal
(c) ELISA
(d) Western

**97. McBerney's point tenderness is present in acute:**
(a) Tonsillitis
(b) Cholecystitis
(c) Appendicitis
(d) Gastritis

**98. The average weight gain during pregnancy for a women of average weight is about:**
(a) 5 to 6 kg
(b) 15 to 16 kg
(c) 19 to 20 kg
(d) 12 to 13 kg

**99. Lifestyle modification is an example for:**
(a) Tertiary prevention
(b) Secondary prevention
(c) Primary prevention
(d) Primordial prevention

**100. Excessive body hair growth in women is termed as:**
(a) Hirsutism
(b) Galactorrhea
(c) Gynecomastia
(d) Varicocele

## ANSWERS

| Part I | | Part II | | | | | | | | | | | |
|---|---|---|---|---|---|---|---|---|---|---|---|---|---|
| **1.** | (d) | **1.** | (b) | **21.** | (d) | **41.** | (c) | **61.** | (c) | **81.** | (a) |
| **2.** | (b) | **2.** | (d) | **22.** | (a) | **42.** | (c) | **62.** | (a) | **82.** | (b) |
| **3.** | (b) | **3.** | (d) | **23.** | (a) | **43.** | (d) | **63.** | (c) | **83.** | (b) |
| **4.** | (b) | **4.** | (d) | **24.** | (d) | **44.** | (a) | **64.** | (c) | **84.** | (c) |
| **5.** | (b) | **5.** | (b) | **25.** | (a) | **45.** | (b) | **65.** | (a) | **85.** | (c) |
| **6.** | (a) | **6.** | (a) | **26.** | (b) | **46.** | (c) | **66.** | (b) | **86.** | (b) |
| **7.** | (b) | **7.** | (a) | **27.** | (c) | **47.** | (c) | **67.** | (a) | **87.** | (c) |
| **8.** | (b) | **8.** | (c) | **28.** | (c) | **48.** | (d) | **68.** | (c) | **88.** | (a) |
| **9.** | (b) | **9.** | (d) | **29.** | (d) | **49.** | (c) | **69.** | (b) | **89.** | (c) |
| **10.** | (d) | **10.** | (d) | **30.** | (a) | **50.** | (c) | **70.** | (c) | **90.** | (d) |
| **11.** | (d) | **11.** | (d) | **31.** | (c) | **51.** | (b) | **71.** | (b) | **91.** | (b) |
| **12.** | (a) | **12.** | (c) | **32.** | (b) | **52.** | (b) | **72.** | (b) | **92.** | (d) |
| **13.** | (b) | **13.** | (b) | **33.** | (c) | **53.** | (c) | **73.** | (a) | **93.** | (c) |
| **14.** | (b) | **14.** | (d) | **34.** | (b) | **54.** | (a) | **74.** | (b) | **94.** | (b) |
| **15.** | (b) | **15.** | (a) | **35.** | (a) | **55.** | (a) | **75.** | (c) | **95.** | (a) |
| **16.** | (a) | **16.** | (a) | **36.** | (a) | **56.** | (b) | **76.** | (c) | **96.** | (d) |
| **17.** | (b) | **17.** | (c) | **37.** | (c) | **57.** | (d) | **77.** | (b) | **97.** | (c) |
| **18.** | (a) | **18.** | (b) | **38.** | (d) | **58.** | (c) | **78.** | (b) | **98.** | (d) |
| **19.** | (d) | **19.** | (a) | **39.** | (b) | **59.** | (a) | **79.** | (c) | **99.** | (d) |
| **20.** | (d) | **20.** | (b) | **40.** | (c) | **60.** | (b) | **80.** | (d) | **100.** | (a) |

# PGIMER 2016 (Chandigarh)

## MULTIPLE CHOICE QUESTIONS

1. **A characteristic of infant and young children who has experienced maternal deprivation is:**
   (a) Tendency towards overeating
   (b) Responsiveness towards stimulus
   (c) Proneness to illness
   (d) Extreme activities
2. **Which of the following is an appropriate nursing action when caring a patient who has radium implant for cervical cancer?**
   (a) Restrict the visitors to a 10-minute stay
   (b) Store urine in a lead container
   (c) Wear lead apron when giving care
   (d) Avoid giving IM injections to gluteal region.
3. **Caput succedaneum is:**
   (a) Birth mark
   (b) Swelling on the face of the baby
   (c) Collection of fluid under scalp
   (d) Swelling will not cross suture line
4. **When a patient is in liver failure, which of the following behavior change is most important assessment to report?**
   (a) Shortness of breath (b) Lethargy
   (c) Fatigue (d) Nausea
5. **Under integrated management of neonatal and childhood illness care is rendered to:**
   (a) Only newborn
   (b) Under 5 children
   (c) 2 months to 5 year old children
   (d) Age upto 2 months and 2 months to 5 years old children.
6. **Which of the following clinical finding indicates the patient is experiencing hypokalemia?**
   (a) Edema
   (b) Muscle spasm
   (c) Kussmaul breathing
   (d) Abdominal distention
7. **A 20 months old is to receive isolyte–p 240 mL IV in 6 hrs. The drop factors to the minidropper is 60 drop/mL. The nurse regulate IV at the rate of:**
   (a) 36 drop/min (b) 40 drop/min
   (c) 32 drop/min (d) 20 drop/min
8. **Total blood volume in newborn at birth is:**
   (a) 80 mL/kg (b) 100 mL/kg
   (c) 125 mL/kg (d) 150 mL/kg
9. **The enzyme released by the sperm which allows penetration of ovum is called:**
   (a) Amylase (b) Hyaluronidase
   (c) Lipase (d) Trypsin
10. **Proteins are required for:**
    (a) Weight reduction
    (b) Absorption of calcium
    (c) Maintenance of body tissue
    (d) Synthesis of steroid hormone
11. **A patient's physician orders nuclear cardiography and makes an appointment for a thallium scan. The purpose of injecting a radioisotope into the blood stream is to detect:**
    (a) Normal versus abnormal tissue
    (b) Damage in area of the heart
    (c) Ventricular functioning
    (d) Myocardial scarring and perfusion
12. **The reason for using parenteral route to administer medication includes:**
    (a) Parenteral medication last longer than an oral medication
    (b) It is least expensive method
    (c) It is easier to measure accurate dose
    (d) The parenteral route allows more rapid absorption than an oral route.
13. **A skin infection that can be a sequel of a staphylococcal infection is:**
    (a) Herpes simple (b) Scabies
    (c) Intertrigo (d) Impetigo
14. **The concept of 'multipurpose health worker' was given by:**
    (a) Kartar Singh committee
    (b) Srivastav committee
    (c) Chadha committee
    (d) National health policy
15. **The principal features of kwashiorkor is:**
    (a) Visible muscle wasting
    (b) Severe fat wasting
    (c) Usually good appetite
    (d) Edema on lower legs and face
16. **The safest method of termination of pregnancy before 12 weeks is:**
    (a) Suction evacuation (b) Dilation and curettage
    (c) Laminaria tent (d) Prostaglandins

**17. Inadequate intake of which vitamin by pregnant women may cause neural tube defect:**
(a) Niacin (b) Riboflavin
(c) Folic acid (d) Thiamine

**18. India accounts for nearly ____ of the global incidence of tuberculosis.**
(a) 50% (b) 25%
(c) 20% (d) 33%

**19. Major cause of blindness in India is:**
(a) Glaucoma (b) Refractive error
(c) Cornea blindness (d) Cataract

**20. Involution of uterus is completed by:**
(a) 6 weeks (b) 8 weeks
(c) 12 weeks (d) 16 weeks

**21. In a normal Indian women the average weight gain per week during later months of pregnancy is:**
(a) 0.25 kg (b) 0.5 kg
(c) 1.0 kg (d) 1.5 kg

**22. Specificity is an ability of screening test to identify:**
(a) True positive (b) True negative
(c) False positive (d) False negative

**23. Which is not freeze dried vaccine:**
(a) BCG (b) Yellow fever
(c) DPT (d) Measles

**24. A patient needs an intradermal injection for Mantoux test, but he currently has bilateral caste in place. Which of the following would be the best alternative site?**
(a) Abdomen (b) Lateral upper arm
(c) Middle upper thigh (d) Antecubital space

**25. A woman has been pushing effectively for 1 hour, a nurse should need at this time is to:**
(a) Change position frequently
(b) Ambulate
(c) Consume oral food and fluids
(d) Rest between contractions

**26. To evaluate a patient's condition following cardiac catheterization, the nurse will palpate the pulse:**
(a) In all extremities
(b) At the insertion site
(c) Distal to catheter insertion
(d) Above catheter insertion

**27. The uterine blood flow at term:**
(a) 50 mL/min (b) 100–150 mL/min
(c) 350–375 mL/min (d) 500–750 mL/min

**28. The mean cardiac output of fetus is:**
(a) 100 mL/kg/min (b) 225 mL/kg/min
(c) 350 mL/kg/min (d) 415 mL/kg/min

**29. Which of the following is a preparation of choice for a patient who has been admitted in ED with an open contaminated injury and no recent history of tetanus immunization?**
(a) DPT vaccine
(b) Tetanus toxoid
(c) Tetanus antitoxin
(d) Tetanus immunoglobulin

**30. Normally newborn lose weight in first week of life is:**
(a) 1% of birth weight (b) 5% of birth weight
(c) 10% of birth weight (d) 20% of birth weight

**31. The immunity developed as a result of infection by pathogenic organism is:**
(a) Active immunity (b) Passive immunity
(c) Natural immunity (d) Acquired immunity

**32. Anti D should be given following Rh+ delivery within:**
(a) 6 hours (b) 24 hours
(c) 72 hours (d) 7 hours

**33. ART-DOTS linkage are being established at all ______.**
(a) Health centers
(b) ART centers under AIDS control program
(c) Hospitals
(d) TB centers

**34. The population served by a subcenter in plain area is:**
(a) 1000 (b) 5000
(c) 30000 (d) 80000

**35. The vaccine used in prevention of cervical cancer is:**
(a) BCG (b) IgG
(c) Hep B (d) HPV

**36. The first person becoming sick in an epidemic is called:**
(a) Primary case (b) Secondary case
(c) Contact case (d) Index case

**37. Most appropriate age for early primary immunization against TB, Diphtheria, whooping cough, tetanus, polio, measles and Hep B is:**
(a) Birth to 6 months (b) Birth to 9 months
(c) Birth to 1 year (d) Birth to 18 months

**38. EPI includes all vaccines except:**
(a) DPT (b) MMP
(c) Polio (d) BCG

**39. A 28 years old male patient is admitted to the hospital for a suspected brain tumor. While assessing the patient, the nurse would keep in mind that the most reliable index of cerebra; status is:**
(a) Pupil response (b) Deep tendon reflexes
(c) Muscle strength (d) Level of consciousness

**40. Pain felt in calf muscle when the foot is dorsiflexed with the leg extended at the knee is called as:**
(a) Kernig's sign (b) Spalding's sigh
(c) Human sigh (d) Goodell's sign

**41. A young patient who was hit by a car was fortunate because the level of his injury did not interrupt his respiratory function. The cord segments involved in maintaining respiratory function are:**
(a) Thoracic level 5 and 6
(b) Thoracic level 2 and 3
(c) Cervical level 7 and 8
(d) Cervical level 3 and 4

**42. Physiological anemia in pregnant women is a result of:**
(a) Poor dietary intake of iron
(b) Increased erythropoiesis
(c) Increased blood volume of women
(d) Increased detoxification demands

**43. Strawberry spot vagina is seen in:**
(a) Candida (b) Trichomonas
(c) CMV (d) Herpes simplex

**44. A way to promote trust with a patient is to:**
(a) Allow family members to visit whenever they want
(b) Assure the patient that her doctor is excellent
(c) Follow through when you say you will do something
(d) Talk to her at length, about her life, likes and dislikes

**45. The first dose of Vit A is given at the age of:**
(a) 1½ years (b) 2 years
(c) 9 months (d) 6 months

**46. Normally by one year of age the birth weight of an infant should increase by:**
(a) 1.5 times (b) 2 times
(c) 3 times (d) 4 times

**47. Tertiary prevention is needed in which stage of the natural history of disease?**
(a) Prepathogenic (b) Pathogenesis
(c) Prodromal (d) Terminal

**48. A non-stress test is prescribed for a pregnant mother. The nurse tells the client about the procedure that:**
(a) The test is an invasive procedure and requires that an informed consent be signed
(b) The test will take about 2 hours and will require close monitoring for 2 hrs after procedure is completed
(c) An ultrasound transducer that record fetal heart activity is secured over the abdomen where fetal heart rate is heard most clearly
(d) The fetus is challenged or stressed by uterine contraction to obtain the necessary information

**49. The physician has ordered a 24 hours urine specimen. After explaining the procedure to the patient the nurse collects the first specimen. This specimen is then:**
(a) Discarded, then the collection begins
(b) Saved as part of the 24 hours collection
(c) Tested, then discarded
(d) Placed in a separate container and later added to the container

**50. Communicability of measles declines:**
(a) After onset of fever
(b) During prodromal period
(c) At the time of eruption
(d) After appearance of rash

**51. The nurse will evaluate for most significant complication in patient undergone chronic peritoneal dialysis, which is:**
(a) Pulmonary embolism
(b) Hypotension
(c) Dyspnea
(d) Peritonitis

**52. BCG, Measles, MMR vaccines should be stored in:**
(a) 10 to 12°C
(b) 20 to 25°C
(c) 2 to 8°C
(d) 15 to 20°C

**53. When a patient's medical record is needed as evidence for legal action, you are aware that the record is the property of:**
(a) The patient (b) The patient's lawyer
(c) The court (d) The healthcare agency

**54. In India which of the following function as First Referral Unit (FRU's)?**
(a) Subcenters
(b) Primary health centers
(c) Community health centers
(d) Regional hospitals

**55. Which of the client would nurse identify as being at most risk for developing disseminated intravascular coagulations (DIC)?**
(a) A 4th gravid delivery 8 hours ago and has lost 500 mL of blood.
(b) A 2nd gravid diagnosed with fetus syndrome
(c) A primigravida with mild pre- eclampsia
(d) A primigravida who has delivered a 3.5 kg baby 3 hours ago

**56. The principal risk of 'at risk' approach is:**
(a) Something for all (b) More for the needy
(c) All for some (d) All for all

**57. A patient has diagnosis of left ventricular failure and high pulmonary capillary wedge pressure (PCWP). The physician ordered dopamine to improve ventricular function. The nurse will know the medication is working if patient's:**
(a) Blood pressure rises
(b) Blood pressure decreases
(c) Cardiac index fails
(d) PCWP rises

**58. The main objectives of intensive IEC activities for leprosy program is:**
(a) Cure of illness (b) Reduction of stigma
(c) Case identification (d) Eradication of disease

**59. Promotion of infant and young child feeding practice is encompassed along with continuation of complementary feeding up to:**
(a) One year of life (b) Two years of life
(c) Three years of life (d) Four years of life

**60. Thrombophlebitis is common complication following vascular surgery. Which of the following sign indicate that the possible thrombus has occurred?**
(a) Kernig's sign (b) Hegar's sign
(c) Homan's sign (d) Brudzinski's sign

**61. During retention catheter insertion or bladder irrigation, the nurse must use:**
(a) Sterile equipment and wear sterile gloves
(b) Clean equipment and maintain surgical asepsis
(c) Sterile equipment and maintain medical asepsis
(d) Clean equipment and technique

**62. Saffron colored meconium seen in:**
(a) Post maturity (b) TB
(c) Breech (d) Normal appearance

**63. The extra calories needed by a women having singleton pregnancy:**
(a) 100 kcal (b) 200 kcal
(c) 300 kcal (d) 500 kcal

**64. Which of the following principles guides nurse's priorities at a disaster caused by a collapsed building in a earthquake?**
(a) Hemorrhage necessitates immediate care to save most lives
(b) Those with head injuries are treated first so that their care more complex
(c) Those requiring minimal care are treated first so that they can help others
(d) Children should get highest priority because they have the greatest life expectancy

**65. Mantoux test is done to diagnose:**
(a) Malaria (b) Filarial
(c) Tuberculosis (d) Typhoid

**66. Bitot's spots are due to the deficiency of:**
(a) Vit B (b) Vit A
(c) Vit D (d) Carbohydrates

**67. A 45 years old patient Mrs. Bhagavati Devi has just been admitted to the hospital for an abdominal hysterectomy following a diagnosis of uterine cancer. Result of lab test indicates that the patient's WBC is 9800/cumm. The most appropriate intervention is to:**
(a) Call the operating room and cancel the surgery
(b) Notify the surgeon immediately
(c) Take no action as this is a normal value
(d) Call the lab and have the test repeated

**68. The result of Mantoux test are read after:**
(a) 6 hours (b) 24 hours
(c) 48 hours (d) 72 hours

**69. Chikungunya is a non-fatal _____ illness.**
(a) Viral (b) Bacterial
(c) Protozoan (d) Plasmodium

**70. Following liver biopsy, the highest priority assessment of the patient's condition is to check for:**
(a) Pulmonary edema
(b) Uneven respiratory pattern
(c) Hemorrhage
(d) Pain

**71. Strongest stimulus for lactation is by:**
(a) Metoclopramide (b) PPH
(c) Bromocriptine (d) Sucking

**72. The number of death per 1,000 population per year in a given community is known as:**
(a) Crude death rate (b) Infant death rate
(c) Neonatal death rate (d) Perinatal death rate

**73. A pregnant woman admitted in labor is attached to external electronic fetal monitor, nurse should do initial nursing assessment which of the following?**
(a) Identify types of acceleration
(b) Assessing baseline fetal heat rate
(c) Determining frequency of the contraction
(d) Determining intensity of the contraction

**74. When serum bilirubin rises on 3rd and 4th day after birth of the baby due to inefficient hepatic function is known as:**
(a) Pathological jaundice
(b) Physiological jaundice
(c) Obstructive jaundice
(d) Viral hepatitis

**75. A female patient Mrs Seema Gupta has cesium needle implanted in her cervix. She asked the nurse if she may get out of the bed to go to the bathroom. The appropriate response is to tell her:**
(a) She may not get out of bed while the needle is implanted
(b) She may get out of bed with the nurse's help
(c) The nurse will have to get a physician's order for her to get out of bed
(d) She must stay in bed, but she can move around to be more comfortable while the needle is implanted

**76. Rice water stool is typical sign of:**
(a) Cholera (b) Hepatitis A
(c) Hepatitis B (d) Dysentery

**77. The assessment finding that should be reported immediately if developed in the patient with acute pancreatitis is:**
(a) Nausea and vomiting
(b) Abdominal pain
(c) Decreased bowel sounds
(d) Shortness of breath

**78. A nurse is assessing a child for dehydration. The nurse determines that the child is moderately dehydrated if which of the following symptoms is noted:**
(a) Flat fontanels
(b) Moist mucus membrane
(c) Pale skin color
(d) Oliguria

**79. The nurse knows that the most informative measurement for determining Cardiogenic shock is:**
(a) Arterial blood pressure
(b) Central venous pressure
(c) Pulmonary artery pressure
(d) Cardiac index

**80. Which of the following is the appropriate nursing intervention for a patient with a terminal illness who is passing through the acceptance stage?**
(a) Allowing patient to cry
(b) Encouraging unrestricted visiting
(c) Explain the patient what is being done
(d) Being around though not speaking

**81. A female patient has laparoscopic cholecystectomy this morning. She is now complaining of right shoulder pain. The nurse would explain to the patient this symptom is:**
(a) Common following this operation
(b) Expected after general anesthesia
(c) Unusual and will be reported to the surgeon
(d) Indicative of need to use the incentive spirometer

**82. Which immunization produces a permanent scar?**
(a) DPT
(b) BCG
(c) Measles vaccination
(d) Hepatitis B vaccination

**83. To disinfect 20 liters of water, one should use chlorine tablet of:**
(a) 0.5 g
(b) 1.5 g
(c) 2.5 g
(d) 3.5 g

**84. A patient was in an automobile accident and sustained a head injury. Following admission to the hospital, a diagnosis of increased intracranial pressure was made. The nursing intervention appropriate in the care of this patient is to:**
(a) Teach controlled coughing and deep breathing
(b) Provide a quiet and brightly lightened environment
(c) Elevate the head 15 to 30 degree
(d) Encourage the intake of clear fluid

**85. Expenditure in health sector on Public health is about _____ of GDP.**
(a) 1%
(b) 2%
(c) 5%
(d) 6%

**86. Which of the following system of medicine is of Indian origin?**
(a) Homeopathy
(b) Siddha
(c) Unani-tibb
(d) Acupuncture

**87. Normal crown-rump length at birth is:**
(a) 20 to 25 cm
(b) 38 to 50 cm
(c) 72 to 80 cm
(d) 78 to 85 cm

**88. Immunity by antibody formation during the course of disease is:**
(a) Active natural immunity
(b) Active artificial immunity
(c) Passive natural immunity
(d) Passive artificial immunity

**89. Dyspnea associated with congestive heart failure is primarily due to:**
(a) Blockage of pulmonary artery by an embolism
(b) Accumulation of fluid in the interstitial spaces and alveoli of the lungs
(c) Blockage of bronchi by mucus secretions
(d) Compression of lung by the dilated heart

**90. Which of the following antituberculosis drug is bacteriostatic?**
(a) Rifampicin
(b) Ethambutol
(c) INH
(d) Streptomycin

**91. Which of the following statements best describes health?**
(a) A relative state of being
(b) The total state of physical and psychological wellness
(c) A state of functioning well physically mentally and socially
(d) Being free of sick or infirmity

**92. Tertiary level of prevention of disease is related to:**
(a) Vaccination
(b) Good nutrition
(c) Rehabilitation to normal physical, mental and social health
(d) Good test and sleep

**93. Major route of transmission of hepatitis A is:**
(a) Feco-oral route
(b) Parenteral route
(c) Sexual transmission
(d) Perinatal transmission

**94. Placental bed blood circulates through:**
(a) Villi
(b) Spiral arteries
(c) Chorionic membrane
(d) Umbilical artery

**95. The danger of convulsion in a women with pre-eclampsia ends:**
(a) After labor begins
(b) After delivery occurs
(c) 24 hours postpartum
(d) 48 hours postpartum

**96. All of the following are the mosquito born diseases except:**
(a) Malaria
(b) Kala-azar
(c) KFD
(d) Dengue

**97. Herd immunity does not protect any individual in:**
(a) Diphtheria
(b) Polio myelitis
(c) Smallpox
(d) Tetanus

**98. Isoniazid (INH) is prescribed for a 2 yrs old child with a positive Mantoux test. The mother of the child asks the nurse how long the child will need to take the medication. The nurse tells the mother that the medication will need to be taken for:**
(a) 6 months
(b) 9 months
(c) 12 months
(d) 18 months

**99. Which of the following assessment finding is typical of extracellular fluid loss?**
(a) Distended jugular veins
(b) Elevated Hematocrit level
(c) Rapid thready pulse
(d) Increased serum sodium level

## ANSWERS

| | | | | | | | | | |
|---|---|---|---|---|---|---|---|---|---|
| 1. | (d) | 21. | (a) | 41. | (d) | 61. | (a) | 81. | (a) |
| 2. | (b) | 22. | (a) | 42. | (c) | 62. | (a) | 82. | (b) |
| 3. | (c) | 23. | (b) | 43. | (b) | 63. | (d) | 83. | (c) |
| 4. | (b) | 24. | (a) | 44. | (c) | 64. | (d) | 84. | (c) |
| 5. | (b) | 25. | (d) | 45. | (a) | 65. | (c) | 85. | (b) |
| 6. | (d) | 26. | (d) | 46. | (d) | 66. | (a) | 86. | (b) |
| 7. | (b) | 27. | (c) | 47. | (d) | 67. | (c) | 87. | (a) |
| 8. | (b) | 28. | (d) | 48. | (c) | 68. | (c) | 88. | (a) |
| 9. | (b) | 29. | (b) | 49. | (a) | 69. | (a) | 89. | (b) |
| 10. | (c) | 30. | (b) | 50. | (c) | 70. | (d) | 90. | (a) |
| 11. | (a) | 31. | (d) | 51. | (d) | 71. | (d) | 91. | (c) |
| 12. | (d) | 32. | (c) | 52. | (c) | 72. | (a) | 92. | (c) |
| 13. | (b) | 33. | (b) | 53. | (d) | 73. | (b) | 93. | (a) |
| 14. | (a) | 34. | (b) | 54. | (a) | 74. | (a) | 94. | (a) |
| 15. | (d) | 35. | (d) | 55. | (c) | 75. | (c) | 95. | (c) |
| 16. | (d) | 36. | (d) | 56. | (a) | 76. | (a) | 96. | (c) |
| 17. | (c) | 37. | (a) | 57. | (a) | 77. | (b) | 97. | (d) |
| 18. | (d) | 38. | (b) | 58. | (d) | 78. | (d) | 98. | (a) |
| 19. | (d) | 39. | (a) | 59. | (a) | 79. | (a) | 99. | (b) |
| 20. | (a) | 40. | (a) | 60. | (a) | 80. | (b) | | |

# DSSSB 2016 (Delhi)

## MULTIPLE CHOICE QUESTIONS

1. **Vaccination to be given after completion of 9 months of birth is:**
(a) MMR (b) DPT
(c) BCG (d) OPV

2. **Which of the following may increase in pregnancies complicated by anemia in the second trimester?**
(a) Urinary tract infection
(b) Gestational diabetes
(c) Pregnancy-induced hypertension
(d) Preterm birth

3. **Which assessment finding is associated with diabetic ketoacidosis?**
(a) Hunger and Hypertension
(b) Cold, clammy skin and irritability
(c) Fruity breath odor and decreasing level of consciousness
(d) Sweating and Tremors

4. **Tuberculosis is a/an:**
(a) Airborne disease (b) Foodborne disease
(c) Arthropod disease (d) Waterborne disease

5. **The IQ level of Moderate Mental Retardation:**
(a) below 20 (b) 35–50
(c) 20–35 (d) 50–70

6. **To administer IV fluids to the children, the nurse should know:**
(a) To do the physical examination
(b) To take history
(c) To calculate the fluid requirement
(d) To calculate the oxygen level

7. **Islets of Langerhans produce:**
(a) Bile (b) Insulin
(c) Trypsin (d) Renin

8. **Which food item is avoided in a patient with hypertension?**
(a) Steamed (b) Apples
(c) Smoked sausages (d) Bananas

9. **Fatty acids can be transported into and out of cell membrane by:**
(a) Facilitated transport (b) Osmosis
(c) Active transport (d) Diffusion

10. **Drug of choice for the prevention of mother to child HIV infection:**
(a) Didanosine (b) Tomoxifen citrate
(c) Indinavir (d) Navilopine

11. **Referring the patients main thought as he expressed:**
(a) Suggesting (b) Restating
(c) Informing (d) Reflection

12. **The position of the uterus is:**
(a) Retroverted and retroflexed
(b) Anteverted and anteflexed
(c) Retroverted and anteflexed
(d) Anteverted and retroflexed

13. **Kellys suture is done in:**
(a) Genito-urinary prolapse
(b) Cervical incontinence
(c) Stress incontinence
(d) Vaginoplasty

14. **Kangaroo mother care means:**
(a) It is not related to human care
(b) Only mother to child
(c) Only father or child
(d) Skin to skin holding of Infants

15. **Peg cells are seen in:**
(a) Fallopian tubes (b) Valva
(c) Ovary (d) Vagina

16. **When performing chest compressions on an adult in CPR, the sternum should be depressed for at least:**
(a) ½ to ¼ inch (b) ¾ to 1 inch
(c) 2½ to 3 inches (d) 1½ to 2 inches

17. **Which of the following is an example of neurotransmitter?**
(a) Acetylcholine (b) Tetrase
(c) Cholecystokinin (d) Cholinesterase

18. **The stage of disease cycle in which signs and symptoms are noticed:**
(a) Incubation period (b) Defecation
(c) Defervescence (d) Fastigium

19. **Projective technique is:**
(a) Indirect measure of data that is unlikely to be obtained
(b) A method of conducting a study
(c) A method of research plan
(d) A method of qualitative research

20. **Community health center covers the population of:**
(a) 50,000–60,000
(b) 5,000–6,000
(c) 1,00,000–1,20,000
(d) 15,000–18,000

21. **Which model states that most frequently occurring behavior as normal?**
(a) Statistical (b) Ideal mental health
(c) Social (d) Biochemical

22. **To diagnose dysthymia, the mood disturbance should last for at least:**
(a) 2 years (b) 1½ years
(c) 1 year (d) 6 months

23. **Causes of high infant mortality rate is:**
(a) All of these (b) Six killer diseases
(c) Low birth weight (d) Diarrheal disease

24. **Antiseptic methods were first introduced by:**
(a) Edward Jenner (b) Beijerwick
(c) Iwoanowski (d) Lord Lister

25. **Umbilical cord consists of:**
(a) 3 veins and 2 arteries (b) 3 arteries and 2 veins
(c) 2 veins and 2 arteries (d) 2 arteries and 1 vein

26. **Which bacilli is responsible for the acidic medium in vaginal secretion?**
(a) Proteus
(b) Doderlein's bacilli
(c) Staphylococci
(d) E coli

27. **Formula to calculate the degree of nutrition for 4 year old baby:**
(a) Age in year × 3 + 4
(b) Age in years × 2 + 8
(c) As per BMI
(d) Age in years × 2 + 5

28. **Features of good unit planning are:**
(a) Its aim should be clear and well
(b) It should be comprehensive
(c) It provides place for beginning and ending.
(d) All of these

29. ______ **refers to the decreased psychoactive effect of drug resulting from repeated exposure.**
(a) Withdrawal (b) Harmful use
(c) Tolerance (d) Dependence

30. **Which is a deviant behavior in marriage?**
(a) All of these
(b) Not observing caste rules in marriage
(c) Widow remarriage
(d) Marriage between the forbidden degrees of relation

31. **Weaning should start from the month of:**
(a) 8th month (b) 7th month
(c) 12th month (d) 6th month

32. **Soiled waste can be disposed by which method?**
(a) Incineration (b) Chemical treatment
(c) Autoclaving (d) Disinfection

33. **Indian Lunacy Act was enacted in the year:**
(a) 1985 (b) 1912
(c) 1987 (d) 1992

34. **Incontinence is observed in ______ stage of dementia.**
(a) Second (b) Initial
(c) Third (d) First

35. **What is the normal score in mini mental status examination?**
(a) 15–20 (b) 20–25
(c) 10–15 (d) 25–30

36. **Normal head circumference of newborn:**
(a) 40–50 cm (b) 33–35 cm
(d) 50 cm (d) 20–25 cm

37. **Which of the following might help the pregnant client to overcome first-trimester morning sickness?**
(a) Have two small meals a day with a snacks at noon
(b) Increase fat intake before bedtime
(c) Eat dry crackers before arising
(d) Drink high-carbohydrate fluids with meals

38. **Examples of housefly borne disease are except:**
(a) Trench fever (b) Cholera
(c) Gastroenteritis (d) Diarrhea

39. **Yellow color is the coding for:**
(a) Animal waste
(b) Human anatomical waste
(c) Human anatomical waste, animal waste, biotechnological waste and soiled waste
(d) Biotechnological waste

40. **Thick white mucous discharge from the female genitalia is:**
(a) Labia (b) Hymen
(c) Estrogen (d) Smegma

41. **Causative organism of AIDS is:**
(a) Orthomyxovirus (b) Rhabdovirus
(c) Retrovirus (d) Paramyxovirus

42. **The stage that designs curriculum is:**
(a) Directive (b) Evaluative
(c) Formative (d) Functional

43. **The cranial nerve which regulates biting, chewing and swallowing is:**
(a) Facial (b) Oculomotor
(c) Cochlear (d) Trigeminal

44. **BFHI means:**
(a) Baby friendly hospital initiative
(b) Baby friendly home initiative
(c) Breast feeding hospital initiative
(d) Breast feeding home initiative

45. **Main principle in neonatal resuscitation:**
(a) Only pulse
(b) Only airway
(c) Only breathing
(d) Airway breathing and pulse

46. **Validity of tool means:**
(a) It detects changes and differences
(b) It measures consistency
(c) It measures what it is supposed to measure
(d) It is free from bias

47. **Which one of the following conveys the acceptance of the patient exactly as she/he is?**
(a) Reducing physical force
(b) Realistic relationship
(c) Use self understanding
(d) Talk with purpose

**48. Fear of crowded or closed in spaces:**
(a) Hydro phobia (b) Agora phobi
(c) Social phobia (d) Zoo phobia

**49. The treatment therapy used for tuberculosis:**
(a) Phototherapy (b) PPI
(c) MDT (d) DOTs

**50. Tools of measurement in epidemiology are:**
(a) Ratio (b) All of these
(c) Proportions (d) Rates

**51. EBF is:**
(a) Effective breastfeeding
(b) Exclusive bottlefeeding
(c) Efficient breastfeeding
(d) Exclusive breastfeeding

**52. Which size of needle is used to give IM (intramuscular) injection?**
(a) 25–27 gauge (b) 5–7 gauge
(c) 22–23 gauge (d) 18–20 gauge

**53. In a patient receiving Total Parental Nutrition (TPN), which of the signs indicate hyperglycemia?**
(a) Nausea, vomiting and oliguria
(b) Fever, weak pulse and thirst
(c) Sweating, chills and abdominal pain
(d) Weakness, thirst and increased urine output

**54. A plan showing the placement of students in theory and practical area is called**
(a) Lesson plan (b) Clinical rotation plan
(c) Master rotation plan (d) Curriculum

**55. Administration of measles vaccine to child is a measure of:**
(a) Health promotion (b) Treatment
(c) Rehabilitation (d) Specific protection

**56. Principles of IV drugs administration is:**
(a) Should dilute before administration
(b) Should not administer IV for children
(c) Do not have flush volume
(d) No need for dilution

**57. Causative organism of diarrhoea in AIDS patient is:**
(a) Cryptosporidium (b) Rota Virus
(c) E coli (d) Streptococcus aureus

**58. Safe Disposal methods of Bio-medical waste exclude:**
(a) Disposal techniques
(b) Collection and segregation
(c) Classification and treatment
(d) Transportation and storage

**59. Which is the most appropriate time of IUD insertion?**
(a) At any time of menstruation
(b) Just before menstruation
(c) During or within 10 days of menstruation
(d) About the midst of the cycle

**60. _________ is characterized by episode of rapid ingestion of large volume of food followed by induced vomiting.**
(a) Anoxeria nervosa (b) Bulimia nervosa
(c) Obesity (d) Binge eating

**61. An intravenous (IV) site is cool, pale and swollen and the solution is not infusing. Which complication has occurred?**
(a) Thrombosis (b) Infiltration
(c) Phlebitis (d) Infection

**62. Standard deviation summarizes the average amount of deviation of values:**
(a) From the median (b) From Correlation
(c) From the mode (d) From the mean

**63. In India 70% of malaria cases occur due to:**
(a) Plasmodium vivex (b) Plasmodium malariae
(c) Plasmodium ovale (d) Plasmodium falciparum

**64. Which method is used to open the airway in a road traffic accident victim?**
(a) Jaw thrust maneuver (b) Flexed position maneuver
(c) Head tilt-chin lift (d) Modified heat tilt-chin lift

**65. A nurse is planning care for a postpartum client who had a vaginal delivery 2 hours ago. The client had a midline episiotomy and has several hemorrhoids. What is the priority nursing diagnosis for this client?**
(a) Impaired urinary elimination
(b) Acute pain
(c) Risk for imbalanced fluid volume
(d) Disturbed body image

**66. A study that examines data collected in the present:**
(a) Pre-experimental research
(b) Basic research
(c) Non-experimental research
(d) Descriptive research

**67. Which regulatory body is associated with registration nurses in the state?**
(a) IMA (b) SNC
(c) INC (d) SMC

**68. A patient suffering with iron deficiency anemia should include the following food items in the diet:**
(a) Coffee and tea
(b) Oranges and dark green leafy vegetables
(c) Cooked oats
(d) Nuts and milk fish

**69. IMNCI means:**
(a) International Maternal Neonatal Child Immunization
(b) Intramuscular Neonatal Childhood Illness
(c) Integrated Management of Neonatal and Childhood Illness
(d) Intramuscular Neonatal Care Initiative

**70. Gluconeogenesis is decreased by:**
(a) Glucagon (b) Insulin
(c) Glucocorticoids (d) Epinephrine

**71. Excessive urination at night is termed as:**
(a) Dysuria (b) Micturation
(c) Nocturia (d) Pyuria

**72. Which is an example of atypical antipsychotics?**
(a) Lithium (b) Haloperidol
(c) Resperidone (d) Chlorpromazine

**73. What do you mean by incidence?**
(a) Old cases of any disease
(b) Total cases of any disease
(c) All of these
(d) New cases of any disease

**74. ORS means:**
(a) Oral Rehydration therapy
(b) Overall Rehydration Solution
(c) Oral Rehydration syringe
(d) Oral Rehydration Solution

**75. Planned educational activities provided in a job setting is called:**
(a) Job analysis (b) Job description
(c) In-service education (d) Continuing education

**76. Which committee is also known as health survey and development committee?**
(a) Mukherjee Committee
(b) Bhore Committee
(c) Shrivastav Committee
(d) Mudaliar Committee

**77. What should nurse conclude that a client is doing when making up stories to fill in the blank spaces of memory?**
(a) Confabulating (b) Denying
(c) Lying (d) Rationalizing

**78. Phases of counseling does not include:**
(a) Assessment (b) Imagination
(c) Setting goals (d) Diagnosis

**79. Who is acknowledged as father of modern management theory?**
(a) FW Taylor (b) Elton Mayo
(c) Henry Fayol (d) McGregor

**80. The amount of sperm present in seminal fluid is:**
(a) 20 million/mL (b) 60 million/mL
(c) 100 million/mL (d) 1 million/mL

**81. Which of the following food item is rich in Vitamin C?**
(a) Milk (b) Chicken
(c) Oranges (d) Bananas

**82. The absorption of the fats and glycerol takes place in the:**
(a) Large Intestine (b) Stomach
(c) Cecum (d) Ileum

**83. According to Maslow, which is the highest level of need of an individual?**
(a) Basic physiological (b) Safety security
(c) Self actualization (d) Safe esteem

**84. Which of the following IV fluids is prescribed to increase intravascular volume, replace immediate blood loss volume and increase blood pressure?**
(a) 5% dextrose in lactated ringers solution
(b) 0.225% sodium chloride (1/4 normal saline)
(c) 0.45% sodium chloride (1/2 normal saline)
(d) 0.33% sodium chloride (1/3 normal saline)

**85. The reason for urbanization is:**
(a) Growth of Agriculture
(b) Increased means of communication
(c) Movement of population
(d) Industrialization

**86. Asymmetrical enlargement of the uterus when there is lateral implantation, is called:**
(a) Goodell's sign (b) Piskacek's sign
(c) Fernwald's sign (d) Hegar's sign

**87. Most important structure preventing uterine prolapse is:**
(a) Broad ligament (b) Round ligament
(c) Cardinal ligament (d) Uterosacral ligament

**88. Which of the following coagulation factor is not increased during pregnancy?**
(a) Factor VIII (b) Factor IX
(c) Factor XI (d) Factor VII

**89. A home care nurse visits a pregnant client who has a diagnosis of mid pre-eclampsia. Which assessment finding indicates a worsening of the pre-eclampsia and the need to notify the physician?**
(a) Blood pressure reading is at the prenatal baseline
(b) Dependent edema has resolved
(c) Urinary output has increased
(d) The client complains of a headache and blurred vision

**90. A patient requires rapid transfusion of several units of blood. Which device is used to prevent cardiac dysrhythmias?**
(a) Blood-warming device
(b) Cardiac monitor
(c) Infusion controller
(d) Pulse Oximetry

**91. The main clinical symptoms of hiatal hernia is:**
(a) Vomitting
(b) Pain in inguinal area
(c) Burning micturation
(d) Heartburn

**92. The term 'schizophrenia' was coined by:**
(a) Krapelin (b) Bleuler
(c) Freud (d) Blessler

**93. Which is not a direct mode of transmission of communicable diseases?**
(a) Droplet infection
(b) Inoculation into skin
(c) Transplacental
(d) Vector borne transmission

**94. What resting position should a nurse encourage for a client with Pelvic Inflammatory Disease (PID)?**
(a) Fowler
(b) Lithotomy with head elevated
(c) Supine with knees flexed
(d) Sims

**95. The length of the uterine tube is approximately:**
(a) 20 cm (b) 5 cm
(c) 15 cm (d) 10 cm

**96. WHO-ORS packet includes following, except:**
(a) Sodium bicarbonate
(b) Sodium chloride
(c) Calcium carbonate
(d) Potassium chloride

**97. What is the principal erogenous organ in women?**
(a) Labia majora
(b) Clitoris
(c) Vagina
(d) Labia minora

**98. Just before beginning blood transfusion, the nurse assesses which priority item?**
(a) Vital signs (b) Urine output
(c) Skin color (d) Latest hematocrit level

**99. Power obtained because of identification with the leader symbolizes:**
(a) Charismatic power (b) Legitimatic power
(c) Referent power (d) Coercive power

**100. Rational behind play therapy is:**
(a) Social development
(b) Sensorimotor development
(c) Sensorimotor and intellectual development
(d) Intellectual development

## ANSWERS

| | | | | | | | | | |
|---|---|---|---|---|---|---|---|---|---|
| **1.** | (a) | **21.** | (b) | **41.** | (c) | **61.** | (b) | **81.** | (c) |
| **2.** | (b) | **22.** | (a) | **42.** | (c) | **62.** | (a) | **82.** | (d) |
| **3.** | (c) | **23.** | (c) | **43.** | (d) | **63.** | (d) | **83.** | (b) |
| **4.** | (a) | **24.** | (d) | **44.** | (a) | **64.** | (a) | **84.** | (a) |
| **5.** | (b) | **25.** | (d) | **45.** | (d) | **65.** | (b) | **85.** | (d) |
| **6.** | (c) | **26.** | (b) | **46.** | (a) | **66.** | (b) | **86.** | (b) |
| **7.** | (b) | **27.** | (c) | **47.** | (b) | **67.** | (c) | **87.** | (d) |
| **8.** | (c) | **28.** | (d) | **48.** | (c) | **68.** | (b) | **88.** | (d) |
| **9.** | (a) | **29.** | (c) | **49.** | (d) | **69.** | (c) | **89.** | (d) |
| **10.** | (d) | **30.** | (a) | **50.** | (b) | **70.** | (a) | **90.** | (b) |
| **11.** | (b) | **31.** | (d) | **51.** | (d) | **71.** | (c) | **91.** | (c) |
| **12.** | (c) | **32.** | (b) | **52.** | (a) | **72.** | (c) | **92.** | (d) |
| **13.** | (c) | **33.** | (b) | **53.** | (d) | **73.** | (b) | **93.** | (d) |
| **14.** | (d) | **34.** | (c) | **54.** | (c) | **74.** | (d) | **94.** | (c) |
| **15.** | (a) | **35.** | (d) | **55.** | (d) | **75.** | (d) | **95.** | (c) |
| **16.** | (d) | **36.** | (b) | **56.** | (a) | **76.** | (b) | **96.** | (a) |
| **17.** | (a) | **37.** | (c) | **57.** | (c) | **77.** | (a) | **97.** | (b) |
| **18.** | (c) | **38.** | (b) | **58.** | (b) | **78.** | (b) | **98.** | (a) |
| **19.** | (a) | **39.** | (b) | **59.** | (b) | **79.** | (c) | **99.** | (a) |
| **20.** | (c) | **40.** | (d) | **60.** | (a) | **80.** | (a) | **100.** | (c) |

# RRB 2015 (Secundarabad)

## MULTIPLE CHOICE QUESTIONS

**1. The characteristic of enantiomers is:**
(a) Only that they are chemically identical
(b) Only that they are mirror image of each other
(c) Both (a) and (b)
(d) None of the above

**2. The guardian of Indian constitution is the:**
(a) Supreme Court of India
(b) High Court
(c) President of India
(d) Prime Minister of India

**3. Repeated urination while sleeping, even after five years of age is called:**
(a) Enuresis (b) Tic
(c) Stuttering (d) Encopresis

**4. In certain code '253' means "books are old", '546' means "man is old" and '378' means "buy good book". What stands for "and" in that code?**
(a) 2 (b) 4
(c) 5 (d) 6

**5. Atmospheric pressure is important in the process of ________.**
(a) Blood flow (b) Micturition
(c) Reproduction (d) Breathing

**6. In certain code, if BHOPAL is written as EERMDI, then how will POWER be written in same code?**
(a) SLZAHO (b) SRZGHU
(c) NMUBCP (d) NRUGCU

**7. The permanent cessation of menstrual cycle in women is called:**
(a) Menopause (b) Menarche
(c) Dysmenorrheal (d) Amenorrhea

**8. Which of the following Vitamin is soluble in water?**
(a) Vitamin A (b) Vitamin C
(c) Vitamin K (d) Vitamin D

**9. A is 40 meters south-west of B, C is 40 meters south-west of B, then C is in which direction from A?**
(a) South (b) West
(c) East (d) North-East

**10. The Aligarh Muslim University was founded by:**
(a) Dr Saifuddin Kitchlew
(b) Sir Syed Ahmed Khan
(c) Mohammad Ali Jinnah
(d) Maulana Mohammad Ali

**11. Of the following, which is the most common site for metastasis in lung cancer?**
(a) Kidney (b) Stomach
(c) Liver (d) Spleen

**12. Express 45 mins as a fraction of a day**
(a) 1/32 (b) 1/40
(c) 1/60 (d) 1/24

**13. When are the chances of acute endometritis developing in a woman?**
(a) After menopause
(b) After menarche
(c) After child birth or abortion
(d) In childhood

**14. Psychoanalytic therapy was developed by:**
(a) Sigmund Freud (b) Jacobson
(c) Franklin (d) Aristotle

**15. What should be temperature of water used for cold sponging?**
(a) 98°F (b) 105°F
(c) 70°F (d) 0°F

**16. A train is running at the speed of 30 meters/sec. crosses platform 600 meter long in 30 seconds. The length of train is:**
(a) 120 meters (b) 150 meters
(c) 200 meters (d) 300 meters

**17. Which of the following is not found in urine?**
(a) Only glucose (b) Only protein
(c) Only RBC (d) All of the above

**18. Which of the above fraction is largest?**
(a) 6/7 (b) 5/6
(c) 7/8 (d) 4/5

**19. Hallucination are caused by:**
(a) Mental illness
(b) Gastrointestinal disorder
(c) Infectious disorder
(d) Disorder of reproduction

**20. Which artery supply oxygenated blood to the stomach?**
(a) Carotid artery (b) Gastric artery
(c) Celiac artery (d) Cephalic artery

**21. Five words are given below. Four are similar. Choose the word which is not similar to the remaining words: paper, wool, wood, plastic, leather.**
(a) Paper (b) Wool
(c) Wood (d) Plastic

**22. Select the latter-series which follows the rule: 'Number of letter skipped in reverse order in between adjacent letter in the series of constant'.**
(a) SPMLG (b) SPNLJ
(c) SQOLJ (d) WUTRQ

**23. Five words are given below. Four of them are similar. Choose the word which is not similar to remaining words: Ink, paper, pencil, pen, sharpener.**
(a) Ink (b) Paper
(c) Pencil (d) Sharpener

**24. A is brother of B. B is the son of CD is C's father. Then what A of D?**
(a) Brother (b) Grandson
(c) Son (d) Grandfather

**25. Which nutrient is not found in Egg?**
(a) Carbohydrate and Vitamin C
(b) Protein and calcium
(c) Fat and Vitamin D
(d) Protein and Iron

**26. Which of the following is not a symptom of depression?**
(a) Loss of interest in daily activities
(b) Delusion of guilt
(c) Suicidal ideas
(d) Delusion of grandiosity

**27. The goal of management of Glaucoma is:**
(a) Only to increase inflow of aqueous humor
(b) Only to increase outflow of aqueous humor
(c) Only to increase production of aqueous humor
(d) All of these

**28. Which is the best test to detect liver dysfunction?**
(a) Serum albumin (b) Serum bilirubin
(c) SGPT (d) Prothrombin time

**29. Find the next term in the series:**
**A3B, C7D, E11F, G15H, __?__.**
(a) I20J (b) I19K
(c) J19K (d) I19J

**30. Select the letter-series which follows the rule:**
**'Number of letter skipped in between adjacent letter in the series double every time'**
(a) ADIPY (b) BDGLU
(c) EDJOF (d) GJNSY

**31. 8th April 1930 is well-known in Indian History because this date is associated with:**
(a) Dandi March by Mahatma Gandhi
(b) Quit India Movement
(c) Partition of Bengal
(d) Partition of India

**32. Select the pair which has the same relationship as the pair 'Bird:Wing'**
(a) Whale:Water (b) Dog:Lung
(c) Car:Wheel (d) Pen:Paper

**33. Out of the 'chemical forces' or bonds listed below, the strongest one is________.**
(a) Van De Waal's (b) Dipole
(c) Covalent (d) Hydrophobic

**34. Which valve prevents backward flow of blood in left atrium?**
(a) Aortic valve (b) Pulmonary valve
(c) Tricuspid valve (d) Mitral valve

**35. The _______ membrane surrounds lung.**
(a) Pericardial (b) Mediastinal
(c) Pleural (d) Peritoneal

**36. When two numbers are separately divided by 33 the remainders are 21 and 28 respectively. If the sum of the two number is divided by 33 the remainder will be:**
(a) 10 (b) 12
(c) 14 (d) 16

**37. Which complication of IV infusion can cause pulmonary edema or heart failure?**
(a) Infiltration (b) Circulatory overload
(c) Infection (d) Pyogenic reaction

**38. Abnormal communication between urinary and genital tract is called Geneto- urinary _______.**
(a) Fistula (b) Tumor
(c) Atresia (d) Prolapsed

**39. What is the main reason for Angina Pectoris?**
(a) Neurological diseases
(b) Gastric disease
(c) Respiratory diseases
(d) Cardiac diseases

**40. Which division of the nervous system initiates a response known as 'fight or flight' reaction?**
(a) Parasympathetic nervous system
(b) Sympathetic nervous system
(c) Somatic nervous system
(d) None of these

**41. The commonest cause of maternal morbidity in India is:**
(a) Anemia (b) Hemorrhage
(c) Abortion (d) Sepsis

**42. Find the next number in series:**
**11, 16, 23, 32, 43, ______**
(a) 56 (b) 55
(c) 57 (d) 54

**43. Find the next number in the series:**
**885, 870, 855, 840, _____.**
(a) 835 (b) 855
(c) 825 (d) 815

**44. World's first White Tiger Safari is set to come up in which state of India?**
(a) West Bengal (b) Kerala
(c) Madhya Pradesh (d) Gujarat

**45. Out of the following, which medicines are used for intestinal evacuation?**
(a) Cathartics (b) Carminatives
(c) Astringents (d) Antimycotics

**46. The abortion of "Sati" by government regulation was at the time of:**
(a) Warren-Hastings (b) Lord Wellesley
(c) Lord Amherst (d) Lord Bentinck

47. **The destruction of alveolar walls is called:**
(a) Empyema (b) Bronchitis
(c) Emphysema (d) Lung abscess

48. **According to World Health Organization, 'low birth weight' means a weight of less then:**
(a) 2.8 kg (b) 2.7 kg
(c) 2.5 kg (d) 2.3 kg

49. **An agent which kills pathogens bacteria is called:**
(a) Asepsis (b) Disinfectant
(c) Fomites (d) Bacteriostat

50. **Select the pair which has same relation as the pair: Spider : Web**
(a) Ink : Pen (b) Poet : Poetry
(c) Cock : Hen (d) Teacher : Student

51. **Vitamin $B_1$ is called as:**
(a) Niacin (b) Thiamine
(c) Riboflavin (d) Pyridoxine

52. **A bag contains ₹ 90, comprising 50 paisa, 25 paisa and 10 paisa coins. If the ratio of 50 paise, 25 paise and 10 paise is 2 : 3 : 5, then the number of 25 Paisa coins will be:**
(a) 80 (b) 120
(c) 100 (d) 135

53. **In a certain code language, 479 means 'fruit is sweet', 248 means 'very sweet voice' and 637 means 'eat fruit daily'. Which digit stand for 'is' in that language?**
(a) 4 (b) 7
(c) 8 (d) 6

54. **A and B can do job in 72 days. B and C can do same job in 120 days and A and C can do the same job in 90 days. In how many days will all the three take to complete the job?**
(a) 80 days (b) 100 days
(c) 60 days (d) 150 days

55. **If gut motility is increased then:**
(a) Drug absorption is decreased
(b) Drug absorption is increased
(c) Drug absorption is not affected
(d) Nothing definite can be said

56. **Name the Indian participant in Miss World 2014 competition.**
(a) Vanya Mishra (b) Priyanka Chopra
(c) Koyal Rana (d) Navneet Kaur Dhillon

57. **An energy consuming process by which cells of human body absorbs molecules (such as protein) by engulfing them is called ________.**
(a) Lipid diffusion
(b) Aqueous diffusion
(c) Exocytosis
(d) Endocytosis

58. **If the IQ of a child is 45, in which category of mental retardation will he be categorized?**
(a) Mild mental retardation
(b) Moderate mental retardation
(c) Severe mental retardation
(d) Profound mental retardation

59. **Data (information) is stored in computers in the form of:**
(a) Files (b) Directories
(c) Floppies (d) Matter

60. **The device primarily used to provide hard copy is the:**
(a) Hard disk (b) CPU
(c) Printer (d) Card Reader

61. **If the cost price of 10 chairs is equal to the selling price of 16 chairs, the loss percentage is:**
(a) 37.5% (b) 20%
(c) 9.6% (d) 17.5%

62. **Out of the four numbers, the average of first 3 is 15 and the average of last 3 is 16. If the number is 19, the first number is:**
(a) 19 (b) 15
(c) 16 (d) 18

63. **CAD stands for:**
(a) Computer Aided Design
(b) Computer Algorithm for Design
(c) Computer Application for Design
(d) None of the above

64. **Kalyani is mother-in-law of Veena, who is sister-in-law of Ashok. Dheeraj is the father of Sandeep, the only brother of Ashok. How is Kalyani related to Ashok.**
(a) Mother-in-law (b) Mother
(c) Aunt (d) Wife

65. **Stillbirth includes babies dead after:**
(a) 20 week (b) 24 week
(c) 28 week (d) 32 week

66. **In which organ does the maximum absorption of Iron takes place?**
(a) Stomach (b) Small intestine
(c) Colon (d) Liver

67. **A man sold an article at a loss of 20%. If he had sold it for ₹ 50 more, he would have gained 5%. The cost price of the article was:**
(a) ₹ 250 (b) ₹ 300
(c) ₹ 180 (d) ₹ 200

68. **Entomology is the science that studies:**
(a) The behavior of human being
(b) Insects
(c) Behavior of ants
(d) Formation of rocks

69. **In which states is Tehri Hydroelectric project located?**
(a) Uttar Pradesh (b) Himachal Pradesh
(c) Uttaranchal (d) Bihar

70. **Which of the following types of dances is essentially a solo dance?**
(a) Kuchipudi (b) Manipuri
(c) Kathak (d) Mohiniattam

71. **Select the pair which has the same relationship as the pair such as Iodine : Goiter.**
(a) Mango : Anemia
(b) Insulin : Diabetes
(c) Hormones : Cancer
(d) Fat : Obesity

**72. The simple interest on a certain sum at a rate of 5% per annum for 3 years and 4 years differs by ₹ 42. The sum is:**
(a) ₹ 210 (b) ₹ 280
(c) ₹ 750 (d) ₹ 840

**73. Lavani is a:**
(a) Marathi Folk Song (b) Musical Instrument
(c) Indian Language (d) None of these

**74. A 150 meter long train crosses a 500 meter long bridge in 30 seconds. What time will it take to cross platform 370 meter long?**
(a) 36 seconds (b) 30 seconds
(c) 24 seconds (d) 18 seconds

**75. The average age of a husband and wife is 23 years at the beginning of their marriage. After five years they have a one year child. The average age of the family of three, when their child was born is:**
(a) 23 years (b) 18 years
(c) 24 years (d) 20 years

**76. The central point in Ashok's Dharma is:**
(a) Royalty to king (b) Peace and non-violence
(c) Respect the elders (d) Religious tolerance

**77. The 'p' wave on the electrocardiogram correspond to:**
(a) Atrial depolarization
(b) Atrial repolarization
(c) Ventricular depolarization
(d) Ventricular repolarization

**78. Who will take over as Director of Intelligence Bureau in India from Jan 1, 2015 onward?**
(a) Arun Majumdar (b) Nehchal Sandhu
(c) Syed Asif Ibrahim (d) Dineshwar Sharma

**79. Commonest cause of neonatal morbidity in India is:**
(a) Diarrheal disease
(b) Birth Injuries
(c) Congenital Anomalies
(d) Prematurity and Low Birth Weight

**80. The rate of drug absorption is greatest in the ______.**
(a) Large intestine (b) Stomach
(c) Gallbladder (d) Small intestine

**81. The process of taking food into the digestive system is:**
(a) Ingestion (b) Propulsion
(c) Digestion (d) Elimination

**82. A computer program which translate one program instruction at a time into machine language is called**
(a) CPU (b) Compiler
(c) Simulator (d) Interpreter

**83. Which color of light has longest wave length?**
(a) Violet (b) Blue
(c) Red (d) Green

**84. Which of the following is the significant difference between human and cow's milk?**
(a) Proteins and fat
(b) Protein and sugar
(c) Proteins and lactose
(d) Minerals

**85. After menopause in women the chances of her developing osteoporosis increases because of:**
(a) Decrease in estrogen level
(b) Increase in estrogen level
(c) Decrease in LH level
(d) Decrease in FSH level

**86. In certain code, APRIL is written as BQSJM. What is the word whose code is HSFFO?**
(a) INDIA (b) GREAT
(c) TREES (d) GREEN

**87. Find the missing term: PART: TRAP:: POTS : ?**
(a) TOPS (b) OPTS
(c) STOP (d) SPOT

**88. Which of these is an example of a neurotransmitter?**
(a) Only Dopamine (b) Only Norepinephrine
(c) Only Acetylcholine (d) All of these

**89. The reason why lipstick and nail-polish is removed before surgery?**
(a) Surgery becomes easier
(b) Surgery becomes more successful
(c) Psychological benefits to patient
(d) Cyanosis is checked

**90. Which of the following is the main side effect of Intra Uterine Death?**
(a) Vaginal bleeding
(b) Pelvic inflammatory disease
(c) Uterine perforation
(d) Ectopic pregnancy

**91. Which of the following is the fastest, biggest and most expensive computer?**
(a) Personal computer (b) Super computer
(c) Laptops (d) Notebook PC's

**92. 3 men and 5 women can do a job in 12 days. How long will 6 men and 5 women working together take to complete the job?**
(a) 4 days (b) 5 days
(c) 6 days (d) 7 days

**93. Most of the drug have molecular weight between:**
(a) 1–10 (b) 10–100
(c) 250–350 (d) Greater than 500

**94. The main function of kidney is to:**
(a) Eliminate oxygen
(b) Regulate fluid balance and remove waste products
(c) Metabolize vitamins
(d) Eliminate carbon dioxide

**95. Different seasons are formed because:**
(a) Sun is moving around the earth
(b) Earth is moving around the sun
(c) Earth rotates on its own axis
(d) None of these

**96. A man started walking with his back toward sun. After sometime, he turned left, then he turned right and then he turned right and then toward the left again. In which direction is he going now?**
(a) North or South (b) East or West
(c) North or West (d) South or West

**97. Barack Obama will become the _______ President of America to participate in India's Republic Day celebration on January 26, 2015.**
(a) Second (b) First
(c) Third (d) None of these

**98. A sailor goes 12 km downstream in 48 minutes and return in 1 hour and 20 minutes. The speed of the sailor in still water is:**
(a) 12 km/hr (b) 12.5 km/hr
(c) 13 km/hr (d) 15 km/hr

**99. The speed of a boat along the stream is 12 km/hr and against stream is 8 km/hr. The time taken by the boat to sail 24 km in still water is:**
(a) 2 hours
(b) 2.4 hours
(c) 3 hours
(d) 1.2 hours

**100. If X is the brother of son of Y's son, how X is related to Y?**
(a) Son (b) Brother
(c) Cousin (d) Grandson

## ANSWERS

| | | | | | | | | | |
|---|---|---|---|---|---|---|---|---|---|
| **1.** | (c) | **21.** | (d) | **41.** | (b) | **61.** | (a) | **81.** | (a) |
| **2.** | (a) | **22.** | (a) | **42.** | (a) | **62.** | (c) | **82.** | (d) |
| **3.** | (a) | **23.** | (b) | **43.** | (c) | **63.** | (a) | **83.** | (c) |
| **4.** | (a) | **24.** | (b) | **44.** | (c) | **64.** | (b) | **84.** | (c) |
| **5.** | (d) | **25.** | (a) | **45.** | (a) | **65.** | (b) | **85.** | (a) |
| **6.** | (a) | **26.** | (d) | **46.** | (d) | **66.** | (b) | **86.** | (d) |
| **7.** | (a) | **27.** | (b) | **47.** | (c) | **67.** | (d) | **87.** | (c) |
| **8.** | (b) | **28.** | (b) | **48.** | (c) | **68.** | (b) | **88.** | (d) |
| **9.** | (c) | **29.** | (d) | **49.** | (d) | **69.** | (c) | **89.** | (a) |
| **10.** | (b) | **30.** | (b) | **50.** | (b) | **70.** | (d) | **90.** | (b) |
| **11.** | (c) | **31.** | (a) | **51.** | (b) | **71.** | (b) | **91.** | (b) |
| **12.** | (a) | **32.** | (c) | **52.** | (b) | **72.** | (d) | **92.** | (a) |
| **13.** | (c) | **33.** | (c) | **53.** | (c) | **73.** | (a) | **93.** | (c) |
| **14.** | (a) | **34.** | (d) | **54.** | (c) | **74.** | (c) | **94.** | (b) |
| **15.** | (c) | **35.** | (c) | **55.** | (a) | **75.** | (b) | **95.** | (b) |
| **16.** | (d) | **36.** | (d) | **56.** | (c) | **76.** | (b) | **96.** | (a) |
| **17.** | (d) | **37.** | (b) | **57.** | (d) | **77.** | (a) | **97.** | (b) |
| **18.** | (c) | **38.** | (a) | **58.** | (b) | **78.** | (d) | **98.** | (a) |
| **19.** | (a) | **39.** | (d) | **59.** | (a) | **79.** | (d) | **99.** | (b) |
| **20.** | (c) | **40.** | (b) | **60.** | (c) | **80.** | (b) | **100.** | (d) |

# RRB 2015 (Mumbai)

## MULTIPLE CHOICE QUESTIONS

**1. Express 0.7% in terms of fraction:**
(a) 7/10 (b) 7/100
(c) 7/1000 (d) 7/10000

**2. What does electronic spreadsheet consist of?**
(a) Rows (b) Columns
(c) Cells (d) All of these

**3. Identify the part of stomach which connects/joins the esophagus.**
(a) Fundus (b) Cardia
(c) Body (d) Pylorus

**4. Which of the following blood group is universal recipient?**
(a) A (b) O
(c) AB (d) B

**5. Which of the following test is used to detect typhoid bacillus?**
(a) Mantoux test
(b) Schick test
(c) Widal test
(d) VDRL test

**6. Which of the following teeth are used for crushing and grinding of food?**
(a) Canine (b) Incisor
(c) Molar (d) Premolar

**7. Find the sum of square of first eight number, i.e ($1^2 + 2^2 + 3^2 + \ldots\ldots\ldots + 8^2$)**
(a) 184 (b) 194
(c) 204 (d) 72

**8. Mohan and .Sohan, together can do job in 12 days. Sohan alone can do this job in 28 days. In how many days can Mohan do this his job?**
(a) 21 days (b) 16 days
(c) 24 days (d) 20 days

**9. Identify the winner of Nobel prize in 2014.**
(a) Kailash Satyarthi and Malala Yousafzai
(b) B Obama
(c) V Putin
(d) Jean Tirole

**10. Insulin is not administered through oral route because:**
(a) It causes GIT bleeding
(b) It causes nausea and vomiting
(c) It is destroyed in GIT
(d) None of these

**11. Which one of the ion helps in blood clotting?**
(a) $Ca^+$ (b) $Mn^+$
(c) $K^+$ (d) $PO_4^{-2}$

**12. Which of the following is called as power house of cell?**
(a) Nucleus (b) Ribosome
(c) Lysosome (d) Mitochondria

**13. The light of which color is used to treat neonatal jaundice?**
(a) Red light (b) Yellow light
(c) Orange light (d) Blue light

**14. Which of the following test is for Diphtheria?**
(a) VDRL (b) WIDAL
(c) BCG (d) UDRL

**15. Thalassemia is a congenital:**
(a) Defect in bone (b) Blood disorder
(c) Neural defect (d) Muscular defect

**16. In certain code language, 'mink yang pe' means 'fruits are ripen'; 'pe lao may mink' means 'oranges are not ripe' and 'may pe nue mink' means 'mangoes are not ripe' which word in that language means 'mangoes'?**
(a) May (b) Pe
(c) Nue (d) Mink

**17. Which of the following is known as the 'great Circle'?**
(a) Equator (b) Arctic circle
(c) Tropic of cancer (d) Tropic of capricorn

**18. The number of chromosomes in normal human cell is:**
(a) 46 (b) 48
(c) 50 (d) 52

**19. Which of the following Cancer is associated in High Fat diet?**
(a) Ovary cancer (b) Lung cancer
(c) Colon cancer (d) Liver cancer

**20. 18th SAARC Summit was recently held in November, 2014 at:**
(a) Thimpu (b) Dhaka
(c) Kathmandu (d) New Delhi

**21. Which of the following is due to deficiency of Vitamin D?**
(a) Night blindness
(b) Pellagra
(c) Rickets
(d) Kwashiorkor

**22. A boat takes 10 hours to travel 100 km downstream. It takes 15 hours to travel 75 km upstream. Then the speed of boat in still water is:**
(a) 10 km/hr (b) 5 km/hr
(c) 2 ½ km/hr (d) 7 ½ km/hr

**23. The white line formed in lower part of abdomen during pregnancy is called:**
(a) Pregnancy marks (b) Linea nigra
(c) Striae gravidarum (d) None of the above

**24. What is the chemical name of Aspirin (ASA)?**
(a) Acetic salicylic acid (b) Acetyl salicylic acid
(c) Acetone salicylic acid (d) Amide salicylic acid

**25. The feeling of fetus movements by mother is known as:**
(a) Ballottement (b) Palmar sign
(c) Hegar's sign (d) Quickening

**26. Find the compound interest if ₹ 2000 is lent out at rate of 10% per annum, (compounded yearly) for 3 years:**
(a) 600 (b) 200
(c) 662 (d) 680

**27. Who built 'Red fort'?**
(a) Akbar (b) Shahjahan
(c) Jahangir (d) Aurangzeb

**28. Which is the most effective method of disposal of hospital waste?**
(a) By recycling (b) By composting
(c) Dumping (d) Incineration

**29. One side of rectangle is 40 meters and is diagonal is 50 meters. Find parameter of rectangle:**
(a) 180 m (b) 140 m
(c) 70 m (d) 90 m

**30. When we open an internet site we see 'www'. What is the full form of 'www'?**
(a) World wide web (b) World wide word
(c) World wise web (d) None of these

**31. A general side effect of 'Penicillin' is:**
(a) Rash with itching
(b) Fever
(c) Renal calculi
(d) Gastrointestinal disturbance

**32. Snellen's chart is used for measuring:**
(a) Vision (b) Hearing
(c) Smell (d) Touch

**33. Pointing to an old man, Kunal said, 'his son is my son's uncle'. How is the old man related to Kunal?**
(a) Brother (b) Grandfather
(c) Father (d) Brother-in-law

**34. Find the greatest four digit number which is exactly divisible by 13.**
(a) 9991 (b) 9997
(c) 9996 (d) 9993

**35. A full form of 'AMBU' bag is:**
(a) Artificial mouth breathing unit
(b) Artificial manual breathing unit
(c) Airway mouth breathing unit
(d) None of these

**36. The symptoms of pemphigus is:**
(a) Red spots (b) Bluish spots
(c) Small vesicles (d) Large vesicles

**37. The currency of Japan is:**
(a) Yen (b) Pound
(c) Yuan (d) Piso

**38. Who gave this slogan 'Swaraj is my birth right and I shall have it'?**
(a) Mahatma Gandhi
(b) Pandit Nehru
(c) Subhashchandra Bose
(d) Bal Gangadhar Tilak

**39. The 1000 men can do the job in 12 days, in how many days 1200 men can do this job?**
(a) 6 days (b) 8 days
(c) 9 days (d) 10 days

**40. In which of the following year right to information act came into force?**
(a) 2002 AD (b) 2003 AD
(c) 2004 AD (d) 2005 AD

**41. The civil disobedience movement was started in year:**
(a) 1905 AD (b) 1920 AD
(c) 1930 AD (d) 1942 AD

**42. If a 13 meter long iron rod weight 24.7 kg, then what will be the weight of 6 m long iron rod?**
(a) 1.9 kg (b) 11.4 kg
(c) 10.8 kg (d) 11.9 kg

**43. The disorder that affects the memory and cognitive function in older person is called:**
(a) Insomnia (b) Paranoia
(c) Aphasia (d) Dementia

**44. A man is working at a speed of 3.5 kmph find the distance covered by him in 15 mins:**
(a) 875 m (b) 525 m
(c) 850 m (d) 675 m

**45. What are the basic functional units of kidney?**
(a) Renal cortex (b) Nephron
(c) Glomerulus (d) Renal medulla

**46. Chickenpox is caused due to infection by:**
(a) Fungi (b) Bacteria
(c) Virus (d) Protozoa

**47. MMR vaccination is done for protection against:**
(a) Measles, Mumps, Rubella
(b) Measles, Mumps, Rabies
(c) Measles, malaria, rabies
(d) Measles, Meningitis, Rubella

**48. A man is facing East, he turns 100° in clock wise direction and then turns 145° in anti clockwise direction. Which direction is he facing now?**
(a) East (b) North-East
(c) North (d) South-West

**49. The first stool of neonate is called:**
(a) Sebum (b) Lenugo
(c) Meconium (d) Vernix Caseosa

**50. If 1st April 2014 is Tuesday, the 1st June 2014 will be:**
(a) Thursday (b) Friday
(c) Saturday (d) Sunday

**51. Arrange the following fraction in descending order. 1/2 , 3/5, 3/10, 21/15.**
(a) 3/5 > 1/2 > 21/15 > 3/10
(b) 21/15 > 3/5 > 3/10 > 1/2
(c) 1/2 > 3/5 > 3/10 > 21/15
(d) 3/10 > 21/15 > 3/5 > 1/2

**52. Manoj walked for 40 m towards north. Then he takes left turn and walks 20 m. He again take left turn and walk 40 m. How far and in which direction is he from starting point?**
(a) 100 m, North (b) 80 m, East
(c) 60 m, West (d) 20 m, West

**53. Rajan is sixth from left end and Vijay is tenth from right end in a row of boys if there are eight boys in between Rajan and Vijay, how many boys are there in their row?**
(a) 23 (b) 24
(c) 25 (d) 26

**54. Which extension is given for WORD documents by default?**
(a) COM (b) EXT
(c) DOC (d) None of the above

**55. Which of the following is infectious hepatitis?**
(a) Hepatitis A (b) Hepatitis B
(c) Hepatitis C (d) Hepatitis D

**56. Find the simple interest amount if ₹ 1500 is lent out at the rate of 9% per annum simple interest for 6 years:**
(a) ₹ 810 (b) ₹ 900
(c) ₹ 1350 (d) ₹ 675

**57. If the Cost Price is ₹ 120 and Selling Price is ₹ 90, then find the loss percentage:**
(a) 30% (b) 33 1/3%
(c) 25% (d) 75%

**58. Find LCM (Lowest Common Multiple) of 15, 21 and 30:**
(a) 210 (b) 3
(c) 630 (d) 105

**59. The product of two numbers is 7. One of those two number is 3/2. Find the sum of these two numbers:**
(a) 8 1/2 (b) 5 1/2
(c) 7 1/7 (d) 6 1/6

**60. Bulimia Nervosa and Anorexia Nervosa are:**
(a) Sleep disorder (b) Eating disorder
(c) Nervous disorder (d) None of the above

**61. Complete the series 1, 4, 27, 16, ________, 36, 343**
(a) 25 (b) 120
(c) 125 (d) 81

**62. Wilms' tumor affects which of the following?**
(a) Liver (b) Kidney
(c) Uterus (d) Skin

**63. A person spend 1/4th part of his salary on food, 3/8th part of his salary on house rent. He is now left with ₹ 4,800. Find his total salary.**
(a) 7680 (b) 15600
(c) 9600 (d) 12800

**64. The average salary of 15 teacher is ₹ 4500 per month, 5 teachers now leave the school. The average salary of remaining 10 teachers now is ₹ 4200 per month. Find total salary per month of five teacher who left the school:**
(a) 24, 000 (b) 25, 000
(c) 27, 000 (d) 25, 500

**65. Green leafy vegetables are rich source of:**
(a) Vitamin A (b) Vitamin B
(c) Vitamin C (d) Vitamin D

**66. Normal blood pressure of an adult:**
(a) 120/80 (b) 120/100
(c) 150/100 (d) 150/60

**67. Hair color of humans turns white due to absence of which of the following pigment?**
(a) Melanin (b) Melatonin
(c) Bilirubin (d) Biliverdin

**68. The difference between the circumference and the diameter of circle is 30 cms. The area of the circle is:**
(a) 154 $cms^2$ (b) 616 $cms^2$
(c) 308 $cms^2$ (d) 462 $cms^2$

**69. Who is known as 'LADY WITH LAMP'?**
(a) Mother Teresa
(b) Sarojini Naidu
(c) Florence Nightingale
(d) None of these

**70. HCF and LCM of two numbers are 8 and 320 respectively. If one of the number is 64, find the other number.**
(a) 40 (b) 80
(c) 32 (d) 48

**71. Who is the Defense Minister of India? (As per on 01. 12. 2014)**
(a) Rajnath Singh (b) Manohar Parrikar
(c) Arun Jaitley (d) Smriti Irani

**72. What is GOUT?**
(a) A degenerative disorder
(b) A vascular disorder
(c) A renal disorder
(d) A metabolic disorder

**73. There are 40 boys in row. Ramesh is fourteenth from the right of the row. What is his position from left end of row?**
(a) 27th (b) 26th
(c) 25th (d) 24th

**74. International nurses day is observed on:**
(a) May, 12 (b) November, 14
(c) October, 24 (d) December, 22

**75. Primary storage in computer terminology refers to:**
(a) Hard disc drive (b) Random access memory
(c) Read only memory (d) None of above

**76. Rice water stool is symptom of:**
(a) Dengue (b) Malaria
(c) Cholera (d) Typhoid

**77. Which is the largest nerve of human body?**
(a) Femoral nerve (b) Sciatic nerve
(c) Pudendal nerve (d) Thoracic nerve

**78. Who is called as 'Grand old man of India'?**
(a) Dadabhai Naoroji
(b) GK Gokhle
(c) Mahatma Gandhi
(d) Rabindranath Tagore

**79. The State of Jammu and Kashmir was accorded special status under:**
(a) Article 360 of constitution
(b) Article 370 of constitution
(c) Article 380 of constitution
(d) Article 356 of constitution

**80. Fertilization process takes place in:**
(a) Ovary (b) Fallopian tube
(c) Uterus (d) Vagina

**81. Which one of vaccination is necessary for pregnant lady?**
(a) Tetanus (b) BCG
(c) Rubella (d) DPT

**82. If L stand for (+), M stand for (–), N stand for (×) and P stand for (/), then find the value for: 14 N 10 L 42 P 2 M 8 = ?**
(a) 153 (b) 216
(c) 248 (d) 251

**83. At present Reena is twice as old as Sunita. Three year ago, Reena was three times as old as Sunita was. How old is Reena now?**
(a) 6 years (b) 8 years
(c) 10 years (d) 12 years

**84. Which of the following is presentation graphic software?**
(a) MS windows (b) MS word
(c) MS Excel (d) MS power point

**85. Complete the series: 21, 47, 23, 49, 25, 51, 27, ?**
(a) 29 (b) 53
(c) 31 (d) 55

**86. The weight of an infant baby becomes twice the birth at weight at the age of:**
(a) 6 month (b) 1 year
(c) 2 years (d) 3 years

**87. Who is called as 'Indian Napoleon'?**
(a) Samudragupta
(b) Chandragupta II
(c) Ashoka
(d) Skandagupta

**88. In which of the following state is 'Kakrapar Power Station' located?**
(a) Karnataka
(b) Tamil Nadu
(c) Maharashtra
(d) Gujarat

**89. Choose the correct alternative to complete following series: a_ba_b_b_a_b**
(a) Abaab (b) Abbab
(c) Aabba (d) Bbabb

**90. Angiography is X-ray visualization of:**
(a) Heart (b) Lungs
(c) Blood clots (d) Blood vessels

**91. The heartbeat rate of newborn babies is generally:**
(a) 75 beat per min.
(b) 80 beat per min.
(c) 90 beat per min.
(d) 120–140 beat per min.

**92. Indian Standard Time (IST) refers to the local time of the following places in India:**
(a) Delhi (b) Kolkata
(c) Allahabad (d) Jaipur

**93. Paracetamol is not given to those patients who is already suffering from:**
(a) Liver disorder
(b) Kidney disorder
(c) Lung disorder
(d) GIT disorder

**94. Find the value of $(128)^{-2/7}$**
(a) 4 (b) 1/4
(c) 24 (d) 1/16

**95. Which city will host Olympic Games, 2020?**
(a) Madrid (b) Istanbul
(c) Rio de Janeiro (d) Tokyo

**96. Find the 21st term of the following series: 3, 9, 15, 21, ____________ ?**
(a) 123
(b) 129
(c) 117
(d) 135

**97. In certain code, DOG is written as GRJ, then how will CAT be written in that code?**
(a) FEW (b) FEV
(c) FDW (d) EDV

**98. Which of the following is known as Poor Man's meat?**
(a) Milk (b) Fish
(c) Pulses (d) Chicken

**99. Complete the series: 6, 11, 21, 36, ______, 81, 111.**
(a) 46 (b) 51
(c) 56 (d) 71

**100. Disulfiram is a drug used in treatment of:**
(a) Malaria
(b) AIDS
(c) Alcoholism
(d) Mania

## ANSWERS

| | | | | | | | | | |
|---|---|---|---|---|---|---|---|---|---|
| **1.** | (c) | **21.** | (c) | **41.** | (c) | **61.** | (c) | **81.** | (a) |
| **2.** | (d) | **22.** | (a) | **42.** | (b) | **62.** | (b) | **82.** | (a) |
| **3.** | (b) | **23.** | (c) | **43.** | (d) | **63.** | (d) | **83.** | (d) |
| **4.** | (c) | **24.** | (b) | **44.** | (a) | **64.** | (d) | **84.** | (d) |
| **5.** | (b) | **25.** | (d) | **45.** | (b) | **65.** | (a) | **85.** | (b) |
| **6.** | (b) | **26.** | (c) | **46.** | (c) | **66.** | (a) | **86.** | (a) |
| **7.** | (d) | **27.** | (b) | **47.** | (a) | **67.** | (a) | **87.** | (a) |
| **8.** | (c) | **28.** | (d) | **48.** | (b) | **68.** | (a) | **88.** | (d) |
| **9.** | (a) | **29.** | (b) | **49.** | (c) | **69.** | (c) | **89.** | (b) |
| **10.** | (a) | **30.** | (a) | **50.** | (d) | **70.** | (a) | **90.** | (d) |
| **11.** | (c) | **31.** | (d) | **51.** | (a) | **71.** | (b) | **91.** | (d) |
| **12.** | (b) | **32.** | (a) | **52.** | (d) | **72.** | (c) | **92.** | (c) |
| **13.** | (a) | **33.** | (c) | **53.** | (b) | **73.** | (a) | **93.** | (a) |
| **14.** | (d) | **34.** | (b) | **54.** | (c) | **74.** | (a) | **94.** | (a) |
| **15.** | (d) | **35.** | (b) | **55.** | (b) | **75.** | (b) | **95.** | (d) |
| **16.** | (c) | **36.** | (a) | **56.** | (a) | **76.** | (c) | **96.** | (b) |
| **17.** | (a) | **37.** | (a) | **57.** | (a) | **77.** | (b) | **97.** | (c) |
| **18.** | (a) | **38.** | (d) | **58.** | (a) | **78.** | (a) | **98.** | (c) |
| **19.** | (c) | **39.** | (b) | **59.** | (d) | **79.** | (b) | **99.** | (c) |
| **20.** | (c) | **40.** | (d) | **60.** | (b) | **80.** | (b) | **100.** | (c) |

# MPPEB 2015 (Bhopal)

## MULTIPLE CHOICE QUESTIONS

### GENERAL APTITUDE TEST (Q.1 TO 20)

1. **Seventy-five percent of a number is equal to four-fifths of another number. What is the ratio between the first number and second number?**
(a) 5 : 3 (b) 15 : 16
(c) 3 : 5 (d) 16 : 15

2. **In certain code ROME is written as 5913 and DONE is written as 4962. How is MEAN written in that code?**
(a) 5216 (b) 3126
(c) 3216 (d) 9126

3. **Find the odd man out 385, 462, 572, 396, 427, 671, 264:**
(a) 385 (b) 427
(c) 671 (d) 264

4. **What number will come in place of question mark (?) :**
$$\frac{3.6 \times 0.48 \times 2.50}{0.12 \times 0.09 \times 0.5} = (?)$$
(a) 80 (b) 800
(c) 8000 (d) 80000

5. **One third of Ramesh saving in National Saving Certificate is equal to one half of his saving in Public Provident Fund. If he has ₹ 1,50,000 as total saving. How much has he saved in Public Provident Fund?**
(a) 30000 (b) 50000
(c) 60000 (d) 90000

6. **What will come in place of question mark (?) in given number series?**
**124, 228, 436, ? , 1648, 3348**
(a) 844
(b) 852
(c) 872
(d) 834

7. **In college election fought between two candidates, one candidates get 55% of the total valid votes, 15% of the voters were invalid. If the total votes were 15,200, what is the number of valid votes the other candidate got?**
(a) 7106 (b) 8630
(c) 6840 (d) 5814

8. **If the numerator of a fraction is increased by 200% and tube denominator in increased by 400% the resultant fraction is 1 1/20. What is the original fraction?**
(a) 1 1/3 (b) 1 ¾
(c) 6/5 (d) 1 ½

9. **A sum of ₹ 2,236 is distributed among A, B and C such that A receives 25% more than C and C receives 25% less than B. What is A share in the amount?**
(a) ₹ 460 (b) ₹ 890
(c) ₹ 780 (d) ₹ 1,280

10. **The length of rectangle plot is thrice its breadth. If the area of the rectangular plot is 7803 sq. meters, what is the breadth of rectangular plot?**
(a) 51 meters (b) 153 meters
(c) 104 meters (d) 88 meters

11. **If 3 4/5 is subtracted from 6 3/5 and the difference is multiplied by 355 then what will be the final number?**
(a) 1004 (b) 884
(c) 774 (d) 994

12. **A sum of five numbers is 924. The average of first two numbers is 201.5 and the average of the last two numbers is 196. What is the third number?**
(a) 133 (b) 129
(c) 122 (d) 140

13. **Preeti invests an amount of ₹ 39,300 for 4 years at the rate of 4% per annum. What amount of approximate compound interest will she obtain at the end of 4 years?**
(a) ₹ 6,675.44 (b) ₹ 6,650.50
(c) ₹ 6,288.40 (d) ₹ 6,450.25

14. **In one kilometer race A beats B by 28 meters or 7 sec. Find A's time over the course.**
(a) 250 sec (b) 235 sec
(c) 243 sec (d) 260 sec

15. **A boat covers distance of downstream in one hour while it comes back in 1½ hrs. Let the speed of the stream be 3 km/hr, what is the speed of the boat in still water?**
(a) 12 kmph (b) 13 kmph
(c) 14 kmph (d) 15 kmph

16. **'Mustard' is related to 'seed' in the same way carrot is related to:**
(a) Fruit (b) Stem
(c) Flower (d) Root

17. **Mangesh spend 17% of his monthly income on traveling. He spend 25% of his monthly income on household expenses and 36% of his monthly income on medical expenses. He has remaining amount of ₹ 10,032 as cash with him. What is Mangesh annual income?**
(a) ₹ 5,50,300 (b) ₹ 5,36,500
(c) ₹ 5,47,300 (d) ₹ 5,25,000

**18 What number will come in given matrix where (?) question mark is there:**

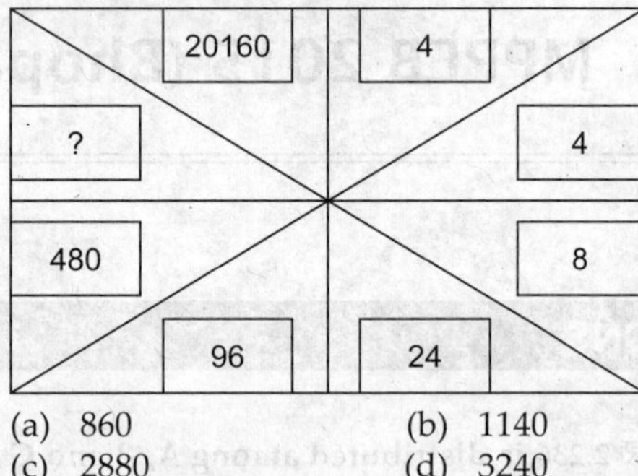


(a) 860 (b) 1140
(c) 2880 (d) 3240

**19. Three of the following four are alike in a certain way and so form a group. Which is the one that does not belong to the group?**

(a) Black (b) Violet
(c) Red (d) Yellow

**20. Three of the following four are alike in a certain way and form a group. Which is the one that does not belong to the group?**

(a) 35 (b) 80
(c) 40 (d) 60

## GENERAL KNOWLEDGE TEST (Q. 21 TO 40)

**21. State flower of Madhya Pradesh is:**

(a) Rose (b) Lotus
(c) Dahlia (d) White Lily

**22. 'Garuda' was insignia of which of the following dynasties?**

(a) Mauryan dynasty (b) Gupta dynasty
(c) Vakataka dynasty (d) Naga dynasty

**23. Which of the following Prime Minister of India was born in Madhya Pradesh?**

(a) Atal Bihari Vajpayee (b) Chaudhary Charan Singh
(c) Indra Kumar Gujral (d) Morarji Desai

**24. Which of the following district has highest female literacy?**

(a) Bhopal (b) Indore
(c) Alirajpur (d) Jhabua

**25. 'Jama Masjid' of Bhopal was built by:**

(a) Nawab Hasrat Khan
(b) Shiraj Khan
(c) Dost Mohammad
(d) Quidsia Begum

**26. The longest river of Madhya Pradesh is:**

(a) Narmada (b) Chambal
(c) Sone (d) Betwa

**27. River 'Sone' originate at:**

(a) Near Multai (b) Amarkantak
(c) Kak Bardi (d) Betul

**28. When did the first radio station came into existence in Madhya Pradesh?**

(a) 1952 (b) 1955
(c) 1961 (d) 1960

**29. 'Kathi' is the folk dance of which region of Madhya Pradesh?**

(a) Malwa (b) Bundelkhand
(c) Nimar (d) Baghelkhand

**30. Who was the leader of 'Narmada Bachao Andolan'?**

(a) JP Narayan
(b) Medha Patkar
(c) P Chidambaram
(d) HN Bahuguna

**31. 'Chausma' is a:**

(a) Bird
(b) Music
(c) Folk dance
(d) Hindi name of rainy season

**32. The number of seats in Lok Sabha for Madhya Pradesh are:**

(a) 29 (b) 30
(c) 31 (d) 32

**33. Who was the first Chief Minister of Madhya Pradesh?**

(a) Shyam Charan Shukla
(b) Kailash Nath Katju
(c) Pt Ravi Shankar Shukla
(d) Bhagawant Rao Mandloi

**34. Where gun carriage factory (GCF) is located in Madhya Pradesh?**

(a) Bhopal (b) Jabalpur
(c) Gwalior (d) Satna

**35. The only tribal sport school of MP is situated at:**

(a) Sehore (b) Jhabua
(c) Alirajpur (d) Petlavad.

**36. Indian Forest Management Institute is situated at:**

(a) Bhopal (b) Indore
(c) Gwalior (d) Jabalpur

**37. The Foundation Day of Madhya Pradesh celebrated on:**

(a) 2nd November
(b) 1st November
(c) 3rd November
(d) 4th November

**38. The state bird of Madhya Pradesh is:**

(a) Owl (b) Parrot
(c) Dudhraj (d) Wood pecker

**39. For contribution in which of the following field is Kalidas Samman is given?**

(a) Art (b) Social service
(c) Medicine (d) Education

**40. With which company is Bhopal gas Tragedy associated?**

(a) Carrboro (b) Seville
(c) Mick (d) Union Carbide

## GENERAL ENGLISH (Q. 41 TO 60)

**41. They loved ________ so much that they thought of no one else.**

(a) Themselves (b) Ourselves
(c) Yourselves (d) Itself

**42. Choose the correct form of indirect speech among the given options.**

**Ram said to Mohan, 'Where do you live'**

(a) Ram asked Mohan where did he lives
(b) Ram told Mohan where he has lived
(c) Ram said Mohan where he lived
(d) Ram asked Mohan where he lived

**43. Choose the correct form of determiners from the given options.**

**_______ of my friend like swimming.**

(a) Either (b) Neither
(c) All (d) Each

**44. Choose the correct form of the tense in the choices given below:**

**She is _______ the soup to see if it needs more salt.**

(a) Been tasting (b) Tasting
(c) Being tasting (d) Tasted

**45. Choose the correct form of the tense in the choices given below:**

**At what temperature _______ into ice.**

(a) Does water turn (b) Do water turns
(c) Do water turned (d) Water turns

**46. Choose the correct form of tenses in the choices given below:**

**_______ get books in library.**

(a) A boy (b) Students
(c) Robert (d) She

**47. Choose the correct form of the tenses in the choices given below:**

**We often _______ each other on our way to office.**

(a) Met (b) Meets
(c) Meeting (d) Meet

**48. Choose the correct form of pronoun to complete the sentence.**

**_______ is the justice of Calcutta High Court.**

(a) He (b) I
(c) They (d) We

**49. Choose the correct form of noun to complete the sentences.**

**_______ were rewarded for their bravery.**

(a) A soldier
(b) Soldier
(c) The soldier
(d) None of these

**50. Choose the correct form of preposition among the given options to complete the sentences.**

**_______ should obey the law of the state.**

(a) Each (b) Either
(c) Neither (d) Everybody

**51. Choose the correct form of preposition among the given options to complete the sentences.**

**The child jumped _______ the river.**

(a) Over (b) Into
(c) In (d) From

**52. Choose the correct form of preposition among the given option to complete the sentences.**

**The soldier fought _______ the courage.**

(a) In (b) By
(c) With (d) From

**53. Tick the correct form of indirect speech among the given options.**

**He said, 'I am working hard for the examination'**

(a) He asked that is working hard for the examination
(b) He said that he was working hard for the examination
(c) He asked that he has been working hard for the examination
(d) He said that he worked hard for the examination

**54. Choose the correct form of determiners from the given options.**

**_______ of them offered to help him.**

(a) No
(b) None
(c) Only
(d) Only certain

**55. Choose the correct form of determiners from the given options.**

**Do you have _____ good book on zoology?**

(a) The (b) Any
(c) All (d) None of these

**56. Choose the correct form of determiners from the given options.**

**_______ children can be naughty sometimes.**

(a) Certain (b) All
(c) A some (d) Half

**57. Tick the correct form of passive voice among the given options.**

**It is now necessary to consult doctors.**

(a) It is now necessary for a doctor to be consulted
(b) It was now necessary for a doctor to be consulted
(c) It is now be necessary for a doctor to be consulted
(d) It would now be necessary for a doctor to be consulted

**58. Choose the correct form of adverb from the option given.**

**I praise him _______ when they deserve it.**

(a) Only (b) For
(c) Ever (d) Never

**59. Choose the right form of pronoun among the given options.**

**This is the man _______ has taken.**

(a) Whom (b) Which
(c) It (d) Who

**60. Choose the correct form of determiners from the given options.**

**_______ I want is a room somewhere.**

(a) Only (b) If
(c) Do (d) All

## MATHEMATICS (Q. 61 TO 80)

**61. What percentage of 64 is 8?**
(a) 12.5 (b) 8
(c) 11 (d) 10

**62. Earning of Ramesh is ₹ 720. After spending 65% of his earning, his saving is:**
(a) 350 (b) 390
(c) 252 (d) 316

**63. Ravi had to secure 36% marks to pass in an examination. He got 24% marks and failed by 9 marks. Then maximum marks for examination was:**
(a) 75 (b) 50
(c) 100 (d) 150

**64. Two candidates contested an election. Total votes casted were 7500, out of them 20% declared invalid. If one of the candidate got 55% of total valid votes then the votes received by the other candidates is:**
(a) 2500 (b) 2700
(c) 1500 (d) 1600

**65. What is percentage of 3% of 5%?**
(a) 60% (b) 50%
(c) 15% (d) None of these

**66. If the annual rate of simple interest increases from 10% to 12.5%, a man annual income increases by ₹ 1250. The principal is:**
(a) 45,000 (b) 60,000
(c) 65,000 (d) 50,000

**67. A sum of money invested for 2 years at certain rate of simple interest is increased by 3% then he would get ₹ 108 more as interest. The principal is:**
(a) ₹ 1,700 (b) ₹ 1,600
(c) ₹ 1,800 (d) ₹ 1,900

**68. A sum of money at simple interest doubles in 10 years. In how many years will it triple at the same rate of interest?**
(a) 25 years (b) 20 years
(c) 30 years (d) 15 years

**69. The compound interest on ₹ 8,000 at 10% per annum for 3 years is:**
(a) ₹ 2,500 (b) ₹ 2,464
(c) ₹ 2,648 (d) ₹ 2,000

**70. Compound interest on ₹ 1,25,000 at 8% per annum for 9 months, compounded quarterly is:**
(a) ₹ 8,460 (b) ₹ 7,651
(c) ₹ 7,842 (d) ₹ 8,000

**71. A sum lent on compound interest amounts to ₹ 30,250 in 2 years and ₹ 33,275 in 3 years. Then rate percent per annum is:**
(a) 10% p. a. (b) 12% p. a.
(c) 11% p. a. (d) 9% p. a.

**72. The percentage worth of ₹ 40,960 due after 3 years at 6 2/3% annual rate of compound interest is:**
(a) ₹ 33,750 (b) ₹ 35,450
(c) ₹ 32,950 (d) ₹ 34,550

**73. If each edge of a cube in 16 cm then its volume is:**
(a) 3296 $cm^3$ (b) 4186 $cm^3$
(c) 3876 $cm^3$ (d) 4096 $cm^3$

**74. How many bricks will be required to construct a wall of 8 m long, 6 m high and 22.5 cm thick, when each brick is of 25 cm long, 11.25 cm wide and 6 cm high?**
(a) 6500 (b) 6400
(c) 7500 (d) 8400

**75. Radii and volume of a cone and a sphere are equal. Then ratio of diameter of the sphere and height of the cone is:**
(a) 1:2 (b) 2:3
(c) 1:3 (d) 3:4

**76. The diameter of copper rod is 1 cm and 8 cm in length. It is melted and recasted into a 18 m long wire of uniform radius. Then radius of the wire is:**
(a) 1/30 cm
(b) 1/15 cm
(c) 2/15 cm
(d) 1/5 cm

**77. There are some solid metallic right circular cones each having radius 3 cm and height 4 cm. These are melted and recasted into a solid sphere of radius 6 cm, the number of these cones is:**
(a) 12
(b) 24
(c) 6
(d) 48

**78. If $2^{x+1} = 8$, then the value of $3^{2x-1}$ is:**
(a) 1
(b) 9
(c) 27
(d) 48

**79. The speed of boat along the stream is 12 km/hr and against the stream is 8 km/hr. The time taken by a boat to sail 24 km in still water is:**
(a) 2 hours
(b) 2.4 hours
(c) 3 hours
(d) 1.2 hours

**80. 3 men and 5 women can do a job in 12 days. How long 6 men and 5 women working together complete the same job?**
(a) 4 days
(b) 5 days
(c) 6 days
(d) 7 days

## ANSWERS

| | | | | | | | |
|---|---|---|---|---|---|---|---|
| **1.** | (d) | **21.** | (d) | **41.** | (a) | **61.** | (a) |
| **2.** | (c) | **22.** | (b) | **42.** | (d) | **62.** | (c) |
| **3.** | (b) | **23.** | (a) | **43.** | (c) | **63.** | (a) |
| **4.** | (b) | **24.** | (a) | **44.** | (b) | **64.** | (b) |
| **5.** | (c) | **25.** | (d) | **45.** | (a) | **65.** | (d) |
| **6.** | (b) | **26.** | (a) | **46.** | (b) | **66.** | (d) |
| **7.** | (d) | **27.** | (b) | **47.** | (d) | **67.** | (c) |
| **8.** | (b) | **28.** | (b) | **48.** | (a) | **68.** | (b) |
| **9.** | (c) | **29.** | (c) | **49.** | (c) | **69.** | (c) |
| **10.** | (a) | **30.** | (b) | **50.** | (d) | **70.** | (b) |
| **11.** | (d) | **31.** | (d) | **51.** | (b) | **71.** | (a) |
| **12.** | (b) | **32.** | (a) | **52.** | (c) | **72.** | (a) |
| **13.** | (a) | **33.** | (c) | **53.** | (b) | **73.** | (d) |
| **14.** | (c) | **34.** | (b) | **54.** | (b) | **74.** | (b) |
| **15.** | (d) | **35.** | (a) | **55.** | (b) | **75.** | (a) |
| **16.** | (d) | **36.** | (a) | **56.** | (b) | **76.** | (a) |
| **17.** | (c) | **37.** | (b) | **57.** | (a) | **77.** | (b) |
| **18.** | (c) | **38.** | (c) | **58.** | (a) | **78.** | (c) |
| **19.** | (a) | **39.** | (a) | **59.** | (d) | **79.** | (b) |
| **20.** | (a) | **40.** | (d) | **60.** | (a) | **80.** | (a) |

# RUHS 2014 (Jaipur) (PB BSc Nursing)

## MULTIPLE CHOICE QUESTIONS

1. **Heat regulating center in body is located in:**
   (a) Thalamus (b) Hypothalamus
   (c) Medulla oblongata (d) Cerebrum
2. **Smallest bone in human body:**
   (a) Stapes (b) Phalanges
   (c) Metacarpal (d) Xiphisternum
3. **The function of fallopian tube is:**
   (a) Secretion of estrogen and progesterone
   (b) Passage way for fetus
   (c) Occurrence of fertilization
   (d) Developing fetus
4. **Normal respiration of healthy person is:**
   (a) 5–10/min (b) 10–15/min
   (c) 15–20/min (d) 20–30/min
5. **Kidney is situated:**
   (a) In abdominal cavity (b) In pelvic cavity
   (c) In thoracic cavity (d) In dorsal cavity
6. **Total numbers of chambers in human heart is:**
   (a) 4 (b) 1
   (c) 3 (d) 2
7. **The only artery which supplies deoxygenated blood:**
   (a) Pulmonary artery (b) Hepatic artery
   (c) Gastric artery (d) Renal artery
8. **To diagnose which type of sample is collected?**
   (a) Urine (b) CSF
   (c) Bone marrow (d) Stool
9. **Thermophilic bacteria grow at following minimum temperature:**
   (a) 20°C (b) 35°C
   (c) 55°C (d) 85°C
10. **Life cycle of malaria parasite was first described by:**
    (a) Ronald Ross (b) Robert Koch
    (c) Louis Pasteur (d) Banting and Best
11. **HIV virus belongs to which of the following group?**
    (a) Flavivirus (b) Retrovirus
    (c) Rhabdovirus (d) Hepadnavirus
12. **In following which is the vector born disease:**
    (a) Diphtheria (b) Dengue
    (c) Tetanus (d) Measles
13. **Which of the following is an antidote for a patient with overdose of heparin?**
    (a) Protamine sulfate (b) Vitamin K
    (c) Atropine slufate (d) Physostigmine
14. **Paracetamol medicine/drug is:**
    (a) Antipyretic (b) Antitussive
    (c) Antiasthmatic (d) Antiemetic
15. **Morphine is contraindicated in:**
    (a) Angina (b) Bronchial asthma
    (c) Pancreatitis (d) MI
16. **Teaspoon medicine is equal to:**
    (a) 2 mL (b) 3 mL
    (c) 5 mL (d) 10 mL
17. **Which of the following medicine is useful for reducing raised intracranial pressure?**
    (a) IV Mannitol (b) IV Phenytoin
    (c) IV Diazepam (d) IV Nitroglycerine
18. **Analgesic are given:**
    (a) To relieve pain
    (b) To give rest
    (c) To induce sleep
    (d) To destroy pathogenic microorganisms
19. **Gullain-Barré syndrome is a disease of which of the following?**
    (a) Brain (b) Spinal cord
    (c) Peripheral nerve (d) All of the above
20. **Which of the following is not a parameter for 'Glasgow coma scale'?**
    (a) Eye opening (b) Papillary response
    (c) Verbal response (d) Motor response
21. **Rice water stool is a typical finding in case of:**
    (a) Cholera (b) Typhoid
    (c) Ulcerative colitis (d) Amebiasis
22. **Full form of CPR:**
    (a) Cardio Pulmonary Resuscitation
    (b) Cardio Pulmonary Relapse
    (c) Cardio Pulmonary restriction
    (d) Chronic Pulmonary Replace
23. **What concentration of NaCl in intravenous fluid is termed as 'Isotonic'?**
    (a) 0.25% (b) 0.45%
    (c) 0.75% (d) 0.90%
24. **A major priority of nursing care of child suspected of having meningitis is to:**
    (a) Check the temperature and give cold sponging
    (b) Isolate the child immediately
    (c) Administer the antibiotic as soon as it is ordered
    (d) Restrain the child to prevent accident

**25. The child's apical pulse is always checked before administering digoxin, the drug is not given is pulse rate is:**
(a) Below 90 beats/min
(b) Above 10 beats/min
(c) Less than 60 beats/min
(d) More than 150 beats/min

**26. During edematous phase of nephritic syndrome an important nursing intervention is to:**
(a) Provide meticulous skin care
(b) Encourage fluid intake
(c) Encourage moderate activity
(d) Weight the child every alternate day

**27. Initial nursing assessment of an infant suffering with acute diarrhea and dehydration reveals:**
(a) Skin turgor (b) Low Hematocrit
(c) Bulging fontanelle (d) Weight gain

**28. The most likely side effect of external radiation to the neck for cancer of larynx is:**
(a) Constipation (b) Dyspnea
(c) Sore throat (d) Diarrhea

**29. When respiratory rate of 12 months old child is 35 breath/minute, the most appropriate nursing action is:**
(a) Notify the physician
(b) Administer oxygen
(c) Reassess respiratory rate in 15 min
(d) Document the finding

**30. Which nursing intervention in thrombophlebitis would be contraindicated?**
(a) Maintaining strict bed rest
(b) Turn the patient form side to side
(c) Apply warm pack to affected site
(d) Massage the affected area

**31. A patient with acute pancreatitis has NG tube for low intermittent suction to prevent:**
(a) Chronic distortion
(b) Gastric reflux
(c) Pancreatic stimulation
(d) Peristalsis

**32. Platelet count decreases in:**
(a) Malaria (b) Filarial
(c) Dengue (d) Typhoid

**33. Eye padding is applied to unconscious patient to prevent:**
(a) Dryness of eye (b) Blinking of eye
(c) Corneal ulcer (d) Eye movement

**34. Hepatitis A is caused:**
(a) Due to infected blood transfusion
(b) Due to use of contaminated water
(c) Due to addiction of drug
(d) Due to dialysis

**35. To priority treatment for ventricular fibrillation includes:**
(a) ECG monitoring (b) Proper positioning
(c) CPR (d) Catheterization

**36. In following which disease occur due to deficiency of thiamine:**
(a) Beri-Beri (b) Pellagra
(c) Anemia (d) Scurvy

**37. To prevent legal implication, what should be done by a nurse during preoperative period:**
(a) Provide psychological support
(b) Obtain written consent
(c) Provide comprehensive nursing care
(d) Explain the patient and his relatives about postoperative complication

**38. Clinical manifestation of anemia includes:**
(a) Low Hb level (b) Fatigue
(c) Hyperactivity (d) Lassitude

**39. Priority basis management of unconscious patient includes:**
(a) IV therapy (b) IV Mannitol
(c) Clearance of airway (d) Pain at McBurney's point

**40. In oliguria volume of urine is:**
(a) Less than 100 mL (b) Less than 400 mL
(c) Less than 800 mL (d) Absence of urine

**41. Management of cardiac arrest includes except:**
(a) Massive infusion of IV infusion
(b) $O_2$ therapy
(c) Clearance of airway
(d) Cardiac compression

**42. During head injury what is the cause of increased body temperature:**
(a) Pons injury (b) Hypothalamus injury
(c) Cerebellum injury (d) Medulla injury

**43. What is the cause of anemia in chronic renal failure?**
(a) Decreased erythropoietin
(b) Hemolysis
(c) Production of immature RBC
(d) Inappropriate renal function

**44. In following which is not a cause of Hypokalemia:**
(a) Vomiting
(b) Potassium wasting diuretics
(c) Aldosteronism
(d) Renal failure

**45. Painful menstruation is termed as:**
(a) Menorrhagia
(b) Dysmenorrheal
(c) Amenorrhea
(d) Decreased production of prostaglandins

**46. Which of the following is not a sexually transmitted disease?**
(a) Chancroid (b) Syphilis
(c) Forbid uterus (d) AIDS

**47. Fault in male that may cause infertility in male:**
(a) Mumps orchitis
(b) Raised scrotal temperature
(c) Undescended testis
(d) All of the above

**48. Secretion from mother's breast during delivery is called:**
(a) Sequestrum (b) Colostrum
(c) Lochia (d) Leukorrhea

**49. During which stage of labor placenta is delivered?**
(a) Stage I (b) Stage II
(c) Stage III (d) Stage IV

**50. 'Pap smear' is used for screening of which of the following?**
(a) Ovarian cancer (b) Endometrial cancer
(c) Cervical cancer (d) Breast cancer

**51. Which abdominal grip is used to assess the descent of head in a pregnant women?**
(a) Fundal grip (b) Lateral grip
(c) Pelvic I (d) Pelvic II

**52. Movement of baby felt by the mother is known as:**
(a) Quickening (b) Lightening
(c) Engagement (d) Ballottement

**53. Bed rest is essential in pre-eclampsia as it:**
(a) Prevent eclampsia
(b) Mobilize tissue fluid there by lowering blood pressure
(c) Improves blood circulation and decreases edema
(d) Prevent premature labor

**54. About 25% maternal death are due to:**
(a) Infection (b) Obstetric hemorrhage
(c) Unsafe abortion (d) Eclampsia

**55. Bleeding after 24 hours of delivery is considered as pastpartum hemorrhage:**
(a) When blood loss is more than 500 mL
(b) When blood loss is more than 700 mL
(c) When blood loss is more than 100 mL
(d) When blood loss is more than 200 mL

**56. Which of the following is highest diameter of pelvis?**
(a) Anterior-posterior (b) Lateral
(c) Oblique (d) All of the above

**57. Total weight gain in pregnancy is about:**
(a) 6 kg (b) 8 kg
(c) 11 kg (d) 14 kg

**58. In following which vaccine is given to a pregnant lady?**
(a) Measles (b) BCG
(c) Tetanus (d) DPT

**59. Primary feature of cervical cancer includes:**
(a) Polyuria (b) Irregular menstruation
(c) Anorexia (d) Headache

**60. The total number of antinatal visit by a pregnant lady should be:**
(a) 2 (b) 3
(c) 1 (d) 5

**61. Commonest complication of IUD insertion is:**
(a) Pain (b) Bleeding
(c) Perforation (d) Ectopic pregnancy

**62. Fertilization occurs in:**
(a) Uterus (b) Fallopian tube
(c) Pelvis (d) Vagina

**63. In following which is the main cause of PID?**
(a) Abruptio placenta
(b) Placenta previa
(c) Ectopic pregnancy
(d) PPH

**64. During +2 station position of fetal head is:**
(a) Below ischial spine (b) Above ischial spine
(c) Behind ischial spine (d) Just above the pelvic inlet

**65. Which of the following is 'fontanels'?**
(a) Frontal (b) Occipital
(c) Sphenoid (d) Mastoid

**66. To calculate a dose of medicine for a child, which of the following formula is used?**
(a) Young's rule (b) Clark's rule
(c) Fried's rule (d) All of the above

**67. The premature labor, which of the following is used for newborn?**
(a) $MgSo_4$ (b) Oxytocin
(c) Dexamethasone (d) Testosterone

**68. A promising treatment for some children suffering from Thalassemia:**
(a) Bone marrow transplantation
(b) Chemotherapeutic agent
(c) Radiation therapy
(d) Steroidal therapy

**69. A child diagnosed with bacterial conjunctivitis, a nurse should educate the mother to do all except:**
(a) Washing hand frequently
(b) Clean eyes as prescribed
(c) Share towel and wash hand
(d) Give eye drops as prescribed

**70. The APGAR scoring is done to appraise the infant for:**
(a) Birth defect (b) Respiratory effort
(c) Rh–sensitization (d) Emotional stability

**71. Wilms' tumor is a tumor of:**
(a) Testis (b) Brain
(c) Kidney (d) Liver

**72. Normal birth weight is:**
(a) 2–2.5 kg (b) 2.2–2.7 kg
(c) 3–3.5 kg (d) 2.5–3 kg

**73. What is the criteria of LBW baby:**
(a) Birth weight less than 2 kg
(b) Birth weight less than 2.5 kg
(c) Birth weight less than 3 kg
(d) Birth weight less than 2.7 kg

**74. At which age a child can start to brush the teeth?**
(a) 2 years (b) 3 years
(c) 4 years (d) 20 months

**75. While taking a temperature from a rectal route in a children thermometer should be inserted about:**
(a) 0.5 inch (b) 1.5 inch
(c) 1 inch (d) 2 inch

**76. MMR vaccine is given by:**
(a) IM route (b) IV route
(c) ID route (d) Sub cute

**77. Deficiency of vitamin D in children may cause:**
(a) Osteomalacia
(b) Pellagra
(c) Ricketsia
(d) Beri-beri

**78. In children which disease occur due to protein deficiency?**
(a) Beri-beri (b) Scurvy
(c) Marasmus (d) Kwashiorkor

**79. After the birth of the baby, breastfeeding should be started:**
(a) Within 2 hours (b) With ½ hour
(c) On second dy (d) After 1 week

**80. When physiological jaundice appear in babies?**
(a) At birth (b) On second week
(c) On second day (d) On first week

**81. In following which is not preventive measures for tetanus neonatorum?**
(a) TT vaccination
(b) Following five clinical rule
(c) TT immunization during reproductive age
(d) Penicillin antibiotic

**82. Causative organism for chickenpox is:**
(a) Paramyxovirus
(b) Varicella zoster virus
(c) Herpes simplex virus
(d) Bordetella pertussis virus

**83. In a patient of fever 'fastigium', treatment is given to which of the following period?**
(a) Onset of fever
(b) When temperature is raised to its maximum and remains constant
(c) When body temperature is gradually returning to normal
(d) When body temperature is suddenly returning to normal

**84. Which of the following disease is not transferred by air droplets?**
(a) Measles (b) Chickenpox
(c) Polio myelitis (d) Tuberculosis

**85. WHO was established on:**
(a) 14th April 1948 (b) 7th April 1948
(c) 7th April 1955 (d) 7th April 1947

**86. What is the full form of UNDP?**
(a) United nations development program
(b) Unique nursing developmental program
(c) United nations developmental project
(d) United nurses developmental project

**87. Typhoid fever is:**
(a) Viral disease (b) Skin disease
(c) Parasitic disease (d) Bacterial disease

**88. Polio vaccine is prepared from:**
(a) Live attenuated organism
(b) Killed organism
(c) Toxoid
(d) Aerobic bacteria

**89. The full form of ICDS is:**
(a) Integrated child developmental services
(b) International children developmental scheme
(c) Internal committee of developmental scheme
(d) Indian child developmental scheme

**90. Community health nursing explains a new diagnosed diabetes mellitus patient that a purpose of medication is to treat:**
(a) Hyperglycemia
(b) Hypoglycemia
(c) Hypocalcemia
(d) Hyperbilirubinemia

**91. Which is the most appropriate time of IUD insertion?**
(a) During or within 10 days of menstruation
(b) About the midst of cycle
(c) Just before a menstruation cycle
(d) At any time of menstruation

**92. A type of BCG vaccine is:**
(a) Killed vaccine
(b) Triple vaccine
(c) Live attenuated
(d) Combined vaccine

**93. Who ORS packet include following except:**
(a) Sodium chloride
(b) Potassium chloride
(c) Sodium bicarbonate
(d) Calcium bicarbonate

**94. Infant mortality rate is expressed in term of:**
(a) Rate/100 live birth
(b) Rate/1000 live birth
(c) Rate/1000 total birth
(d) Rate/100 total birth

**95. On which day international AIDS day is celebrated ever year?**
(a) 1st May
(b) 7th April
(c) 11th April
(d) 1st December

**96. Which of the following disease is caused by Varicella zoster:**
(a) Diphtheria
(b) Smallpox
(c) Syphilis
(d) Chickenpox

**97. Treatment therapy which is used for TB:**
(a) MDT (b) BCG vaccine
(c) ORS (d) DOTS

**98. Polio is mainly infection of:**
(a) Respiratory tract
(b) Central nervous system
(c) Alimentary canal
(d) Reproductive system

**99. What do you mean by incidence?**
(a) New case of any disease
(b) Old case of any disease
(c) Total cases of any cases
(d) All of the above

**100. In following which disease is eradicated from all over the world?**
(a) Chickenpox (b) Smallpox
(c) Cholera (d) Pertussis

## ANSWERS

| | | | | | | | | | |
|---|---|---|---|---|---|---|---|---|---|
| **1.** | (b) | **21.** | (a) | **41.** | (a) | **61.** | (b) | **81.** | (d) |
| **2.** | (a) | **22.** | (a) | **42.** | (b) | **62.** | (b) | **82.** | (b) |
| **3.** | (c) | **23.** | (d) | **43.** | (a) | **63.** | (d) | **83.** | (b) |
| **4.** | (c) | **24.** | (b) | **44.** | (d) | **64.** | (a) | **84.** | (c) |
| **5.** | (a) | **25.** | (a) | **45.** | (b) | **65.** | (b) | **85.** | (b) |
| **6.** | (a) | **26.** | (a) | **46.** | (c) | **66.** | (d) | **86.** | (a) |
| **7.** | (a) | **27.** | (a) | **47.** | (d) | **67.** | (c) | **87.** | (d) |
| **8.** | (b) | **28.** | (c) | **48.** | (b) | **68.** | (a) | **88.** | (a) |
| **9.** | (c) | **29.** | (d) | **49.** | (c) | **69.** | (c) | **89.** | (a) |
| **10.** | (a) | **30.** | (a) | **50.** | (c) | **70.** | (b) | **90.** | (a) |
| **11.** | (b) | **31.** | (c) | **51.** | (d) | **71.** | (c) | **91.** | (a) |
| **12.** | (b) | **32.** | (c) | **52.** | (a) | **72.** | (a) | **92.** | (c) |
| **13.** | (a) | **33.** | (c) | **53.** | (c) | **73.** | (b) | **93.** | (d) |
| **14.** | (a) | **34.** | (b) | **54.** | (b) | **74.** | (b) | **94.** | (b) |
| **15.** | (b) | **35.** | (c) | **55.** | (a) | **75.** | (b) | **95.** | (d) |
| **16.** | (c) | **36.** | (a) | **56.** | (a) | **76.** | (b) | **96.** | (d) |
| **17.** | (a) | **37.** | (b) | **57.** | (c) | **77.** | (c) | **97.** | (d) |
| **18.** | (a) | **38.** | (c) | **58.** | (c) | **78.** | (b) | **98.** | (c) |
| **19.** | (c) | **39.** | (c) | **59.** | (b) | **79.** | (b) | **99.** | (a) |
| **20.** | (b) | **40.** | (b) | **60.** | (b) | **80.** | (c) | **100.** | (b) |

# RUHS 2014 (Jaipur)
# (Medical College Recruitment Exam, Nurse Grade II)

## MULTIPLE CHOICE QUESTIONS

**1. The innermost layer of heart is:**
(a) Epicardium
(b) Endocardium
(c) Myocardium
(d) Pericardium

**2. What is a sociological definition of the word drug?**
(a) A substance that changes mood, behavior or consciousness
(b) A dysfunction
(c) A chemical
(d) Ecology

**3. Hypnotherapy is least effective on people suffering from:**
(a) Anxiety (b) Hypertension
(c) Pain (d) Schizophrenia

**4. Which of the following stain is used to detect *Mycobatctrium* species?**
(a) Gram staining (b) Capsule stain
(c) Acid fast stain (d) Endospore stain

**5. The best method of sterilization of dressing powder is:**
(a) Autoclaving (b) Hot air oven
(c) Inspissations (d) Chemical method

**6. Which of the following results of lab test is invectives of the bacterial infections?**
(a) RBC: 4.0 million
(b) Hemoglobin: 13.2 gm/dl
(c) Platelets: 3,50,000/cmm
(d) WBC: 15,000/cmm

**7. If after surgery the patient's abdomen becomes distended and no bowel sounds appreciated, what would be the most suspected complication?**
(a) Intussusceptions (b) Paralytic Ileus
(c) Hemorrhage (d) Ruptures colon

**8. A registered nurse witnessed an old women hit by motorcycle while crossing train railway. The old women fell at railway. She was rushed at the scene. As a registered nurse, the first thing that needs to be done is:**
(a) Stay with the person, encourage her to remain still and immobilizes the leg while waiting for the ambulance
(b) Leave the person for a few moments to call for help
(c) Reduce the fracture manually
(d) Move the person to a safer place

**9. Good source of vitamin D includes all except:**
(a) Blueberries
(b) Sunlight
(c) Salmon, tuna sardines and mackerel
(d) Fortified milk and other dairy products.

**10. A 48-year-old women present with intermenstrual bleeding for two month occurring any time in the cycle. There is no associated pain. Differential diagnosis for intermenstrual bleeding does not include:**
(a) Endocervical polyp (b) Ovarian teratoma
(c) Cervical malignancy (d) Endometrial polyp

**11. Following are the complications of premenstrual menopause except:**
(a) Osteoporosis
(b) Infertility
(c) Decreased cardiovascular risk
(d) Vasomotor symptoms

**12. Which nursing diagnosis should receive priority in the plan of care for a three month old infant who has a *salmonella* infection?**
(a) Weight loss (b) Fluid volume deficit
(c) Sleeping (d) Shouting and crying

**13. Which of the following is a non-communicable disease?**
(a) Smallpox (b) Tuberculosis
(c) Typhoid (d) Diabetes Mellitus

**14. A new case in population during a fixed period is determined by:**
(a) Prevalence ratio (b) Attack rate
(c) Disability ratio (d) Incidences ratio

**15. Factors affecting parenting behavior does not include a parent's own:**
(a) Personal experiences and trauma
(b) Mental health
(c) Family experience
(d) Dietary habits

**16. A 32-year-old woman is present to the gynecology clinic with infrequent period. A hormone profile is done and all of the following are consistent with polycystic ovarian syndrome except:**
(a) Increased androgen levels
(b) Normal FSH
(c) Normal estradiol
(d) Decreased LH

**17. Which of the drug is responsible for 'Red man syndrome'?**
(a) Vancomycin (b) Linezolid
(c) Cefadroxil (d) Chloramphenicol

**18. A male patient's daughter telephones an adult gerontology primary nurse practitioner to inquire about the patient's illness. The daughter reports that her father relies upon her to explain everything to him. The nurse practitioner's initial response is to:**
(a) Ask the daughter to provide a copy of the patient's advance directive document
(b) Tell the daughter that the nurse practitioner can discuss the information only with the patient
(c) Assure the daughter that the nurse practitioner can disclose the requested information
(d) Inform the daughter that she must come to discuss her father's case

**19. Which of the following is used in bed wetting in children?**
(a) Imipramine (b) Chlorpromazine
(c) Levodopa (d) Tacrine

**20. What is the most common site of rupture of a cerebral aneurysm with resulting subarachnoid hemorrhage?**
(a) Anterior cerebral artery
(b) Middle cerebral artery
(c) Anterior communicating artery
(d) Posterior communicating artery

**21. Which of these used in multidrug resistant tuberculosis?**
(a) Ciprofloxacin (b) Metronidazole
(c) Penicillin (d) Linezolid

**22. When caring for a patient who is on a mechanical ventilator, the nurse should monitor the patient for which of the following complication?**
(a) Pulmonary embolism
(b) Pleural effusion
(c) Flail chest
(d) Pneumothorax

**23. A patient comes to the clinic with report of acute pain and loss of vision in the right eye. The adult-gerontology primary care nurse practitioner informs the patient that these symptoms require:**
(a) Immediate referral to an ophthalmologist
(b) Assessment with split lamp
(c) Examination with otoscope
(d) Treatment with several ophthalmologic agent

**24. Which of the following blood group is universal recipient?**
(a) A (b) B
(c) AB (d) O

**25. Deficiency of which of the following vitamin during pregnancy may cause neural tube defect?**
(a) Folic acid (b) Riboflavin
(c) Niacin (d) Thiamine

**26. During the initial care of rape victim the following are considered by a nurse except:**
(a) Maintain non-judgmental approach
(b) Assure privacy
(c) Touch the client to show acceptance and empathy
(d) Accompany the client in the examination room

**27. Shick test is carried up to determine:**
(a) Polio (b) Pertussis
(c) Meningitis (d) Diphtheria

**28. Which of the following is the most common side effect of 'Aspirin'?**
(a) Gastrointestinal bleeding
(b) Constipation
(c) Nystagmus
(d) Urinary incontinence

**29. The intestinal juice secreted in the intestine containing digestive enzymes is known as:**
(a) Succusenterius (b) Juicy fluid
(c) Succus juices (d) Chime

**30. All are the non-modifiable risk factors of atherosclerosis except:**
(a) High cholesterol intake
(b) Age
(c) Heredity
(d) Gender

**31. The first drug of choice for a patient admitted with status epileptics is:**
(a) Phenytoin (b) Carbamazepine
(c) Diazepam (d) Sodium valproate

**32. Which of the following is not a saturated fatty acid?**
(a) Oleic acid (b) Palmitic acid
(c) Lauric acid (d) Stearic acid

**33. A 69-year-old female patient reports dyspareunia. Physical examination reveals sparse hair, a introitus that admit two finger and a pale dry vagina. The adult gerontology primary care nurse practitioner's initial management is to recommend:**
(a) Daily douching
(b) Topical hormonal cream
(c) Topical antibiotic cream
(d) Topical antifungal cream

**34. Which of the following antibody occurs in pentameric structure?**
(a) IgA (b) IgG
(c) IgE (d) IgM

**35. Which of the following is not a typical antipsychotic and does not have marked extrapyramidal side effect?**
(a) Chlorpromazine
(b) Fluphenazine
(c) Clozapine
(d) Haloperidol

**36. In case of heparin over dose which agent should be used:**
(a) Diltiazem (b) Protamine
(c) Imferon (d) Warfarin

**37. In case of development of urticaria, half hour after the blood transfusion has begun, the first action by the nurse should be:**
(a) To slow down the rate of infusion
(b) To administer the anti histaminic agent
(c) To note vital sign
(d) To stop the infusion

**38. When hemoglobin combines with oxygen it is known as:**
(a) Oxyhemoglobin
(b) Deoxyhemoglobin
(c) Reduced hemoglobin
(d) Oxidized hemoglobin

**39. Which of the following monoclone antibody is approved for the treatment of asthma?**
(a) Bevacizumab (b) Omalizumab
(c) Cetuximab (d) Trastuzumab

**40. A 55-year-old man was admitted after a motor vehicle accident with multiple injuries. His friend reported that he had been seeing psychiatrist for an unknown diagnosis. He stated that patient sometime gets hyper for no reason, and becomes violent and sometime get depressed. Of the following, which general psychiatric disorder is characterized by the pattern of aggression includes irritability, agitation and violent behavior during manic or psychotic episode?**
(a) Schizophrenia (b) Bipolar disorder
(c) Delusion disorder (d) Depression

**41. Which of the following is not filtered out during glomerular filtration?**
(a) Glucose (b) Water
(c) Salt (d) Protein

**42. For a 6 month pregnant lady following is contra-indicated:**
(a) Retinol (b) Tetanus
(c) Folic acid (d) Ferrous sulfate

**43. Recommended site for administration of DPT in infant is:**
(a) Deltoid (b) Gluteal
(c) Forearm (d) Intravenous

**44. Spironolactone produces:**
(a) Hypernatremia (b) Hyperkalemia
(c) Hyponatremia (d) Hypokalemia

**45. The agent contraindicated with warfarin treatment is:**
(a) Aspirin (b) Ranitidine
(c) Codeine (d) Isaphgol

**46. After obtaining 3 L of fluid from a client via paracentesis, the nurse would be alert for which complication?**
(a) Encephalopathy
(b) Bleeding from site
(c) Vascular collapse
(d) Respiratory distress

**47. Which of the following is the most prominent feature of public health nurse?**
(a) Public nurse focus on preventive, not curative services
(b) Services are provided free of charges to people within catchment area
(c) The public health nurse functions as part of team providing a public health nursing services
(d) It involves providing home care to sick people who are not confined in the hospital

**48. The lung function test is determined by:**
(a) Tonometer (b) Spirometer
(c) Barometer (d) Sphygmomanometer

**49. Which of the following part of eye contain rhodopsin pigment?**
(a) Rods (b) Cones
(c) Lens (d) Iris

**50. Which of the following agent causes discoloration of teeth if taken in milk?**
(a) Tetracycline (b) Metronidazole
(c) Penicillin (d) Ciprofloxacin

## ANSWERS

| | | | | | | | | | |
|---|---|---|---|---|---|---|---|---|---|
| **1.** | (b) | **11.** | (c) | **21.** | (d) | **31.** | (c) | **41.** | (d) |
| **2.** | (a) | **12.** | (b) | **22.** | (d) | **32.** | (a) | **42.** | (a) |
| **3.** | (d) | **13.** | (d) | **23.** | (a) | **33.** | (b) | **43.** | (a) |
| **4.** | (c) | **14.** | (d) | **24.** | (c) | **34.** | (d) | **44.** | (b) |
| **5.** | (b) | **15.** | (d) | **25.** | (a) | **35.** | (c) | **45.** | (a) |
| **6.** | (d) | **16.** | (d) | **26.** | (c) | **36.** | (b) | **46.** | (c) |
| **7.** | (b) | **17.** | (a) | **27.** | (d) | **37.** | (d) | **47.** | (a) |
| **8.** | (d) | **18.** | (b) | **28.** | (a) | **38.** | (a) | **48.** | (b) |
| **9.** | (b) | **19.** | (a) | **29.** | (a) | **39.** | (b) | **49.** | (a) |
| **10.** | (b) | **20.** | (c) | **30.** | (a) | **40.** | (b) | **50.** | (a) |

# KEA 2013
# (Bangalore Medical College and Research Institute)

## MULTIPLE CHOICE QUESTIONS

1. **Nurses day is celebrated on:**
   (a) April 1st (b) March 7th
   (c) May 12th (d) December 1st
2. **One-way communication not possesses the following:**
   (a) Past experience (b) Communication skill
   (c) Understand message (d) Understand audience
3. **The scale used to assess the level of consciousness in the patient:**
   (a) Bhore scale (b) Robert scale
   (c) Glasgow coma scale (d) None
4. **Coining new term means:**
   (a) Echolalia (b) Flight of ideas
   (c) Neologism (d) Delusion
5. **The most important step in health education:**
   (a) Community discussion
   (b) Contact with doctor
   (c) Knowledge of local need
   (d) Announcement by loud speaker
6. **Anterior fontanel normally closes between:**
   (a) 2–3 months (b) 3–6 months
   (c) 18–20 months (d) 1–9 months
7. **In hypocalcemia, the most important clinical manifestation is:**
   (a) Chvostek's sign (b) Trousseau's sign
   (c) Inverted ST (d) Both (a) and (b)
8. **After delivery mother should be placed in:**
   (a) Dorsal position (b) Lithotomy
   (c) Left lateral position (d) None
9. **Indian mental health act passed on:**
   (a) 1983 (b) 1987
   (c) 1897 (d) 1899
10. **The first sign of dementia is loss of:**
    (a) Long-term memory (b) Short-term memory
    (c) Complete memory (d) None of the above
11. **An infant begins to sit with support by:**
    (a) 4 months (b) 7 months
    (c) 6 months (d) 9 months
12. **Fat soluble vitamins:**
    (a) Vitamin C (b) Vitamin K
    (c) Vitamin B (d) All the above
13. **The first fetal movement felt by mother is called:**
    (a) Quickening (b) Flexion
    (c) Attitude (d) Lighting
14. **Patient treated in triage 1 is:**
    (a) Vomiting (b) Cardiac arrest
    (c) Fever (d) None
15. **Specific gravity of urine is:**
    (a) 1.010 (b) 1.001
    (c) 1.100 (d) 1.110
16. **Fear of height is known as:**
    (a) Acrophobia (b) Claustrophobia
    (c) Social phobia (d) Echophobia
17. **Positive sign of meningeal irritation:**
    (a) Kerning's sign (b) Opisthotonus position
    (c) Nuchal rigidity (d) All of the above
18. **Lupus erythematosus is an:**
    (a) Immune disease (b) Auto immune disorder
    (c) Self disease (d) Skin disease
19. **CPR ratio chest compression is to breath is:**
    (a) 30:2 (b) 20:2
    (c) 15:3 (d) 20:3
20. **Sleep disorder in children is use to:**
    (a) Loss of appetite (b) Insecurity
    (c) Bright light (d) Constipation
21. **The outermost membrane that helps to form the placenta:**
    (a) Chorion (b) Amnion
    (c) Amniotic sac (d) Peritoneum
22. **MTP act was passed in:**
    (a) 1971 (b) 1972
    (c) 1973 (d) 1974
23. **Protrusion of the stomach content into the thoracic cavity is called:**
    (a) Hernia (b) Hiatal hernia
    (c) Gastro hernia (d) None
24. **The normal infant respiratory rate per minute is:**
    (a) 30 to 60 B/min (b) 10 to 20 B/min
    (c) 40 to 40 B/min (d) 60 to 120 B/min
25. **Removal of entire eye including sclera is:**
    (a) Enucleation (b) Orthoptics
    (c) Evisceration (d) Extenteration
26. **MRI is contraindicated in patient with:**
    (a) Pace maker (b) Metal implant
    (c) Brain tumor (d) Both a and b
27. **The shick test is used to determine:**
    (a) Scarlet fever (b) Diphtheria
    (c) Tuberculosis (d) Typhoid

28. **The systolic murmur associated with diminished second heart rate is seen in:**
(a) Aortic regurgitation (b) Aortic stenosis
(c) Mitral regurgitation (d) Mitral stenosis

29. **Primary health care is meant for:**
(a) Rural health care (b) First level health care
(c) Tertiary health care (d) Second level health care

30. **While blood transfusion, the patient has increased pulse rate. What is nurse role?**
(a) Call the doctor (b) Stop the transfusion
(c) Increased NS flow (d) Continue transfusion

31. **Indication of fetal distress is:**
(a) Decreased in fetal scalp blood pH
(b) Meconium staining
(c) Late deceleration of heart rate
(d) All of the above

32. **A perceptual disorder is called:**
(a) Delusion (b) Hallucination
(c) Phobia (d) Neologism

33. **Aneurysm means dilation of:**
(a) Artery (b) Vein
(c) Skin (d) All of the above

34. **Anti-tuberculosis treatment is given for at least:**
(a) 3 months (b) 6 months
(c) 1 year (d) 8 months

35. **A mentally healthy person:**
(a) Feels reasonably secure and accepts his short mistake
(b) Is unable to concentrate
(c) Lose temper
(d) Always working

36. **Human skeletal system consists of:**
(a) 201 bones (b) 206 bones
(c) 198 bones (d) 105 bones

37. **INC is located in:**
(a) New Delhi (b) Mumbai
(c) Bengaluru (d) Chennai

38. **Graves disease is an autoimmune disease caused due to:**
(a) Hypoparathyroidism
(b) Hypothyroidism
(c) Hyperparathyroidism
(d) Hyperthyroidism

39. **Hormone which helps production of milk is:**
(a) FSH (b) Prolactin
(c) LH (d) Oxytocin

40. **The preferred route of administration of drug in unconscious patient is:**
(a) Sublingual (b) Oral
(c) Intravenous (d) Nasal

41. **Movement of bone towards the midline is:**
(a) Abduction (b) Extension
(c) Adduction (d) Circumduction

42. **Hemoglobin is:**
(a) A polysaccharide (b) A protein
(c) A enzyme (d) A hormone

43. **The patient is prescribed Injection Heparin 2500 IU subcutaneous one dose. You are given vial of 25000 IU in 5 ml. How much mL will you administered?**
(a) 1 mL (b) 2 mL
(c) 0.5 mL (d) 0.2 mL

44. **Booster dose of DPT vaccine is given at:**
(a) 18 weeks (b) 18 months and 4–6 years
(c) 12 months (d) Every 4 months

45. **Observation is method of:**
(a) Assessment (b) Evaluation
(c) Planning (d) Data collection

46. **An agent that has power to kill the micro- organism and its spore:**
(a) Bacteriostatic (b) Phenol
(c) Bacteriocidal (d) Alcohol

47. **A patient comes to emergency with breathlessness. What is its priority?**
(a) Call the doctor
(b) Record vital sign
(c) Provide oxygen mask
(d) Registration

48. **Suction is pressure:**
(a) Equal to atmosphere
(b) Less than atmosphere
(c) More than atmosphere
(d) None of the above

49. **Pace-maker of heart**
(a) AV node (b) AV bundle
(c) Purkinje fiber (d) SA node

50. **Pus in urine is called**
(a) Polyuria (b) Oliguria
(c) Pyuria (d) Anuria

51. **DNR stand for:**
(a) Do not respond (b) Do not resuscitate
(c) Do not read (d) Do not receive

52. **The center for controlling body temperature:**
(a) Hypothalamus (b) Medulla oblongata
(c) Cerebellum (d) Midbrain

53. **Insufficieny of oxygen in tissue is:**
(a) Hypoxemia (b) Hypoxia
(c) Hyponemia (d) Anemia

54. **The amount of solution to be given to evacuate enema for adults:**
(a) 200 mL (b) 300 mL
(c) 500 mL (d) 500–1000 mL

55. **If the room was used for a client with communicable disease, it should be:**
(a) Washed (b) Cleaned
(c) Sterilized (d) Fumigation

56. **Glycogenesis is regulated by the hormone:**
(a) Insulin (b) Cortisol
(c) Glycolysis (d) Enterokinase

57. **Kwashiorkor is caused due to deficiency of:**
(a) Carbohydrate (b) Protein
(c) Fat (d) Vitamin A

**58. In profound mental retardation the IQ is:**
(a) Less than 10 (b) Less than 20
(c) 20–30 (d) 20–50

**59. A drug which dilate pupil:**
(a) Mydriatics (b) Mycotics
(c) Keratolytic (d) Scabicides

**60. In unconscious patient mouth care is given to prevent:**
(a) Aspiration (b) Infection
(c) Mouth odor (d) All of the above

**61. Blind spot is recorded on the:**
(a) Sclera (b) Choroid
(c) Retina (d) Iris

**62. Normal urine output per day is:**
(a) 150 mL (b) 500 mL
(c) 1500 mL (d) 5000 mL

**63. Lithium toxicity range is:**
(a) Above 2 mEq/L (b) 0.8–1.0 mEq/L
(c) 0.6–1.2 mEq/L (d) Above 3 mEq/L

**64. Which among the following is killed vaccine?**
(a) BCG (b) Oral polio
(c) Pertussis (d) Mumps

**65. A cause of sudden death in the major fracture is:**
(a) Fat embolism (b) Bleeding
(c) Pain (d) None of the above

**66. A characteristic radiological finding in neonatal necrotizing enterocololitis is:**
(a) Gas in peritoneum
(b) Gas in the intestinal wall
(c) Pneumoperitonium
(d) Airfluid level

**67. Collection of thick pus in the pleural cavity:**
(a) Emphysema (b) Pleural effusion
(c) Atelectasis (d) All of the above

**68. Which part of brain regulates posture and balance?**
(a) Midbrain (b) Medulla oblongata
(c) Cerebellum (d) Cerebrum

**69. Consent of surgery is duty of:**
(a) Doctor
(b) Nurse
(c) OT technician
(d) Anesthesiologist

**70. Rickets is caused due to deficiency of:**
(a) Vitamin A (b) Vitamin B1
(c) Vitamin C (d) Vitamin D

**71. In kernicterus which is increased?**
(a) Conjugated bilirubin
(b) Conjugated and unconjugated bilirubin
(c) Unconjugated bilirubin
(d) None

**72. The antidote in warfarin overdose is:**
(a) Vitamin C (b) Protamine Sulfate
(c) Vitamin D (d) Vitamin K

**73. The cardinal sign for appendicitis is at:**
(a) String sign (b) Bird beak sign
(c) Mcburney's sign (d) Brudzinski sign

**74. Morphine is contraindicated in head injury because it causes:**
(a) Increased intracranial pressure
(b) Respiratory depression
(c) Vomiting miosis and mental clouding
(d) All the above

**75. Food allergy occurs by immunoglobulin:**
(a) IgM (b) IgE
(c) IgD (d) IgA

**76. An artificial active immunity is:**
(a) DPT (b) BCG
(c) TT (d) None

**77. In Primigravid total duration of labor is:**
(a) 16 hours (b) 20 hours
(c) 12 hours (d) 18 hours

**78. Haloperidol is an:**
(a) Antipsychotic (b) Antiseptic
(c) Antidepressant (d) Antiarrhythmic

**79. If a patient is prescribed for Injection Magnex 750 mg, you have vial of 1 gm with 10 mL of water for injection. How much mL will you administered?**
(a) 5 mL (b) 7.5 mL
(c) 2.5 mL (d) 6 mL

**80. Which is the most effective method to prevent infection?**
(a) Universal precaution
(b) Cap, gloves
(c) Handwashing
(d) Sterilium

**81. Causes of best sore are:**
(a) Friction
(b) Moisture
(c) Presence of pathogenic organism
(d) All of the above

**82. One ounce has:**
(a) 10 gms (b) 20 gms
(c) 35 gms (d) 30 gms

**83. Which position should be given to the client with respiratory diseases?**
(a) Supine position (b) Prone positione
(c) Fowler position (d) Lateral position

**84. Diuretics act as:**
(a) Increases the flow of urine
(b) Decreases the flow of urine
(c) Retention of urine
(d) None of the above

**85. The bone most frequent fracture during delivery is the:**
(a) Radius (b) Humerus
(c) Clavical (d) Ulna

**86. Macewen's sign is clinical manifestation of:**
(a) Delusion (b) Hallucination
(c) Phobia (d) Neologism

**87. Normal value of sodium in blood:**
(a) 120 to 130 mEq/L (b) 100 to 130 mEq/L
(c) 135 to 145 mEq/L (d) 200 to 210 mEq/L

**88. Collection of blood in thoracic cavity:**
(a) Hematoma (b) Hemothorax
(c) Hemopneumothorax (d) Hemorrhage

**89. When counseling about ageing, the nurse should teach that older adults normally have:**
(a) A rigid attitude (b) Slower reacton
(c) Period of confusion (d) Some senile dementia

**90. Optic nerve is:**
(a) 1st cranial nerve (b) 2nd cranial nerve
(c) 3rd cranial nerve (d) 5th cranial nerve

**91. Gastric lavage is contraindicated in case of:**
(a) Food poisoning (b) Corrosive poisoning
(c) Drug poisoning (d) OP poisoning

**92. Inability to carry out certain activity is:**
(a) Impairment (b) Handicap
(c) Retarded (d) Disability

**93. A 12 kg child is prescribed 10 mg/kg/day of injection amox tid. What is the single dosage?**
(a) 120 mg (b) 40 mg
(c) 30 mg (d) 20 mg

**94. Example of dry heat are except:**
(a) Heat pad (b) Sitz bath
(c) Diathermy (d) Hot water bag

**95. Contraindication for nasogastric intubation:**
(a) Gastric surgery (b) Polyps in nose
(c) Fractured jaw (d) Ulcer

**96. Skills required for nurses are:**
(a) Cognitive skill (b) Psychomotor skill
(c) Technical skill (d) All of the above

**97. Legal importance is given to:**
(a) Registration (b) Files
(c) Ordersheets (d) Records

**98. The temperature of sponge bath should be:**
(a) 110–115°F (b) 90–100°F
(c) 100–105°F (d) 100°F

**99. During an ear irrigation in an adult the ear lobe position:**
(a) Lifted upward and outward
(b) Pulled downward and forward
(c) Lifted upward and backward
(d) Pulled downward and blow

**100. Cold chain is used in vaccination for:**
(a) Good appearance
(b) Storage
(c) Potency and efficacy
(d) Carrying

## ANSWERS

| | | | | | | | | | |
|---|---|---|---|---|---|---|---|---|---|
| **1.** | (c) | **21.** | (a) | **41.** | (c) | **61.** | (c) | **81.** | (d) |
| **2.** | (a) | **22.** | (a) | **42.** | (b) | **62.** | (c) | **82.** | (d) |
| **3.** | (c) | **23.** | (b) | **43.** | (c) | **63.** | (a) | **83.** | (c) |
| **4.** | (c) | **24.** | (a) | **44.** | (b) | **64.** | (c) | **84.** | (a) |
| **5.** | (c) | **25.** | (a) | **45.** | (a) | **65.** | (b) | **85.** | (c) |
| **6.** | (c) | **26.** | (d) | **46.** | (c) | **66.** | (c) | **86.** | (b) |
| **7.** | (d) | **27.** | (b) | **47.** | (c) | **67.** | (a) | **87.** | (c) |
| **8.** | (a) | **28.** | (a) | **48.** | (b) | **68.** | (c) | **88.** | (b) |
| **9.** | (b) | **29.** | (b) | **49.** | (d) | **69.** | (a) | **89.** | (d) |
| **10.** | (b) | **30.** | (b) | **50.** | (c) | **70.** | (d) | **90.** | (b) |
| **11.** | (a) | **31.** | (d) | **51.** | (b) | **71.** | (c) | **91.** | (b) |
| **12.** | (b) | **32.** | (b) | **52.** | (a) | **72.** | (d) | **92.** | (a) |
| **13.** | (a) | **33.** | (a) | **53.** | (b) | **73.** | (c) | **93.** | (b) |
| **14.** | (b) | **34.** | (b) | **54.** | (d) | **74.** | (d) | **94.** | (b) |
| **15.** | (a) | **35.** | s | **55.** | (d) | **75.** | (b) | **95.** | (b) |
| **16.** | (a) | **36.** | (b) | **56.** | (a) | **76.** | (b) | **96.** | (d) |
| **17.** | (a) | **37.** | (a) | **57.** | (b) | **77.** | (c) | **97.** | (d) |
| **18.** | (b) | **38.** | (d) | **58.** | (b) | **78.** | (a) | **98.** | (b) |
| **19.** | (a) | **39.** | (b) | **59.** | (a) | **79.** | (b) | **99.** | (c) |
| **20.** | (b) | **40.** | (c) | **60.** | (d) | **80.** | (c) | **100.** | (b) |

# Questions Frequently Asked in All Different Examinations

## MULTIPLE CHOICE QUESTIONS

1. **While giving NG tube feeding which of the following nursing action prevents complications? (DSSSB 2013)**
   (a) Advance tube 2 cm
   (b) Flush with 20 mL air
   (c) Provide high Fowler's position
   (d) Plug the air vent during feeding
2. **Which of the following is an indication of portal hypertension? (DSSSB 2013)**
   (a) Asterixis (b) Hematemesis
   (c) Confusion (d) Elevated blood pressure
3. **A patient's GRBS is 40 mg% the immediate management is to administer: (DSSSB 2013)**
   (a) 5% dextrose
   (b) 50% dextrose
   (c) 10 units human actrapid insulin
   (d) Normal saline
4. **Goniometer is used to assess: (DSSSB 2013)**
   (a) Auditory acuity
   (b) Muscle strength
   (c) Range of motion of joints
   (d) Visual acuity
5. **Color coding for nitrous oxide cylinder is: (DSSSB 2013)**
   (a) Black (b) Black with white shoulder
   (c) Light blue (d) Gray
6. **The most appropriate time for nurse to obtain a sputum specimen for the culture is: (DSSSB 2013)**
   (a) Early in the morning
   (b) After the patient eats a light breakfast
   (c) After aerosol therapy
   (d) After chest physiotherapy
7. **Which of the following needed to be done before radial arterial cannulation to evaluate radial and ulnar arterial patency? (DSSSB 2013)**
   (a) Allen's test (b) Angiography
   (c) Buergors test (d) Capillary refill test
8. **Apical pulse is assessed by placing the diaphragm of the stethoscope at the area of: (DSSSB 2013)**
   (a) Aortic area (b) Pulmonic area
   (c) Mitral area (d) Tricuspid area
9. **The size of intravenous cannula used for neonates is: (DSSSB 2013)**
   (a) 18 (b) 20
   (c) 22 (d) 24
10. **Normal serum potassium level in meq/L is: (DSSSB 2013)**
    (a) 2.5 to 3.5 (b) 3.5 to 5
    (c) 5.5 to 6.5 (d) 6.5 to 7.5
11. **Bleeding from nose is known as: (DSSSB 2013)**
    (a) Epistaxis (b) Hemoptysis
    (c) Hematemesis (d) Hematuria
12. **Which of the following is used to assess the level of consciousness? (DSSSB 2013)**
    (a) Apgar score (b) Braden scale
    (c) Glasgow coma scale (d) Snellen's chart
13. **Lateral curvature of spine I known as: (DSSSB 2013)**
    (a) Kyphosis (b) Lordosis
    (c) Scoliosis (d) Pectus Excavatum
14. **Sensitivity and reaction is tested by administering the drug: (DSSSB 2013)**
    (a) Intradermally (b) Intramuscularly
    (c) Intravenously (d) Subcutaneous
15. **Which of the following is used to assessing the pain in children? (DSSSB 2013)**
    (a) Brief pain inventory
    (b) Numerical rating
    (c) Visual analogue scale
    (d) Wong baker face pain rating scale
16. **Medication used for nausea and vomiting is known as: (DSSSB 2013)**
    (a) Analgesic (b) Antipyretic
    (c) Antiemetic (d) Antibiotics
17. **The equipment used for examination of ear: (DSSSB 2013)**
    (a) Laryngoscope (b) Ophthalmoscope
    (c) Otoscope (d) Proctoscope
18. **The normal cholesterol level: (DSSSB 2013)**
    (a) 100–150 mg/dL (b) 150–200 mg/dL
    (c) 200–250 mg/dL (d) 250–300 mg/dL
19. **Which of the following is used to assess the function of brain stem? (DSSSB 2013)**
    (a) Cold calorie test (b) Glasgow coma scale
    (c) Braden scale (d) Intracranial pressure
20. **While installing ear drop, ear canal an adult is straightened by pulling the pinna: (DSSSB 2013)**
    (a) Down and back
    (b) Up and back
    (c) Straight down
    (d) Straight back

**21. The solution used to disinfect the bed linen of HIV positive patient is: (DSSSB 2013)**
(a) Dettol (b) Lysol
(c) Savlon (d) Sodium hypochlorite

**22. While measuring central venous pressure the zero point of the manometer is adjusted to: (DSSSB 2013)**
(a) Anterior axillary line
(b) Mid axillary line
(c) Posterior axillary line
(d) Shoulder level

**23. Which of the following is the preferred site for intramuscular injection in infants? (DSSSB 2013) (Rajasthan RRB 96)**
(a) Deltoid (b) Rectus femoris
(c) Vastus lateralis (d) Ventrogluteal

**24. The appropriate needle size for insulin injection is: (DSSSB 2013)**
(a) 18 G, 1½″ long (b) 22 G, 1″ long
(c) 22 G, 1½″ long (d) 25 G, 5/8″ long

**25. While performing tracheotomy suctioning, suctioning time should be not more than: (DSSSB 2013)**
(a) 10 sec (b) 20 sec
(c) 30 sec (d) 45 sec

**26. Braden scale is used for assessing the risk for: (DSSSB 2013)**
(a) Decubitus ulcer (b) Diabetes mellitus
(c) Hypertension (d) Urinary tract infection

**27. The percentage and the flow of air in red color venture mask is: (DSSSB 2013)**
(a) 31% and 6 lit/min (b) 35% and 8 lit/min
(c) 40% and 10 lit/min (d) 60% and 15 lit/min

**28. Inflammation of tongue is known as: (DSSSB 2013)**
(a) Gingivitis (b) Glossitis
(c) Parotids (d) Stomatitis

**29. Which of the following intervention can best prevent bed sore? (DSSSB 2013)**
(a) Massage reddened area with lotion or oils
(b) Change the position every one hour
(c) Use special water mattress
(d) Keep skin clean and dry

**30. Which of the following position is given to a patient with severe breathing difficulty? (DSSSB 2013)**
(a) Dorsal recumbent (b) Fowler
(c) Supine (d) Trendelenberg

**31. Antidote for heparin: (DSSSB 2013)**
(a) Vitamin K (b) Protamine sulfate
(c) Aminocaproic acid (d) Amiodarone

**32. Which of the following is used in the management of hyperkalemia? (DSSSB 2013)**
(a) Insulin with glucose (b) Sodium bicarbonate
(c) Potassium chloride (d) Magnesium sulfate

**33. The normal intraocular pressure: (DSSSB 2013)**
(a) 8–21 mm of Hg (b) 16–25 mm of Hg
(c) 20–35 mm of Hg (d) 19–38 mm of Hg

**34. Which of the ECG finding indicates the presence of hypokalemia? (DSSSB 2013)**
(a) Tall, peak T wave
(b) ST segment depression
(c) Widening of QRS complex
(d) Prolonged PR interval

**35. Which of the following part of pharynx have both respiratory and digestive function? (Bangalore PSC 2001)**
(a) Nasopharynx and oropharynx
(b) Oropharynx
(c) Oropharynx and laryngopharynx
(d) Laryngopharynx

**36. Which of the following is used as antidote organophosphrus poisoning? (DSSSB 2013)**
(a) Atropine
(b) Adrenaline
(c) Avil
(d) Amiodarone

**37. A patient receiving antibiotic therapy complaint of ringing in the ear. This ototoxicity is damage to: (DSSSB 2013)**
(a) 4th CN (b) 8th CN
(c) 7th CN (d) 9th CN

**38. Severe allergic reaction to drug is known as: (DSSSB 2013)**
(a) Anaphylactic (b) Interaction
(c) Adverse (d) Toxicity

**39. Lead poisoning is known as: (DSSSB 2013)**
(a) Asterixis
(b) Plumbism
(c) Plummer-Vinson syndrome
(d) Prader-Willi syndrome

**40. The drug of choice for pre-eclampsia is: (DSSSB 2013)**
(a) Magnesium sulfate
(b) Sodium bicarbonate
(c) Sodium nitroprusside
(d) None of the these

**41. Which of the following drug is administered sublingually for managing angina pectoris? (DSSSB 2013)**
(a) Aspirin (b) Betaloc
(c) Nitroglycerine (d) Warfarin

**42. Which of the following listed drug is a proton pump inhibitor? (DSSSB 2013)**
(a) Pantoprazole (b) Ranitidine
(c) Sucralfate (d) Famotidine

**43. Which of the following drug is withhold if the patients pulse is less than 60/min? (DSSSB 2013)**
(a) Digoxin (b) Dopamine
(c) Dobutamine (d) Phenytoin

**44. Ondansetron 8 mg IV given before chemotherapy is to prevent: (DSSSB 2013)**
(a) Alopecia (b) Fatigue
(c) Vomiting (d) Pain

**45. All of the following are the side effects of phenytoin, except: (DSSSB 2013)**
(a) Ataxia (b) Hirsutism
(c) Hypoglycemia (d) Gum hypertrophy

**46. The ideal place to record the temperature in dead body is from: (AIIMS PG 2001)**
(a) Axilla (b) Groin
(c) Rectum (d) Mouth

**47. In fetus insulin secretion begins with: (AIIMS 1998)**
(a) 3rd month (b) 5th month
(c) 7th month (d) 9th month

**48. Which of the following condition leads to tissue hypoxia without alteration of oxygen content of blood? (ESI 2008 )**
(a) CO poisoning (b) Met Hb
(c) Cyanide poisoning (d) Respiratory acidosis

**49. Which of the following statement is true about BCG vaccination? (AIIMS PG 2004)**
(a) Distilled water is used as diluent for BCG vaccine
(b) The site for injection should be cleaned thoroughly with spirit
(c) Mantoux test becomes positive after 48 hours
(d) WHO recommends Danish 1331 strain for vaccine production

**50. Which of the following pulses has highest content of iron? (PGIMER 2004)**
(a) Bengal gram (b) Black gram
(c) Red gram (d) Soybean

**51. Which of the following is the National level system that provides annual national as well as state level reliable estimate of fertility and mortality? (Kearla PSC 2004)**
(a) Civil registration system
(b) Census
(c) Adhoc survey
(d) Sample registration system

**52. The most common side effect of chemotherapy is: (PGIMS)**
(a) Nausea (b) Myelosuppression
(c) Alopecia (d) Renal dysfunction

**53. The function of 8th cranial nerve is related to: (RPSC)**
(a) Smell (b) Taste
(c) Touch (d) Balance

**54. Dengue shock syndrome is characterized by all of the following except: (ESI)**
(a) Hepatomegaly (b) Plural effusion
(c) Thrombocytopenia (d) Decreased hemoglobin

**55. Which complication of cardiac catheterization should the nurse monitor for initial 24 hours after procedure? (RPSC)**
(a) Angina at rest (b) Thrombus formation
(c) Dizziness (d) Falling blood pressure

**56. Which finding is persistent with pernicious anemia? (ESI Delhi)**
(a) Strawberry tongue (b) Current jelly stool
(c) Beefy red tongue (d) Pale (hypochromic) RBC

**57. Vitamin taken along with isoniazid to prevent peripheral neuritis: (AIIMS Delhi)**
(a) Vitamin B1 (b) Vitamin B2
(c) Vitamin B3 (d) Vitamin B6

**58. Breathing that is normal in rate and depth: (RPSC)**
(a) Eupnea (b) Bradypnea
(c) Tachypnea (d) Apnea

**59. In human corneal transplant, the donor tissue is: (AIIMS PG 2002)**
(a) Synthetic polymer
(b) Donated human cadaver eye
(c) Donated eye from live human being
(d) Monkey eye

**60. When teaching a client with coronary artery disease about nutrition, the nurse should emphasize: (ESI)**
(a) Eating number of balance meal in a day
(b) Adding complex carbohydrate
(c) Avoid very heavy meals
(d) Limiting sodium to 7 gms per day

**61. Which laser is used in management of cataract? (AIIMS PG)**
(a) Argon (b) Krypton
(c) Nd-YAG (d) Excimer

**62. A client is 1 day postoperative after total hip replacement. The client should be placed in which of the following position? (RAK MSc)**
(a) Supine (b) Semi Fowler
(c) Orthopneic (d) Trendelenburg

**63. Which of the following devices provides fixed performance oxygen therapy? (AIIMS 1988)**
(a) Nasal cannula (b) Venture mask
(c) Oxygen by T piece (d) Edinburgh mask

**64. A 16-year-old male is found to have a mental age of 9 years on IQ testing. He has: (AIIMS PG 2002)**
(a) Mild mental retardation
(b) Moderate mental retardation
(c) Severe mental retardation
(d) Profound mental retardation

**65. Which nursing intervention is appropriate for client with skeletal traction? (RAK MSc)**
(a) Pin care
(b) Prone positioning
(c) Intermittent weights
(d) 5 lb weight

**66. The nurse teaches the client with COPD to assess for sign and symptoms of right sided heart failure, which includes: (ESI 2006)**
(a) Clubbing of nail beds
(b) Hypertension
(c) Ankle edema
(d) Increased edema

**67. Defect in which of the following factor result in hemophilia B? (RPSC 2000)**
(a) Factor V (b) Factor VIII
(c) Factor IX (d) Factor X

**68. In the occurrence of SARS and other pandemics, which of the following is the most vital role of a nurse in epidemiology? (PGIMS 1996)**
(a) Health promotion (b) Disease prevention
(c) Surveillance (d) Case finding

**69. Euthanasia is: (AIIMS PG)**
(a) Preservation of the body
(b) Postmortem
(c) Putting into painless death
(d) None of the above

**70. According to WHO, which of the following is the most frequent cause of death in children under five worldwide in the 2003 WHO Survey? (AIIMS PG 2004)**
(a) Neonatal (b) Pneumonia
(c) Diarrhea (d) HIV/AIDS

**71. For treatment of class III dog bite all of them are correct except: (AIIMS 2001)**
(a) Give immunoglobulins for passive immunity
(b) Give ARV
(c) Immediately stitch wound under antibiotic coverage
(d) Immediately wash wound with soup and water

**72. Which of the following intervention demonstrate the nurse understands about the newborn's thermoregulatory abilities? (RPSC)**
(a) Placing newborn under a radiant warmer
(b) Suctioning with bulb syringe
(c) Obtaining Apgar score
(d) Inspecting newborn umbilical cord

**73. The umbilical vein carrying the blood from the placenta enters the fetus with: (RAK MSc)**
(a) Oxygenated blood by 80% saturation
(b) Oxygenated blood by 25% saturation
(c) Deoxygenated blood
(d) Both (a) and (c)

**74. Medication that is contraindicated during breastfeeding includes all except: (PGIMER 2004)**
(a) Bromocriptine (b) Cyclosporine
(c) Methotrexate (d) Prednisolone

**75. The antidote of choice in paracetamol poisoning is: (RMI)**
(a) Flumazenil (b) Sodium bicarbonate
(c) N-Acetyl cystine (d) Methylene blue

**76. Language development in autistic child resemble: (AIIMS PG)**
(a) Scanning speech (b) Speech lag
(c) Shuttering (d) Echolalia

**77. An 80-year-old women has sudden onset of right-sided paresis, short term memory loss, depression, right visual field defect and mild expressive aphasia, indicating a possible stroke. The most likely part of brain affected is the: (RRB)**
(a) Right hemisphere (b) Left hemisphere
(c) Brain stem (d) Cerebellum

**78. Low set ears are seen in: (ESI 2008)**
(a) Down syndrome (b) Renal disorder
(c) Kwashiorkor (d) Marasmus

**79. A client continuously repeat phrase that others have just said. The nurse recognizes this behavior as: (AIIMS 2005)**
(a) Autistic (b) Echopraxia
(c) Echolalic (d) Catatonic

**80. What is the color coding of bag in hospital to dispose off human anatomical wastes such as body part? (AIIMS)**
(a) Yellow (b) Black
(c) Red (d) Blue

**81. A form of aversion therapy where rather than actually experience the pairing of sexual stimuli with aversion outcome the client imagine these associations during controlled treatment session is known as: (AIIMS PG)**
(a) Overt conditioning (b) Operant conditioning
(c) Covert conditioning (d) Classical conditioning

**82. The world health day is celebrated on: (ESI 2007)**
(a) 7th April (b) 21st May
(c) 2nd August (d) 31st December

**83. Long acting insulin preparations are frequently administered by: (PGIMS 2009)**
(a) Oral route (b) Intramuscular route
(c) Intradermal route (d) Subcutaneous route

**84. The vaccine administered as nose drops: (PGIMS 2009)**
(a) Rubella (b) Poliomyelitis
(c) Influenza (d) Measles

**85. MTP is done up to: (RPSC)**
(a) 12 weeks (b) 16 weeks
(c) 20 weeks (d) 10 weeks

**86. Which committee is known as health survey and development committee? (RAK MSc)**
(a) Bhore Committee
(b) Mudalier Committee
(c) Shrivastav Committee
(d) Mukharji Committee

**87. Administration of readymade antibody creates:**
(a) Active acquired immunity
(b) Passive acquired immunity
(c) Active natural immunity
(d) Passive natural immunity

**88. Which of the danger sign should be informed promptly during the antepartum period? (RPSC)**
(a) Constipation (b) Breast tenderness
(c) Nasal stiffness (d) Leaking amniotic fluid

**89. Aspermia is the term used to describe: (AIIMS PG 1997)**
(a) Absence of semen
(b) Absence of sperm in ejaculation
(c) Absence of sperm motility
(d) Occurrence of abnormal sperm

**90. The client present with severe rectal bleeding, 16 diarrheal stool a day, severe abdominal pain, tenesmus and dehydration. Because of these symptoms the nurse should be alert for other problem associated with what disease? (PGIMER)**
(a) Crohn's disease (b) Ulcerative colitis
(c) Diverticulitis (d) Peritonitis

**91. Which of the following cells are involved in bone resorption? (RPSC 2000)**
(a) Chondrocytes (b) Osteoblast
(c) Osteoclast (d) Osteocytes

**92. A team of nurse was assign to teach the community regarding hazards of smoking/alcoholism, which method of teaching is most useful? (RRB)**
(a) Seminar (b) Demonstration
(c) Puppet show (d) Lecture method

**93. The ICDS (Integrated Child Development Scheme) was started in India on: (RPSC 2008)**
(a) October 2, 1975 (b) August 15, 1947
(c) January 26, 1950 (d) January 30, 1948

**94. Sunset eye is typical feature of: (AIIMS PG 2004)**
(a) Encephalitis (b) Hydrocephalous
(c) Hirschspung disease (d) Congenital heart disease

**95. After suctioning of tracheotomy, the nurse evaluate the effectiveness of procedure by monitoring: (ESIC 1994)**
(a) Temperature (b) Pulse rate
(c) BP (d) Breath sound

**96. The following is the example for total prenateral nutrition: (AIIMS 2009)**
(a) Colloids (b) 5% dextrose
(c) 25% dextrose (d) None of the above

**97. A patient who has hypertension attends clinic. Because of the diagnosis, the nurses should assess the patient for which of these symptoms? (ESI 2007)**
(a) Episode of dizziness
(b) Bleeding gums
(c) Bradycardia
(d) Near sightedness

**98. A freshly prepared ORS should not be used after: (PGIMES)**
(a) 4 hours (b) 6 hours
(c) 12 hours (d) 24 hours

**99. A structure composed of two or more tissue is termed as: (ESI)**
(a) Organ
(b) Serous membrane
(c) Organ system
(d) Complex tissue

**100. A homeostatic imbalance: (AIIMS 2004)**
(a) Must be restored by negative feedback mechanism
(b) Is considered the cause of most disease
(c) Is when the internal condition of body becomes more stable
(d) Only occurs when positive feedback mechanisms are overwhelmed.

## ANSWERS

| | | | | | | | | | |
|---|---|---|---|---|---|---|---|---|---|
| 1. | (b) | 21. | (d) | 41. | (c) | 61. | (c) | 81. | (c) |
| 2. | (b) | 22. | (b) | 42. | (a) | 62. | (b) | 82. | (a) |
| 3. | (b) | 23. | (c) | 43. | (a) | 63. | (b) | 83. | (a) |
| 4. | (c) | 24. | (d) | 44. | (c) | 64. | (a) | 84. | (c) |
| 5. | (c) | 25. | (a) | 45. | (c) | 65. | (a) | 85. | (c) |
| 6 | (a) | 26. | (a) | 46. | (c) | 66. | (a) | 86. | (a) |
| 7. | (a) | 27. | (c) | 47. | (c) | 67. | (a) | 87. | (b) |
| 8. | (c) | 28. | (b) | 48. | (c) | 68. | (c) | 88. | (d) |
| 9. | (d) | 29. | (b) | 49. | (d) | 69. | (c) | 89. | (a) |
| 10. | (b) | 30. | (b) | 50. | (d) | 70. | (a) | 90. | (b) |
| 11. | (a) | 31. | (b) | 51. | (d) | 71. | (c) | 91. | (c) |
| 12. | (c) | 32. | (a) | 52. | (a) | 72. | (a) | 92. | (c) |
| 13. | (c) | 33. | (a) | 53. | (d) | 73. | (a) | 93. | (a) |
| 14. | (a) | 34. | (b) | 54. | (d) | 74. | (a) | 94. | (b) |
| 15. | (d) | 35. | (c) | 55. | (b) | 75. | (c) | 95. | (d) |
| 16. | (c) | 36. | (a) | 56. | (c) | 76. | (d) | 96. | (a) |
| 17. | (c) | 37. | (b) | 57. | (d) | 77. | (b) | 97. | (a) |
| 18. | (b) | 38. | (a) | 58. | (a) | 78. | (a) | 98. | (d) |
| 19. | (a) | 39. | (b) | 59. | (b) | 79. | (c) | 99. | (a) |
| 20. | (b) | 40. | (b) | 60. | (c) | 80. | (a) | 100. | (b) |